Complications in Surgery

SECOND EDITION

EDITORS

Michael W. Mulholland, MD, PhD

Frederick A. Coller Distinguished Professor of Surgery and Chairman; Surgeon-in-Chief, Department of Surgery, University of Michigan, Ann Arbor, Michigan

Gerard M. Doherty, MD

N.W. Thompson Professor of Surgery; Vice-Chair, Department of Surgery, University of Michigan, Ann Arbor, Michigan

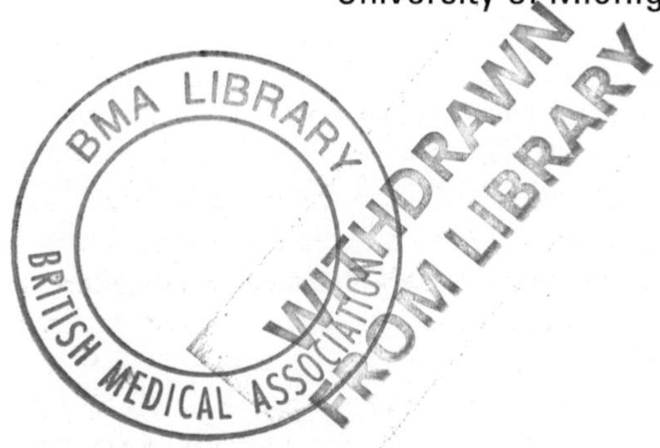

Wolters Kluwer | Lippincott Williams & Wilkins
Health

Philadelphia • Baltimore • New York • London
Buenos Aires • Hong Kong • Sydney • Tokyo

Acquisitions Editor: Brian Brown
Product Manager: Brendan Huffman
Production Manager: Bridgett Dougherty
Senior Manufacturing Manager: Benjamin Rivera
Marketing Manager: Lisa Lawrence
Design Coordinator: Doug Smock
Production Service: Aptara Inc.

Two Commerce Square
2001 Market Street
Philadelphia, PA 19103, USA
LWW.com

Printed in China

Library of Congress Cataloging-in-Publication Data

Complications in surgery / editors, Michael W. Mulholland, Gerard M. Doherty. – 2nd ed.
p. ; cm.
Includes bibliographical references and index.
ISBN 978-1-60547-530-1 (hardback : alk. paper)
1. Surgery–Complications. I. Mulholland, Michael W. II. Doherty, Gerard M.
[DNLM: 1. Intraoperative Complications. 2. Postoperative Complications. 3. Surgical Procedures, Operative–adverse effects. WO 181]
RD98.C63 2011
617'.01—dc22

2011004679

To purchase additional copies of this book, call our customer service department at (800) 638-3030 or fax orders to (301) 223-2320. International customers should call (301) 223-2300.

Visit Lippincott Williams & Wilkins on the Internet at LWW.com. Lippincott Williams & Wilkins customer service representatives are available from 8:30 AM to 6:00 PM, EST.

10 9 8 7 6 5 4 3 2 1

CCS0411

To our wives, Patricia and Faith

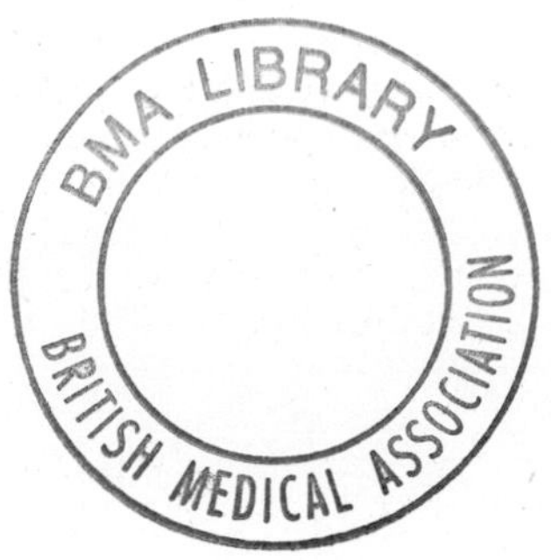

Sanjeev Aggarwal, MD
Director, Mechanical Circulatory Support
Associate Director, Cardiac Transplantation
Mid America Heart Institute
Saint Luke's Hospital of Kansas City
Kansas City, Missouri

Gorav Ailawadi, MD
Assistant Professor
Department of Surgery
University of Virginia
Charlottesville, Virginia

Ahmad Azari, MD
Clinical Instructor
Department of Surgery and OB-GYN
University of Michigan
Ann Arbor, Michigan

Richard J. Battafarano, MD, PhD
Assistant Professor of Surgery
Chief, Division of Thoracic Surgery
Washington University School of Medicine
Saint Louis, Missouri

John D. Birkmeyer, MD
George D. Zuidema Professor of Surgery
Department of Surgery
University of Michigan
Director of Bariatric Surgery
University Hospital
Ann Arbor, Michigan

Imad F. Btaiche, PharmD, BCNSP
Clinical Associate Professor
Department of Clinical, Social and Administrative Sciences
University of Michigan College of Pharmacy
Program Director, Critical Care Residency
Clinical Pharmacist, Surgery and Nutrition Support
University of Michigan Hospitals and Health Centers
Ann Arbor, Michigan

Richard E. Burney, MD
Professor
Department of Surgery
University of Michigan
Ann Arbor, Michigan

Darrell A. Campbell Jr., MD
H. King Ransom Professor of Surgery
Chief of Staff
Office of Clinical Affairs
University of Michigan
Ann Arbor, Michigan

Andrew C. Chang, MD
Assistant Professor
Department of Surgery
University of Michigan
Ann Arbor, Michigan

Craig M. Coopersmith, MD, FCCM, FACS
Assistant Professor
Departments of Surgery and Anesthesiology
Washington University School of Medicine
Attending Physician, Barnes-Jewish Hospital
Saint Louis, Missouri

Traves D. Crabtree
Assistant Professor
Department of Surgery
Washington University
Barnes Jewish Hospital
St. Louis, Missouri

Niraj M. Desai, MD
Department of Surgery
Johns Hopkins University
Balitimore, Maryland

Justin B. Dimick, MD, PhD
Assistant Professor
Department of Surgery
University of Michigan
Ann Arbor, Michigan

Gerard M. Doherty, MD
N.W. Thompson Professor of Surgery
Vice-Chair
Department of Surgery
University of Michigan
Ann Arbor, Michigan

James M. Donahue, MD
Assistant Professor of Surgery
General Thoracic Surgery
Greenebaum Cancer Center
University of Maryland
Maryland

Jessica S. Donington, MD
Assistant Professor
Department of Cardiothoracic Surgery
NYU School of Medicine
New York, New York

Kim A. Eagle, MD
Albion Walter Hewitt Professor of Internal Medicine
Department of Internal Medicine/Cardiovascular Medicine
Director, Cardiovascular Center
University of Michigan
Ann Arbor, Michigan

Matthew J. Eagleton, MD
Assistant Professor
Department of Vascular Surgery
Cleveland Clinic Lerner College of Medicine of Case Western Reserve University
Staff, Vascular Surgery
The Cleveland Clinic Foundation
Cleveland, Ohio

Jonathan L. Eliason, MD
Assistant Professor
Department of Surgery
University of Michigan
Ann Arbor, Michigan

Michael J. Englesbe, MD
Assistant Professor of Surgery
Department of Surgery
University of Michigan
Ann Arbor, Michigan

Jonathan F. Finks, MD
Assistant Professor
Department of Surgery
University of Michigan
Ann Arbor, Michigan

Emily Finlayson, MD
Assistant Professor
Division of General Surgery
University of California, San Francisco
San Francisco, California

Michael G. Franz, MD
Associate Professor of Surgery
Department of Surgery
University of Michigan
Ann Arbor, Michigan

Bradley D. Freeman, MD, FACS
Professor
Department of Surgery
Washington University School of Medicine
Attending Surgeon
Barnes Jewish Hospital
St. Louis, Missouri

Kevin Fung, BA, MD, FRCS(C)
Assistant Professor
Department of Otolaryngology
Department of Oncology
Director of the Vocal Health Clinic
Director of Undergraduate Affairs
Royal College of Physicians and Surgeons of Canada
American Board of Otolaryngology
London Health Sciences Centre
Westminster Campus, London
Ontario Canada

Samir K. Gadepalli, MD, MBA
Fellow, Pediatric Surgery
University of Michigan
C.S. Mott Children's Hospital
Ann Arbor, Michigan

Paul G. Gauger, MD
William J. Fry Professor of Surgery
Departments of Surgery and Medical Education
University of Michigan
Ann Arbor, Michigan

James D. Geiger, MD
Professor of Surgery
Department of Surgery
University of Michigan
Ann Arbor, Michigan

Alicia Growney, MD
Clinical Instructor
Department of Surgery
University of Michigan
Ann Arbor, Michigan

Richard Van Harrison, PhD
Professor
Department of Medical Education
University of Michigan
Ann Arbor, Michigan

Linnea S. Hauge, PhD
Assistant Professor and
Departments of Surgery and Medical Education
University of Michigan
Ann Arbor, Michigan

Awori Hayanga, MD
Resident in Thoracic Surgery
University of Washington
Seattle, Washington

Mark J. Hemmila, MD
Associate Professor
Department of Surgery
University of Michigan
Ann Arbor, Michigan

Peter K. Henke, MD
Associate Professor
Department of Surgery
University of Michigan
Ann Arbor, Michigan

Sara A. Hennessy, MD
Resident in Surgery
Department of Surgery
University of Virginia
Charlottesville, Virginia

Ronald B. Hirschl, MD
Arnold G. Coran Professor of Pediatric Surgery
University of Michigan
Surgeon-in-Chief
C.S. Mott Children's Hospital
Ann Arbor, Michigan

Norman D. Hogikyan, MD, FACS
Professor, Department of Otolaryngology—Head and Neck Surgery
Chief, Division of Laryngology, Rhinology and General Otolaryngology
University of Michigan
Ann Arbor, Michigan

Mark D. Iannettoni, MD
Johann L. Ehrenhaft Professor and Chairman
Department of Cardiothoracic Surgery
University of Iowa Hospitals and Clinics
Iowa City, Illinois

Paul Kanzanjian, MD
Assistant Professor
Department of Anesthesiology
University of Michigan
Ann Arbor, Michigan

Dixon B. Kaufman, MD
Professor
Department of Surgery
Feinberg School of Medicine
Northwestern University
Chicago, Illinois

Christina L. Klein, MD
Assistant Professor
Department of Medicine
Washington University in St. Louis School of Medicine
St. Louis, Missouri

Mary E. Klingensmith, MD
Professor of Surgery
Washington University School of Medicine
St. Louis, Missouri

James A. Knol, MD
Associate Professor
Department of Surgery
University of Michigan
Ann Arbor, Michigan

Terry C. Lairmore, MD
Professor of Surgery
Director, Division of Surgical Oncology
Texas A&M University Health Science Center, College of Medicine
Scott & White Hospital
Temple, Texas

Christine L. Lau, MD
Associate Professor
University of Virginia Health System
Division of Thoracic and Cardiovascular Surgery
Charlottesville, Virginia

Jennifer S. Lawton, MD
Associate Professor
Department of Surgery
Division of Cardiovascular Surgery
Washington University
Cardiothoracic Surgeon
Barnes Jewish Hospital
St. Louis, Missouri

Cortney Youens Lee, MD
Surgery
Endocrine Surgery Fellow
Department of Surgery
Texas A&M University/Scott and White Clinic
Temple, Texas

Spencer J. Melby, MD
Fellow, Division of Cardiothoracic Surgery
Washington University in St. Louis/ Barnes Jewish Hospital
St. Louis, Missouri

Robert M. Merion, MD
Professor of Surgery
Department of Surgery
University of Michigan
Ann Arbor, Michigan

Bryan F. Meyers, MD
Williamson Professor of Surgery
Washington University School of Medicine
Saint Louis, Missouri

Rebecca M. Minter, MD
Associate Professor Surgery
Assistant Professor of Medical Education
Departments of Surgery and Medical Education
University of Michigan
Ann Arbor, Michigan

Eiichi Miyasaka, MD
Research Fellow
Department of Surgery
University of Michigan
Ann Arbor, Michigan

Jeffrey F. Moley, MD
Professor, Surgery
Division of General Surgery
Washington University School of Medicine
Saint Louis, Missouri

Marc R. Moon, MD
Joseph C. Bancroft Professor of Surgery
Department of Surgery
Washington University School of Medicine
Saint Louis, Missouri

Arden M. Morris, MD
Associate Professor
Department of Surgery
University of Michigan
Ann Arbor, Michigan

Debabrata Mukherjee, MD, FACC
Chief, Cardiovascular Medicine
Professor of Internal Medicine
Vice Chairman, Department of Internal Medicine
Texas Tech University
El Paso, Texas

Michael W. Mulholland, MD, PhD
Frederick A. Coller Distinguished Professor
Surgeon-in-Chief
Chairman, Department of Surgery
University of Michigan
Ann Arbor, Michigan

Lisa A. Newman, MD, MPH, FAC
Professor of Surgery and Director
University of Michigan
Ann Arbor, Michigan

Francis D. Pagani, MD, PhD
Otto Gago, MD, Professor in Cardiac Surgery
Director, Heart Transplant Program
Director, Center for Circulatory Support
Department of Surgery
University of Michigan
Ann Arbor, Michigan

Pauline K. Park, MD, FACS, FCCM
Associate Professor, Surgery
Co-Director, Surgical Intensive Care Unit
Ann Arbor, Michigan

Harvey I. Pass, MD
Professor, Department of Surgery and Cardiothoracic Surgery
Vice-Chairman for Research and Division Chief, Thoracic Surgery
Department of Cardiothoracic Surgery
NYU Langone Medical Center
New York, New York

Shawn J. Pelletier, MD
Assistant Professor
Department of Surgery
University of Michigan
Ann Arbor, Michigan

John E. Rectenwald, MD
Professor of Surgery
Section of Vascular Surgery
University of Michigan
Ann Arbor, Michigan

Alvin H. Schmaier, MD
Robert W. Kellermeyer Professor of Hematology and Oncology
Department of Medicine
Case Western Reserve University
Director of the Ireland Cancer Center Laboratory and Hemophilia Program
Department of Medicine
University Hospital Case Medical Center
Cleveland, Ohio

Diane M. Simeone, MD
Lazar J. Greenfield Professor of Surgery and Molecular & Integrative Physiology
Department of Surgery
University of Michigan
Ann Arbor, Michigan

Michael A. Smith, MD
Assistant Professor
Cardiothoracic Surgery
Keck School of Medicine
University of Southern California
Los Angeles, California

Christopher J. Sonnenday, MD, MHS
Assistant Professor
Department of Surgery
University of Michigan
Ann Arbor, Michigan

Robert E. Southard, MD
Assistant Professor
Division of General Surgery
Section of Acute and Critical Care Surgery
Washington University School of Medicine
Saint Louis, Missouri

Sunita D. Srivastava, MD
Assistant Professor
Section of Vascular Surgery, Department of Surgery
Cleveland Clinic Lerner College of Medicine of Case Western Reserve University
Staff, Department of Vascular Surgery
The Cleveland Clinic Foundation
Cleveland, Ohio

James C. Stanley, MD
Professor of Surgery
Section of Vascular Surgery
Co-director, Cardiovascular Center
University of Michigan
Ann Arbor, Michigan

Randall S. Sung, MD
Associate Professor
Department of Surgery
University of Michigan
Ann Arbor, Michigan

Daniel H. Teitelbaum, MD
Professor of Surgery
Department of Surgery
University of Michigan
Ann Arbor, Michigan

Gilbert R. Upchurch Jr., MD
Professor of Surgery
Department of Surgery
University of Virginia
Charlottesville, VA

Wendy Wahl, MD
Professor
Department of Surgery
University of Michigan
Ann Arbor, Michigan

Thomas W. Wakefield, MD
S. Martin Lindenauer Professor of Surgery
Department of Surgery
University of Michigan
Ann Arbor, Michigan

Stewart Wang, MD, PhD
Professor of Surgery
Associate Chairman of Surgery
University of Michigan
Ann Arbor, Michigan

Christina H. Wei, MD
General Surgeon
San Francisco, California

Theordore H. Welling, MD
Assistant Professor
Department of Surgery
University of Michigan
Ann Arbor, Michigan

Alliric I. Willis, MD
Assistant Professor of Surgery
University of Pennsylvania School of Medicine
Philadelphia

Sandra L. Wong, MD, MS
Assistant Professor
Department of Surgery
University of Michigan
Ann Arbor, Michigan

Preface

Surgical therapy is inherently risky. All surgeons seek to balance an operation's potential benefit and risk with the disease being treated. The best surgeons display a combination of knowledge, technical skill, and clinical judgment. Knowledge begins with a thoughtful appraisal of the medical literature. Operative technical ability develops from an understanding of the process of surgery with comprehension of both the operation's objectives and the steps needed to meet them. Clinical judgment may be developed individually from experience, but it is also acquired from the distilled experience of others. Surgical judgment and understanding crucially depend on a detailed reading of the surgical literature and the expertise of others.

In recent years, it has become clear that surgical results depend not only on individual technical facility and judgment but also on the system in which a surgeon treats patients. Institutional parameters, the organization of clinical care, and teamwork play key roles in assuring that patients receive care that is both safe and efficacious. In many instances, the setting of care is as important in clinical outcomes as the individual surgeon.

Complications in Surgery is organized to cover both the broad concepts of surgical care and the complications relevant to operations on specific organs. Surgical epidemiology, operative technique, and disease pathophysiology are each essential in contemporary surgical practice; each is emphasized in this new textbook. In selecting contributors to *Complications in Surgery*, the editors sought surgeons who had significant clinical experience with the diseases and the operations described. In addition, the authors chosen are active contributors to new clinical knowledge and to the contemporary practice of surgery. The editors believe that the second edition of *Complications in Surgery* makes a truly unique contribution to the surgical literature—unique in its concept, focus, and breadth. We hope that our readers will find that the book combines unique perspectives and information on modern surgical practice. Our ultimate goal, of course, is to positively affect the lives of the patients we are honored to serve.

Acknowledgments

We are very grateful to the outstanding group of contributors who we believe are unchallenged in their understanding and experience in these areas of surgery. We appreciate their precious time and effort on this project. We are privileged to have worked with Holly Fischer, M.F.A., who did the original drawings. Her carefully detailed drawings clarify and add detail to the contributors' text. We have enjoyed wonderful support for Jenny Koleth and Brian Brown at Lippincott, Williams & Wilkins who gently guided this process. It has been a pleasure for us to work with such a dedicated group of individuals.

CONTENTS

PART

I

Institutional Issues

CHAPTER

1

Surgical Complications

Michael W. Mulholland and Gerard Doherty

A surgical complication is any undesirable, unintended, and direct result of an operation affecting the patient that would not have occurred had the operation gone as well as could reasonably be hoped (1).

Surgical care has always focused on balancing risk and benefit. In traditional surgical teaching, risk is represented by operative complications, while benefit is equated with cure rates or palliation of symptoms. In the second half of the past century, surgical attention was directed to avoiding complications by developing meticulous operative techniques and through early detection of postoperative problems with rapid efforts to minimize undesirable events. While surgical complications are often obvious and clearly tied to the act of surgical intervention, issues of risk have traditionally been regarded as a private matter addressed between an individual surgeon and a single patient.

This traditional view of surgical risk and benefit is no longer adequate. Risk, still, properly begins with an assessment of intraoperative problems and postoperative events. Surgical risk in contemporary practice also includes consideration of balancing complementary, sometimes competing, techniques and achieving results that optimize physical, occupational, and societal goals. Modern surgeons must appreciate the appropriate sequence and combination of operative and nonoperative therapy. Judicious utilization of resources is now a consideration. Patient engagement and satisfaction, in addition to physical healing, are required.

The relationship of an individual surgeon with an individual patient, still central to surgical care, has become overlaid with increased scrutiny and with additional societal expectations. Standards of expected outcomes for groups of patients require evidence-based practice and have made both seniority and individual experience less important. Surgical care must be provided within financial constraints. Societal interest in surgical outcomes is expressed in the now-familiar Institute of Medicine report, "To Err Is Human," which detailed "unnecessary" deaths resulting from surgical complications (2).

Investment in the health care sector by the American society is enormous and continues to grow. In 1997, approximately 14% of the country's gross domestic product (GDP), \$1.1 trillion, was spent on health services. By 2007, this figure increased to \$2.2 trillion, amounting to 16.2% of GDP or \$7421 per person, and health care reforms became a major factor in American electoral politics (3,4). The Agency for Healthcare Research and Quality has identified the top priority conditions: cancer, diabetes mellitus, emphysema, human immunodeficiency virus (HIV) infection, hypertension, ischemic heart disease, stroke, and gallstones. Many of these conditions are highly relevant to contemporary surgical practice. In treating patients with these conditions, the 21st century health care system must adapt and focus increasingly upon provision of care that is

safe,
effective,
patient-centered,
timely,
efficient, and
equitable (5).

Patient safety has become a major issue for American patients and has prompted increasing efforts to promote a culture of hospital safety. As detailed in Chapter 9 of this second edition, safety means "freedom from harm"; in the context of patient care safety means freedom from harm associated with any medical action or treatment. Quality is a more global term referring to a "degree of excellence." It is theoretically possible for a hospital to be safe but offer average or poor quality. However, it is not possible for a hospital to be of high quality and unsafe.

New knowledge related to the practice of surgery has increased exponentially during the past decade. Surgical studies are also increasingly sophisticated, requiring of the reader knowledge of patient selection, statistical analysis, and molecular biology. The number of drugs, surgical devices, and technological support systems has expanded as well. In this context, it is not possible for any one clinician to synthesize all of the information necessary for effective, evidence-based practice. No surgeon can read, organize, and recall the current volumes of clinically important information (5). Chapter 6, "Understanding variation in surgical outcomes," is designed to provide a framework for this new field of inquiry.

Michael W. Mulholland, Gerard M. Doherty: University of Michigan, Ann Arbor, MI 48109.

The revolution in information technology has the potential to greatly accelerate changes in surgical care, to make that care both more effective and safer. Reduction in surgical complications will require effective use of the available scientific database. Evidence must be instantly available to clinicians from laboratory experiments, clinical trials, epidemiology, and health services research. The Institute of Medicine has identified five major areas in which information technology could contribute to safer health care delivery: (a) access to the medical knowledge base; (b) computer-aided decision support systems; (c) collection and sharing of clinical information; (d) reduction in errors; and (e) enhanced patient and clinician communication (5). With the proper application of new tools, fruitful strategies can be developed for improvement in surgical outcomes, which is discussed further in Chapter 8.

The Internet has led to a great surge in medical consumerism. An estimated 70 million Americans sought health care information online in 2000 (6). These numbers continue to increase. Medical IT users demand both sound information and convenience in all areas of health commerce. Medical information systems hold great promise for reduction in surgical complications. An informed patient is a safer patient.

Knowledge, technical skill, and judgment are the foundations of safe surgical care, but do not always prevent complications. Patients are frequently injured because of flaws in the design of medical systems. Recognition of the importance of the system in which care is received has led to a reexamination of surgical culture. Increasingly, improvement is a result of team efforts in the form of surgical collaboratives, rather than individual technical brilliance. Chapter 9 of the second edition, "Building successful quality improvement collaborative," explicitly recognizes the power of group effort and cooperation.

The ethics of surgical complications can be described in the framework of the "Four Principles" approach to medical ethics, including respect for patient autonomy, beneficence, nonmaleficence and justice (7,8). The stress of responsibility for patient outcomes including complications has also been emphasized. Importantly, for both the surgeon and the patient, a system of surgical accountability that focuses on blaming individuals has a poor prospect of significant improvement. Contemporary surgical morbidity and mortality conferences must reflect this realization. The prevention, reporting, analysis, and minimization of surgical harm can only occur in learning environments, not those of blame and reprisal. The moral imperative to improve patient care to the extent humanly possible implies that surgical complications will remain a major focus area for surgeons. These changes also mean that new texts on this subject must include new perspectives to remain relevant to contemporary practice.

REFERENCES

1. Sokol DK, Wilson J. What is a surgical complication? [see comment]. *World J Surg* 2008;32(6):942–944.
2. Linda TK, Janet MC, Molla SD, eds. *To err is human: building a safer health system*. Washington, DC: National Academy Press; 2000.
3. Smith S, Freeland M, Heffler S, et al. The next ten years of health spending: what does the future hold? The Health Expenditures Projection Team [see comment]. *Health Aff* 1998;17(5):128–140.
4. Hartman M, Martin A, McDonnell P, et al. National health spending in 2007: slower drug spending contributes to lowest rate of overall growth since 1998. *Health Aff* 2009;28(1):246–261.
5. Committee of on Quality of Health Care in America. *Crossing the quality chasm*. Washington, DC: Institute of Medicine National Academy Press; 2003.
6. Cain M, Mittman R, Sarasohn-Kahn J. *Health e-people: the online consumer experience*. Oakland, CA: Institute for the Future, California Health Care Foundation; 2000.
7. Adedeji S, Sokol DK, Palser T, et al. Ethics of surgical complications [see comment]. *World J Surg* 2009;33(4):732–737.
8. Angelos P. Complications, errors, and surgical ethics [comment]. *World J Surg* 2009;33(4):609–611.

CHAPTER

2

Learning from Unanticipated Outcomes and Error

Linnea S. Hauge

INTRODUCTION

Inherent to the study of surgical complications is the challenge of learning from them. Surgery encompasses layers of complexity that represent the human systems involved. It is these complex layers that create unmatched learning opportunities. It is these layers that raise expectations for performance excellence.

Expectations for productive team dynamics, decision-making accuracy, technical precision, effective communication, and compassionate, quality patient care create a unique learning and performance environment. Each surgical performance presents an opportunity to learn. The purpose of this chapter is to optimize how we learn from error. This chapter will address the following points:

1. factors that affect how surgeons learn from unanticipated outcomes, especially those that involve error,
2. recommendations for enhancing learning experiences that involve error,
3. strategies for communicating about error with peers, learners, and patients, and
4. methods for coping with the stressors that accompany error and recovery from error.

Like many surgical learners, one of my earliest—and most memorable—experiences observing how a surgical team manages error was at Morbidity and Mortality (M&M) Conference. As the educational faculty "expert" in the department, I frequently attended M&M Conferences to observe the learning environment and methods. On the morning's list was a complication in an appendectomy where a Fallopian tube was mistaken for the appendix. The resident's recounting of a procedure gone horribly wrong—a Fallopian tube unintentionally removed having been mistaken for an appendix, and the patient communication that followed—elicited palpable silence from the room of attending surgeons and trainees. My lack of clinical training and my inclination as a relative layperson to understand the patient's perspective more often than the physician's made me curious about the lessons of the case. Confused by the silence of the room when there appeared to be much to learn, I turned to the senior resident seated and inquired about the silence. His explanation still reverberates: "it's relief that it wasn't any of us." There, but for the grace of God, go I . . . not an uncommon response. Loud chastising of the responsible attending surgeon after the results of their operation became known by administration predicted the absence of that surgeon from the conference. The experience made me (and others) very concerned that we had progress to make on how we learn from error in surgery.

The tenuous nature of health, healthcare systems, and the humanity of those who provide health care predict that patient outcomes are not always anticipated, planned, or satisfactory. It is widely recognized that making mistakes is a natural part of learning on the path to becoming a competent physician and surgeon, and that errors are sure to happen during one's career. The discipline of surgery embraces a long-held tradition of performance review in the M&M, unmatched by other disciplines in its history and method. Messages of excellence and superiority color the educational experience of those acquiring surgical acumen—reasonably so, the stakes are high and professional tradition and the public would allow nothing else. It is this intersection of expected perfection and certain fallibility that creates a cultural challenge in addressing error in surgery—one that is often felt deeply and personally by all involved. These cultural challenges have been studied and described by sociologists and surgeons (1–4).

The process of learning from error is often implicit, which tends to inhibit effective learning, communication, and coping. An increased awareness of how physician reflection can improve patient care and safety reinforces the need for the surgical community to explicitly address the process of learning from error and unanticipated outcomes.

DEFINING ERROR

The definitions of an adverse event, near miss, error, and mistake are critical to learning from error. One of the barriers to learning from error is the failure to recognize it (5,6). The definitions presented below are those frequently utilized by researchers in error education and error management.

An adverse event is defined as "an unintended injury caused by medical management rather than the underlying disease or condition of the patient" (7).

Linnea S. Hauge: University of Michigan Medical School, Ann Arbor, MI 48109.

A near miss is "any event or situation that could have resulted in an accident, injury or illness, but did not, either by chance or through timely intervention" (8).

An error is "an unintended act, either of omission or commission, or an act that does not achieve its intended outcome" (9). An error of execution is defined as "the failure of a planned action to be completed as intended," and an error of planning is "the use of a wrong plan to achieve an aim" (9).

A mistake is defined by Wu and colleagues as "a commission or an omission with potentially negative consequences for the patient that would have been judged wrong by skilled and knowledgeable peers at the time it occurred, independent of whether there were negative consequences" (10).

LEARNING FROM ERROR

Most medical students' and residents' exposure to error is casual or distant observation and frequently occurs without debriefing or discussion with an attending physician. Students rarely have the option to directly observe or participate in team debriefing about error or error disclosure conversations with patients. Some institutions have begun to include formal learning experiences in their student or resident curricula (11–15). These courses are in their infancy and tend to be classroom-based with little opportunity for guided practice, real or simulated. The standard approaches for implicitly learning from error via observation are not sufficient to provide constructive experience in this domain. Less than one-fifth of U.S. and Canadian physicians surveyed had themselves received formal education on disclosing errors to patients, and 86% were interested in receiving training in error disclosure (16). The risk of implicit lessons about error that come from unguided observation is that maladaptive behaviors and error management strategies may develop. Without skilled attending surgeon guidance or modeling, our surgical learners may adopt behaviors and strategies that are barriers to future practice (6,17).

Another concern about allowing surgical learners to be responsible for independently identifying appropriate lessons about error is echoed in the findings of Arora and colleagues (18). They studied attending surgeons' and residents' perceptions of what performance domains contribute to competency as a surgeon. Junior residents placed a lower value on a surgeon's roles as communicator and collaborator. This finding suggests that a lack of role models or learning opportunities exist. Or that residents may not place an appropriate priority on seeking learning experiences to develop effective communication skills, especially if residents are overextended on their clinical responsibilities.

The M&M Conference, "the golden hour" of surgery (19), is the primary, formal method for learning from error in surgery. Results of a review of M&M Conferences in Medicine and Surgery indicate that error is more frequently addressed in surgery proceedings than in medicine proceedings (20). Traditional surgery conference proceedings call for residents to present their surgical patients whose course of disease or injury resulted in surgical complications and/or death. These cases are often selected, in advance by the conference leader, for their learning opportunities. The case presentation typically includes an overview of the patient's course of diagnosis and treatment, a literature review of the disease or procedure, categorization of the behavior(s) that led to the complication or death, and questions and discussion by audience members. The M&M Conference meets Joint Commission on Accreditation of Healthcare Organizations (JCAHO) quality assurance requirements and requirements of the Residency Review Committee for Surgery.

The discipline and profession of surgery is respected for its long tradition of learning from suboptimal outcomes in M&M Conferences. The challenge of capitalizing on these learning opportunities that involve individual, team, and system failures is particularly difficult because of the individual and social factors affecting how failures are experienced, defined, and addressed in surgery (2,3). This challenge has led surgical educators to identify the need to enhance the dynamics and format of the traditional M&M Conference (21–27).

Surgical educators have documented conference improvements that include abbreviating presentations and literature reviews to increase the number of cases presented during a session; identifying faculty moderators to enhance audience engagement; increasing the interactions and questions during conference; and encouraging resident presenters to meet with their attending surgeon in advance of the conference to discuss their case (22,27) Others have attempted to improve the conference by employing anonymous systems for rating different aspects of M&M case presentations, including participants' ratings of complication severity in trauma (28), peer reviewers' perceptions about surgeon and system performance (23), and quantifying the efficacy of case presentations (24).

Since the Accreditation Council on Graduate Medical Education's (ACGME) 2001 mandate for residency programs to implement competency-based curriculum and assessment (also known as "the competencies"), the M&M Conference is frequently noted as a means of ensuring that residents learn practice-based learning and improvement. Optimally, M&M Conferences offer this potential, although this goal must be part of the conference design.

National initiatives on improving patient care have yielded methods for performance review and benchmarking, and surgeons have incorporated these methods into the M&M review process. Researchers at Massachusetts General Hospital utilized the American College of Surgeons' National Surgical Quality Improvement Program (NSQIP) database to study reporting accuracy of complications at their M&M Conference (29), and found significant under-reporting of deaths and complications in their M&M process. Approximately one of two deaths and three of four complications reported in the NSQIP database were not reported in the M&M conference. Their results led the department to adopt use of an M&M database that is modeled after the NSQIP database. A consistent finding in error disclosure research demonstrates that, following an error, many physicians are not likely to tell peers about their error, nor are they likely to confront peers about error (5,10,16,30). This finding suggests that departments that chose to compare their M&M and NSQIP databases would discover a similar trend of under-reporting, an indication that we have progress to make in the design and conduct of our M&M Conferences if our goal is to constructively learn from our errors.

Antonacci and colleagues created a classification system for postsurgical adverse events that they used as part of their M&M Conference review (25). Their purpose was to standardize the manner in which surgical performance was quantified for the department. They followed up that endeavor with the creation of individualized report cards that were used in conjunction with their M&M Conference proceedings (26). Fabri and Zayas-Castro also created and studied the validity of an instrument to classify medical errors by frequency, type, and severity, to determine the cause of errors that led to surgical complications in their department (31).

The process of learning from adverse events and near misses in surgery M&M Conference is affected not only by the culture of surgery, but by the culture of the conference, department and institution. Role modeling is perhaps the most dominant educational force for learning about professionalism (17). M&M Conferences are opportunities for surgeons, especially senior faculty, to model error recognition, error disclosure, and "constructive responses to their own errors" (32). The manner in which M&M Conferences are conducted are wide-ranging and contribute significantly to the opportunities to learn and recover from error. Effective conference management and faculty modeling reinforces more thorough and accurate reporting of errors and near misses, and will result in enhanced learning opportunities. The use of anonymous, problem- and system-focused approaches for reporting complications and reviewing surgical team performance has promise for enhancing the opportunity to learn and improve as a result of M&M conference participation. Surgeons can draw on the wisdom offered by a principle from the negotiation literature: be hard on the problem, easy on the people (33).

PREDISPOSITIONS TO ERROR

Learning from error requires reflection on past performance and identifying when we are most vulnerable to making an error. Many researchers in surgery, medical education, and human factors have studied the conditions that set the stage for error. These conditions include fatigue and overwork, stress, work interruptions, team discord and conflict, inexperience, self-assessment inaccuracy, and cognitive bias.

Cognitive bias

Being part of a surgical team that has dealt with a bad complication can leave a surgeon with memories about the experience and the patient that can unduly influence decision-making on the next similar patient. Learning from past performance is a critical aspect of learning from error. However, it is these most memorable experiences that can create biases that may negatively affect decision-making in the next similar patient care experience. Croskerry has summarized more than 30 types of predispositions to decision-making error as "cognitive dispositions to respond" (CDRs) (34). CDRs are biases that have the potential to impact how physicians make decisions and arrive at diagnoses. Examples of CDRs, each taken from Croskerry's CDR List (34) are given below:

"*Anchoring*: The tendency to perceptually lock onto salient features in the patient's initial presentation too early in the diagnostic process, and failing to adjust this initial impression in the light of later information" (34).

"*Confirmation bias:* The tendency to look for confirming evidence to support a diagnosis rather than look for disconfirming evidence to refute it, despite the latter often being more persuasive and definitive" (34).

"*Hindsight bias:* Knowing the outcome may profoundly influence the perception of past events and prevent a realistic appraisal of what actually occurred. . . . it may compromise learning through either an underestimation (illusion of failure) or overestimation (illusion of control) of the decision maker's abilities" (34).

"*Order effects:* Information transfer is a U-function: we tend to remember the beginning part (primacy effect) or the end (recency effect). Primacy effect may be augmented by anchoring. In transitions of care, in which information transferred from patients, nurses, or other physicians in being evaluated, care should be taken to give due consideration to all information, regardless of the order in which it was presented" (34).

Croskerry reviewed the literature on the CDR phenomena to raise awareness and to provide strategies for reducing error. He refers to these strategies as "cognitive debiasing" and advises physicians to seek timely feedback, use memory aids, reflect on the thinking process used in decision-making, and consider alternative diagnoses (34). He also recommends reviewing the list of CDRs and writing about one's own clinical examples to help determine how each CDR may predispose one to error.

Fatigue

Since the introduction and implementation of duty hours regulations in graduate medical education, the relationship between fatigue and medical error has received increased interest. Although the link between patient care and physician fatigue has not been well-established (35), the potentially devastating effect that fatigue can have on physician performance has (36). Surveys of physicians indicate that their fatigue has contributed to error and near misses in patient care (37). Well-designed studies yield consistent findings that fatigue has a detrimental effect on cognitive and psychomotor performance in surgery, manifested by increased error and slower performance on technical tasks (38–41). Finally, an oft-cited cause of error in surgery, especially the operating room (OR), is communication failure (42–47). The research on fatigue yields consistent findings that fatigue is a common contributor to physicians' and medical students' communication failure (5,35,37,48). Details are forgotten, hand-off protocols are truncated, patience wanes, and communication failure occurs. One of the greatest challenges in dealing with fatigue in surgery is that many surgeons believe that they are not susceptible to fatigue the way that others are. A study of surgical and nonsurgical residents was conducted to investigate trainees' perceptions about the impact that sleep deprivation has on their performance, and the results demonstrate that surgery residents may be less willing to recognize their performance limitations that are due to fatigue (49). The culture of surgery contributes to the maintenance of these misbeliefs—making it difficult to implement strategies for fatigue-caused error reduction, and reinforcing silence among surgical learners when they recognize that they are in a risky, fatigued state.

Inexperience is an expected cause of medical error, and heightened supervision of the least experienced surgeons is standard in medical and surgical education. The arrival of more than 20,000 inexperienced interns and the departure of the most experienced trainees in the United States on July 1 create a supervisory challenge. The transition time between the end of an academic year and the start of a new academic year has been the focus of attention for individual and team predisposition to performance deficits. The onslaught of new physicians at the beginning of the academic year raises concern about relative novices' vulnerabilities to error in patient care. Studies of the "July phenomenon" (50) have yielded mixed results, although researchers utilizing large databases have identified increased rates of undesirable events at the beginning of the surgical trainees' academic year in Europe (51,52) and the United States (53,54).

Self-assessment inaccuracy

Self-assessment inaccuracy, the misjudgment one makes about one's own abilities, can contribute to an individual's susceptibility to error. In surgery, this is often described as "not knowing one's limits." All humans are susceptible to inaccuracy in self-assessment—we tend to overestimate our positive traits and abilities, and underestimate our weaknesses. It is the intersection of this human flaw with high-demand, high-risk work environments that can become a problem. Physicians frequently work in solo, reducing the opportunities for comparison or discussion with peers and increasing the propensity for self-assessment inaccuracies. The problem of self-assessment inaccuracy is compounded by one's inability and varies by task. Higher-level performers tend to be most accurate in their self-assessments, often making slight underestimations of their performance. On the other hand, the lowest-level performers tend to greatly overestimate their performance (55,56). All levels of surgical performers are vulnerable to self-assessment inaccuracies or misjudgment about their own specific abilities. However, those surgeons with the least experience are at particular risk of self-assessment inaccuracy due to their lack of knowledge and skill that serve as the basis for self-assessment. Furthermore, the least experienced, in efforts to preserve professional credibility, are often hesitant to ask for help when they recognize it is needed (57).

Stress

Stress is a predisposing factor for error in surgery, and surgeons generally recognize how it can affect performance in the OR (47,58). LeBlanc describes the manner in which stress can impact memory and negatively impact retrieval, memory consolidation, and retention (59). For example, remembering details of patient care that occurred during a highly stressful event such as a code may be difficult. The working memory becomes less reliable in situations stressful enough that a performer produces stress cortisol. In conditions of high stress, quick recall of patient details may be compromised. Another example of how stress affects the working memory is derived from one of LeBlanc's earlier works using simulation to study paramedics' drug calculations under low-stress and simulated high-stress conditions (60). The paramedics working under the simulated, high-stress condition made significantly more calculation errors than the paramedics working in low-stress conditions, despite their level of experience. The increase in errors was attributed to the working memory's vulnerability to stress. Similar to fatigue, the challenges in addressing this predisposition to error in surgery are the cultural beliefs that surgeons are immune to the effects of stress. This environment makes it difficult for trainees to admit their vulnerabilities and to recognize errors that are related to stress-induced memory failure.

Interruptions

Interruptions to work and workflow predispose a healthcare team to error. These may occur during conversations about patient care, handover between team members, or in surgery, during an operation or resuscitation. Effectively managing interruptions, especially during critical steps of a difficult operation, is a skill that must be acquired early in surgical training, as the work of interns is frequently interrupted. Clinical hand-offs and operating are each susceptible to error caused by interruptions (47,61,62).

Communication breakdown

Breakdown in team communication is a major cause of error and near misses in medicine and surgery (42–47). A breakdown in communication may occur due to absence of communication, communication of misinformation, or exchanges between team members that cause team discord. Rogers and Lingard have described conflict in surgery and strategies for managing conflict (63). Task conflict is disagreement about how to complete a task or solve a problem, such as management of a patient's postoperative care. Interpersonal conflict is dissension that develops between two or more individuals and manifests itself in anger, frustration, or friction. In the OR, common "causes of interpersonal conflict include time, resources, roles, safety, and situation control" (63). Either of these types of conflict has the potential to make a healthcare team more susceptible to error. Team dynamics that prohibit active listening, an open exchange of ideas, and subordinates' participation create an environment for communication failures that result in error. Managing conflict requires a surgeon be able to effectively respond to it and control emotions, avoid reactionary responses, problem-solve, listen without interrupting, and negotiate in an expedited manner (63).

STRATEGIES FOR REDUCING RISK AND SUSCEPTIBILITY

One of the best strategies for reducing risk is to be aware of situations that make one more vulnerable to error and these may vary for every individual. Identify the error-related variables that your behaviors influence (e.g., OR environment, reporting complications). Be aware of your CDRs and your predispositions due to past experiences. Employ strategies such as self-monitoring, reflection, seeking feedback, and engaging peers in discussing cases. Self-monitoring is "awareness, in the moment, of whether or not the current situation is going well" (64). Moulton's description of expert surgeon behavior termed as "slowing down when you should" is an example of self-monitoring and describes an expert surgeon's cognitive and psychomotor action when they recognize that they need to reassess or prepare for a difficult part of an operation (65). Reflection is deliberate use of cognitive energy to exploring and elaborating how one understands a problem (64). A reflection about a patient with a surgical infection that became septic would elicit questions about how the patient acquired the infection and how it deteriorated.

Preparing for the OR is a critical aspect of surgical performance, and each surgeon develops their own routine of preparation. In addition to clinical requirements related to the patient, review steps of the cases, by reading or by verbal or mental rehearsal. If one is not yet experienced in a procedure or time has passed since the last performance, a combination of reading and verbal or mental rehearsal should be done. Verbal rehearsal entails listing the steps of the procedure in correct order. Mental rehearsal or practice involves imaging, where one sees himself performing the steps of the procedure in order. Mental rehearsal of the procedure and contingency plans relevant to the procedure is recommended. Additionally, technical warm-ups have been shown to yield better surgical performance (66).

Managing intraoperative stress, especially in crises, is important to safe performance in the OR (47,58,67,68). Recognition of stress is the first step in successfully applying coping techniques. Experienced surgeons use a range of techniques that they develop over the course of their careers. It would be beneficial to design programs to learn about stress during residency training (47). Music and humor are commonly used means of allaying stress and because both are shared with other team members, consideration should be given to team dynamics in selection of music and use of humor. Stretching, progressive muscle relaxation, mental rehearsal, and positive self-talk are strategies successfully employed in other arenas and may be useful to mitigate stress in surgery.

Effectively reducing the risk imposed by communication breakdowns will require communication between healthcare team members that is "against the authority gradient" (69). Discourse between attending surgeons and residents and nurses would forego the hierarchical traditions in surgery, so that all team members, despite their authority, could ask questions and offer observations and suggestions about the procedure or case, without the fear of intimidation or retribution. This manner of discourse is key to safe team communication in and out of the OR. Communication strategies to maintain and enhance effective team performance can be displayed in the following ways:

1. Be willing to engage others' opinions and ideas.
2. Use problem-solving to manage conflict.
3. Prioritize interruptions and use colleagues to help manage them and recover from them.
4. Be an active listener.
5. Employ checklist-driven briefing protocols before every operation.
6. Debrief after surgical procedures especially if you have student or resident learners or new staff. Address critical events. Provide and invite feedback about what went well and what could be improved.
7. Learn and use healthcare team members' names. Introduce team members in the OR.
8. If you are working with residents or students in the OR, ask them—before the case—about how they feel about the case, their experience, and their preparation for it. If this question does not elicit a useful response, ask them to verbally rehearse the key steps of the procedure. This "self-efficacy check" will provide insight about the extent of guidance, prompts, and supervision that will be needed.

LEARNING ABOUT ERROR THROUGH OBSERVATION

Performing an anastomosis, diagnosing an insulinoma, managing hypovolemic shock . . . the methods that surgeons most frequently employ to learn these skills are observation, practice in simulated situations, supervised practice with patients, instruction and guidance from an experienced surgeon. Unfortunately, the lessons about learning from error and coping with error are not typically as explicit or supervised. The nature of learning from error is unique, and observation, if directed, can be an effective teaching method. Surgeons learn about professionalism through observing role models (17) and Bandura's social learning theory posits, "most human behavior is learned observationally through modeling: from observing others, one forms an idea of how new behaviors are performed, and on later occasions this coded information serves as a guide for action" (70). The conditions that are necessary for *effective* modeling and teaching are relevant for learning some of the most important lessons in surgery—learning from and coping with error. There are many examples of theory-based teaching strategies that one can use:

1. Direct learners' attention toward critical yet level-appropriate aspects of an error situation.
2. Allow learners the opportunity to observe or be directly involved in discussion of error, when appropriate.
3. Give learners the opportunity to verbally review and critique observations of performances.
4. Create a blame-free, team approach to reviewing and learning from error.
5. Debrief about your own experiences, past or present, with learning from and coping with error.

COPING AND RECOVERY FROM ERROR

Errors in medicine are both "inevitable and reducible" (71). Results of a survey of more than 3,000 physicians about their experience with medical error depict the negative effect that error has on physicians' well-being and continued practice (16). Physicians "experienced increased stress about future errors, loss of confidence, sleep difficulties, and reduced job satisfaction" (16). The majority (90%) of physicians felt that they did not have adequate support in coping with medical error, and perceived several barriers to obtaining counseling. More than other specialties, surgeons reported that a barrier to obtaining counseling after medical error was that it was not likely to be helpful (16), a finding that may be attributable to the culture of surgery and the current state of support systems.

Perceived and actual availability of physician and healthcare team support systems are important for resolution and recovery in the wake of an error. One model of finding resolution includes recognizing an error, disclosing it, apologizing for it, and making amends (32). Physician feelings of remorse, guilt, fear, humiliation, and inadequacy commonly accompany recognition of an error (72–74). Coping with the range of emotions is an important step in resolution, and support from a confidante or through an established group process can be helpful in this process. It is recommended that a physician identify a confidante who is knowledgeable about error but has no role in evaluation of the individual's performance. This confidante would be selected, advisably in advance of need, for the purpose of having a trusted individual with whom to confidentially discuss an error, when one occurs. A confidante would be available to review decision-making and provide reassurance. Physicians affected by error often report feeling uncomfortable talking with colleagues about mistakes (6,30,74) and identifying a confidante in advance of need increases the options for coping after an error and perhaps the likelihood that recovery will be less stressful.

Open, honest disclosure of the error to colleagues, learners, and the patient is another important step in the process of resolution as it prevents isolation and initiates the beginning of learning from the error. Fear of litigation often inhibits disclosure. However, as error disclosure policies and procedures are adopted, there is growing evidence that fewer lawsuits occur at institutions where error disclosure is part of the institution's norms and practices (75–78).

An apology through which the physician accepts responsibility and affirms to a patient that there was no intent to err is an important aspect of resolution for the physician and the patient. A physician should, however, maintain reasonable expectations for patient response to disclosure and apology. Patient responses vary from gratitude to anger, and being prepared to hear and allow those responses can help to ensure a meaningful, productive conversation. The Harvard Full Disclosure Working Group outlines the "4 Steps to Full Communication" and recommends the following:

"Tell the patient and family what happened.
Take responsibility.
Apologize.
Explain what will be done to prevent future events" (79).

Initiating honest communication and providing compassionate patient care in the event of an error will go a long way to facilitate physician recovery from an adverse event. However, there is much progress to be made to ensure that the needs of the "second victim" of medical error, the physician, are met (16,72,73). Institutions need to provide accessible resources beyond risk management for coping and recovery from error. Additionally, faculty development programs in recognizing error, error disclosure, and coping with the stress of error are clearly warranted.

SUMMARY

Error in medicine is inevitable. It is our responsibility to learn from it, and to do so in ways that maintain a productive learning and work environment. Constructive team- and system-based approaches to learning from error are important to effective learning and error reduction. The M&M Conference is an opportunity to improve how we learn from error. Being aware of predispositions to error facilitates efforts to address systems issues—systems issues that unnecessarily allow humans to err. Modeling professional behaviors, such as self-monitoring and compassionate honesty in disclosure, will serve us and our learners well.

REFERENCES

1. Katz P. *The scalpel's edge: the culture of surgeons*. Needham Heights, MA: Allyn & Bacon; 1999.
2. Bosk C. *Forgive & Remember*, 2nd ed. Chicago: University of Chicago Press; 2003.
3. Gawande A. *Complications: a surgeon's notes on an imperfect science*. New York, NY: Picador; 2002.
4. Gawande A. *Better: a surgeon's notes on performance*. New York, NY: Picador; 2007.
5. Wu AW, Folkman S, McPhee SJ, et al. Do house officers learn from their mistakes? *Qual Saf Health Care* 2003;12:221–228.
6. Hobgood C, Hevia A, Tamayo-Sarver JH, et al. The influence of the causes and contexts of medical errors on emergency medicine residents' responses to their errors: an exploration. *Acad Med* 2005;80: 758–764.
7. Brennan T, Leape L, Laird N. The nature of adverse events in hospitalized patients: results from the Harvard medical practice study. *N Engl J Med* 1991;324:2377–2384.
8. Kohn KT, Corrigan JM, Donaldson MS. *To err is human: building a safer health system*. Washington, DC: National Academy Press; 1999.
9. Reason J. *Human Error*. New York, NY: Cambridge University Press, 1990.
10. Wu AW, Cavanaugh TA, McPhee SJ, et al. To tell the truth: ethical and practical issues in disclosing medical mistakes to patients. *J Gen Int Med* 1997;12:770–775.
11. Brannick MT, Fabri PJ, Zayas-Castro J. Evaluation of an error-reduction training program for surgical residents. *Acad Med* 2009;84:1809–1814.
12. Paxton JH, Rubinfeld IS. Medical errors education for students of surgery: a pilot study revealing the need for action. *J Surg Educ* 2009; 66:20–24.
13. Newell P, Harris S, Aufses A Jr, et al. Student perceptions of medical errors: incorporating an explicit professionalism curriculum in the third-year surgery clerkship. *J Surg Educ* 2008;65:117–119.
14. Keller DR, Bell CL, Dottl SK. An effective curriculum for teaching third-year medical students about medical errors and disclosure. *WMJ* 2009;108:27–29.
15. Halbach JL, Sullivan LL. Teaching medical students about medical errors and patient safety: evaluation of a required curriculum. *Acad Med* 2005;80:600–606
16. Waterman AD, Garbutt J, Hazel E, et al. The emotional impact of medical errors on practicing physicians in the United States and Canada. *Jt Comm J Qual Patient Saf* 2007;33:467–476.
17. Park J, Woodrow SI, Reznick RK, et al. Observation, reflection, and reinforcement: surgery faculty members' and residents' perceptions of how they learned professionalism. *Acad Med* 2010;85:134–139.
18. Arora S, Sevdalis N, Suliman I, et al. What makes a competent surgeon? experts' and trainees' perceptions of the roles of a surgeon. *Am J Surg* 2009;198:726–732.
19. Gordon LA. *Gordon's guide to the surgical morbidity and mortality conference*. Philadelphia, PA: Hanley & Belfus; 1994.
20. Pierluissi E, Fischer MA, Campbell AR, et al. Discussion of medical errors in morbidity and mortality conferences. *JAMA* 2003;290:2838–2842.
21. Harbison SP, Regehr G. Faculty and resident opinions regarding the role of morbidity and mortality conference. *Am J Surg* 1999;177: 136–139.
22. Prince JM, Vallabhaneni R, Zenati MS, et al. Increased interactive format for morbidity and mortality conference improves educational value and enhances confidence. *J Surg Educ* 2007;64:266–272.
23. Bender LC, Klingensmith ME, Freeman BD, et al. Anonymous group peer review in surgery morbidity and mortality conference. *Am J Sur* 2009;198:270–276.
24. Risucci DA, Sullivan T, DiRusso S, et al. Assessing educational validity of the morbidity and mortality conference: a pilot study. *Curr Surg* 2003;60:204–209.
25. Antonacci AC, Lam S, Lavarias V, et al. A morbidity and mortality conference-based classification system for adverse events: surgical outcome analysis: part I. *J Surg Res* 2008;147:172–177.
26. Antonacci AC, Lam S, Lavarias V, et al. A report card system using error profile analysis and concurrent morbidity and mortality review: surgical outcome analysis: part II. *J Surg Res* 2008;153:95–104.
27. Murayama K, Derossis A, DaRosa D, et al. A critical evaluation of the morbidity and mortality conference. *Am J Surg* 2002;183:246–250.
28. Dissanaike S, Berry M, Ginos J, et al. Variations in the perception of trauma-related complications between attending surgeons, surgery residents, critical care nurses, and medical students. *Am J Surg* 2009; 197:764–768.
29. Hutter MM, Rowell KS, Devaney LA, et al. Identification of surgical complications and deaths: an assessment of the traditional surgical morbidity and mortality conference compared with the American College of Surgeons-National Surgical Quality Improvement Program. *J Am Coll Surg* 2006;203:618–624.
30. Gallagher TH, Waterman AD, Ebers A, et al. Patients' and physicians' attitudes regarding the disclosure of medical errors. *JAMA* 2003;289: 1001–1007.
31. Fabri PJ, Zayas-Castro JL. Human error, not communication and systems, underlies surgical complications. *Surgery* 2008;144:557–563; discussion 563–565.
32. Pollack C, Bayley C, Mendiola M, et al. Helping clinicians find resolution after a medical error. *Camb Q Healthc Ethics* 2003;12:203–207.
33. Fisher R, Ury W. *Getting to yes*. New York, NY: Penguin Books; 1991.
34. Croskerry P. The importance of cognitive errors in diagnosis and strategies to minimize them. *Acad Med* 2003;78:775–780.
35. Fletcher KE, Davis SQ, Underwood W, et al. Systematic review: effects of resident work hours on patient safety. *Ann Intern Med* 2004;141:851–857.
36. Lockley SW, Barger LK, Harvard Work Hours, Health and Safety Group et al. Effects of health care provider work hours and sleep deprivation on safety and performance. *Jt Comm J Qual Patient Saf* 2007;33: 7–18.
37. West CP, Tan AT, Habermann TM, et al. Association of resident fatigue and distress with perceived medical errors. *JAMA* 2009;302:1294–1300.
38. Gawande A, Zinner MJ, Studdert DM, et al. Analysis of errors reported by surgeons at three teaching hospitals. *Surgery* 2003;133:614–621.
39. Gerdes J, Kahol K, Smith M, et al. The effect of fatigue on cognitive and psychomotor skills of trauma residents and attending surgeons. *Am J Surg* 2008;196:813–819.
40. Kahol K, Satava RM, Ferrara J, et al. Effect of short-term pretrial practice on surgical proficiency in simulated environments: a randomized trial of the 'preoperative warm-up' effect. *J Am Coll Surg* 2009;208:255–268.
41. Eastridge BJ, Hamilton EC, O'Keefe GE, et al. Effect of sleep deprivation on the performance of simulated laparoscopic surgical skill. *Am J Surg* 2003;186:169–174.
42. ElBardissi AW, Wiegmann DA, Henrickson S, et al. Identifying methods to improve heart surgery: an operative approach and strategy for implementation on an organizational level. *Eur J Cardiothorac Surg* 2008;34:1027–1033.
43. Rogers SO, Gawande AA, Kwaan M, et al. Analysis of surgical errors in closed malpractice claims at 4 liability insurers. *Surgery* 2006;140:25–33.
44. Greenberg CC, Regenbogen SE, Studdert DM, et al. Patterns of communication breakdowns resulting in injury to surgical patients. *J Am Coll Surg* 2007;204:533–540.
45. Christian CK, Gustafson ML, Roth EM, et al. A prospective study of patient safety in the operating room. *Surgery* 2006;139:159–173.
46. Lingard L, Espin S, Whyte S, et al. Communication failures in the operating room: an observational classification of recurrent types and effects. *Qual Saf Health Care* 2004;13:330–334.
47. Arora S, Hull L, Sevdalis N, et al. Factors compromising safety in surgery: stressful events in the operating room. *Am J Surg* 2010;199:60–65.
48. Brown R, Dunn S, Brnes K, et al. Doctors' stress responses and poor communication performance in simulated bad-news consultations. *Acad Med* 2009;84:1595–1602.
49. Woodrow SI, Park J, Murray BJ, et al. Differences in the perceived impact of sleep deprivation among surgical and non-surgical residents. *Med Educ* 2008;42:459–467.
50. Nash R. The "killing season": does inexperience cost lives? (Comment). *Lancet* 2009;347:1313–1314.

51. Haller G, Myles PS, Taffe P, et al. Rate of undesirable events at beginning of academic year: retrospective cohort study. *BMJ* 2009;339: b3974.
52. Jen MH, Bottle A, Majeed A, et al. Early in-hospital mortality following trainee doctors' first day at work. *PLoS One* 2009;4:e7103.
53. Englesbe MJ, Pelletier SJ, Magee JC, et al. Seasonal variation in surgical outcomes as measured by the American College of Surgeons-National Surgical Quality Improvement Program (ACS-NSQIP). *Ann Surg* 2007; 246:456–462.
54. Inaba K, Recinos G, Teixeira P, et al. Complications and death at the start of the new academic year: is there a "July phenomenon"? *J Trauma* 2010;68:19–22.
55. Ehrlinger J, Johnson K, Banner M, et al. Why the unskilled are unaware: further explorations of (absent) self-insight among the incompetent. *Organ Behav Hum Decis Process* 2008;105:98–121.
56. Kruger J, Dunning D. Unskilled and unaware of it: how difficulties in recognizing one's own incompetence lead to inflated self-assessments. *J Pers Soc Psychol* 1999;77(6):1121–1134.
57. Kennedy TJ, Regehr G, Ross Baker G, et al. Preserving professional credibility: grounded theory study of medical trainees' requests for clinical support. *BMJ* 2009;338:b138.
58. Wetzel CM, Kneebone RL, Woloshynowych M. The effects of stress on surgical performance. *Am J Surg* 2006;191:5–10.
59. LeBlanc VR. The effects of acute stress on performance: implications for health professions education. *Acad Med* 2009;84:S25–S33.
60. LeBlanc VR, McArthur B, King K, et al. Paramedic performance in calculating drug dosages following stressful scenarios in a human patient simulator. *Prehosp Emerg Care* 2005;9:439–444.
61. Liu D, Grundgeieger T, Sanderson PM, et al. Interruptions and blood transfusion checks: lessons from the simulated operating room. *Anesth Analg* 2009;108:219–222.
62. Williams RG, Silverman R, Schwind C. Surgeon information transfer and communication: factors affecting quality and efficiency of inpatient care. *Ann Surg* 2007;245:159–169.
63. Rogers D, Lingard L. Surgeons managing conflict: a framework for understanding the challenge. *J Am Coll Surg* 2006;203:568–574.
64. Eva KW, Regehr G. "I'll never play professional football" and other fallacies of self-assessment. *J Contin Educ Health Prof* 2008;28:14–19.
65. Moulton CA, Regehr G, Lingard L, et al. 'Slowing down when you should': initiators and influences of the transition from the routine to the effortful [published online ahead of print March 23, 2010]. *J Gastrointest Surg* 2010;14(6):1019–1026.
66. Kahol K, Leyba MJ, Deka M, et al. Effect of fatigue on psychomotor and cognitive skills. *Am J Surg* 2008;195:195–204.
67. Arora S, Sevdalis N, Nestel D, et al. Managing intraoperative stress: what do surgeons want from a crisis training program? *Am J Surg* 2009;197:537–543.
68. Yule S, Flin R, Paterson-Brown S, et al. Non-technical skills for surgeons in the operating room: a review of the literature. *Surgery* 2006;139:140–149.
69. Etchells E, O'Neill C, Bernstein M. Patient safety in surgery: error detection and prevention. *World J Surg* 2003;27:936–941.
70. Bandura A. *Self-efficacy: the exercise of control*. New York, NY: W. H. Freeman; 1997.
71. Pilpel D, Schor R, Benbassat J. Barriers to acceptance of medical error: the case for a teaching program. *Med Educ* 1998;32:3–7.
72. Wu AW. Medical error: The second victim (editorial). *BMJ* 2000;320: 726–727.
73. Schwappach DL, Boluarte TA. The emotional impact of medical error involvement on physicians: a call for leadership and organizational accountability. *Swiss Med Wkly* 2008;138(1–2):9–15.
74. Christensen JF, Levinson W, Dunn PM. The heart of darkness: the impact of perceived mistakes on physicians. *J Gen Intern Med* 1992;7: 424–431.
75. Clinton HR, Obama B. Making patient safety the centerpiece of medical liability reform. *N Engl J Med* 2006;354:2205–2208.
76. Boothman RC, Blackwell A, Campbell D Jr, et al. A better approach to medical malpractice claims? The University of Michigan experience. *J Health Life Sci Law* 2009;2:125–159.
77. Kraman SS, Hamm G. Risk management: extreme honesty may be the best policy. *Ann Int Med* 1999;131:963–967.
78. Gallagher TH. A 62-year-old woman with skin cancer who experienced wrong-site surgery: review of medical error. *JAMA* 2009;302:669–677.
79. Harvard Full Disclosure Working Group. *When things go wrong: responding to adverse events*. Burlington, MA: Massachusetts Coalition for the Prevention of Medical Errors; 2006.

CHAPTER

3

Surgical Training: Present and Future

Rebecca M. Minter and Paul G. Gauger

INTRODUCTION

Three prominent themes characterize American medicine today. There has been an explosive increase in the basic knowledge underlying clinical practice. There is a crisis in the manner in which we deliver health care. And recent technologic advances are so fundamentally complex as to require major reassessment and change in accepted educational paradigms (1). All these factors have affected the long-standing model of American surgical training to create a unique crisis in surgical education. Table 3.1 contains an incomplete assessment of the factors contributing to this crisis.

Although every generation laments change, it is not an overstatement to say that surgical training is undergoing more changes and challenges than ever before. As a field steeped in tradition and inherited wisdom, surgery has been slow to embrace change; however, viewed from the proper perspective, much of the change is welcome and necessary. Change must be managed to ensure that the values of the profession are preserved. To do so, it is critically important to understand the internal and external forces that have led to this point. Selected influences are examined below within the context of surgical training, and the manner in which educational programs will have to adapt are delineated.

FORCES AFFECTING SURGICAL TRAINING

Increase in number and complexity of procedures

Remarkable advances have been made in the last few decades in the understanding of diseases and in the options available for treatment. For some diseases, surgical intervention is less common (e.g., peptic ulcer disease); but for many others, factors such as earlier detection have rendered some operations more common (e.g., colon cancer). For nearly all examples, the breadth of therapeutic options has increased significantly. The emergence of laparoscopic and endoscopic technologies has greatly amplified this trend. The present-day graduating surgical resident is responsible for demonstrating exposure to an ever-increasing list of procedures, leading to a potentially diffuse and superficial experience. Without careful attention, exposure may become the rule, rather than demonstration of proficiency and competency within a given domain. Current competency-based curricular initiatives led by the Surgical Council on Resident Education (SCORE) consortium and the American College of Surgeons (ACS) and the Association of Program Directors of Surgery (APDS) will hopefully reverse this trend in the coming years.

The emergence of general surgery subspecialty practice

General surgery has gradually changed from a broad and flexible specialty responsible for "the skin and its contents" to a more limited definition. Many of the operations formerly performed by the general surgeon are now being performed by a general surgeon with additional fellowship training or declared interest. The rise in vascular, endocrine, and colorectal surgery practices is an example of this increase in subspecialization. These changes have a bearing on the curriculum redesign required to facilitate specialization and fellowship training, while preserving the critical experiences required for General Surgery training.

As surgical training represents a microcosm of medical practice, it was to be expected that the sweeping changes of the last 30 to 40 years have had downstream effects. Medical practice has been transformed into medical industry. Declining professional reimbursement, an increased pace of clinical practice, and dehumanization of the physician–patient relationship have taken their toll on practicing physicians. The medical professional is occasionally demoralized, confused, and cynical. Perhaps amplified by the perception that surgeons are working harder and being paid less than those in other specialties, dissatisfaction and frustration might be vocally and visibly expressed during the daily routine. As a result, young, enthusiastic, impressionable medical students and trainees find themselves analyzing their interactions with established surgeons and asking, "Why would I want to do what they do when they don't even want to do what they do?"

Rebecca M. Minter, Paul G. Gauger: University of Michigan, Ann Arbor, MI 48109.

Table 3.1 **Medical education issues, influences, and responsibilities**

General Educational Issues
Explosive increase in medical knowledge
Competitive imbalance between workload and educational opportunity
Need for new training paradigms
ACGME outcome project (competencies)
Changing expectations of patients and society
Changes in educational techniques and technology (Internet, simulation, etc.)
Sources of innovation outside academic medicine (industry R&D)
Focus on documentation instead of delivery of care
Policy, Administrative, and Financial Issues
Decreased number of applicants for training
Changes in applicant quality
Changing demographics of applicant pool
Increased medical school dependence on clinical revenue
Decreased reimbursement for graduate medical education
Decreased faculty professional reimbursement
Length of training programs
Increased indebtedness of trainees
Increased fraction of foreign medical graduates in training programs
Specific Surgical Training Issues
Ensuring broad exposure to surgical subspecialties
Increased technologic sophistication and dependency on procedures
Assessing surgical competency
RRC mandates/standards for case volume during training
Continuity of care/workload
Disenchantment with specialty among practitioners
Personal Issues for Trainees
Increased indebtedness of graduates
Low pay
Lack of overtime compensation
Lack of retirement benefits
Length and intensity of training
Balance between workload and personal time
Decreased income as practitioner to repay loan burden

ACGME, Accreditation Council for Graduate Medical Education; R&D, research and development; RRC, Residency Review Committee.
From Zelenock GB. Presidential address: medical education: thoughts on the training of physicians and surgeons. *J Vasc Surg* 2003;37:921–929, with permission.

The business of medicine can be so all-consuming that surgeons might find themselves more concerned with the business of coding, billing, and reimbursement than with taking care of patients. Patients sense this, and accordingly, trust is eroded (2). Media exploitation, public perception and dissatisfaction, and the medical liability crisis further test this relationship. This strain is often visible to medical students.

Although trends suggesting declining interest in surgical careers 7 to 10 years ago (2000–2002) appeared to portend significant problems, recent match statistics suggest that the trend might be reversing, with 99.5% to 99.9% of all positions being filled over the last 5 to 7 years (Table 3.2). It has been hypothesized that limitations on duty hours are attracting students who previously may have been too concerned about lifestyle issues to pursue surgical training. In addition, in many segments of the profession, this trend was noted, analyzed, and specifically addressed with interventions intended to demonstrate the pleasure, reward, and satisfaction associated with a surgical career (3).

An evolution in the way we learn and teach

Advances in medical practice, especially those that depend on advanced technologies, require skills neither selected for nor taught in medical schools and residencies. In contrast to the prodigious increase in medical knowledge that occurs every year, our ability to comprehend and then assimilate this knowledge into medical practice is constrained. Even the evolution of clinical practice has been driven by technology. Consider the incorporation of endoscopic, laparoscopic, and robotic technology into current surgical practice. It has been a challenge for practicing surgeons to learn and master the requisite new skills and more difficult to decide how best to teach these skills to surgeons in training. Academic medicine no longer has a monopoly on innovation and research. Many technological advances are driven by industry, which changes the dynamics of education and requires an ongoing interaction with commercial entities, and recent national attention regarding both perceived and real conflicts of interest between medical professionals and industry has made these relationships even more complicated.

Because declining reimbursement exacerbates the economic crisis in surgical practice, a nearly constant attention to one's practice is required. Dedicating time for education and self-improvement is increasingly difficult. In addition, surgical departments are the clinical engines that drive the financial mission of the hospital—especially in academic health centers. As such, the pace of surgical practice is often breakneck and the time for learning,

Table 3.2 **Percentage of open surgical residency slots filled[a,b]**

	2002 Positions[c]		2006 Positions		2007 Positions		2008 Positions		2009 Positions	
	% U.S.	% Total	% U.S.	% Total	% U.S.	% Total	% U.S.	% Total	% U.S.	% Total
Categorical	75.3	94.4	83.3	99.9	78.1	99.8	83.1	99.8	77.4	99.5
Preliminary	38.6	58.1	38.9	60.6	38.1	61.9	41.4	64.0	34.8	58.9

[a]The % U.S. columns indicate the % of positions filled by U.S. medical graduates.
[b]The % total columns indicate the % of positions filled by U.S. and foreign medical graduates.
[c]Indicates nadir of surgical residency positions filled.

teaching, reflection, and innovation is critically diminished. This pace hurts both faculty members and residents. As the educational environment has changed, so has educational technology. As computer-based and Internet-enabled educational programs continue to improve, it is clear that they will soon be the means to provide educational content at an individualized pace, document content exposure, and evaluate content mastery. The ability to simulate both patients and procedures has exponentially increased educational opportunities for the present and the future.

External regulation of the profession and the educational process

When external forces regulate a profession, it nearly always means that the profession has not adequately managed to do so itself. Surgeons have done an inadequate job of articulating why the practice of surgery and the implicit training are different and must remain different from other specialties. Therefore, surgical training is now subject to the same group of regulations as all other specialties. In the wake of frequent and often poorly coordinated regulation from agencies such as the Accreditation Council for Graduate Medical Education (ACGME), the Residency Review Committee (RRC), and the American Board of Surgery (ABS), many program directors find themselves mired in regulations and pressing changes.

Work hour regulations have become highly politicized. This issue has grown in the public eye to center around concerns of sleep deprivation and inadequate supervision. The 2000 Institute of Medicine (IOM) report, To *Err Is Human: Building a Safer Health System*, claimed that medical errors resulted in >1 million patient injuries and nearly 100,000 patient deaths each year (4). Although many possible contributors to medical errors were considered, this report implied a relationship to physician workload, fatigue, lack of alertness, and sleep deprivation, and laid the groundwork for the 2003 duty-hour policy issued by the ACGME. In 2008, another report titled *Resident Duty Hours: Enhancing Sleep, Supervision, and Safety* (5) was issued by the IOM. In this report, further significant restrictions on duty hours were recommended for all residents in training, regardless of specialty. While we currently await ACGME's deliberations and response to this report, it is anticipated that further restrictions will be coming, adding even greater strain on the system. Unfortunately, education has become a casualty of this public and political discourse, such that the time that residents spend engaged in sanctioned educational activities is counted against the duty-hours limit, which only further exacerbates the educational dilemma.

A health care system in crisis

It is an accepted observation that the crisis environment is especially severe in the academic health centers (6). For this reason, the crises more directly impact undergraduate, graduate, and continuing medical education. The Balanced Budget Act of 1997 exacerbated these problems—especially for graduate medical education (GME)—and has severely curtailed educational resources (7). Still, direct and indirect federal funds flow to hospitals—in part to support and subsidize GME. The impact the Affordable Care Act of 2010 will have on GME funding is yet to be determined.

The social contract of medicine and changes in the doctor–patient relationship

The pressures that have led to a perturbed relationship between physicians and patients are complicated. A few decades ago, patients covered under Medicare and Medicaid understood that their care might be provided by physicians in training under the supervision of senior physicians. This relationship was an accepted part of the social contract of medicine. Patients knew that they were participants in the educational process of the profession (8). Increasing affluence and consumerism, dissatisfaction with the insurance industry and the "medical machine," and a general increase in a sense of entitlement and empowerment in the American patient population have altered these expectations. Many patients are no longer interested or willing to participate in the educational process. Many expect their care to be delivered by the most highly skilled practitioner available at all times. Some might misunderstand the process of supervision and question or refuse the participation of trainees in the provision of their care.

Personal economic factors

The definition of residents' jobs is ambiguously mired in a no-man's land between student and employee. This confusion is used as justification for low salaries, lack of retirement benefits, and inadequate work facilities and support systems. For decades the residency years served as a rite of passage and these conditions were tolerated. It was understood that the prestige and affluence afforded to physicians in practice would act as eventual compensation. An increasing number of current medical school graduates do not seek additional training and instead leverage their M.D. degree for success in related fields. As college friends find early success and happiness in fields that require only a fraction of the education and dedication that medicine does, it becomes even more difficult to run the gauntlet of surgical training.

An especially difficult factor in this economic equation is medical school graduate indebtedness. Many students continue to carry loan debt from undergraduate education. The average debt level of graduating American medical students is over $100,000. Because most residents do not accrue retirement savings, each additional year of training threatens lifetime earning potential. Surgical residents, by virtue of extensive training and decreasing remuneration, are disproportionately disadvantaged.

Generational values and lifestyle considerations

It is the archetype of the surgeon to be dedicated to patients at any expense. Most of the great surgeons of the last century had an unflagging dedication to their patients and their careers. However, such dedication, while benefiting patients, often penalized surgeons' marriage and family life. The current generation of men and women pursuing a career in surgery has begun to reject some of these values. It is the pervasive sentiment of this generation that personal happiness is a right to be claimed. Where happiness cannot be guaranteed from one's career alone, it might be found in leisurely pursuit of other interests and in a fulfilling family life. These characteristics are influencing the growth of "lifestyle" specialties such as dermatology and anesthesiology and will be reflected in the workstyles of the next generation of surgeons. While this balance is positive in most regards, it serves to further alter the culture of Surgery, which is currently struggling with an identity crisis related to many simultaneous shifts in practice and evolving expectations of trainees and patients as compared with generations past.

Threats to patient safety and the quality and continuity of care

Society, through its regulatory agencies, has determined that surgical training must change to protect patients from overly tired physicians and medical errors. The consequences of these externally managed changes might not be fully apparent for years (9). The limitation of duty hours and the resulting increase in information transfer (patient handoffs), and the possible emergence of a surgical workforce with a "shift work" mentality, may create a decrease in patient satisfaction from further dilution of the physician–patient relationship as well as in patient safety, as defined by an increase in "near-misses" or medical errors. The field of error analysis has clearly shown that errors occur in systems that are designed in a way that unintentionally enables the error. Although residents previously were largely responsible for the longitudinal care of patients, this care now occurs in spurts and intervals. This care model necessitates frequent transfer of encapsulated medical information and simultaneously discourages individual reassessment of the patient when called upon for intervention or judgment of some sort. Patient rounds now may serve as occasions in which latent errors are enabled.

A recent survey of surgeons in training indicated that the majority felt that they should be allowed to work >80 hours per week (10). Perhaps this response indicates some discomfort with interrupted continuity of care and challenges to professional values. Threshold limitations of work hours, no matter whether they are well reasoned or completely arbitrary, undercut the importance of continuity of care, a principle highly valued by surgeons and one that is absolutely critical to inculcate in future practitioners. Temporal restraints have no place in the definition of a profession or professional behaviors. It is paradoxical that duty-hour regulations are being assimilated into the structure of surgical residency at the same time that professionalism is one of the ACGME Educational Outcomes (Competencies) to be separately taught and measured (11). This juxtaposition of values will require major attention and vigilance in the structure and practice of surgical training in the future, and this strain between professional values may become even further exacerbated if additional constraints are placed on the work and duty-hour environment as a result of the most recent IOM report (5).

Many developed nations have restrictions on the duty hours of physicians in training. It is impossible to completely extrapolate these experiences to American surgery because of differences in patient and societal expectations, as well as differences in traditions and values. In general, maintaining excellent quality surgical training appears to be possible, largely because of an increase in the number of educational resources and technologies, which can facilitate more efficient content assimilation and skill mastery (12). In Sweden, the duty-hour limit has been 40 hours per week for 30 years, and patient outcomes appear not to have suffered as a result. Because of the limited hours and thus, ultimately, limited exposure, the training period has become structured around time-targeted competency goals (13). Curricula have been tightly tailored for specific training programs. The full impact of the European Working Time Directive is yet to be appreciated, however, as many countries have only recently begun to implement these rules.

Decreased operative experience of graduating surgical residents

With the increased breadth of operative procedures to master during graduate medical training, decreasing the work hours in which to be exposed to these procedures is inopportune. Novel solutions will be required. A very practical question is whether the hours off duty are hours lost from mastering operations and preoperative and postoperative care. Several studies that characterize the time and workflow of surgical residents have discovered a large amount of time spent in noneducational activities (14). There is a large opportunity to streamline and redesign surgical residency. "Hours worked" is a poor surrogate for determining "work done," and a large fraction of the traditional duties of residents needs to be transferred to nonphysician clinicians and ancillary staff, or be offset by more efficient models of health care delivery. If it is not accurate to say that residents have been the engine of the academic health center, they traditionally have been the drivetrain. As residents learn to work smarter rather than harder, hospitals must also readjust.

Although limitation of duty hours for surgical training in Sweden appears to not have damaged patient outcomes, it has changed the level of experience and the end product of surgical training. A period of junior specialist practice follows residency training to enhance skills, and subspecialization is very common. Perhaps this factor has preserved excellent patient outcomes, but emergency general surgery operations have suffered because few broadly trained surgeons remain (15). It seems likely that our own system might eventually come to mimic these changes and adjustments. Without an accompanying overhaul of the national (GME) administrative and reimbursement structure and limitations, patient outcomes may ultimately suffer.

Another question centers on how to determine competency. The assumption inherent in the current model of American surgical training is that repeated exposure to patient care and specific operations ensures competency. Competency is a relative concept, and objective determination of proficiency and competency remains elusive. How many cholecystectomies are enough? Should the goal be to do as many operations as possible? Can one perform too many operations before ideal learning no longer occurs? Should these definitions be individualized for different residents? The overarching question is whether the graduating resident meeting RRC requirements is truly prepared for independent surgical practice, and how do we create metrics by which we can reliably make this determination?

Threats to professional values

For many years the nature of surgical training was a paradox. The fact that surgical training was so hard, both mentally and physically punishing, so relentless and lengthy, was the thing that made it so unique, so valuable, and so worthy. Surgeons were imbued with professional values such as altruism and lifetime learning and continuous self-improvement. Most illustrative of this value system was the continuity of care, which permeated surgical practice. Surgeons knew it, patients knew it, and other physicians knew it. As the current model of training involves limitation of work hours and shifts in clinical practice toward outpatient and short-stay procedures, surgical residents are increasingly operating on patients whom they have not previously met or evaluated. Similarly, other residents and faculty address complications when they occur. Aside from losing the opportunity to learn about the continuum of disease and healing, the overall doctor–patient relationship becomes compartmentalized, and as such, is likely diminished. As care is more frequently provided in shifts, it will be challenging and critically important to identify innovative means by which these professional qualities can be inculcated into surgical trainees of today and into the future.

HOW WILL SURGICAL TRAINING CHANGE?

Early specialization programs

In 2003, the ABS approved a pilot training scheme called the Early Specialization Program (ESP). This program is meant to enable residency directors in general surgery, pediatric surgery, and vascular surgery (but not thoracic surgery) to create specific curricular tracks, which lead to dual certification in 6 instead of 7 years. In concept, the fourth clinical year serves as a general surgery chief year and the last 2 years have a concentrated experience in the subspecialty. Both portions of the program need to take place at a single institution, and the pilot requires both a carefully defined curriculum and specific metrics to determine whether the ESP is a success or failure. The American Board of Thoracic Surgery (ABTS) approved a similar pilot program in 2001. This latter resolution determined that certification by the ABS is optional and that other pathways to ABTS certification could be developed. Specifically, the Thoracic Surgery Directors Association would develop categorical integrated 6-year programs for primary certification in Thoracic Surgery. While there has been the development of a handful of ESP Cardiothoracic Surgery programs, these early ESP pilot programs have been largely supplanted with the development of primary integrated residency programs in Vascular and Thoracic Surgery.

While these changes are meant to redefine the training of vascular, pediatric, and thoracic surgeons, the standard curriculum of the general surgery residency will also need to be rearranged to provide a consistent core exposure for those residents who track into specialties from an initial core of general surgery, while redefining the fourth- and fifth-year curricula for residents remaining in general surgery. In addition, for institutions that have integrated vascular and cardiothoracic residencies, core experiences will need to be carved out for the General Surgery residents as well. Although many are concerned about the further disintegration of general surgery that this change may cause, it is conceivable that it could reaffirm general surgery as a destination instead of an in-transit experience. If the final years are to be preserved as advanced experiences in general surgery (complex hepatobiliary cases, oncology cases, endocrine procedures, etc.), careful attention will need to be paid to the redesign of the curriculum required to facilitate the ESPs and integrated residency training programs in order to preserve experiences for those pursuing a career in general surgery. At present, approximately 85% of general surgery trainees are pursuing fellowship training for an additional 1 to 2 years to gain expertise within a given field of general surgery. This is a message from our trainees that cannot be ignored, and it is unclear whether there will be opportunities for this tracking and final training to occur within the context of general surgery training in the future or not.

Length of training issues

The trend to support earlier specialization and consolidation of surgical training could not have come at a more awkward time. The impact of the 80-hour workweek on resident education is not yet completely defined, and the workweek may become even more constrained in the near future. On the basis of the experience in New York State over the last decade, it seems possible to provide solid surgical training in the setting of limited work hours. If the ESP is to succeed in the context of limited work hours, the program director position will become even more challenging. All rotation experiences will need to be planned and provided with the education–service balance clearly tipped toward the former.

It has been suggested that if surgical experience is meant to stay the same, then limitation of the weekly work schedule would require additional years of training. This calculus is oversimplified. If our current federal reimbursement for GME continues, training extension will almost certainly not occur because of the limits of the current GME funding structure that dictates the maximum term of reimbursable training to be 5 years. If, however, further restrictions are placed on duty hours, additional years of training are likely to be required as has occurred in Europe. Some would argue that this has already occurred with the proliferation of fellowships, which many refer to as the "new Chief resident year."

Novel residency structures and physician extenders

If residencies could be redesigned to form the ideal training system with unlimited financial and political support, they would likely look vastly different. However, the immediately necessary changes must be made within the matrix of current resources and restrictions. A number of reengineering solutions have been suggested that manage immediate regulatory issues while variably balancing educational needs (15). An Apprenticeship Model is built around sequential close working relationships with mentor faculty who are chosen for both their skills as teachers and the educational value of their practice. This model theoretically minimizes in-house time on call and results in early intensive technical skills training. The Mastery (Case-Based) Model proposes that residents develop knowledge and skills associated with predefined diseases and operations. A logistical challenge, this type of program would assign cases to residents on the basis of individual educational needs. This type of residency would potentially be most flexible in terms of advancement, "job-sharing," and overall training time. Another proposed model is based on the Night Float System. This is a more traditional team-based system in which some residents provide patient care only during the night shift (on a rotating basis). This schedule obviously is meant to facilitate most of the other residents going home, but, admittedly, it sublimates the educational value of the rotation to the service component. Because it is a temporary and equally distributed experience, it might be a legitimate trade-off.

As the pace of clinical practice increases with the aging of the population and the impending shortage in physicians and as the overall length of training is very unlikely to change, it is clear that many new members of the patient care team will be required. Nurse practitioners and physician assistants have already added substantially to both inpatient and outpatient settings. Often the cost of these practitioners is borne by the hospitals that have long benefited from a seemingly inexhaustible and inexpensive workforce in the resident pool. It will take careful attention by program directors and chairmen to deploy these additional professionals in duties that decrease the "service" expectations of physicians in training while increasing the "education" opportunities. In short, we have a responsibility to ensure that physician extenders do not become physician replacements. However, the model in which physician assistants are charged only with dictations and paperwork while surgical residents spend all day operating carries an inherent danger that we will be breeding a generation of "incomplete" surgeons or "technicians," which will eventually decrease our respect and stature as a profession. Incorporation of these nonphysician clinicians will eventually lead to reforms in the inadequate pay and benefit structure of residents as the differences in their training and their level of commitment will become more evident.

New methods of feedback and assessment

One of the basic premises of surgical training is that facts must be learned. Those residents most successful in surgical training are often not those with the largest selection of facts at the ready but those who are facile at finding accurate information when knowledge deficiencies are encountered. In response to the growing body of medical knowledge and practical limits to the capacity to learn and memorize, technology has fostered robust and available decision support. Surgical decision making increasingly utilizes handheld computing and electronic resources for access to the best evidence for clinical practice. Residency programs will become less focused on teaching residents what to know and think and more on how to find the answers they need from trusted sources when a gap in their knowledge and experience is encountered. This approach is a much more appropriate andragogical model for lifelong learning and for the continual quest for improvement that defines the surgical profession.

The ways that residents and practicing physicians are evaluated will change substantially. Surgical training has long used a model of evaluation that assessed skills globally and assumed transfer of competency from one skill set to another. The ACGME outcomes project has already changed this issue by requiring a much more specific and granular way of rating competency in defined domains. The final format of the related evaluation instruments and methods is still unsettled. The level of feedback will be increased to close the loop between education and assessment. One can imagine that the steep slope of the learning curve during surgical residency can be increased even further by individualized, supportive, and specific feedback provided in defined areas. Computers will provide some of this feedback during exercises in decision analysis and in procedural simulations.

No longer will subjective assessment of skills, knowledge, and attitude be sufficient for evaluation during residency training. Competency will be defined by measurable criteria, and these data will be used for decisions regarding graded responsibility and for promotions and advancement through the training schemes. If these strategies are adequately operationalized, residencies might eventually be competency-driven (and relatively time-independent) instead of time-driven (and relatively competency-independent). For this change to occur, the rigid limitations of GME funding need to be redesigned significantly. Implementation will ultimately require accurately defining the key elements of surgical training, establishing quantifiable metrics, stringently measuring performance against criteria, and reporting outcomes throughout the career of a surgeon (15).

Educational integration

A shift in where and by whom residents are trained will likely occur. There is very likely to be a shortage of qualified physicians in the years to come (16). It is probable that the total number of slots for training will increase, and these will most likely be incremental additions at larger, better-coordinated programs. This will require, however, concessions made in the Balanced Budget Act of 1997 which has currently capped the total number of trainees in a given institution at the level present in 1997. As the complexity of the surgical field and the prevalence of subspecialty practice increases, and residents increasingly pursue fellowship training, it is inevitable that the operative experience of fellows will compete with that of residents. Successful management of this competition will require an increase in the coordination that occurs within and between training programs, especially in light of the curricular implications of the ESPs and primary subspecialty integrated programs. For example, programs with an active vascular surgery fellowship or residency might choose to have general surgery residents rotate at active sites where the vascular surgery fellow or resident do not rotate.

Another aspect of educational coordination will involve taking full advantage of scientific and clinical expertise, where and when it exists. Distance learning via the Internet and live telesurgery transmissions make this a very tangible possibility. As the body of surgical knowledge increases, and as the multidisciplinary aspect of clinical care becomes more prominent, better coordination between undergraduate, graduate, and continuing medical curricula will need to be defined. Because the advanced technology aspects of surgical practice impact the spectrum of caregivers, the educational process will often involve teams. Because of patient-safety issues, the costs of this education will likely be shifted to hospitals.

Simulation training

To fully develop the skills of surgeons, live patients are absolutely necessary. Of course, there is an obligation to provide optimal treatment and ensure patient safety and best outcomes. Balancing these two needs represents a fundamental ethical tension in surgical education (17). Other professions that are typified by long stretches of routine shattered infrequently by high-hazard, high-acuity crises, such as the aviation industry, the military, and the nuclear power industry, have long ago institutionalized simulation-based training. Medical education has been slow to embrace simulation for reasons of cost, complacency, and lack of rigorous determination of reliability and construct validity. Focused by the patient safety movement, the face validity of simulation education is overwhelming. Many recent articles in the ethics literature have condemned the use of sedated or dying patients for training in examinations or basic procedures, again highlighting the role for simulation-based training (18).

The first attempted surgical simulations utilizing virtual reality took place a decade ago. Since then, computer power has rapidly improved, as has the quality of procedural simulation both in terms of visual fidelity and enhancements such as haptic feedback. The digital aspect of these computer-based simulations allows robust data capture to provide immediate performance assessment and feedback. Although the literature establishing the construct validity and the reliability of these education and assessment tools is relatively limited, it is growing exponentially. Professional organizations have begun to seriously consider the potential of these tools to revolutionize the surgical training and certification processes, and at present all surgery training programs are required by the ACGME to have access to some level of simulation for general surgery training (19,20).

Although the advent and diffusion of laparoscopic surgery was soon followed by curricula and guidelines for training, the specific metrics of evaluation were lacking. Owing to efforts in such diverse locations as Scotland, Canada, and the United States, sophisticated analyses of psychomotor skills have led to objective structured assessments for technical skills. Currently, there is no standardized threshold level that residents are expected to attain, and there is no consensus on metrics of performance, methods of evaluation, or the significance of these measurements when applied to clinical outcomes (20,21). This experience in teaching standard surgical skills has not been fully realized in surgical simulation technology. For a curriculum based on accepted criteria in the training and evaluation of technical skills on a simulator, Satava has recommended the following steps: (i) development of standardized definitions/taxonomy of technical skills (e.g., metrics); (ii) definitions/taxonomy of errors; (iii) establishment of core outcomes/results reporting; and (iv) development of a comprehensive curriculum. The curriculum

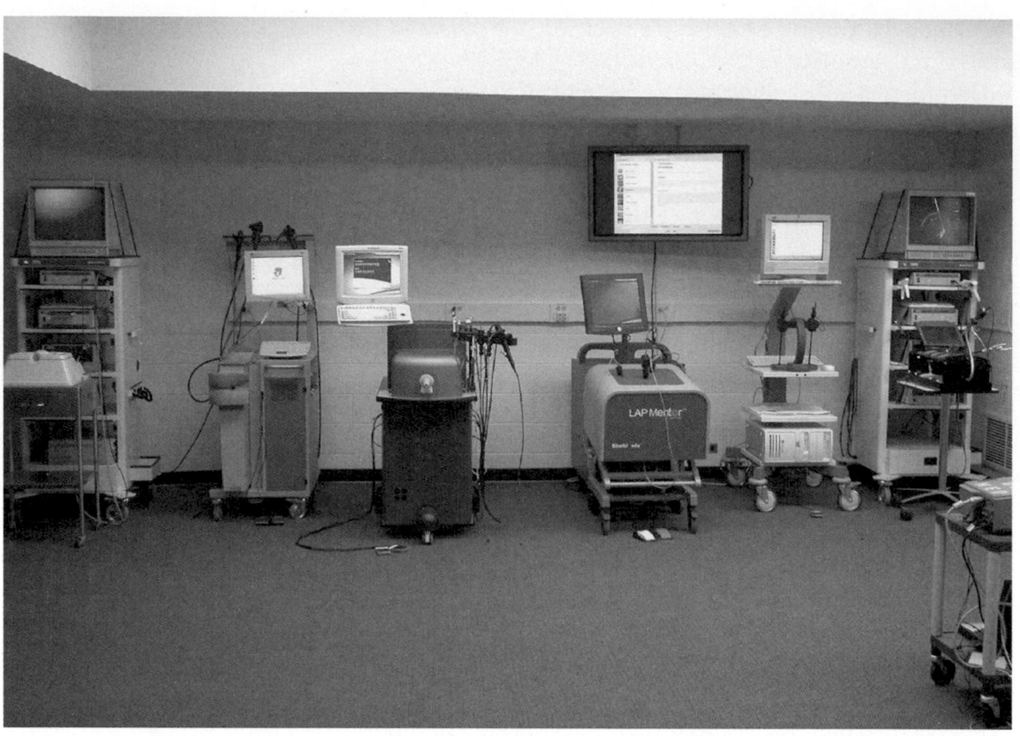

FIGURE 3.1. Simulators are available for many procedures.

should include (i) didactic information (lecture, multimedia, etc.) of the relevant anatomy and correct performance of the skills being taught; (ii) definition and description of the errors the simulator will detect; (iii) pretest documentation that the student understands the information; (iv) performance of the simulation with immediate feedback after errors; (v) a final report on performance; and (vi) a longitudinal record of the performances over time as well as comparison to peer levels (21).

Currently, simulation-based training and assessment is available for such diverse procedures as general laparoscopy, laparoscopic cholecystectomy, hysteroscopy, bronchoscopy, esophagoduodenoscopy, endoscopic retrograde cholangiopancreatography, endoscopic ultrasound, arthroscopy, endoscopic sinus surgery, endovascular surgery, and others (Fig. 3.1). For most of these applications, the procedure being simulated requires interaction with an image. The image serves as the basis for the simulation. For that reason, simulation of open operations, where the interaction with tissue uses many senses, is years away—or perhaps unattainable. As impressive as some of the currently available simulators are, it is fascinating to consider that the field is generally at the same stage of development as the first flight simulator (20). It took nearly 20 years for the field of flight simulation to develop into a standard part of flight training and certification, so we will likely continue to see significant advances in surgical simulation. In addition, the ability to simulate interactive environments with technologies such as the CAVE (Cave Automatic Virtual Environment) (Fig. 3.2) and the geowall stereoscopic

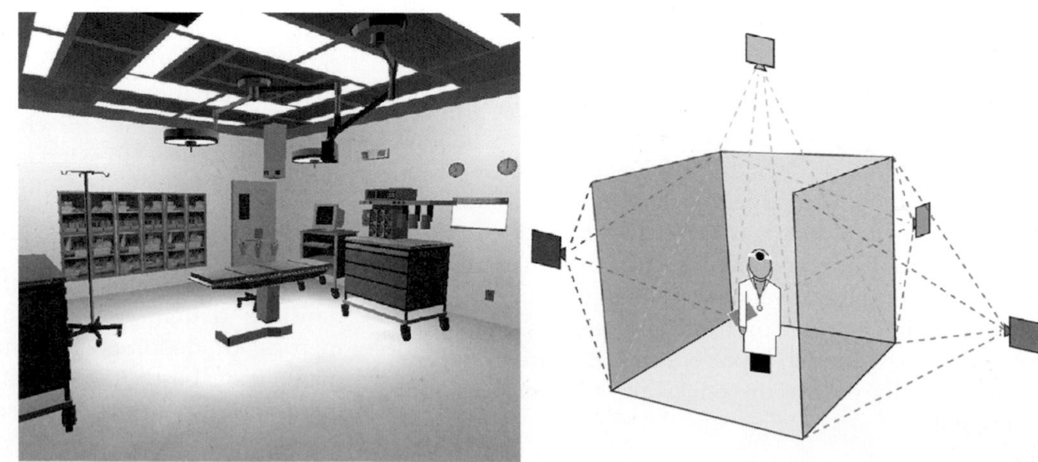

FIGURE 3.2. Simulated environments may be important to increase the fidelity (sense of realism) when interacting with simulated patients or procedures. Interactive virtual reality environments such as the operating room (left panel) can be projected into the CAVE (Cave Automatic Virtual Environment) environment (right panel) to create an immersive virtual environment.

projection system will have the potential to increase fidelity and to enhance evaluation of performance under stress.

CONCLUSION

Change is upon us and the opportunities are numerous to further improve the system of surgical training in the United States. We must now be proactive in order to improve the field and enhance the aspects of surgery that we cherish. As characterized by an improvement in the ratio of resident education to resident service and the incorporation of physician extenders into the clinical enterprise, and as enhanced by computer-based learning and simulation, the future of surgical training is quite bright.

REFERENCES

1. Zelenock GB. Presidential address: medical education: thoughts on the training of physicians and surgeons. *J Vasc Surg* 2003;37:921–929.
2. Russell TR. What is the future of surgery? *Arch Surg* 2003;138:825–831.
3. Mulholland MW. Program increases medical student interest in surgical careers. *Bull Am Coll Surg* 2003;88:25–27.
4. Kohn L, Corrigan J, Donaldson ME. *To err is human: building a safer health system*. Washington, DC: National Academic Press; 2000.
5. Ulmer C, Wolman D, Johns M. *Resident duty hours: enhancing sleep, supervision, and safety*. Washington, DC: National Academic Press; 2009.
6. Kassirer JP. Academic medical centers under siege. *N Engl J Med* 1994; 331:1370–1371.
7. Inglehart JK. Medicare's declining payments to physicians. *N Engl J Med* 2001;346:1924–1930.
8. Ludmerer KM. *A time to heal*. New York: Oxford University Press; 1999.
9. Russell RCG. Limitations of work hours: the U.K. experience. *Surgery* 2003;134:19–22.
10. Underwood W, Boyd AJ, Fletcher KE, The Executive Committee of the American College of Surgeons-Candidate Associate Group, Lypson ML. Viewpoints from generation X. A survey of candidate and associate viewpoints on resident duty-hour regulations. *J Am Coll Surg* 2004; 198:989–993.
11. Fischer JE. Continuity of care: a casualty of the 80-hour work week. *Acad Med* 2004;79:381–383.
12. Romanchuk K. The effect of limiting residents' work hours on their surgical training: a Canadian perspective. *Acad Med* 2004;79:384–385.
13. Ihse I, Haglund U. The Swedish 40-hour workweek: how does it affect surgical care? *Surgery* 2003;134:17–18.
14. Brasel KJ, Pierre AL, Weigelt JA. Resident work hours. What they are really doing. *Arch Surg* 2004;139:490–494.
15. DaRosa DA, Bell RH, Dunnington GL. Residency program models, implications, and evaluation: results of a think tank consortium on resident work hours. *Surgery* 2003;133:13–23.
16. Cooper RA, Getzen TE, McKee JH, et al. Economic and demographic trends signal an impending physician shortage. *Health Aff* 2002;21: 140–154.
17. Ziv A, Wolpe PR, Small SD, et al. Simulation-based medical education: an ethical imperative. *Acad Med* 2003;78:783–788.
18. Rosenson J, Tabas JA, Patterson P. Teaching invasive procedures to medical students. *JAMA* 2004;291:119–120.
19. Seymour NE, Gallagher AG, Roma SA, et al. Virtual reality training improves operating room performance. *Ann Surg* 2002;236:458–464.
20. Satava RM. Accomplishments and challenges of surgical simulation. Dawning of the next-generation surgical education. *Surg Endosc* 2001; 15:232–241.
21. Satava RM. Disruptive visions. Surgical education. *Surg Endosc* 2004; 18:779–781.

CHAPTER

4

Continuing Education for Practicing Surgeons

Richard E. Burney and R. Van Harrison

Continuing medical education (CME) consists of educational activities that serve to maintain, develop, or increase the knowledge, skills, and professional performance and relationships that a physician uses to provide services to patients, the public, or the profession. The content of CME is the body of knowledge and skills generally recognized and accepted by the profession as within the basic medical sciences, the discipline of clinical medicine, and the provision of health care to the public (1).

In the broadest sense, CME for surgeons is the acquisition of new knowledge and skills after completing residency or fellowship training. Once beyond the structured environment of postgraduate training, all surgeons face the ongoing challenge of maintaining their general medical knowledge base, keeping up with changes in basic pathophysiology of disease, learning about new pharmacotherapeutic agents, becoming acquainted with new or improved surgical techniques, improving day-to-day medical and surgical care practices, acquiring new technical skills, and learning how to use new devices and apply new technology in their daily lives. Physicians today also need to learn how to put new medical knowledge and new aspects of surgical care into practice in collaboration with other health care team members, within their health care systems, consistent with national health care policies. All these things are part of CME and continued professional development (also referred to as "life-long learning"). Continued learning is a prerequisite to good practice and to the prevention of complications that can occur when education or practices are deficient. Surgeons have a professional obligation to continue their education and to maintain competence throughout their surgical careers (2).

A narrower view of CME is that it is the enterprise overseen by the Accreditation Council for Continuing Medical Education (ACCME). The ACCME's mission is to identify, develop, and promote standards for quality of CME. ACCME accredits eligible institutions by reviewing the processes that CME providers follow in developing and producing CME activities. Accredited CME providers can designate American Medical Association Physician Recognition Award (AMA-PRA) Category 1 Credit™ for their activities. Physicians participating in these activities are awarded this credit. Various state and local administrative entities mandate that physicians obtain this formal credit for relicensure and other regulatory requirements. CME may also be mandated as a requirement for credentialing within a hospital or health care organization. The primary purpose for seeking continuing education is to improve patient care, not to satisfy licensing and other mandates, but the latter provides incentive for participating in CME activities. For those motivated to learn, the accumulation of CME credits presents less of a problem than does the proper recording and documentation of that CME for administrative and reporting purposes.

Richard E. Burney, R. Van Harrison: University of Michigan, Ann Arbor, MI 48109.

BRIEF HISTORY OF CME

At the turn of the 20th century, on July 3, 1900, Sir William Osler gave an address in London entitled "The Importance of Post-Graduate Study," in which he emphasized the importance of lifelong learning for professional competence. This event is generally accepted as the birth of CME (3). Since then the importance of advancing the profession by providing opportunities for individual practitioners to acquire new information and improve skills has never been questioned. The American College of Surgeons (ACS) was founded in 1913 to develop, among other goals, a broad and continuing program for postgraduate surgical education. One of the chief purposes of medical societies, surgical associations, and specialty societies has been to sponsor journals in which to publish and disseminate new information. University-based postgraduate courses were developed in the 1930s. In the past 50 years, academic medical centers and medical and surgical specialty organizations have played increasingly larger roles in providing continuing education programs that offer learning opportunities for practicing physicians. More recently, specialty societies and device manufacturers have sponsored courses to assist surgeons to learn how to use new technologies, such as ultrasound, laparoscopic and robotic surgery.

In the early 1970s, several trends made CME a focus of additional attention. First, the expansion of scientific information made medical practice more complex while offering hope for cure of previously untreatable medical problems. Second, patients and their advocates began to call attention to errors and failures in medical practice, and the costs associated with medical malpractice actions began to rise and be recognized as a major societal problem. Third, educational psychologists began to define and analyze adult educational processes more scientifically and to identify those that are most effective. Finally, the American Medical Association, in response to these pressures and making the assumption that lack of information was a remediable cause of physician failure, proposed that physicians voluntarily obtain 50 hours of CME per year in order to maintain proficiency. Physicians who did so became eligible for the PRA from the AMA.

Another response to these pressures was the introduction of new regulations by state governments. By 1978, 13 states, beginning with New Mexico and Michigan, had passed laws that made 50 hours per year of CME mandatory for relicensure. Most other states have passed similar laws—currently 44 states require CME for relicensure (4). This new, mandatory CME requirement led to an expansion of entrepreneurial CME offerings. Time and money were swiftly invested in providing education opportunities for physicians, sometimes in vacation settings and often of questionable practical or educational value. At the same time, mandatory CME had the salutary effect of encouraging hospitals to devote funds and attention to providing CME for medical staff members.

SOURCES AND CHARACTERISTICS OF HIGH-QUALITY, EFFECTIVE CME

Diffusion and acquisition of new knowledge occur through a variety of mechanisms and stimuli, both formal and informal. A list of the most common, readily available sources of continuing education is shown in Table 4.1. Only a small number of these are formal CME offerings. The most common and frequently unacknowledged source of new information is informal discussion with professional colleagues. Most surgeons obtain new information by asking questions of their medical and surgical colleagues. In the right circumstance, this is one of the chief sources of reliable, practical information.

Regular gathering of general information through reading of relevant journals and reports is a simple yet basic way to expand one's knowledge base. Every surgeon must set aside time to read a selection of journals and other sources of written information. Computer- and Internet-based educational materials are proliferating and are readily available from a variety of sources, as well.

Also important is attending a selection of local, regional, or national professional meetings at which a broad range of information is offered and at which one can share information with colleagues and ask questions. Becoming aware of new knowledge induces one to ask questions that lead to more directed or focused learning and is the first step toward the application of this new knowledge into practice. High-quality skill acquisition courses offered through universities, professional societies, and industry facilitate the skill acquisition needed to apply new knowledge.

Table 4.1 Readily available sources of continuing medical education (CME)

Source
Informal discussion or consultation with colleagues
Textbooks and journals
Reading only
Reading + CME quiz
Hospital/Intramural conferences and committees
Teaching conferences
Morbidity and mortality conferences
Multidisciplinary committees (e.g., Tumor Board)
Journal club
Quality assurance/quality improvement committees
Computer- (CD/DVD) and Internet-based educational programs
Hospital/medical school sponsored
Specialty society-provided (e.g., Society of Colon and Rectal Surgeons)
Industry-sponsored and commercial sites
Professional meetings
Surgical association meetings (e.g., American College of Surgeons)
Clinical Congress
Postgraduate courses
Regional meetings
Special certification courses (e.g., Advanced Trauma Life Support)
Specialty society meetings
University-sponsored postgraduate courses
Skills/Technology acquisition courses (with or without commercial funding)
University-based (e.g., sentinel node biopsy)
Professional society-based (e.g., ultrasound)
Industry-sponsored (e.g., advanced laparoscopy)
Simulation centers

PRINCIPLES OF ADULT EDUCATION AND LEARNING

An understanding of how adults learn will help one select a balance of learning activities that will be most efficient and effective. A number of models have been developed for the complex processes involved in learning (5). Most education models suggest at least four prerequisites for effective continuing education and learning to occur.

- **Motivation:** The first and most important prerequisite is the intrinsic motivation to question oneself, to learn, and to improve. The student who has a question to be answered, or is aware of a deficiency or an inadequacy in need of correction, will have a strong motivation to learn or change behavior. Dilemmas and questions encountered in daily practice are prime sources of motivation, but not the only ones. Competitive pressures and changes in services arising from strategic planning can also be motivating.

- **Objective:** The student must have a clear goal or objective in mind for applying that new knowledge or skill, i.e., know how and when the new information will be put to use.
- **Practice:** The student must have the opportunity not only to read and hear about what is to be learned but also to apply or practice the new behavior in an appropriate simulation context or environment, both to gain familiarity with it and to gain insight into it.
- **Application and feedback:** Finally, the student must apply the new behavior or practice it promptly on a regular basis and there must be timely evaluation or feedback, through data collection and analysis of outcomes, on its success or failure.

For an individual, the phases of learning that bring about behavioral change may be summarized as awareness, agreement, adoption, and adherence (6).

- **Awareness:** Individuals become aware of new ideas through reading, browsing Internet sites, attending meetings, discussing matters with colleagues, and confronting clinical dilemmas on a daily basis.
- **Agreement:** Individuals must intellectually agree that new information is appropriate and worthwhile. Sometimes new and important information is not accepted rapidly, particularly when it calls for a change in behavior. New pain-management approaches and techniques have been available for over a decade, but surgeons are only now slowly accepting them.
- **Adoption:** Having agreed that new information is valid, individuals must decide to adopt that information into their practices. Adopting a new idea might require making changes in day-to-day practices and in the related practices of those around them.
- **Adherence:** The cycle of learning is complete when individuals regularly apply the changes in practice, examine the outcomes over time, and make modifications that improve practice.

Table 4.2 displays four types of continuing education activity in the form of a continuum, the level of personal engagement required for each, how each relates to the general prerequisites for adult learning and to the individual phases of learning outlined above, and some of the advantages and disadvantages of each. The types of CME activity may be summarized as follows:

- **General awareness:** A surgeon's intrinsic motivation to increase knowledge leads to scanning journals and attending weekly lectures, annual update programs, and general review courses. These passive activities are important in providing an awareness of new knowledge but are the least likely to bring insight into

Table 4.2 Types of CME activities and their characteristics

Type of Activity	Level of Engagement	General Prerequisites for Learning	Phases of Individual Learning	Advantages and Limitations
General Awareness				
General reading Informal discussion Listening at conference Viewing a video	Passive learning Unfocused	Motivation	Awareness	Broad content covered Introduces unknown issues Limited expense Limited likelihood of producing change by itself
Answering Questions				
Consultation with colleague Literature search Problem-based learning activities Interaction with others	Active learning More focused	Motivation Objective	Awareness Agreement	Focus on practical issues Must be aware of issue already Limited expense Somewhat likely to produce change
Skill Training				
Preparation and interaction Role playing or simulation Skill practice/demonstration Testing/evaluation	Interactive learning Skill acquisition	Motivation Objective Practice	Awareness Agreement Adoption	Focus on priority skills Often meaningful Likely to produce specific change May carry high direct or indirect expense
Performance Review				
Regular data collection, analysis, and evaluation Regular feedback regarding performance or outcome Prompt application of change or skill into daily practice with feedback	Participation in research or clinical trial Organized change initiative	Motivation Objective Practice Application and feedback	Awareness Agreement Adoption Adherence	Focus on specific activities Often requires supporting infrastructure and related expense Very likely to produce specific change

current problems or by themselves to induce change in behavior.

- **Answering questions:** Settings that demand active participation, presentation, discussion, or argument help the surgeon determine the usefulness of new information and decide whether to accept it. Active participation includes directed reading or a literature search designed to answer specific questions.
- **Skill training:** Having a specific goal and participating in a course that offers a setting for learning and practice under expert monitoring and assistance provide excellent in-depth learning, including practice and adoption of new skills. Highly successful postgraduate courses, such as the ACS Advanced Trauma Life Support course, embody the characteristics of active learning and participation by motivated participants. Courses that teach new surgical techniques, such as laparoscopic and robotic surgery, are also commonly available. Simulation centers now assist physicians to acquire specific new skills as well.
- **Performance review:** Reviews of practice through morbidity and mortality conferences, examination of complication rates, personal databases, or case logs that record outcomes, and other methods of feedback help assure ongoing improvement in practice.

An organized plan for continuing education and professional development must have a balance across the various types of CME activities. Time, location, and practicality demand that much CME time will be devoted to broad, information-gathering activities, such as scanning for new information in discussions, reading, conferences, and regular meetings. In so doing, one continuously gathers information that is potentially applicable to all aspects of one's surgical practice. This broader information gathering helps identify gaps in knowledge and motivates in-depth study of a few areas each year. Skill acquisition courses, although highly effective, are expensive, time consuming, and resource intensive. They should be carefully selected to fill in known gaps or to improve clinical practice in which a scan of the environment suggests it is deficient. Only a limited amount of time and resources can be devoted to these, and they should, therefore, fit carefully into one's overall plan for professional development. Ordinarily, one can learn, adopt, implement, and evaluate new skills only one at a time. Ideally, at the end of each year, one should be able to record the learned items that have improved one's clinical practices and patient care.

TRANSLATING KNOWLEDGE INTO PRACTICE

Social and financial pressures on the U.S. health care system have increased expectations for CME—not simply to instill new biomedical knowledge but also to facilitate the implementation of that knowledge into practice. In 2006 the ACCME adopted new criteria for accreditation that require CME providers to demonstrate that overall their programs of CME result in changes in competence (ability to implement), performance, and/or patient outcomes (7). CME is expected to also foster participation in systems-based practice and practice-based learning. CME should support practice improvement, which is part of new requirements for recertification (see next section), evolving Joint Commission on Accreditation of Healthcare Organizations (JCAHO) requirements, and national quality improvement efforts to identify and address performance "gaps."

Future high quality CME activities will increasingly balance two types of knowledge: (1) information about new biomedical processes and treatments and (2) information about how to translate that biomedical knowledge into practice. The "translation" process requires consideration of barriers and facilitating factors affecting patients, other members of the health care team, and the institutional setting.

Surgeons who plan, participate in and/or attend CME activities are going to be asked to enhance the "translational" content of those activities. Didactic sessions that typically begin with the presentation of new methods of care and evidence for those methods will need to go beyond that content. Ways to implement those methods should also be introduced and discussed, i.e., translate the changes in knowledge into operationally improving patient care. Attention should be given to changes needed in the care environment (the "system" of care, e.g., people, processes, physical arrangements) that will facilitate successful implementation. The session should conclude by helping participants formulate plans for taking the next steps needed to bring about desired changes. These requirements are consistent with the primary purpose for seeking continuing education, which is to improve actual patient care.

PREPARING FOR RECERTIFICATION AND RECREDENTIALING REQUIREMENTS

Public demand for more evidence of competence in practice has led to new professional efforts to develop broader, more reliable, reproducible methods to demonstrate clinical competence and appropriate performance. The American Board of Medical Specialties (ABMS) in 1999 adopted a new description of the "competent physician." The general competencies defined by the ABMS are

- medical knowledge
- patient care
- interpersonal and communication skills
- professionalism
- practice-based learning and improvement
- systems-based practice.

As a functional complement to this new definition, the ABMS adopted in September 2002 a new program for "maintenance of certification" (8,9). The four components of this program are

CHAPTER 5

Surgical Credentials

Mary E. Klingensmith

INTRODUCTION

The processes leading to board certification and hospital credentialing are often confusing to surgical trainees or those new to the American health care system. This chapter will seek to outline these two areas, pointing out where they overlap and how they relate to the requirements for residency training in surgery. Evolving issues in credentialing and the certification process will also be discussed with regard to the maintenance of certification initiative.

BOARD CERTIFICATION

The American Board of Surgery (ABS) is a member of the American Board of Medical Specialties (ABMS). The ABMS is the umbrella organization for 24 medical specialty boards. In early 2009, more than 85% of all licensed physicians in the United States were certified by at least one ABMS member board (1). Thus, board certification status is clearly recognized as a critical component of the professional dossier of all physicians in the United States, surgeons included.

The ABS was founded in 1937 as a private, voluntary, nonprofit organization with three primary purposes:

1. To conduct examinations of acceptable candidates who seek certification or maintenance of certification by the board;
2. To issue certificates to all candidates meeting the board's requirements and satisfactorily completing its prescribed examinations;
3. To improve and broaden the opportunities for graduate education and training of surgeons (2).

According to ABS definitions, "general surgery" is a discipline that encompasses the following content areas (2):

1. alimentary tract
2. abdomen and its contents
3. breast, skin, and soft tissue
4. endocrine system
5. head and neck surgery
6. organ transplantation
7. pediatric surgery
8. surgical critical care
9. surgical oncology
10. trauma/burns and acute care surgery
11. vascular surgery.

The ABS goes on to state that the expected knowledge and performance of a certified surgeon includes

1. a comprehensive clinical knowledge within the content areas, including epidemiology, anatomy, physiology, clinical presentation, and pathology (including neoplasia);
2. knowledge of the scientific foundations of wound healing, infection, fluid management, shock/resuscitation, immunology, antibiotic usage, metabolism, and nutrition;
3. experience in clinical evaluation including the appropriate use of imaging, indications for surgery and nonsurgical treatment, preoperative, operative and postoperative care, and management of comorbidities and complications;
4. extensive experience in minimally invasive surgery for diagnosis and treatment in the essential content areas, including basic and advanced laparoscopic procedures;
5. substantial experience in diagnostic and therapeutic endoscopy, including colonoscopy, esophagogastroduodenoscopy, and bronchoscopy;
6. resuscitation of critically ill patients, including trauma victims;
7. airway intubation;
8. conscious sedation;
9. diagnostic ultrasonography;
10. noninvasive diagnostic evaluation of the vascular system;
11. sentinel lymph node mapping for breast cancer and melanoma;
12. team-based interdisciplinary care of
    a. terminally ill patients, to include palliative care and the management of pain
    b. morbid obesity, to include metabolic derangements and weight-loss surgery
    c. geriatric surgical patients.

Mary E. Klingensmith: Washington University School of Medicine, Saint Louis, MO 63110.

It is also noted by the ABS that the certified surgeon is expected to be familiar with common diseases and operations in thoracic surgery, plastic and reconstructive surgery, and urgent/emergent problems in gynecologic, neurologic, orthopedic, and urologic surgery (2).

To be admitted to the board certification process, the residency program director must endorse a candidate's application, adding a statement that attests to an applicant's appropriate educational experience in the above areas and that signifies the applicant has the judgment, knowledge, and skills to be considered for board certified status.

STEPS LEADING TO BOARD CERTIFICATION

Prerequisites

Candidates for board certification must have completed training in an accredited general surgery residency program. Accredited programs must meet standards set forth by the Accreditation Council for Graduate Medical Education (ACGME). Within the ACGME, each specialty has its own Residency Review Committee (RRC). Individual RRCs collaborate with the specialty board (i.e., ABS) to determine the components that shall be deemed essential for a program to be accredited. Accredited programs produce graduates that are potentially board eligible.

As part of a process overseen by both the ABS and RRC, a minimum number of cases in each of the essential content areas listed above is determined for board examination admissibility. Residents must keep track of the operations they perform during training, as they count toward these minimum numbers. Upon completion of training, these case logs must be submitted to the ABS as part of the initial application for board examination. This application also includes areas in which the trainee must list the rotation schedules for the 5 years of general surgery training to demonstrate that the trainee has acquired adequate experience in each of the essential content areas. Additionally, the board specifies minimum numbers of weeks and months that must be completed in various academic years and various content and leadership areas; these too must be specified in the application for examination (2). Further, beginning with applicants who complete training in 2009–2010 (and thereafter), all applicants will be required to have successfully completed Advanced Cardiovascular Life Support (ACLS), Advanced Trauma Life Support (ATLS), and Fundamentals of Laparoscopic Surgery (FLS) at any time during training (2).

Other requirements for certification in surgery include "satisfactory ethical, professional, and moral standing," active practice in surgery with admitting privileges in an accredited health care organization (or currently in pursuit of additional graduate education in surgery or a surgical subspecialty), and permanent licensure to practice medicine in a state or jurisdiction of the United States or Canada. All of these prerequisite components are represented on the initial application for board certification.

The examination process

After the ABS has accepted the initial application, the applicant is eligible for the examination process. This has two parts. A written examination (called the *Qualifying Examination*) is to be taken in August of the year following completion of training. If the candidate passes this exam, an oral exam (the *Certifying Examination*) follows. This exam is held in several cities around the United States, with examinees directed to the nearest test site. If the examinee passes the oral exam, a certificate signifying board certification in surgery and designating the examinee as a diplomat of the ABS is issued.

(For updated information and any revisions in Board examination admissibility requirements, see www.absurgery.org. The Web site is updated annually.) Readers are encouraged to access this information frequently during surgical training to stay abreast of any changes in Board examination admissibility requirements that might occur.

MAINTENANCE OF CERTIFICATION

The certificate issued by the board is valid for up to 10 years. In order to maintain certification, a recertification exam is required, in addition to additional components that comprise "Maintenance of Certification" (MOC). This recertification exam can be taken as early as 7 years following certificate issuance but no later than 10. This examination is only one component of the MOC process.

The ABMS has led an effort termed the Maintenance of Certification © (MOC) program, an initiative that has been several years in the making. The process has evolved as the member boards of the ABMS have collectively agreed that the "snapshot" evaluation of physicians that is available through the current system of certification and recertification does not capture a physician's true competency and efforts at practice assessment and improvement (1). The ABS has reported that current recertification exam statistics indicate that recertification examinees who are roughly 30 years out of training fail the recertification exam at much higher rates than do those closer to their training (3). MOC will allow additional aspects of a practitioner's qualifications to be considered as proof of competency.

MOC has four primary components (1):

1. Evidence of professional standing
2. Evidence of a commitment to lifelong learning and involvement in periodic self-assessment processes
3. Evidence of cognitive expertise (currently the written recertification examination)
4. Evidence of evaluation of performance in practice.

These components are based on the six competency areas defined by the ACGME for residency training (medical knowledge, patient care, interpersonal and communication skills, professionalism, practice-based learning and improvement, and systems-based practice). Eventually, evaluation based on the six competency areas will be a

DENIAL OF PRIVILEGES

Individuals applying for privileges in a given area should be certain they possess the qualifications for work in that area. If privileges are denied, the appeals process outlined by the hospital credentials committee should be followed. However, applicants should be aware that if a formal denial of privileges is returned, such information is reported to the National Practitioner Databank and kept as part of that practitioner's permanent file.

REFERENCES

1. ABMS Web site. Available at: www.abms.org. Accessed February 16, 2009.
2. *Booklet of information, 2008–2009.* The American Board of Surgery; 2009. Available at: www.absurgery.org. Accessed February 16, 2009.
3. Buyske J. For the protection of the public and the good of the specialty. *Arch Surg* 2009;144(2):101–103.
4. Joint Commission on Accreditation of Health Care Organizations (JCAHO). The credentialing process. *CAMH: Comprehensive accreditation manual for hospitals.* Oakbrook Terrace, IL: JCAHO; 2000:MS5–MS7.
5. American College of Surgeons. Recommendations for facilities performing bariatric surgery. *Bull Am Coll Surg* 2000;85(9):20–23.

CHAPTER

6

Understanding Variation in Surgical Outcomes

Justin B. Dimick and John D. Birkmeyer

There is growing recognition that the risk of death after surgery is determined in large part by the place of surgery and the person who performs the procedure.

Seminal studies in cardiac surgery, conducted more than two decades ago, documented wide variation in mortality rates across both hospitals and surgeons (1,2). More recent studies have suggested similar variations in performance with general and vascular surgery (3,4). A growing body of evidence also documents that outcomes vary according to a number of provider attributes, especially provider volume and subspecialty training (5,6). These studies on "variations" in outcomes suggest substantial opportunities for improving the outcomes of surgical care.

UNDERSTANDING VARIATION IN OUTCOMES

Surgeons often make the mistake of attributing variations in surgical outcomes as variations in quality. Traditional morbidity and mortality conferences often encourage this view by expecting surgeons to accept blame for all adverse outcomes. However, in reality surgical outcomes may vary for other reasons. In a more complete conceptual model, the so-called "Calculus of quality," variation in surgical outcomes can be attributed to three contributing factors: chance, case mix (i.e., patient factors), and quality of care (7). Although the main themes in this review apply to all outcomes, we focus primarily on surgical mortality, reflecting the predominance of this measure in existing literature and ongoing policy initiatives.

CHANCE

Surgical outcomes can vary across providers simply due to chance (i.e., good or bad luck). Hospital-specific outcome measures are often based on small numbers of adverse events and surgical cases, resulting in statistically imprecise or "noisy" estimates of performance. Chance is particularly important when the event rate is low (e.g., mortality rate after cholecystectomy) or the procedure is uncommon (e.g., pancreatectomy).

Justin B. Dimick, John D. Birkmeyer: University of Michigan, Ann Arbor, MI 48109.

Chance can cause two types of errors in quality measurement. First, extreme outcomes may be attributed to quality when they are really due to chance alone (Type I errors). With many quality measurement platforms, for example, hospitals are labeled as "outliers" if their outcomes are statistically different from expected (e.g., when the 95% confidence intervals around their outcome rates fail to overlap the population average). Depending on where the statistical threshold for outliers is set, some hospitals will be labeled outliers based on chance alone.

Conceptual Type I errors are often made when evaluating a hospital or surgeon with no deaths ("zero mortality") in a particular procedure. While having no deaths is considered a sign of quality, it is also possible that such providers have no deaths simply due to chance (i.e., good luck), especially if they perform a low number of surgeries. A recent study using national Medicare data on five surgical procedures, demonstrated that zero mortality hospitals (no deaths during 3 years) had the same or higher mortality during the following year (8). This so-called "Zero Mortality Paradox" was most striking for pancreatic resection, where a history of no deaths over a 3-year period was associated with a 30% increased risk of death in the subsequent year. This paradoxical finding—that hospitals with no deaths are actually lower quality—is likely due to the well-known relationship between low volume and high mortality for pancreatic resection. In other words, for this operation, hospitals with no deaths are more likely to be "lucky" than "good" (8).

Type II errors occur when chance obscures real differences in quality. One recent study examined seven surgical procedures for which hospital mortality rates had been recommended as quality indicators by the Agency for Healthcare Quality & Research (AHQR) (9). For only one operation, coronary artery bypass grafting (CABG), did the majority of U.S. hospitals perform enough cases over a 3-year period to detect with statistical confidence mortality rates at least twice the national average (Fig. 6.1). For most procedures, few hospitals had sufficient caseloads to meet this low bar of statistical power.

There is growing interest in the use of statistical techniques for better dealing with chance. Reliability adjustment, an application of hierarchical modeling, reduces statistical "noise" in provider-specific outcome measures

efficient approaches to risk adjustment. For example, emphasis could be placed on data collection of the most important variables (e.g., 5–10 risk factors) rather than the 70 to 80 variables presently collected (13). Further, since chance (i.e., "noise") seems to be a more important driver than patient severity, reliability adjustment (as discussed in the previous section) should be given at least as much emphasis as risk adjustment.

QUALITY OF CARE

Mechanisms underlying variation in outcomes

Variation in surgical outcomes not attributable to chance or case mix can be reasonably attributed to differences across providers in the quality of care. In considering mechanisms underlying variation in provider outcomes, it is useful to consider a conceptual model that describes surgical quality in terms of structure, process of care, and outcomes (14) (Fig. 6.5).

STRUCTURE OF CARE

Structural variables are hospital-level resources (e.g., hospital volume, ICU staffing, RN staffing levels) or attributes of individual providers (e.g., surgeon volume, subspecialty training). Structural variables impact outcomes indirectly by influencing process of care. Procedure volume is by far the most visible structural variable and has been linked to surgical outcomes for a broad range of operations. Although there remains relatively little debate about the general importance of procedure volume, the strength of volume-outcome relationships varies widely by procedure (15). Hospital volume is more important for high risk but relatively uncommon procedures (e.g., esophagectomy and pancreatectomy). Conversely, with other procedures (including coronary bypass, carotid endarterectomy), differences in operative mortality rates at low volume and high volume hospitals are much smaller. Finally, for some operations (e.g., colon resection) outcomes are the same at high and low volume hospitals. Similarly, the proportion of variation in hospital mortality rates explained by procedure volume also varies by procedure. In our recent analyses of national Medicare data, volume accounted for 69% of nonrandom variation in hospital mortality with pancreatectomy, 58% with abdominal aortic aneurysm repair, and only 7% with coronary bypass surgery (16).

Many studies have also explored associations between surgeon volume and outcomes. In one large study of Medicare patients, surgeon volume was inversely related to mortality with each of eight different cardiovascular procedures and cancer resections (17). Besides demonstrating the importance of surgeon volume, this study also provided insight into mechanisms underlying the hospital volume-outcome relationship. Specifically, this study showed that surgeon volume explains a large proportion of the apparent hospital volume effect for some operations, but it explains almost none of the hospital volume effect for others. With carotid endarterectomy, for example, surgeon volume explained 100% of the apparent hospital volume effect. In contrast, with lung resection, only 24% of the hospital volume effect was attributable to surgeon volume. For procedures where outcomes are closely related to surgeon volume, quality depends primarily on surgeon-dependent processes, such as good judgment (i.e., who to operate on) or technical proficiency. For other procedures, patient outcomes may depend more on hospital-level resources, including nursing care and management in the intensive care unit.

PROCESS OF CARE

Processes of care refer to the details of clinical care delivered to patients. Important processes include those related to patient selection and evaluation before surgery, the procedure itself, and other aspects of peri- and post-operative care. Process of care influences the frequency of initial "seminal" complications (e.g., quality of operation itself, use of appropriate prophylaxis), "domino" complications (e.g., timeliness and effectiveness of managing postoperative problems), and ultimately patient death (Fig. 6.5).

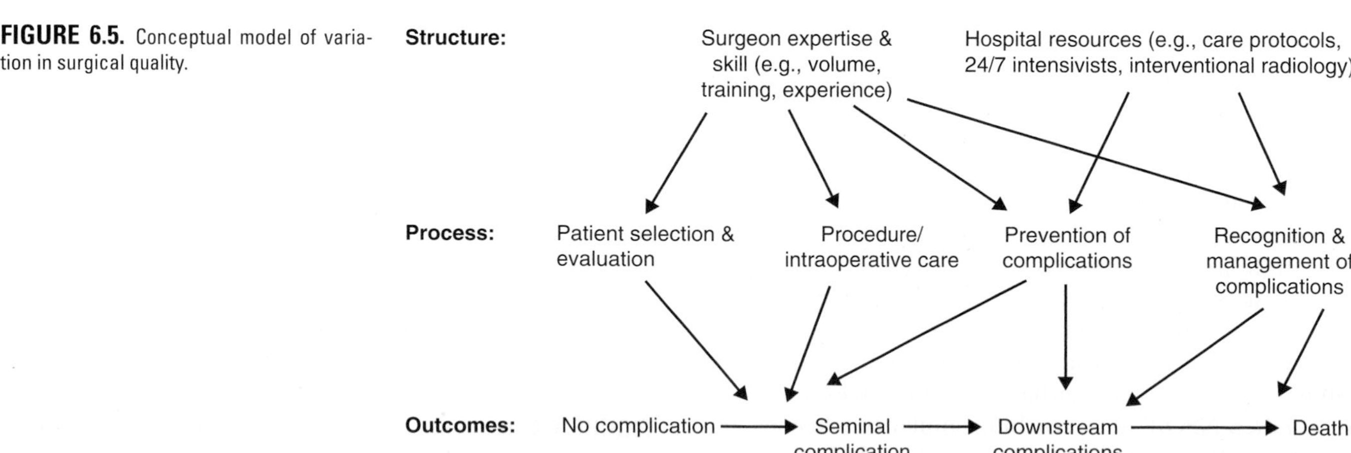

FIGURE 6.5. Conceptual model of variation in surgical quality.

Although a list of processes potentially linked to the outcomes of different surgical procedures would be extensive, payers and policy makers are currently focusing on a narrow set of perioperative care practices in their ongoing quality measurement initiatives. These include measures aimed at reducing risks of surgical site infection (e.g., prophylactic antibiotic administration within 60 minutes prior to surgery), venous thromboembolism, cardiac events, and ventilator-acquired pneumonia. These processes were selected because of high-level evidence linking them to surgical outcomes and perceptions that many were underutilized by providers.

However, it remains uncertain whether increasing compliance with this narrow set of processes will substantially reduce variation in surgical outcomes. Providing good surgical care involves innumerable, interrelated processes of care, many of which are unknown or immeasurable. Previous studies focusing on nonsurgical conditions have demonstrated the limited ability of individual process measures to explain variation in the end result. For example, Bradley et al. studied relationships between the seven Centers for Medicare and Medicaid Services/Joint Commission on the Accreditation of Healthcare Organizations (CMS/JCAHO) core process measures and mortality after acute myocardial infarction in a national study of 962 hospitals (18). Several of these process measures were statistically significant predictors of mortality at the patient level. However, the seven measures collectively explained only 6% of variation in hospital mortality rates.

The perioperative processes of care on which Surgical Care Improvement Project (SCIP) and other pay-for-performance plans are focusing may suffer from similar limitations. Moreover, they relate to complications that likely have little bearing on hospital mortality rates. For example, perioperative care processes highlighted by the SCIP have to date focused largely on superficial surgical site infection and venous thromboembolism. Although the latter can be life-threatening, it only accounts for a small proportion of postoperative deaths. The next chapter provides detailed data showing no association between hospital compliance with SCIP measures and surgical outcomes, including risk-adjusted mortality, surgical infections, and thromboembolism.

Given the nature of surgical care, processes relating to the operation itself, rather than to perioperative care, may be more important in explaining variation in outcomes. For example, Hannan et al. studied outcomes in 2644 patients undergoing carotid endarterectomy in New York State between 1997 and 1999. Consistent with prior work, the investigators found that high volume surgeons and board-certified vascular surgeons (vs. general surgeons and neurosurgeons) had significantly lower rates of perioperative stroke and death. However, they also identified four processes of care strongly associated with patient outcomes: protamine use, placement of intra-arterial shunts during cross clamp, use of eversion endarterectomy techniques, and use of prosthetic patches for closing the arteriotomy. Better outcomes for high volume surgeons and vascular surgeons were no longer statistically significant after accounting for their more consistent adoption of these four practices (19).

Such data do not imply that process of care is unimportant in understanding and improving surgical mortality. Rather, they suggest that many of the most important processes may be difficult to measure (e.g., good judgment in selecting patients for surgery, technical skill in the operating room). In addition, they underscore the complexity of clinical care and the innumerable processes of care that collectively determine good outcomes after surgery. For many procedures, focusing on a limited set of individual processes will not be sufficient for understanding or reducing variation in outcomes.

OUTCOMES

Patient outcomes are obviously the end results of clinical care. In the context of our conceptual model (Fig. 6.5), the relevant outcomes are the initial "seminal" complication, downstream "domino" complications, and mortality. A better understanding of this pathway will provide important insights into reducing variations in surgical outcomes across providers.

It is clinically intuitive that providers with high mortality rates simply have higher complication rates than low mortality hospitals. Although appealing, this hypothesis is refuted in part by previous studies describing relatively weak correlations between hospitals' complication rates and mortality (20). In other words, how hospitals rank on complication rates with a given procedure has little relationship with their mortality rates.

An alternative explanation is that low mortality hospitals and surgeons may be better at rescuing patients once they have a complication, rather than at avoiding them in the first place. Nearly two decades ago, initial studies by Silber et al. suggest that while complication incidence rates seem to be influenced by patient factors, failure to rescue rates (the likelihood of mortality given a complication) are predominantly determined by hospital factors (20–22). These findings were confirmed in a rigorously conducted study by Ghaferi et al., which used detailed, clinically rich data from the ACS-NSQIP (23). In this study, hospitals were ranked according to risk-adjusted mortality and grouped into quintiles (five equal-sized groups). When comparing the "best" to "worst" quintiles, there were no significant differences in overall (24.6% vs. 26.9%) or major (18.2% vs. 16.2%) complication rates. However, "failure to rescue" was almost twice as high in hospitals with very high mortality as in those with very low mortality (21.4% vs. 12.5%, $p<0.001$). The findings held up when stratified by individual operations, such as colon resection and abdominal aortic aneurysm repair (Fig. 6.6).

Another explanation for the lack of hospital-level correlation in complications and mortality is that we have been studying the wrong complications. In the study by

CHAPTER

7

Strategies for Reducing Variation in Surgical Outcomes

John D. Birkmeyer and Justin B. Dimick

INTRODUCTION

As described in the preceding chapter, surgical outcomes vary widely. In addition to variation among individual providers, (1,2) a growing body of evidence suggests that risks of adverse events after surgery vary widely according to a number of provider attributes, including procedure volume, surgeon subspecialty training, and other factors (3–5). Apparent variation in surgical outcomes can be attributed partly to chance and, to a lesser extent, to case mix differences across providers. Nonetheless, there remains little doubt that variation in surgical outcomes also reflects real differences in quality among hospitals and surgeons and thus suggests substantial opportunities for quality improvement.

In response, payers, policymakers, and professional organizations have implemented a variety of different strategies aimed at reducing variation and improving surgical quality (6). Selective referral initiatives, which aim to steer surgical patients to hospitals or surgeons likely to have the best results, have been particularly popular among private payers and purchaser coalitions. Other efforts are instead hoping to improve outcomes at all hospitals, particularly those with subpar results. These include pay-for-performance programs and "checklists" aimed at increasing hospital and surgeon compliance with evidence-based processes related to perioperative care (7). Others are instead offering providers rigorous feedback on their outcomes relative to those of their peers, but letting hospitals and surgeons determine how to improve at the local level. Such strategies are particularly popular among professional organizations in surgery, including the American College of Surgeons and its National Surgical Quality Improvement Program (ACS-NSQIP) (8,9).

In this chapter, we review these three different models for reducing variation in surgical outcomes: selective referral, process compliance, and outcomes measurement. In addition to examining their strengths and weaknesses, we consider how recent advances in the science of quality measurement and improvement might ultimately enhance the real world effectiveness of each strategy. (Table 7.1)

John D. Birkmeyer, Justin B. Dimick: Department of Surgery, University of Michigan Medical School, Ann Arbor, MI 48104.

SELECTIVE REFERRAL

With this approach, payers (usually) identify hospitals with the best results in the selected procedures and direct care to these facilities. Toward this end, they can use selective contracting, tiered health plans, and benefits packages that give patients financial incentives (e.g., lower co-pays) to use preferred providers. These levers are often supplemented with public reporting of volume or outcomes data, in the hopes that patients themselves will "shop for quality."

Among current examples of selective referral, the Leapfrog Group, a large coalition of public and private employers and purchasers, is promoting "evidence-based hospital referral" for seven surgical procedures, based on minimum procedure volume criteria and, for some procedures, risk-adjusted mortality rates (10). Cardiac surgery, bariatric surgery, and breast cancer care are becoming increasingly popular targets for payers' Centers of Excellence programs.

To date, such efforts have been effective in concentrating some high risk procedures in high volume centers. We used national Medicare claims data to assess longitudinal trends in market concentration, that is, the proportion of total cases performed in the top 10% of the busiest hospitals. While there was little evidence of trends toward increased market concentration in cardiovascular surgery, major cancer resections are being increasingly directed to high volume hospitals (Fig. 7.1). With pancreatic resection, for example, the proportion of patients undergoing surgery in very high volume hospitals increased from 22% to 54% between 1997 and 2007.

Among their advantages, selective referral efforts often rely on relatively simple structural measures of quality (e.g., procedure volume) and thus can be implemented expediently and inexpensively. They also reflect the natural response of many payers and patients when confronted with the problem of variation in provider performance with surgery. On the other hand, from the perspective of providers, selective referral strategies are highly polarizing, dividing hospitals and surgeons into winners and losers. In alienating the latter, a price of selective referral may be lost opportunities for engaging physicians in other types of quality improvement efforts.

A fundamental problem with selective referral is that it is hard to know which hospitals and surgeons are truly best.

Table 7.1 Characteristics of three different models for reducing variation and improving surgical mortality

	Selective Referral	Process Compliance	Outcomes Measurement
Goal/mechanism	Steer patients to best hospitals or surgeons	Improve care in all settings by increasing hospital compliance with evidence-based processes of perioperative care	Improve care in all settings by providing feedback on surgical outcomes; hospitals and surgeons implement improvement efforts at local level
Examples	Leapfrog Group evidence-based hospital referral program Payers' Centers of Excellence programs in cardiac and bariatric surgery	Surgical Care Improvement Project (SCIP), other pay-for-performance programs Surgical checklists	Society of Thoracic Surgery database for cardiothoracic surgery American College of Surgeons-National Surgical Quality Improvement Program
Advantages	Inexpensive, expedient Traction with patients and payers	Likely to achieve rapid improvements in many aspects of perioperative care	Measurement alone may be effective in improving outcomes ("Hawthorne effort")
Disadvantages	Highly polarizing (for providers) Hard to identify best providers (at individual level)	Current process measures not strongly linked with mortality and other important outcomes	No insights about how best to improve; may limit ultimate extent of improvement Expensive

Although volume- or mortality-based quality indicators can reliably identify groups of providers with better results on average, they do not reliably discriminate performance among individuals (in part due to statistical power limitations). For example, Krumholz et al. used clinical data from the Cooperative Cardiovascular Project to assess the usefulness of *Healthgrades'* hospital ratings for acute myocardial infarction (based primarily on risk-adjusted mortality rates from Medicare data) (11). Relative to 1-star (worst) hospitals, 5-star (best) hospitals had significantly lower mortality (16% vs. 22%, $p < 0.001$) after risk adjustment with clinical data. However, the *Healthgrades'* ratings poorly discriminated among any two individual hospitals. In only 3% of head-to-head comparisons did 5-star hospitals have statistically lower mortality rates than 1-star hospitals.

PROCESS COMPLIANCE

Another approach to reducing variation is to encourage hospitals and surgeons to increase their compliance with processes of care linked to improved surgical outcomes. This model is perhaps best represented by the ongoing pay-for-performance programs of both public and private payers. For example, payers are linking hospital reimbursement to satisfactory adherence to evidence-based practices related to perioperative care, as defined by the Surgical Care Improvement Project (SCIP), a joint effort of the Centers for Medicare and Medicaid Services (CMS) and the Centers for Disease Control (12). These include specific processes aimed at reducing rates of surgical site infection, postoperative cardiac events, venous thromboembolism, and ventilator-associated pneumonia.

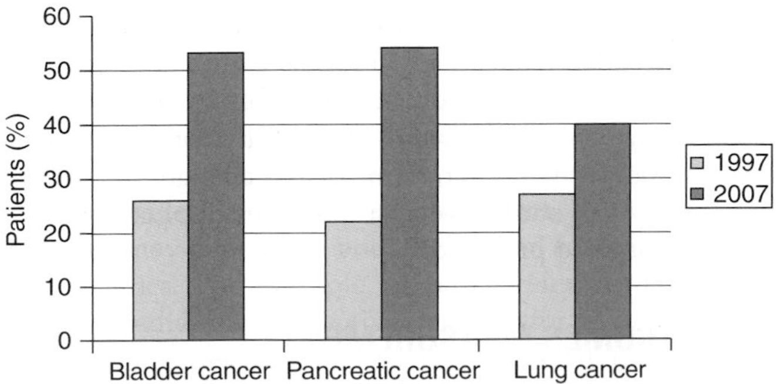

FIGURE 7.1. Proportion of patients undergoing cancer surgery in very high volume hospitals (as defined previously (26)), 1997 vs. 2007. Based on analysis of national Medicare population (Nicholas Osborne, MD, personal communication).

Long standard in the safety-conscious aviation industry, surgical "checklists," including preoperative time-outs, represent another increasingly popular application of the process compliance model. Their initial dissemination in U.S. hospitals had been motivated primarily by desires to reduce risks of so-called "never events," including wrong site and wrong patient surgery. At many centers, however, surgical checklists have been substantially broadened in clinical scope, aiming to reduce much more common adverse events, such as surgical site infection. Interest in checklists received a considerable boost when a highly publicized study by Pronovost et al. demonstrated their effectiveness in markedly reducing rates of blood stream infections in patients with central venous lines (13).

Among their advantages, process compliance strategies are considerably less polarizing than those based on selective referral. In theory, anyone can "win." To the extent that surgeons can "play to the quiz," process-based pay-for-performance programs have the potential to achieve rapid and significant improvements in many aspects in perioperative care. At the University of Michigan Hospital, for example, the proportion of colorectal surgery patients receiving an appropriate antibiotic within 60 minutes prior

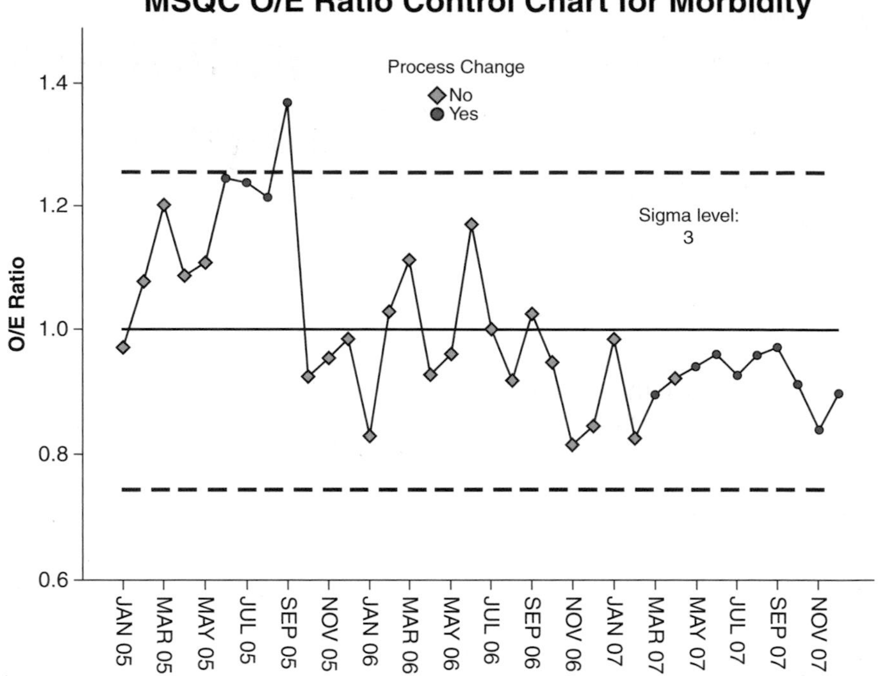

FIGURE 8.1. Shewart control-chart demonstrating changes in the Michigan Surgical Quality Collaborative (MSQC) observed to expected morbidity rates (O/E ratio) over time. The observed morbidity rates are adjusted for patient characteristics. The expected morbidity rates are calculated based on a national sample from the ACS-NSQIP. (• represents a process change where a run of eight or more points are on one side of the center line).

potential quality improvement and cost implications of any initiative to improve care.

Quality collaboratives can be expensive. For example, the ACS-NSQIP (covering only general and vascular surgery) costs participating institutions approximately $135,000 per year (26,27). This includes the costs of database management, statistical analysis, data collection, and auditing for data accuracy. The collection of high quality clinical data requires a highly trained individual, and in the case of the ACS-NSQIP, this is generally a full-time nurse reviewer. High quality data does have significant value for a collaborative. First, it provides robust risk-adjusted center-specific outcomes. Second, it facilitates surgeon trust in reported outcomes. In contrast to the ACS-NSQIP, other quality collaboratives have developed highly efficient and inexpensive data collection methodologies (3,26,28). For example, in the state of Washington, the Surgical Clinical Outcomes Assessment Program (SCOAP) relies upon claims data, limited primary data collection, and a highly selective case mix. Though SCOAP is more limited in its breadth, this highly focused collaborative functions at a small fraction of the costs of the ACS-NSQIP.

Participation in quality improvement initiatives, whether voluntary or required, can become overwhelming for hospitals. Numerous state and federal agencies have significant data collection and reporting requirements which occupy substantial hospital resources. In addition, hospitals are invited to participate in numerous voluntary quality improvement initiatives. Participation requires resources and as a result hospitals must carefully consider the potential return on the investment for each quality improvement program. If a surgeon feels strongly about a quality improvement initiative, he or she must communicate the potential clinical benefits to hospital administrators. In addition, the surgeon must work closely with hospital officers to develop a viable business plan for participation.

Within this context, there is a significant amount of data that reports the financial benefits of quality improvement for both payers and hospitals in the United States (9–12). Understanding this relationship requires a brief description of how hospitals are generally paid for surgery. A high proportion of the costs of surgery are from payments to hospitals for the procedure-specific diagnosis related group (DRG). DRG payments were devised under the Prospective Payment System to bundle payments for hospitals for the care of a patient with a particular diagnosis. This DRG payment can generally be adjusted for illness severity and/or case complexity. The DRG payment system is used by Medicare and many large private payers. Importantly, hospitals may receive additional payments for readmissions and outlier payments, both of which are

- Develop a business case for the collaborative
  - In general, quality improvement is associated with significant cost savings for payers. Within this context, large payers are potential partners in quality collaboratives.
- Have a standardized outcomes infrastructure
  - Surgeons and hospitals must feel accountable for reported outcomes. For this to occur, they must trust the data and analysis.
- Strong leadership by surgeons
  - Collaborative leaders should be surgeons with significant clinical credibility
- Collegial atmosphere
  - The collaborative must foster an environment in which participants feel comfortable sharing outcomes, both good and bad.

FIGURE 8.2. Key components to a successful surgical quality collaborative.

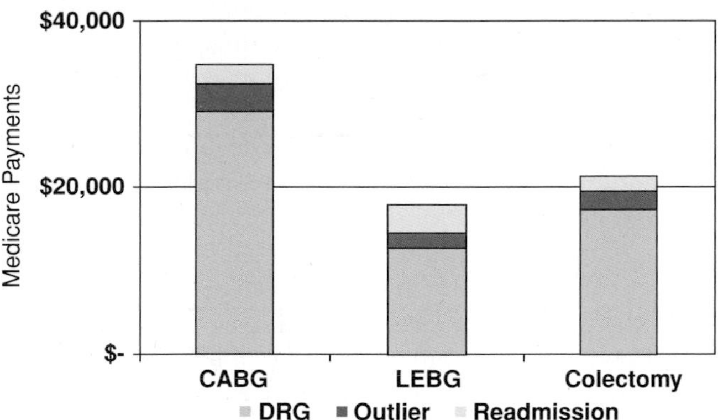

FIGURE 8.3. Medicare payments for major surgery (MEDPAR 2002). Mean hospital payments for the surgical event (within 30 days of the operation or during the initial hospital admission) are classified into DRG payments, outlier payments, and payments for readmissions within 30 days of the surgical event. CABG, coronary artery bypass grafting; LEBG, lower extremity bypass grafting.

associated with adverse outcomes. Medicare identifies outlier cases by comparing the estimated costs for the case to a fixed loss threshold that is specific to the case DRG. Once a case qualifies as an outlier, the hospital is reimbursed as a fixed percentage of submitted charges. Outlier payments and payments for 30-day readmissions can represent a significant proportion of total payments for a surgical event. (Fig. 8.3) For example, when only considering coronary artery bypass grafting (CABG), lower extremity bypass grafting, and colectomy, Medicare paid hospitals $1.5 billion in outlier payments and 30-day readmissions payments in 2002. Additional sources of payment potentially related to surgical complications include payment for home health and nursing home care. Little is known about how much these sources of payments contribute to the total costs of surgery.

Improvements in quality are associated with financial incentives for hospitals. Fewer surgical complications result in shorter length of stay. Prolonged bed occupancy is associated with significant opportunity costs for hospitals, as bed turnover is profitable for hospitals. Insurance carriers look favorably upon centers with a commitment to quality improvement and cost reduction. In addition, voluntary programs in quality improvement may reduce third party regulation and oversight. Characterization of relative patient acuity and exemplary outcomes provide leverage for hospital administration when negotiating with insurance companies.

On a more granular level, both the hospital and the payers have a financial stake in surgical complications. With respect to colectomy, our group has evaluated the financial implications of surgical complications for our institution and for a large private payer. We note that a complication following colectomy is associated with $12,137 of additional reimbursement to the hospital (payer costs) while a complication is associated with $20,486 of additional costs to the hospital (Table 8.1) (11). As a result, the hospital loses $8,349 in profit on colectomy cases with a complication. Further, the hospital actually has a negative financial margin of $1460 on colectomy cases that involve a complication. Similar financial relationships between hospital margin, payer reimbursement, and surgical complications have been noted following kidney transplantation, liver transplantation, and hepatobiliary surgery (10,29).

The development of a successful quality collaboration requires careful consideration of finances. This includes the costs of administering the program in addition to the potential cost savings associated with quality improvement goals. This return on investment analysis must be done prior to initiating a collaborative. Both clinical and financial benchmarks must be considered as the collaboratives progresses (26,30). Frequent reporting of quality improvement as well as cost savings will facilitate ongoing financial support for the collaboratives and opportunities for expansion.

In the development of the MSQC, the need for careful consideration of the costs implications was appreciated early in the process. As mentioned, the MSQC was created on the foundation of the ACS-NSQIP. Participation was funded by Blue Cross Blue Shield Michigan/Blue Care Network (BCBSM). The officers of BCBSM were wholeheartedly engaged in efforts to improve the care of patients. Nonetheless, they made it very clear that any broad clinical initiative would be carefully scrutinized by

Table **8.1** **The financial implications of surgical complications following colon surgery for the payer and the hospital (11)**[a]

Course Following Colectomy	Reimbursement to Hospital	Hospital Costs	Hospital Profit: (Reimbursements Minus Costs)
Complications	$34,490	$35,950	($1,460)
No complications	$22,353	$15,464	$6,889
Change in reimbursement	$12,137	Loss in profit	($8,349)

[a]Note that not only does the payer have increased costs following complications, but the hospital loses profit and actually has a negative financial margin following colectomy cases with surgical complications.

their large clients (such as General Motors). As a result, at the initiation of the MSQC, specific quality improvement (QI) goals were established in order to assure that BCBSM would have a reasonable financial return on the investment. More specifically, we determined that if the MSQC could achieve a 1.8% reduction in complications per year over a 3-year pilot program, BCBSM would fully recoup the $5 million investment in the program (26). Based on previous experiences with the ACS-NSQIP, our goal was a 3% reduction in complications over the 3-year pilot program (31). If we had achieved this clinical goal, we calculated a $2.5 million savings to BCBSM. Importantly, as the initial hospitals that joined the MSQC reached their third year of participation, the program has significantly exceeding the proposed quality improvement benchmarks. Because of this excellent communication between the MSQC leadership and BCBSM, both clinical and financial goals are clearly stated and aligned.

STANDARDIZED DATA INFRASTRUCTURE

Participants in a collaborative must feel accountable for their hospital's outcomes data. Surgeon and nurse participants drive the quality improvement within their institutions. The collaborative provides a bounty of potential quality improvement initiatives for each institution. Within this context, it is paramount that surgeons within the collaborative trust both the analytic and data collection methods. When faced with poor outcomes, surgeons and hospitals frequently will assume that this is related to case mix complexity within their institution or problems with data. For example, at the University of Michigan we assumed that our high rates of surgical site infection (SSI) were related to the fact that we had the most obese patients in Michigan. When we looked at the data, our patients were actually slightly thinner than the average patient at other institutions. With this observation it became clear to us that excuses for high SSI rates were no longer appropriate, and action was aggressively taken, with remarkable success.

Clinical outcomes data shared within a collaborative essentially drive the agenda of the collaborative. As mentioned previously, high quality data can be complex and expensive to collect. This is particularly true when collecting data on clinically complex outcomes such as surgical complications. When determining the data to be collected for a QI initiative, careful consideration must be given to the definition of the complication. Significant work has been done on this issue by other groups (32,33). This data must be collected by a highly trained individual, usually a nurse with significant clinical experience. Data collection must be audited to ensure accuracy across participating hospitals. Considering the efforts required to ensure high quality data collection, determination of specific variables for collection must be carefully considered. In addition, collection of any new data must be tested to ensure accuracy before widespread rollout. Unfortunately, the collection of high quality data is expensive. Hospitals collect large amounts of data, some of which are quite reliable, as requirements for other mandatory reporting mechanisms. Quality collaboratives that take advantage of some of this data collection can potentially function with much lower costs (27).

Analytic methods used within a collaborative must be valid and broadly accepted in order to ensure that participants feel accountable for reported outcomes. A frequently reported anecdote involving inadequate data analysis involves cardiac surgery in the state of New York (4,34,35). When the state began releasing, and newspapers began publishing, unadjusted mortality rates following heart surgery for hospitals within New York State, it had a profound effect on patients, surgeons, and hospitals. To the uninitiated, a higher percent mortality was bad, and a lower percentage was good. But the raw percentages left out any consideration of the involved patient population, something of no small nuance to surgeons. At that time, there was no system for statistical covariate adjustment in place. Not only did surgeons not feel accountable for these outcomes, but the public reporting of these data had long-term and profound effects, both good and bad, on future quality improvement efforts.

Clearly, the analytic methods used in a quality collaborative must be broadly accepted by all members of the collaborative. This can be a challenge considering the diverse background of members of the collaborative. Methodologies must be understood not only by the small number of surgeons and analysts overseeing the outcomes reporting, but also by the nurses and surgeons participating in the collaborative. The majority of these individuals will have no expertise in health services research. In short, collaborative participants must trust the data and the individuals overseeing data management. As has been discussed elsewhere, this observation favors a locally based collaborative. In addition, it also favors an administrative and analytic infrastructure of the collaborative rooted in surgeon members, not payers or nonsurgeon researchers.

Overall, fair metrics of accountability are critical. With a foundation of strict definitions, rigorous data collection, and standardized endpoints, a reliable predictive model for outcomes can be developed. Importantly, operations that are compared between hospitals must be relatively common, with relatively high rates of complications, otherwise reliable comparisons are not possible due to inadequate statistical power (36). Within this context, the collaborative should focus on hospital-level outcomes and not surgeon-level outcomes. Surgeon-level outcomes are difficult to reliably measure, and focusing on these outcomes may alienate participants (37,38).

SURGEON LEADERSHIP

Leadership of quality collaboratives is critical. The leadership of the collaborative needs expertise and clinical credibility. In short, the collaborative needs to be led by a surgeon. Though support from nurses, statisticians, and health services researchers is important, surgeons are less likely to actively participate in collaboratives led by these individuals. Every surgeon knows the importance of clinical credibility when trying to influence the opinions of other surgeons. Influential surgeons are generally respected in the operating room. Overall, collaborative leadership by a single or a small group of prominent senior surgeons, though not mandatory, has many advantages.

Collaboratives generate ideas for quality improvement. The information disseminated at the collaborative must be not only appreciated but implemented. Implementation of improvement initiatives within hospitals can be challenging. Some of the success of the MSQC is likely related to the fact that participating surgeons are senior institutional leaders. More specifically, most of the participating surgeons lead the department of surgery within their hospitals. These individuals are well suited to influence important initiatives at their institution. As we developed the MSQC, there was some concern about too much senior surgeon participation. We were worried that the senior surgeons would be less open to sharing outcomes and more resistant to change. Fortunately, this has not been the experience.

Collegial atmosphere

It is imperative that surgeon leaders of the collaborative set a tone of collegiality. We all know that local surgical markets can be competitive. Within the MSQC, there was an early appreciation for the deleterious impact of potential competition among surgeons and institutions. This was addressed at the onset with all potential participants. The MSQC by-laws state that any institution using MSQC outcome data for competitive advantage will be expelled from participation. Similarly, every effort must be made to facilitate a comfortable environment for sharing outcomes, both good and bad. This requires trust in the leadership and other members of the collaborative. It also requires trust in data confidentiality. For example, though the MSQC is funded by BCBSM, BCBSM does not have access to hospital-specific data. In addition, only the leadership of the collaborative has access to hospital-specific data. Both BCBSM and the participating centers have made a commitment not to seek the outcomes data from other hospitals. Initially, potential participants were concerned that BCBSM might try to use the data for selective contracting within the state. This has not happened. In fact, when we surveyed the nurses and surgeons at a quarterly meeting, 100% reported that BCBSM was a reliable partner.

Local professional organizations, such as state chapters of the American College of Surgeons (ACS), can provide the core leadership of new collaboratives. Active members of such societies tend to be senior surgeons. The surgeons will likely have already developed a collegial relationship among themselves. It is critical that collegiality among the surgeon leadership sets the tone for the entire collaborative. For example, much of the leadership of the MSQC, and a similarly formatted collaborative within Tennessee, came from the leadership of the state chapter of the ACS. These individuals had known each other for a long time and already had a mutually respectful and collegial relationship. In all, local professional societies play an important role in the genesis of regional quality collaboratives.

SUCCESSFUL QUALITY COLLABORATIVES

Traditionally in surgery, clinical improvements in care have come from weekly morbidity and mortality conferences. During these interactive meetings, cases are presented and clinicians discuss clinical decision-making, technique, and relevant clinical literature. Though not often considered collegial, the strengths of such conferences include face-to-face communication and broad understanding of processes of care within an institution. Though surgeons were the first to have regular structured quality improvement efforts such as these, in recent years it has become clear that additional efforts are needed. This realization was fueled primarily by the observation that there was broad variation across hospitals in outcomes, indicating significant opportunity for improvement (4–6,39). Within this context, numerous surgical quality collaboratives have been developed. We will briefly discuss three highly successful collaboratives.

Northern New England Cardiovascular Disease Study Group

Among the first groups to recognize the power of regional collaboration was the Northern New England Cardiovascular Disease Study Group (6). Starting in 1987, this remarkable group attempted to determine whether an organized intervention including data feedback, site visits, and continuous quality improvement efforts would improve hospital mortality rates following CABG. This study included 23 cardiac surgeons in Maine, Vermont, and New Hampshire and resulted in a 24% reduction in hospital mortality rate in 6488 consecutive operations. This study set the stage for multi-institutional, regional collaboration for surgical quality improvement.

American College of Surgeons-National Surgical Quality Improvement Program

The most prominent nationally based quality collaborative is the ACS-NSQIP. The ACS-NSQIP was developed by Shukri Khuri in response to a call from the Congress regarding fears of low quality care within the Veterans Health Administration. The NSQIP established methods for reliable data collection and risk-adjusted assessment of center-specific performance. Presumably related to this work, remarkable reductions in surgical complications were noted within Veterans Affairs (VA) Medical Centers (5,40,41). More recently, the NSQIP has partnered with the

ACS and has been successfully implemented in private sector hospitals (31). Currently, there are approximately 200 private sector hospitals enrolled in the ACS-NSQIP.

The ACS-NSQIP provides high quality comparative data to hospitals to facilitate internal quality improvement efforts. The early success of the ACS-NSQIP is largely related to acceptance by surgeons of the quality of the data and analysis. As a tool for quality improvement, many questions surrounding its utility. In order to maximize the benefits of the ACS-NSQIP, there needs to be a medium in which data can be evaluated and turned to quality improvement. It had been assumed that this would occur at the hospital level, but may not be occurring. This is where a regional collaborative may provide important supplementation to ACS-NSQIP participation.

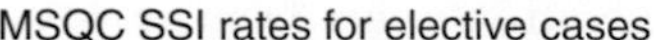

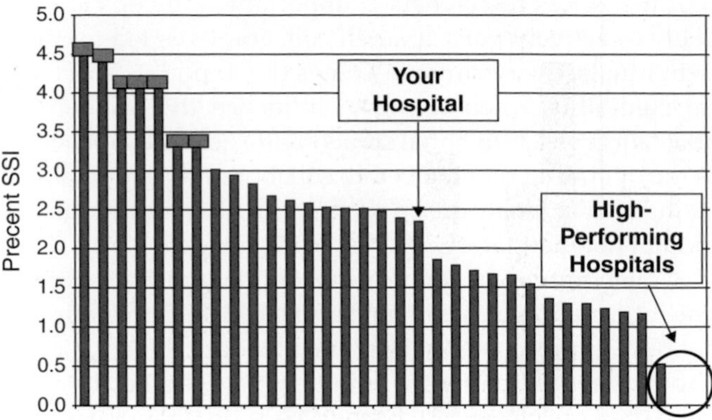

FIGURE 8.4. As an example of data feedback received by participating hospitals, this Pareto chart compares surgical site infection (SSI) rates for elective cases among MSQC hospitals. Red bars on left represent high outliers or "poor performers." With our quality improvement efforts, we focus on the right side of the figure or "high performing hospitals." We identify these hospitals and they share best practices.

Michigan Surgical Quality Collaborative

Our experience in Michigan with a successful quality collaborative has been with the MSQC. This is a group of 34 mostly community hospitals within Michigan that was established in 2005. Based on the work of others, we recognized an opportunity for partnership with a large private payer within the state. Similarly, it became clear that the best way to overcome strong institutional biases that may stifle quality improvement was to collaborate with other hospitals throughout the state (3,6,20,22,32,42,43). The results showed a significant reduction in surgical complication rates within Michigan (Fig. 8.1).

Each participating hospital is enrolled in the ACS-NSQIP. The collaborative is based on the structure and data of the ACS-NSQIP. In addition, the MSQC also has its own data coordinating center at the University of Michigan which facilitates rapid and focused analyses that are germane to the participants. Hospitals receive quarterly reports comparing their risk-adjusted outcomes to both national averages and to the other participating hospitals within Michigan. The reports clearly indicate an individual center's performance, as well as high and low performing hospitals (Fig. 8.4). Significant efforts are made to make these reports easily understood by all surgeons, nurses, and quality improvement professionals. In addition, we discuss how to best communicate these data with hospital administration.

A key aspect of the MSQC is its quarterly meetings. At these meetings, hospital reports are distributed to surgeons, nurses, and other members of hospital team. Attendance is a requirement for participation. Incentive payments to institutions will be withheld from any institution that does not actively participate and attend the meetings.

Each meeting has a theme related to a specific QI initiative. For example, in a recent meeting we noticed a 10-fold variation in SSI rates among diabetic patients following elective surgery. We always make an effort to focus on high performing hospitals. We asked these hospitals why they had such good results. One hospital brought in their perioperative insulin protocol to share with the group. Another hospital talked about the importance of intraoperative glucose monitoring. Discussions of complications centered on the high performing hospitals in an effort not to alienate poor performing hospitals. Continuing with our theme of SSI, we then had a national expert in SSI review evidence-based practices and participate in a question and answer session. Overall, surgeon and nursing leaders throughout Michigan were able to hear granular quality improvement approaches by other institutions within the state and balance these efforts with the best available data on SSI. High quality data indicating poor performance is very influential with hospital administrations. These surgeons and nurses, armed with this data and knowledge, are uniquely well suited to lead quality improvement efforts within home institutions.

Within the MSQC, some unique initiatives have garnered significant enthusiasm among participants. We have created a number of QI videos on YouTube™. Some videos have experts within the collaborative explain their successful processes of care. For example, one institution with remarkable outcomes following colectomy specifically detailed their preoperative assessment, operative management, and postoperative care. In addition, we frequently invite prominent national experts to our quarterly meetings. We interview these individuals and post the video. Links to these videos are readily available on the MSQC website. We have encouraged surgeons and clinical nurse reviewers to bring QI officers and administrators from their institutions. These are the individuals that will be actively participating in the grassroots effort to improve quality within member institutions, and their involvement in the quarterly meetings is critical. During recent quarterly meetings, we have used real-time audience responses to better understand current processes of care. We will

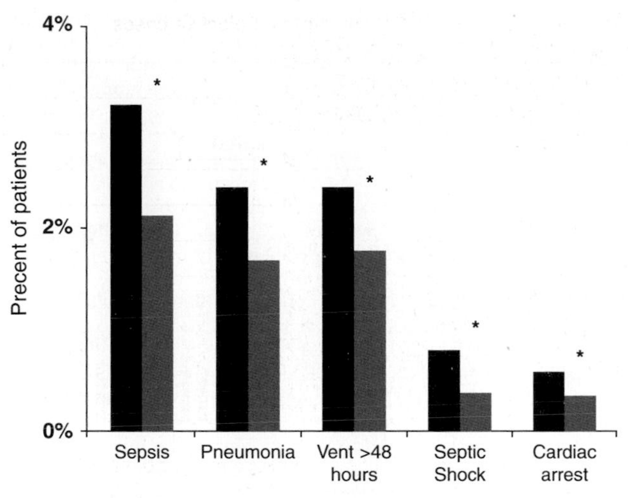

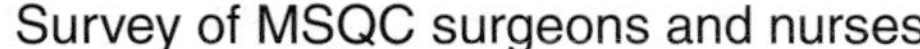

FIGURE 8.5. Changes in rates of major postoperative complications between the first 2 years of the MSQC (MSQC Time Period 1) and the third year (MSQC Time Period 2). *$p < 0.05$

choose 10 specific questions regarding processes of care and have attendees respond in real time. Attendees will be able to compare their hospital's processes of care to those of other hospitals within Michigan. This can provide significant insights, particularly to hospitals with poor outcomes and in an anonymous, nonthreatening way.

The focus of the MSQC stands in stark contrast to recently implemented Center for Medicare and Medicaid Services (CMS) policies for nonpayment for hospital acquired conditions, otherwise known as "never events." Clearly, certain clinical events, such as wrong patient or wrong side surgery, should be considered "never events." Unfortunately, such policies focusing on poor outcomes within an institution may detract from real QI by driving clinical problems underground. The focus should remain on high performers, rewarding their efforts and outcomes.

Unlike many national initiatives, the collegial atmosphere within the collaborative is critical to foster detailed and honest discussions of outcomes, good or bad. BCBSM has supported the collaborative approach to QI within their broad-based QI "pay-for-participation" programs. There been significant reductions in the rate of complications following major surgery. In addition, there have been reductions in the rates of serious postoperative complications such as sepsis, pneumonia, and cardiac arrest. (Fig. 8.5) Hopefully this trend toward QI will continue.

SUMMARY

Surgical quality collaboratives offer significant opportunities for QI and cost savings. There are several core components to a successful collaborative. In Michigan, largely because of the support from BCBSM, we have had significant success with the MSQC. In order to get a better understanding of the perceptions of participating surgeons and nurses, we recently surveyed MSQC nurses and surgeons. (Fig. 8.6) The results of this survey highlight critical components of a quality collaborative. Importantly, 100% of respondents reported that there is a high degree of collegiality within the group. Similarly, 100% of respondents reported that BCBSM is a reliable partner in the collaborative. The importance of financial support by BCBSM for participation is clear, with 77% of respondents reporting that it is necessary. Finally, only 2% of the respondents reported that they felt reluctant to discuss quality problems within the home institution.

Obviously, the development of the quality collaboratives must rely upon the strengths of the potential participants. Most successful collaboratives have been regional and have had a narrow clinical focus. In addition, quality collaboratives frequently have their genesis within local professional societies such as state chapters of the ACS. Hopefully, surgical collaboratives will continue to expand

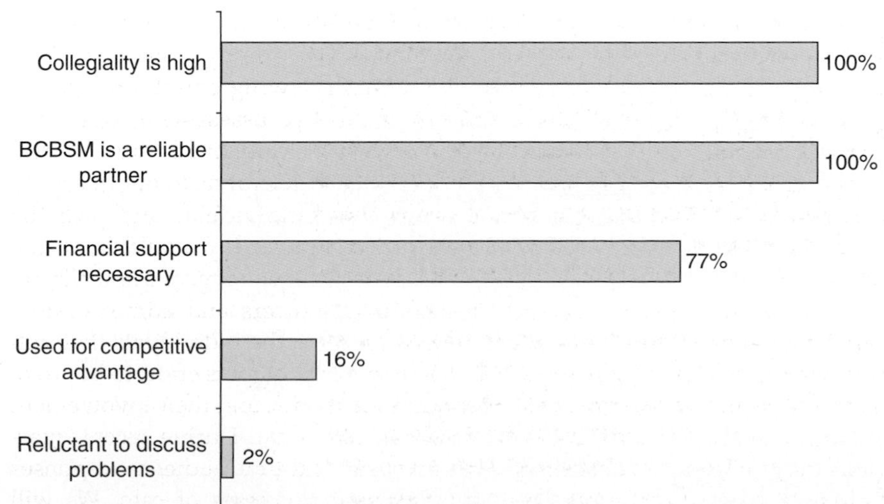

FIGURE 8.6. Results of a survey of MSQC nurses and surgeons. The results of this survey highlight critical components for all the quality collaboratives.

throughout the United States. This offers the opportunity for surgeons to lead efforts to improve surgical care. In addition and most importantly, it will lead to better care for our patients.

REFERENCES

1. Birkmeyer JD, Siewers AE, Finlayson EV, et al. Hospital volume and surgical mortality in the United States. *N Engl J Med* 2002;346(15): 1128–1137.
2. Birkmeyer JD, Stukel TA, Siewers AE, et al. Surgeon volume and operative mortality in the United States. *N Engl J Med* 2003;349(22): 2117–2127.
3. Flum DR, Fisher N, Thompson J, et al. Washington State's approach to variability in surgical processes/Outcomes: Surgical Clinical Outcomes Assessment Program (SCOAP). *Surgery* 2005;138(5):821–828.
4. Hannan EL, Kilburn H Jr, O'Donnell JF, et al. Adult open heart surgery in New York State. An analysis of risk factors and hospital mortality rates. *JAMA* 1990;264(21):2768–2774.
5. Khuri SF, Daley J, Henderson W, et al. The National Veterans Administration Surgical Risk Study: risk adjustment for the comparative assessment of the quality of surgical care. *J Am Coll Surg* 1995;180(5):519–531.
6. O'Connor GT, Plume SK, Olmstead EM, et al. A regional intervention to improve the hospital mortality associated with coronary artery bypass graft surgery. The Northern New England Cardiovascular Disease Study Group. *JAMA* 1996;275(11):841–846.
7. Neumayer L, Mastin M, Vanderhoof L, et al. Using the Veterans Administration National Surgical Quality Improvement Program to improve patient outcomes. *J Surg Res* 2000;88(1):58–61.
8. Polk HC Jr, Birkmeyer J, Hunt DR, et al. Quality and safety in surgical care. *Ann Surg* 2006;243(4):439–448.
9. Englesbe MJ, Dimick JB, Fan Z, et al. Case mix, quality and high-cost kidney transplant patients. *Am J Transplant* 2009;9(5):1108–1114.
10. Englesbe MJ, Dimick J, Mathur A, et al. Who pays for biliary complications following liver transplant? A business case for quality improvement. *Am J Transplant* 2006;6(12):2978–2982.
11. Dimick JB, Weeks WB, Karia RJ, et al. Who pays for poor surgical quality? Building a business case for quality improvement. *J Am Coll Surg* 2006;202(6):933–937.
12. Dimick JB, Chen SL, Taheri PA, et al. Hospital costs associated with surgical complications: a report from the private-sector National Surgical Quality Improvement Program. *J Am Coll Surg* 2004;199(4):531–537.
13. Galvin RS, Delbanco S, Milstein A, et al. Has the leapfrog group had an impact on the health care market? *Health Aff (Millwood)* 2005;24(1): 228–233.
14. Milstein A, Galvin RS, Delbanco SF, et al. Improving the safety of health care: the leapfrog initiative. *Eff Clin Pract* 2000;3(6):313–316.
15. Rosenthal MB, Dudley RA. Pay-for-performance: will the latest payment trend improve care? *JAMA* 2007;297(7):740–744.
16. Rosenthal MB. Beyond pay for performance–emerging models of provider-payment reform. *N Engl J Med* 2008;359(12):1197–1200.
17. Fung-Kee-Fung M, Goubanova E, Sequeira K, et al. Development of communities of practice to facilitate quality improvement initiatives in surgical oncology. *Qual Manag Health Care* 2008;17(2):174–185.
18. Fung-Kee-Fung M, Watters J, Crossley C, et al. Regional collaborations as a tool for quality improvements in surgery: a systematic review of the literature. *Ann Surg* 2009;249(4):565–572.
19. Pronovost P, Needham D, Berenholtz S, et al. An intervention to decrease catheter-related bloodstream infections in the ICU. *N Engl J Med* 2006;355(26):2725–2732.
20. Moscucci M, Rogers EK, Montoye C, et al. Association of a continuous quality improvement initiative with practice and outcome variations of contemporary percutaneous coronary interventions. *Circulation* 2006; 113(6):814–822.
21. Khuri SF, Henderson WG. The patient safety in surgery study. *J Am Coll Surg* 2007;204(6):1087–1088.
22. Chassin MR. Achieving and sustaining improved quality: lessons from New York State and cardiac surgery. *Health Aff (Millwood)* 2002;21(4): 40–51.
23. Bratzler DW, Hunt DR. The surgical infection prevention and surgical care improvement projects: national initiatives to improve outcomes for patients having surgery. *Clin Infect Dis* 2006;43(3):322–330.
24. Campbell DA, Englesbe MJ, Kubus JJ, et al. Accelerating the pace of surgical quality improvement: the power of hospital collaboration. *Arch Surg* 2010;145(10):985–991.
25. *Producer price index for the direct health and medical insurance carriers industry*. U. S. Department of Labor, Bureau of Labor Statistics; 2007. Available at: www.bls.gov. Accessed June 19, 2009.
26. Englesbe MJ, Dimick JB, Sonnenday CJ, et al. The Michigan surgical quality collaborative: will a statewide quality improvement initiative pay for itself? *Ann Surg* 2007;246(6):1100–1103.
27. Birkmeyer JD, Shahian DM, Dimick JB, et al. Blueprint for a new American College of Surgeons: National Surgical Quality Improvement Program. *J Am Coll Surg* 2008;207(5):777–782.
28. Cuschieri J, Florence M, Flum DR, et al. Negative appendectomy and imaging accuracy in the Washington State Surgical Care and Outcomes Assessment Program. *Ann Surg* 2008;248(4):557–563.
29. Cohn JA, Englesbe MJ, Ads YM, et al. Financial implications of pancreas transplant complications: a business case for quality improvement. *Am J Transplant* 2007;7(6):1656–1660.
30. Moscucci M, Muller DW, Watts CM, et al. Reducing costs and improving outcomes of percutaneous coronary interventions. *Am J Manag Care* 2003;9(5):365–372.
31. Khuri SF, Henderson WG, Daley J, et al. Successful implementation of the Department of Veterans Affairs' National Surgical Quality Improvement Program in the private sector: the patient safety in surgery study. *Ann Surg* 2008;248(2):329–336.
32. Moscucci M, Share D, Kline-Rogers E, et al. The Blue Cross Blue Shield of Michigan Cardiovascular Consortium (BMC2) collaborative quality improvement initiative in percutaneous coronary interventions. *J Interv Cardiol* 2002;15(5):381–386.
33. Khuri SF, Daley J, Henderson W, et al. The Department of Veterans Affairs' NSQIP: the first national, validated, outcome-based, risk-adjusted, and peer-controlled program for the measurement and enhancement of the quality of surgical care. National VA Surgical Quality Improvement Program. *Ann Surg* 1998;228(4):491–507.
34. Hannan EL, Kumar D, Racz M, et al. New York State's Cardiac Surgery Reporting System: four years later. *Ann Thorac Surg* 1994;58(6): 1852–1857.
35. Hannan EL. Report cards: are they passing or failing? One New Yorker says they're passing. *Clin Perform Qual Health Care* 1996;4(4): 218–219.
36. Dimick JB, Welch HG, Birkmeyer JD. Surgical mortality as an indicator of hospital quality: the problem with small sample size. *JAMA* 2004; 292(7):847–851.
37. Hall BL, Campbell DA Jr, Phillips LR, et al. Evaluating individual surgeons based on total hospital costs: evidence for variation in both total costs and volatility of costs. *J Am Coll Surg* 2006;202(4): 565–576.
38. Hall BL, Hirbe M, Waterman B, et al. Comparison of mortality risk adjustment using a clinical data algorithm (American College of Surgeons National Surgical Quality Improvement Program) and an administrative data algorithm (Solucient) at the case level within a single institution. *J Am Coll Surg* 2007;205(6):767–777.
39. O'Connor GT, Quinton HB, Traven ND, et al. Geographic variation in the treatment of acute myocardial infarction: the Cooperative Cardiovascular Project. *JAMA* 1999;281(7):627–633.
40. Daley J, Khuri SF, Henderson W, et al. Risk adjustment of the postoperative morbidity rate for the comparative assessment of the quality of surgical care: results of the National Veterans Affairs Surgical Risk Study. *J Am Coll Surg* 1997;185(4):328–340.
41. Brown RS Jr, Ascher NL, Lake JR, et al. The impact of surgical complications after liver transplantation on resource utilization. *Arch Surg* 1997;132(10):1098–1103.
42. Shroyer AL, Coombs LP, Peterson ED, et al. The Society of Thoracic Surgeons: 30-day operative mortality and morbidity risk models. *Ann Thorac Surg* 2003;75(6):1856–1864; discussion 1864–1855.
43. Bratzler DW. The Surgical Infection Prevention and Surgical Care Improvement Projects: promises and pitfalls. *Am Surg* 2006;72(11): 1010–1016; discussion 1021–1030, 1133–1048.

CHAPTER

9

Patient Safety

Darrell A. Campbell

IMPORTANT DEFINITIONS: SAFETY VERSUS QUALITY

The terms quality and safety have important bearings on any discussion of patient care. These are related subjects but have different meanings, and these differences should be underscored before any dialogue about patient safety begins. Safety means "freedom from harm"; in the context of patient care, "safety" means freedom from harm associated with any medical action or treatment. Quality is a more global term referring to a "degree of excellence." It is theoretically possible for a hospital to be safe, but for quality to be average or poor. It is not possible, however, for a hospital to be of high quality and unsafe. In this chapter we focus primarily on the subject of patient safety, but admit that some aspects of the subject drift into the area of quality as well.

THE PROBLEM

By now all are familiar with the report issued by the Institute of Medicine (IOM) in 2000 entitled, "To Err is Human" (1). The report was an exhaustive review of the status of safety in our nation's hospitals. The bottom line—which served as a "burning platform" for the patient safety movement—was the astonishing calculation that between 44,000 and 98,000 Americans died annually in hospital as the result of preventable medical error. The report produced a flurry of outrage from consumer groups, and denials and refutations from medical groups, but when the dust settled what was left was the recognition, by all groups, that something was seriously wrong in our medical care delivery system.

Comparisons are often made between the safety of airline travel and medical care. One airline disaster every two or three years produces calls for new regulation, better airports, more frequent mechanical checks, and earlier retirement for pilots. But consider medical care. If even the lower number of preventable deaths extrapolated by the IOM report (44,000 annually) were seen as accurate, and one accepted that an average of 350 passengers were on board every major commercial aircraft flight, deaths from medical error would be equivalent of 63 separate mid-air collisions per year in the airline industry or five per month. Imagine the public outcry this would produce, the laws that would be quickly passed, and the boon to travel on Amtrak that would result. But this is not what has happened in medicine. The government response has been weak at best, and the medical community has been slow to acknowledge and even slower to respond to the safety imperative.

Darrell A. Campbell: University of Michigan Health Systems, Ann Arbor, MI 48109.

CULTURE

Culture is defined as "how we do things around here." That is, there is a certain level of acceptance for what goes on in a given hospital. That acceptance is based on two precepts that in the past have not been challenged. One precept is that medical errors exist because "humans will always make mistakes." While superficially true, this statement fails to acknowledge that modern human factors engineering strategies can militate against commonly encountered errors. A concrete example of how human factors engineering can be brought into play involves something as simple as a connector for medical tubing. If the connector is designed such that it is not possible to connect an O_2 line to a CO_2 valve, a potentially catastrophic mistake becomes impossible. More globally, work hour restrictions for medical trainees, which reduce fatigue, could be expected to result in fewer errors by exhausted and stressed doctors. To date, human factors engineering has not been brought into the delivery of medical care effectively. While humans will always be capable of making mistakes, the number of mistakes will be reduced if design is targeted to what we know about human fallibilities.

The second precept accounting for complacency is the notion that a medical error is the result of poor individual performance rather than an imperfect system of care. If an individual made the error, in isolation, the only corrective step would be to dismiss the hapless caregiver or immerse him or her in intensive remedial education. The problem with this approach is that it does not apply to the next hapless caregiver faced with the same situation. And so, since there is a high turnover in most medical environments, mistakes continue to happen, caregivers continue to be dismissed, and nothing really changes. This sequence has been ingrained in the medical culture, and it is why the medical community has been slow to respond to the safety crisis.

SWISS CHEESE AND MEDICAL ERRORS

A popular paradigm in the medical safety area is the "Swiss cheese" model, introduced by James Reason (2). (Fig. 9.1) This model is a visual representation of the multiple system layers that could prevent a medical error from occurring. A beam of light representing a latent error passes through a hole in the cheese representing a system of vulnerability. The latent error passing through the system via vulnerability will result in a medical error. If enough systems are set up with vulnerabilities, but in different locations, it becomes progressively harder for the latent error to become manifest clinically. The point here is that, while we recognize that humans have vulnerabilities and systems of care have vulnerabilities, the prevention of error lies at the door of hospital leadership. Positive results come from the establishment of effectively redundant systems of error prevention. This concept is a major paradigm shift in the patient safety movement.

Even though the system should be constructed to backup human fallibilities, it is instructive to recognize the fallibilities. This subject is hard to quantify, but a good list, developed in a family practice environment, reads as follows: hurry, distraction, lack of knowledge, premature closure of the diagnostic process, and inadequate aggressiveness in patient management (3). The first three issues are probably obvious, but premature closure of the diagnostic process is a problem needing emphasis. Humans often fall into this trap. We see issues as black and white, in an attempt to make sense out of complex circumstances. Hurry, distraction, and lack of knowledge contribute. Relevant pieces of Swiss cheese, which could counteract this tendency, include electronic diagnosis and decision-making aids, an institutional policy fostering physician interactions, teamwork, and second opinions, and setting and adhering to reasonable workload standards.

Depending on the environment, other fallibilities are exposed. In the acute hospital setting, as opposed to the outpatient environment in family practice, safety problems typically involve poor handoffs, failures of teamwork, excess workload, and fatigue (4).

But what about the concept of individual responsibility? One can not show up for work with a careless attitude, engage in irresponsible actions, and expect to be held immune from poor performance because of the emphasis on systems. This is a delicate balance for any healthcare system. The underlying principle here is that most employees of a hospital wake up each morning wanting to do a good job and to avoid mistakes, and hence (with exceptions) the general philosophy should be that a major improvement in safety will be at the level of system engineering rather than individual fallibility. When the onus of individual fallibility is lessened (not entirely), there emerges a new sense of system responsibility, with increased willingness to identify system errors and to participate in safety enhancement as a group. This collaborative participation does not occur when one is worried about punitive consequences for reporting and the possibility of job loss.

LEADERSHIP AND POLICY

How to change a culture? This is not done easily. There are two crucial elements which, if effective, can change the culture direction positively. The first element is set by the example of hospital leadership. When the rank and file sees that the hospital CEO places patient safety at the top of the list and backs this priority up with funding, a number of good things happen. When the CEO emphasizes a change in hospital policy with an emphasis on safety, the change is reinforced. We introduced two policies that serve as examples of this point. The first, the "full disclosure" policy, stipulated that employees were obligated (not just encouraged) to disclose fully to patients important errors made in rendering their care. Remarkably, this policy resulted in fewer malpractice claims against the system, but more importantly, it underscored for employees the institutional emphasis on openness and honesty (5). The second policy change implemented was the "speak up with safety concerns" policy, which stipulated that no caregiver could be punished for voicing a concern involving patient safety, regardless of feelings hurt or hierarchy violated. Again, this written

FIGURE 9.1. Systems failures (Reproduced with permission from Mulholland, MW, et al., eds. Greenfield's Surgery: Scientific Principles and Practice, Fifth Edition. Philadelphia: Lippincott Williams & Wilkins, 2010; Figure 16.1).

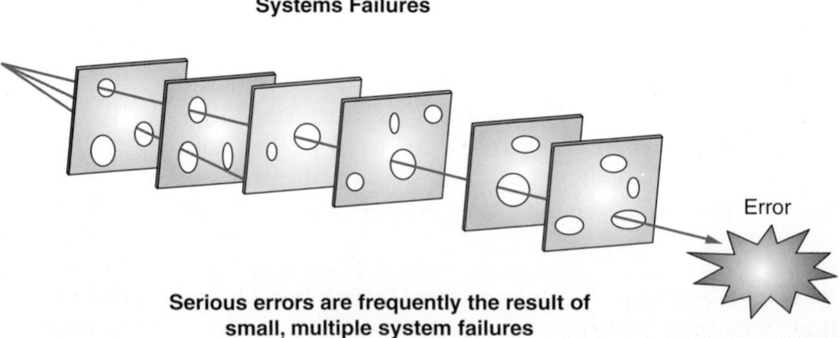

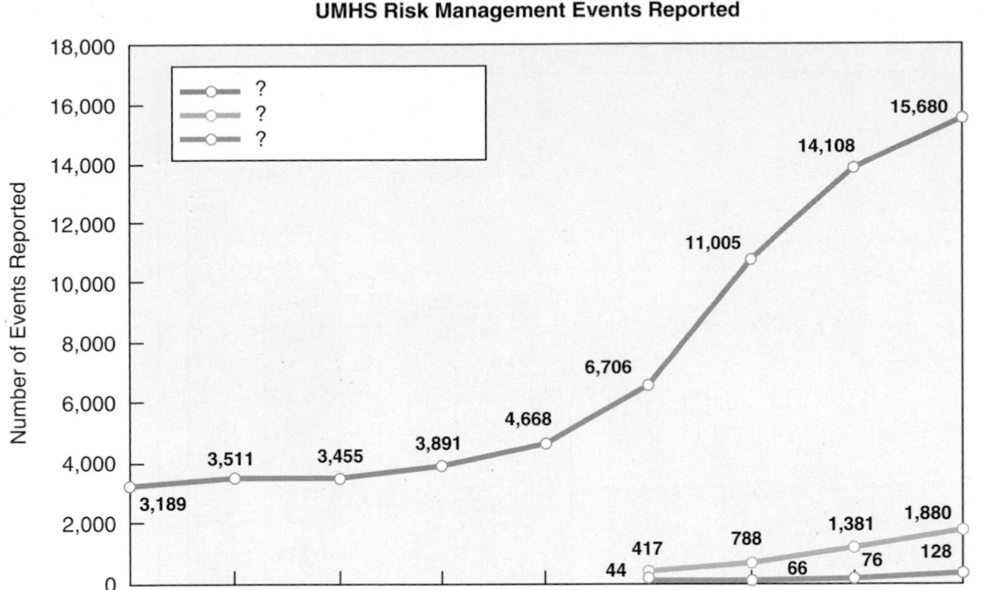

FIGURE 9.2. Overview of the reporting system (Reproduced with permission from Mulholland, MW, et al., eds. Greenfield's Surgery: Scientific Principles and Practice, Fifth Edition. Philadelphia: Lippincott Williams & Wilkins, 2010; Figure 16.2).

policy clearly articulated a health system goal—that patient safety trumped all other considerations.

One manifestation of an improved safety culture is an increased error reporting rate. Clearly the error reporting rate will not go up if there exists widespread fear of retribution for reporting. What is desired is an increased rate of error reporting, but a decreasing rate of events resulting in temporary or permanent harm. This pattern suggests that caregivers are vigilant, care about safety, and are reporting on "near misses." The data from "near misses" represent a treasure chest of information that can be used to prevent actual mistakes. We have seen increased reporting in association with the purchase of a new electronic reporting format. Whether a change in culture or a change in reporting format is responsible for the increased level of reports is hard to say, but we believe that it is a combination of both (Fig. 9.2).

ASSESSING THE CULTURE

If one places priority on "improving" a safety culture, it is necessary for the "culture" to be measured. Validated culture surveys exist, which, if applied periodically in a hospital environment, give important insight into the success of the safety culture initiatives. We use the Agency for Healthcare Research and Quality (AHRQ) safety culture instrument primarily, and survey all caregivers at approximately two-year intervals. We use the resulting information in three ways. First, we use the aggregate response to answer the question "are we improving the safety culture" and, if not, what are the areas that need to be addressed institutionally. In our last survey, a clear sore point at our institution was difficulty with "hand offs" or the transfer of information between caregivers and teams. We then developed a task force focused on fixing the problem, over both short and long term. The long-term solution is an electronic one, but we also needed a short term solution. A paper-based hand off tool designed to address the hand off issue in the short term was quickly developed. This effort was a direct result of information gained from the safety culture survey.

A second way we use the safety culture survey data is to identify specific hospital units that are struggling with a dispirited or complacent attitude toward the safety effort. Such problems often result from poor nurse leadership, disruptive physicians, or a lack of perceived resources. Armed with information about the safety culture (or lack of it), the institution can implement a focused strategy customized to the problem. Figure 9.3 shows results from our survey arranged by an individual nursing unit, demonstrating certain units in need of help with error reporting, and conversely, units where the culture is good and institutional resources are not needed. A third source of information derived from the survey comes from narrative comments entered by individual caregivers. This is a very rich source of information and, since it is anonymous, often draws a fine line under issues that are hard to talk about in any other forum. Issues of suspected physician

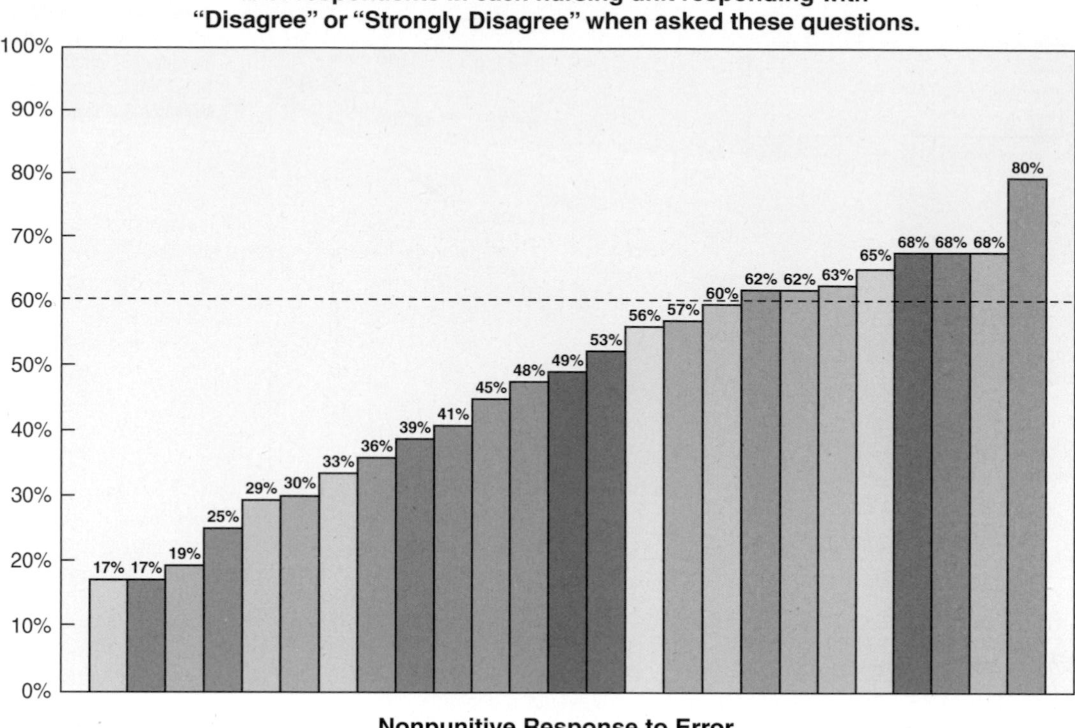

FIGURE 9.3. Nonpunitive response to error (Reproduced with permission from Mulholland, MW, et al., eds. Greenfield's Surgery: Scientific Principles and Practice, Fifth Edition. Philadelphia: Lippincott Williams & Wilkins, 2010; Figure 16.3).

impairment, abusive behavior, or lack of leadership skills are sometimes identified.

Two important questions regarding safety culture and our efforts to improve it remain. First, using the AHRQ tool, have we seen an aggregate improvement over the past two survey intervals? Many safety initiatives have been instituted over this period of time, and yet the aggregate culture data has not shown much change. We interpret this information to mean that much more work needs to be done and that changing a culture is a hard thing to do, akin to changing direction of an aircraft carrier. Also, over the period of time we have been studying our culture, we have observed that our institutional activity has gone up dramatically, the complexity of our patients has increased, and nursing turnover has been high. Under these circumstances no change in the safety culture data might be viewed more optimistically.

A second question is "are there individual strategies we have used that influence the safety culture positively?" If so, we could use these strategies more broadly. The answer to this question is yes. Patient safety rounds have been an important strategy that has improved the safety culture. Over the course of the past several years, we have made safety rounds on over 125 occasions, at two week intervals. Safety rounds are carried out by leadership (Chief of Staff, Chief of Nursing, CEO, etc.) and a pointed 45-minute discussion ensues with the unit caregivers, including nurses, aides, clerks, and transporters. The culture effects of this endeavor are profound. When caregivers believe that leadership is willing to listen, takes safety very seriously, and will put resources behind the articulated concerns, an overall feeling of confidence and support of the safety effort follows. Figure 9.4 demonstrates that caregivers having participated in patient safety rounds viewed the patient safety environment much more positively than those who had not.

But is a positive safety culture actually associated with improved safety? The assumption is yes, but data were hard to come by until recently. In Michigan, a multihospital collaborative was initiated (The Keystone Project), the object of which was to implement evidence-based practices known to decrease the incidence of blood stream infections (BSI) (6). One hundred seven hospitals were involved, and caregivers responded to the Safety Attitudes Questionnaire (SAQ), similar to the AHRQ tool described previously. Results (incidence of BSI) were correlated with answers to the SAQ. The results are seen in Figure 9.5. There was an important association noted between the best results (% reduction in BSI) and the most positive answers to SAQ questions. This is only an association, (and subject to the usual caveats about associations vs. cause and effect) but important nonetheless. These results support the underlying

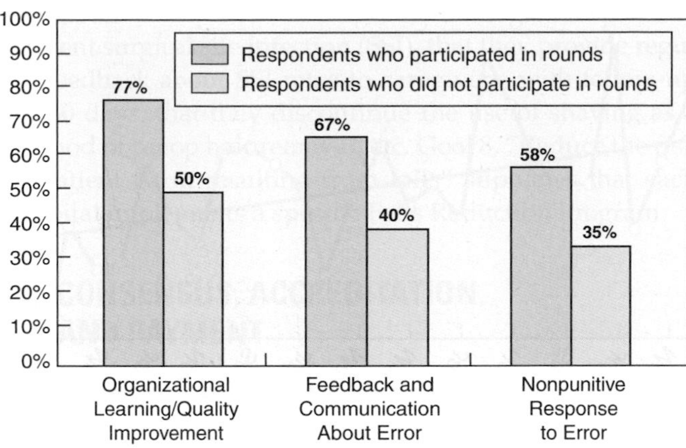

FIGURE 9.4. Comparison of 2007 AHRQ data participants vs. nonparticipants in patient safety rounds (Reproduced with permission from Mulholland, MW, et al., eds. Greenfield's Surgery: Scientific Principles and Practice, Fifth Edition. Philadelphia: Lippincott Williams & Wilkins, 2010; Figure 16.4).

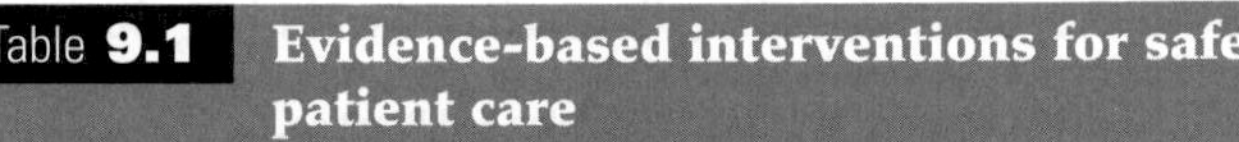

Table 9.1 Evidence-based interventions for safe patient care

- Appropriate use of prophylaxis to prevent venous thromboembolism.
- Use of perioperative beta-blockers in appropriate patients to prevent perioperative morbidity and mortality.
- Use of maximum sterile barriers while placing central intravenous catheters to prevent infections.
- Asking that patients recall and restate what they have been told during the informed consent process.
- Continuous aspiration of subglottic secretions to prevent ventilator-associated pneumonia.
- Use of pressure relieving bedding materials to prevent pressure ulcers.
- Use of real-time ultrasound guidance during central line insertion to prevent complications.
- Patient self-management for warfarin to achieve appropriate outpatient anticoagulation and prevent complications.
- Appropriate provision of nutrition, with a particular emphasis on early enteral nutrition in critically ill and surgical patients.
- Use of antibiotic impregnated central venous catheters to prevent catheter-related infections.

hypothesis that when leadership prioritizes safety and implements actions to support safety, caregivers reflect this in their answers to the SAQ, and this is associated with improved patient safety.

THE EVIDENCE BASE FOR PATIENT SAFETY

As important as it is to lay a strong foundation in safety culture, the energy and enthusiasm of caregivers to provide safe patient care must be rooted in activities that have been found to be effective. Unfortunately there does not exist, at this point, a large base of evidence in patient safety, largely because the field is relatively young. Recently, the World Health Organization (WHO) convened a group to carefully analyze existing studies and highlight effective strategies with an evidence base (7). These are listed in Table 9.1. Comments about specific evidence-based actions follow.

With regard to the administration of perioperative β-blockers to prevent postoperative myocardial ischemia, it is very clear that patients already on such medications must be given these postoperatively. However, an initial interest in β-blocker administration for patients never having received them previously declined rapidly as the result of the POISE trial (8). This was an international randomized controlled trial focusing on this specific issue, and the result, after analyzing many thousands of patients, was that giving β-blockers perioperatively to naïve patients caused more harm than good. Specifically, treated patients developed more troublesome bradycardia and hypotension than controls, and this resulted in a higher incidence of stroke, obviating the potential benefit of the drug in preventing myocardial ischemia.

Using maximum sterile barriers for central venous pressure (CVP) catheter insertion, in order to prevent BSI may

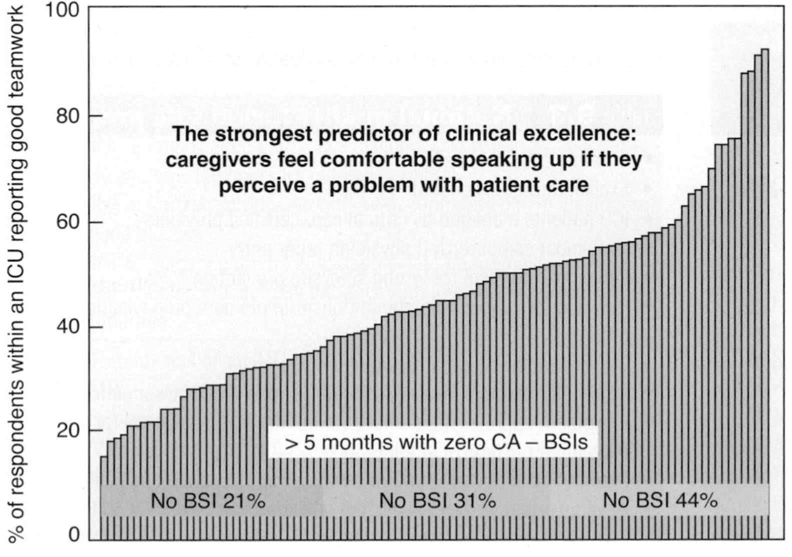

FIGURE 9.5. Teamwork climate across Michigan ICUs (Reproduced with permission from Mulholland, MW, et al., eds. Greenfield's Surgery: Scientific Principles and Practice, Fifth Edition. Philadelphia: Lippincott Williams & Wilkins, 2010; Figure 16.5).

useful information can be obtained from this system, a disadvantage is that the data is obtained from medical billing coders and may not accurately reflect whether a complication was actually preventable for not. An example might be the PSI labeled "accidental puncture and laceration." An enterotomy made during the course of a difficult dissection in an irradiated and multiple-operated abdomen would fit into this category, and be interpreted by nonsurgeons as an "accident." The surgeon who was carefully dissecting under these circumstances would definitely not agree. Despite such limitations, the AHRQ PSIs will be publicly reported as a safety indicator by the government next year. They already form the basis of certain proprietary safety indices, such as those put forth by HealthGrades.com or the University Health System Consortium.

EFFORTS FROM THE WORLD HEALTH ORGANIZATION

Recognizing that patient safety should be a global imperative, the WHO, working with JCO, has embarked on an ambitious project to reduce the incidence of medical errors internationally. One effort, known as the "high 5's" initiative, focuses on reducing five prevalent types of medical errors, over a five-year period, in at least seven countries. The identified problem areas are (1) managing concentrated injectable medicines, (2) assuring medication accuracy at transitions of care, (3) improved communication during patient care handovers, (4) improved hand hygiene, and (5) performance of the correct procedure at the correct body site.

The WHO has focused on surgical care specifically through a separate effort referred to as the "Safe Surgery Saves Lives" campaign. One very tangible result of this effort is the Surgical Safety Checklist, shown in Table 9.6 (9). Now being tested in eight countries, the vision is that a standardized forum for intraoperative communication will be adopted internationally, much in the same way that the international aviation community has endorsed standardized flight checklists.

IMPLEMENTATION STRATEGIES

While establishing a safe culture and emphasizing an evidence base and consensus guidelines are important, ensuring implementation of what is known to be safe practice is critical and may be the most difficult of all safety strategies to accomplish. Several strategies have been helpful in our environment.

ADDING PHARMACISTS TO ROUNDS

Our medical center is a tertiary care referral center; the complexity of cases is high and always increasing.

Table 9.6 World Health Organization (WHO) surgical safety checklist

Before Induction of Anesthesia	Before Skin Incision	Before Patient Leaves Operating Room
SIGN IN	**TIME OUT**	**SIGN OUT**

• Patient Has Confirmed
  • Identity
  • Site
  • Procedure
  • Consent
• Site Marked/Not Applicable
• Anesthesia Safety Check Completed
• Pulse Oximeter on Patient and Functioning
Does Patient Have a: Known Allergy?
• No
• Yes
Difficult Airway/Aspiration Risk?
• No
• Yes
Risk of >500 ml Blood Loss (7 ML/KG in Children)?
• No
• Yes, and Adequate Intravenous Access and Fluids Planned
	• Confirm All Team Members Have Introduced Themselves by Name and Role
	• Surgeon, Anesthesia Professional, and Nurse Verbally Confirm
	  • Patient
	  • Site
	  • Procedure
	Anticipated Critical Events
	• Surgeon Reviews: What Are the Critical or Unexpected Steps, Operative Duration, Anticipated Blood Loss?
	• Anesthesia Team Reviews: Are There Any Patient-Specific Concerns?
	• Nursing Team Reviews: Has Sterility (Including Indicator Results) Been Confirmed? Are There Equipment Issues or Any Concerns?
	Has Antibiotic Prophylaxis Been Given Within the Last 60 Minutes?
	• Yes
	• Not Applicable
	Is Essential Imaging Displayed?
	• Yes
	• Not Applicable
		Nurse Verbally Confirms with the Team
		• The Name Of The Procedure Recorded
		• That Instrument, Sponge and Needle Counts Are Correct (Or Not Applicable)
		• How The Specimen Is Labeled (Including Patient Name)
		• Whether There Are Any Equipment Problems to be Addressed
		• Surgeon, Anesthesia Professional, and Nurse Review the Key Concerns for Recovery and Management of This Patient

From World Health Organization. *World Alliance for Patient Safety Progress Report 2006–2007.* Geneva, Switzerland: WHO Press; 2008.

Transplants, complex oncologic problems, extracorporeal membrane oxygenation (ECMO) patients, and others with multisystem organ failure fill a large portion of our beds. The pharmacologic aspects of these cases are complex. Adding to the difficulty of managing such patients is the educational aspect of our enterprise, which guarantees a constant supply of new faces on rounds. To address these issues, and to prevent errors, we have implemented a policy of adding a clinical pharmacist to each of our high complexity services. The role of this individual is to suggest appropriate drugs, screen for allergies and incompatibilities, and monitor for important side effects. The program has been invaluable in improving patient safety at our institution and at others (10).

RAPID RESPONSE TEAM

Mortality rates for in-hospital cardiac arrest have been high for decades, despite advances in cardiopulmonary resuscitation (CPR) techniques and cardiotropic medications. This is true particularly for "floor arrests," those cases of arrest occurring outside of the intensive care unit. In our center, and many others, analysis of CPR cases has led to allegations that insufficient attention had been paid to the patient's condition in the hours prior to the arrest, at a time when interventions could conceivably have been very helpful.

One approach to this problem has been to develop a "rapid response team" (RRT), which is activated when certain physiologic parameters fall outside a specified range. Such parameters identified at our center are heart rate (<40 or >140 with new symptoms), respiratory rate (<8 or >36), blood pressure (BP systolic <80 or >220, BP diastolic >110 with symptoms) and unexplained change in cognition or neurologic status of adult inpatients. A key feature of the RRT activation is that it is seen as mandatory for nursing; no judgment is required. If the parameters are exceeded, the RRT is activated. This relieves some of the anxieties experienced by nursing in the past about communication with physicians, particularly at odd hours. In our center, activation of RRT results in the timely arrival of an experienced surgical intensive care unit (SICU) nurse and a respiratory therapist. If the conditions are found to warrant it, a hospitalist is called. This occurs in 15% of cases. There is controversy in the literature as to whether the RRT effort actually is effective (11). However, the concept has so much face validity that most hospitals have accepted it as an important strategy to promote a safety culture.

An interesting and entirely unexpected offshoot of the RRT has been the process, by the RRT team, of visiting nursing floors on a shift-by-shift basis prior to any RRT activation. This process lets the team become more familiar with patients who might subsequently warrant RRT activation. Visits often foster a discussion among caregivers and family as to whether any intervention is appropriate or warranted.

CREW RESOURCE MANAGEMENT

Another approach to the implementation of safe practices is to educate and train physicians and nurses within the context of a team. The team is defined, goals are set, and individual responsibilities are assigned. The completion of tasks (or omission) is apparent to members of the team, which provides a fail-safe structure. There has been considerable interest in crew resource management in the area of medicine since it has been conclusively shown to add value to aviation cockpit training. Crew resource management is probably best applied in small well-defined areas, with relatively consistent staffing patterns, such as an operating room. In one report a perioperative crew resource management training program consisted of an e-learning module, the development of laminated checklists and pocket-sized cards, briefing scripts, a communication whiteboard, and a hands-on training program facilitated by experienced personnel. Even with focused effort at crew resource management, perioperative safety practice implementation was found to be less than perfect, (12) but the field, at least in medicine, is in its infancy, and it will probably be an important part of safety strategies in years to come.

DEVELOPING COLLABORATIVE GROUPS OF HOSPITALS

When motivated hospitals join forces to discuss safety, the result is often a more consistent implementation of safety practices and better results. The development of a collaborative group directed at safety and/or quality allows for comparative evaluation of quality and safety and often results in a spirit of friendly competition, which improves the aggregate level of safety.

A prominent example of such collaboration was mentioned previously, the Michigan Hospital Association sponsored Keystone Initiative. Here evidence-based practice for the care of patients in the intensive care unit (ICU) was monitored and found to be low across the state. A protocol was adopted for over 100 ICU groups which included elevation of the head of the bed to 30° angle, ulcer prophylaxis, regular respiratory weaning trials, and a central line insertion protocol with line maintenance involving chlorhexidine patches. When the latter protocol was implemented a profound drop in the incidence of BSI across the state was seen, and the estimated cost savings exceeded 160 million dollars (6).

In a different example, 34 Michigan hospitals formed the Michigan Surgical Quality Collaborative. These hospitals, using the American College of Surgeons-National Surgical Quality Improvement Project (ACS-NSQIP) as a quality reporting infrastructure, convene at 3-month intervals to share information about surgical results. Hospitals with the fewest complications in a specific area discuss why they feel they have been successful. "Best practices" are then distributed in a network including the Internet, a

PART

II

Management of Surgical Complications

CHAPTER

10

Assessment of Perioperative Cardiac Risk

Debabrata Mukherjee and Kim A. Eagle

INTRODUCTION

In the United States, approximately 25 million patients undergo noncardiac surgery annually. Of these, nearly 50,000 patients suffer perioperative myocardial infarction (MI), and more than half of 40,000 perioperative deaths are caused by cardiac events (1,2). Most perioperative cardiac morbidity and mortality is related to myocardial ischemia, congestive heart failure, or arrhythmias. Therefore, preoperative evaluation and management to reduce morbidity and mortality rates emphasize the detection, characterization, and treatment of coronary artery disease, left ventricular (LV) systolic dysfunction, abnormal valve function, and significant arrhythmias. The purpose of preoperative evaluation is not to "clear" patients for surgery but to assess medical status and cardiac risks posed by the surgery planned, and recommend strategies to reduce risk. There are two goals of the preoperative evaluation: first, to identify patients at increased risk of an adverse perioperative cardiac event and, second, to modify cardiac risk to improve short-term and long-term clinical outcomes. This chapter reviews preoperative identification of risk markers, opportunities for modifying risk, early identification of post-operative complications, and management of such complications. Its primary focus is on coronary artery and coronary heart disease since these problems dominate the clinical landscape.

IDENTIFICATION OF RISK MARKERS

The majority of patients at increased risk of adverse perioperative cardiac events can be identified using a simple bedside or office assessment. A careful history, physical examination, and review of the resting 12-lead electrocardiogram (ECG/EKG) are usually sufficient to allow stratification of most patients into low, intermediate, or high-risk categories for an adverse perioperative cardiac event. Risk markers for adverse post-operative outcomes can be stratified as major, intermediate, and minor (Table 10.1) (3). Greater weight is given for active than for quiescent problems, and the severity of disease is used to modify its importance. Risk markers recognized as predictive of increased perioperative risk (4–7) include poor functional capacity, and prior history or electrocardiographic evidence of coronary artery disease, congestive heart failure, arrhythmia, valvular heart disease, diabetes mellitus, uncontrolled systemic hypertension, renal insufficiency, and stroke.

Identifying several features on physical examination may be useful in assessment of perioperative risk. Patients with uncontrolled systemic hypertension should be identified and treated. Because congestive heart failure and valvular heart disease are associated with increased risk, physical findings suggestive of these diagnoses should be sought. The physical examination should cover general appearance (cyanosis, pallor, dyspnea during conversation/minimal activity, Cheyne-Stokes respiration, poor nutritional status, obesity, skeletal deformities, tremor, and anxiety), blood pressure in arms, carotid pulses, extremity pulses, and ankle-brachial indices. Jugular venous pressure and positive hepatojugular reflex are reliable signs of volume overload in chronic heart failure, and pulmonary rales and chest X-ray evidence of pulmonary congestion correlate better with acute heart failure. Patients with aortic stenosis can be identified by a typical murmur and when accompanied by a diminished and delayed upstroke of the carotid or brachial pulse. Finally, the presence of carotid or other vascular bruits helps identify patients at increased risk of harboring occult coronary artery disease.

The type of surgery also has important implications for cardiac risk, and surgical procedures generally can be classified as having high, intermediate, and low cardiac risk based upon the likely degree and duration of hemodynamic stress during surgery and the potential correlation of the operation (e.g. vascular surgery) with concomitant coronary or other heart disease (Table 10.2). Patients at very low clinical risk and those at high clinical risk of an adverse perioperative cardiac event typically can be identified using clinically available features described above. Patients at low clinical risk generally require no additional testing prior to noncardiac surgery. Among patients undergoing elective noncardiac surgery in whom risk is determined to be intermediate or high, additional testing may be useful to better define risk (3). It is useful to employ a stepwise approach to the preoperative assessment of cardiac risk as

Debabrata Mukherjee: Texas Tech University Health Sciences Center, EL Paso, TX 79905.

Kim A. Eagle: University of Michigan, Ann Arbor, MI 48109.

Table **10.1** **Clinical predictors of increased perioperative cardiovascular risk**

- Major predictors
- Unstable coronary syndromes
  - Unstable or severe angina (CCS class III or IV)[a]
  - Recent MI[b]
- Decompensated HF (NYHA functional class IV; worsening or new-onset HF)
- Significant arrhythmias (High-grade atrioventricular block; Mobitz II atrioventricular block; Third-degree atrioventricular heart block; Symptomatic ventricular arrhythmias; Supraventricular arrhythmias (including atrial fibrillation) with uncontrolled ventricular rate (Heart rate >100 bpm at rest); Symptomatic bradycardia; Newly recognized ventricular tachycardia
- Severe valvular disease (Severe aortic stenosis [mean pressure gradient greater than 40 mm Hg, aortic valve area less than 1.0 cm^2, or symptomatic]; Symptomatic mitral stenosis (progressive dyspnea on exertion, exertional presyncope, or HF)
- Intermediate predictors
- History of ischemic heart disease
- History of compensated or prior HF
- History of cerebrovascular disease
- Diabetes mellitus
- Renal insufficiency (Creatinine ≥ 2.0 mg/dL)
- Minor predictors
- Advanced age
- Abnormal ECG (left ventricular hypertrophy, left bundle branch block, ST–T abnormalities)
- Rhythm other than sinus (e.g., atrial fibrillation)
- Uncontrolled systemic hypertension

MI, myocardial infarction; HF, heart failure; ECG, electrocardiogram; CCS, Canadian cardiovascular class; NYHA, New York Heart Association.

[a]May include stable angina in patients who are usually sedentary.

[b]Recent myocardial infarction is defined as occurring within a period greater than seven days but less than or equal to one month; acute myocardial infarction is within seven days.

Adapted from Fleisher LA, Beckman JA, Brown KA, et al. ACC/AHA 2007 Guidelines on perioperative cardiovascular evaluation and care for noncardiac surgery: executive summary: a report of the American College of Cardiology/American Heart Association Task Force on Practice Guidelines (Writing Committee to Revise the 2002 Guidelines on Perioperative Cardiovascular Evaluation for Noncardiac Surgery): developed in collaboration with the American Society of Echocardiography, American Society of Nuclear Cardiology, Heart Rhythm Society, Society of Cardiovascular Anesthesiologists, Society for Cardiovascular Angiography and Interventions, Society for Vascular Medicine and Biology, and Society for Vascular Surgery. *Circulation* 2007;116:1971–1996.

suggested by the American College of Cardiology/American Heart Association (ACC/AHA) guidelines (Fig. 10.1).

Management of specific cardiovascular conditions

Valvular Heart Disease

Severe aortic stenosis [valve area ≤1.0 cm (2) or mean pressure gradient greater than 40 mm Hg] presents the greatest valve-associated cardiovascular risk for patients undergoing noncardiac surgery (3). The presence of a fixed obstruction to LV outflow dramatically limits functional cardiac reserve and may be associated with intracavitary LV pressures in excess of 300 mm Hg. Accompanying LV hypertrophy predisposes the patient to diastolic dysfunction and pulmonary congestion. In general, severe and/or symptomatic aortic stenosis should be addressed prior to the patient undergoing elective noncardiac surgery. In most cases, aortic valve replacement is indicated as the definitive therapy of choice (8). If cardiac surgery is contraindicated, percutaneous aortic balloon valvotomy can be used to mitigate a LV outflow obstruction, even if only as a temporizing measure. When neither surgery nor percutaneous aortic valvotomy is considered feasible, noncardiac surgery with careful hemodynamic assessment may still be appropriate, albeit with a heightened risk of perioperative death with a mortality risk of approximately 10% (9,10).

Mitral stenosis can usually be medically managed with heart rate control, when mild and asymptomatic. Severe mitral stenosis should be corrected to prolong survival and patient complications, unrelated to the proposed noncardiac surgery, in accordance with ACC/AHA guidelines on management of vascular heart disease. In general, aortic and mitral regurgitation lesions are better tolerated perioperatively than stenotic lesions. Medical regimens for these individuals should be optimized pre-operatively with diuretics and afterload reduction with vasodilators. Appropriate prophylaxis for bacterial endocarditis is indicated in patients with valvular heart disease and prosthetic heart valves. Appropriate perioperative antithrombotic therapy for patients with prosthetic heart valves is outlined in Table 10.3.

Cardiac Arrhythmias

In individuals with arrhythmias, a metabolic profile and the list of medications should be carefully reviewed and corrected. Even mild hypokalemia should be corrected in these individuals. Sustained or symptomatic ventricular arrhythmias should be treated with suppressive therapy.

Table 10.2 Cardiac risk[a] stratification for different types of surgical procedures

- **High risk**, Vascular (Reported cardiac risk[a] >5%)
  - Aortic and other major vascular surgery
  - Peripheral vascular surgery
- **Intermediate risk** (Reported cardiac risk 1%–5%)
  - Intraperitoneal and intrathoracic
  - Carotid endarterectomy
  - Head and neck surgery
  - Orthopedic surgery
  - Prostate surgery
- **Low risk**[b] (Reported cardiac risk < 1%)
  - Endoscopic procedures
  - Superficial biopsy
  - Cataract
  - Breast surgery

[a]Combined incidence of cardiac death and nonfatal myocardial infarction.
[b]Do not generally require further preoperative cardiac testing
Adapted from Fleisher LA, Beckman JA, Brown KA, et al. ACC/AHA 2007 Guidelines on perioperative cardiovascular evaluation and care for noncardiac surgery: executive summary: a report of the American College of Cardiology/American Heart Association Task Force on Practice Guidelines (Writing Committee to Revise the 2002 Guidelines on Perioperative Cardiovascular Evaluation for Noncardiac Surgery): developed in collaboration with the American Society of Echocardiography, American Society of Nuclear Cardiology, Heart Rhythm Society, Society of Cardiovascular Anesthesiologists, Society for Cardiovascular Angiography and Interventions, Society for Vascular Medicine and Biology, and Society for Vascular Surgery. *Circulation* 2007;116:1971–1996.

Patients with symptomatic bradyarrhythmias should be treated with temporary pacing and a permanent pacemaker implanted when indicated. If an individual already has a permanent pacemaker, this should be checked prior to surgery. Electrocautery should be minimized in patients who are totally pacemaker dependent and pacemakers checked again after surgery to ensure settings are optimal. Typically, implanted defibrillators are turned off during surgery and turned back on after surgery.

Hypertension

Mild to moderate hypertension should be managed with medical therapy and closely monitored during surgery. Individuals with severe hypertension (diastolic >110 mm) need control prior to surgery. For urgent surgery in patients with severe hypertension, intravenous agents may be used to achieve control of blood pressure. Abrupt withdrawal of beta-blockers and clonidine should be avoided to prevent rebound hypertension.

Cardiomyopathy

Pulmonary artery catheters may be beneficial in patients with severe LV dysfunction. Close monitoring of the volume status, heart rate, and systemic vascular resistance in indicated in patients with hypertrophic cardiomyopathy. Intravascular volume depletion is poorly tolerated in these patients and may result in cardiogenic shock.

Diagnostic testing

Routine laboratory tests such as serum creatinine, hemoglobin, platelet count, potassium level, liver profile, and oxygen saturation are important in risk stratification. Arterial blood gas analysis is useful in patients with advanced pulmonary disease. A 12-lead ECG provides important prognostic information. Patients who are at low risk based on history, physical examination, and routine laboratory tests may not need further evaluation. Noninvasive testing is primarily useful in intermediate risk patients. The perioperative guidelines are straightforward on recommendations for patients about to undergo emergency surgery, the presence of prior cardiac revascularization, and the occurrence of major cardiac predictors. However, the majority of patients have either intermediate or minor clinical predictors of increased perioperative cardiovascular risk. Table 10.4 presents the currently recommended approach for noninvasive testing before noncardiac surgery. In a patient with an intermediate clinical predictor, the presence of either a low functional capacity or high surgical risk should lead the physician to consider noninvasive testing. In the absence of intermediate clinical predictors, noninvasive testing should be considered when both the surgical risk is high and the functional capacity is low. Clinical predictors are defined in Table 10.1.

In most ambulatory patients, the test of choice is exercise ECG testing, which can provide an estimate of both functional capacity and detect myocardial ischemia through changes in the ECG and hemodynamic response. The ability to exercise moderately beyond 4 to 5 metabolic equivalents (METs) without symptoms defines low risk. Patients who can achieve >85% of maximum predicted heart rate without EKG changes are at lowest risk. Patients with an abnormal EKG response at greater than 70% of predicted heart rate are at intermediate risk and those with abnormal EKG response at less than 70% of predicted heart rate are at highest risk. It must be emphasized that although routine EKG stress testing has the sensitivity to identify one vessel coronary artery disease (CAD) of just 55% to 60%, its sensitivity for left main or advanced three vessel disease is far higher, in the 85% to 90% range. Thus, for the purposes of identifying the highest risk population, it is quite reasonable.

In patients with important abnormalities on their resting ECG (e.g., left bundle-branch block, LV hypertrophy with "strain" pattern, or digitalis effect), other techniques such as exercise echocardiography, exercise myocardial perfusion imaging, or pharmacological stress imaging may be indicated. Pharmacological stress or perfusion imaging is indicated in patients undergoing orthopedic, neurosurgical, or vascular surgery who are unable to exercise or have left bundle branch block (LBBB)/paced rhythm. The sensitivity and specificity of exercise thallium scans in the presence of left bundle-branch block are low, and overall diagnostic accuracy varies from 36% to 60% (11,12). In contrast, the use of vasodilator [dipyridamole/adenosine]

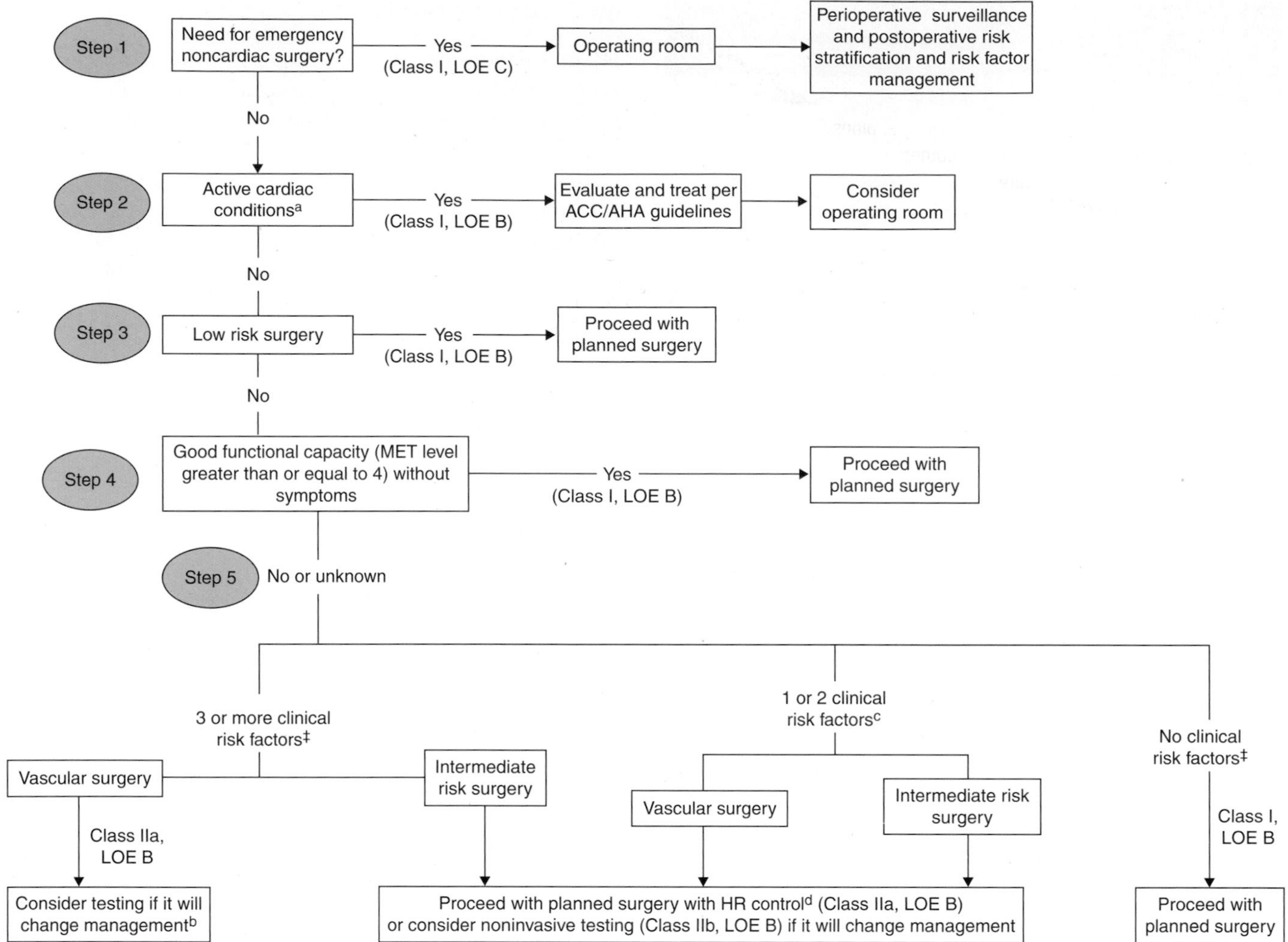

FIGURE 10.1. Cardiac evaluation and care algorithm for noncardiac surgery based on active clinical conditions, known cardiovascular disease, or cardiac risk factors for patients 50 years of age or greater. [a]See Table 10.1 for active clinical conditions. [b]Noninvasive testing may be considered before surgery in specific patients with risk factors if it will change management. [c]Clinical risk factors include ischemic heart disease, compensated or prior heart failure, diabetes mellitus, renal insufficiency, and cerebrovascular disease. [d]Consider perioperative beta blockade for populations in which this has been shown to reduce cardiac morbidity/mortality. ACC/AHA, American College of Cardiology/American Heart Association; HR, heart rate; LOE, level of evidence; MET, metabolic equivalent. Adapted from Fleisher LA, Beckman JA, Brown KA, et al. ACC/AHA 2007 Guidelines on perioperative cardiovascular evaluation and care for noncardiac surgery: executive summary: a report of the American College of Cardiology/American Heart Association Task Force on Practice Guidelines (Writing Committee to Revise the 2002 Guidelines on Perioperative Cardiovascular Evaluation for Noncardiac Surgery): developed in collaboration with the American Society of Echocardiography, American Society of Nuclear Cardiology, Heart Rhythm Society, Society of Cardiovascular Anesthesiologists, Society for Cardiovascular Angiography and Interventions, Society for Vascular Medicine and Biology, and Society for Vascular Surgery. *Circulation* 2007;116:1971–1996.

nuclear stress testing in such patients has a sensitivity of 98%, a specificity of 84%, and a diagnostic accuracy of 88% to 92% (13–15). Thus, in patients with LBBB, dipyridamole or adenosine-thallium imaging is the preferred method.

In patients unable to perform adequate exercise as with most patients with peripheral vascular disease (PVD), a nonexercise stress test should be used. In this regard, dipyridamole myocardial perfusion imaging testing and dobutamine echocardiography are the most commonly used tests. Intravenous dipyridamole should be avoided in patients with significant bronchospasm, critical carotid disease, or a condition that prevents withdrawal from theophylline preparations. Dobutamine should not be used as a stressor in patients with serious arrhythmias or severe hypertension or hypotension. For patients in whom echocardiographic image quality is likely to be poor, a myocardial perfusion study is more appropriate. If there is an additional question about valvular diseases, the echocardiographic stress test may be more useful. In many instances, either stress perfusion or stress echocardiography is appropriate. In a meta-analysis of dobutamine stress echocardiography, ambulatory electrocardiography, radionuclide ventriculography, and dipyridamole thallium scanning in predicting adverse cardiac outcome after vascular surgery, all tests had a similar predictive value, with overlapping confidence intervals (16). Another meta-analysis of 15 studies

Table 10.3 Antithrombotic therapy in the perioperative setting in patients with prosthetic heart valves

- Very low risk surgery (dental work, superficial biopsy)
  - Briefly reduce the INR to low or subtherapeutic range and resume normal dose post-procedure
- High risk for thrombosis [recent (<1 year) thromboembolism, Bjork Shiley valve especially in mitral position, or ≥3 of the following risk factors: A Fib, previous embolism, hypercoagulable condition, mechanical prosthesis and LVEF <30%]
  - Stop warfarin 72 hours prior to procedure
  - Start heparin when INR ≤2.0
  - Stop heparin 6 hours after the procedure
  - Restart heparin within 24 hours and continue until INR ≥2.0
- Approach for patients between these two extremes
  - Physicians must assess the risk and benefit of reduced anticoagulation versus perioperative heparin therapy

A Fib, atrial fibrillation; LVEF, left ventricular ejection fraction INR, International Normalized Ratio.
Adapted from Eagle KA, Berger PB, Calkins H, et al. ACC/AHA guideline update for perioperative cardiovascular evaluation for noncardiac surgery–executive summary: a report of the American College of Cardiology/American Heart Association Task Force on Practice Guidelines (Committee to Update the 1996 Guidelines on Perioperative Cardiovascular Evaluation for Noncardiac Surgery). *J Am Coll Cardiol* 2002;39:542–553.

demonstrated that the prognostic value of noninvasive stress imaging abnormalities for perioperative ischemic events is comparable for the available techniques but the accuracy varies with CAD prevalence (17). The expertise of the local laboratory in identifying advanced coronary disease is quite important in choosing the appropriate test.

Dipyridamole thallium stress testing to risk-stratify patients with suspected CAD is particularly effective before vascular surgery. Boucher et al. (18) reported on the utility of dipyridamole thallium imaging in the preoperative assessment of cardiac risk in patients with peripheral vascular disease. Forty-eight patients with suspected CAD were evaluated before they underwent vascular surgery; sixteen of these patients had thallium redistribution. All eight perioperative cardiac events occurred in patients who had preoperative thallium redistribution. Leppo et al. (19) performed dipyridamole thallium imaging in 100 consecutive patients admitted for elective peripheral vascular surgery and determined that the presence of thallium redistribution was the most significant predictor of serious nonfatal MI or cardiac death. The odds for a serious cardiac event were 23 times greater in a patient with thallium redistribution than in a patient without redistribution, strongly suggesting that myocardial imaging may be used as a primary screening test before elective vascular surgery (19). The findings of these early papers have been confirmed by many subsequent studies. A meta-analysis by Shaw et al. (17) analyzed the results of 10 articles and 1,994 vascular surgery candidates over a 9 year period. Cardiac death or nonfatal MI occurred in 1%, 7%, and 9% of patients with normal results, fixed defects, and reversible defects on thallium scans, respectively, demonstrating the utility of dipyridamole-thallium scintigraphy for preoperative risk stratification.

The extent and severity of perfusion defects play a significant role in adverse perioperative events, as the more extensive the perfusion abnormalities or the finding of cavity dilation or thallium lung uptake, the worse the perioperative prognosis. Although the immediate purpose of preoperative examination is to assess the risk associated with the planned surgical procedure, the determination of a long-term prognosis may be valuable in the overall management of a patient with known or suspected coronary

Table 10.4 Guide to noninvasive testing in preoperative patients

- ***Class I (is recommended)***
  1. Patients with active cardiac conditions (see Table 10.1) in whom noncardiac surgery is planned should be evaluated and treated before noncardiac surgery.
- ***Class IIa (is reasonable)***
  1. Noninvasive stress testing of patients with 3 or more clinical risk factors and poor functional capacity (less than 4 METs) who require vascular surgery is reasonable if it will change management.
- ***Class IIb (may be considered)***
  1. Noninvasive stress testing may be considered for patients with at least 1 to 2 clinical risk factors and poor functional capacity (less than 4 METs) who require intermediate-risk or vascular surgery if it will change management.
- ***Class III (not recommended)***
  1. Noninvasive testing is not useful for patients with no clinical risk factors undergoing intermediate-risk noncardiac surgery.
  2. Noninvasive testing is not useful for patients undergoing low-risk noncardiac surgery.

METs, metabolic equivalents; Emergency major operations may require immediately proceeding to surgery without sufficient time for noninvasive testing or preoperative interventions.
Adapted from Fleisher LA, Beckman JA, Brown KA, et al. ACC/AHA 2007 Guidelines on perioperative cardiovascular evaluation and care for noncardiac surgery: executive summary: a report of the American College of Cardiology/American Heart Association Task Force on Practice Guidelines (Writing Committee to Revise the 2002 Guidelines on Perioperative Cardiovascular Evaluation for Noncardiac Surgery): developed in collaboration with the American Society of Echocardiography, American Society of Nuclear Cardiology, Heart Rhythm Society, Society of Cardiovascular Anesthesiologists, Society for Cardiovascular Angiography and Interventions, Society for Vascular Medicine and Biology, and Society for Vascular Surgery. *Circulation* 2007;116:1971–1996.

artery disease. By using adenosine-sestamibi stress imaging, clinicians can assess both perfusion as well as regional and overall LV function. Thus, this form of nuclear cardiac imaging has largely superseded thallium imaging.

Dobutamine stress echocardiography has also been used successfully to identify patients at risk for cardiac complications of surgery, with very high negative predictive values. In a meta-analysis, patients with no dobutamine-induced wall motion abnormalities had a very low event rate (0.4%), compared with a 23.4% event rate in patients who developed new wall motion abnormalities during dobutamine infusion. Dobutamine stress echocardiography has also been shown to have prognostic value for predicting late events after vascular surgery. Furthermore, as for dipyridamole thallium imaging, the most useful role for stress echocardiography appears to be in patients at intermediate clinical risk.

For patients at high risk, it may be appropriate to proceed with coronary angiography rather than perform a noninvasive test. For high-risk patients with contraindications to angiography or coronary revascularization, medical therapy with aggressive beta-blockade may be the correct approach (20). In patients with unstable angina or evidence of residual ischemia after recent MI, direct coronary angiography may be indicated. In general, indications for preoperative coronary angiography are similar to those identified for the nonoperative setting (Table 10.5).

Combined clinical and scintigraphic assessment

Although the sensitivity of dipyridamole thallium imaging for detecting patients at increased risk is excellent, one of its limitations for preoperative screening is its low specificity and positive predictive value. In order to improve the value of risk stratification, many reports have suggested utilization of the combination of clinical markers and noninvasive test results. Eagle et al. (21) first reported on using assessment of clinical markers (history of angina, MI, congestive heart failure, diabetes, and Q wave on ECG) and thallium redistribution to identify a low risk subset of patients. The authors demonstrated that patients without any of these clinical markers did not require dipyridamole thallium testing. However, thallium redistribution had a significant predictive value in patients with—one or two clinical risk factors. Within this group, two of 62 (3.2%; 95% CI, 0% to 8%) patients without thallium redistribution had events compared with 16 events in 54 patients (29.6%; 95% CI, 16% to 44%) with thallium redistribution (21). L'Italien et al. (22) reported the results of a Bayesian model for perioperative risk assessment which combined clinical variables with dipyridamole thallium findings. This analysis examined the type of procedure, specific institutional complication rates, and other clinical factors in a sequential manner followed by the addition of the dipyridamole-thallium findings. The addition of dipyridamole-thallium

Table 10.5 American College of Cardiology/American Heart Association recommendations regarding coronary angiography before/after non-cardiac surgery

Class I: Patients With Suspected or Known CAD (strongly recommended)
- Evidence for high risk of adverse outcome based on noninvasive test results
- Angina unresponsive to adequate medical therapy
- Unstable angina, particularly when facing intermediate-risk or high-risk noncardiac surgery
- Equivocal noninvasive test results in patients at high-clinical risk undergoing high-risk surgery

Class IIa (Weight of evidence/opinion is in favor of usefulness/efficacy)
- Multiple markers of intermediate clinical risk and planned vascular surgery (noninvasive testing should be considered first)
- Moderate to large ischemia on noninvasive testing but without high-risk features and lower LVEF
- Nondiagnostic noninvasive test results in patients of intermediate clinical risk undergoing high-risk noncardiac surgery
- Urgent noncardiac surgery while convalescing from acute MI

Class IIb (Usefulness/efficacy is less well established by evidence/opinion)
- Perioperative MI
- Medically stabilized class III or IV angina and planned low-risk or minor surgery

Class III (contraindicated)
- Low-risk noncardiac surgery with known CAD and no high-risk results on noninvasive testing
- Asymptomatic after coronary revascularization with excellent exercise capacity ($\geq$ to 7 METs)
- Mild stable angina with good left ventricular function and no high-risk noninvasive test result.
- Noncandidate for coronary revascularization owing to concomitant medical illness, severe left ventricular dysfunction (e.g., LVEF less than 0.20), or refusal to consider revascularization

Candidate for liver, lung, or renal transplant more than 40 years old as part of evaluation for transplantation, unless noninvasive testing reveals high risk for adverse outcome.

CAD, coronary artery disease; LVEF, left ventricular ejection fraction; MI, myocardial infarction; MET, metabolic equivalents.
Adapted from Eagle KA, Berger PB, Calkins H, et al. ACC/AHA guideline update for perioperative cardiovascular evaluation for noncardiac surgery–executive summary: a report of the American College of Cardiology/American Heart Association Task Force on Practice Guidelines (Committee to Update the 1996 Guidelines on Perioperative Cardiovascular Evaluation for Noncardiac Surgery). *J Am Coll Cardiol* 2002;39:542–553.

data reclassified >80% of the moderate risk patients into low (3%) and high (19%) risk categories ($p < 0.0001$) but provided no stratification for patients classified as low or high risk according to the clinical model.

MODIFYING PREOPERATIVE RISK FACTORS

CAD is responsible for the majority of life-threatening perioperative cardiac complications. Once recognized, specific therapy should be instituted to minimize the risk of perioperative myocardial ischemia, MI, or death. Several studies have addressed the effect of anti-ischemic medical therapy on perioperative prognosis (23).

Medical therapy

Beta-Blockers

The effectiveness of beta-blockers in reducing perioperative cardiac risk has been evaluated in several studies. The first randomized, placebo-controlled study used atenolol in 200 high-risk patients scheduled to undergo noncardiac surgery including vascular, orthopaedic, intra-abdominal and neurosurgical procedures (24). Atenolol was administered either intravenously or orally two days preoperatively and continued for seven days postoperatively. The incidence of perioperative ischemia was significantly lower in the atenolol group than in the placebo group (24,25). There was no difference in the incidence of perioperative MI or death from cardiac causes, but the rate of event-free survival at six months was higher in the atenolol group.

Poldermans et al. studied the perioperative use of bisoprolol in elective major vascular surgery (20). Bisoprolol was started at least 7 days preoperatively, and the dose adjusted to achieve a resting heart rate of less than 60 beats per minute and continued for 30 days postoperatively. The study was confined to patients who had at least one cardiac risk factor (a history of congestive heart failure, prior MI, diabetes, angina pectoris, heart failure, age >70 years, or poor functional status) and evidence of inducible myocardial ischemia on dobutamine echocardiography. Patients with extensive regional wall-motion abnormalities were excluded. Bisoprolol was associated with a 91% reduction in the perioperative risk of MI or death from cardiac causes from 34% to 4% in this high-risk population. Because of the selection criteria used in this trial, the efficacy of bisoprolol in the group at very highest risk, those in whom coronary revascularization or modification would be considered or for whom the surgical procedure might ultimately be cancelled, cannot be determined. The rate of events in the standard-care group of 34% suggests that all but the patients at highest risk were enrolled in the trial. Urban et al. evaluated the role of prophylactic beta-blockers in patients undergoing elective total knee arthroplasty (26). One hundred and seven patients were preoperatively randomized into two groups, control and beta-blockers, who received postoperative esmolol infusions on the day of surgery and metoprolol for the next 48 hours to maintain a heart rate less than 80 bpm. The number of ischemic events (control, 50; beta-blockers, 16) and total ischemic time (control, 709 minutes; beta-blocker, 236 minutes) were significantly lower with esmolol compared to those for the control group. In this study prophylactic beta adrenergic blockade administered after elective total knee arthroplasty was associated with a reduced prevalence and duration of postoperative myocardial ischemia detected with Holter monitoring (26). The PeriOperative ISchemic Evaluation (POISE) trial randomly assigned 8351 patients with, or at risk of, atherosclerotic disease who were undergoing noncardiac surgery to receive extended-release metoprolol succinate ($n = 4174$) or placebo ($n = 4177$) (27). In this large study, perioperative extended-release metoprolol reduced the risk of MI, cardiac revascularization, and clinically significant atrial fibrillation 30 days after randomization compared with placebo; the drug also resulted in a significant excess risk of death, stroke, and clinically significant hypotension and bradycardia (27). The results of this trial suggest that the addition of perioperative beta-blockers has both potential benefits and risks. Table 10.6 lists current guideline recommendations for appropriate use of beta-blockers in the preoperative setting.

Alpha 2-Adrenergic Agonists

The effect of α 2-adrenergic agonists has also been studied in the perioperative period. Several small, randomized studies comparing clonidine with placebo failed to demonstrate that clonidine was effective in reducing the rates of MI and death from cardiac causes (16,28). Mivazerol, an intravenous α 2-adrenergic agonist administered by continuous infusion, was compared with placebo in patients with known coronary disease or risk factors who underwent major vascular or orthopedic procedures. Mivazerol was found to have no overall effect on the rates of cardiac complications (29). However, in the predefined subgroup of patients with known CAD who underwent major vascular surgery, mivazerol was associated with a significantly lower incidence of MI and death from cardiac causes. This agent is used by some institutions in Europe but has not been available in the United States.

Calcium Channel Blockers and Nitrates

There are no large randomized trials of either nitrates or calcium channel antagonists in terms of reducing perioperative MI or cardiac death. Therefore their use in the perioperative setting should mirror that in the general cardiology practice. They are second line agents to beta-blockers for the control of angina or stress induced ischemia. If a patient has required either or both to control ischemia, then they should be continued perioperatively.

Statins

HMG CoA reductase inhibitors [statins] have been shown to reduce ischemic events, stroke, and cardiac death in patients with established atherosclerosis. In patients

Table 10.6 Recommendations for beta-blocker medical therapy

Class I

1. Beta blockers should be continued in patients undergoing surgery who are receiving beta blockers to treat angina, symptomatic arrhythmias, hypertension.
2. Beta blockers should be given to patients undergoing vascular surgery who are at high cardiac risk owing to the finding of ischemia on preoperative testing

Class IIa

1. Beta blockers are probably recommended for patients undergoing vascular surgery in whom preoperative assessment identifies coronary heart disease.
2. Beta blockers are probably recommended for patients in whom preoperative assessment for vascular surgery identifies high cardiac risk, as defined by the presence of more than one clinical risk factor.
3. Beta blockers are probably recommended for patients in whom preoperative assessment identifies coronary heart disease or high cardiac risk, as defined by the presence of more than one clinical risk factor, who are undergoing intermediate-risk or vascular surgery.

Class IIb

1. The usefulness of beta blockers is uncertain for patients who are undergoing either intermediate-risk procedures or vascular surgery, in whom preoperative assessment identifies a single clinical risk factor.
2. The usefulness of beta blockers is uncertain in patients undergoing vascular surgery with no clinical risk factors who are not currently taking beta blockers.

Class III

1. Beta blockers should not be given to patients undergoing surgery who have absolute contraindications to beta blockade.

Adapted from Fleisher LA, Beckman JA, Brown KA, et al. ACC/AHA 2007 Guidelines on perioperative cardiovascular evaluation and care for noncardiac surgery: executive summary: a report of the American College of Cardiology/American Heart Association Task Force on Practice Guidelines (Writing Committee to Revise the 2002 Guidelines on Perioperative Cardiovascular Evaluation for Noncardiac Surgery): developed in collaboration with the American Society of Echocardiography, American Society of Nuclear Cardiology, Heart Rhythm Society, Society of Cardiovascular Anesthesiologists, Society for Cardiovascular Angiography and Interventions, Society for Vascular Medicine and Biology, and Society for Vascular Surgery. *Circulation* 2007;116:1971–1996.

undergoing vascular surgery, several recent reports suggest statins may reduce perioperative coronary events (30). Since stains are known to reduce atherosclerotic plaque formation and growth and potentially stabilize plaques that have been preexistent, it is not entirely surprising that they could reduce the risk of coronary plaque rupture and thrombosis during or after the stresses of vascular surgery. Hindler et al. (31) conducted a meta-analysis to evaluate the overall effect of preoperative statin therapy and reported a 44% reduction in mortality. Le Manach et al. demonstrated that postoperative statin withdrawal (more than four days) was an independent predictor of postoperative myonecrosis (32). Further studies are needed to determine how long the statins must be given before a perioperative benefit can be realized. Based on current evidence, patients taking statins, and scheduled for noncardiac surgery, should continue statins. For patients undergoing vascular surgery with or without clinical risk factors, statin use is reasonable and may be considered in patients with at least one clinical risk factor who are undergoing intermediate-risk procedures (3).

Revascularization

Percutaneous Revascularization

Percutaneous coronary intervention (PCI) utilizing primarily balloon angioplasty has been evaluated in three studies involving patients who were undergoing noncardiac surgery (33–35). The indications for PCI were not well described in the studies but most likely included the need to relieve symptomatic angina or reduce the perioperative risk of ischemia identified by noninvasive testing. All three studies had a low incidence of cardiac complications after noncardiac surgery, but no comparison groups were included.

One study used an administrative database of patients who were undergoing noncardiac surgery in the State of Washington. As compared with patients who did not undergo PCI preoperatively, those who did undergo the procedure had a lower incidence of perioperative cardiac complications (36). The benefit of revascularization was most apparent in the group that underwent PCI at least 90 days before noncardiac surgery. In contrast, when revascularization was performed within 90 days before noncardiac surgery, PCI was not associated with an improved outcome. The Coronary Artery Revascularization Prophylaxis (CARP) trial prospectively assessed the long-term benefit of preoperative coronary-artery revascularization among patients with stable CAD who are scheduled for elective vascular surgery. In this trial, coronary-artery revascularization before elective vascular surgery did not significantly alter the long-term outcome (37). These findings would suggest that PCI should not be used solely as a means of reducing perioperative risk.

Coronary stents are now used in more than 80% of PCI, and use of stents during PCI presents unique challenges because of the risk of coronary thrombosis and bleeding during the initial recovery phase. In a cohort of 40 patients who received stents within 30 days of noncardiac surgery, all eight deaths and seven MIs, as well as eight of 11 bleeding episodes, occurred in patients who had undergone surgery within 14 days of stent placement (38). The complications appeared to be related to serious bleeding resulting from postprocedural anticoagulant therapy or to coronary thrombosis in those who did not receive four full weeks of antithrombotic therapy after stenting. In general, one should wait at least 14 days after balloon angioplasty, 30–45 days after bare metal coronary stenting and 365 days after drug eluting stents to perform noncardiac surgery in order to allow complete endothelization and a full course of dual antiplatelet therapy to be given (3,39). Drug eluting stents should not be implanted in individuals who will undergo noncardiac surgery within a year of implantation.

Coronary-Artery Bypass Grafting

Coronary artery bypass grafting (CABG) has also been recommended to reduce the incidence of perioperative cardiac complications in highly selected patients. Evidence of a potential protective effect of preoperative coronary-artery bypass grafting comes from follow-up studies of randomized trials and/or registries comparing medical and surgical therapy for coronary artery disease. The largest study to date included 3,368 noncardiac operations performed within a 10-year period among patients assigned to medical therapy or coronary-artery bypass grafting in the Coronary Artery Surgery Study (40). Prior successful coronary-artery bypass grafting had a cardio-protective effect among patients who underwent high-risk noncardiac surgery (abdominal, thoracic, vascular, or orthopaedic surgery) (40). The perioperative mortality rate was nearly 50 percent lower in the group of patients who had undergone coronary-artery bypass grafting than in those who received medical therapy (3.3% vs. 1.7%, $p < 0.05$). There was no difference in the outcome of patients undergoing low-risk procedures such as breast and urologic surgery. Fleisher et al. used Medicare claims data to assess 30-day and 1-year mortality after noncardiac surgery according to the use of cardiac testing and coronary interventions such as CABG and PCI within the year before noncardiac surgery (41). Preoperative revascularization significantly reduced the 1-year mortality rate for patients undergoing aortic surgery but had no effect on the mortality rate for those undergoing infrainguinal surgeries. Finally, an analysis of the Bypass Angioplasty Revascularization Investigation (BARI) evaluated the incidence of postoperative cardiac complications after noncardiac surgery among patients with multivessel coronary disease who were randomly assigned to undergo PCI or CABG for severe angina (42). At an average of 29 months after coronary revascularization, both groups had similar, low rates of postoperative MI or death from cardiac causes (1.6% in each group). These data suggest that prior successful coronary revascularization, when accompanied by careful follow-up and therapy for subsequent coronary symptoms or signs, is associated with a low rate of cardiac events after noncardiac surgery (42). The CARP trial randomly assigned 510 patients with significant coronary artery stenosis to either coronary artery revascularization before surgery or no revascularization before surgery. Routine coronary revascularization in patients with stable cardiac symptoms before elective vascular surgery did not significantly alter the long-term outcome or short-term risk of death or MI in this study (37). The DECREASE-V pilot study identified a high-risk cohort of patients scheduled for vascular surgery who were randomized to best medical therapy and revascularization or best medical therapy alone before vascular surgery. There was no difference in the combined outcomes of death or MI at 30 days or 1 year between the revascularization and medical therapy groups (43). Based on recent studies, routine prophylactic coronary revascularization with either PCI or CABG should not be performed in patients with stable CAD before noncardiac surgery.

IDENTIFICATION OF POSTOPERATIVE COMPLICATIONS

Perioperative MI can be documented by assessing clinical symptoms, serial ECGs, and cardiac-specific biomarkers. On the basis of current evidence, in patients without documented CAD, surveillance should be restricted to those patients who develop perioperative signs of cardiovascular dysfunction. Postoperative troponin measurement is recommended in patients with ECG changes or chest pain typical of acute coronary syndrome (3). Perioperative surveillance for acute coronary syndromes with routine ECG and cardiac serum biomarkers is unnecessary in clinically low-risk patients undergoing low-risk operative procedures.

MANAGEMENT OF COMPLICATIONS

Despite optimal perioperative management, some patients will experience perioperative MI, which is associated with 40%–70% mortality. The reason for the high mortality is multifactorial and largely related to substantial comorbidity in such patients. Patients who develop ST-elevation MI should be considered for urgent coronary reperfusion whereas patients with non ST-elevation MI should undergo risk stratification after initial stabilization with intensive medical therapy. Individuals who develop heart failure after surgery should be evaluated for the etiology of heart failure and treated based on the precipitating or underlying cause. Immediate coronary angioplasty is feasible and beneficial in patients with ST-elevation MI. However, time to reperfusion is a critical determinant of outcome in acute MI, and any hope of benefiting patients who have a perioperative acute MI due to an acute coronary occlusion requires that revascularization be rapidly performed (i.e., within 12 hours of symptom onset). Since fibrinolytics are usually contraindicated in this circumstance, and dual antiplatelet therapy may not be ideal either, balloon angioplasty without stenting is often the best strategy.

Although immediate reperfusion therapy is an important therapy in acute ST-segment-elevation MI, the emphasis on reperfusion therapy should not detract from pharmacological therapy, which is also very important and has been shown to reduce adverse events in such patients, as well as in patients with non-ST-elevation acute coronary syndromes. Therapy with aspirin, a beta blocker, and often an angiotensin-converting enzyme inhibitor, particularly for patients with low ejection fractions or anterior infarctions, should be administered where possible. Patients who sustain acute myocardial injury in the perioperative or postoperative period should receive careful medical evaluation for residual ischemia and overall LV function. In all cases, the appropriate evaluation and management of complications and coronary risk factors such as angina, heart failure, hypertension, hyperlipidemia, cigarette smoking, diabetes (hyperglycemia), and other cardiac abnormalities should commence before hospital discharge. Most post-MI patients should also receive a statin at discharge.

CONCLUSIONS

Appropriate preoperative evaluation and therapy may significantly improve periprocedural and long-term outcomes. Successful management of high-risk patients requires an integrated "team" approach between surgeons, anesthesiologists, cardiologists, and generalists. In general, indications for further cardiac testing and revascularization are the same as in the nonoperative setting. Beta-blocker therapy should be considered in appropriate patients at high risk for coronary events with the understanding that these agents have both benefits and risks. For many patients, evaluation prior to noncardiac surgery may be the first comprehensive assessment of their short-term and long-term cardiac risk and provides an opportunity to not only decrease their immediate periprocedural risk but also to improve their long-term outcomes with appropriate evidence based therapies. Early identification and appropriate management of post-operative complications is important and may prevent fatality.

REFERENCES

1. National Center for Health Statistics. *Vital statistics of the United States: 2003*. Washington, DC: NCHS U.S. Public Health Services; 2003, 2004.
2. Mangano DT. Perioperative cardiac morbidity. *Anesthesiology* 1990;72: 153–184.
3. Fleisher LA, Beckman JA, Brown KA, et al. ACC/AHA 2007 Guidelines on perioperative cardiovascular evaluation and care for noncardiac surgery: executive summary: a report of the American College of Cardiology/American Heart Association Task Force on Practice Guidelines (Writing Committee to Revise the 2002 Guidelines on Perioperative Cardiovascular Evaluation for Noncardiac Surgery): developed in collaboration with the American Society of Echocardiography, American Society of Nuclear Cardiology, Heart Rhythm Society, Society of Cardiovascular Anesthesiologists, Society for Cardiovascular Angiography and Interventions, Society for Vascular Medicine and Biology, and Society for Vascular Surgery. *Circulation* 2007;116:1971–1996.
4. Eagle KA, Berger PB, Calkins H, et al. ACC/AHA guideline update for perioperative cardiovascular evaluation for noncardiac surgery–executive summary: a report of the American College of Cardiology/American Heart Association Task Force on Practice Guidelines (Committee to Update the 1996 Guidelines on Perioperative Cardiovascular Evaluation for Noncardiac Surgery). *J Am Coll Cardiol* 2002;39:542–553.
5. Mukherjee D, Eagle KA. A common sense approach to perioperative evaluation. *Am Fam Physician* 2002;66:1824–1826.
6. Mukherjee D, Eagle KA. Cardiac risk in noncardiac surgery. *Minerva Cardioangiol* 2002;50:607–619.
7. Mukherjee D, Eagle KA. Perioperative cardiac assessment for noncardiac surgery: eight steps to the best possible outcome. *Circulation* 2003; 107:2771–2774.
8. Logeais Y, Langanay T, Roussin R, et al. Surgery for aortic stenosis in elderly patients. A study of surgical risk and predictive factors. *Circulation* 1994;90:2891–2898.
9. Raymer K, Yang H. Patients with aortic stenosis: cardiac complications in non-cardiac surgery. *Can J Anaesth* 1998;45(9):855–859.
10. Torsher LC, Shub C, Rettke SR, et al. Risk of patients with severe aortic stenosis undergoing noncardiac surgery. *Am J Cardiol* 1998;81(4): 448–452.
11. DePuey EG, Guertler-Krawczynska E, Robbins WL. Thallium-201 SPECT in coronary artery disease patients with left bundle branch block. *Q J Nucl Med* 1988;29(9):1479–1485.
12. Larcos G, Gibbons RJ, Brown ML. Diagnostic accuracy of exercise thallium-201 single-photon emission computed tomography in patients with left bundle branch block. *Am J Cardiol* 1991;68(8):756–760.
13. Rockett JF, Wood WC, Moinuddin M, et al. Intravenous dipyridamole thallium-201 SPECT imaging in patients with left bundle branch block. *Clin Nucl Med* 1990;15(6):401–407.
14. O'Keefe JH Jr, Bateman TM, Barnhart CS. Adenosine thallium-201 is superior to exercise thallium-201 for detecting coronary artery disease in patients with left bundle branch block. *J Am Coll Cardiol* 1993;21(6): 1332–1338.
15. Hirzel HO, Senn M, Nuesch K, et al. Thallium-201 scintigraphy in complete left bundle branch block. *Am J Cardiol* 1984;53(6):764–769.
16. Ellis JE, Drijvers G, Pedlow S, et al. Premedication with oral and transdermal clonidine provides safe and efficacious postoperative sympatholysis. *Anesth Analg* 1994;79(6):1133–1140.
17. Shaw LJ, Eagle KA, Gersh BJ, et al. Meta-analysis of intravenous dipyridamole-thallium-201 imaging (1985 to 1994) and dobutamine echocardiography (1991 to 1994) for risk stratification before vascular surgery. *J Am Coll Cardiol* 1996;27(4):787–798.
18. Boucher CA, Brewster DC, Darling RC, et al. Determination of cardiac risk by dipyridamole-thallium imaging before peripheral vascular surgery. *N Engl J Med* 1985;312(7):389–394.
19. Leppo J, Plaja J, Gionet M, et al. Noninvasive evaluation of cardiac risk before elective vascular surgery. *J Am Coll Cardiol* 1987;9(2):269–276.
20. Poldermans D, Boersma E, Bax JJ, et al. The effect of bisoprolol on perioperative mortality and myocardial infarction in high-risk patients undergoing vascular surgery. Dutch Echocardiographic Cardiac Risk Evaluation Applying Stress Echocardiography Study Group. *N Engl J Med* 1999;341(24):1789–1794.
21. Eagle KA, Coley CM, Newell JB, et al. Combining clinical and thallium data optimizes preoperative assessment of cardiac risk before major vascular surgery. *Ann Intern Med* 1989;110(11):859–866.
22. L'Italien GJ, Paul SD, Hendel RC, et al. Development and validation of a Bayesian model for perioperative cardiac risk assessment in a cohort of 1,081 vascular surgical candidates. *J Am Coll Cardiol* 1996;27(4):779–786.
23. Pasternack PF, Grossi EA, Baumann FG, et al. Beta blockade to decrease silent myocardial ischemia during peripheral vascular surgery. *Am J Surg* 1989;158(2):113–116.
24. Mangano DT, Layug EL, Wallace A, et al. Effect of atenolol on mortality and cardiovascular morbidity after noncardiac surgery. Multicenter Study of Perioperative Ischemia Research Group. *N Engl J Med* 1996; 335(23):1713–1720.
25. Wallace A, Layug B, Tateo I, et al. Prophylactic atenolol reduces postoperative myocardial ischemia. McSPI Research Group. *Anesthesiology* 1998;88(1):7–17.
26. Urban MK, Markowitz SM, Gordon MA, et al. Postoperative prophylactic administration of beta-adrenergic blockers in patients at risk for myocardial ischemia. *Anesth Analg* 2000;90(6):1257–1261.
27. Devereaux PJ, Yang H, Yusuf S, et al. Effects of extended-release metoprolol succinate in patients undergoing non-cardiac surgery (POISE trial): a randomised controlled trial. *Lancet* 2008;371(9627):1839–1847.

28. Stuhmeier KD, Mainzer B, Cierpka J, et al. Small, oral dose of clonidine reduces the incidence of intraoperative myocardial ischemia in patients having vascular surgery. *Anesthesiology* 1996;85(4):706–712.
29. Oliver MF, Goldman L, Julian DG, et al. Effect of mivazerol on perioperative cardiac complications during non-cardiac surgery in patients with coronary heart disease: the European Mivazerol Trial (EMIT). *Anesthesiology* 1999;91(4):951–961.
30. Poldermans D, Bax JJ, Kertai MD, et al. Statins are associated with a reduced incidence of perioperative mortality in patients undergoing major noncardiac vascular surgery. *Circulation* 2003;107(14):1848–1851.
31. Hindler K, Shaw AD, Samuels J, et al. Improved postoperative outcomes associated with preoperative statin therapy. *Anesthesiology* 2006;105(6):1260–1272 and 1289–1290.
32. Le Manach Y, Godet G, Coriat P, et al. The impact of postoperative discontinuation or continuation of chronic statin therapy on cardiac outcome after major vascular surgery. *Anesth Analg* 2007;104(6): 1326–1333.
33. Allen JR, Helling TS, Hartzler GO. Operative procedures not involving the heart after percutaneous transluminal coronary angioplasty. *Surg Gynecol Obstet* 1991;173(4):285–288.
34. Elmore JR, Hallett JW Jr, Gibbons RJ, et al. Myocardial revascularization before abdominal aortic aneurysmorrhaphy: effect of coronary angioplasty. *Mayo Clin Proc* 1993;68(7):637–641.
35. Gottlieb A, Banoub M, Sprung J, et al. Perioperative cardiovascular morbidity in patients with coronary artery disease undergoing vascular surgery after percutaneous transluminal coronary angioplasty. *J Cardiothorac Vasc Anesth* 1998;12(5):501–506.
36. Posner KL, Van Norman GA, Chan V. Adverse cardiac outcomes after noncardiac surgery in patients with prior percutaneous transluminal coronary angioplasty. *Anesth Analg* 1999;89(3):553–560.
37. McFalls EO, Ward HB, Moritz TE, et al. Coronary-artery revascularization before elective major vascular surgery. *N Engl J Med* 2004;351(27): 2795–2804.
38. Kaluza GL, Joseph J, Lee JR, et al. Catastrophic outcomes of noncardiac surgery soon after coronary stenting. *J Am Coll Cardiol* 2000;35(5): 1288–1294.
39. Wilson SH, Fasseas P, Orford JL, et al. Clinical outcome of patients undergoing non-cardiac surgery in the two months following coronary stenting. *J Am Coll Cardiol* 2003;42(2):234–240.
40. Eagle KA, Rihal CS, Mickel MC, et al. Cardiac risk of noncardiac surgery: influence of coronary disease and type of surgery in 3368 operations. CASS Investigators and University of Michigan Heart Care Program. Coronary Artery Surgery Study. *Circulation* 1997;96(6):1882–1887.
41. Fleisher LA, Eagle KA, Shaffer T, et al. Perioperative and long-term mortality rates after major vascular surgery: the relationship to preoperative testing in the medicare population. *Anesth Analg* 1999;89(4):849–855.
42. Hassan SA, Hlatky MA, Boothroyd DB, et al. Outcomes of noncardiac surgery after coronary bypass surgery or coronary angioplasty in the Bypass Angioplasty Revascularization Investigation (BARI). *Am J Med* 2001;110(4):260–266.
43. Poldermans D, Schouten O, Vidakovic R, et al. A clinical randomized trial to evaluate the safety of a noninvasive approach in high-risk patients undergoing major vascular surgery: the DECREASE-V Pilot Study. *J Am Coll Cardiol* 2007;49(17):1763–1769.

CHAPTER

11

Assessment of Noncardiac Perioperative Risk

Pauline K. Park

INTRODUCTION

Determination of perioperative risk is a critical step in preventing complications in surgery. Surgical patients often present with multisystem disease separate from the process requiring operation; the surgeon must weigh not only the risk attributable to the surgical procedure, but also the additional contributions of underlying medical comorbidities. Variations in preoperative status have been associated with operative outcomes (1), hospital length of stay (2), and hospital costs (3).

Risk assessment in general surgery has advanced greatly over the past two decades. The most comprehensive effort to date has been the National Surgical Quality Improvement Program (NSQIP) (1). Since 1991, the Department of Veterans Affairs (VA) has systematically collected and analyzed risk-adjusted surgical data in VA hospitals. Trained nurse reviewers at each VA site regularly abstract demographic information, baseline physiologic status, medical comorbidity, laboratory values, and operative characteristics in surgical patients. By measuring and analyzing patient level data, the VA has been able to implement changes based on observed hospital variations in outcome. The program is credited with increasing patient satisfaction and reducing complications, 30-day mortality and hospital length of stay in a broad range of surgical patients (4).

The NSQIP provides an important, validated tool for risk assessment. The program has been adopted by the American College of Surgeons (ACS-NSQIP) and this initiative supplements initial NSQIP data derived from the primarily older, male population seen in the VA system. Data collection was successfully mirrored in the private-sector hospital environment in a validation cohort of 14 academic medical centers (5). The most predictive preoperative risk factors for mortality and morbidity in private sector, noncardiac surgery patients are summarized in Tables 11.1 and 11.2. Similar to the VA experience, implementation of the ACS-NSQIP demonstrated reductions in postoperative morbidity, surgical site infections, renal complications, and 30-day postoperative morbidity (5).

The majority of preoperative risk variables identified by NSQIP and ACS-NSQIP relate to underlying systemic disease and acuity of presenting illness. The impact of "optimizing" any of these single parameters is not known and some of the variables, such as age, are fixed. Recent evaluation of the ACS-NSQIP database found that while rates of individual complications did not vary significantly among hospitals with differing mortality rates, mortality in patients with major complications was almost twice as high in hospitals with very high overall mortality as in those with very low overall mortality (21.4% vs. 12.5%, $P<0.001$)(6). This suggests that the quality of perioperative care provided once complications occur may be as important as the efforts to prevent them. Nevertheless, the ability to systematically identify patients at higher risk, analyze variations in practice, and reliably change hospital level process has resulted in improvement in overall outcomes.

Risk assessment aids the surgeon in appropriately advising patient expectations and in developing strategies to potentially reduce postoperative complications (7). As the occurrence of postoperative complications remains one of the strongest predictors of long term outcomes after major surgery (8,9), the time spent evaluating and optimizing the patient preoperative status can directly facilitate the best outcomes.

ELECTIVE SURGERY

Preoperative evaluation for elective surgery is most commonly performed in the outpatient setting. Centralized centers facilitate registration, anesthesia evaluation, and preoperative teaching, resulting in decreased costs as well as improved laboratory utilization and rates of cancellation on the date of surgery (10–12). Patient education is critical in ensuring that patients understand expectations of care to be delivered. Performing this in the preoperative setting not only ensures cooperation with postoperative interventions but also improves patient satisfaction (13). Ideally, appointments should be scheduled well ahead of the actual date of surgery, to allow for complete assessment and to allow patients time to assimilate the information and instructions given to them.

A standard medical history is performed to identify medication allergies, current medications (including prescription, over-the-counter, and alternative medications), prior or familial disorders with anesthetics, prior history of bleeding disorder and prior medical history. A complete physical examination is performed to identify other concurrent findings separate from the planned surgical procedure, determine nutritional status, and ascertain the

Pauline K. Park: University of Michigan, Ann Arbor, MI 48109

Table 11.1 Logistic regression models for prediction of 30-day operative mortality using preoperative variables

Variable	Odds Ratio
ASA class 4/5 vs. 1/2	8.1
ASA 3 vs. 1/2	3.5
Serum albumin (per gram)	0.62
Emergency operation	2.6
Age (per year)	1
Platelet count <150,000	1.9
Disseminated cancer	2.9
Dyspnea at rest vs. none	1.6
Dyspnea with minimal exertion vs. none	1.3
DNR	3.9
BUN >40 mg/dL	1.3
Work RVU (per unit)	1.02

Derived from private sector hospitals, $n = 54{,}450$ patients.
ASA, American Society of Anesthesiologist's Patient Severity Score; BUN, blood urea nitrogen; DNR, do not resuscitate; RVU, relative value unit; COPD, chronic obstructive pulmonary disease; WBC, white blood cell count k/cmm.
From Khuri SF, Henderson WG, Daley J, et al. Successful implementation of the Department of Veterans Affairs' National Surgical Quality Improvement Program in the private sector: the Patient Safety in Surgery study. *Ann Surg* 2008;248(2):329–336.

Table 11.2 Logistic regression models for prediction of 30-day operative morbidity using preoperative variables

Variable	Odds Ratio
ASA 4/5 vs. 1/2	2.1
ASA 3 vs. 1/2	1.6
Albumin (per gram)	0.73
Work RVU (per unit)	1.05
Emergency operation	1.7
Dyspnea at rest vs. none	1.7
Dyspnea with minimal exertion vs. none	1.2
Wound infection	1.6
Patient on ventilator prior to surgery	1.9
Bleeding disorder	1.5
WBC > 11,000/mL^3	1.2
Age (per year)	1.01

Derived from private sector hospitals, $n = 54{,}450$ patients.
ASA, American Society of Anesthesiologist's Patient Severity Score; BUN, blood urea nitrogen; DNR, do not resuscitate; RVU, relative value unit; COPD, chronic obstructive pulmonary disease; WBC, white blood cell count k/cmm.
From Khuri SF, Henderson WG, Daley J, et al. Successful implementation of the Department of Veterans Affairs' National Surgical Quality Improvement Program in the private sector: the Patient Safety in Surgery study. *Ann Surg* 2008;248(2):329–336.

presence of acute infection. Formal evaluation by anesthesiology is performed for suitability for regional and general anesthesia (see Chapter 12).

A significant number of patients take prescription medications which require individual management perioperatively (14). The majority can be administered until the day of surgery, but certain medications should be discontinued prior to surgery, with consideration given to risk of continuation versus the risk of intra-operative complications (Table 11.3).

Herbal medications and supplements are increasingly popular (15). Specific inquiry as to their use should be included in the preoperative history, as the patient may not

Table 11.3 Common prescription medications that may require special perioperative management

Steroids	May require perioperative stress dose steroids
Metformin	Risk of lactic acidosis, withhold at least 2 days prior to surgery
Insulin	Adjust dose prior to surgery
Anticoagulants	May require bridge therapy with unfractionated or LMW heparin
Aspirin, thienopyridines (clopidogrel, Ticlid) or dipyridamole (Persantine)	Withhold seven days prior to surgery with increased bleeding risk
NSAIDs	Withhold prior to surgery with risk of renal complications
Angiotensin converting enzyme inhibitors, angiotensin receptor blockers	Renal risk
Potassium sparing diuretics	Renal risk, potential for hyperkalemia
Lithium	Potential prolongation of neuromuscular blockade, sedative action, cardiac arrhythmia, withhold at least 1 day prior to surgery
Monoamine oxidase inhibitors	Anesthetic interactions
Butyrophenone	Pain management
Oral contraceptives, conjugated estrogen	Increase hypercoagulable state, consider holding 4 weeks prior to surgery, DVT prophylaxis

LMW, low molecular weight; NSAIDs, nonsteroidal anti-inflammatory drugs; DVT, deep venous thrombosis.

Table 11.4 Potential interactions for some common herbal medicines

Common Name of Herb	Potential Interactions	Preoperative Recommendations
Echinacea	Allergic reactions; decreased effectiveness of immunosuppressants; potential for immunosuppression with long-term use, potential hepatotoxicity	No data
Ephedra	Risk for myocardial ischemia and stroke from tachycardia and hypertension; ventricular arrhythmias with halothane; long-term use depletes endogenous catecholamines and may cause intra-operative hemodynamic instability; life-threatening interaction with monoamine oxidase inhibitors	Discontinue at least 24 hr before surgery
Dong Quai Vitamin E Evening Primrose Oil Fish Oil Feverfew Garlic Ginkgo Ginger Ginseng Guarana Goldenseal	Potential to increase risk for bleeding, especially when combined with other medications that inhibit platelet aggregation	Consider discontinuation 7 days before surgery (36 hours for ginkgo)
Ginseng	Hypoglycemia; potential to increase risk for bleeding; potential to decrease anticoagulative effect of warfarin	Discontinue at least 7 days before surgery
Kava	Potential to increase sedative effect of anesthetics; potential for addiction, tolerance, and withdrawal after abstinence unstudied	Discontinue at least 24 hr before surgery
St. John's wort	Induction of cytochrome P-450 enzymes, with effect on cyclosporine, warfarin, steroids, protease inhibitors, and possibly benzodiazepines, calcium channel blockers, and many other drugs; decreased serum digoxin levels	Discontinue at least 5 days before surgery
Valerian	Potential to increase sedative effect of anesthetics; benzodiazepine-like acute withdrawal; potential to increase anesthetic requirements with long-term use	No data

Adapted from Ang-Lee MK, Moss J, Yuan CS. Herbal medicines and perioperative care. *JAMA* 2001;286(2):208–216 and Halaszynski TM, Juda R, Silverman DG. Optimizing postoperative outcomes with efficient preoperative assessment and management. *Crit Care Med* 2004;32(4, Suppl):S76–S86.

consider these to be "medications" or they may be reluctant to report using nontraditional therapy (16). The quality of preparations, content of actual ingredients, and consistency are not always known and an exact mechanism of action cannot always be cited. Nevertheless, multiple drug-herbal preparation interactions have been reported, including effects on platelet aggregation, p450 cytochrome function, and drug metabolism (15) (Table 11.4)

The added value and cost-effectiveness of routine preoperative laboratory and chest x-ray testing has been disputed and the practice has been largely discounted (10,17). Evidence suggests that results are often normal, and even when abnormal, they do not alter the course of treatment (18,19). Recommendations for preoperative testing should be based on patient history and physiologic status and performed selectively (20) (Table 11.5).

Prophylaxis for surgical site infection and venous thromboembolism should also be ordered appropriately. The Surgical Care Improvement Project (SCIP) is a national quality partnership committed to improving safety of surgical care by significantly reducing surgical complications. The national goal of the organization is to reduce preventable surgical complications by 25% by 2010 (21). Practice recommendations are focused on four areas: surgical site infection, venous thromboembolism prophylaxis, cardiac surgery, and ventilator associated pneumonia. SCIP core datasets have broad administrative support. Hospital data submission and analysis is currently required for Joint Commission accreditation, national and state regulatory compliance as well as insurance plan initiatives. Process and outcome measures in infection and venous thromboembolism prophylaxis are depicted in Table 11.6.

EMERGENCY SURGERY

Emergency procedures are often performed in acute situations with limited opportunities to optimize preoperative status. The need for emergent intervention has been

Table **11.5** **Suggestions for adult preoperative testing**

	BASIC MINOR SURG. IN HEALTHY PATIENT (w/in 90 days)				ADDITIVE SURGICAL AND MEDICAL FACTORS: SURGICAL PROCEDURES (within 90 days)								ADDITIVE SURGICAL AND MEDICAL FACTORS: CLINICALLY SIGNIFICANT AND CHANGING DISORDERS AND/OR MEDICATIONS (white = w/in 90 days; grey = given test for given disorder likely should be w/in 30 days)																					
TEST	**Healthy Adult <45**	**45-54 y/o**	**55-69 y/o**	**≥ 70 y/o**	**Cardiac/Thoracic**	**Vascular**	**Maj. Intraperit/abd**	**Antic > 2u EBL**	**Intracranial**	**Ortho Prothesis**	**TURP, Hysteros**		**Hypertension**	**Smoking**	**Morbid Obesity**	**h/o Stoke**	**Cancer (?metastatic)**	**Seizure Meds**	**Cardiovascular**	**Respiratory**	**Diabetes**	**Hepatic**	**Renal**	**Fluid or Lyte Loss**	**Autoimmune/Lupus**	**EtoH/DrugAbuse**	**Steroids/Cushings**	**HIV**	**Parathyroid**	**Unstable Thyroid**	**Anticoag/Bleeding**	**Suspected Pregnan.**		
ECG		M	Y	Y	Y	Y	Y	Y	Y				Y	Y	Y	Y	Y		Y	Y	Y	Y	Y	±	Y	Y	Y	Y	Y	Y				
CBC+ platelets			Y	Y	Y	Y	Y	Y	Y	Y	Y				Y	Y	Y	Y	Y	Y	Y	Y	Y	Y	Y	Y	Y	Y	Y	Y	Y			
Lytes				Y	Y	Y	Y	Y	Y	Y	Y		Y		Y	Y	Y		Y	Y	Y	Y	Y	Y	Y	Y	Y	Y	Y	Y				
BUN/Creat				Y	Y	Y	Y	Y	Y	Y	Y		Y			Y	Y		Y	Y	Y	Y	Y		Y	Y	Y	Y	Y	Y				
Glucose				Y	Y	Y	Y	Y	Y	Y	Y				Y	Y	Y		Y		Y	Y	Y			Y	Y	Y	Y	Y				
LFTs							±										Y	Y				Y				Y		Y						
Calcium																													Y					
PT/PTT					Y			Y	Y													Y	Y		Y	Y					Y			
U/A (?culture)										S																								
CXR					Y												S			Y								S						
Hormone Level																														Y				
Bleed Time									S																						±			
Pregnancy																																Y		
Drug Levels									S									S								±								
Tumor Markers																	S																	
Clot	Depends primarily on extensiveness of proposed surgery, as per Blood Bank MSBOS guidelines																																	

Legend: Y = usually indicated; **M** = usually indicated for male; **S** = may be requested (and reviewed) by surgeon as part of surgical w/u; ± = if situation acute/severe.
From Halaszynski TM, Juda R, Silverman DG. Optimizing postoperative outcomes with efficient preoperative assessment and management. *Crit Care Med* 2004;32(4, Suppl): S76–S86.

Table **11.6** **Surgical Care Improvement Project (SCIP) process and outcome measures: infection and venous thromboembolism prophylaxis**

	Guideline
SCIP INF 1	Prophylactic antibiotic received within 1 hour before surgical incision
SCIP INF 2	Prophylactic antibiotic selection for surgical patients
SCIP INF 3	Prophylactic antibiotics discontinued within 24 hours after surgery completion time (48 hours for cardiac patients)
SCIP INF 4	Cardiac surgery patients with controlled 6 AM postoperative serum glucose
SCIP INF 5	Postoperative wound infection diagnosed during index hospitalization (outcome)
SCIP INF 6	Surgery patients with appropriate hair removal
SCIP INF 7	Colorectal surgery patients with immediate postoperative normothermia
SCIP VTE 1	Surgery patients with recommended venous thromboembolism prophylaxis ordered
SCIP VTE 2	Surgery patients who received appropriate venous thromboembolism prophylaxis within 24 hours prior to surgery to 24 hours after surgery

repeatedly demonstrated to confer additional risk of morbidity and mortality (1,8). In addition to baseline medical status, additional physiologic derangements must be evaluated and treated, including the presence of shock, altered volume status, electrolyte abnormalities, and anemia. Prompt resuscitation, stabilization, and infectious source control comprise the basis of treatment. In the presence of acute infection, appropriate antibiotics should be given as soon as is feasible.

In some cases, the risk of delaying surgery for further medical stabilization is higher than any potential gains. The natural history of the disease and timing of surgical intervention must be considered. In an analysis of small bowel obstruction, morbidity increased in patients requiring small bowel resection in addition to adhesiolysis, suggesting that timing of intervention potentially impacted care (22). In management of acute appendicitis, improved outcomes were achieved by facilitating time to definitive surgery (23).

SPECIFIC ORGAN SYSTEMS

Robust literature exists regarding preoperative cardiac and airway evaluation, and these are addressed in individual chapters in the text. The majority of evidence in other areas is less well developed, although the body of supporting literature is increasing. In many cases, data regarding risk of specific disease entities is accrued from organ-specific surgery and extrapolated to more general situations. A generally accepted principle is that medical management of acute single-system compromise prior to and during the perioperative period should improve the patient's overall condition and lower operative risk. The following sections review specific recommendations for pulmonary, renal, and hepatic risk assessment and management.

Pulmonary

Postoperative pulmonary complications are among the most frequent and costly postsurgical events. In noncardiac surgery, pulmonary complications occur with similar prevalence, and lead to similar increases in morbidity, mortality, and length of stay as cardiac complications (24). In addition, the occurrence of pulmonary complications may be more likely to predict long term mortality after surgery in elderly patients (9).

In order to address the relative lack of structured recommendations for preoperative pulmonary evaluation, the American College of Physicians issued a summary guideline in 2006 (25). Certain patient-related characteristics, operative factors, and a low serum albumin were identified as risk factors for postoperative pulmonary complications. NSQIP additionally identified elevated blood urea nitrogen (BUN) as a risk factor for postoperative pulmonary complications (26) and dyspnea at rest or low levels of activity as risk factors for increased morbidity and mortality (Table 11.7).

Table 11.7 Risk assessment for pulmonary complications in noncardiothoracic surgery

Patient Related Factors
Age >60
ASA class II, or greater
Chronic obstructive pulmonary disease
Functional dependence
Congestive heart failure
Dyspnea at rest or minimal exertion
Operative Factors
Prolonged surgery (>3 hours)
Abdominal surgery
Thoracic surgery
Neurosurgery
Head and neck surgery
Vascular surgery
Emergency surgery
Use of general anesthesia
Laboratory Values
Serum albumin <3.5
BUN >40

Modified from Khuri SF, Henderson WG, Daley J, et al. Successful implementation of the Department of Veterans Affairs' National Surgical Quality Improvement Program in the private sector: the Patient Safety in Surgery study. *Ann Surg* 2008;248(2):329–336 and Qaseem A, Snow V, Fitterman N, et al. Risk assessment for and strategies to reduce perioperative pulmonary complications for patients undergoing noncardiothoracic surgery: a guideline from the American College of Physicians. *Ann Intern Med* 2006;144(8):575–580.

Patient-Related Risk Factors

Chronic lung disease is the most commonly identified risk factor for postoperative pulmonary complications. Chronic lung disease is common, occurs in all ages and may be asymptomatic. A history of pulmonary symptoms including chronic cough, exercise intolerance, dyspnea, change in sputum production or prior pulmonary complications, cigarette smoking, recurrent pneumonia, chronic obstructive lung disease, reactive airway disease, systemic disease with potential pulmonary involvement, occupational exposures, or prior lung surgery should be assessed further. Physical examination findings may include abnormal auscultation, anatomic abnormalities such as morbid obesity, scoliosis, or chest wall deformities, and signs of chronic hypoxia and accessory muscle respiration.

ASA Classification. The American Society of Anesthesiologists (ASA) classification is a measure of comorbidity aimed at predicting perioperative mortality rates, but has also demonstrated strong correlation with postoperative pulmonary complication. Substantial increases in pulmonary complication risk occurred with increasing ASA class greater than II.

Age. Age-related decreases in pulmonary function are associated with increased postoperative complications. Increasing age is an independent risk factor for postoperative complications, even after adjustment for comorbid conditions (25). Patients aged 60 to 69 were twice as likely and patients aged 70 to 79 were three times as likely to develop postoperative pulmonary complications when compared to younger patients less than 60 years old. Nevertheless, age alone should not be considered a contraindication to surgery in otherwise healthy patients.

Congestive Heart Failure. Congestive heart failure has been identified as an important predictor for postoperative pulmonary complications, with odds ratio of 2.93 (25).

Functional Dependence. Total or partial dependence on others for performing activities of daily living is a significant risk factor for the development of postoperative pulmonary complications.

Restrictive Chest Wall Disease. Specific studies to evaluate the impact of restrictive chest wall disease, neuromuscular disorders, or pulmonary vascular disease are insufficient to draw conclusions. These patients may have an impaired ventilatory reserve as a result of weak muscles or abnormal mechanics of ventilation and many physicians will consider these to impart additional risk.

Obesity and Obstructive Sleep Apnea. Obesity was not identified as carrying specific increased risk for pulmonary complications, but may be associated with obstructive sleep apnea, postoperative atelectasis, and delayed mobilization. An ASA task force observed that the prevalence of sleep disordered breathing was 9% in women and 24% in men and concluded that perioperative risk increases in proportion to the severity of sleep apnea (27). The literature is insufficient to draw conclusions on its impact on specific complications; however, patients with obstructive sleep apnea may have associated difficult airway management and preoperative status may be improved with the application of continuous positive airway pressure (CPAP), noninvasive positive pressure ventilation, mandibular advancement devices, oral appliances, and preoperative weight loss. Intraoperative sedative administration should be carefully monitored and neuromuscular blockade fully reversed prior to extubation.

Reactive Airway Disease. Asthma was not confirmed to be an independent risk factor for postoperative pulmonary complications. Nevertheless, poorly controlled asthmatics are at increased risk for pulmonary complications, and risk may be reduced by preoperative management aimed at eliminating wheezing and targeting peak expiratory flows >80% of predicted or the patient's personal best (28). Stepwise guidance for management based on severity of asthma has been published by the National Asthma Education and Prevention Program (NAEPP).

Operative Factors

Risk assessment in elective surgery can be modified by adjusting operative variables: site, duration, and choice of anesthesia. Emergency procedures significantly increase odds of pulmonary complications.

Surgical Site. The site of surgery influences risk for postoperative pulmonary complications. Aortic aneurysm, thoracic surgery, abdominal surgery, upper abdominal surgery, neurosurgery, prolonged surgery, head and neck surgery, vascular surgery, and emergency surgery have been identified as procedures carrying additional risk of pulmonary complications. Thoracotomy and upper abdominal surgery are associated with the most marked changes in functional residual capacity after surgery.

Risk factors for postoperative complications after laparotomy include ASA class > II, upper abdominal procedures, residual intraperitoneal sepsis, age greater than 59 years, body mass index (BMI) higher than 25 kg/m^2, preoperative stay for longer than 4 days, and colorectal or gastroduodenal surgery (29).

Minimally invasive approaches have demonstrated reductions in operative pain and musculoskeletal dysfunction but do not clearly lead to reduction in pulmonary complications. Physiologic alterations due to anesthesia, intraperitoneal CO_2 insufflation, and underlying disease process may reduce the potential impact of these approaches and further studies are needed (30).

Planned Thoracic Surgery. The American College of Chest Physicians (ACCP) recently updated recommendations for evaluation of patients with lung cancer being considered for resection (31) (Fig. 11.1). Initial pulmonary function testing should be performed with the patient on optimal bronchodilator therapy. Findings of significant reduction in Forced Expiratory Volume in 1 second (FEV_1) (<80%) or values below thresholds for safe resection (2.0 L for pneumonectomy, 1.5 L for lobectomy) or a history suggesting dyspnea on minimal exertion or chest radiograph demonstrating diffuse parenchymal abnormalities should direct additional pulmonary function testing. Further risk stratification is based on measurement of the diffusing capacity of the lung for carbon dioxide ($DLCO_2$), estimation of cardiopulmonary exercise tolerance, and calculation of the postoperative expected FEV_1 and $DLCO_2$ (see Fig. 11.1). Concurrent epidural anesthesia in conjunction with general anesthesia has been utilized to blunt intra-operative shunting and preemptively address postoperative pain (32).

Duration of Surgery. The duration of surgery, defined as greater than 3 to 4 hours is an independent predictor of postoperative pulmonary complications (25).

General Anesthesia. General anesthesia may decrease the functional residual capacity (FRC) for up to 1 to 2 weeks postoperatively. Endotracheal intubation, inhalational anesthetic, and neuromuscular blockade may contribute to pulmonary dysfunction. A meta-analysis of 141 randomized controlled trials of general anesthesia suggested that the incidence of pneumonia and respiratory failure decreased with the use of spinal or regional anesthesia (33). It has been proposed but not proven that the use of shorter acting neuromuscular blocking agents may further reduce risk from general anesthesia (30).

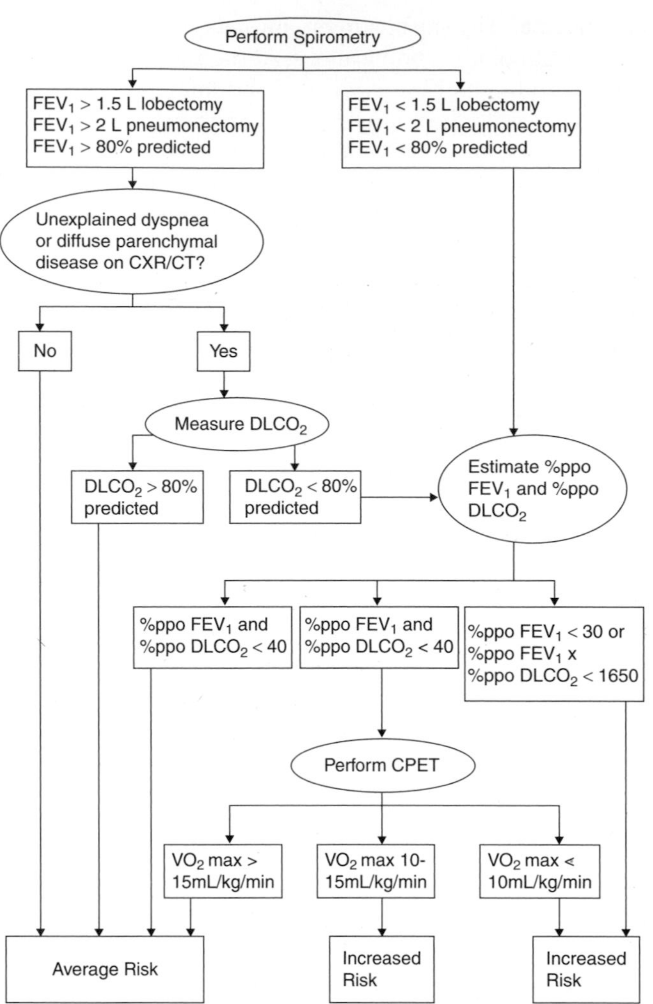

FIGURE 11.1. Preoperative evaluation of patients with lung cancer prior to resection (Adapted from Colice GL, Shafazand S, Griffin JP, et al. Physiologic evaluation of the patient with lung cancer being considered for resectional surgery: ACCP evidenced-based clinical practice guidelines (2nd edition). *Chest* 2007;132(3, Suppl):161S–177S.) FEV_1 = Forced Expiratory Volume in 1 second; CXR = Chest X-Ray; CT = Computed Tomography; $DLCO_2$ = Diffusing capacity of the lung for carbon dioxide; %ppo = percent of predicted postoperative; CPET = Cardiopulmonary exercise testing; $\dot{V}O_2max$ = Maximal oxygen consumption.

Preoperative Testing

The utility of preoperative pulmonary function tests, arterial blood gas analysis, and routine chest radiography in preventing postoperative complications is debatable. Routine preoperative spirometry is not recommended in extrathoracic surgery. In patients with planned thoracic procedures, with or without pulmonary resection, acute symptoms, or chronic lung disease, these should be considered as adjuncts to the evaluation.

Perioperative Interventions

Lung expansion modalities have been extensively studied and are the only maneuvers demonstrated to reduce pulmonary risk (29). Incentive spirometry and deep-breathing exercises are inspiratory maneuvers to recruit alveoli and counteract the postoperative reduction in FRC. CPAP has been demonstrated to improve postoperative pulmonary outcomes (34). A few controlled studies in elective surgical patients have demonstrated that reduction in pulmonary complications is obtained when high-risk patients are identified and interventions are initiated preoperatively (35,36). Concentrated efforts during preoperative sessions may result in increased patient compliance.

Cigarette smoking is directly toxic to respiratory ciliary epithelium and impairs normal intratracheal mucus transport. In addition, impaired wound healing and vasospasm increase postoperative local complications. Despite evidence in the cardiothoracic surgery population, surprisingly little evidence is available in the noncardiac population. Conflicting evidence exists regarding timing of discontinuation of smoking prior to surgery based on reports of increased airway reactivity following cessation (37,38). A general recommendation is that smoking should be stopped at least 6 to 8 weeks preceding elective surgery.

General management to improve preoperative pulmonary status includes the use of short-acting aerosolized beta2-agonists, leukotriene inhibitors, steroids, and bronchodilators when necessary to improve pulmonary function. Patients with acute bronchitis, increased secretions, or change in character of sputum production should be treated with a course of antibiotics and elective surgery delayed until symptom resolution.

Measures aimed at avoiding limited mobilization secondary to pain include use of minimally invasive videoscopic procedures and the use of thoracic epidural anesthesia, particularly in patients with associated chronic obstructive pulmonary disease (COPD) (39). Postural drainage and chest physiotherapy are useful in mobilizing secretions but should be reserved for patients with lobar collapse or high sputum production, as they may exacerbate bronchospasm.

Renal

Chronic renal disease commonly reflects end organ damage from systemic conditions such as hypertension, diabetes mellitus, and atherosclerosis, and, once established, is associated with accelerated development of cardiovascular disease (40). The overall condition of the patient is related to the extent of renal impairment as well as the presence of the underlying disease. Renal function is directly related to the glomerular filtration rate (GFR), traditionally estimated by the Cockcroft-Gault equation (Fig. 11.2) (41). Electrolyte homeostasis, volume status, anemia, and medication excretion may be significantly altered when GFR approaches <30% of baseline.

Preoperative Assessment

Acute interventions such as surgery may worsen already compromised renal function. Preexisting chronic kidney disease is a strong risk factor for the development of postoperative acute kidney injury (AKI) (42), which is in turn strongly associated with increased mortality (43–45). Preoperative renal risk assessment centers on detection of unsuspected underlying renal failure and institution of measures to minimize further renal insult.

The prevalence of chronic kidney disease in the adult population is estimated at 13% (46) and the incidence of postoperative renal failure in a noncardiac general surgical population may be as high as 1% (44). Analysis of a large

Cockcroft and Gault estimation of creatinine clearance
CrCl = (140 − age) × IBW/(Cr × 72)   (× 0.85 for females)
CrCl = creatinine clearance; IBW = ideal body weight, kg; Cr = serum creatinine
IBW: Males = 50 kg + 2.3 kg for each inch over 5 feet. Females = 45.5 kg + 2.3 kg for each inch over 5 feet.

FIGURE 11.2. Cockcroft and Gault equation estimating creatinine clearance (mL/min) (40).

operative dataset identified risk factors for the development of AKI in noncardiac surgical patients (Table 11.8). Based on this, the authors developed an AKI scoring system which correlated the occurrence of AKI in stepwise fashion with increasing scores (Table 11.9).

Comparison of studies of postoperative renal failure have been hampered by historical lack of a consistent definition and the limitations of serum creatinine in detecting acute injury. In 2004, the Acute Dialysis Quality Initiative group developed a consensus definition of acute renal failure, referred to as the RIFLE (Risk, Injury, Failure, Loss, End-Stage) criteria (47) (Table 11.10). These criteria have been utilized in the critical care setting and are being validated in evaluation of cardiac, general, and vascular surgical outcomes (45,48). A single episode of AKI as defined by RIFLE criteria has been found to be associated with long-term mortality in proportion to severity of the insult. Even small changes in creatinine are associated with increased long-term risk of death, even though renal function is observed to have returned to normal at the time of discharge in the vast majority of patients (45).

Perioperative Interventions

Strategies for prevention of postoperative renal failure are aimed at avoidance of intra-operative hypotension and maintenance of adequate renal perfusion. Specific nephrotoxic medications such as nonsteroidal anti-inflammatory drugs (NSAIDS), aminoglycosides, ace-inhibitors, and intravenous contrast dye should be avoided. Abdominal compartment syndrome associated with prerenal oliguria that fails to respond to medical management requires treatment with decompressive laparotomy (49).

To date, no pharmacologic intervention has successfully improved renal outcomes. Efforts to preserve urinary flow, including low dose dopamine and furosemide have been demonstrated to improve oliguria but not renal function (50). A large body of literature concerns attempts to minimize acute tubular damage from intravenous contrast dye. Preemptive sodium bicarbonate administration has been associated with reduced renal failure, but was not demonstrably superior to saline hydration alone (51). Results of prophylactic or therapeutic acetylcysteine administration are variable (52). Calcium channel blockers have been associated with renoprotection in transplant surgery (53), but have been associated with increased renal failure rates after cardiac surgery (54). Atrial natriuretic peptide (ANP) (55) and insulin-like growth factor (56) have demonstrated no improvement in renal failure rates. Fenoldopam (57,58) has shown some promise in cardiac surgery and further studies are awaited.

Perioperative management is aimed at stabilization of homeostatic imbalance, adjustment of medications, and prevention of postoperative renal failure. Careful evaluation for intravascular volume overload, electrolyte abnormalities, and anemia should be performed.

Hyperkalemia may exist preoperatively in up to 38% of patients with chronic renal failure (59). Administration of intravenous calcium is immediately indicated in the presence of acute EKG changes. Intracellular shift may be achieved with sodium bicarbonate or insulin and glucose; however, removal of excess potassium stores will require administration of exchange resins or acute dialysis.

Anemia is well tolerated in patients with chronic renal failure. Erythropoietin-stimulating agents are commonly utilized when the GFR is less than 60% and may be associated with increased thrombotic state. This is often offset by uremic coagulopathy related to platelet dysfunction. Desmopressin, conjugated estrogens, blood product transfusion, or dialysis may be utilized to minimize coagulopathy.

Altered metabolism and excretion in renal failure mandates adjustment of drug dosages. The elevated half-life of sedatives and muscle relaxants must be taken into consideration. Prolonged neuromuscular blockade may occur with agents that extend drug action at the neuromuscular junction. Succinylcholine administration leads to increases in serum potassium and is contraindicated in hyperkalemia. Atracurium undergoes peripheral Hoffman degradation and may be utilized preferentially in the face of renal dysfunction.

Table **11.8** General surgery acute kidney injury risk index

Risk Factor
Age ≥ 56 yr
Male sex
Active congestive heart failure
Ascites
Hypertension
Emergency surgery
Intraperitoneal surgery
Renal insufficiency–mild or moderate*
Diabetes mellitus–oral or insulin therapy

General Surgery Acute Kidney Injury Risk Index classes are based on the number of risk factors the patient possesses: class I (zero, one or two risk factors), class II (three risk factors), class III (four risk factors), class IV (five risk factors), and class V (six or more risk factors).
*Preoperative serum creatinine value > 1.2 mg/dl.
From Kheterpal S, Tremper KK, Heung M, et al. Development and validation of an acute kidney injury risk index for patients undergoing general surgery: results from a national data set. *Anesthesiology* 2009;110(3):505–515.

Table **11.9** General surgery acute kidney injury risk index classification system

Preoperative Risk Class	Derivation Cohort, N = 57,080			Validation Cohort, N = 18,872		
	Total Patients, n	Acute Kidney Injury Incidence, % (n)	Hazard Ratio (95% Confidence Interval)	Total Patients, n	Acute Kidney Injury Incidence, % (n)	Hazard Ratio (95% Confidence Interval)
Class I (0–2 risk factors)	31,500	0.2 (66)		10,301	0.2 (25)	
Class II (3 risk factors)	12,576	0.8 (104)	4.0 (2.9–5.4)	4,218	0.8 (32)	3.1 (1.9–5.3)
Class III (4 risk factors)	7,933	1.8 (144)	8.8 (6.6–11.8)	2,625	2.0 (53)	8.5 (5.3–13.7)
Class IV (5 risk factors)	3,615	3.3 (118)	16.1 (11.9–21.8)	1,244	3.6 (45)	15.4 (9.4–25.2)
Class V (6+ risk factors)	1,456	8.9 (129)	46.3 (34.2–62.6)	484	9.5 (46)	46.2 (26.3–70.9)

Patients are assigned to a risk class based on the number of preoperative risk factors they possess: age ≥ 56 yr, male sex, active congestive heart failure, ascites, hypertension, emergency surgery, intraperitoneal surgery, renal insufficiency (serum creatinine > 1.2 mg/dl), and diabetes mellitus (oral or insulin therapy).
From Kheterpal S, Tremper KK, Heung M, et al. Development and validation of an acute kidney injury risk index for patients undergoing general surgery: results from a national data set. *Anesthesiology* 2009;110(3):505–515.

Renal replacement therapy is usually indicated once the GFR falls below 5 to 10 mL/min. Routine dialysis should be undertaken 24 hours before elective surgery to allow the patient to stabilize after treatment. More emergent treatment is indicated for correction of acidosis, hyperkalemia, severe volume overload, and pericarditis or prior to emergent surgery. Continuous venovenous hemodialysis may be indicated to relieve volume overload in the hemodynamically unstable patient. Subclavian access should be avoided in patients who will need permanent access because of the unacceptably high incidence of subclavian vein stenosis.

Hepatic

The liver plays a protean role in metabolism and its central anatomic location in the mesenteric circulation further increases the impact of intra-abdominal surgical procedures on hepatic function. Risk assessment is based on the severity of underlying liver disease, the type of surgery, and the anesthetic used.

Patients with chronic liver disease may be asymptomatic and liver function tests may not correlate with the extent of underlying hepatic dysfunction. The history and physical examination is critical in detecting unsuspected disease. Prior history of alcohol or substance abuse, hepatitis, transfusion, variceal bleeding, prior anesthetic hepatotoxicity, bleeding disorders, biliary stone disease, family history of enzyme deficiencies and prior malignancy should trigger further investigation. Physical examination findings of jaundice, ascites, hepatosplenomegaly, palmar erythema, abdominal varices, and asterixis may be signs of severe hepatic derangement. Compromised synthetic function may manifest as elevations in prothrombin time and international normalized ratio (INR). Thrombocytopenia secondary to splenic sequestration may be an early sign of previously undiagnosed portal hypertension. If liver disease is suspected on initial evaluation, elective surgery should be deferred for further workup (60).

Acute Hepatitis

Acute hepatitis may develop secondary to alcohol or other drug ingestion or viral infection. Mortality rates for surgery are high: older reports cite 10% following open liver biopsy in viral hepatitis and 55% to 100% in patients with acute alcoholic hepatitis undergoing open liver biopsy or laparotomy. Considerable recovery may occur following the initial insult and elective surgery should be deferred until several weeks after normalization of liver function tests. For acute alcoholic hepatitis, abstinence from alcohol for 12 weeks before elective surgery has been recommended.

Table **11.10** The RIFLE classification for acute renal failure

	Urine Output Criteria	CFR Criteria
Risk (R)	<0.5 mL/kg/hr × 6 hrs	Increased [creat] × 1.5 or GFR decrease of >25%
Injury (I)	<0.5 mL/kg/hr × 12 hrs	Increased [creat] × 2 or GFR decrease of >50%
Failure (F)	<0.3 mL/kg/hr × 24 hrs or anuria for 12 hrs	Increased [creat] × 3 or GFR decrease of >75% or [creat] >4 mg/dL
Loss (L)	N/A	Persistent ARF ("F") for >4 wks but <3 mos
End-stage renal disease (E)	N/A	Persistent renal failure ("F") for >3 mos

GRF, glomerular filtration rate; [creat], serum creatinine concentration; N/A, not applicable; ARF, acute renal failure.
From Kellum JA, Bellomo R, Ronco C. Classification of acute kidney injury using RIFLE: What's the purpose? *Crit Care Med* 2007;35(8):1983–1984.

Modified Child-Turcotte-Pugh (CTP) Score			
	Score		
	1 point	2 points	3 points
Total serum bilirubin (umol/dL)	<3.4	3.4 – 5.0	>5.0
Serum albumin (g/dL)	> 3.5	2.8 – 3.5	<2.8
International normalized ratio	<1.7	1.7 – 2.2	>2.2
Ascites	None	Controlled with medication	Treatment refractory
Encephalopathy	None	Grade I–II or controlled with medication	Grade III–IV or treatment refractory

Sum total points for each component:

	Total Points	Surgical Mortality
Class A	5–6	10%
Class B	7–9	30%
Class C	10–15	80%

FIGURE 11.3. Modified Child-Turcotte-Pugh score (Adapted from Child CG, Turcotte JG. Surgery and portal hypertension. *Major Probl Clin Surg* 1964;1:1–85; Pugh RN, Murray-Lyon IM, Dawson JL, et al. Transection of the oesophagus for bleeding oesophageal varices. *Br J Surg* 1973;60:646–649.)

Chronic Liver Disease

Risk assessment in chronic liver disease is largely based on studies of outcome in patients undergoing surgery for portal hypertension (Modified Child-Turcotte-Pugh score, Fig. 11.3) (61,62) and survival models for patients with end-stage liver disease (Model for End Stage Liver Disease, MELD score, Fig. 11.4) (63–65). Surgical risk in cirrhotic patients appears to correlate with these scoring systems, with the presence of infection, preoperative upper gastrointestinal bleeding, intra-operative hypotension, associated renal failure or COPD, emergency or abdominal procedures correlating with poorer outcomes (66). A preoperative risk assessment algorithm based on these scores has been suggested (Fig. 11.5)

In general, patients with compensated chronic liver disease can tolerate most surgical procedures well; patients with decompensated cirrhosis have significant surgical morbidity and mortality proportional to the degree of hepatic dysfunction. Intra-abdominal (67,68) and cardiac surgery (69) have been associated with high mortality rates in cirrhotics. In one series, patients with cirrhosis undergoing surgery had a 30-day mortality of 11.6% and an overall complication rate of 30%, most frequently pneumonia (66). Complications included bleeding, hepatic decompensation, sepsis, and renal failure.

MELD Score
MELD score = $(9.6 \times \log_e[\text{creatinine mg/dL}]) + (3.8 \times \log_e[\text{bilirubin mg/dL}]) + (11.2 \times \log_e[\text{international normalized ratio}]) + 6.4$
Minimum laboratory value is 1.0 (for laboratory values less than 1.0, use value of 1.0) Maximum creatinine is 4.0 (for creatinine >4.0, use value of 4.0) if patient has had dialysis twice within the previous week, use value of 4.0
Round final score to nearest whole number
Maximum score is 40

90-day mortality for hospitalized patients	
MELD score	**Mortality**
>40	100%
30–39	83%
20–29	76%
10–19	27%
<10	4%

FIGURE 11.4. Model end-stage liver disease score (Adapted from Kamath PS, Wiesner RH, Malinchoc M, et al. A model to predict survival in patients with end-stage liver disease. *Hepatology* 2001;33:464–470.)

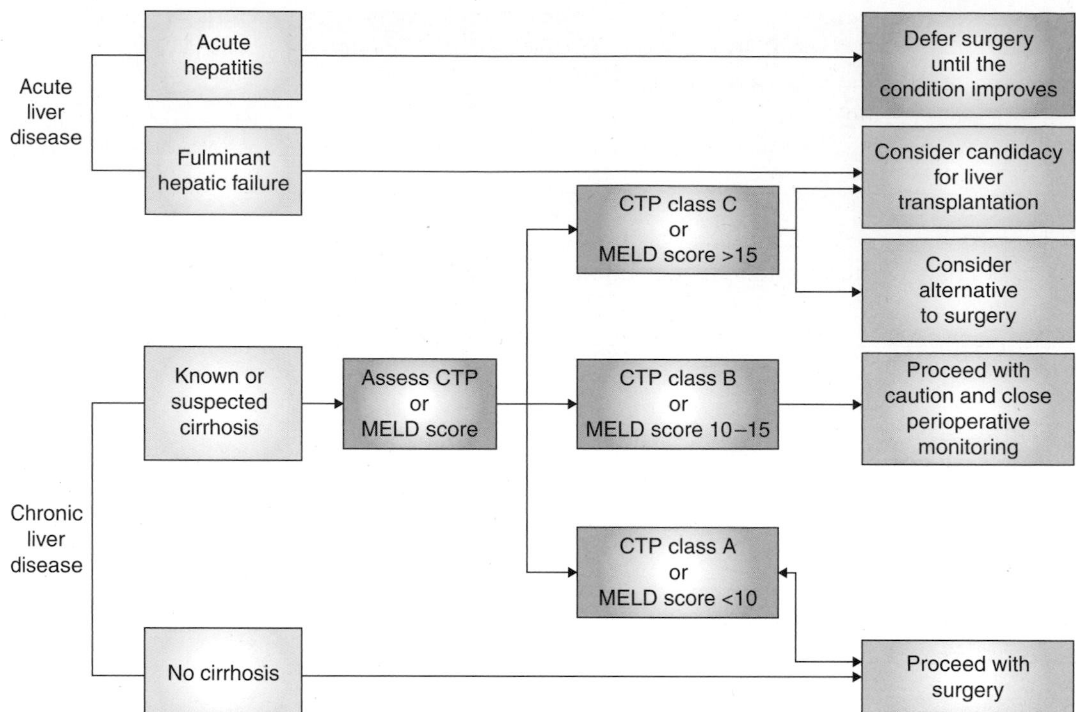

FIGURE 11.5. Proposed algorithm for evaluation of patients with liver disease (Adapted from Hanje AJ, Patel T. Preoperative evaluation of patients with liver disease. *Nat Clin Pract Gastroenterol Hepatol* 2007;4:266–276.)

Cholestasis

Cholestasis has been associated with increased operative risk, particularly in the presence of biliary tract infection. Cholangitis should be treated promptly with decompression and systemic antibiotics. Risk factors reported for postoperative complications in patients with obstructive jaundice include anemia, bilirubin >11 mg/dL, malignancy, hypoalbuminemia, infection, and azotemia (70). Acute renal failure with renal tubular dysfunction has been reported in approximately 9% of postoperative patients (71) with the risk being apparently related to degree of hyperbilirubinemia and the presence of infection. Empiric preoperative biliary drainage, either percutaneously or endoscopically has been recommended for patients with biliary obstruction, but management should be individualized.

Other

NASH. Nonalcoholic steatohepatitis (NASH) is an often silent disease affecting 2% to 5% of Americans, particularly middle-aged and overweight or obese patients. The etiology is unclear and the course may progress silently to cirrhosis. The incidence of fatty liver in patients undergoing bariatric surgery is high and unsuspected cirrhosis is found in 6% (72). No specific measures to prevent or treat the dysfunction have been identified. Surgical risk appears to be linked to the degree of cirrhosis present.

Hepatic resection. There is little formal guidance regarding estimation of ability to tolerate hepatic resection in cirrhotic patients. MELD and Child-Turcotte-Pugh (CTP) scores correlate with postoperative mortality and may be utilized in decision-making. Patients with significant steatohepatitis may have higher mortality following major anatomic resection.

Perioperative Interventions

Preoperative measures directed at minimizing surgical complications secondary to liver dysfunction include management of portal hypertension, cholestasis, and coagulopathy, and prevention of further hepatic compromise. Evidence that modifying risk category affects outcome is not strong, but medical management inherently seems important.

Intra-operative management is directed at maintaining perfusion to avoid precipitating further ischemic injury. Inhalational anesthetics reduce cardiac output and hepatic blood flow; isoflurane may be the preferred agent to minimize this. Direct hepatotoxicity may occur, historically with halothane, but with less frequency with newer agents such as sevoflurane. Sedative and narcotic metabolism may be altered in severe hepatic dysfunction. As the degree of hepatic dysfunction is not easily quantified, dose adjustment is often titrated to effect.

The presence of portal hypertension mandates meticulous surgical technique. Management of portal hypertension may include beta-blockade, octreotide, and transvenous intrahepatic portosystemic shunting. Volume management is complicated by high output cardiac failure, peripheral arteriovenous shunting, and disturbed salt-conservation secondary to hyperaldosteronemia. Postoperative volume shifts superimposed on the underlying vasodilatory state of liver disease may lead to progressive renal failure.

Careful monitoring with judicious resuscitation may improve outcomes.

The coagulopathy of liver failure is multifactorial; decreased absorption of fat soluble vitamin K associated with obstructive jaundice, poor nutritional intake, and failure of synthetic function in patients with parenchymal disease all may contribute. Concomitant thrombocytopenia may be present secondary to splenic sequestration in portal hypertension. Disseminated intravascular coagulation (DIC) may be present secondary to low grade biliary sepsis. Treatment is supportive and includes vitamin K administration, fresh frozen plasma, and platelet transfusion. DDAVP and inhibitors of fibrinolysis may also be utilized. Successful correction of severe coagulopathy has been reported with off-label use of Factor rVIIa, but enthusiasm is waning in the wake of reports of adverse thrombotic events (73).

Delayed wound healing and wound infection are likely to be exacerbated by associated malnutrition, malignancy, and sepsis. Nutritional deficiencies may include hypomagnesemia and hypophosphatemia as well as protein-calorie deficits. Postoperative nutritional supplementation may be hampered by the development of encephalopathy and intolerance of enteral protein loading. Ascites should be managed with volume restriction, active diuresis, and paracentesis to reduce intra-abdominal pressure and the incidence of abdominal wound disruption.

Encephalopathy may be precipitated by surgical stress, sepsis, and volume shifts and aggravated by analgesic medication. No specific prophylaxis is recommended other than careful medical management and judicious sedation use. Exacerbations are managed with lactulose titrated to 2 to 3 loose stools daily and oral antimicrobial agents such as neomycin or rifaximin to reduce fecal flora and minimize bacterial translocation.

Acute severe alcohol withdrawal, delirium tremens (DTs), is classically seen 72 hours after cessation of alcohol use, but may be seen earlier. Despite treatment, mortality remains 5% to 15%. The hallmark is autonomic instability, with hypertension, tachycardia, sweating, anxiety, and visual hallucinations. The mainstay of treatment is benzodiazepines, with symptomatic treatment with beta-blockers or clonidine. Symptom-triggered medication regimens are associated with reduction in total medication dose compared to standing regimens (74); pharmacologic DT prophylaxis is not indicated except in high-risk cases. Other supportive therapy includes thiamine, folate, and multivitamin administration, intravenous fluid and electrolyte replacement.

REFERENCES

1. Khuri SF, Daley J, Henderson W, et al. The Department of Veterans Affairs' NSQIP: the first national, validated, outcome-based, risk-adjusted, and peer-controlled program for the measurement and enhancement of the quality of surgical care. National VA Surgical Quality Improvement Program. *Ann Surg* 1998;228(4):491–507.
2. Collins TC, Daley J, Henderson WH, et al. Risk factors for prolonged length of stay after major elective surgery. *Ann Surg* 1999;230(2):251–259.
3. Davenport DL, Henderson WG, Khuri SF, et al. Preoperative risk factors and surgical complexity are more predictive of costs than postoperative complications: a case study using the National Surgical Quality Improvement Program (NSQIP) database. *Ann Surg* 2005;242(4):463–468; discussion 68–71.
4. Khuri SF. The NSQIP: a new frontier in surgery. *Surgery* 2005;138(5):837–843.
5. Khuri SF, Henderson WG, Daley J, et al. Successful implementation of the Department of Veterans Affairs' National Surgical Quality Improvement Program in the private sector: the Patient Safety in Surgery study. *Ann Surg* 2008;248(2):329–336.
6. Ghaferi AA, Birkmeyer JD, Dimick JB. Variation in hospital mortality associated with inpatient surgery. *N Engl J Med* 2009;361(14):1368–75.
7. Napolitano LM. Standardization of perioperative management: clinical pathways. *Surg Clin North Am* 2005;85(6):1321–1327, xiii.
8. Khuri SF, Henderson WG, DePalma RG, et al. Determinants of long-term survival after major surgery and the adverse effect of postoperative complications. *Ann Surg* 2005;242(3):326–341; discussion 41–43.
9. Manku K, Bacchetti P, Leung JM. Prognostic significance of postoperative in-hospital complications in elderly patients. I. Long-term survival. *Anesth Analg* 2003;96(2):583–589, table of contents.
10. Halaszynski TM, Juda R, Silverman DG. Optimizing postoperative outcomes with efficient preoperative assessment and management. *Crit Care Med* 2004;32(4, Suppl):S76–S86.
11. Fischer SP. Development and effectiveness of an anesthesia preoperative evaluation clinic in a teaching hospital. *Anesthesiology* 1996;85(1):196–206.
12. Pollard JB, Zboray AL, Mazze RI. Economic benefits attributed to opening a preoperative evaluation clinic for outpatients. *Anesth Analg* 1996;83(2):407–410.
13. Brumfield VC, Kee CC, Johnson JY. Preoperative patient teaching in ambulatory surgery settings. *AORN J* 1996;64(6):941–946, 948, 951–952.
14. Kluger MT, Gale S, Plummer JL, et al. Peri-operative drug prescribing pattern and manufacturers' guidelines. An audit. *Anaesthesia* 1991;46(6):456–459.
15. Ang-Lee MK, Moss J, Yuan CS. Herbal medicines and perioperative care. *JAMA* 2001;286(2):208–216.
16. Kaye AD, Clarke RC, Sabar R, et al. Herbal medicines: current trends in anesthesiology practice–a hospital survey. *J Clin Anesth* 2000;12(6):468–471.
17. Schein OD, Katz J, Bass EB, et al. The value of routine preoperative medical testing before cataract surgery. Study of Medical Testing for Cataract Surgery. *N Engl J Med* 2000;342(3):168–175.
18. Perez A, Planell J, Bacardaz C, et al. Value of routine preoperative tests: a multicentre study in four general hospitals. *Br J Anaesth* 1995;74(3):250–256.
19. Dzankic S, Pastor D, Gonzalez C, et al. The prevalence and predictive value of abnormal preoperative laboratory tests in elderly surgical patients. *Anesth Analg* 2001;93(2):301–308, 2nd contents page.
20. American Society of Anesthesiologists Task Force on Preanesthesia Evaluation. Practice advisory for preanesthesia evaluation: a report by the American Society of Anesthesiologists Task Force on Preanesthesia Evaluation. *Anesthesiology* 2002;96(2):485–496.
21. Griffin FA. Reducing surgical complications. *Jt Comm J Qual Patient Saf* 2007;33(11):660–665.
22. Margenthaler JA, Longo WE, Virgo KS, et al. Risk factors for adverse outcomes following surgery for small bowel obstruction. *Ann Surg* 2006;243(4):456–464.
23. Earley AS, Pryor JP, Kim PK, et al. An acute care surgery model improves outcomes in patients with appendicitis. *Ann Surg* 2006;244(4):498–504.
24. Smetana GW, Lawrence VA, Cornell JE. Preoperative pulmonary risk stratification for noncardiothoracic surgery: systematic review for the American College of Physicians. *Ann Intern Med* 2006;144(8):581–595.
25. Qaseem A, Snow V, Fitterman N, et al. Risk assessment for and strategies to reduce perioperative pulmonary complications for patients undergoing noncardiothoracic surgery: a guideline from the American College of Physicians. *Ann Intern Med* 2006;144(8):575–580.
26. Arozullah AM, Daley J, Henderson WG, et al. Multifactorial risk index for predicting postoperative respiratory failure in men after major noncardiac surgery. The National Veterans Administration Surgical Quality Improvement Program. *Ann Surg* 2000;232(2):242–253.
27. Gross JB, Bachenberg KL, Benumof JL, et al. Practice guidelines for the perioperative management of patients with obstructive sleep apnea: a report by the American Society of Anesthesiologists Task Force on Perioperative Management of patients with obstructive sleep apnea. *Anesthesiology* 2006;104(5):1081–1093; quiz 117–118.

28. Sweitzer BJ, Smetana GW. Identification and evaluation of the patient with lung disease. *Med Clin North Am* 2009;93(5):1017–1030.
29. Hall JC, Tarala RA, Hall JL, et al. A multivariate analysis of the risk of pulmonary complications after laparotomy. *Chest* 1991;99(4):923–927.
30. Lawrence VA, Cornell JE, Smetana GW. Strategies to reduce postoperative pulmonary complications after noncardiothoracic surgery: systematic review for the American College of Physicians. *Ann Intern Med* 2006;144(8):596–608.
31. Colice GL, Shafazand S, Griffin JP, et al. Physiologic evaluation of the patient with lung cancer being considered for resectional surgery: ACCP evidenced-based clinical practice guidelines (2nd edition). *Chest* 2007;132(3, Suppl):161S–177S.
32. Von Dossow V, Welte M, Zaune U, et al. Thoracic epidural anesthesia combined with general anesthesia: the preferred anesthetic technique for thoracic surgery. *Anesth Analg* 2001;92(4):848–854.
33. Rodgers A, Walker N, Schug S, et al. Reduction of postoperative mortality and morbidity with epidural or spinal anaesthesia: results from overview of randomised trials. *BMJ* 2000;321(7275):1493.
34. Zarbock A, Mueller E, Netzer S, et al. Prophylactic nasal continuous positive airway pressure following cardiac surgery protects from postoperative pulmonary complications: a prospective, randomized, controlled trial in 500 patients. *Chest* 2009;135(5):1252–1259.
35. Torrington KG, Henderson CJ. Perioperative respiratory therapy (PORT). A program of preoperative risk assessment and individualized postoperative care. *Chest* 1988;93(5):946–951.
36. Hulzebos EH, Helders PJ, Favie NJ, et al. Preoperative intensive inspiratory muscle training to prevent postoperative pulmonary complications in high-risk patients undergoing CABG surgery: a randomized clinical trial. *JAMA* 2006;296(15):1851–1857.
37. Barrera R, Shi W, Amar D, et al. Smoking and timing of cessation: impact on pulmonary complications after thoracotomy. *Chest* 2005; 127(6):1977–1983.
38. Nakagawa M, Tanaka H, Tsukuma H, et al. Relationship between the duration of the preoperative smoke-free period and the incidence of postoperative pulmonary complications after pulmonary surgery. *Chest* 2001;120(3):705–710.
39. Licker MJ, Widikker I, Robert J, et al. Operative mortality and respiratory complications after lung resection for cancer: impact of chronic obstructive pulmonary disease and time trends. *Ann Thorac Surg* 2006;81(5):1830–1837.
40. Sarnak MJ, Levey AS, Schoolwerth AC, et al. Kidney disease as a risk factor for development of cardiovascular disease: a statement from the American Heart Association Councils on Kidney in Cardiovascular Disease, High Blood Pressure Research, Clinical Cardiology, and Epidemiology and Prevention. *Circulation* 2003;108(17):2154–2169.
41. Cockcroft DW, Gault MH. Prediction of creatinine clearance from serum creatinine. *Nephron* 1976;16(1):31–41.
42. Waikar SS, Liu KD, Chertow GM. Diagnosis, epidemiology and outcomes of acute kidney injury. *Clin J Am Soc Nephrol* 2008;3(3):844–861.
43. Chertow GM, Levy EM, Hammermeister KE, et al. Independent association between acute renal failure and mortality following cardiac surgery. *Am J Med* 1998;104(4):343–348.
44. Kheterpal S, Tremper KK, Heung M, et al. Development and validation of an acute kidney injury risk index for patients undergoing general surgery: results from a national data set. *Anesthesiology* 2009;110(3): 505–515.
45. Bihorac A, Yavas S, Subbiah S, et al. Long-term risk of mortality and acute kidney injury during hospitalization after major surgery. *Ann Surg* 2009;249(5):851–858.
46. Coresh J, Selvin E, Stevens LA, et al. Prevalence of chronic kidney disease in the United States. *JAMA* 2007;298(17):2038–2047.
47. Bellomo R, Ronco C, Kellum JA, et al. Acute renal failure – definition, outcome measures, animal models, fluid therapy and information technology needs: the Second International Consensus Conference of the Acute Dialysis Quality Initiative (ADQI) Group. *Crit Care* 2004;8(4): R204–R212.
48. Kuitunen A, Vento A, Suojaranta-Ylinen R, et al. Acute renal failure after cardiac surgery: evaluation of the RIFLE classification. *Ann Thorac Surg* 2006;81(2):542–546.
49. Cheatham ML, Malbrain ML, Kirkpatrick A, et al. Results from the International Conference of Experts on Intra-abdominal Hypertension and Abdominal Compartment Syndrome. II. Recommendations. *Intensive Care Med* 2007;33(6):951–962.
50. Mahesh B, Yim B, Robson D, et al. Does furosemide prevent renal dysfunction in high-risk cardiac surgical patients? Results of a double-blinded prospective randomised trial. *Eur J Cardiothorac Surg* 2008; 33(3):370–376.
51. Brar SS, Shen AY, Jorgensen MB, et al. Sodium bicarbonate vs sodium chloride for the prevention of contrast medium-induced nephropathy in patients undergoing coronary angiography: a randomized trial. *JAMA* 2008;300(9):1038–1046.
52. Fishbane S. N-acetylcysteine in the prevention of contrast-induced nephropathy. *Clin J Am Soc Nephrol* 2008;3(1):281–287.
53. Wagner K, Albrecht S, Neumayer HH. Prevention of posttransplant acute tubular necrosis by the calcium antagonist diltiazem: a prospective randomized study. *Am J Nephrol* 1987;7(4):287–291.
54. Young EW, Diab A, Kirsh MM. Intravenous diltiazem and acute renal failure after cardiac operations. *Ann Thorac Surg* 1998;65(5):1316–1319.
55. Allgren RL, Marbury TC, Rahman SN, et al. Anaritide in acute tubular necrosis. Auriculin Anaritide Acute Renal Failure Study Group. *N Engl J Med* 1997;336(12):828–834.
56. Hirschberg R, Kopple J, Lipsett P, et al. Multicenter clinical trial of recombinant human insulin-like growth factor I in patients with acute renal failure. *Kidney Int* 1999;55(6):2423–2432.
57. Bove T, Landoni G, Calabro MG, et al. Renoprotective action of fenoldopam in high-risk patients undergoing cardiac surgery: a prospective, double-blind, randomized clinical trial. *Circulation* 2005;111(24):3230–3235.
58. Landoni G, Biondi-Zoccai GG, Tumlin JA, et al. Beneficial impact of fenoldopam in critically ill patients with or at risk for acute renal failure: a meta-analysis of randomized clinical trials. *Am J Kidney Dis* 2007;49(1):56–68.
59. Krishnan M. Preoperative care of patients with kidney disease. *Am Fam Physician* 2002;66(8):1471–1476, 1479.
60. O'Leary JG, Yachimski PS, Friedman LS. Surgery in the patient with liver disease. *Clin Liver Dis* 2009;13(2):211–231.
61. Child CG, Turcotte JG. Surgery and portal hypertension. *Major Probl Clin Surg* 1964;1:1–85.
62. Pugh RN, Murray-Lyon IM, Dawson JL, et al. Transection of the oesophagus for bleeding oesophageal varices. *Br J Surg* 1973;60(8): 646–649.
63. Kamath PS, Wiesner RH, Malinchoc M, et al. A model to predict survival in patients with end-stage liver disease. *Hepatology* 2001;33(2): 464–470.
64. Northup PG, Wanamaker RC, Lee VD, et al. Model for End-Stage Liver Disease (MELD) predicts nontransplant surgical mortality in patients with cirrhosis. *Ann Surg* 2005;242(2):244–251.
65. Farnsworth N, Fagan SP, Berger DH, et al. Child-Turcotte-Pugh versus MELD score as a predictor of outcome after elective and emergent surgery in cirrhotic patients. *Am J Surg* 2004;188(5):580–583.
66. Ziser A, Plevak DJ, Wiesner RH, et al. Morbidity and mortality in cirrhotic patients undergoing anesthesia and surgery. *Anesthesiology* 1999;90(1):42–53.
67. Meunier K, Mucci S, Quentin V, et al. Colorectal surgery in cirrhotic patients: assessment of operative morbidity and mortality. *Dis Colon Rectum* 2008;51(8):1225–1231.
68. Lehnert T, Herfarth C. Peptic ulcer surgery in patients with liver cirrhosis. *Ann Surg* 1993;217(4):338–346.
69. Suman A, Barnes DS, Zein NN, et al. Predicting outcome after cardiac surgery in patients with cirrhosis: a comparison of Child-Pugh and MELD scores. *Clin Gastroenterol Hepatol* 2004;2(8):719–723.
70. Friedman LS. The risk of surgery in patients with liver disease. *Hepatology* 1999;29(6):1617–1623.
71. Wait RB, Kahng KU. Renal failure complicating obstructive jaundice. *Am J Surg* 1989;157(2):256–263.
72. Brolin RE, Bradley LJ, Taliwal RV. Unsuspected cirrhosis discovered during elective obesity operations. *Arch Surg* 1998;133(1):84–88.
73. O'Connell KA, Wood JJ, Wise RP, et al. Thromboembolic adverse events after use of recombinant human coagulation factor VIIa. *JAMA* 2006;295(3):293–298.
74. Jaeger TM, Lohr RH, Pankratz VS. Symptom-triggered therapy for alcohol withdrawal syndrome in medical inpatients. *Mayo Clin Proc* 2001;76(7):695–701.
75. Kellum JA, Bellomo R, Ronco C. Classification of acute kidney injury using RIFLE: what's the purpose? *Crit Care Med* 2007;35(8):1983–1984.
76. Hanje AJ, Patel T. Preoperative evaluation of patients with liver disease. *Nat Clin Pract Gastroenterol Hepatol* 2007;4(5):266–276.

CHAPTER

12

Anesthesia Complications

Paul E. Kazanjian

INTRODUCTION

There are a wide variety of complications in anesthesiology ranging from relatively frequent and minor adverse events to rare but disastrous outcomes, including brain damage and death. The anesthesiologist's expertise in management of the airway is crucial to the safe conduct of anesthesia care. Unfortunately, airway complications are a major source of serious morbidity and mortality. Anesthetic medications play a crucial role in rendering patients insensate, immobile, and unconscious but they also account for a number of adverse effects and complications. Machines are used to administer drug infusions, ventilate the lungs, measure the blood pressure, and deliver volatile anesthetics and oxygen. Machines can breakdown or be misused, sometimes resulting in patient injury. Like surgery, anesthesiology is a procedure-oriented field and some complications result from technical mishaps or untoward patient-device interactions.

Whole textbooks are devoted to the subject of complications in anesthesia and this one chapter cannot cover the entire subject. This chapter serves as a starting point for surgeons interested in an introduction to the gamut of complications due to anesthesia. Also, the references at the end of the chapter are good resources for those interested in more information about individual types of anesthesia-related complications.

Throughout this chapter, there are references to The American Society of Anesthesiologists Closed Claims Database. The Closed Claims Project was begun in 1984 in response to rising professional liability premiums. The intention was to identify anesthetic-related complications, improve patient safety, and improve the insurance problem for anesthesiologists. The project is an ongoing evaluation and in-depth analysis of nearly 9000 closed claims from 35 professional liability insurance companies covering 60% of the anesthesiologists in the United States. Each case is described by a brief narrative summary describing the claim, patient information, surgical procedure and positioning, preanesthetic evaluation, anesthetic technique, events leading to the injury or claim, type and severity of injury, and the outcome of litigation. A physician reviews the case, rates the severity of injury, and determines the potential for prevention and appropriateness of anesthesia care. Claims are separated into two categories: damaging events and complications. The damaging event is the specific incident that leads to the complication, while the complication is the injury that the patient sustained. The findings are reported in the scientific literature and a number of these articles have been referenced in this chapter. More information about the project and a complete bibliography is available on the American Society of Anesthesiologists' (ASA) Closed Claims Project Web site (1).

There are limitations to closed claims analysis including lack of data regarding the total population at risk for injury and nonrandom, retrospective data collection. For several reasons, it is not possible to provide numerical estimates of risk or establish true incidence rates based on closed claims analysis. All adverse outcomes do not result in a malpractice claim and 40% of practicing anesthesiologists are not included in the analysis because their insurance companies do not participate in the Closed Claims Project. It is not possible to determine whether increases or decreases in cases over time represent actual changes in the rate of complications, a more or less litigious patient population or both.

AIRWAY COMPLICATIONS

Management of the airway is a central activity of daily anesthetic practice and it involves a variety of maneuvers and devices designed to support or maintain adequate oxygenation and ventilation while the patient is not fully capable of doing so himself. Techniques range from simple maneuvers to maintain airway patency during spontaneous ventilation to fiberoptic intubation of the trachea in patients who are difficult to intubate. Problems occurring during management of the airway are the most important cause of major anesthetic-related morbidity and mortality. In an analysis of closed claims in the American Society of Anesthesiologists Closed Claims Project, respiratory events are the single largest class of incidents leading to injury, accounting for 30% of claims in adults and 43% of claims in pediatric patients (2). Most of the adverse respiratory events were due to difficulty managing the airway, including inadequate ventilation, esophageal intubation, and failure to intubate the trachea.

Paul E. Kazanjian: Department of Anesthesiology, University of Michigan Medical School, Ann Arbor, MI 48109-5861.

One of the most critical and potentially dangerous portions of an operation occurs at induction of, and emergence from, general anesthesia (GA). During induction of GA, the anesthetist transitions the patient from conscious and spontaneously breathing to unconscious and apneic. As a patient emerges from anesthesia, he or she passes through several stages of anesthesia, each of which has certain implications for management of the airway. Emergence from anesthesia is not an all-or-none phenomenon and proper timing of endotracheal extubation is critical to avoid airway obstruction, aspiration, and hypoxemia. The attention of the entire operating room team should be focused on the patient, the anesthetist, and his or her assistant during these two phases of GA. Potentially life-threatening problems can develop quickly, in which case, the anesthetist will require rapid, competent assistance. Emergent cricothyrotomy may be necessary and the surgeon, regardless of his or her specialty, must be prepared to perform this life-saving technique on a moment's notice.

Oral intubation with an endotracheal tube (ETT) is usually performed after induction of anesthesia with a short-acting intravenous (IV) anesthetic like thiopental or propofol. Alternatively, anesthesia can be induced by inhalation of nitrous oxide and steadily higher concentrations of a volatile anesthetic. Mask ventilation is established and anesthesia maintained with inhaled anesthetic such as isoflurane. Muscle relaxants facilitate intubation by ablating reflexive resistance to laryngoscopy and intubation. Successful direct laryngoscopy and intubation then depends on patient characteristics including adequate mouth opening, sufficient pharyngeal space, compliant submandibular tissue, and unimpaired atlantooccipital extension. If any one or more of these basic characteristics are abnormal then visualization and intubation may be difficult (3,4).

Induction of anesthesia, laryngoscopy, and tracheal intubation is very stimulating and can be associated with marked hemodynamic changes, which can be of concern in certain subsets of patients, such as those with ischemic heart disease, acute aortic syndrome or intracranial aneurysm. The hemodynamic response depends on a variety of factors, including the method of induction, the technique used for intubation, and the combination of anesthetic medications used to attenuate these responses. For example, a study comparing several induction regimens demonstrated that induction with thiopental alone resulted in undesirable hemodynamics (tachycardia and hypertension) and elevations of plasma catecholamines while thiopental supplemented with fentanyl (6 μg/kg) attenuated this response (5). Barak et al. compared two methods of intubating anesthetized patients, direct laryngoscopy and fiberoptic bronchoscopy, and found that both methods resulted in similar hemodynamic changes (6). Heart rate and blood pressure increased after intubation but not during laryngoscopy or bronchoscopy.

There are alternatives to oral intubation with an ETT. For example, certain operations are best served by nasotracheal intubation. Many patients do not need tracheal intubation and mechanical ventilation during GA and placement of a laryngotracheal mask airway (LMA) is sufficient. If tracheal intubation is required, then there are alternatives to direct laryngoscopy under anesthesia. Awake intubation using fiberoptic technique, retrograde intubation, or surgical tracheostomy are alternative methods available for patients who are difficult to ventilate, difficult to intubate, or both (3,7–9).

A difficult airway is defined as a clinical situation where an anesthesiologist experiences difficulty with face mask ventilation of the upper airway, difficulty with tracheal intubation, or both. If it is difficult or impossible to visualize the glottis despite proper positioning of the head and neck, then laryngoscopy is difficult. Difficulty with an airway may be *anticipated* when preoperative evaluation reveals a history of, or physical exam suggestive of, difficult intubation. While a number of very complex clinical and radiographic factors that suggest potential difficulty with laryngoscopy and intubation have been described, most anesthesiologists rely on a more straightforward examination combined with clinical experience. Factors suggesting difficulty include a short muscular neck, full set of teeth, receding lower jaw, high arched palate, limited mouth opening, limited cervical extension, chin-to-thyroid cartilage distance of less than 7 cm, and a Mallampati score of 3 or 4 (Table 12.1) (4). The Mallampati test classifies the ability to see the faucial pillars and uvula when the patient opens his or her mouth as wide as possible (10). When combined, the latter two criteria have a specificity of almost 98% (11,12). At other times, difficulty is *unanticipated* because there are no predisposing factors suggesting difficulty and intubation is expected to be uncomplicated. The latter situation can be especially problematic if it is difficult or impossible to *ventilate* the patient by mask after induction of anesthesia. The American Society of Anesthesiologists Task Force on Management of the Difficult Airway has developed and refined practice guidelines for managing these various clinical situations (8). The guidelines include an algorithm, which is reproduced in Figure 12.1. The practice guidelines and algorithm describe a set of strategies that may be executed in the acute situation of unfolding difficulty. A recent survey of anesthesiologists revealed that when confronted with a difficult airway scenario, most chose to approach the airway with direct laryngoscopy or fiberoptic techniques (13). All other methods were much less frequently used.

The lips, teeth, tongue, buccal mucosa, palate and permanent dental appliances can be injured or damaged during laryngoscopy or by any one of a number of foreign objects (oral airway, bite block, ETT, or laryngeal mask airway) placed in the airway during GA. Injury to the lips, both upper and lower, is common during intubation using a laryngoscope, especially when performed by inexperienced practitioners. Serious consequences are rare and the injury can be treated conservatively. Dental injury requiring repair or extraction occurs in approximately 1 in

Table **12.1** **Components of the preoperative airway physical examination**

Airway Examination Component	Nonreassuring Findings
Length of upper incisors	Relatively long
Relation of maxillary and mandibular incisors during normal jaw closure	Prominent "overbite" (maxillary incisors anterior to mandibular incisors)
Relation of maxillary and mandibular incisors during voluntary protrusion of mandible	Patient cannot bring mandibular incisors anterior to (mandible in front of) maxillary incisors
Interincisor distance (mouth opening)	Less than 3 cm
Visibility of uvula	Not visible when tongue is protruded with patient in sitting position (e.g., Mallampati class greater than II)
Shape of palate	Highly arched or very narrow
Compliance of mandibular space	Stiff, indurated, occupied by mass, or nonresilient
Thyromental distance	Less than three ordinary finger breadths
Length of neck	Short
Thickness of neck	Thick
Range of motion of head and neck	Patient cannot touch tip of chin to chest or cannot extend neck

Adapted from Society of Anesthesiologists Task Force on Management of the Difficult Airway. Practice guidelines for management of the difficult airway: an updated report by the American Society of Anesthesiologists Task Force on Management of the Difficult Airway. *Anesthesiology* 2003;98(5):1269–1277.

4500 cases and usually involves the upper incisors (14). Preexisting poor dentition and difficulty intubating the patient increases the risk of damage to the teeth. Tongue trauma and swelling can be the result of prolonged compression by an ETT oral airway, or surgical retractor, or it can be the result of positioning the head in extreme flexion, especially when the patient is positioned head-up for posterior neurosurgical procedures. In contrast to other oral and dental injuries, injuries to the temporomandibular joint almost always occur in young, female, ASA physical status 1 and 2 patients although patients with facial skeletal abnormalities are also at risk (Table 12.2). The dislocated temporomandibular joint should be reduced immediately after the condition is recognized.

The topics of esophageal injury and laryngotracheal trauma are covered in a recent review (15).

Improper manipulation of an unstable cervical spine may cause fracture or subluxation of the osseous components of the spine resulting in cord compression and neurologic injury. Establishing a mask airway for ventilation, and positioning the head and neck for intubation, involves positioning the head and neck in the sniffing position by flexing the lower cervical spine and extending the occipital atlantoaxial complex. The majority of motion during laryngoscopy and intubation in anesthetized, paralyzed patients with intact cervical spines occurs at the occiput-C1 junction (16). Theoretically, a person performing tracheal intubation could create or exacerbate a spinal cord injury, especially during difficult laryngoscopy, but there are very little data to support this occurrence (17).

In the acute setting of a known or suspected spinal cord injury and a compromised airway, establishing an airway and supporting breathing takes precedence (17). Current Advanced Trauma Life Support guidelines recommend orotracheal intubation with manual in-line cervical spine stabilization, but the value of this and other stabilization maneuvers is not proven (16). In a study using cadavers, Lennarson et al. demonstrated that manual in-line stabilization did not prevent motion of the injured or intact cervical spine during laryngoscopy and intubation (16). Still, current teaching and guidelines advocate that all effort should be made to minimize cervical spine motion during laryngoscopy and intubation. With careful technique, the risk of causing or worsening a spinal cord injury is low, regardless of the technique used to intubate the patient. During elective intubation, the patient's anatomic configuration or halo cervical stabilization may suggest difficulty with direct laryngoscopy and in these cases alternate techniques for intubation (fiberoptic) may be necessary.

A variety of conditions are associated with potential immobility and/or instability of the cervical spine, including Down's syndrome, rheumatoid arthritis, ankylosing spondylitis and trauma (see Table 12.3). High-risk rheumatoid patients are those with neck symptoms, advanced age, longstanding disease, erosive disease, and subcutaneous nodules. These patients should have lateral cervical spine x-rays performed in neutral position, flexion, and extension prior to GA.

Nasal intubation is a safe and useful technique when performed by experienced persons (Table 12.4). The most common complication is epistaxis, which is usually self-limited but can be serious in anticoagulated patients or those patients with a coagulopathy. Nasal bruising is also quite common, but frank mucosal tears, lacerations, and false submucosal passage are uncommon. Nasal intubation is potentially very hazardous in certain conditions such as facial trauma and skull fracture where inadvertent intubations of the cranium and orbit have been reported (18). The

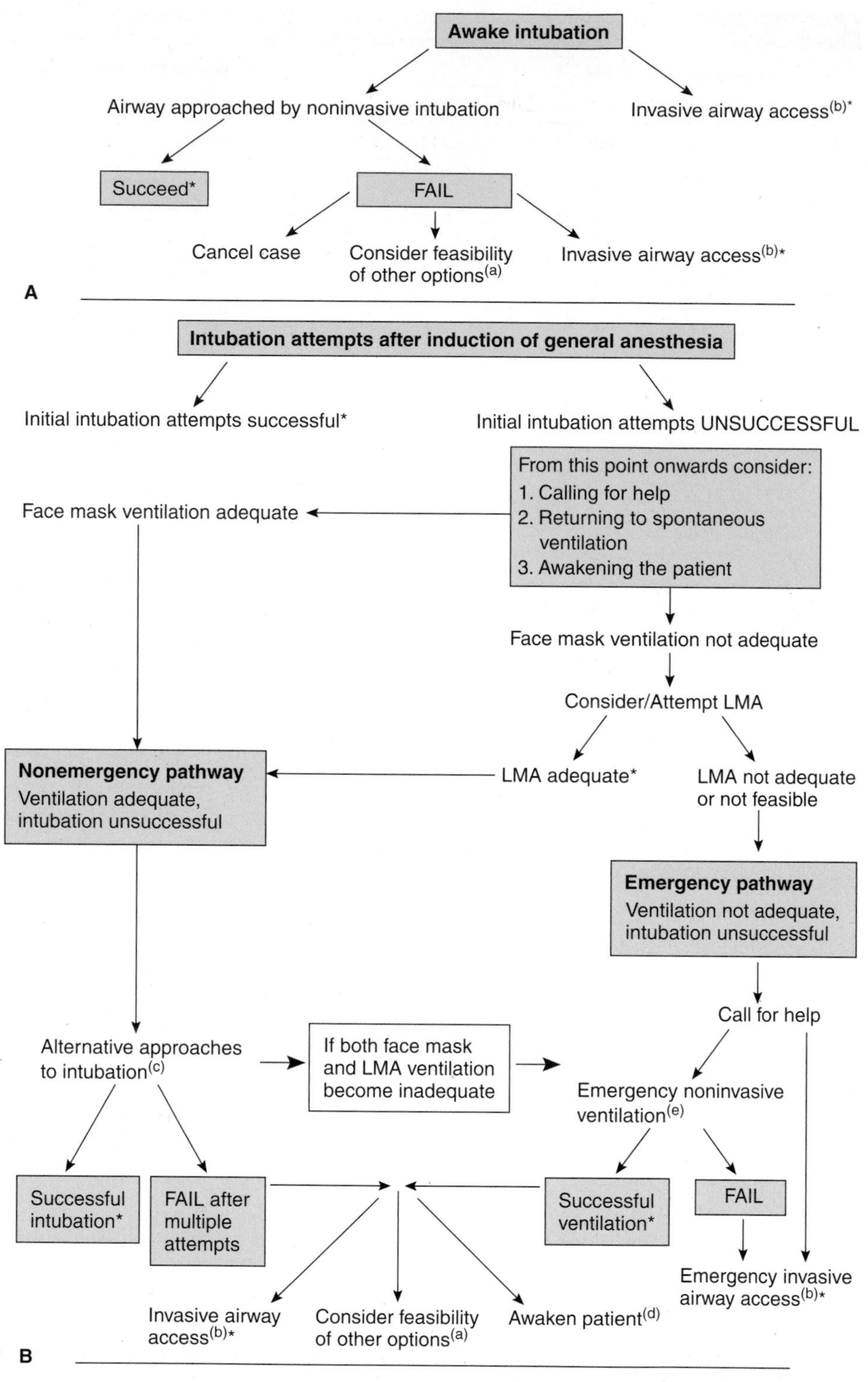

FIGURE 12.1. The ASA Difficult Airway Algorithm. [a]Other options include (but are not limited to) surgery utilizing face mask or LMA anesthesia, local anesthesia infiltration or regional nerve blockade. Pursuit of these options usually implies that mask ventilation will not be problematic. Therefore, these options may be of limited value if this step in the algorithm has been reached in the Emergency Pathway. [b]Invasive airway access includes surgical or percutaneous tracheostomy or cricothyrotomy. [c]Alternative noninvasive approaches to difficult intubation include (but are not limited to): use of different laryngoscope blades. LMA as an intubation conduit (with or without fiberoptic guidance), fiberoptic intubation, intubating stylet or tube changer, light wand, retrograde intubation, and blind oral or nasal intubation. [d]Consider re-preparation of the patient for awake intubation or canceling surgery. [e]Options for emergency noninvasive airway ventilation include (but are not limited to): rigid bronchoscope, esophageal-tracheal Combitube ventilation, or transtracheal jet ventilation. (Adapted from Society of Anesthesiologists Task Force on Management of the Difficult Airway. Practice guidelines for management of the difficult airway: an updated report by the American Society of Anesthesiologists Task Force on Management of the Difficult Airway. *Anesthesiology* 2003;98(5):1269–1277.)

technique is generally contraindicated in these situations unless absolutely necessary and performed carefully with the assistance of fiberoptic bronchoscopy.

The technique of nasal intubation has been recently and thoroughly reviewed (19). The authors emphasize several aspects of the technique in order to reduce the incidence of common complications, including careful preoperative assessment, preparation of the nasal mucosa with lubricating jellies and vasoconstrictors, selection of a supple, uncuffed tube, and careful insertion of a well-lubricated tube. Once the tube is beyond the nasopharynx, it can be guided into the trachea either blindly, under direct laryngoscopic visualization, or with the assistance of fiberoptic bronchoscopy. Once in place, the tube must be carefully

Table 12.2 ASA physical classification

P1	A normal healthy patient
P2	A patient with mild systemic disease
P3	A patient with severe systemic disease
P4	A patient with severe systemic disease that is a constant threat to life
P5	A moribund patient who is not expected to survive without the operation
P6	A declared brain-dead patient whose organs are being removed for donor purposes

Table 12.4 Indications for nasal intubation (19)

Head and neck surgery	Dental surgery Intraoral and oropharyngeal surgery Rigid laryngoscopy and microlaryngeal surgery Jaws wired or fixed shut at end of operation
General indications	Intra-oral pathology including obstructive lesions Cervical spine instability or degenerative spine disease Obstructive sleep apnea

secured to prevent inadvertent extubation and to avoid pressure on the nasal ala, which can cause tissue ischemia or necrosis.

Inadvertent intubation of the esophagus can occur when direct visualization of the glottis is difficult but it can also occur when visualization is ideal. Esophageal intubation and ventilation of the stomach is of little consequence, *as long as the condition is rapidly recognized and corrected.* The presence of carbon dioxide (CO_2) in exhaled gases can be detected by end-tidal CO_2 monitoring and is the most accurate and reliable method of confirming proper placement of the ETT in the trachea. Clinical signs such as bilateral breath sounds, condensation in the ETT, chest wall movement, and absence of gastric sounds cannot be relied upon for confirmation because they are all potentially misleading. If the esophagus is intubated, the ETT should be left in place until the trachea is correctly intubated (12). Leaving the ETT in the esophagus helps protect the trachea from regurgitated gastric contents and helps identify the proper orifice for intubation.

Perhaps one of the most common causes of intra-operative arterial oxygen desaturation in an otherwise healthy patient is bronchial intubation. An ETT that is placed too deeply will most likely intubate the right mainstem bronchus, resulting in hypoventilation of the left lung. Clinical evidence of this phenomenon (unilateral decreased breath sounds, increased inflation pressure, asymmetric chest expansion during inhalation) should be obvious. An otherwise normally placed ETT may "migrate" into a bronchus for a variety of reasons. A steep Trendelenburg position can force the abdomen, diaphragm, and chest organs to move cephalad toward the ETT. Flexion of the head will move the ETT deeper into the airway (20).

An endobronchial injury can be the result of misplaced ETTs, tube guides, tube changers or properly placed double-lumen ETTs. Severe endobronchial injury almost always results in pneumothorax, which can rapidly progress to tension pneumothorax in patients receiving positive pressure ventilation (18).

The laryngeal mask airway is an invaluable tool for management of the airway in elective operations and certain emergency situations. In fact, the laryngeal mask airway has emerged as a very important component of the difficult airway algorithm and is frequently successful in salvaging ventilation in patients who are difficult to intubate and difficult to ventilate by face mask (21,22). While many anesthesiologists and surgeons regard placement of an LMA as "less invasive" and less traumatic than direct laryngoscopy followed by endotracheal intubation, use of the LMA is not without complication. In one review of airway complications in pediatric patients, the rate of complications was actually higher with the LMA than with endotracheal intubation but they were clinically less significant (23). Complications with the LMA can be broadly divided into pharyngolaryngeal and neurovascular complications.

One disadvantage of the LMA is that it cannot provide complete protection against aspiration of gastric contents or secretions. The incidence of subclinical aspiration may be as high as 25% but the incidence of serious aspiration appears to be much lower (18). The occurrence of mild hoarseness (12%), sore throat (10%), and dysphagia (4%) all appear to be related to malposition or excess cuff pressure. Pharyngeal abrasions and ulcers of the soft palate and uvula are usually associated with difficult placement of the device.

A variety of nerve injuries have been reported with use of the LMA, including lingual, recurrent laryngeal, and hypoglossal nerve damage (18). In general, serious nerve

Table 12.3 Conditions associated with atlantoaxial subluxation (230)

Congenital	Down syndrome Odontoid anomalies Mucopolysaccharidoses
Acquired	Still's disease Ankylosing spondylitis Psoriatic arthritis Enteropathic arthritis (Crohn's disease, ulcerative colitis) Reiter's syndrome Trauma (odontoid fracture, ligamentous disruption)

injuries seem to be related to neurovascular compression from excess pressure on pharyngeal structures. Excess pressure on adjacent structures may be a result of malposition of the device, or excessive cuff inflation, especially in the presence of nitrous oxide. Thus, some injuries may be avoided by monitoring cuff pressure and keeping it at the lowest level that allows for adequate gas exchange. In a prospective, randomized trial in 200 patients, Seet et al. demonstrated that maintaining LMA intracuff pressure to less than 44 mm Hg lowers the incidence of postoperative pharyngolaryngeal complications. The investigators suggest that LMA cuff pressures should be measured routinely using manometry, and deflating the intracuff pressure to less than 44 mm Hg should be recommended as anesthetic best practice (24). Malposition, on the other hand, may be hard to recognize because adequate ventilation may be possible even when the device is not properly seated. The only way to accurately confirm proper positioning is with fiberoptic examination of the glottis from within the LMA but fiberoptic confirmation is not performed routinely (18).

As mentioned earlier, extubation is another critical phase (stage) in the conduct of GA and it can be complicated by a variety of events including, but not limited to, aspiration, laryngospasm, negative pressure pulmonary edema (NPPE), and airway compression.

Tracheomalacia leading to tracheal collapse may produce upper airway obstruction following extubation. Tracheomalacia is usually secondary to thyroid goiter where the cartilaginous rings of the trachea may be weakened or destroyed. In these cases, removal of the goiter further compromises the structural integrity of the trachea and collapse can occur shortly after tracheal extubation. Reintubation is required. Subsequent treatment options include tracheostomy, tracheoplasty, or placement of external or internal tracheal support (25).

Laryngospasm is normally a protective reflex where the glottis is occluded by contraction of the intrinsic laryngeal muscles. Usually laryngospasm occurs to prevent aspiration of foreign material into the trachea and is mediated by the vagus nerve. The reflex can occur in response to the presence of airway irritants (secretions, blood, ETT) during a light plane of anesthesia. During this light plane of anesthesia, referred to as stage II, the level of anesthesia is insufficient to prevent the laryngospasm reflex but is too deep to allow a normal cough reflex (26). If laryngospasm occurs after tracheal extubation, then upper airway obstruction may ensue. Laryngospasm is the most common cause of upper airway obstruction after tracheal extubation and is especially frequent in children after upper airway surgery (27). Ideally, all attempts should be made to avoid precipitating laryngospasm by removing potential irritants by thorough suctioning of the mouth and throat prior to extubation. Extubation should occur while the patient is deeply anesthetized or after the patient has passed out of stage II anesthesia and is following simple commands. Applying positive pressure during extubation can clear potentially irritating material from the cords. If laryngospasm develops, then the precipitating irritating material should be removed while administering 100% oxygen by positive pressure ventilation. Occasionally, it is necessary to deepen the anesthesia or administer a small dose of succinylcholine to "break" the spasm and sometimes reintubation is required.

Pulmonary edema may occur after acute upper airway tract obstruction, in which case it is termed NPPE. The pulmonary edema occurs within minutes of the onset of airway obstruction and radiological findings demonstrate perihilar infiltrate with diffuse pulmonary edema. The pathogenesis of NPPE is multifactorial but the predominant mechanism is generation of markedly negative intrapleural pressures by forceful inspiration against an obstructed airway (28). The differential diagnosis includes acid aspiration, cardiogenic pulmonary edema, and iatrogenic volume overload, but the temporal relation of pulmonary edema to clinically obvious airway obstruction in an otherwise healthy patient strongly suggests NPPE. The most frequent cause of airway obstruction leading to NPPE is postextubation laryngospasm but acute airway obstruction occurring anytime during management of the airway can be followed by NPPE (29). The first priority in managing NPPE is reestablishing a patent airway and assuring adequate oxygenation. Most cases resolve spontaneously without further complication although some patients may require reintubation followed by a brief period of mechanical ventilation with positive end-expiratory pressure (PEEP) (28).

GENERAL ANESTHESIA

The term "anesthesia" signifies insensibility to surgical pain. Other components of anesthesia include amnesia, hypnosis (unconsciousness), muscle relaxation, inhibition of movement, and blunting of the autonomic response in response to noxious stimuli. A variety of drugs provide some or all of these components of anesthesia. The gamut of pharmacologic agents used in GA has been thoroughly reviewed elsewhere (30). Recent development of anesthetic medications has focused on those compounds with a rapid onset and recovery with minimal side effects and drug-drug interactions.

A fundamental premise of GA is that the state of unconsciousness and unresponsiveness produced by anesthetics is reversible and that the brain and spinal cord are neurophysiologically the same before and after anesthesia. Recent studies have questioned the complete reversibility of anesthesia, suggesting that anesthesia and/or anesthetics may have long-lasting detrimental or toxic effects. This concept will be discussed below.

Potent inhaled anesthetics

Potent inhaled anesthetics (PIAs) are halogenated hydrocarbons and ether compounds that render patients amnestic and immobile to noxious stimuli. Current theories on the mechanisms of action of the PIAs have been recently reviewed (31). Their amnestic and hypnotic affects are mediated in the brain while their action to inhibit movement in response to noxious stimuli is secondary to depression of spinal cord function. There are separate molecular targets for each of these actions. While the volatile anesthetics can cause cardiopulmonary depression and death at concentrations near those that produce deep anesthesia, this is extremely rare, largely due to reliable gas delivery systems, agent analyzers, and hemodynamic monitors. Rather, adverse side effects are usually mild and include nausea, vomiting, and delirium.

The clinical effects of inhaled anesthetics, ranging from euphoria to profound cardiopulmonary depression, depend on the inhaled concentration. A number of scales are used to assess anesthetic potency and they are based on the relation between alveolar concentration and a certain behavioral endpoint. The median alveolar concentration (MAC) is one of these scales and is defined as the median end-tidal concentration of inhaled anesthetic that ablates movement in response to surgical incision in 50% of the test population.

All of the volatile anesthetics decrease blood pressure in a dose-dependent manner and all are myocardial depressants. The effect of halothane and enflurane is greater than isoflurane, sevoflurane, and desflurane in this regard. Halothane sensitizes the myocardium to the arrhythmogenic effects of epinephrine. Isoflurane and desflurane decrease blood pressure and peripheral vascular resistance while increasing heart rate. Animal studies suggest that isoflurane promotes "coronary steal" by dilating nondiseased coronary vessels and diverting blood flow to normal areas away from ischemic areas (32). Clinically, the effect is not apparent and, if factors affecting myocardial oxygen consumption are controlled, isoflurane anesthesia does not cause a greater incidence of ischemia than any other technique (33–35). In fact, there is substantial evidence that isoflurane actually protects the myocardium, effectively limiting infarct size and improving functional recovery following myocardial ischemia through a mechanism similar to ischemic preconditioning (36,37).

PIAs are respiratory depressants and depress the normal response to hypercarbia in a dose-dependent manner. The PIAs irritate the airways and may produce coughing or laryngospasm during inhalation induction of GA. Sevoflurane and halothane are the least irritating while desflurane is the most irritating.

In a discussion of halothane-associated liver failure from 1970, halothane is regarded as close to an ideal anesthetic agent, despite many reports of halothane-induced hepatitis (38). Today, this assessment is not valid because other agents are available that have a much better margin of safety. Halothane-associated liver damage presents as one of two clinical syndromes (39). Mild hepatic damage, moderately increased transaminase levels, occasional transient jaundice, and low morbidity characterize the first syndrome, which may have an incidence as high as 20%. The second syndrome is very rare, occurs after repeated exposure to halothane, and is characterized by fulminant hepatic failure with high mortality. Even in 1970, an allergic type reaction was hypothesized despite the relatively inert nature of halothane. Hepatotoxicity resulting in fulminant liver failure involves a humoral response that is directed toward hepatocyte cytochromes that have been altered by an oxidative reactive metabolite of halothane (40,41).

When the body metabolizes methoxyflurane, enflurane, and sevoflurane, fluoride ions are produced, which may be toxic to the kidneys resulting in impairment of concentrating ability and acute renal failure. The metabolism of halothane, isoflurane, and desflurane does not produce significant levels of fluoride ions and there is little potential for nephrotoxicity with these compounds (41).

Sevoflurane reacts with the material in CO_2 absorbers to form a vinyl chloride called Compound A, which produces renal tubular necrosis in laboratory animals (41). The majority of human studies show that there is no clinical degradation in renal function even after prolonged exposure to low-flow sevoflurane anesthesia (42,43). In patients with impaired renal function, it would seem prudent to limit exposure to sevoflurane and use high fresh gas flow rates, which will "wash out" the compound from the anesthesia breathing circuit.

PIAs and nitrous oxide are known triggering agents for malignant hyperthermia. Epinephrine, beta-adrenergic receptor agonists, and theophylline can cause arrhythmias in the presence of halothane. The myocardial depressant activity of inhaled anesthetics is increased in the presence of beta-blockers and calcium channel blockers.

Nitrous oxide

Nitrous oxide is a relatively insoluble gas that is primarily used to supplement the PIAs in GA. It is used alone for analgesia in labor and outpatient procedures such as flexible sigmoidoscopy, colonoscopy, and dental procedures (44,45). The primary danger in using nitrous oxide is *hypoxia* that results from either using excess amounts of nitrous oxide or through diffusion. During recovery from anesthesia using nitrous oxide, large amounts of the gas exit the blood and "flood" the alveoli, displacing alveolar oxygen and CO_2. The patient can become hypoxic if supplemental oxygen is not provided along with adequate ventilatory support. The hypoxic ventilatory drive is blunted.

Nitrous oxide usually produces mild sympathetic stimulation when used with the PIAs but it can cause profound cardiovascular depression when used in an anesthetic technique primarily based on opioids. It may also cause myocardial depression and hypotension in patients with coronary artery disease (46). Nitrous oxide raises pulmonary vascular resistance and may increase pulmonary artery pressure in patients with pulmonary hypertension.

Nitrous oxide inactivates vitamin B_{12}, which is an important component of two biochemical reactions. In the first reaction, vitamin B_{12} acts as a cofactor in the formation of methionine, which is essential to DNA synthesis and to the maintenance of the myelin sheath in nerves. In the second reaction, a form of vitamin B_{12} functions as a cofactor in a reaction that forms succinyl coenzyme A, which is important for lipid and carbohydrate synthesis via the Krebs cycle. Patients can develop megaloblastic anemia, bone marrow depression, and neurologic problems after either prolonged exposure to or chronic inhalation of nitrous oxide (47,48). Persons who have vitamin B_{12} deficiency from any cause, including pernicious anemia, terminal ileum resection, or subtotal gastrectomy, are especially at risk of serious neurological deterioration even after a single anesthetic with nitrous oxide. Neurological manifestations are similar to vitamin B_{12} deficiency and may be reversed by vitamin B_{12} therapy (47). Patients who intentionally abuse the gas are also at risk of anemia and neurologic disease. Nitrous oxide exposure is an occupational hazard to operating room personnel but the exact extent of the risk is not well established (49).

Nitrous oxide diffuses into gas filled spaces in the body more quickly than nitrogen diffuses out. Thus, it can cause expansion of these spaces and cavities. Animal studies performed 40 years ago demonstrated that anesthesia with nitrous oxide caused expansion of air pockets within the pleural space (50). Bowel distension, tension pneumothorax, blindness after vitrectomy, venous air embolism, and hearing loss have all been reported to occur during, and owing to, anesthesia with nitrous oxide (51–53). Interestingly, there is very little literature to support the contention that nitrous oxide definitely causes clinically significant bowel distention. In fact, one randomized trial comparing operative conditions with and without nitrous oxide for laparoscopic cholecystectomy failed to demonstrate any detectable difference (54).

Anesthesia delivery systems

The anesthesia machine consists of several components that are specified in the current anesthesia gas machine (workstation) standard ASTM F1850 promulgated by the American Society for Testing and Materials. At a minimum, the machine functions as a gas delivery system by providing a method of metering and delivering oxygen, dosing and delivering PIAs, and delivering controlled mechanical ventilation. In addition, the modern machine incorporates a wide variety of safety mechanisms, monitors, and alarms that are designed to alert the anesthetist to malfunction or operation that is out normal parameters. A variety of physiologic monitors, computers, cabling, drug delivery systems, suction devices, and other adjuvants may be attached or incorporated into the machine (Fig. 12.2).

The gas delivery system controls the flow of oxygen, air, and nitrous oxide from wall connections or gas cylinders. The vaporizers meter vapor from PIAs and blend the vapors with the fresh gas flow. The fresh gas flow enters the breathing circuit, which may or may not recirculate exhaled gases through a CO_2 scavenging system. During controlled ventilation, a mechanical ventilator controls delivery of gas to the patient. Thus, the gas delivery system in the anesthesia machine serves a critical function in delivering oxygen and anesthetic gases to the patient while also providing adequate ventilation and CO_2 removal.

Serious patient injuries, including death and brain injury, have resulted from misuse or failure of anesthesia gas delivery equipment. Other potential injuries include awareness, cardiovascular collapse, delayed recovery, and pneumothorax. In a study of closed claims, the breathing circuit was the most common source of injury followed by the vaporizers, ventilator, and the gas supply tank or line (55). Misconnect and disconnect of the breathing circuit were the most frequent initiating events. The two most common sites of disconnect were between the ETT and the circuit, and the ventilator and the breathing circuit. Half of the cases involved inadequate oxygenation as a result of disconnects, oxygen supply errors, and failures to turn on the ventilator. Misuse of equipment, defined as fault or error associated with the preparation, maintenance, or deployment of a medical device, was much more frequent than equipment failure.

Contemporary monitoring guidelines now mandate the use of devices to assure adequate oxygenation and ventilation. Some of the cases included in the analysis of closed claims occurred well before the widespread adoption of pulse oximetry and end-tidal CO_2 detection and 53% of claims were judged to be preventable if pulse oximetry, capnography, or both had been used (55). Therefore, minimal monitoring should reduce the incidence of these events, if appropriately applied.

Medications

Intravenous Anesthetics, Sedatives

The ideal IV anesthetic should provide hypnosis, amnesia, and analgesia with rapid onset, rapid elimination with minimal or no side effects. Unfortunately, an ideal IV anesthetic does not exist but several medications play an important role as adjuncts in balanced anesthesia. Several of the IV anesthetics are also used at lower doses for short-term or long-term sedation.

The barbiturates (thiopental, methohexital, and thiamylal) have a rapid and short action. They are some of the standard drugs used to induce anesthesia. They enhance and mimic the action of gamma amino butyric acid (GABA) at the GABA receptor in the central nervous system (CNS). The primary cardiovascular effect is venodilation and pooling of blood in the periphery. Blood pressure and cardiac output can drop due to decreased venous return (56). Hypotension can be severe in patients with impaired cardiac function, hypovolemia, adrenocortical insufficiency, uremia, or sepsis. The barbiturates are potent respiratory depressants; the degree of respiratory depression depends on the dose and rate of injection and presence of other medications. An induction dose that renders a patient unconscious will cause apnea. Smaller doses may leave the patient in a light plane of anesthesia and susceptible

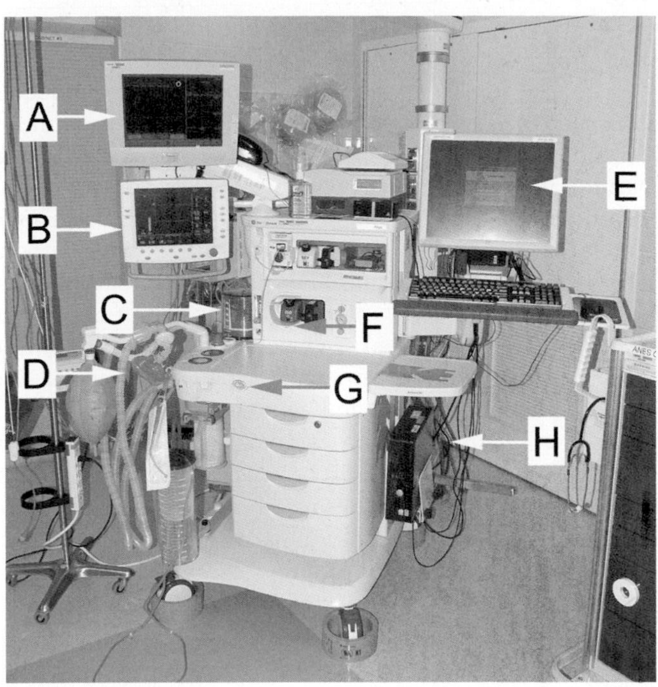

FIGURE 12.2. The anesthesia machine. It is almost always located at the head of the operating room table on the patient's right-hand side. A modern anesthesia workstation ("machine") typically includes the following components (letters in parenthesis correspond with labeled arrows on the photograph).

- **Pipeline gas supply (H)**—Gases from the hospital medical gas system provide oxygen, nitrous oxide, and air. The machine must preferentially use pipeline gas as long as pipeline pressure is greater than 345 kPa (50 psi).
- **Oxygen flush (C)**—A high-flow oxygen flush is present, which does not proceed through any vaporizers and provides pure oxygen at 35–75 L/min.
- **Flow meters (rotameters) for oxygen, air, and nitrous oxide (B)**—The flow meters allow the anesthetist to provide accurate mixtures of medical gases to the patient. Increasingly, flow meters, which were previously mechanical and pneumatic, are digital, electromagnetic devices.
- **Anesthetic vaporizers (F)**—The anesthetic vaporizer is concentration calibrated for a specific agent. It is filled with liquid anesthetic via a keyed-filler device. The vaporizer accurately adds volatile anesthetic vapor in a precise amount to the fresh gas flow.
- **Ventilator (C)**—Modern ventilators are capable of providing a number of ventilation modes. The breathing circuit can also be manually inflated by a handbag.
- **Physiological monitors (A)**—These systems display, monitor, and record the patient's heart rate, ECG, noninvasive blood pressure and oxygen saturation, end-tidal CO_2, temperature. In addition, arterial blood pressure, central venous pressure, pulmonary artery pressure, cardiac output, bispectral index, etc., can be displayed and monitored.
- **System monitors (B)**—A number of other parameters are monitored continuously including the exhaled volume, inflation pressure, inspired oxygen concentration, the composition of the gases delivered to the patient (and breathed out).
- **Breathing circuit (D)**—The breathing circuit is commonly a circle system that incorporates one-way valves and a CO_2 absorber. The circle system passes exhaled gas through the CO_2 absorber and back into the inspiratory limb allowing for conservation of anesthetic vapor (gas).
- **Suction apparatus**
- **Anesthesia information system (E)**—This optional system provides automated record keeping, rules-based prompts, and access to other hospital information systems.

Other (safety) features not illustrated

- **Reserve gas cylinder(s)**—The machine must have at least one reserve gas cylinder of oxygen connected by a pin-indexed (specific) hanger yoke. Newer machines may only have oxygen reserve cylinders but many other machines have cylinders of nitrous oxide and air as well.
- **Scavenging system**—Scavenging systems remove expired anesthetic gases from the operating room. Scavenged gases are usually vented to the outside atmosphere.
- **Alarm systems**—There are numerous alarms built into the machine and grouped into high, medium, and low priority. Mandatory alarms that are automatically enabled include breathing circuit pressure, oxygen concentration, exhaled volume, and/or exhaled CO_2. Other alarms include disconnect, oxygen supply failure, and low inspired oxygen concentration.
- **Hypoxic guard system**—It protects against less than 21% inspired oxygen if nitrous oxide is in use.
- **Pressure gauges, regulators, and "pop-off" valves**—These components protect the patient and machine from high pressure.
- **Checklist**—The machine checklist guides the operator through a series of steps designed to check the machine for proper set up and function. The checklist may be electronic or on paper, to be filled out manually by the user.
- **Digital interface**—The digital interface transfers data about the operating parameters of the system to the electronic medical record and/or diagnostic equipment.
- **Battery backup**—It is capable of providing several minutes of operation in the absence of electricity from a wall connection.

to laryngospasm, coughing, or bronchospasm during airway stimulation, such as placement of an oral airway or mask ventilation.

The barbiturates can cause serious tissue damage if the medication extravasates during IV injection or is accidentally injected intra-arterially. Thiobarbiturates induce release of histamine from mast cells; an urticarial rash on the upper body and arms is not uncommon but true anaphylactic reactions are unusual (57). Patients may experience delirium, prolonged somnolence and recovery, and headache after their anesthetic especially if they are given high doses of barbiturates during short procedures. Barbiturates can precipitate acute abdominal pain, vomiting, tachycardia, hypertension, fever, confusion, seizures, paralysis, and even death in patients with various types of porphyria (58). In general, barbiturates are contraindicated in patients with porphyria and there are several alternatives available.

Benzodiazepines are a mainstay in contemporary anesthesia because of their hypnotic and amnestic properties combined with a low incidence of side effects. Midazolam is probably the most frequently used drug in the class. Midazolam causes a mild decrease in blood pressure, peripheral vascular resistance, and cardiac output when used alone. When midazolam is combined with other medications, especially the synthetic opioids, hypnosis, respiratory depression, and hypotension can be profound (59,60). The synergistic effect of midazolam and fentanyl or alfentanil has been exploited for induction of anesthesia in day surgery (61). Even when used alone for conscious sedation, midazolam alone can cause respiratory depression.

Etomidate is a substituted imidazole, like ketoconazole, that is used as an IV sedative-hypnotic to induce anesthesia. It can cause pain on injection, phlebitis, myoclonic movements, nausea, vomiting, and adrenocortical suppression. Nausea and vomiting are especially common (62). A major disadvantage of etomidate is its inhibition of cortisol and mineralocorticoid synthesis in the adrenal glands. This was first noted in the mid-1980s when increased mortality was reported in patients sedated with continuous infusions of etomidate (63). Both a single dose and continuous infusion of etomidate inhibit two mitochondrial cytochrome P-450-dependent enzymes, which, in turn, inhibits adrenal steroid production (64,65). On the other hand, etomidate is generally associated with cardiovascular stability and preserved blood pressure during induction (66). Unfortunately, cardiovascular stability is not assured in all patients (67).

Propofol can cause pain on injection, cough, hiccups, involuntary skeletal muscle movements, and seizure-like episodes. Propofol causes less nausea and vomiting than thiopental. Like the barbiturates, propofol is a respiratory depressant and causes apnea with induction and decreased tidal volume with preserved respiratory rate during maintenance (68). Propofol usually causes a drop in blood pressure during induction of anesthesia due to vasodilation and decreased cardiac output from myocardial depression (69–71). In patients with coronary artery disease, propofol can cause cardiovascular depression and hypotension. Propofol is supplied as an aqueous emulsification of soybean oil, glycerol, and egg phosphatide and it supports microbial growth at room temperature (72). Originally, propofol was preservative-free but it now comes in formulations that retard microbial growth. Epidemiologic studies have suggested that propofol, poor aseptic technique, and mishandling of this medication have contributed to postoperative infections but there is considerable controversy over whether there is a true causal relationship (73–76). In response to these case reports, studies and concerns, the manufacturer and the FDA conducted an extensive education campaign and the package insert was changed. The insert now warns about the potential for infection and provides recommendations for proper methods to reduce this risk (77). Unfortunately, infectious complications related to propofol continue to occur. In 2010, a Las Vegas jury awarded plaintiffs a $500 million judgment against the manufacturers of propofol for an alleged outbreak of hepatitis C related to improper reuse of single-dose vials of propofol across multiple patients. This outbreak was attributed to unsafe injection practices on the part of anesthesia personnel who were administering propofol to patients undergoing sedation for endoscopy procedures (78,79).

The term "propofol infusion syndrome" has been used to describe a rare syndrome of cardiac failure, rhabdomyolysis, severe metabolic acidosis, and renal failure occurring in critically ill children and adults receiving high dose, long-term propofol infusions (80). It is likely that propofol impairs free fatty acid utilization and mitochondrial activity leading to an imbalance between energy demand and utilization. In some patients with critical illnesses, propofol, along with glucocorticoids and catecholamines, can lead to necrosis of cardiac and skeletal muscle.

Ketamine is a unique IV anesthetic because it provides sedation, amnesia, analgesia, and anesthesia. Ketamine is classified as an antagonist of the N-methyl-D-aspartate (NMDA) receptor but it also binds to opioid receptors. In vivo, ketamine increases heart rate, blood pressure, and pulmonary artery pressure by increasing sympathetic tone (81). Ketamine produces its sympathomimetic action through direct stimulation of CNS structures. Administration of ketamine can result in hypotension and myocardial depression in chronically ill patients with depleted catecholamine stores. Airway reflexes are usually maintained but obstruction and apnea can occur. Oropharyngeal secretions can be increased. Ketamine is a potent cerebral vasodilator that can increase intracranial pressure (ICP). Ketamine is notorious for causing psychic disturbances and emergence delirium, which can occur in 15% to 30% of patients. These disturbances are described as extracorporeal (out-of-body) experiences, floating sensations, vivid dreams, and frank delirium (82). Administering benzodiazepines along with ketamine reduces the incidence of postanesthesia emergence reactions and adverse cardiovascular reactions.

Neuromuscular Blocking Agents

Muscle relaxation during anesthesia can be accomplished with a variety of methods and medications. Inhalational anesthesia works at the level of the spinal cord to inhibit movement to noxious stimulation. Local anesthetics are used during neuraxial blockade at the level of the spinal cord or peripherally with nerve blocks to block transmission along motor nerves as well as sensory nerves. Finally, neuromuscular blocking (NMB) drugs work at the level of the neuromuscular junction to interrupt transmission between the nerve ending and the muscle. NMB drugs are indicated to facilitate endotracheal intubation, and to decrease muscle tone during GA to improve surgical working conditions.

It must be emphasized that NMB drugs have no intrinsic analgesic, hypnotic, or amnestic properties. These medications cause complete apnea and cessation of spontaneous breathing. Use of NMB drugs is indicated only if a means of artificial ventilation is available and feasible.

There are two major classes of muscle relaxants: depolarizing and nondepolarizing muscle relaxants. Regardless of their classification, all muscle relaxants work by binding to, and interacting with, prejunctional and postjunctional nicotinic acetylcholine receptors at the neuromuscular junction. NMB drugs also bind to rare extrajunctional nicotinic receptors, which are located on the muscle fibers away from the neuromuscular junction. Depolarizing muscle relaxants mimic acetylcholine at the postjunctional receptors, causing prolonged depolarization. Depolarization of the postjunctional receptors causes muscle contractions that are quickly replaced by flaccid paralysis, called phase I block. There is only one depolarizer in clinical use today, succinylcholine. It has a rapid onset and brief duration of action making it a good drug in situations where tracheal intubation must be performed rapidly after induction of anesthesia or where brief relaxation is desirable.

Succinylcholine generally causes an increase in the serum potassium of 0.5 to 1.0 mEq/L. There are certain pathologic conditions where the rise in potassium can be much greater. In certain conditions, like upper motor neuron disease (stroke, spinal cord injury), lower motor neuron disease, muscle disease (disuse atrophy, certain muscular dystrophies), muscle injury, and burns, there can be a proliferation of extrajunctional receptors. If succinylcholine is administered to a patient with one of these conditions, hyperkalemia may result from efflux of potassium through depolarized extrajunctional receptors. Schow et al. retrospectively reviewed the records from 40,000 anesthetics to evaluate the outcome following the administration of succinylcholine to hyperkalemic patients. The found no increased morbidity or mortality despite a consistent rise in the serum potassium (83). Thapa and Brull thoroughly reviewed the issue of use of succinylcholine in the setting of renal failure and concluded that it could be used safely as long as the preoperative potassium level was within normal range, there was no neuropathy, and the dose of succinylcholine was not repeated (84).

Some patients do not metabolize succinylcholine normally and they have a prolonged response to the drug. Four percent of patients have an abnormal gene that controls the quantity and quality of the enzyme that degrades succinylcholine, plasma cholinesterase. About 0.04% of patients are homozygous for this atypical gene and will have a very prolonged neuromuscular block following administration of succinylcholine. Decreased levels of plasma cholinesterase and prolonged blockade may also be seen in patients with severe liver disease and in peripartum patients.

Patients who receive succinylcholine may report postoperative myalgias and generalized muscle pain, which has been described as being similar to the pain experienced after intense physical exercise. The incidence of succinylcholine-induced myalgias is varyingly reported from 1.5% to 89% (85). It usually appears on the first postoperative day and is located in the neck, shoulders, and upper abdominal muscles. Although it would seem that intense fasciculations are the direct cause of myalgias, the exact etiology of the discomfort is unknown and probably complex (85). A number of strategies have been tried in efforts to reduce or abolish this adverse effect of succinylcholine include pretreatment with lidocaine or a small dose nondepolarizing neuromuscular blocking agent (NMBA). A meta-analysis of a large number of studies revealed that the most effective therapy was pretreatment with 1.5 mg/kg of lidocaine (86).

Succinylcholine causes a mean intraocular pressure (IOP) increase of 4 to 7 mm Hg due to tonic contraction of extraocular muscles. Crying, Valsalva maneuvers, coughing, and cricoid pressure all raise the IOP at least as much and perhaps more (87). It is a common belief among many anesthesiologists that succinylcholine is relatively contraindicated for induction in patients with open globe injury because of the fear of causing extrusion of vitreous contents (87). Yet, there are no reports of eye damage after rapid sequence induction of anesthesia with thiopental and succinylcholine. Furthermore, a variety of studies have compared the change in IOP after succinylcholine with other nondepolarizing muscle relaxants and found little or no difference (88,89). A group of investigators developed a trauma model in the cat eye to investigate the effects of succinylcholine and they found that the only observable effect of succinylcholine administration was forward displacement of the lens and iris and that no intraocular content was lost in any case (90). Thus, the proscription against the use of succinylcholine in open globe emergencies appears to be based more on theoretical concerns than evidence. As one editorialist wrote, "The benefits (of succinylcholine) are real, the risks unproven" (91). The origin and history of this dogma have been recently reviewed (92).

Other side effects of succinylcholine include increased ICP, increased intragastric pressure, and bradycardia (93). Succinylcholine is a trigger of malignant hyperthermia in susceptible patients.

cardiac arrest with electrical standstill as a part of bupivacaine toxicity. Many of these cases were reported in young healthy parturients receiving bupivacaine epidural anesthesia and/or analgesia for labor and were associated with difficult, prolonged, and occasionally futile resuscitation (132). Development and recovery from block differs between bupivacaine and lidocaine, helping to explain the greater cardiac toxicity with bupivacaine (135). Lidocaine blocks channels in a "fast-in, fast-out" fashion, allowing recovery of the sodium channel for a portion of the cardiac cycle. Bupivacaine, on the other hand, blocks sodium channels in a "slow-in, slow-out" manner at low concentrations, and a "fast-in, slow-out" manner at high concentrations. Thus, bupivacaine blocks the sodium channels throughout the cardiac cycle leaving no opportunity for sodium channel recovery.

Clinically, tachycardia and hypertension accompany CNS toxicity. As blood levels of local anesthetics continue to rise, there is myocardial depression, hypertension, and decreased cardiac output. At even higher blood levels, peripheral vasodilation, profound hypotension, conduction abnormalities, sinus bradycardia and ventricular arrhythmias lead to cardiovascular collapse. Hypoxemia and acidosis often accompany seizures and cardiovascular collapse and can potentiate local anesthetic-induced myocardial depression.

Cardiovascular toxicity is influenced by a number of factors. The ratio between doses that cause cardiovascular toxicity and central nervous toxicity varies with each local anesthetic (136). For example, the cardiovascular toxicity to CNS toxicity ratio is lower with bupivacaine than for lidocaine. Interestingly, the mechanisms of lethal toxicity appear to differ among local anesthetics in both conscious and anesthetized subjects. For example, IV bupivacaine is more likely to produce death by the sudden onset of lethal dysrhythmias, while IV lidocaine is more likely to produce death through progressive myocardial depression and contractile failure. In animals, IV ropivacaine and levobupivacaine have produced fatalities by either mechanism, and it is not yet clear what makes one outcome more likely than the other in individual cases (137).

Both the CNS effects and cardiovascular effects are primarily associated with high levels of local anesthetic in the blood. Besides the specific local anesthetic and total local anesthetic dose, a variety of other factors influence the likelihood and severity of LAST, including individual patient risk factors, concurrent medications, location and technique of the block, timeliness of detection, and adequacy of treatment. LAST can occur secondary to tissue absorption of a large amount of local anesthetic. Acute toxicity can also be caused by accidental intravascular injection of a submaximal dose, occasionally intra-arterial but more commonly IV. Unfortunately, it is very difficult to establish a maximal dose for each local anesthetic even though such information is available in textbooks (Table 12.7) (138,139). Furthermore, many episodes of LAST are due to unintentional intravascular injection of a submaximal dose rather than uptake of excessive doses from regional blockade

Table **12.7** Toxicity of local anesthetics

Drug	Maximum Dose	Equieffective Concentration	Toxic Plasma Concentration (μg/mL)
Lidocaine	4 mg/kg 300–500 mg	1% (10 mg/mL)	>5
Bupivacaine	2 mg/kg 175–200 mg	0.25% (2.5 mg/mL)	1.5

Note: A 1% solution contains 10 milligrams per milliliter.

(140). For example, even a small amount of drug injected into an artery supplying the brain will cause seizures. The site of injection and the presence of vasoconstrictors affect toxicity, also. In general, epinephrine decreases the peak plasma concentration of local anesthetic after it is injected but the magnitude of this affect depends on both the local anesthetic and the site of injection (141). Finally, there are variations in the response of individual patients to different doses of local anesthetics. Readers are referred to an excellent review on this topic (139).

The current American Society of Regional Anesthesia (ASRA) practice advisory emphasizes the importance of prevention in reducing the frequency and severity of LAST (Table 12.8). The practice advisory lists a number of methods to reduce the likelihood of LAST, recognizing that there is not a single measure that can prevent LAST in clinical practice. The lowest effective dose of local anesthetic should be used, and the injection of relatively large volumes of local anesthetic should be done in increments reducing the potential toxic dose if it is inadvertently injected intravascularly. Avoiding, or rapidly detecting, an unintentional intravascular injection is central to preventing serious toxicity. Intravascular injection may be detected by incremental aspiration after positioning the needle or catheter and by adding an intravascular marker to the local anesthetic. An intravascular "test dosing" remains the most reliable marker of intravascular injection. Ten to fifteen micrograms per milliliter of epinephrine added to the local anesthetic has a positive predictive value and a sensitivity of 80% in detecting intravascular injection in adults. Epinephrine test doses are unreliable in patients who are elderly, taking β-blockers, sedated, or anesthetized (132).

Ultrasound guidance of injection of local anesthetics and placement of infusion catheters may reduce the frequency of complications from regional anesthesia including intravascular injection but there are no trials that confirm or refute and actual reduction in the incidence of LAST (142).

Treatment priorities for LAST are outlined in the ASRA practice advisory and include airway management, circulatory support, and reducing the systemic effects of local anesthetics. Clearly, the success of any resuscitation effort depends on adequate preparedness that includes the

Table 12.8 Local Anesthetic Systemic Toxicity

For Patients Experiencing Signs or Symptoms of Local Anesthetic Systemic Toxicity (LAST)

- **Get Help**
- **Initial Focus**
  - **Airway management:** ventilate with 100% oxygen
  - **Seizure suppression:** benzodiazepines are preferred
  - **Basic and Advanced Cardiac Life Support (BLS/ACLS)** may require prolonged effort
- **Infuse 20% Lipid Emulsion (values in parenthesis are for a 70 kg patient)**
  - **Bolus 1.5 mL/kg** (lean body mass) intravenously over 1 min (~100 mL)
  - **Continuous infusion at 0.25 mL/kg/min** (~18 mL/min)
  - Repeat bolus once or twice for persistent cardiovascular collapse
  - Double the infusion rate to 0.5 mL/kg per minute if blood pressure remains low
  - **Continue infusion** for at least 10 min after attaining circulatory stability
  - Recommended upper limit: approximately 10 mL/kg lipid emulsion over the first 30 min
- **Avoid** vasopressin, calcium channel blockers, β-blockers, or local anesthetic
- **Alert** the nearest facility having cardiopulmonary bypass capability
- **Avoid propofol** in patients having signs of cardiovascular instability
- **Post LAST events** at www.lipidrescue.org and report use of lipid to www.lipidregistry.org

Adapted from the ASRA Practice Advisory on Treatment of Local Anesthetic Systemic Toxicity. For more complete recommendations, see Table 4 of reference (142).

availability of properly trained staff and equipment to provide basic and advanced life support. Systemic toxicity must be rapidly diagnosed recognizing that CNS and cardiac toxicity may present simultaneously or cardiac toxicity may occur in the absence of prodromal signs and symptoms of CNS toxicity. Isolated CNS toxic responses are best treated with rapid administration of supplemental oxygen, benzodiazepines or barbiturates, and supportive measures. Intubation and ventilation is rarely necessary for isolated CNS toxicity.

Cardiac toxicity usually requires aggressive and prolonged resuscitation measures and pharmacological support in accordance with Advanced Cardiac Life Support (ACLS) protocols. The practice advisory emphasizes the importance of immediate restoration of oxygenation and ventilation in facilitating successful resuscitation and halting the progression to cardiovascular collapse. Local anesthetic induced cardiac arrest requires rapid restoration of coronary perfusion pressure to improve myocardial contractility and maintain cardiac output. The practice advisory also recognizes the efficacy of lipid emulsion therapy in facilitating resuscitation, most probably by acting as a "lipid sink" that lowers the concentration of lipid-soluble local anesthetic within cardiac tissue thereby improving contractility, conduction, and coronary perfusion (142).

Lipid Emulsion Therapy for LAST

In addition, the advisory describes the use of intralipid as an antidote to LAST. Recently, numerous case reports and many animal studies have supported the use of IV lipid emulsion in cardiac toxicity that is refractory to conventional therapy. While studying the metabolic effects of bupivacaine, Weinberg et al. made the serendipitous observation that rats pretreated with a lipid soy bean emulsion were more resistant to the cardiac effects of bupivacaine than nontreated rats. Subsequent studies were performed to specifically investigate the effect of lipid emulsions on resuscitation from bupivacaine-induced cardiac toxicity. Cardiac arrest was induced in animals with a toxic dose of bupivacaine. Animals treated with a lipid emulsion during resuscitation were more likely to recover cardiac function. Small animal studies were supported by subsequent work in dogs. A large dose of bupivacaine (10 mL/kg) was injected as a bolus into dogs while under GA. Cardiac arrest was treated with open chest massage alone or in combination with an infusion of 20% lipid emulsion, given as a bolus followed by continuous infusion. All dogs developed cardiac toxicity as manifested by severe hypotension and bradycardia. All lipid treated animals were successfully resuscitated to normal hemodynamics while all control dogs died (143).

These encouraging results in animal studies have been supported by a number of case reports of successful resuscitation from refractory cardiac arrest after the administration of lipid emulsion. In one such case, a middle-aged man with heart disease suffered cardiac arrest shortly after placement of a brachial plexus block using bupivacaine and mepivacaine. The patient remained in asystole with intermittent ventricular tachycardia and ventricular fibrillation despite 20 minutes of standard ACLS, which included several countershocks and multiple doses of epinephrine, atropine, amiodarone, and vasopressin. Within minutes of an infusion of 100 mL of 20% Intralipid, the patient's heart started beating, and this was followed almost immediately by return of normal sinus rhythm and blood pressure. The patient recovered without neurological deficit.

Subsequent studies in animal models have shown conflicting results. For example, administration of lipid emulsion actually diminished the return of spontaneous circulation in rats subjected to nondrug-induced, hypoxic cardiac arrest. Mayr et al. compared the combination of vasopressin and epinephrine versus lipid emulsion in a porcine model of asphyxial, cardiac arrest following bupivacaine infusion. In their model, pigs received an infusion of 5 mg/kg of a 0.5% bupivacaine solution IV and ventilation was interrupted for approximately 2 minutes until asystole developed. After 2 minutes of cardiopulmonary resuscitation (CPR), 10 animals received, every 5 minutes, either vasopressin combined with epinephrine or 4 mL/kg of a 20% lipid emulsion. Vasopressor therapy resulted in higher coronary perfusion pressure during CPR and higher survival rates as compared to treatment with lipid emulsion. These studies suggest that hypoventilation and asphyxia resulting in hypoxemia, hypercarbia, and acidosis may blunt or negate the efficacy of lipid emulsion to reverse lipophilic drug-induced cardiac toxicity.

The exact mechanism of action of lipid emulsion in the reversal of local anesthetic toxicity is unknown. The two major proposed mechanisms of action are that the lipid emulsion may extract lipophilic local anesthetics from aqueous plasma or tissues or that it may counteract local anesthetic inhibition of myocardial fatty acid oxidation. Other advantages of lipid emulsion include apparent rapid reversal of cardiotoxicity (within 5 to 10 minutes), accessibility, and low cost. Many institutions and organizations have adopted guidelines that incorporate the use of lipid emulsion in these cases. The use of propofol, which is formulated in a lipid emulsion, as an antidote for local anesthetic-induced cardiac toxicity is now discouraged because of the myocardial depressant effects of propofol. Finally, it should be noted that lipid emulsion may have efficacy in treating cardiac toxicity from other medications including, clomipramine, propranolol, and verapamil.

Local Anesthetic Tissue Toxicity

In addition to systemic toxicity, local anesthetics (LAs) are implicated in local injury to the central and peripheral nervous system from direct exposure of these tissues to injected formulation. There are a variety of proposed mechanisms for LA-induced neurotoxicity including increased permeability of the mitochondrial membrane, collapse of mitochondrial membrane potential, and decrease in adenosine triphosphate production by either uncoupling of oxidative phosphorylation or inhibition of complex I of the mitochondrial respiratory chain (144). Clinically, the spinal cord and nerve roots appear to be more prone to the toxic effects of LAs than the peripheral nerves. Animal studies suggest that lidocaine and tetracaine may be especially neurotoxic in a dose-dependent fashion. On the other hand, *in vitro* experiments with human neuroblastoma cells demonstrated that bupivacaine and ropivacaine had greater killing potency than lidocaine (144). Transient neurologic symptoms (TNSs) after spinal anesthetic likely represent a variation of LA-induced neurotoxicity.

Experimentally, all local anesthetics, including cocaine, are potentially myotoxic. Experimental myotoxic effects of local anesthetics are characterized by hypercontracted myofibrils, followed by lytic degeneration of striated muscle sarcoplasmic reticulum, myocyte edema, and finally necrosis (145). These effects are intense and reproducible. Of the local anesthetics studied, bupivacaine and levobupivacaine produce the most severe muscle injury (146,147). Many anesthesiologists and pain physicians recognize that intramuscular injections of local anesthetics can result in clinically inapparent myonecrosis. The clinical impact of myotoxicity remains controversial. Most clinically relevant cases of myopathy and myonecrosis have been described in the setting of continuous peripheral nerve blocks, infiltration of wound margins, trigger-point injections, and periorbital and retrobulbar blocks. Transient or persistent diplopia can occur after cataract surgery when performed using a retrobulbar or peribulbar nerve block. While there are a number of potential mechanisms for this complication, in some cases diplopia is believed to be due to direct damage to the inferior rectus muscle from local anesthetic (148).

Postarthroscopic glenohumeral chondrolysis is a devastating, noninfectious complication of arthroscopic shoulder surgery. In addition to radiofrequency ablation, this complication is associated with intra-articular injection of bupivacaine via a pain pump. Presumably, bupivacaine is chondrotoxic although research on this matter is unclear (149).

Complications of neuraxial anesthesia

Neuraxial anesthesia (also known as central neuraxial blockade) includes spinal, epidural, and caudal techniques. These techniques involve deposition of local anesthetics, opioids, and/or other adjuvant medications in the spinal canal, epidural space, or caudal epidural space. Various techniques may or may not utilize a catheter for prolonged or continuous drug administration.

Postdural Puncture Headache

Postdural puncture headache (PDPH), ocular disturbances, and auditory difficulties constitute a syndrome associated with cerebrospinal fluid leak and decreased ICP following dural puncture (150). The most prominent and common symptom of this syndrome is bilateral, frontal, or occipital headache that is relieved when the patient is supine. Needle penetration of the dura results in a leak of cerebrospinal fluid, which leads to intracranial hypotension. Loss of cerebrospinal fluid allows the brain to drop caudad when the patient is upright, resulting in traction on the dura, which causes pain. The size of the defect and the incidence of PDPH are related to needle gauge, bevel design, orientation of the bevel, and angle of approach on insertion (151). Other factors that increase the incidence of PDPH include youth, female sex, pregnancy, dehydration, and prior history of PDPH (152). The use of small-gauge, noncutting spinal needles and refinement in technique has reduced the incidence of PDPH to 0.4% from 2% (153).

PDPH is usually benign and self-limited but in severe cases, the headache may be incapacitating and treatment is indicated. Many treatments have been proposed for PDPH but the most effective by far is the epidural blood patch, which provides relief in 90% of patients after one patch (154,155). A second patch provides relief in another 8% of patients. The epidural blood patch is performed by aseptically transferring 8 to 15 mL of autologous blood to the epidural space at the level of the dural puncture. Magnetic resonance imaging of the lumbar region after a blood patch confirms that the hematoma causes a mass effect around the injection site that compresses the thecal sac (156). Mass effect was present at 30 minutes and 3 hours but the clot had resolved by 7 hours. There was extensive extravasation of blood into the surrounding subcutaneous tissues, which may explain the most common side effect of blood patch, backache.

Backache

Transient minor backache is common after epidural (incidence of 30%) and spinal anesthesia (incidence of 21%) but is not necessarily causally related to the anesthetic technique (157). A prospective evaluation of women found that postpartum back pain was associated with antepartum back pain, greater weight, and younger age (158). The incidence was essentially the same (45%) in women who had received epidural anesthesias and in those who had not. An magnetic resonance imaging (MRI) study on volunteers demonstrated two potential sources for back pain in the lithotomy position, flattening of the lumbar lordosis, and added tension on the lumbosacral nerve roots (159). Serious, protracted back pain is rare after central neuraxial blockade and is most often due to trauma from needle insertion. Spinal or epidural needles may injure the intraspinous ligament or patients may develop spasm of the paraspinous muscles. Abrupt, postoperative onset of back pain with a radicular component or neurologic signs may indicate the development of spinal hematoma and immediate investigation is warranted.

Urinary Retention

Postoperative urinary retention is very common and is associated with all types of anesthesia and surgery (160). Difficulty in urinating can be from any number or combination of causes including overdistention of the bladder, pain-induced reflex spasm of the urethral sphincters, trauma to the pelvic nerves or bladder, and pharmacologic effects. It is more common in elderly men and in patients receiving opiates (161). In a large review of published studies of urinary retention in inguinal hernia surgery, the authors found that the incidence is lower with local anesthesia (0.4%) than with regional (2.4%) or general (3.0%) (162). Spinal anesthesia rapidly eliminates the micturition reflex and it does not return until after motor and most sensory function has recovered. Patients should be monitored for return of bladder function, especially with long-acting local anesthetics. Urinary retention after epidural anesthesia seems to be related more to the epidural administration of opioids than the LA.

Transient Neurologic Symptoms

TNSs, consisting of a back pain or dysesthesia with bilateral radiation into the buttocks or legs, have been described as a complication of spinal anesthesia, especially when performed with lidocaine (150). Symptoms begin after total recovery from spinal anesthesia and within 24 hours of surgery. The incidence of this complication may be as high as 36% depending on the type of surgery performed; the incidence is highest for procedures performed in the lithotomy position and lowest for those performed while the patient is supine (163). Incidence does not vary with the concentration of lidocaine used in the spinal anesthetic (164). While the etiology of TNS is not known, most authorities feel that symptoms are due primarily to a direct toxic effect of the local anesthetic. An important contributing factor may be local ischemia from nerve stretch. The clinical implications of TNS are still unclear but some practitioners avoid using lidocaine for spinal anesthetics, especially if the procedure will be performed in the lithotomy position (157).

Spinal Hematoma and Abscess

The most dreaded complication of neuraxial blockade, paraplegia from spinal hematoma or epidural abscess, is extremely rare (165). Meta-analysis of data from large retrospective studies suggests an incidence of spinal hematoma of 1:150,000 after epidural anesthesia and 1:220,000 after spinal anesthesia (166). In a comprehensive analysis of case reports between 1906 and 1994, Vandermeulen et al. found only 61 published cases of epidural and/or subdural hematoma involving central neuraxial blockade and 42 of these occurred in patients with a clotting disorder or who were using anticoagulants (165). Risk factors for hematoma formation following neuraxial blockade include full anticoagulation at the time of the procedure, coagulopathy (factor deficiency, thrombocytopenia, disseminated intravascular coagulopathy), and difficult needle or catheter placement (165). Epidural hematomas can occur spontaneously (the most common cause) or after diagnostic lumbar puncture followed by anticoagulation.

The most common site for hematoma formation is the epidural space, presumably because of traumatic disruption of the epidural venous plexus. Early symptoms include back pain or radicular pain but muscle weakness may be the first complaint (165). Neurologic symptoms of lower extremity weakness and bowel and bladder dysfunction develop once enough blood has accumulated to create a mass effect and compress the spinal cord or nerve roots. Vigilance, regular neurologic assessment, and expeditious diagnostic studies are necessary to detect spinal hematoma early enough to avoid permanent neurologic damage. Recovery of neurologic function is possible if decompressive laminectomy is performed within 8 hours of the onset of paraplegia.

The reported incidence of epidural abscess in neuraxial anesthesia varies widely depending on the study method but is generally low, between 1 in 2000 and 1 in 5000 catheters (167,168). Like spontaneous spinal hematoma, epidural abscess is more commonly reported from sources not related to epidural or spinal anesthesia. Abscess formation related to neuraxial blockade is believed to be due to introduction of bacteremic blood into the epidural space. Risk factors for infection and abscess formation include immunosuppression, bacteremia, caudal anesthesia, and breaks in aseptic technique. One recent survey of epidural abscesses found that half of incidents were associated with low molecular weight heparin (LMWH) therapy (168). In addition to back pain and neurological symptoms, patients with epidural abscess usually present with fever, leukocytosis, meningeal signs, and signs of localized infection. Not surprisingly, *Staphylococcus aureus* was the most common etiologic agent in one large series (167). Once the diagnosis has been established, prompt therapy with antibiotics and surgical evacuation should be performed in order to maximize the likelihood of neurologic recovery.

Anticoagulation and Neuraxial Blockade

A number of large case series in a variety of operative settings have established the safety of systemic anticoagulation following neuraxial blockade in select patients using strict guidelines (153,169). In general, patients without preexisting coagulopathy can receive IV heparin 60 minutes following atraumatic insertion of an epidural catheter without significant risk of hematoma. On the other hand, there is an increased risk for spinal hematoma in those patients where there was less than a 60-minute time interval between the administration of heparin and lumbar puncture, traumatic needle placement, and concomitant use of other anticoagulants (aspirin). In addition, there have been numerous reports of spinal hematoma developing after spinal or epidural anesthesia in patients receiving LMWH for perioperative thromboprophylaxis (166,170,171). Most of these cases involved epidural anesthesia and some were related to removal of the epidural catheter while receiving LMWH (172). The risk of fatal pulmonary embolus without prophylaxis is greater than the risk of spinal hematoma but that does not mean that effective thromboprophylaxis takes precedence over, and excludes, regional anesthesia (173). A consensus statement from the ASRA states that spinal or epidural anesthesia can be administered in the setting of heparinization or LMWH administration as long as certain precautions are heeded (174). A complete description of the current recommendations for evaluating and managing patients for regional anesthesia while receiving antithrombotic or thrombolytic therapy is available on the ASRA web site.

Nerve Injury

Several large retrospective studies have confirmed that permanent injury to the spinal cord or nerve roots is very uncommon (175). The most common neurologic complication of central blockade is damage to a nerve root from needle or catheter placement. Injury to the lumbosacral nerve root and the spinal cord accounted for 16% and 13% of closed claims related to nerve injuries, respectively, in the ASA's Closed Claims Project (176). In a prospective, multicenter study of serious complications of regional anesthesia, Auroy et al. found a low incidence of radiculopathy following spinal and epidural anesthesia (175). Needle insertion or drug injection was associated with pain or paresthesias in most cases. In contrast to the midline approach, the paramedian (oblique lateral) approach to the epidural and subarachnoid space directs the needle toward the dural cuff region of the nerve root, increasing the risk of injury.

Reynolds reported on a cluster of seven cases with persistent unilateral sensory loss, foot drop, and urinary symptoms (three patients) following spinal or combined spinal-epidural anesthesia. All had a painful lumbar puncture and six had MRI showing a syrinx in the conus. The authors pointed out that the termination of the conus is variable and emphasized the importance of performing the lumbar puncture at the correct level (177).

Spinal Cord Ischemia

The anterior portion of the spinal cord is supplied by the anterior spinal artery, which has poor vertical anastomotic connections between radicular branches that supply it. The anterior spinal cord is susceptible to ischemic injury if the segmental blood supply is compromised either through trauma or due to systemic reasons. The anterior spinal artery syndrome is characterized by a dense motor paralysis, variable sensory impairment, and preservation of position and vibratory sense. Injury to the anterior spinal artery has been reported with epidural catheter or needle placement but surgical disruption of the blood supply and/or systemic hypotension is much more likely a cause (178).

Bradycardia, Hypotension, and Cardiac Arrest

Hypotension is extremely common during neuraxial anesthesia and is better regarded as a side effect than a complication. Hypotension results from the preganglionic sympathetic block that reduces systemic vascular resistance and increases venodilation. Decreased venous return enhances vagal tone. High sympathectomy also results in bradycardia through blockade of the cardiac accelerator fibers, which arise from spinal levels T1 to T4. Decreased venous return, systemic hypotension and bradycardia can reduce cardiac output. Moderate and severe bradycardia occurs in about 10% and 1% of neuraxial anesthetics, respectively, and can develop at any time during the anesthetic (179). Risk factors for the development of hypotension and bradycardia during spinal and epidural anesthesia have been identified in large-scale prospective studies (Table 12.9) (180,181).

In the 1980s, review of closed insurance claims revealed a set of cases involving cardiac arrest during spinal anesthesia in otherwise healthy patients (182). The outcome in these cases was catastrophic; most patients died or had severe neurologic injury. Further evaluation of these cases suggested that sedation and respiratory insufficiency might

Table **12.9** **Risk factors for bradycardia and hypotension during central neuraxial blockade**

Technique	Risk Factors for Hypotension	Risk Factors for Bradycardia
Epidural anesthesia	• Epidural fentanyl • Increased spread of sensory blockade • Lack of tourniquet use • Use of carbonated lidocaine	• Female sex • Use of tourniquet
Spinal Anesthesia	• Sensory block higher than the fifth thoracic dermatome • Age older than 40 years • Baseline systolic blood pressure less than 120 mm Hg • Use of combined spinal and general anesthesia • Dural puncture cephalad to the L2–L3 interspace • Addition of phenylephrine to the local anesthetic spinal block	• Baseline heart rate less than 60 beats/min • ASA physical status I • Use of beta-adrenergic blocking agents • Sensory block higher than the fifth thoracic dermatome

have contributed to the cardiac arrest. Cardiopulmonary resuscitation in these witnessed cardiac arrests might have been ineffective due to the sympathetic blockade during high spinal anesthesia and delayed administration of potent vasoconstrictors. In large, prospective surveys of complications of regional anesthesia, cardiac arrest during spinal anesthesia occurred with an incidence of 2.7 to 7.0 per 10,000 (175,183,184). The incidence of cardiac arrest during spinal anesthesia is higher than that seen with GA and epidural anesthesia. Survivors of cardiac arrest were younger and were healthier as measured by ASA classification. Sedation, respiratory insufficiency, and especially severe bradycardia have been implicated as major contributing factors to cardiac arrest. Studies in human volunteers given spinal anesthetics have shown that hypovolemia potentiates the vagally mediated bradycardia and can even precipitate cardiac arrest (184). Other cases of bradycardia and cardiac arrest during spinal anesthesia have occurred after the addition of potent vasodilators such as sodium nitroprusside. Studies in dogs show that spinal anesthesia suppresses the catecholamine response to cardiac arrest and reduces the coronary perfusion pressure (CPP) that is obtained during CPR (185,186). The CCP achieved during CPR in spinal anesthetized dogs was significantly below the threshold for predicting successful resuscitation, and relatively high doses (0.1 mg/kg) of epinephrine were required to restore CPP (185). These studies help to explain why CPR may be ineffective in patients suffering cardiac arrest during spinal anesthesia and they suggest that high doses of vasopressors (epinephrine, norepinephrine, and/or vasopressin) may be required to restore CPP during CPR. In summary, severe bradycardia with hypotension should be treated rapidly with volume infusion, atropine, and vasopressors, preferably epinephrine (184). If cardiac arrest develops, CPR should be accompanied by early and aggressive administration of vasopressors.

Failed Block

Perhaps one of the most frequent "complications" of regional anesthesia is failure of the blockade. Entry into the epidural space is confirmed by tactile loss of resistance to pressure on the plunger of a syringe. This endpoint is subject to misinterpretation. Even with the visual clues of spinal technique (return of cerebrospinal fluid), failures occur in 4% to 17% of spinal anesthetics. The other extreme is total spinal anesthesia when an excessive dose of local anesthetic is delivered into the subarachnoid or subdural space. Patients are rendered apneic, unconscious, and hypotensive and require intubation, mechanical ventilation, and vasopressor support.

MISCELLANEOUS COMPLICATIONS OF ANESTHESIA

Postoperative nausea and vomiting

Postoperative nausea and vomiting (PONV) is anesthesiology's "big little problem" and a great deal of effort is focused on strategies to reduce the frequency of this problem. Nausea is an unpleasant sensation in the epigastrium that is associated with an urge to vomit while vomiting is the forceful expulsion of gastric contents. The incidence of nausea and vomiting varies depending on the patient population and setting but generally affects 10% of patients in the postoperative anesthesia care unit (PACU) and 30% of patients during the first 24 hours (187) (Fig. 12.5).

Vomiting is controlled by emetic centers that receive afferent input from many sources inside and outside the CNS. A major input is from the chemoreceptor trigger zone. Structures involved in vomiting are rich in dopaminergic, muscarinic, serotonergic, histaminic, and opioid receptors, which explains the basic approach of antagonizing various neurotransmitter receptors in order to control vomiting.

Recently, a multidisciplinary panel of experts published consensus guidelines on PONV based on a structured review of the medical literature (188). A great deal of useful information can be drawn from the conclusions reached by the expert panel and other authors who have reviewed this topic (187). A variety of factors are suspected to influence the occurrence of PONV including patient characteristics, site of surgery, duration of surgery, and type of anesthetic. A combination of factors may contribute to the occurrence of nausea, vomiting,

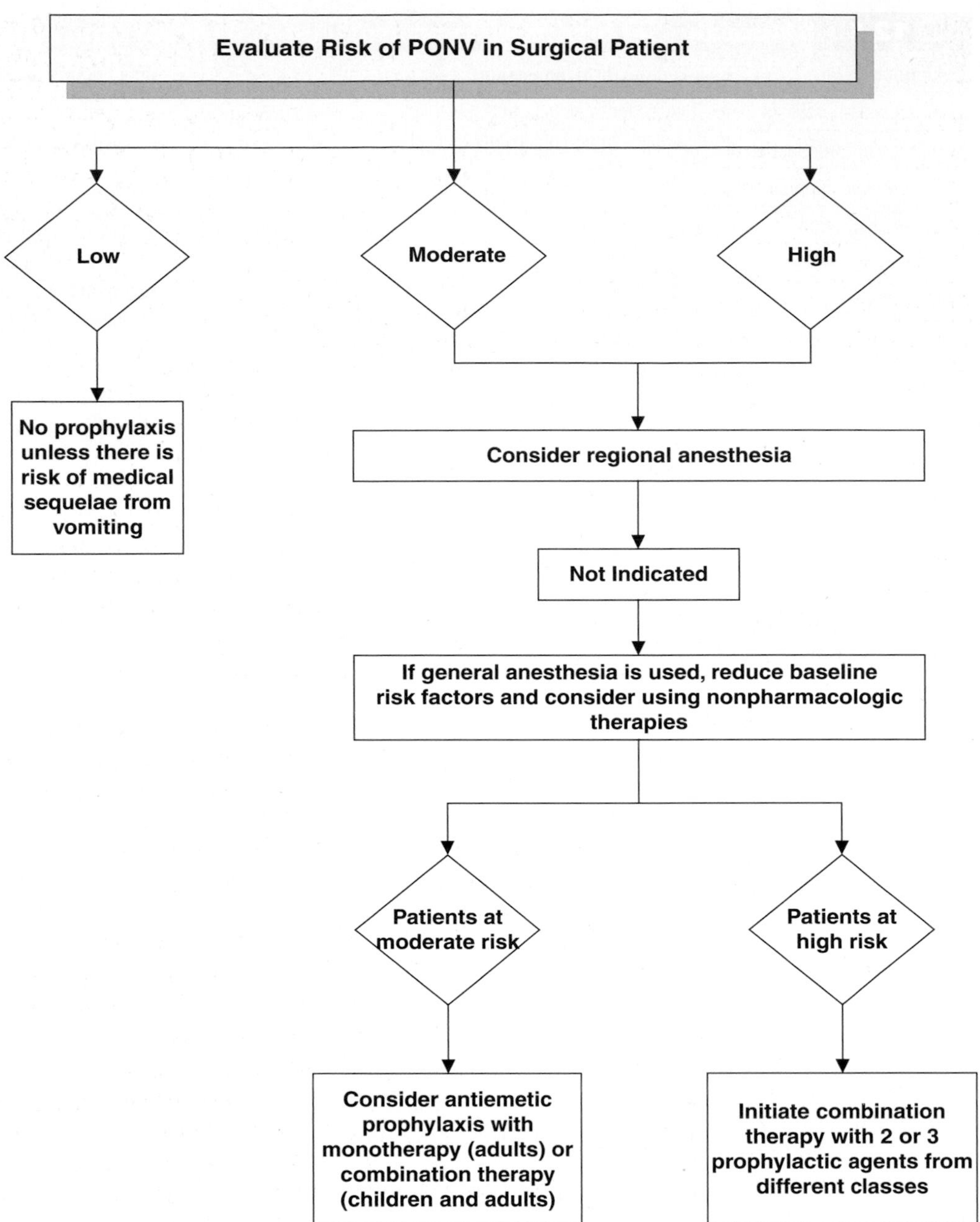

FIGURE 12.5. Algorithm for the management of postoperative nausea and vomiting. (Reprinted with permission from Gan TJ, Meyer T, Apfel CC, et al. Consensus guidelines for managing postoperative nausea and vomiting. *Anesth Analg* 2003;97(1):62–71.)

or both. For example, volatile anesthetics appear to be the most important cause of early vomiting in both children and adults but late vomiting seems to be due to postoperative opioids (189). The guidelines stress identifying patients at high risk for PONV. Risk factors for PONV in adults include female sex, nonsmoking status, a history of PONV or motion sickness, duration of surgery, type of surgery (laparoscopy, ear-nose-throat, neurosurgery, breast, strabismus, laparotomy, plastic surgery), use of volatile anesthetics, use of nitrous oxide, and use of opioids. Risk factors in children are similar to adults with the following differences, vomiting is twice as frequent in children, the risk increases as children age but decreases after puberty and sex differences are not seen before puberty. Surprisingly, smoking protects against PONV, perhaps through increased clearance of anesthetic drugs due to enzyme induction (190). Apfel et al. have created a simplified risk score based on identifying four primary risk factors: female sex, nonsmoking status, history of PONV, and opioid use (191). The incidence of PONV increases with the presence of one or more of these risk factors.

Strategies to reduce the baseline risk of PONV are listed in Table 12.10. There is no single "magic bullet" and the most effective strategy may be one that encompasses many or all of the methods listed. In certain high-risk patients, a multimodal approach consisting of anxiolysis, hydration, supplemental oxygen, prophylactic antiemetics, total IV anesthesia without nitrous oxide, and ketorolac, may be effective. The consensus guidelines suggest antiemetic therapy for prophylaxis in patients at moderate or high risk of PONV. There is no difference in the efficacy and safety profiles of the various serotonin (5-HT_3) receptor antagonists in the prophylaxis of PONV. These drugs have

Table **12.10** Strategies to reduce baseline risk of postoperative nausea and vomiting
Use regional anesthesia instead of general anesthesia
Use propofol for induction and maintenance of anesthesia
Intra-operative supplemental oxygen
Adequate hydration
Avoid nitrous oxide
Avoid volatile anesthetics
Minimize intra-operative and postoperative opioids
Minimize or eliminate use of neostigmine

a favorable side effect profile; the most common problems are headache, constipation, and increased liver function tests. To be most effective, 5-HT_3 receptor antagonists, like ondansetron, should be given at the end of surgery. Small doses of dexamethasone (2.5 to 5 mg) are effective in reducing PONV when given prior to induction of anesthesia. Although adverse events have not been reported in humans after a single bolus dose of dexamethasone, there is some evidence that a single dose can impair wound healing in rats (192). Droperidol is equally effective as ondansetron for prophylaxis of PONV and, like the 5-HT_3 receptor antagonists, is most effective when given at the end of surgery. The Food and Drug Administration (FDA) has issued a "black box" warning that droperidol may cause death or life-threatening events associated with QT prolongation and torsade de pointes but the warning is not well substantiated by the medical literature. The expert panel authoring the consensus guidelines expressed considerable concern about the validity of the FDA warning. Importantly, metoclopramide is not effective for PONV prophylaxis and has considerable side effects. Antiemetics should be given to those patients who develop PONV and were not given prophylaxis or in whom prophylaxis failed. Treatment doses of the 5-HT_3 receptor antagonists are one quarter of those used for prophylaxis. In those patients failing prophylaxis, drugs used to treat PONV should be from another class than the drugs used for prophylaxis. Interestingly, a small, subhypnotic dose of propofol (20 mg) is effective in treating PONV (193).

Obesity and morbid obesity

Obesity has now reached epidemic proportions in the United States and the health concerns of an obese population are being addressed in the lay press as well as the medical literature (194). The body mass index (BMI) is a measure of the relationship between height and weight and it is calculated by the formula:

$$\text{BMI} = \frac{\text{body weight (in kg)}}{\text{height}^2\text{ (in meters)}}$$

A BMI of <25 kg/m is normal while a person with a BMI of 25 to 30 kg/m is overweight. Persons with a BMI of >30, >35, and >55 kg/m are considered obese, morbidly obese, and super-morbidly obese, respectively, and have an increased risk of medical complications and increased mortality. Physiologic changes associated with obesity and morbid obesity lead to an increased incidence of comorbid conditions, such as gall bladder disease, diabetes, hypertension, heart disease, osteoarthritis, and obstructive sleep apnea (OSA) (195). Persons with a BMI >30 have an increased rate of mortality especially if they have an android (central or male) pattern of fat distribution or rapid weight gain after age 20.

Many of the pathophysiologic changes in obesity combine to increase the risk of complications during induction of anesthesia, maintenance of the airway, mask ventilation, intubation and extubation. A fat face and cheeks, a fat, short neck, large tongue, excess pharyngeal tissue, restricted mouth opening, and large breasts may make mask ventilation and intubation difficult or impossible. Mask ventilation and intubation are also difficult in many patients with OSA. While only 5% of morbidly obese patients have OSA, the majority of patients with OSA are obese (196). In obese patients with OSA, the pharyngeal area is reduced due to deposition of fat in the pharyngeal tissues and the airway is compressed externally by fat masses in the superficial neck area. All central depressants and muscle relaxants will promote pharyngeal collapse in obese patients with OSA by diminishing the action of the pharyngeal dilator muscles. Thus, obese patients with or without OSA are at risk of airway obstruction when given sedatives, anesthetics, or muscle relaxants. In a retrospective study of patients being surgically treated for OSA, the complication rate was 13%. Seventy-seven percent of these complications were airway problems (197). Patients with problems with intubation were heavier while patients experiencing problems following extubation had received more narcotic analgesia.

It is commonly believed that obese patients have increased intragastric volumes, increased intra-abdominal pressures, increased incidence of hiatal hernia, and increased incidence of gastroesophageal reflux, all of which may put them at higher risk of gastric regurgitation and aspiration during mask ventilation, intubation and extubation. Difficult mask ventilation may result in gastric insufflation, which further increases the risk of regurgitation and aspiration. Although the evidence for these risk factors is conflicting, many authors recommend taking routine precautions to prevent acid aspiration in obese patients (194).

In a large multicenter study of adverse outcomes after GA, obesity was one of several predictors of severe respiratory outcomes (198). Obesity causes abnormalities of both lung volumes and gas exchange that are exacerbated by the supine position and anesthesia. Functional residual capacity (FRC) and expiratory reserve volume (ERV) are reduced so that tidal volume may occur at or below closing capacity leading to closure of small airways, ventilation-perfusion mismatching, atelectasis, and arterial desaturation (194,199).

Pelosi et al. studied the effects of BMI on respiratory function during anesthesia in 24 patients (8 normal weight patients, 8 moderately obese patients, and 8 morbidly obese patients) (199). With increasing BMI, there was an exponential decline in FRC, an exponential decline in compliance of the respiratory system, an increase in resistance, an exponential decline in the oxygenation index (PaO_2/PAO_2) and an increase in the work of breathing (199). Increased basal metabolic rate and high resting oxygen consumption decreased FRC and altered oxygenation work in combination to drastically reduce the time it takes obese patients to desaturate during periods of hypoventilation or apnea. In general, obese patients desaturate rapidly after induction of anesthesia despite preoxygenation. In summary, morbidly obese patients may be very difficult to ventilate by mask, prone to rapid desaturation during apneic periods, difficult to intubate, and be at increased risk of acid aspiration. Therefore, many authorities recommend awake fiberoptic intubation for GA (194). Desaturation due to atelectasis during GA and mechanical ventilation is better treated with moderate levels of PEEP than with excessive tidal volumes.

Obese patients are prone to hypertension, and obesity is recognized as an independent risk factor for ischemic heart disease, especially in patients with a central, android distribution of fat. Obesity-induced cardiomyopathy refers to a condition where volume and pressure overload lead to heart failure, which is often biventricular. Increased blood volume and high cardiac output result in left ventricular enlargement and increased wall stress. Persistent, abnormally high wall stress promotes the development of eccentric hypertrophy, which results in left ventricular (LV) systolic dysfunction, diastolic dysfunction, and clinical heart failure. Pulmonary hypertension secondary to OSA may cause right ventricular enlargement, hypertrophy, and failure, as well. In an autopsy study of morbidly obese patients dying of sudden cardiac death, 10 of 22 patients had dilated cardiomyopathy, six had severe coronary artery disease, and four had LV hypertrophy without dilation (200).

Finally, obese patients may present challenges with respect to IV access, patient positioning, monitoring, and regional anesthesia. For example, noninvasive blood pressure cuffs often do not fit properly even if they are large size and it may be difficult or impossible to obtain an accurate blood pressure reading without direct arterial cannulation.

Independent of additional comorbid conditions, the physical state of obesity implies that patients are at increased risk of perioperative complications because of their excess weight and obese body habitus although there are few studies available to establish the precise impact of obesity on anesthesia and surgery (201). Of the studies that have looked at the question of whether or not obesity is an independent risk factor for adverse outcomes after surgery, few actually confirm any additional serious risk. In a multivariate single center study of 2299 patients undergoing cardiac surgery, 25% of patients were obese and 13% were severely obese, and, with the exception of superficial wound infections and atrial dysrhythmias, obesity was not a significant multivariate risk factor for adverse outcomes (202). In a similar study, Fasol et al. found that there was no difference in operative mortality between obese and nonobese cardiac surgery patients, but the former had higher rates of infection, sternal dehiscence, arrhythmias, and myocardial infarction (203). Choban and Flancbaum reviewed the literature for a number of elective surgical procedures and concluded that there was only a modest increase in perioperative complications, and these were mostly wound problems (201). Mortality was not increased and operative results were not adversely affected. On the other hand, obese patients had higher morbidity and mortality following trauma and burn surgery.

Hypothermia

While the human thermoregulatory system normally maintains a core body temperature near 37°C, anesthesia and exposure to a cold environment often result in perioperative hypothermia. Hypothermia has been implicated as an important factor in numerous perioperative complications including coagulopathy, surgical wound infection, and cardiac morbidity (204). A number of afferent receptors throughout the body terminate in the CNS, which normally responds to small variations in temperature to maintain thermal homeostasis within a narrow range. Besides obvious behavioral response to changes in temperature, effector responses to cold include vasoconstriction and shivering while effector responses to warmth include cutaneous vasodilation and sweating. Normally, the threshold for response to warmth is narrowly maintained only 0.2°C above the response to cold. Thermoregulatory vasoconstriction and vasodilation occurs in arteriovenous shunts located primarily in the fingers and toes.

GA and muscle relaxants abolish the most important behavioral responses to perturbations in temperature, and they also prevent shivering (205). GA, opioids, and IV anesthetics lower the threshold for cold responses and widen the range of temperatures where thermoregulatory responses are not triggered. Thus, anesthesia decreases the patient's response to cold and renders the patient poikilothermic over an extended range of temperatures (~4°C). During the first hour of GA, core temperature drops by 1 to 5°C resulting from redistribution of body heat from the core to the periphery due to opening of peripheral arteriovenous shunts. After the first hour, temperature continues to decline due to loss of body heat in excess of metabolic production, although at a slower rate. Most heat is lost through the skin by convection. The core temperature stops declining after 3 to 5 hours. This thermal plateau, or steady state, may be secondary to effective insulation or warming measures, or it may be due to intense thermoregulatory vasoconstriction in patients not well protected against heat loss.

Hypothermia affects patients who receive epidural or spinal anesthesia as well (205). Regional anesthesia blocks afferent and efferent neural components of the thermoregulatory response. Regional anesthesia has a surprising central effect on thermoregulation, also, so that the CNS erroneously judges the skin temperature in blocked areas to be abnormally high. Undetected hypothermia is relatively common during spinal or epidural anesthesia because patients feel warmer and anesthetists seldom monitor temperature during regional anesthesia.

Hypothermia is used to protect the heart and CNS from potential periods of ischemia during cardiac surgery and neurosurgery. On the other hand, mild hypothermia reduces the resistance to wound infection by decreasing cutaneous blood flow and impairing immune function. Maintenance of normothermia has been shown to reduce the incidence of wound infections in patients undergoing colon resection (206). Hypothermia impairs platelet function and hinders activation of the coagulation cascade resulting in coagulopathy, increased blood loss, and increased need for blood transfusion (207). The incidence of ventricular dysrhythmias and cardiac morbidity is increased by hypothermia. Decreased metabolism and clearance of drugs can prolong postoperative recovery (204).

Normothermia is best maintained using a variety of measures to prevent heat loss and actively warm the patient (204). Both cold blood and room-temperature IV fluid can significantly decrease body temperature and, when given in large amounts, these fluids should be warmed to prevent further decline in temperature. Warming these fluids, however, will not actively increase a patient's body temperature. Skin is the major source of heat loss and increasing the ambient temperature will reduce convective heat losses. Forced air warming blankets can also prevent convective losses. In addition, forced air warming is the most effective method of actively warming a patient. Despite some concerns about the increased turbulent airflow created by these warming devices, they do not appear to increase the risk of infections; in fact, these devices may reduce the incidence of wound infections (206). Skin is relatively vulnerable to injury from heat especially when pressure is applied to the skin. Circulating-water mattresses are relatively ineffective in warming the patient and can be a source of pressure-thermal injury. Patients at the extremes of age, who are debilitated, and/or who are undergoing major operations, may be especially at risk of burns from circulating-water mattresses (208).

Hyperthermia

There are numerous causes of perioperative hyperthermia, and increased body temperature may be due to iatrogenic causes or it may be secondary to any one of a number of diseases (209). A list of etiologies appears in Table 12.11. Iatrogenic intra-operative hyperthermia may occur during long procedures where the patient is almost completely covered by surgical drapes and the operative area is small. Excessive active warming can cause mild hyperthermia, especially in pediatric patients.

Table 12.11 Differential diagnosis of intra-operative hyperthermia

1. Iatrogenic causes
   a. Active warming of patients (particularly pediatric patients)
   b. Application of tourniquets to upper or lower extremities for prolonged periods of time (especially in children)
   c. Injection of sclerosing solutions into arteriovenous malformations
   d. Long procedures where patient is mostly covered with drapes
2. Hyperthermia secondary to diseases
   a. Thyrotoxicosis and thyroid storm
   b. Riley-Day syndrome (dopamine β-hydroxylase deficiency)
   c. Osteogenesis imperfecta
   d. Central nervous system dysfunction (status epilepticus, hypoxic encephalopathy)
   e. Infectious agents (surgical manipulation of infected tissue, head trauma, prolonged surgery on urinary tract)
3. Drug-induced hyperthermia
   a. Malignant hyperthermia
   b. Neuroleptic malignant syndrome

Malignant Hyperthermia

Malignant hyperthermia is a serious condition that develops in genetically predisposed patients who are exposed to certain "triggering agents," namely the PIAs and/or succinylcholine. Nonspecific signs and symptoms of malignant hyperthermia include tachycardia, tachypnea, diaphoresis, and fever. More specific signs include skeletal muscle rigidity, myoglobinuria, myoglobinemia, hyperkalemia, hypercalcemia, and mixed acidosis (209). The most sensitive indicator of potential malignant hyperthermia is an unanticipated increase (e.g., doubling or tripling) of the end-tidal CO_2 concentration while minute ventilation is kept constant. While the exact cause of malignant hypothermia is not known, the pivotal role of increased intracellular calcium is well established (210). The consequences of increased intracellular calcium include activation of ATPases with depletion of adenosine triphosphate (ATP), actin-myosin interaction causing muscle contraction, consumption of glucose, glycogen and oxygen, and generation of heat. As ATP is depleted, membrane integrity is compromised and potassium, myoglobin, creatine kinase, and tissue thromboplastin are released extracellularly. The treatment of malignant hyperthermia is outlined in Table 12.12.

Anaphylactic and anaphylactoid reactions in the perioperative period

Unfortunately, allergic reactions are one of the major factors contributing to morbidity and mortality during anesthesia (211). Of the various types of allergic reactions, anaphylactic and anaphylactoid reactions are the most serious. This topic has been reviewed recently in the anesthesiology literature (212,213). Anaphylaxis is an immune-mediated allergic reaction and usually occurs on

Table 12.12 Suggested treatment of malignant hyperthermia (MH)

- Call for experienced help.
- Stop potent inhaled agents and succinylcholine.
- Hyperventilate with 100% oxygen at two to three times the predicted minute ventilation.
- Prepare and administer IV dantrolene 2.5 mg/kg. Repeat as often as necessary to control clinical signs of MH.
- Treat acidosis with sodium bicarbonate.
- Avoid calcium channel blockers. Treat arrhythmias with other medications as needed.
- Obtain blood gases, electrolytes, creatine kinase (CK), blood, and urine for myoglobin, coagulation profile. Measure CKs every 6 hours until decreased. Follow coagulation profile to monitor for disseminated intravascular coagulation (DIC).
- Treat hyperkalemia with glucose, insulin, and calcium.
- Monitor core temperature and begin cooling measures, if hyperthermic (nasogastric lavage, rectal lavage and/or surface cooling). Avoid over cooling.
- Continue intravenous dantrolene for at least 24 hours after control of the episode (approximately 1 mg/kg q 6 hours). Continue dantrolene administration for at least 36 hours after an event. Watch for recrudescence by monitoring in an ICU for at least 24 hours.
- Ensure adequate urine output by hydration and diuretics.
- Report patients who have had acute MH episodes to the North American MH Registry of the Malignant Hyperthermia Association of the United States: 1-412-692-5464

For consultation to help with patient management, call the MH Hotline: 1-800-MH-HYPER (1-800-644-9737) or 1-315-464-7079 if outside the United States.

reexposure to a specific antigen but can occur on first exposure. The reaction involves (Ig)E-mediated release of pro-inflammatory mediators (histamine, prostacyclin, leukotrienes) from mast cells and basophils. Histamine acts on type 1 receptors to increase mucus production, increase heart rate, and cause flushing. Type 2 receptors are responsible for increasing vascular permeability, increasing gastric acid secretion and airway mucus production. Histamine and other inflammatory mediators increase the production of nitric oxide. Prostaglandins and leukotriene receptors are present in bronchial smooth muscle, the skin, and the vascular bed. Activation of these receptors causes bronchoconstriction, cutaneous wheal, and increased vascular permeability. Anaphylactoid reactions are due to nonimmune release of inflammatory mediators and are clinically indistinguishable from anaphylactic reactions.

Anaphylaxis is an unanticipated, severe allergic reaction manifested by cardiovascular symptoms (tachycardia, hypotension, shock), cutaneous symptoms (urticaria, flushing, pruritus, angioedema), and respiratory symptoms (bronchospasm, wheezing, dyspnea, hypoxemia). In rare cases, acute coronary events can occur in conjunction with a hypersensitivity reaction, a condition referred to as Kounis syndrome, allergic angina, or allergic myocardial infarction (214). Perioperative anaphylaxis can occur within minutes of exposure to the offending medication or compound, which is often a medication given during induction of anesthesia. In the patient covered by drapes with GA already well underway, the early cutaneous signs may be overlooked and the diagnosis can be delayed or missed. In addition, atypical presentations have been described so the absence of cutaneous vasodilatory signs and/or bradycardia instead of tachycardia should not preclude the diagnosis of anaphylaxis.

The most frequent class of anesthetic medications causing anaphylaxis is the muscle relaxants with an estimated incidence of 1 in 6,500 administrations of NMBAs (215). Even patients who have never been exposed to NMBAs can have an allergic reaction to these medications. Recent work has implicated the quaternary ammonium ion as the allergenic determinant in NMBAs. A number of medicines and commonly used chemicals, such as toothpastes, detergents, shampoos, and cough medicines, share these determinants with NMBAs and may account for allergic reactions in patients not previously exposed to the drug (213,216). Natural rubber latex is the second most common cause followed by antibiotics and anesthetic induction agents. During cardiac surgery, patients are exposed to large doses of a variety of antigenic medications including heparin, protamine, and occasionally aprotinin. Yet, antibiotics, muscle relaxants, and blood products account for the majority of allergic reactions during cardiac cases (217). Table 12.13 reviews a number of medications used in the perioperative period and their allergic reactions.

Natural rubber latex is a ubiquitous material found in a wide variety of medical products, although latex-free alternatives are becoming more widely available. Expanding use of universal precautions has led to an increase in the use of gloves containing latex. This high demand for gloves resulted in rapid manufacture of products with increased protein content, which led to an increase in the incidence of latex anaphylaxis (218). Recent improvements in latex production and the increased use of low-protein, powder-free gloves have reduced the incidence of reactions. Not all reactions to latex are anaphylactic in nature. The most common reaction associated with latex is an irritant contact dermatitis that is probably due to the alkaline pH of latex gloves. Healthcare workers, patients with a history of multiple

Table 12.13 Medications and allergic reactions

Local anesthetics	• Anaphylactic reactions to amide local anesthetics are extremely rare • True allergic reactions to esters account for <1% of reactions to local anesthetics • Allergic reactions are usually due to paraaminobenzoic acid metabolite of esters or methylparaben preservative
Muscle relaxants	• Muscle relaxants account for most anaphylactic reactions during anesthesia • Incidence: succinylcholine > benzylisoquinoliniums > aminosteroids • Rocuronium: possible increased incidence when compared to other muscle relaxants • Benzylisoquinolinium compounds can cause direct mast cell degranulation
Opioids	• Allergic reactions to opioids are rare • Morphine causes nonimmunologic histamine release
Propofol	• Current evidence suggest that egg-allergic patients are not more likely to develop anaphylaxis
Inhaled anesthetics	• Immune mediated hepatic injury
Aprotinin (serine protease inhibitor used to decrease blood loss and transfusion during certain cardiac surgical procedures)	• Antigenic, derived from bovine lung • 2.5%–2.8% incidence of anaphylaxis on re-exposure
Heparin (232)	• Antigenic, derived from bovine or porcine intestine • Heparin induced thrombocytopenia is the most common nonanaphylactic reaction
Protamine (233,234)	• Antigenic, derived from salmon sperm • Slightly increased risk on reexposure and in diabetic patients exposed to neutral protamine hagedorn or protamine zinc insulin • Increased risk in vasectomized patients and those with fish allergies is controversial
Vancomycin	• "Red man" syndrome of hypotension, pruritus, flushing and rash in 5%–14%; due to nonimmunologic histamine release • very rare cases of (Ig)-E mediated hypersensitivity reactions
Penicillins, cephalosporins	
Isosulfan blue dye	• Approved for intra-operative lymphatic mapping and sentinel node biopsy procedures for breast cancer and melanoma • 1%–2% incidence of allergic reactions including severe, anaphylactic reactions

surgical procedures, spina bifida, atopic individuals, and those with fruit or food allergy (kiwi, chestnut, avocado, passion fruit, banana) are at increased risk of having a latex allergy. Parenteral or mucus membrane exposure is most likely to lead to a severe reaction but a reaction can develop in response to inhalation of airborne latex particles.

Avoidance of latex containing products is the only effective management option in most cases (218). Latex allergic patients should be scheduled early in the day in order to reduce their exposure to aeroallergens. Prophylactic administration of steroids and antihistamines is not effective and is not recommended. Certain desensitization techniques may be effective in some cases.

When intra-operative anaphylaxis is suspected, the following initial treatment measures should be applied whenever possible: (a) withdraw the suspected offending drug; (b) when the anaphylactic event occurs during induction, immediately discontinue anesthetic drugs; (c) maintain the airway with 100% oxygen; (d) in severe reactions, provide early administration of epinephrine and call for help; (e) place the patient supine in the Trendelenburg position; and (f) abbreviate the surgical procedure if possible when it occurs during surgery. A first priority is restoration of cardiovascular homeostasis primarily through early administration of epinephrine and restoration/expansion of circulating intravascular volume. Poor outcomes following anaphylaxis are associated with late or absent administration of epinephrine. Bronchospasm should be treated with inhaled and/or IV β_2 agonist. Corticosteroids and/or H1 receptor antagonists are often recommended in the management of anaphylaxis, but their effects have never been established in placebo-controlled trials. Likewise, the role of arginine vasopressin and methylene blue remains controversial.

Positioning and peripheral nerve injury

A complete, thorough discussion of patient positioning is outside the scope of this chapter and the reader is referred to textbooks and chapters dedicated to this subject. In most textbooks and chapters covering positioning during surgery, a major portion of the discussion is devoted to methods aimed at reducing postoperative complications of positioning. As pointed out in the ASA's practice advisory on prevention of perioperative peripheral neuropathies, there is scant evidence of a causal relation between intraoperative positioning and postoperative neuropathy (219).

Peripheral nerve injury can be caused by metabolic derangement, ischemia, excessive stretch, compression or pressure, direct trauma, or other unknown factors (220). Improper positioning of the patient is presumed to cause peripheral nerve injury through one or more of these mechanisms. Other causative factors have been associated with nerve injury including automated blood pressure cuffs, subclinical diabetes, induced or prolonged hypotension, and stretch or compression during operative manipulation. Nerves with a preexisting injury are much more susceptible to permanent injury from a second, possibly subclinical, insult in the operating room. Patients may come to the operating room with a preexisting nerve injury from trauma or compressive syndromes, such as carpal tunnel syndrome or thoracic outlet syndrome.

Ulnar neuropathy represents one third of all nerve injuries reported in the Closed Claims Project. The ulnar nerve appears to be especially vulnerable to injury at the elbow as it courses near the medial epicondyle of the humerus (221). The nerve can be constricted by the cubital tunnel retinaculum especially during flexion of the elbow. Yet, it is disconcerting that several studies suggest that perioperative measures to protect the ulnar nerve from injury do not prevent postoperative ulnar neuropathy, and the cause of ulnar neuropathy may be beyond the control of the anesthesiologist. In fact, most cases of ulnar neuropathy may not be related to positioning at all. In a large retrospective study of ulnar nerve injuries following diagnostic and noncardiac surgical procedures, persistent ulnar neuropathies were identified in 414 cases, for an incidence of 1 per 2,729 patients (222). Seventy percent of the 414 patients with ulnar neuropathy were male, 9% had bilateral neuropathies, and many occurred even when precautions and padding were documented. Univariate analysis revealed the following risk factors: male gender, extremes of weight (BMI >37 or less than 24), and a hospital stay greater than 14 days. No association was found with the duration of surgery, type of anesthetic, or patient position during surgery. Most cases presented greater than 24 hours after the completion of the operation. Interesting studies in normal conscious male volunteers reveal that patients may not perceive paresthesias of ulnar nerve compression even when somatosensory evoked potentials document impaired electrophysiologic function (221). Finally, ulnar neuropathy occurs in equal frequency in medical and surgical patients who are hospitalized for more than two days. Thus, patients, especially sedated and narcotized elderly men, who are in the supine position for a prolonged period of time may be vulnerable to ulnar neuropathy whether or not they have had on operation.

A variety of other complications of positioning are listed in Table 12.14.

Ocular injury

Injury to the eye is a potentially disastrous complication. Ocular injury may occur during either ophthalmologic surgery or nonophthalmic surgery and can range from relatively minor corneal abrasion to permanent loss of vision. The broad category of ocular injury is comprised of various types of injuries including corneal abrasion, vitreous loss and hemorrhage, and damage to the retina or visual pathway. The overall incidence of ocular injury appears to be low (0.06% to 0.17%) but may be greater in selected groups such as patients undergoing operations with cardiopulmonary bypass (223,224). In a closed claims analysis of eye injury associated with anesthesia, the most frequent complication resulting in a claim was corneal abrasion (225). The other subset of injury identified in the closed claims analysis was characterized by patient movement during ophthalmologic surgery resulting in blindness.

Corneal Abrasions

Risk factors for corneal abrasion include long surgical procedures, lateral positioning, operation on the head or neck, and GA (224). In most cases of corneal abrasion, the exact mechanism of injury is unknown. Postulated mechanisms include prolonged exposure or contact with foreign bodies. GA reduces tear production predisposing the eye to desiccation and GA impairs or obliterates protective behaviors and reflexes. Corneal abrasions can occur despite taping the eyelids closed and/or applying ointments. Injury prior to the placement of tapes has been described. After induction and prior to the placement of eye tapes, the patient is at risk of injury from a variety of foreign bodies including wristwatch bands, name badges, stethoscopes, IV tubing, and monitoring cables. Exposure keratitis can still occur if the eyelids are not well approximated after taping. Likewise, inclusion of eyelashes under the eyelids during taping, or contact of the adhesive tape with the cornea, can lead to injury. Once the tapes are removed, the patient is at risk once again of corneal abrasion. During emergence, patients have been observed to injure their own eyes by reaching up to rub their face with an index finger that has a pulse oximeter on it. The anesthetist can also cause injury to the cornea at this time by dragging objects across the patient's face.

Damage to the Retina or Visual Pathway

The retina can be damaged through occlusion of the central retinal artery or its branches. Central retinal artery occlusion (CRAO) is thought to be due to direct pressure on the globe, emboli, or low perfusion pressure. Visual loss is usually unilateral and permanent. Ischemic optic neuropathy (ION) results from damage to, or impairment of, the circulatory supply to the optic nerve. The etiology of ION is unknown but it has been associated with large blood loss, hypotension, anemia, the prone position, and preexisting cardiovascular disease. Visual impairment is bilateral and may improve with time in some cases (226).

The incidence of visual loss due to CRAO and ION is low and most information is derived from analysis of case reports and closed claims (223,225). In July 1999, the Postoperative Visual Loss (POVL) Registry was established to collect and analyze information on closed claims cases of visual loss (227). The majority of cases in this analysis have

Table **12.14** **Complications of various patient positions during operations and diagnostic procedures**

Position	Complications	Possible Mechanism	Potentially Protective Measures
Supine, head-down tilt	Decreased pulmonary compliance, increased work of breathing, increased inspiratory pressures, increased intracranial pressure, increased intracranial vascular congestion		
	Compression of subclavian neurovascular bundle or neurovascular structures emerging from the area of the scalene musculature	Shoulder brace malpositioned	Place shoulder brace over the acromioclavicular joint
Dorsal decubitus	Postural hypotension with head-elevated posture		Volume loading, vasopressors
	Pressure alopecia		Turn head frequently and/or use padded head support
	Pressure point reaction (heels, elbows, sacrum)	Prolonged pressure while immobile	Proper padding
	Brachial plexus injuries	Shoulder brace	Place shoulder brace over the acromioclavicular joint
		Lateral displacement of head Sternal retraction	Secure head in neutral position
	Long thoracic nerve dysfunction	(etiology and prevention unclear)	
	Axillary trauma of the humeral head		Avoid excess abduction of the arm
	Radial nerve compression	Pressure from vertical bar of anesthesia screen, sternal retraction, excessive cycling of blood pressure cuff	Avoid prolonged pressure
			Avoid excessive cycling of automated blood pressure cuff
	Ulnar nerve at the elbow	See text	Use a padded armboard
			Arm abduction should be limited to 90° in supine patients
			Position arm to decrease pressure on the postcondylar groove of the humerus
			Padded armboards and/or padding at the elbow may decrease the risk of upper extremity neuropathy
	Backache	Ligamentous relaxation during general and regional anesthesia	Maintain lumbar lordosis Place support under knees
Lateral decubitus	Ocular injury (corneal abrasion, displacement of lens, retinal ischemia)	Direct contact	Protect (tape) eyes before turning
		Pressure on eye Systemic hypotension	Avoid direct pressure to eyes
	Ear injury	Dependent ear folded or compressed	Palpate ear to check padding
	Neck pain	Excessive lateral flexion, ventral flexion, extension or rotation	Secure head in neutral position
	Suprascapular injury	Ventral circumduction of the dependent shoulder	Supporting pad under the thorax just caudad to the axilla
	Long thoracic syndrome		
	Compartment syndrome of down-side upper extremity	Mediad compression or circumduction of down-side shoulder	Supporting pad under the thorax just caudad to the axilla
	Aseptic necrosis of the upside femoral head	Pressure compression of arterial blood supply	Place restraining tapes across up-side on the soft tissue between head of femur and iliac crest

(continued)

Table 12.14 Complications of various patient positions during operations and diagnostic procedures *(continued)*

Position	Complications	Possible Mechanism	Potentially Protective Measures
Ventral decubitus (prone)	Ocular injury (corneal abrasion, displacement of lens, retinal ischemia)	Direct contact	Protect (tape) eyes before turning
		Pressure on eye Systemic hypotension	Avoid direct pressure to eyes
	Neck pain	Lateral rotation of head	Keep head secured in sagittal plane
	Ulnar and radial nerve injuries	See text	See supine position
	Thoracic outlet syndrome (severe pain)	Compression of brachial plexus and subclavian vessels near first rib	Avoid overhead arm position in patients with preoperative signs and symptoms of thoracic outlet syndrome
Head-elevated	Postural hypotension		Volume loading, vasopressors, decrease inhaled anesthetics, change patient position incrementally
	Air embolism	Incised vein above the level of the heart	
	Pneumocephalus	Air trapped in superior regions of cranium	
	Midcervical tetraplegia	Marked flexion of neck with stretching of spinal cord compromising its vasculature in midcervical area	
	Edema of face, tongue (macroglossia) and neck	Venous and lymphatic obstruction by prolonged neck flexion	

ophthalmologic diagnoses of ION and CROA and are associated with spine surgery (67%) followed by cardiopulmonary bypass procedures (10%). Interestingly, the POVL analysis has revealed strong evidence that ION occurs in the absence of direct pressure on the globe, in contrast to a commonly held perception.

CONCLUSION

Most anesthesiologists would like to believe that the delivery of anesthesia is relatively safe and that recent advances in monitoring, pharmacology, anesthesia delivery systems, resident training, and information technology have made our practice even safer. Despite significant biases and limitations, the Closed Claims Project has provided information suggests that anesthesia care is becoming safer. Studies based on the Closed Claims Project have influenced anesthetic practice and stimulated research in problem areas (228). For example, the Closed Claims Project has identified that three damaging events account for nearly half of all claims of injury: respiratory system events, cardiovascular system events, and problems with equipment. The three most common complications or injuries are death (30%), brain damage (12%) and nerve damage (18%). Thus, management strategies directed at these few areas of clinical practice may have large results on decreasing injury leading to claims. Cheney et al. found that respiratory events accounted for a third of claims and that 85% of these claims involved brain damage or death (229). Most of these adverse events were due to inadequate ventilation, esophageal intubation, and difficult tracheal intubation. Furthermore, most of these claims were thought to be preventable by pulse oximetry and capnography monitoring. Based partly on these findings, the ASA formulated new standards for perioperative monitoring that stress the use of pulse oximetry and capnography, and the ASA created practice guidelines for management of the difficult airway. While the Closed Claims Project cannot determine whether the actual incidence of severe injuries is decreasing, there are trends in outcomes that suggest that this is so (228).

The administration of anesthesia invokes remarkable physiologic changes that are sometimes subtle but often profound. The neurological system is greatly affected, either regionally or globally. The state of anesthesia and the effects of the medications used to block the response to noxious stimuli likewise impact the cardiovascular and respiratory systems. Anesthesia converts a relatively hardy, independent, and resilient person into a patient who is dependent, vulnerable, and barely a few moments away from jeopardy, damage, or demise. Modern anesthetic practice has made the process seem routine, but with each anesthetic, there is a risk of complications or adverse outcome. Unfortunately, every surgeon will become familiar with some of the more common adverse events and may have a brush with some of the rare ones as well. Hopefully, the increasing complexity of surgical operations, presence of multiple comorbid conditions, and advancing age of the patient population will not negate the positive impact of improvements in anesthesia safety.

REFERENCES

1. Posner K. *ASA Closed Claims Project*. 2004. Available at: http://depts.washington.edu/asaccp. Accessed January 20, 2010.
2. Caplan RA, Posner KL, Ward RJ, et al. Adverse respiratory events in anesthesia: a closed claims analysis. *Anesthesiology* 1990;72(5):828–833.
3. Behringer EC. Approaches to managing the upper airway. *Anesthesiol Clin North America* 2002;20(4):813–832, vi.
4. Rose DK, Cohen MM. The airway: problems and predictions in 18,500 patients [comment]. *Can J Anaesth* 1994;41(5, Pt 1):372–383.
5. Chraemmer-Jorgensen B, Hertel S, Strom J, et al. Catecholamine response to laryngoscopy and intubation. The influence of three different drug combinations commonly used for induction of anaesthesia [comment]. *Anaesthesia* 1992;47(9):750–756.
6. Barak M, Ziser A, Greenberg A, et al. Hemodynamic and catecholamine response to tracheal intubation: direct laryngoscopy compared with fiberoptic intubation. *J Clin Anesth* 2003;15(2):132–136.
7. Society of Anesthesiologists Task Force on Management of the Difficult Airway. Practice guidelines for management of the difficult airway. A report by the American Society of Anesthesiologists Task Force on Management of the Difficult Airway. *Anesthesiology* 1993;78(3): 597–602.
8. Society of Anesthesiologists Task Force on Management of the Difficult Airway. Practice guidelines for management of the difficult airway: an updated report by the American Society of Anesthesiologists Task Force on Management of the Difficult Airway. *Anesthesiology* 2003;98(5):1269–1277.
9. Stern Y, Spitzer T. Retrograde intubation of the trachea. *J Laryngol Otol* 1991;105(9):746–747.
10. Mallampati SR, Gatt SP, Gugino LD, et al. A clinical sign to predict difficult tracheal intubation: a prospective study. *Can Anaesth Soc J* 1985; 32(4):429–434.
11. Frerk CM. Predicting difficult intubation [comment]. *Anaesthesia* 1991; 46(12):1005–1008.
12. Hagberg C, Boin MH. Management of the airway: complications. In: Benumof JL, Saidman LJ, eds. *Anesthesia and perioperative complications*, 2nd ed. St. Louis: Mosby; 1999:3–24.
13. Rosenblatt W, Wagner P, Ovassapian A, et al. Practice patterns in managing the difficult airway by anesthesiologists in the United States. *Anesth Analg* 1998;87(1):153–157.
14. Warner ME, Benenfeld SM, Warner MA, et al. Perianesthetic dental injuries: frequency, outcomes, and risk factors. *Anesthesiology* 1999; 90(5):1302–1305.
15. Loh KS, Irish JC. Traumatic complications of intubation and other airway management procedures. In: Bogetz MS, ed. *The upper airway and anesthesia*. Philadelphia, PA: W.B. Saunders; 2002:953–969.
16. Lennarson PJ, Smith D, Todd MM, et al. Segmental cervical spine motion during orotracheal intubation of the intact and injured spine with and without external stabilization. *J Neurosurg* 2000;92(2, Suppl): 201–206.
17. Dutton RP. Anesthetic management of spinal cord injury: clinical practice and future initiatives. *Int Anesthesiol Clin* 2002;40(3):103–120.
18. Weber S. Traumatic complications of airway management. In: Weber S, ed. *Anesthesia-related complications*. Philadelphia, PA: W.B. Saunders; 2002:265–274, v–vi.
19. Hall CE, Shutt LE. Nasotracheal intubation for head and neck surgery [comment]. *Anaesthesia* 2003;58(3):249–256.
20. Conrardy PA, Goodman LR, Lainge F, et al. Alteration of endotracheal tube position. Flexion and extension of the neck. *Crit Care Med* 1976; 4(1):7–12.
21. Parmet J, Colonna-Romano P, Horrow J, et al. The laryngeal mask airway reliably provides rescue ventilation in cases of unanticipated difficult tracheal intubation along with difficult mask ventilation. *Anesth Analg* 1998;87(3):661–665.
22. Benumof JL. Laryngeal mask airway and the ASA difficult airway algorithm [comment]. *Anesthesiology* 1996;84(3):686–699.
23. Bordet F, Allaouchiche B, Lansiaux S, et al. Risk factors for airway complications during general anaesthesia in paediatric patients. *Paediatr Anaesth* 2002;12(9):762–769.
24. Seet E, Yousaf F, Gupta S, et al. Use of manometry for laryngeal mask airway reduces postoperative pharyngolaryngeal adverse events: a prospective, randomized trial. *Anesthesiology* 2010;112(3):652–657. DOI:10.1097/ALN.0b013e3181cf4346.
25. Geelhoed GW. Tracheomalacia from compressing goiter: management after thyroidectomy. *Surgery* 1988;104(6):1100–1108.
26. Rex MA. A review of the structural and functional basis of laryngospasm and a discussion of the nerve pathways involved in the reflex and its clinical significance in man and animals. *Br J Anaesth* 1970;42(10):891–899.
27. Hartley M, Vaughan RS. Problems associated with tracheal extubation [comment]. *Br J Anaesth* 1993;71(4):561–568.
28. Lang SA, Duncan PG, Shephard DA, et al. Pulmonary oedema associated with airway obstruction [comment]. *Can J Anaesth* 1990;37(2): 210–218.
29. Deepika K, Kenaan CA, Barrocas AM, et al. Negative pressure pulmonary edema after acute upper airway obstruction. *J Clin Anesth* 1997;9(5):403–408.
30. Hug CC Jr. New perspectives on anesthetic agents [Review]. *Am J Surg* 1988;156(5):406–415.
31. Campagna JA, Miller KW, Forman SA. Mechanisms of actions of inhaled anesthetics. *N Engl J Med* 2003;348(21):2110–2124.
32. Buffington CW, Romson JL, Levine A, et al. Isoflurane induces coronary steal in a canine model of chronic coronary occlusion. *Anesthesiology* 1987;66(3):280–292.
33. Tuman KJ, McCarthy RJ, Spiess BD, et al. Does choice of anesthetic agent significantly affect outcome after coronary artery surgery? *Anesthesiology* 1989;70(2):189–198.
34. Cason BA, Verrier ED, London MJ, et al. Effects of isoflurane and halothane on coronary vascular resistance and collateral myocardial blood flow: their capacity to induce coronary steal. *Anesthesiology* 1987;67(5):665–675.
35. Pulley DD, Kirvassilis GV, Kelermenos N, et al. Regional and global myocardial circulatory and metabolic effects of isoflurane and halothane in patients with steal-prone coronary anatomy. *Anesthesiology* 1991;75(5):756–766.
36. Agnew NM, Pennefather SH, Russell GN. Isoflurane and coronary heart disease [comment]. *Anaesthesia* 2002;57(4):338–347.
37. Tanaka K, Ludwig LM, Kersten JR, et al. Mechanisms of cardioprotection by volatile anesthetics. *Anesthesiology* 2004;100(3):707–721.
38. Aach R. Halothane and liver failure. *JAMA* 1970;211(13):2145–2147.
39. Elliott RH, Strunin L. Hepatotoxicity of volatile anaesthetics. *Br J Anaesth* 1993;70(3):339–348.
40. Hubbard AK, Roth TP, Gandolfi AJ, et al. Halothane hepatitis patients generate an antibody response toward a covalently bound metabolite of halothane. *Anesthesiology* 1988;68(5):791–796.
41. Kenna JG, Jones RM. The organ toxicity of inhaled anesthetics. *Anesth Analg* 1995;81(6, Suppl):S51–S66.
42. Conzen PF, Kharasch ED, Czerner SF, et al. Low-flow sevoflurane compared with low-flow isoflurane anesthesia in patients with stable renal insufficiency [comment]. *Anesthesiology* 2002;97(3):578–584.
43. Kharasch ED, Frink EJ Jr, Artru A, et al. Long-duration low-flow sevoflurane and isoflurane effects on postoperative renal and hepatic function. *Anesth Analg* 2001;93(6):1511–1520, table of contents.
44. Forbes GM, Collins BJ. Nitrous oxide for colonoscopy: a randomized controlled study [comment]. *Gastrointest Endosc* 2000;51(3):271–277.
45. Harding TA, Gibson JA. The use of inhaled nitrous oxide for flexible sigmoidoscopy: a placebo-controlled trial. *Endoscopy* 2000;32(6): 457–460.
46. Eisele JH, Reitan JA, Massumi RA, et al. Myocardial performance and N2O analgesia in coronary-artery disease. *Anesthesiology* 1976;44(1): 16–20.
47. Flippo TS, Holder WD Jr. Neurologic degeneration associated with nitrous oxide anesthesia in patients with vitamin B12 deficiency. *Arch Surg* 1993;128(12):1391–1395.
48. Louis-Ferdinand RT. Myelotoxic, neurotoxic and reproductive adverse effects of nitrous oxide. *Adverse Drug React Toxicol Rev* 1994; 13(4):193–206.
49. Suruda A. Health effects of anesthetic gases. *Occup Med* 1997;12(4): 627–634.
50. Eger EI II, Saidman LJ. Hazards of nitrous oxide anesthesia in bowel obstruction and pneumothorax. *Anesthesiology* 1965;26(1):61–66.

51. Ohryn M. Tympanic membrane rupture following general anesthesia with nitrous oxide: a case report. *AANA J* 1995;63(1):42–44.
52. Seaberg RR, Freeman WR, Goldbaum MH, et al. Permanent postoperative vision loss associated with expansion of intraocular gas in the presence of a nitrous oxide-containing anesthetic. *Anesthesiology* 2002; 97(5):1309–1310.
53. Astrom S, Kjellgren D, Monestam E, et al. Nitrous oxide anesthesia and intravitreal gastamponade. *Acta Anaesthesiol Scand* 2003;47(3): 361–362.
54. Taylor E, Feinstein R, White PF, et al. Anesthesia for laparoscopic cholecystectomy. Is nitrous oxide contraindicated? *Anesthesiology* 1992; 76(4):541–543.
55. Caplan RA, Vistica MF, Posner KL, et al. Adverse anesthetic outcomes arising from gas delivery equipment: a closed claims analysis [comment]. *Anesthesiology* 1997;87(4):741–748.
56. Anagnostou JM, Stoelting RK. Complications of drugs used in anesthesia. In: Benumof JL, Saidman LJ, eds. *Anesthesia and perioperative complications*. St. Louis: Mosby; 1999:161–191.
57. Hirshman CA, Edelstein RA, Ebertz JM, et al. Thiobarbiturate-induced histamine release in human skin mast cells. *Anesthesiology* 1985;63(4):353–356.
58. Harrison GG, Meissner PN, Hift RJ. Anaesthesia for the porphyric patient [comment]. *Anaesthesia* 1993;48(5):417–421.
59. Ben-Shlomo I, abd-el-Khalim H, Ezry J, et al. Midazolam acts synergistically with fentanyl for induction of anaesthesia. *Br J Anaesth* 1990; 64(1):45–47.
60. Heikkila H, Jalonen J, Arola M, et al. Midazolam as adjunct to high-dose fentanyl anaesthesia for coronary artery bypass grafting operation. *Acta Anaesthesiol Scand* 1984;28(6):683–689.
61. Vinik HR, Bradley EL Jr, Kissin I. Midazolam-alfentanil synergism for anesthetic induction in patients. *Anesth Analg* 1989;69(2):213–217.
62. Zacharias M, Dundee JW, Clarke RS, et al. Effect of preanaesthetic medication on etomidate. *Br J Anaesth* 1979;51(2):127–133.
63. Wagner RL, White PF, Kan PB, et al. Inhibition of adrenal steroidogenesis by the anesthetic etomidate. *N Engl J Med* 1984;310(22):1415–1421.
64. Wagner RL, White PF. Etomidate inhibits adrenocortical function in surgical patients. *Anesthesiology* 1984;61(6):647–651.
65. Crozier TA, Beck D, Schlaeger M, et al. Endocrinological changes following etomidate, midazolam, or methohexital for minor surgery. *Anesthesiology* 1987;66(5):628–635.
66. Gooding JM, Corssen G. Effect of etomidate on the cardiovascular system. *Anesth Analg* 1977;56(5):717–719.
67. Price ML, Millar B, Grounds M, et al. Changes in cardiac index and estimated systemic vascular resistance during induction of anaesthesia with thiopentone, methohexitone, propofol and etomidate [comment]. *Br J Anaesth* 1992;69(2):172–176.
68. Goodman NW, Black AM, Carter JA. Some ventilatory effects of propofol as sole anaesthetic agent. *Br J Anaesth* 1987;59(12):1497–1503.
69. Lepage JY, Pinaud ML, Helias JH, et al. Left ventricular performance during propofol or methohexital anesthesia: isotopic and invasive cardiac monitoring. *Anesth Analg* 1991;73(1):3–9.
70. Claeys MA, Gepts E, Camu F. Haemodynamic changes during anaesthesia induced and maintained with propofol. *Br J Anaesth* 1988; 60(1):3–9.
71. Prys-Roberts C, Davies JR, Calverley RK, et al. Haemodynamic effects of infusions of diisopropyl phenol (ICI 35 868) during nitrous oxide anaesthesia in man. *Br J Anaesth* 1983;55(2):105–111.
72. Sosis MB, Braverman B. Growth of Staphylococcus aureus in four intravenous anesthetics. *Anesth Analg* 1993;77(4):766–768.
73. Bennett SN, McNeil MM, Bland LA, et al. Postoperative infections traced to contamination of an intravenous anesthetic, propofol [comment]. *N Engl J Med* 1995;333(3):147–154.
74. Veber B, Gachot B, Bedos JP, et al. Severe sepsis after intravenous injection of contaminated propofol. *Anesthesiology* 1994;80(3):712–713.
75. Nichols RL, Smith JW. Bacterial contamination of an anesthetic agent [comment]. *N Engl J Med* 1995;333(3):184–185.
76. Bach A, Geiss HK. Propofol and postoperative infections [comment]. *N Engl J Med* 1995;333(22):1505–1506; discussion 1507.
77. Sklar GE. Propofol and postoperative infections. *Ann Pharmacother* 1997;31(12):1521–1523.
78. Gutelius B, Perz JF, Parker MM, et al. Multiple clusters of hepatitis virus infections associated with anesthesia for outpatient endoscopy procedures. *Gastroenterology* 2010;139(1):163–170.
79. Labus B. *Outbreak of hepatitis C at outpatient surgical centers.* Las Vegas: Southern Nevada Health District; 2009.
80. Vasile B, Rasulo F, Candiani A, et al. The pathophysiology of propofol infusion syndrome: a simple name for a complex syndrome. *Intensive Care Med* 2003;29(9):1417–1425.
81. Gooding JM, Dimick AR, Tavakoli M, et al. A physiologic analysis of cardiopulmonary responses to ketamine anesthesia in noncardiac patients. *Anesth Analg* 1977;56(6):813–816.
82. White PF, Way WL, Trevor AJ. Ketamine–its pharmacology and therapeutic uses. *Anesthesiology* 1982;56(2):119–136.
83. Schow AJ, Lubarsky DA, Olson RP, et al. Can succinylcholine be used safely in hyperkalemic patients? *Anesth Analg* 2002;95(1):119–122.
84. Thapa S, Brull SJ. Succinylcholine-induced hyperkalemia in patients with renal failure: an old question revisited. *Anesth Analg* 2000;91(1): 237–241.
85. Wong SF, Chung F. Succinylcholine-associated postoperative myalgia [comment]. *Anaesthesia* 2000;55(2):144–152.
86. Pace NL. The best prophylaxis for succinylcholine myalgias: extension of a previous meta-analysis. *Anesth Analg* 1993;77(5):1080–1081.
87. Cunningham AJ, Barry P. Intraocular pressure–physiology and implications for anaesthetic management. *Can Anaesth Soc J* 1986;33(2): 195–208.
88. Mitra S, Gombar KK, Gombar S. The effect of rocuronium on intraocular pressure: a comparison with succinylcholine. *Eur J Anaesthesiol* 2001;18(12):836–838.
89. Zimmerman AA, Funk KJ, Tidwell JL. Propofol and alfentanil prevent the increase in intraocular pressure caused by succinylcholine and endotracheal intubation during a rapid sequence induction of anesthesia. *Anesth Analg* 1996;83(4):814–817.
90. Moreno RJ, Kloess P, Carlson DW. Effect of succinylcholine on the intraocular contents of open globes [comment]. *Ophthalmology* 1991; 98(5):636–638.
91. McGoldrick KE. The open globe: is an alternative to succinylcholine necessary? [comment]. *J Clin Anesth* 1993;5(1):1–4.
92. Vachon CA, Warner DO, Bacon DR. Succinylcholine and the open globe. Tracing the teaching. *Anesthesiology* 2003;99(1):220–223.
93. Cook DR. Can succinylcholine be abandoned? *Anesth Analg* 2000; 90(Suppl 5):S24–S28.
94. Sparr HJ, Beaufort TM, Fuchs-Buder T. Newer neuromuscular blocking agents: how do they compare with established agents? *Drugs* 2001;61(7):919–942.
95. Moore EW, Hunter JM. The new neuromuscular blocking agents: do they offer any advantages? *Br J Anaesth* 2001;87(6):912–925.
96. Cammu G. Interactions of neuromuscular blocking drugs. *Acta Anaesthesiol Belg* 2001;52(4):357–363.
97. Fodale V, Santamaria LB. Laudanosine, an atracurium and cisatracurium metabolite. *Eur J Anaesthesiol* 2002;19(7):466–473.
98. Murphy GS, Vender JS. Neuromuscular-blocking drugs. Use and misuse in the intensive care unit. *Crit Care Clin* 2001;17(4):925–942.
99. Prielipp RC, Coursin DB, Wood KE, et al. Complications associated with sedative and neuromuscular blocking drugs in critically ill patients. *Crit Care Clin* 1995;11(4):983–1003.
100. Douglass JA, Tuxen DV, Horne M, et al. Myopathy in severe asthma. *Am Rev Respir Dis* 1992;146(2):517–519.
101. Segredo V, Caldwell JE, Matthay MA, et al. Persistent paralysis in critically ill patients after long-term administration of vecuronium. *N Engl J Med* 1992;327(8):524–528.
102. Coursin DB, Prielipp RC. Prolonged paralysis with atracurium infusion. *Crit Care Med* 1995;23(6):1155–1157.
103. Prielipp RC, Coursin DB, Scuderi PE, et al. Comparison of the infusion requirements and recovery profiles of vecuronium and cisatracurium 51W89 in intensive care unit patients. *Anesth Analg* 1995;81(1):3–12.
104. Murray MJ, Cowen J, DeBlock H, et al. Clinical practice guidelines for sustained neuromuscular blockade in the adult critically ill patient. *Crit Care Med* 2002;30(1):142–156.
105. Flacke JW, Flacke WE, Bloor BC, et al. Histamine release by four narcotics: a double-blind study in humans. *Anesth Analg* 1987;66(8): 723–730.
106. Simopoulos TT, Smith HS, Peeters-Asdourian C, et al. Use of meperidine in patient-controlled analgesia and the development of a normeperidine toxic reaction. *Arch Surg* 2002;137(1):84–88.
107. Michelsen LG, Hug CC Jr. The pharmacokinetics of remifentanil. *J Clin Anesth* 1996;8(8):679–682.
108. Patel P, Sun L. Update on neonatal anesthetic neurotoxicity: insight into molecular mechanisms and relevance to humans [comment]. *Anesthesiology* 2009;110(4):703–708.

109. Cottrell JE, Cottrell JE. We care, therefore we are: anesthesia-related morbidity and mortality: the 46th rovenstine lecture. *Anesthesiology* 2008;109(3):377–388.
110. Jevtovic-Todorovic V, Olney JW. PRO: Anesthesia-induced developmental neuroapoptosis: status of the evidence. *Anesth Analg* 2008; 106(6):1659–1663.
111. Olney JW, Young C, Wozniak DF, et al. Anesthesia-induced developmental neuroapoptosis: does it happen in humans? [Editorial]. *Anesthesiology* 2004;101(2):273–275.
112. Jevtovic-Todorovic V, Hartman RE, Izumi Y, et al. Early exposure to common anesthetic agents causes widespread neurodegeneration in the developing rat brain and persistent learning deficits. *J Neurosci* 2003;23(3):876–882.
113. Fredriksson A, Ponten E, Gordh T, et al. Neonatal exposure to a combination of N-methyl-D-aspartate and gamma-aminobutyric acid type A receptor anesthetic agents potentiates apoptotic neurodegeneration and persistent behavioral deficits. *Anesthesiology* 2007;107(3): 427–436.
114. Yon J-H, Carter LB, Reiter RJ, et al. Melatonin reduces the severity of anesthesia-induced apoptotic neurodegeneration in the developing rat brain. *Neurobiol Dis* 2006;21(3):522–530.
115. Kalkman CJMDPD, Peelen LMS, Moons KGPD, et al. Behavior and development in children and age at the time of first anesthetic exposure. *Anesthesiology* 2009;110(4):805–812.
116. Wilder RTMDPD, Flick RPMDMPH, Sprung JMDPD, et al. Early exposure to anesthesia and learning disabilities in a population-based birth cohort. *Anesthesiology* 2009;110(4):796–804.
117. Mellon RD, Simone AF, Rappaport BA. Use of anesthetic agents in neonates and young children. *Anesth Analg* 2007;104(3):509–520.
118. Moller JT, Cluitmans P, Rasmussen LS, et al. Long-term postoperative cognitive dysfunction in the elderly: ISPOCD1 study. *Lancet* 1998; 351(9106):857–861.
119. Monk TG, Weldon BC, Garvan CW, et al. Predictors of cognitive dysfunction after major noncardiac surgery. *Anesthesiology* 2008;108(1): 18–30.
120. Newman MF, Kirchner JL, Phillips-Bute B, et al. Longitudinal assessment of neurocognitive function after coronary-artery bypass surgery. *N Engl J Med* 2001;344(6):395–402.
121. Matthey P, Finucane BT, Finegan BA. The attitude of the general public towards preoperative assessment and risks associated with general anesthesia. *Can J Anaesth* 2001;48(4):333–339.
122. Kerssens C, Klein J, Bonke B. Awareness: Monitoring versus remembering what happened. *Anesthesiology* 2003;99(3):570–575.
123. Sandin RH, Enlund G, Samuelsson P, et al. Awareness during anaesthesia: a prospective case study. *Lancet* 2000;355(9205):707–711.
124. Bailey AR, Jones JG. Patients' memories of events during general anaesthesia. *Anaesthesia* 1997;52(5):460–476.
125. Russell IF. Midazolam-alfentanil: an anaesthetic? An investigation using the isolated forearm technique. *Br J Anaesth* 1993;70(1):42–46.
126. Tempe DK, Siddiquie RA. Awareness during cardiac surgery. *J Cardiothorac Vasc Anesth* 1999;13(2):214–219.
127. Osterman JE, Hopper J, Heran WJ, et al. Awareness under anesthesia and the development of posttraumatic stress disorder. *Gen Hosp Psychiatry* 2001;23(4):198–204.
128. Domino KB, Posner KL, Caplan RA, et al. Awareness during anesthesia: a closed claims analysis. *Anesthesiology* 1999;90(4):1053–1061.
129. Bergman IJ, Kluger MT, Short TG. Awareness during general anaesthesia: a review of 81 cases from the Anaesthetic Incident Monitoring Study. *Anaesthesia* 2002;57(6):549–556.
130. Ghoneim MM, Block RI, Haffarnan M, et al. Awareness during anesthesia: risk factors, causes and sequelae: a review of reported cases in the literature. *Anesth Analg* 2009;108(2):527–535.
131. Kurosawa S, Kato M, Kurosawa S, et al. Anesthetics, immune cells, and immune responses. *J Anesthesia* 2008;22(3):263–277.
132. Mulroy MF. Systemic toxicity and cardiotoxicity from local anesthetics: incidence and preventive measures. *Reg Anesth Pain Med* 2002; 27(6):556–561.
133. Liu PL, Feldman HS, Giasi R, et al. Comparative CNS toxicity of lidocaine, etidocaine, bupivacaine, and tetracaine in awake dogs following rapid intravenous administration. *Anesth Analg* 1983;62(4):375–379.
134. Covino BG. Toxicity of local anesthetic agents. *Acta Anaesthesiol Belg* 1988;39(3, Suppl 2):159–164.
135. Clarkson CW, Hondeghem LM. Mechanism for bupivacaine depression of cardiac conduction: fast block of sodium channels during the action potential with slow recovery from block during diastole. *Anesthesiology* 1985;62(4):396–405.
136. Morishima HO, Pedersen H, Finster M, et al. Bupivacaine toxicity in pregnant and nonpregnant ewes. *Anesthesiology* 1985;63(2):134–139.
137. Mather LE, Copeland SE, Ladd LA. Acute toxicity of local anesthetics: underlying pharmacokinetic and pharmacodynamic concepts. *Reg Anesth Pain Med* 2005;30(6):553–566.
138. Scott DB. "Maximum recommended doses" of local anaesthetic drugs. *Br J Anaesth* 1989;63(4):373–374.
139. Rosenberg PH, Veering BT, Urmey WF. Maximum recommended doses of local anesthetics: a multifactorial concept. *Reg Anesth Pain Med* 2004;29(6):564–575.
140. Brown D, Ransom D, Hall J, et al. Regional anesthesia and local anesthetic-induced systemic toxicity: seizure frequency and accompanying cardiovascular changes. *Anesth Analg* 1995;81(2):321–328.
141. Braid DP, Scott DB. Effect of adrenaline on the systemic absorption of local anaesthetic drugs. *Acta Anaesthesiol Scand Suppl* 1966;23:334–346.
142. Neal JM, Bernards CM, Butterworth JFIV, et al. ASRA practice advisory on local anesthetic systemic toxicity. *Reg Anesth Pain Med* 2010; 35(2):152–161.
143. Weinberg GL, Ripper R, Feinstein DL, et al. Lipid emulsion infusion rescues dogs from bupivacaine-induced cardiac toxicity [see comment]. *Reg Anesth Pain Med* 2003;28(3):198–202.
144. Perez-Castro R, Patel S, Garavito-Aguilar ZV, et al. Cytotoxicity of local anesthetics in human neuronal cells. *Anesth Analg* 2009;108(3): 997–1007.
145. Zink W, Graf BM. Local anesthetic myotoxicity. *Reg Anesth Pain Med* 2004;29(4):333–340.
146. Zink W, Seif C, Bohl JR, et al. The acute myotoxic effects of bupivacaine and ropivacaine after continuous peripheral nerve blockades. *Anesth Analg* 2003;97(4):1173–1179, table of contents.
147. Zink W, Bohl JRE, Hacke N, et al. The long term myotoxic effects of bupivacaine and ropivacaine after continuous peripheral nerve blocks. *Anesth Analg* 2005;101(2):548–554.
148. Gomez-Arnau JI, Yanguela J, Gonzalez A, et al. Anaesthesia-related diplopia after cataract surgery. *Br J Anaesth* 2003;90(2):189–193.
149. Busfield BT, Romero DM. Pain pump use after shoulder arthroscopy as a cause of glenohumeral chondrolysis. *Arthroscopy* 2009;25(6): 647–652.
150. Liu SS, McDonald SB. Current issues in spinal anesthesia [comment]. *Anesthesiology* 2001;94(5):888–906.
151. Lambert DH, Hurley RJ, Hertwig L, et al. Role of needle gauge and tip configuration in the production of lumbar puncture headache. *Reg Anesth* 1997;22(1):66–72.
152. Lybecker H, Moller JT, May O, et al. Incidence and prediction of postdural puncture headache. A prospective study of 1021 spinal anesthesias. *Anesth Analg* 1990;70(4):389–394.
153. Gerancher JC, Liu SS. Complications of neuraxial (spinal/epidural/caudal) anesthesia. In: Benumof JL, ed. *Anesthesia and perioperative complications*, 2nd ed. St. Louis: Mosby; 1999:50–65.
154. Vercauteren MP, Hoffmann VH, Mertens E, et al. Seven-year review of requests for epidural blood patches for headache after dural puncture: referral patterns and the effectiveness of blood patches. *Eur J Anaesthesiol* 1999;16(5):298–303.
155. Safa-Tisseront V, Thormann F, Malassine P, et al. Effectiveness of epidural blood patch in the management of post-dural puncture headache [comment]. *Anesthesiology* 2001;95(2):334–339.
156. Beards SC, Jackson A, Griffiths AG, et al. Magnetic resonance imaging of extradural blood patches: appearances from 30 min to 18 h [comment]. *Br J Anaesth* 1993;71(2):182–188.
157. Gupta S, Tarkkila P, Finucane BT. Complications of central neural blockade. In: Finucane BT, ed. *Complications of regional anesthesia*. Philadelphia, PA: Churchill Livingstone; 1999:184–212.
158. Breen TW, Ransil BJ, Groves PA, et al. Factors associated with back pain after childbirth. *Anesthesiology* 1994;81(1):29–34.
159. Hirabayashi Y, Igarashi T, Suzuki H, et al. Mechanical effects of leg position on vertebral structures examined by magnetic resonance imaging. *Reg Anesth Pain Med* 2002;27(4):429–432.
160. Pertek JP, Haberer JP. [Effects of anesthesia on postoperative micturition and urinary retention]. *Ann Fr Anesth Reanim* 1995;14(4):340–351.
161. Petros JG, Rimm EB, Robillard RJ. Factors influencing urinary tract retention after elective open cholecystectomy. *Surg Gynecol Obstet* 1992;174(6):497–500.
162. Jensen P, Mikkelsen T, Kehlet H. Postherniorrhaphy urinary retention–effect of local, regional, and general anesthesia: A review. *Reg Anesth Pain Med* 2002;27(6):612–617.
163. Pollock JE. Transient neurologic symptoms: etiology, risk factors, and management [comment]. *Reg Anesth Pain Med* 2002;27(6):581–586.

CHAPTER

13

Complications of Wound Healing

Michael G. Franz

Wound healing failure is the mechanism of many surgical complications. Incomplete tissue repair leads to incisional hernias and anastomotic leaks, while excessive tissue repair results in burn wound contractures and luminal strictures. Dysregulated wound healing, therefore, is a common cause of poor surgical outcomes. Although wounds are most frequently understood to mean injuries to the skin, practicing surgeons appreciate the importance of wounds and wounding to all types of tissue. The cellular and molecular pathways by which all types of injured tissues heal share common integrated components. A basic understanding of the biologic mechanisms of tissue repair is necessary to prevent or treat the complications of wound healing.

NORMAL WOUND HEALING

A wound initially is tissue that has lost normal structure and functions following the transfer of internal or external kinetic, chemical, or thermal energy. Wound healing is the sequence of cellular and molecular events activated at the time of injury resulting in a time-dependent pattern of tissue repair (1). The integration of each component pathway along the continuum of the host response to injury results in complete wound healing (Fig. 13.1). Classically, the phases of wound healing are described as hemostasis, inflammation, fibroproliferation, and remodeling (maturation).

Hemostasis

The cellular and molecular structure of the acute wound matrix changes continuously through wound maturation and remodeling. The dynamic process involves molecular and cellular interactions during which the initial fibrin-rich clot is transformed into a collagen-rich scar. Before a wound can heal it must stop bleeding. Therefore, the earliest phase of wound healing following injury is characterized by the deposition of fibrinogen, a soluble plasma protein synthesized by the liver and secreted into the systemic circulation. Fibrinogen extravasates from disrupted blood vessels and fills the gap of the wound. The coagulation cascade is activated and sustained through thrombin-mediated cleavage of fibrinogen, leading to the formation of fibrin monomers that polymerize into an insoluble fibrin clot to prevent further bleeding. The fibrin network also establishes the provisional matrix that allows migration of monocytes, fibroblasts, and endothelial cells into the wound. Fibroblasts within the fibrin clot synthesize collagen, and the fibrin matrix is progressively degraded and replaced with a collagen-rich scar (2). Fibrinogen has also been reported to induce angiogenesis. Other mediators activated during hemostasis such as platelet-derived growth factor (PDGF) and thrombin peptides have overlapping regulatory effects on many of the cellular elements of early tissue repair, such as fibroblasts and endothelial cells (3).

Inflammation

The cellular and humoral inflammatory phase is activated soon after wounding, and an immune barrier is established against pathologic microorganisms. Although most acute surgical wounds are sterile, chronic wounds may be colonized or infected with bacteria. Wound healing will be significantly impaired if wound tissue bacterial levels exceed 10^5 organisms per gram of tissue (4). The redundancy of the signals for the wound inflammatory response and wound healing is beginning to be described. Necrotic tissue locally releases cellular breakdown products capable of maintaining and amplifying the early inflammatory response following injury. Eicosanoids, 20-carbon metabolites of arachidonic acid derived from cell-membrane fatty acids, function as primary mediators in the wound healing scheme. Macrophages are tissue leukocytes fundamental to the inflammatory response following injury, which provides an abundant reservoir of potent tissue growth factors necessary for repair, such as transforming growth factor-β (TGF-β). The intensity of the early inflammatory response is greater in adult wound healing, in which protection against microbial insult supports tissue repair. During fetal wound healing until midgestation, the intensity of this tissue inflammatory response is significantly reduced. One proposed mechanism is immaturity of the cellular immune

Michael G. Franz: University of Michigan, Ann Arbor, MI 48109.

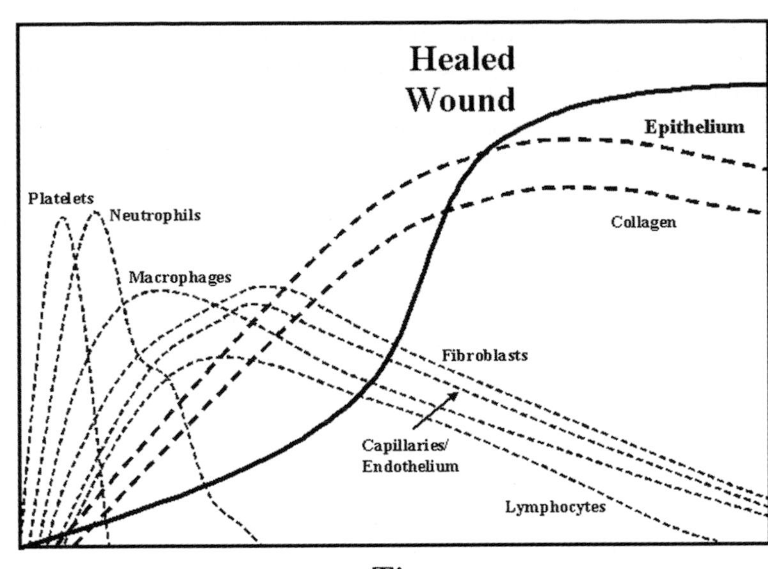

FIGURE 13.1. Functional acute wound healing requires the coordinated activation of cellular and molecular repair pathways beginning at the moment of injury. Each component must then be integrated into a continuum during the host response. For surgical incisions, it is the rate of recovery in breaking strength that determines the outcome of the acute wound.

system and reduced growth factor production (5). The blunted immediate tissue inflammatory response *in utero* is one potential explanation for the phenomenon of scarless fetal healing.

Over the past decade, the free radical nitric oxide (NO) has emerged as a fundamental signaling molecule for many biologic processes (6,7). NO has proven especially important in physiologic responses important to surgeons, such as following traumatic injury and during sepsis. NO level and activity is central to the regulation of vascular tone during shock and is equally important as a metabolite that can establish a host barrier against microorganism invasion.

NO is synthesized by one of three isoforms of nitric oxide synthase (NOS). Inducible NOS (iNOS) is upregulated following tissue injury. Most data suggest that local NO production promotes normal wound healing. NOS inhibitors delay the healing of acute excisional wounds, while supplemental NO provided via molecular donors accelerates acute wound healing. The recovery of incisional wound breaking strength is also delayed following NOS blockade. Knockout mice missing the iNOS gene exhibit marked impairment of acute healing that can be reversed by iNOS gene transfer. It appears that NO contributes to acute tissue repair by promoting collagen synthesis and angiogenesis (8).

Once bleeding is controlled, the increased permeability of vessels adjacent to the injury facilitates the migration of inflammatory cells into the wound. Polymorphonuclear leukocytes (neutrophils) are the predominant initial inflammatory cell population to enter the wound site. The rise in wound neutrophil number begins almost immediately following injury and peaks by postinjury day 2. The primary function of acute wound neutrophils appears to be phagocytosis of invading microbes and release of cytochemoattractants to further propagate the cellular inflammatory response. In neutrophil-depleted animal models, it has been shown that neutrophils are not mandatory for the progression of normal tissue repair (3). However, it is also well known that if a wound infection develops, healing will be delayed. In patients with chronic granulomatous disease in which an absence of the enzyme NADPH-oxidase occurs, the intracellular killing of bacteria and fungi within neutrophils is impaired. This defect results in chronic infections, which retard the repair process.

Following burns, there is delayed tissue necrosis secondary to vascular occlusion caused by thrombi deposition in the vascular bed surrounding the burn wound. The absence of blood flow through these vessels results in extended tissue necrosis and an increase in the wound surface area. Preventing the infiltration of circulating neutrophils into a burn wound using blocking antibodies directed against neutrophil surface antigens has been shown in animal models to prevent the development of secondary burn necrosis. Observations such as these demonstrate that a balance between wound benefit and wound detriment exists and that excessive neutrophil-derived factors such as oxygen radicals can actually impede tissue repair.

Circulating monocytes enter the wound in a second wave of inflammatory cells within 24 hours after the appearance of neutrophils (1). Monocytes terminally differentiate into tissue macrophages upon exiting the vasculature and entering the wound site. Macrophages are clearing houses for many important molecular signals for the propagation of the wound repair process, such as oxygen free radicals, inflammatory cytokines, and tissue growth factors. Tissue macrophages also have the capacity to undergo cell division within the wound site and, like the neutrophils, can clear the wound of contaminating microbes as well as nonviable tissue. Macrophage synthesis and release of tissue growth factors is a predominant signal mechanism for the initiation of the proliferative

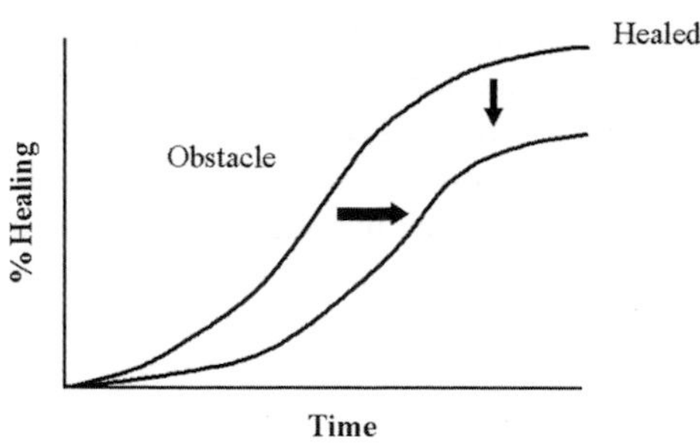

FIGURE 13.2. Wound healing failure occurs when an impediment to normal repair pathways results in an abnormality in the quality or duration of the sequential components of tissue repair. The obstacles to normal wound healing might be biologic or mechanical in origin and might derive from the wounded host or from external forces.

Table 13.1 Impediments to wound healing

Systemic	Local
Malnutrition	Contamination and infection
Chronic diseases	Repeated trauma
Drugs	Tissue hypoperfusion
Shock	Irradiation
Age	Neoplasm
Genetic repair defects	Factitious wounding

the wound surface area is small, regenerative reepithelialization might occur with little or no scar formation.

Contraction is a metabolically active mechanism by which wound volume is mechanically diminished. Although the mechanism of wound contraction is complex, it appears to involve tractional forces generated by repair fibroblasts transmitted to the wound extracellular matrix via cellular adhesion molecules (13). The early wound matrix is composed in large part of collagen, fibrin, fibronectin, and vitronectin. Intracellular fibroblast cytoskeletal polymerization, an energy requiring process, is the source of the tractional forces. Some evidence also suggests that terminally differentiated wound fibroblasts, called *myofibroblasts*, are involved. These cells express cytoplasmic smooth muscle actin and are contractile.

Wound failure occurs when there is an abnormality in the magnitude or duration of the sequential components of tissue repair. Inadequate hemostasis due to platelet dysfunction or poor technique results in hematoma formation with ensuing mechanical disruption of the provisional wound matrix. Delayed or deficient inflammatory responses increase the risk of wound contamination or infection. A *prolonged* inflammatory response due to foreign material delays the progression of tissue repair into the fibroproliferative phase in which rapid gains in breaking strength and wound contraction should occur. Impaired fibroblast activation in turn impedes the establishment of the early wound matrix and synthesis of immature scar. Epithelialization requires an underlying functional bed of granulation tissue. Obstacles to normal wound healing therefore shift the wound healing trajectory and result in wound complications (Fig. 10.2).

PREOPERATIVE RISK FACTORS FOR WOUND COMPLICATIONS

Contamination and infection

The risk factors for surgical wound complications can be broadly categorized as local or systemic wound healing impediments (Table 13.1). The most common local risk factor is wound contamination or infection. The risk for wound contamination and infection can be predicted by categorizing surgical wounds according to clinical circumstances. In increasing order of risk for wound infection, they are operating in (i) a clean field, (ii) a clean-contaminated field, (iii) a contaminated field, and (iv) an infected or dirty field (Table 13.2). A clean operative field minimizes wound bacterial exposure by operating upon otherwise normal and healthy soft tissue usually breaching only the skin. The bacterial organisms normally colonizing skin surfaces are predominantly Gram-positive *Staphylococcus* and *Streptococcus* species. Following standard operative field sterile preparation, expected wound infection rates in this setting are 1% to 3% (18,19). Examples include breast biopsies and inguinal hernia repair. An operation is classified

Table 13.2 Risk for wound contamination and infection according to clinical circumstances

Wound Classification	Examples	Risk for Wound Infection (%)
Dirty/infected with necrotic debris	Infected traumatic wound	60
Contaminated	Gunshot wound to left colon	33
Clean-contaminated	Elective colon resection	5
Clean	Breast biopsy or hernia repair	1

clean contaminated if an organ that is colonized with high numbers of potentially pathologic bacteria is exposed to the wound. Common examples are colorectal and pulmonary resections. In this setting, expected wound infection rates are reduced to 10% with appropriate preoperative preparation and prophylaxis. A procedure is classified as contaminated if high-level, uncontrolled bacterial contamination occurs, especially when associated with local tissue necrosis or ischemia. Examples of these procedures include repair of gunshot wounds of the colon or severe burn injuries. Wound infection rates in these settings are 33% to 60% (18).

Necrotic tissue exacerbates defective wound repair. Bacteria use necrotic debris as a nutrient source, increasing the likelihood of invasive wound infection. Metabolites of cell-membrane arachidonic acid released from dying cells are toxic to adjacent normal cells. Necrotic debris within the wound also establishes a mechanical barrier against the influx of wound repair cells, such as fibroblasts and keratinocytes. Tissue proteases released by necrotic cells degrade wound growth factors, preventing the initiation of growth factor-dependent repair pathways.

Tissue hypoperfusion

Operating during periods of shock increases the risk of surgical wound failure. Wound infection and dehiscence rates increase threefold when operating during profound hypotension and acidosis (20). Tissue perfusion is impaired as a consequence of other disorders, including peripheral vascular disease, edema, hypothermia, vasospastic disease, and venous hypertension. Irradiated tissue is also hypoperfused as the result of microangiopathy. Previously irradiated tissue might be especially susceptible to wound necrosis given its reduced capillary blood supply and increased fibrosis, which results in an abnormal wound inflammatory response.

Reduced capillary perfusion results in a low tissue oxygen tension, which is associated with collagen defects and increased wound infections (21). Severe ischemia and hypoxia can directly inhibit other wound healing processes such as angiogenesis and epithelialization. Transcutaneous tissue oxygen monitors provide a clinically available means for measuring wound oxygen levels. Chronic wounds like pressure ulcers and diabetic foot ulcers do not heal when tissue oxygen levels fall below 30 mm Hg.

Malnutrition

Severely malnourished or catabolic patients, as during the systemic inflammatory response syndrome, demonstrate impaired healing (22). The deleterious effects of malnutrition are expressed in each of the phases of wound healing. An altered inflammatory response might result from the effects of malnutrition on immune function. Animals fed protein-free diets develop reduced levels of fibronectin and complement, both important chemotactic factors for fibroblasts and macrophages. Decreased polymorphonuclear leukocyte activity against fungi and bacteria has been measured in children suffering kwashiorkor protein deficiency (23). Prolonged protein malnutrition limits collagen synthesis, fibroblast proliferation, and neovascularization.

Although nutritional status is difficult to measure in most clinical settings, a serum albumin <3 g per dL increases the risk of wound infection and incisional hernia formation. A large Veterans Administration cooperative study of perioperative risk factors found that a low preoperative serum albumin level was the single most significant variable for predicting surgical morbidity (20). Wound infection and acute wound failure were among the most commonly observed complications. Protein synthesis and cell division are stimulated at wound sites, and an abundant supply of amino acids is necessary to sustain repair. Fatty acid deficiencies are known to cause delayed dermal healing. Cancer cachexia is associated with profound delays in wound repair. Elevated circulating cytokine levels, such as tumor necrosis factor-α, contribute through disturbances in the normal wound inflammatory response.

Micronutrient deficiency can also impair wound healing. Vitamin A is a cofactor for normal cell differentiation and epithelial keratinization. Vitamin C is critical for strength gain in healing wounds, catalyzing the hydroxylation of proline and lysine residues during collagen cross-linking. Vitamin K is required for the synthesis of several coagulation proteins, including prothrombin. Deficiencies are therefore associated with excessive bleeding from wounded tissue and abnormal provisional matrix formation. Trace mineral deficiencies can develop in surgical patients, especially those treated with prolonged parenteral nutrition and in patients with chronic conditions such as alcoholism, GI disorders, and diabetes. Zinc acts as a cofactor to many enzymatic reactions involved in DNA synthesis, protein synthesis, mitosis, and cellular proliferation. Reduced zinc levels result in delayed epithelialization and fibroblast proliferation. Iron is a cofactor in collagen synthesis, and low iron levels indirectly impair healing because of reduced oxygen transport.

Chronic diseases

Underlying disease in the injured host can complicate wound healing. Diabetes mellitus is known to delay the closure of dermal foot ulcers, but it is not clear that incisional healing is delayed in diabetic patients. Diabetic patients are more susceptible to wound infection because of impaired neutrophil chemotaxis and phagocytosis. The clean wound infection rate is higher in diabetic patients (11%) than in the general patient population (24).

Increasing patient age is not a consistent risk factor for global wound healing complications. There appears to be a minor defect in epidermal-dermal repair that is the result of changes in tissue extracellular matrix structure and resultant elasticity of aged skin, but this does not appear to affect myofascial, GI, or vascular repair. In specific models, increased host age is associated with impaired wound healing. Fibroblast proliferation and activity are diminished and collagen production and wound contraction are slowed down (23). Tissue repair observed in the elderly is often complicated by an increased incidence of comorbid conditions and polypharmacy.

Immunodeficiency states have been associated with delayed wound healing. In the presence of an impaired immune defense, wound bacterial loads might rise to uncontrolled levels and delay healing trajectories. Although polymorphonuclear leukocytes are not absolutely required for wound healing, the absence or reduction in wound macrophage number or activity leads to significant impairment of tissue repair (1).

Acute and chronic liver diseases are associated with delays in wound healing. In animal models, acute jaundice caused a 25% to 50% reduction in abdominal incision bursting strength after 1 week (1). Long-standing jaundice had less of an inhibitory effect on healing incisions. Clinically, increased fascial dehiscence has been reported following laparotomy performed in jaundiced patients, especially those with malignant causes for jaundice. Acute wound failure rates of 60% have been observed in small series.

Drugs

Cytotoxic and metabolically active pharmacologic agents should always be considered when managing a wound. The active cellular components of wound healing, such as macrophages, fibroblasts, and epithelial cells, are targets for undesirable inhibitory side effects. Although there are not many class one data sets proving the impairment of tissue repair by most pharmacologic agents, clinical experience and pharmacologic mechanisms should alert all clinicians managing wounds to the possibility of drug-induced wound complications.

It is not clear that corticosteroid use delays most soft tissue repair following surgical wounding. Category II evidence suggests that epidermal repair is delayed, but there is no solid evidence that myofascial or GI healing is impaired (25). Steroids have been shown to inhibit fibroblast function *in vitro*. Although the recovery of dermal tensile strength is delayed in rodents treated with corticosteroids at the time of incision, the effects of corticosteroids on human clinical wound healing have not been well studied. Mechanistically, it is likely that corticosteroids impair tissue repair through their inhibitory effects on inflammation and structural gene expression. The inhibitory effect of cortisone on skin wound strength in rodents is negated if vitamin A is given concurrently. No data are available on the treatment of patients on steroids with vitamin A prior to surgical wounding, although empirical therapy might be reasonable.

Cytotoxic agents can induce profound delays in wound repair by inhibiting cell proliferation, DNA, and protein synthesis. Chemotherapeutic drugs might suppress the normal wound inflammatory response as well as inhibit fibroblast proliferation and collagen deposition. Clinically, it is usual to delay administration of an antineoplastic agent in a postoperative cancer patient until the acute wound healing phases are completed because of concern for adverse drug effects on wound healing (usually 3 to 6 weeks).

Genetic defects

The classic genetic disorder with an abnormal wound healing phenotype is the Ehlers–Danlos syndrome. Variable penetrance of the defective structural protein genes might cause subtle clinical presentations. There are at least 12 distinct subtypes of Ehlers–Danlos, and although it is infrequent, encountering such a patient occurs in most surgical careers. Ehlers–Danlos syndrome is often associated with fragile skin, weakened scar and wound disruption, spontaneous aneurysms in major blood vessels, and bleeding disorders. A careful personal and family history as well as physical exam should alert the observant surgeon to these disorders. Other frequently encountered patients with disordered wound healing include Marfan's syndrome patients. Newer genetic and biochemical evidence suggests that spontaneous abdominal aortic aneurysm patients might also express abnormal content or collagen protease activity contributing to both arterial wall weakness and defective wound healing. Abdominal aortic aneurysm patients are commonly encountered in surgical practices. Once a clinical diagnosis associated with defective tissue repair is made, great care must be exercised in wound closure and management, since there are no known methods for correcting the defective biochemical pathways.

MODIFICATION OF PREOPERATIVE RISK FACTORS

Minimize contamination

Minimization of microbial wound contamination lowers the incidence of wound infection and wound failure. Antiseptic preparation of the surgical site is known to reduce the incidence of wound infection following clean cases. In the case of GI surgery, preoperative luminal mechanical and antibiotic preparation may reduce exposure to enteric bacteria and lower wound infection rates, although some studies show no clinically significant benefit (18). Sharp debridement of necrotic tissue from acute and chronic wounds increases the incidence of complete wound healing (4). In the case of gross wound contamination, the wound should be copiously irrigated at the time of the operation to clear necrotic tissue and foreign material.

Antibiotics

Therapeutic tissue antibiotic levels at the surgical site during incision reduce the incidence of wound infection following clean and clean-contaminated cases. This requires that a bolus dose of the appropriate antibiotic be given just prior to the time of wounding. Antibiotics with a spectrum of coverage for Gram-positive skin organisms are indicated for clean cases (e.g., first-generation cephalosporin). An antibiotic class with broader Gram-negative coverage is indicated for clean-contaminated GI cases (e.g., second-generation cephalosporin). It is not clear that antibiotic administration following grossly contaminated traumatic injuries lowers the incidence of postoperative wound infections. Because of the high incidence of wound infection following contaminated cases, antibiotics are typically begun empirically.

Resuscitation

Transcutaneous oxygen tension is the optimal method for measuring nutritive skin perfusion and has a direct correlation with the success of dermal healing. Molecular oxygen is necessary for mature collagen formation, and optimized collagen fibril cross-linking fails as tissue oxygen pressure (PO_2) levels fall below 40 mm Hg. When periwound PO_2 falls below 30 mm Hg, healing may be impaired. Below 10 mm Hg, oxygen is deficient and growth factors have little chance of inducing healing mechanisms for these wounds. In most models, hyperbaric oxygen (HBO) therapy has been found to improve wound oxygen delivery and to induce angiogenesis in ischemic wounds (21).

Wound closure technique

Primary wound closure is defined as the surgical closure of a wound within several hours after the wound is made. Primary wound closure results in low infection and wound failure rates for clean and clean-contaminated wounds. Whenever possible, incisions should be placed in lines of minimal tension to prevent hypertrophic scarring. This is especially true in locations of cosmetic importance such as the face. For example, on the forehead, the lines of minimal tension are transverse, so that a transverse incision will heal with a thinner and finer scar-line than a perpendicular, vertical incision.

Following gross wound contamination, secondary closure (healing by secondary intent) will reduce wound infection rates. Secondary intention occurs in an open, full-thickness wound that heals by the host biologic mechanisms of epithelialization, contraction, collagen deposition, and granulation tissue formation. Although better than wound infection, the drawback of this approach is that open wounds require more nursing care and result in a worse cosmetic result.

Delayed primary closure provides an alternative. This technique involves leaving a contaminated wound open with moist dressing changes until bacterial balance is achieved. When quantitative wound culture levels fall to $\leq 10^5$ colony forming units per gram of wound tissue, the wound healing success rate following closure approaches that of primary closure (1). Delayed primary closure also provides the time necessary for the cellular and molecular elements of tissue repair to enter the wound prior to wound closure. Delayed primary closure is usually performed 24 hours to several days following injury.

Tertiary wound closure involves the transfer of viable autologous tissue from a distant site to the wound. Partial thickness skin grafting is a frequently used example. The technique can accelerate epithelialization when wound contraction has stopped or there is a large surface area of granulation tissue.

The choice of suture material does not significantly affect wound healing. In principle, the suture should provide approximation of the injured tissue and maintain bursting strength until wound mechanics recover. A very rapidly absorbed suture material would therefore be appropriate for a low load wound repair in which wound tensile strength rapidly recovers, such as following corneal keratotomy. In contrast, wound closure following abdominal wall laparotomy requires a stout suture material that maintains its mechanical integrity for the 6 to 12 weeks necessary for recovery of maximal wound bursting strength. Class 2 and 3 data suggest that braided suture materials are associated with higher suture abscess rates, especially when used in contaminated wounds. Bacteria lodge within the interstices of braided suture and escape wound immune cell phagocytosis.

Acute wound failure is most often due to suture pulling through adjacent tissue and not suture fracture or knot slippage (25). Tissue failure occurs in the biochemically active zone adjacent to the acute wound edge in which proteases activated during normal tissue repair result in a loss of native tissue integrity. This is especially true for GI anastomoses in which a fall in wound tensile strength has been measured during the first 3 days following repair (26–30). The breakdown of the tissue matrix adjacent to the wound appears to be part of the mechanism for mobilizing the many cellular elements of acute tissue repair.

Improve nutritional status

Preoperative nutritional repletion has been shown to improve surgical wound outcomes only in cases of severe malnutrition (31). In fact, some studies suggest that aggressive preoperative nutritional supplementation increases wound complications and surgical morbidity and mortality, especially in oncology patients. The additional procedures required for peripheral and enteral access as well as delays in surgical therapy contribute to the disappointing results of

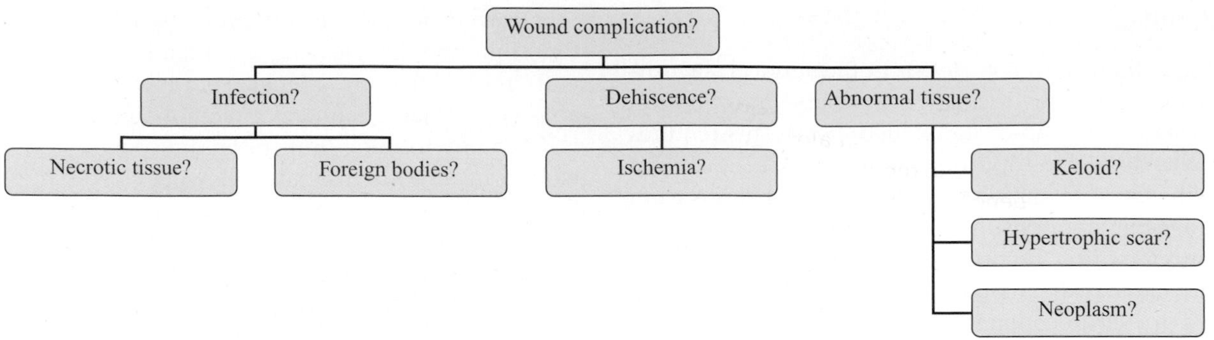

FIGURE 13.3. Most wound complications might be clinically categorized as infections, mechanical failure (dehiscence), or abnormal tissue (neoplasia). A systematic approach to wound complications can guide accurate diagnosis and therapy.

aggressive preoperative attempts at nutritional therapy. If possible, operations should be performed when the serum albumin level is >3 g.

DIAGNOSIS OF POSTOPERATIVE WOUND COMPLICATIONS

A healing wound should remain structurally and functionally intact and display no signs of inflammation. There should be no intense redness, warmth, swelling, or pain (rubor, calor, tumor, and dolor). Progressive fibroplasia should result in a prominent midwound "healing ridge" (Fig. 13.3).

Wound infections

A wound infection exists when $>10^5$ invasive organisms per gram of wound tissue or any level of β-hemolytic streptococcus are present. This manifests clinically as wound cellulitis, drainage, odor, and/or pain.

Accurate diagnosis of wound infections requires precise anatomical localization (Fig. 13.4). Complicated deep wound infections might progress to fasciitis or myonecrosis, as in Fournier's gangrene. Surrounding skin bullae should always raise concern for an invasive wound infection, as should unexplained fevers occurring near the fifth postoperative day. If the clinical presentation is confusing or if empiric therapy fails, wound biopsy for histology and quantitative wound cultures provide the most definitive diagnosis of wound infection. Surface wound cultures might suggest a pathogenic organism and guide antimicrobial therapy, but a wound infection is not defined until tissue invasion occurs with associated tissue inflammation (32).

Dehiscence and acute wound failure

Acute wound failure can present as mechanical wound separation or dehiscence. Dermal wound separation worsens cosmetic results but is unlikely to cause significant harm. Abdominal wall, GI, and vascular anastomosis wound failure can have life-threatening outcomes and will be discussed in later chapters. Wound dehiscence occurs when the distractive forces exerted perpendicular to a wound edge exceeds the recovery of wound mechanical properties (33).

Hypertrophic scars and keloids

Hypertrophic scars are raised and often inflamed but confined to the area of the original wound. Most will resolve slowly over 1 to 2 years without surgical intervention. There is some evidence that steroid derivative injections

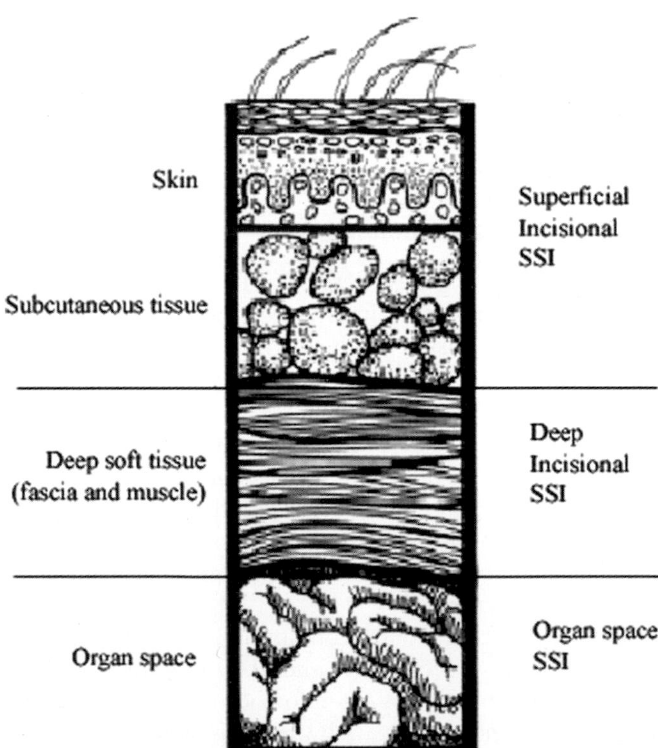

FIGURE 13.4. The accurate diagnosis and therapy of wound infections requires precise anatomical localization. Tracking of uncontrolled soft tissue infections along fascial planes might progress to myonecrosis, as in Fournier's gangrene. The development of bullae in the skin surrounding a wound should always raise concern for an invasive wound infection. Wound tissue biopsies provide the most definitive diagnosis of wound infection.

(triamcinolone) can inhibit the prolonged inflammatory phase of scar formation and induce remodeling. Keloids, in contrast, extend beyond the boundaries of the original wound and do not regress spontaneously. Keloids tend to recur following excision, and excision alone is rarely adequate therapy to prevent recurrence. Intralesional steroid therapy has shown benefit. Any steroid therapy must be used with close surveillance to avoid tissue atrophy and skin depigmentation. Antihistamine therapy might improve the burning and itching often associated with keloids and might help to avoid cyclical attempts at surgical excision.

Neoplasms

Malignancy should be considered in a nonhealing wound and a biopsy performed in any open area that is difficult to debride and is failing to heal.

MANAGEMENT OF WOUND COMPLICATIONS

Wound dressings

Most wound complications can be managed nonoperatively. Appropriately dressing and protecting a wound can reduce the incidence of wound complications. Basic wound healing studies and clinical research have confirmed that wound healing is optimized in a moist environment (34). The ideal wound dressing therefore should protect a wound against desiccation (hydrophobic dressing). In addition, dressings should keep a wound clean, protect against repeated wound trauma, absorb exudates, and minimize wound pain (Fig. 13.5).

Specific types of wounds have unique requirements for optimized tissue repair. Pressure ulcers need off-loading to improve capillary perfusion of the wound and surrounding skin and to minimize traumatic shear forces. Venous stasis ulcers heal best when lower extremity sequential compression is used, in part, to improve capillary perfusion and tissue oxygen delivery (35).

Antibiotics

Antibiotic chemotherapy improves outcomes for the treatment of wound infections. Therapeutic wound and periwound tissue levels are required for antimicrobial efficacy. For antibiotic therapy to be successful, a wound must first be adequately prepared. This most commonly means debridement of necrotic tissue and the excision of foreign material.

Therapeutic wound tissue antibiotic levels can be achieved both topically and systemically. Often, infected nonhealing wounds are hypoperfused, limiting the delivery of systemically administered antibiotics. Burn eschars, venous stasis ulcers, and pressure ulcers are common examples. In these settings, topically applied antimicrobials such as silver sulfadiazine and Sulfamylon preparations might be efficacious. Systemically applied antibiotics will improve wound healing rates only if minimum inhibitory concentrations are reached in the wounded and infected tissue. Regardless of the route of wound antibiotic therapy, the anti-infectives used will be most effective if directed to the organisms infecting the wound. This can be achieved by performing quantitative wound cultures. In general, first-generation penicillins and cephalosporins provide a spectrum of coverage for most Gram-positive skin surface organisms, while second-generation and third-generation cephalosporins and modified, later-generation penicillins increase Gram-negative and enteric coverage at the expense of anti–Gram-positive activity.

Wound adjuvants

The high prevalence of nonhealing wounds has stimulated the development of novel adjuvants designed to improve wound-healing outcomes. Vacuum-assisted wound closure can improve closure rates. The most common design allows maintenance of a moist wound environment, drainage of wound exudates, and continuous negative pressure to the open wound surface. This arrangement has been shown to accelerate the appearance of repair fibroblasts in the wound

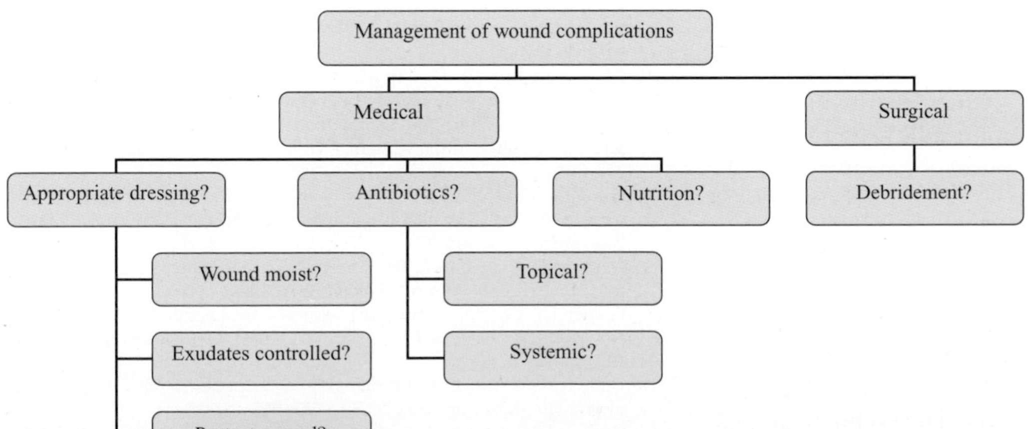

FIGURE 13.5. The management of wound complications may apply nonoperative and operative principles. The optimum dressing protects the wound from repeat trauma and maintains a moist wound environment. Topical antibiotic therapy might be effective when the infection is confined to the wound, especially when wound blood supply is compromised. Surgical therapy is fundamental to the successful management of complicated wounds.

and to improve wound perfusion (36). HBO therapy has also been shown to improve the healing rates of difficult wounds. When transcutaneous tissue oxygen levels of <30 mm Hg are achieved, reported wound closure rates have been accelerated by 50% (21).

Debridement

A skin wound should be reopened when wound infection is suspected or if surrounding cellulitis does not respond to antibiotics. This allows a quantitative wound culture to be performed for more accurate diagnosis. In addition, an open wound can be debrided with moist gauze dressing changes several times a day. Dressing debridement lowers wound bacterial counts directly and by removing from the wound necrotic tissue that acts as a nutrient supply for invasive organisms.

Necrotic wounds might need more aggressive surgical intervention. Necrotic wound tissue is by definition without a blood supply and will not heal. Necrotic tissue should therefore always be debrided from wounds. The most reliable way to debride any wound is sharply using standard surgical principles. Necrotic tissue should be excised back to healthy appearing soft tissue with obvious blood supply. All foreign material-like asphalt or retained sutures should also be debrided from a nonhealing wound. Debridement might be limited by extension to a nonhealing surface or structure such as tendon sheath or bone. In these cases, a viable tissue transfer might be indicated. Chemical enzymatic wound debridement is efficacious when surgical debridement is not available, but it remains a second-line alternative to complete surgical excision. Protease compounds of papain and collagenases are often applied. Chemical debridement is effective only for the removal of necrotic soft tissue and biofilms. Enzymatic treatment cannot replace surgical debridement of complicating foreign materials.

Seromas and hematomas can impede wound healing. These fluid collections mechanically distract wound edges and reduce capillary perfusion. Wound fluid collections also increase the risk of wound infection. Whenever possible, wound seromas or hematomas that are not spontaneously resolving or that are associated with a wound complication like infection or dehiscence should be aspirated or drained through the open incision. If the wound fluid collection is associated with a nearby implanted device, it might be best to attempt needle aspiration of the fluid collection under sterile conditions to minimize the risk of a foreign body infection.

Scar revision

Scars resulting in poor cosmetic results can be surgically revised. The broad goal of scar revision is to reorient the scar into lines of tension so that the dimension of the scar is oriented into lines of relaxation. The techniques most often used for dermal scars are Z-plasties or W-plasties. Stricture plasties of GI strictures apply the same principles in an effort to redirect scar forces.

REFERENCE

1. Robson MC, Steed DL, Franz MG. Wound healing: biologic features and approaches to maximize healing trajectories. *Curr Probl Surg* 2001; 38(2):77–89.
2. Henry G, Garner WL. Inflammatory mediators in wound healing. *Surg Clin North Am* 2003;83:491–497.
3. Clark RAF. *The molecular and cellular biology of wound repair*, 2nd ed. New York: Plenum Publishing; 1995.
4. Robson MC, Hill DP, Woodske ME, et al. Wound healing trajectories as predictors of effectiveness of therapeutic agents. *Arch Surg* 2000;135: 773–777.
5. Ferguson MW, Whitby DJ, Shah M, et al. Scar formation: the spectral nature of fetal and adult wound repair. *Plast Reconstr Surg* 1996;97: 854–860.
6. Tzeng E, Billiar TR. Nitric oxide and the surgical patient: identifying therapeutic targets. *Arch Surg* 1997;132:977–982.
7. Yamasaki K, Edington HD, McClosky C, et al. Reversal of impaired wound repair in iNOS-deficient mice by topical adenoviral-mediated iNOS gene transfer. *J Clin Invest* 1998;101: 967–971.
8. Leibovich SJ, Polverini PJ, Fong TW, et al. Production of angiogenic activity by human monocytes requires an L-arginine/nitric oxide synthase-dependent effector mechanism. *Proc Natl Acad Sci USA* 1994;91: 4190–4194.
9. Rappolee DA, Mark D, Banda MJ, et al. Wound macrophages express and other growth-factors in vivo: analysis by mRNA phenotyping. *Science* 1988;241:708–712.
10. Pajulo OT, Pulkki KJ, Lertola KK, et al. Hyaluronic acid in incision wound fluid: a clinical study with the Cellstick device in children. *Wound Repair Regen* 2001;9(3):200–204.
11. Gosiewska A, Yi CF, Brown LJ, et al. Differential expression and regulation of extracellular matrix-associated genes in fetal and neonatal fibroblasts. *Wound Repair Regen* 2001;9(3):213–222.
12. Morgan CJ, Pledger WJ. Fibroblast proliferation. In: Cohen IH, Diegelmann RF, Lindblad WJ, eds. *Wound healing: biochemical and clinical aspects*. Philadelphia, PA: WB Saunders; 1992:63–76.
13. Ballas CB, Davison JM. Delayed wound healing in aged rats is associated with increased collagen gel remodeling and contraction by skin fibroblasts, not with differences in apoptotic or myofibroblast cell populations. *Wound Repair Regen* 2001;9(3): 223–237.
14. Prockop DJ, Kivirikko KI, Tuderman L, et al. The biosynthesis of collagen and its disorders. *N Engl J Med* 1979;301:13–23.
15. Jorgensen LN, Kellehave F, Karlsmark T, et al. Reduced collagen accumulation after major surgery. *Br J Surg* 1996;83:1591–1594.
16. Robson MC, Mustoe TA, Hunt TK. The future of recombinant growth factors in wound healing. *Am J Surg* 1998;176 (Suppl 2A): 80–82.
17. Friedman DW, Boyd CD, Norton P, et al. Increases in type III collagen gene expression and protein synthesis in patients with inguinal hernias. *Ann Surg* 1993;218:754–760.
18. Culver DH. Surgical wound infection rates by wound class, operative procedure and patient risk index. *Am J Med* 1991;91(Suppl 3B):152–157S.
19. Horan TC, Gaynes RP, Martone WJ, et al. CDC definitions of nosocomial surgical site infections, 1992: a modification of CDC definitions of surgical wound infections. *Am J Infect Control* 1992;20:271–274.
20. Best WR, Khuri SF, Phelan M, et al. Identifying patient preoperative risk factors and postoperative adverse events in administrative databases: results from the Department of Veterans Affairs National Surgical Quality Improvement Program. *J Am Coll Surg* 2002;194(3): 257–266.
21. Hunt TK. Physiology in wound healing. In: Clowes GHA, ed. *Trauma, sepsis and shock: the physiological basis of therapy*. New York: Marcel Dekker Inc; 1988:443–471.
22. Demling RH, DeSanti L. The stress response to injury and infection: the role of nutritional support. *Wounds* 2000;12:3.
23. Leaper DJ, Gottrup F. Surgical wounds. In: Leaper DJ, Harding KG, eds. *Wounds: biology and management*. Oxford: Oxford University Press; 1998:23–40.
24. Gibbons GW. Lower extremity bypass in patients with diabetic foot ulcers. *Surg Clin North Am* 2003;83:659–669.
25. Carlson MA. Acute wound failure. Wound healing. *Surg Clin North Am* 2001;77(3):607–635.

26. Folli S, Morgagni P, Bazzocchi F, et al. An alternative repair technique for anastomotic leakage after total gastrectomy. *J Am Coll Surg* 2000;190(6):757–759.
27. Vignali A, Fazio WV, Lavery I, et al. Factors associated with the occurrence of leaks in stapled rectal anastomosis: review of 1,014 cases. *J Am Coll Surg* 1997;185:105–113.
28. Irvin TT, Hunt TK. Pathogenesis and prevention of disruption of colonic anastomoses in traumatized rats. *Br J Surg* 1974;61: 437–439.
29. Tadros T, Wobbes T, Hendriks T. Blood transfusion impairs the healing of experimental intestinal anastomoses. *Ann Surg* 1992;215: 276–281.
30. Tani T, Tsutamoto Y, Eguchi Y, et al. Protease inhibitor reduces loss of tensile strength in rat anastomosis with peritonitis. *J Surg Res* 2000;88: 135–141.
31. Williams JG, Barbul A. Nutrition and wound healing. *Surg Clin North Am* 2003;83:571–596.
32. Robson MC, Shaw RC, Heggers JP. The reclosure of postoperative incisional abscesses based on bacterial quantification of the wound. *Ann Surg* 1970;171:279.
33. DuBay DA, Franz MG. Acute wound healing: the biology of acute wound failure. *Surg Clin North Am* 2003;83:463–481.
34. Bolton L, Pirone L, Chen J. Dressings' effects on wound healing. *Wounds* 1990;2:126–134.
35. Macdonald JM, Sims N, Mayrovitz HN. Lymphedema, lipedema and the open wound: the role of compression therapy. *Surg Clin North Am* 2003;83:639–658.
36. Lionelli GT, Lawrence WT. Wound dressings. *Surg Clin North Am* 2003; 83:631–633.

Thus, the careful consideration of these issues is important to minimizing the risk of this complication.

National healthcare safety network

The NHSN (http://www.cdc.gov/nhsn/) was developed in 2005 to combine the work of three legacy efforts: the NNIS, the Dialysis Surveillance Network, and the National Surveillance System for Healthcare Workers. The NNIS was established in 1970 in selected hospitals within the United States (11). These hospitals began routinely reporting their nosocomial infection surveillance data to a national database that is now reported as NHSN data (1). Greater than 1500 acute care adult or children's hospitals participate; their identities are confidential. The NHSN data are collected according to standardized protocols, and include separate components for adult and pediatric intensive care unit infection rates, high-risk nursery infection rates, and surgical infection rates. The SSI statistics are mainly contained within this third component.

The NHSN surgical patient surveillance data are categorized according to the procedures performed. Records for every patient include information on risk factors such as wound class, duration of operation, American Society of Anesthesiologists (ASA) score, inpatient or outpatient status, and the use of laparoscopy or endoscopy to perform the procedure. These data are then combined to create risk index categories. The risk index category is calculated by counting the number of risk factors that the patient has. The risk factors are an ASA score greater than or equal to 3, a duration of operation greater than the 75th percentile for that procedure, or a wound class of contaminated or dirty. There are nominally four risk index categories for SSIs, representing patients who have 0, 1, 2, or 3 of the risk factors. However, if two risk index categories are similar, then those two categories are combined into a single category (Table 14.2). For example, in Table 14.2, while there are four separate risk categories for colon operations, in the cholecystectomy category there are only three reported risk index categories, as 2 and 3 are combined into 2,3. For other data sets, there were insufficient patients within some categories to perform statistical analysis, and so those risk index categories are not reported.

Table 14.2 shows some of the NHSN data for the 2006–2008 period regarding mean infection rate per 100 procedures for all hospitals (1). The data are then separated by percentile of hospitals to demonstrate the spread in infection rate across institutions. More detailed data are available in the reference. These data provide very reliable and well-defined information regarding SSI rates for commonly performed procedures across the United States. This allows benchmarking and comparison of hospital infection rates. Hospital infection rates can be compared to these only if the data is collected completely and in accordance with the CDC definitions. If these definitions are followed, then the demonstration of a high rate of infection for some procedure may help to identify an area that should be investigated further, as it may indicate some specific or systemic problem within the institution that is creating a discrepancy. Similarly, a rate substantially lower than the national benchmark data may indicate either an exceptional level of practice or a failure to detect infections by the surveillance program that is in place. The institution of some hospital infection control program to define these rates, such as the NHSN system, is an important component of quality systems-based patient care.

Microbiology of surgical site infection

The microbiology of SSIs has not changed significantly during the last decade (1,4,12). The most commonly isolated pathogens include *Staphylococcus aureus*, coagulase negative staphylococci, enterococcus species, and *Escherichia coli*. However, there has been an increasing incidence of SSIs caused by antibiotic resistance pathogens, such as methicillin-resistant *S. aureus* (MRSA) (6,12). This increased proportion of SSIs caused by resistant pathogens may be due to the increased and widespread use of broad spectrum antibiotics.

Most SSIs are caused by pathogens that are identified on the skin of the patient (Table 14.3). Thus most operations can be complicated by infection with *S. aureus* or coagulase-negative staphylococci. However, a violation of the respiratory or gastrointestinal tract or other sites that are colonized with bacteria, may lead to infection with specific organisms. Examples of this include gram-negative bacilli anaerobic bacteria or enterococci that may complicate operations on the gastrointestinal tract. Operations that traverse the oropharyngeal mucosa may contaminate the wound with oropharyngeal anaerobic bacteria, which can cause infections in these wounds.

Knowledge of the specific pathogen that is likely to cause SSIs is necessary to appropriately select prophylactic antimicrobial therapy for those patients at risk.

Specific risk factors

Effect of Laparoscopy on Risk

One of the important features in the risk of SSI is the use of laparoscopy to perform the procedure (4,11). Laparoscopy may be expected to decrease the risk of SSI because of decreased tissue trauma, decreased dead space in the subcutaneous tissue that might provide a site for surgical infection, and more limited tissue trauma overall. The occurrence of SSI is significantly decreased by the use of the laparoscope to do similar procedures. This advantage may be offset if the laparoscopic procedure takes significantly longer (>75th percentile for that procedure). In general, the decreased tissue trauma for laparoscopy appears to have a beneficial effect on the SSI risk.

Tobacco use

The use of tobacco may increase the risk of SSI by delaying primary wound healing (13–15). This has been clearly demonstrated for sternal or mediastinal SSIs after cardiac

Table **14.2** **Percentile distributions of hospital risk of surgical site infection (SSI) by procedure and NHSN risk index**

Procedure	NNIS Risk Index	Duration Cutpoint (Minutes)	No. of Hospitals	Mean Rate[a]	Mean Rate for percentile of Hospitals 10%	25%	50%	75%	90%
Cardiac	0, 1	306	150	1.10	0	0	0.49	1.64	2.60
Cardiac	2, 3		145	1.84	0	0	1.24	3.25	4.71
CABG[b]	0	301	135	0.35					
CABG[b]	1		292	2.55	0	0.65	1.90	3.45	5.37
CABG[b]	2		285	4.26	0	1.33	3.08	5.81	8.70
CABG	3		48	8.49					
Thoracic	0, 1	188	15	0.76					
Thoracic	2, 3		14	2.04					
Appendectomy	0, 1	81	31	1.15	0	0	0.60	1.23	2.76
Appendectomy	2, 3		27	3.47					
Cholecystectomy	0	99	96	0.23	0	0	0	0	0.86
Cholecystectomy	1		95	0.61	0	0	0	0.97	2.06
Cholecystectomy	2, 3		92	1.72	0	0	0	3.23	4.73
Cholecystectomy (Outpatient)	0	65	71	0.11	0	0	0	0	0.13
Cholecystectomy (Outpatient)	1, 2, 3		71	0.34	0	0	0	0	0.47
Colon	0	187	278	3.99	0	1.58	3.49	5.56	8.73
Colon	1		292	5.59	0	2.06	4.48	7.43	11.16
Colon	2		277	7.06	0	2.38	5.06	9.09	13.78
Colon	3		207	9.47					
Gastric	0, 1	160	40	1.72	0	0.70	1.21	2.57	3.58
Gastric	2, 3		37	4.23	0	1.04	2.30	5.00	8.16
Small bowel	0	192	29	3.44					
Small bowel	1, 2, 3		32	6.75					
Herniorrhaphy	0	124	89	0.74	0	0	0	1.77	2.42
Herniorrhaphy	1		88	2.32	0	0	1.02	3.15	5.63
Herniorrhaphy	2.3		72	5.25					
Thyroid/Parathyroid	0, 1, 2, 3	150	11	0.26					
Splenectomy	0, 1, 2, 3	217	15	2.33					
Exploratory Laparotomy	0, 1	199	29	1.67	0	0	0	1.08	1.91
Exploratory Laparotomy	2, 3		21	2.82	0	0.78	1.54	2.54	3.79

[a]Per 100 procedures.
[b]Coronary artery bypass graft, includes vein harvest site.

has a higher risk of infection than no hair removal at all. It is clear that if the hair is to be removed, it should be clipped in as atraumatic a fashion as possible immediately prior to the operation (28–31). Alternatively, removing no hair at all appears acceptable (32).

Operating Room Skin Preparation

The preparation of the skin in the operating room is designed to remove as much of the bacterial load as possible from the operative site prior to incision (4). The skin should be free of gross contamination prior to the initiation of the skin preparation. The antiseptic is applied in concentric circles beginning at the area of the proposed incision and working out to the periphery of the field. The area prepared should be wide and should include room to extend the incision, place drains, or create new incisions if necessary. There are a variety of antiseptic agents that can be used to decrease the bacterial counts on the skin. These include povidone iodine, chlorhexidine, and alcohol containing products as the most frequently utilized agents. There are some data to suggest superiority of chlorhexidine-based skin preparation (33).

Operating room environment

The operating room is designed as a sterile environment to try to minimize the contamination of the operative wound by environmental bacteria. For this reason, the operating suite has features designed to limit the available bacteria.

Ventilation

Room air can contain bacteria laden dust, lint, exfoliated skin, or respiratory droplets. To try to limit this, operating rooms are maintained at a positive pressure relative to corridors and adjacent areas (34). This prevents airflow from less clean areas into the operating rooms. The ventilation systems for the operating room should have at least two filter beds in series and be designed to produce a minimum of 15 air changes per hour (35). This helps to clear any airborne contamination created by personnel in the room.

The amount of airborne contamination in the room is affected by the number of people moving around in the room as well as the number of times that the door to the room is opened. Limitation of these activities to only those necessary is important.

Additional mechanisms to try to decrease the airborne contamination in operating rooms can include the use of laminar airflow designs. This moves particle-free air over the aseptic operating field at a uniform velocity sweeping away any particles in its path (34). These systems have been studied only in orthopedic procedures where there does seem to be some small but real further decrease in SSI risk beyond the use of other efforts. Another strategy that has been used is intraoperative ultraviolet radiation to try to sterilize the air within the operating room; this does not appear to decrease overall SSI risk based on prospective data (4).

Room Surfaces

The surfaces in the operating room (including tables, floors, walls, ceilings, and lights) must be cleansed routinely to re-establish a clean environment for each operation (4). There are no data to support routine disinfection of these surfaces between operation in the absence of gross contamination or visible soiling. If such contamination does occur, then a disinfectant agent should be used prior to the next operation (36). Wet vacuuming of the floor with a hospital disinfectant should be performed routinely after the last operation of the day or night. There are no data to support the use of special disinfectant procedures or periodic closing of an operating room if a dirty operation has been performed. Sticky mats on the floor at the entrance to operating rooms do not reduce the number of organisms on shoes, stretcher wheels, or flat surfaces in the operating room, and do not reduce the incidence of SSI (4).

Instrument Sterilization

Surgical instruments should be sterilized prior to use to limit the introduction of bacteria into the wounds. Surgical instruments can be sterilized by steam under pressure, dry heat, or ethylene oxide (37). The quality of sterilization must be routinely monitored to ensure adequate elimination of microbial contamination. A biological indicator must be used for microbial monitoring of steam autoclave performance.

Flash sterilization of surgical instruments is the use of rapid steam sterilization for immediate instrument use (4,38). This immediate sterilization is often used during an operation for instruments that have not been sterilized, or that have been dropped or otherwise contaminated during the procedure. Flash sterilization is not recommended for routine sterilization because it does not allow for timely biological indicators to monitor the performance of the sterilizer. These approaches also typically use minimal sterilization cycle parameters designed to sterilize the instruments in the shortest period of time. Flash sterilization should generally not be used as an alternative to purchasing additional instrument sets or merely to save time between operations (4). In addition, flash sterilization is not recommended for implantable devices because of the potential for serious infection. Thus, all surgical instruments should be conventionally sterilized prior to routine use, and flash sterilization should be limited to the truly urgent or emergent need for sterilization or resterilization of equipment.

Operating room personnel

Specific rituals in the operating room are established to protect the patient from contamination by bacteria carried by the healthcare workers and also to protect the healthcare workers from contaminants carried by the patient. Attention to these activities is important to maintain a safe environment.

Surgical Scrub

Members of the surgical team who are directly involved in the operation and the handling of the sterile instruments used in the field must perform some surgical scrub prior to covering with surgical gown and gloves. The purpose of the surgical scrub is to decrease or eliminate bacteria from the hands and arms to limit the possibility of transmission to the operative wound (39). Currently in the United States, most surgical personnel skin preparation is done using either povidone iodine solutions or chlorhexidine gluconate solution (40). Outside of the United States, the use of alcohol-based agents is the standard, although this is gaining use in the United States (41). Any of these approaches appear to have the capability of decreasing the hand bacterial colony counts (40,42). It is important that, whatever skin preparation is selected, it be used in accordance with its instructions to obtain optimal effect.

Scrubbing technique, the duration of the scrub and the techniques used for drying and gloving can all affect the colony counts on the hands (39). Recent data show that a shorter (e.g., two minute) hand preparation is as effective as the traditional ten-minute hand scrub to reduce bacterial colony counts (43,44). It is also clear that the initial scrub of an operating day should include thorough cleaning underneath the fingernails as this is a site of entrapped bacterial load.

Surgical Garb and Gloves

Operating room personnel typically wear a work uniform including scrub pants, shirts, or dress (45,46). These are frequently maintained and laundered by the hospital. There are no studies that evaluate the wearing or handling of the scrub suit as it relates to SSI risk. However, Occupational Safety and Health Administration (OSHA) regulations require that soiled or contaminated scrub suits be changed for the protection of the wearer. Many institutions have policies regarding the laundering of the scrub suits, and the wearing of the suits outside of the operating room or outside of the facility (45). There are not data to support any particular policies.

Similarly, surgical masks have been worn to try to limit bacteria from the operative personnel from contaminating the air in the operating room (45). However, the efficacy of this is unproven. The main benefit of the surgical mask may be in protecting the wearer from exposure to blood or body fluids that may splash during the procedure. In addition, OSHA regulations require that not only the mask be worn to protect the wearer but that eye protection be worn to protect the eyes from splashes (36). For patients with special infectious risks, more densely filtering masks may be useful, to protect the healthcare personnel from exposure to tuberculosis, for example.

Surgical caps and hoods are worn by surgical personnel to decrease the contamination of the field by hair or dead skin from the scalp (45). These are inexpensive methods that appear to be effective in preventing this problem. There have been SSI outbreaks traced to bacteria carried in the hair.

Shoe covers do not decrease the risk of SSI or decrease the bacteria counts on the operating room floor (45). However, OSHA regulations recommend shoe covers whenever gross contamination of the wearer is likely (36).

Sterile Gloves and Gown

After the surgical scrub, the operating room personnel who will be in direct contact with the operating room field don a surgical gown and sterile gloves (39,46). These are worn to minimize transmission of microorganisms from the hands and arms of team members to the patient, as well as to prevent contamination of the team members with the patient's blood and body fluids (36). If the glove is punctured or torn, it should be changed promptly. Wearing two pairs of gloves decreases the incidence of healthcare worker contact with patients' blood or body fluids, when compared to only wearing a single pair of gloves (47). Similarly, the sterile gown creates a barrier between the surgical field and the healthcare workers' arms and torso. The role of the gowns is also to protect the healthcare workers from exposure to the patient's blood and body fluids.

Antibiotic prophylaxis

Antibiotic prophylaxis is best delivered as a very short course of effective antimicrobial agent delivered just prior to operative incision. This course is not attempted to sterilize tissues, but if timed correctly can decrease the dose of wound contaminant experienced by the patient. It is important to provide the antimicrobial shortly before incision so that effective concentrations are obtained at the incision site.

There are four important principles that may maximize the effectiveness of an antimicrobial prophylaxis plan (4). First, the chosen agent must be used for every patient in whom there are data that the use of antimicrobial prophylaxis is effective, or for those procedures after which an infection would be a catastrophic event. Second, the chosen antibiotic agent should ideally be safe, inexpensive, and bactericidal for the likely microbiologic wound contaminants for the planned operation. Third, the course of antibiotics should be very brief but timed to provide a bactericidal concentration of drug in the serum and tissues at the moment of incision and through the operation. Fourth, the therapeutic levels of the antimicrobial agent should be maintained until just a few hours following the closure of the incision. Continuation of antibiotics beyond that time is not necessary and does not further decrease the wound infection rate.

The selection of antimicrobial agents can be guided by the likely infections that can occur with the procedure (Table 14.3). The options listed in the table are commonly recommended, but are not exclusively effective. Any antibiotic choices and regimens that conform to the principles noted above should be useful.

The soluble mediators produced are proinflammatory cytokines, chemokines, prostanoids, as well as reactive oxygen and nitrogen species (7). Elevated circulating levels of these mediators lead to progressive endothelial dysfunction and microvascular injury. Macrophage-produced cytokines induce endothelial cell expression of adhesion markers that in turn mediate neutrophil attachment, recruitment, and persistence at inflammatory sites. Activated leukocytes, as well as bacterial products themselves, also activate the coagulation cascade. Tissue factor is released in response to proinflammatory cytokines such as and interleukin-1 (IL-1) and leads to the formation of thrombin and fibrin clots. Concurrently, many endogenous fibrinolytic mechanisms are impaired because of the release of plasminogen-activator inhibitor-1, production of thrombin-activatable fibrinolysis inhibitor, and decreased conversion of protein C to the serine protease-activated protein C. Activated protein C exerts important antithrombotic, anti-inflammatory, and profibrinlytic properties by inactivating factors Va and VIIIa, which limits thrombin generation and reduces its procoagulant and antifibrinolytic properties. Activation of protein C normally occurs by thrombin bound to endothelial thrombomodulin, but thrombomodulin expression becomes markedly impaired with progressive endothelial dysfunction. Altered local coagulation and progressive microvascular thrombosis, in conjunction with hypotension, lead to tissue hypoperfusion and shock.

Sepsis can be thought of as a process comprising two major components, infectious and inflammatory. The clinical inflammatory response extends from infection to sepsis, severe sepsis, and septic shock, with clinical outcome progressively worsening with advancing stages. In a large study examining the natural history of patients with SIRS, 48% were found to have infections: 26% had sepsis only, 18% developed severe sepsis, and 4% developed septic shock (10). Bacteremia was increased with the severity of the clinical response. Positive blood cultures were found in 17% of patients with sepsis and in 69% of patients with septic shock.

Patients with sepsis have a lower mortality rate compared with patients with severe sepsis or septic shock (11–13). The mortality rate from septic shock is between 35% and 40% in the month following onset of septic shock. The mortality from hypovolemic shock varies greatly and depends on the etiology as well as the rapidity with which it is recognized and treated (14–16).

EVALUATION

Shock is the physiologic condition in which there is inadequate oxygen delivery. This leads to cellular hypoxia and disruption of necessary biochemical processes with resultant tissue and organ dysfunction. In the early phases, these alterations can be reversed, but they rapidly become irreversible, leading to cell death, end-organ damage, multiple organ failure (MOF), and death. Shock is broadly divided into three categories: (a) hypovolemic, (b) cardiogenic, and (c) distributive.

Hypovolemic shock results from inadequate intravascular volume and decreased cardiac preload that lead to decreased cardiac output (CO) and end-organ perfusion. Hypovolemic shock is generally due to either loss of blood or fluid. Blood loss can be secondary to trauma, GI bleeding, ruptured aortic aneurysm, or other causes. Fluid loss can be due to intestinal obstruction, pancreatitis, burns, diarrhea, as well as other causes. Cardiogenic shock is due to failure of the heart as a pump. The four major causes of cardiogenic shock are arrhythmias, cardiomyopathies, mechanical abnormalities, and obstructive disorders. Arrhythmias such as atrial fibrillation can suppress CO by disrupting normal coordination of atrial and ventricular filling and pumping. Bradyarrhythmias and heart block can markedly decrease CO and end organ perfusion. Cardiomyopathies, whether due to ischemic, viral infection, or other reasons, can cause severe deficits in myocardial contractility and CO. Mechanical causes of pump failure are valvular insufficiency or chordae tendineae rupture. Obstructive causes such as pericardial tamponade, massive pulmonary embolism, and tension pneumothorax can also disrupt the heart's ability to function as a pump. Abnormally low systemic vascular resistance causes distributive shock and can be due to a variety of causes. Septic shock is generally classified within the distributive shock category, although it can present with components of the other two categories. Aside from septic shock, other types of distributive shock are neurogenic shock after central nervous system (CNS) or spinal cord injury, Addisonian crisis, myxedema coma, anaphylaxis, and drug or toxin reactions.

HISTORY

Patients presenting with septic shock might be in such dire condition as to be unable to provide a clear history. Nonetheless, it is important to elicit a history of current and recent complaints from the patient or the patient's family. Pre-existing conditions such as diabetes, malignancy, and immunosuppression are important to consider. Current medication regimens as well as recent alterations in medication might provide important clues with regard to the patient's underlying pathophysiology. In surgical patients presenting with shock, a detailed surgical history is essential. This surgical history must include not only a list of past and planned surgical procedures but also the underlying pathology requiring surgical intervention. The nature, extent, and outcome of recent surgical procedures and the patient's perioperative course must be taken into consideration as they might shed considerable light on why the patient is presenting with shock. Was the operation elective or emergent? Which body cavities were opened? Was it a clean, contaminated, or dirty operation? Was a hollow viscus opened? Is there an anastomosis? Does the patient have an indwelling catheter? What is the patient's underlying condition? What are the locations of the patient's symptoms? What is the nature of the patient's complaints? To which organ systems are the complaints most attributable? The differential diagnosis for a patient presenting with septic shock following recent emergency operation for colonic perforation would differ greatly from that of a patient presenting with septic shock 1 year after lung transplantation.

CLINICAL ASSESSMENT

The physical examination should focus on rapid assessment of the patient's current clinical conditions, differentiating the types of shock and determining the etiology of the patient's shock. Clinical signs of decreased global perfusion are oliguria, delayed capillary refill, cool skin, and decreased level of consciousness in addition to hypotension. Patients presenting with shock must be continuously monitored in an ICU setting. For patients in shock, arterial catheterization provides a more accurate measure of blood pressure than noninvasive techniques.

Although elevated lactate levels can be due to causes other than septic shock, efforts to normalize lactate levels by means of hemodynamic optimization should be considered (17). The prognostic value of blood lactate concentration has been established in septic shock patients (18,19). Gastric tonometry has been shown to be a predictor of multiorgan dysfunction syndrome and mortality in patients with septic shock (20,21). However, resuscitation of critically ill patients on the basis of gastric tonometry failed to significantly improve outcome (22).

Hemodynamic measurements can be made in septic shock patients using pulmonary artery catheterization. Parameters such as CO, pulmonary artery occlusion pressure, and systemic vascular resistance can be useful in differentiating septic shock from other forms of shock. Pulmonary artery catheterization can also provide useful information about the adequacy of fluid resuscitation, the effectiveness of vasopressors and inotropes, and the effect of mechanical ventilatory support on hemodynamics (23). However, pulmonary artery catheterization may be frequently associated with inaccurate measurements (24) and one retrospective analysis suggested a worsened clinical outcome with pulmonary artery catheterization (25). At this time, there is no conclusive clinical evidence about the utility and potential benefit of pulmonary artery catheterization in septic shock. There is a growing popularity of the Esophageal Doppler Monitor (EDM) with its demonstrable clinical utility and efficacy in estimating fluid status and CO in the critically ill population using noninvasive techniques (26).

LABORATORIES AND STUDIES

Laboratory tests are helpful to assess the patient's condition and evidence of organ dysfunction as well as response to treatment. They can help identify the etiology of the patient's shock. Basic tests include arterial blood gas, lactate level, complete blood count (CBC) with differential, basic chemistries, amylase and lipase, liver function tests, cardiac enzymes, coagulation profile, fibrinogen, and fibrin split products. An urinalysis and toxicology screen might also provide helpful information. Cosyntropin challenge or cortisol levels can be used to detect adrenal insufficiency. It is essential to identify the causative microbial pathogen and the sites of infection. Although sepsis and septic shock can result from infections at many sites, the most common sites are the lungs, abdomen, urinary tract, and skin (27). Blood, sputum, and urine cultures can be helpful in identifying the source of sepsis. Routine cultures drawn on patients on Continuous Renal Replacement Therapy (CRRT) have not proven such therapy to be efficacious in the absence of clinical suggestion of infection (28). No clinical difference in outcome has been shown between bronchoalveolar lavage with quantitative culture of the bronchoalveolar-lavage fluid and endotracheal aspiration with nonquantitative culture of the aspirate in the diagnosis of ventilator associated pneumonia (VAP) (29). Additionally, the growing clinical menace posed by Clostridium difficile warrants consideration as a cause of presumed sepsis in the critically ill surgical patient (30). For patients in shock, a chest x-ray and electrocardiogram are essential for basic assessment of the cardiopulmonary system. Imaging studies should also be promptly performed to identify the potential source of infection (31). Plain or contrast radiographs and radionuclide studies can be used to determine the presence of surgical complications such as visceral perforation or obstruction and anastomotic disruption. Computed tomography or magnetic resonance imaging scans might help detect the presence of infectious foci or fluid collections.

MANAGEMENT

The essential steps in the management of septic shock are the same as those used to treat patients with mild or moderate sepsis: (a) timely resuscitation, (b) timely diagnosis of the infectious focus, (c) prompt antibiotic therapy, and (d) expeditious infectious source control. Because of the severity of the disease process, these steps must be undertaken concurrently (Fig. 15.1). Identification of the infectious foci and institution of the appropriate antibiotic treatment and source control are discussed in greater detail in Chapter 14; hence, the current focus will be on resuscitative measures for septic shock.

SHOCK

Shock is a medical emergency and must be treated immediately. As with any critical patient, treatment must first address the ABCs—airway, breathing, and circulation. First, the airway must be assessed and supported. Patients in septic shock may have a depressed level of consciousness or encephalopathy and require intubation for airway protection. Second, ventilation and oxygenation should be

or patients requiring surgery (63,64). More recently, hypertonic saline has been shown to be a fluid with significant modulation of systemic inflammatory response to reperfusion injury, which may be beneficial in patients with shock (65). Early hypertonic saline administration may attenuate innate immune response to injury, such as macrophage, neutrophil, and endothelial cell activation, and decrease the risk of future organ dysfunction syndrome (66–68).

Clinical trials to evaluate the outcome for patients in shock following blunt traumatic injury, randomized to receive 250 ml of 7.5% hypertonic saline/6% dextran followed by lactated Ringers versus lactated Ringers alone, were recently suspended due to lack of demonstrable improved outcomes despite positive results in animal models (69). Currently, hypertonic saline is not routinely used and further research is ongoing in isolated head injury patients to define the timing, amount, and if this trauma subpopulation may benefit from hypertonic saline resuscitation (70).

Lactated Ringers is the solution used by most surgeons for resuscitation of hypovolemic patients. Lactated Ringers is physiologically balanced with similar electrolyte concentrations as plasma with 130 mEq Na^+, 4 mEq K^+, 3 mEq Ca^{++}, 109 mEq Cl^-, and 28 mEq of HCO_3^- per liter. Due to the presence of potassium, lactated Ringers should not be given to patients with hyperkalemia or renal failure. Lactated Ringers has been routinely used for massive resuscitation for trauma and burn patients. However, recent studies have demonstrated a potential association between lactated Ringers resuscitation and modulation of leukocyte function (71,72). Most commercially available lactated Ringers is a racemic mixture of D and L stereoisomers. While the L isomer is associated with low toxicity, the D isomer, which is normally only produced by gastrointestinal flora, has been associated with clinical toxicity and potentially harmful changes in leukocyte function (71,73). Further studies of the effect of lactated Ringers resuscitation in surgical patients are in progress. Meanwhile, lactated Ringers remains a clinically acceptable solution for resuscitation of surgical patients.

SUMMARY

Hypovolemic shock remains a common entity in surgical patients. Early recognition and prompt resuscitation are the major cornerstones for positive outcomes. Restoration of circulating volume, dependent on the etiology of fluid loss, is crucial. Stabilization of the patient may require airway control to allow for adequate fluid replacement. Attention to acid-base, electrolyte, and coagulation abnormalities is also central to successful resuscitation from hypovolemic shock.

REFERENCES

1. American College of Surgeons. *Advanced Trauma Life Support: instructor manual*. 6th ed. Chicago: American College of Surgeons; 1997.
2. Assadi F, Copelovitch L. Simplified treatment strategies to fluid therapy in diarrhea. *Pediatr Nephrol* 2003;18(11):1152–1156.
3. Sack DA, Sack RB, Nair GB, et al. Cholera. *Lancet* 2004;363(9404): 223–233.
4. Buchman TG, Jacobsohn E. Shock. In: Greenfield LJ, Mulholland MW, Oldham KT, Zelenock GB, Lillemoe KD, eds. *Surgery: Scientific principle and practice*. Philadelphia, PA: Lippincott Williams & Wilkins; 2001: 202–217.
5. Groeneveld ABJ. Hypovolemic shock. In: Parrillo JE, Dellinger RP, eds. *Critical care medicine*, 2nd ed. St. Louis, MO: Mosby; 2002:465–500.
6. Rose B, Post TW. *Clinical physiology of acid-base and electrolyte disorders*. New York, NY: McGraw-Hill; 2001.
7. American Burn Association. *Advance Burn Life Support Course: Provider manual*. Chicago: American Burn Association; 2001.
8. Magnuson DK. Neonatal and pediatric physiology. In: Greenfield LJ, Mulholland MW, Oldham KT, Zelenock GB, Lillemoe KD, eds. *Surgery: Scientific principle and practice*, 3rd ed. Philadelphia, PA: Lippincott Williams & Wilkins; 2001:1901–1931.
9. Miller TR, Anderson RJ, Linas SL, et al. Urinary diagnostic indices in acute renal failure: a prospective study. *Ann Intern Med* 1978;89(1): 47–50.
10. *Clinical manifestations and diagnosis of volume depletion*. Post TW, Rose BD. Available at: http://www.utdol.com/application/topic.asp?file=c_neph/6291&type=A&selectedTitle=2~19. UptoDate Online 18.2 accessed November 22, 2010.
11. Dossetor JB. Creatininemia versus uremia. The relative significance of blood urea nitrogen and serum creatinine concentrations in azotemia. *Ann Intern Med* 1966;65(6):1287–1299.
12. Cohn JN. Blood pressure measurement in shock. Mechanism of inaccuracy in ausculatory and palpatory methods. *JAMA* 1967;199(13):118–122.
13. Baskett PJ. ABC of major trauma. Management of hypovolaemic shock. *BMJ* 1990;300(6737):1453–1457.
14. Sauaia A, Moore FA, Moore EE, et al. Epidemiology of trauma deaths: a reassessment. *J Trauma* 1995;38:185–193.
15. Capone AC, Safar P, Stezoski W, et al. Improved outcome with fluid restriction in treatment of uncontrolled hemorrhagic shock. *J Am Coll Surg* 1995;180:49–56.
16. Bickell WH, Wall MJ Jr, Pepe PE, et al. Immediate versus delayed fluid resuscitation for hypotensive patients with penetrating torso injuries. *N Engl J Med* 1994;331(17):1105–1109.
17. Silbergleit R, Satz W, McNamara RM, et al. Effect of permissive hypotension in continuous uncontrolled intra-abdominal hemorrhage. *Acad Emerg Med* 1996;3(10):922–926.
18. Solomonov E, Hirsh M, Yahiya A, et al. The effect of vigorous fluid resuscitation in uncontrolled hemorrhagic shock after massive splenic injury. *Crit Care Med* 2000;28(3):749–754.
19. Holcomb JB, Jenkins D, Rhee P, et al. Damage control resuscitation: directly addressing the early coagulopathy of trauma. *J Trauma* 2007; 62:307–310.
20. Gonzalez EA, Moore FA, Holcomb JB, et al. Fresh frozen plasma should be given earlier to patients requiring massive transfusion. *J Trauma* 2007;62:112–119.
21. Borgman MA, Spinella PC, Perkins JG, et al. The ratio of blood products transfused in patients receiving massive transfusions at combat support hospitals. *J Trauma* 2007;63:805–813.
22. Gajic O, Rana R, Winters JL, et al. Transfusion-related acute lung injury in the critically ill. *Am J Respir Crit Care Med* 2007;176:88–91.
23. Kashuk JL, Morre EE, Johnson JL, et al. Post-injury life threatening coagulopathy: is 1:1 fresh frozen plasma packed red blood cells the answer? *J Trauma* 2008;65(2):261–270.
24. Teboul JL, Pinsky MR, Mercat A, et al. Estimating cardiac filling pressure in mechanically ventilated patients with hyperinflation. *Crit Care Med* 2000;28(11):3631–3636.
25. Diebel LN, Myers T, Dulchavsky S. Effects of increasing airway pressure and PEEP on the assessment of cardiac preload. *J Trauma* 1997; 42(4):585–590; discussion 590–581.
26. Luecke T, Roth H, Herrmann P, et al. Assessment of cardiac preload and left ventricular function under increasing levels of positive end-expiratory pressure. *Intensive Care Med* 2004;30(1):119–126.
27. Cheatham ML, Nelson LD, Chang MC, et al. Right ventricular end-diastolic volume index as a predictor of preload status in patients on positive end-expiratory pressure. *Crit Care Med* 1998;26(11):1801–1806.
28. Durham R, Neunaber K, Vogler G, et al. Right ventricular end-diastolic volume as a measure of preload. *J Trauma* 1995;39(2):218–223; discussion 223–214.
29. Sandham JD, Hull RD, Brant RF, et al. A randomized, controlled trial of the use of pulmonary-artery catheters in high-risk surgical patients. *N Engl J Med* 2003;348(1):5–14.

30. Bernard GR, Sopko G, Cerra F, et al. Pulmonary artery catheterization and clinical outcomes: National Heart, Lung, and Blood Institute and Food and Drug Administration Workshop Report. Consensus Statement. *JAMA* 2000;283(19):2568–2572.
31. Robin ED. The cult of the Swan-Ganz catheter. Overuse and abuse of pulmonary flow catheters. *Ann Intern Med* 1985;103(3):445–449.
32. Seoudi HM, Perkal MF, Hanrahan A, et al. The esophageal Doppler monitor in mechanically ventilated surgical patients: does it work? *J Trauma* 2003;55(4):720–725; discussion 725–726.
33. Velmahos GC, Demetriades D, Shoemaker WC, et al. Endpoints of resuscitation of critically injured patients: normal or supranormal? A prospective randomized trial. *Ann Surg* 2000;232(3):409–418.
34. McKinley BA, Kozar RA, Cocanour CS, et al. Normal versus supranormal oxygen delivery goals in shock resuscitation: the response is the same. *J Trauma* 2002;53(5):825–832.
35. Shoemaker WC. Monitoring and therapy for young trauma patients. *Crit Care Med* 1994;22(4):548–549.
36. Waxman K, Annas C, Daughters K, et al. A method to determine the adequacy of resuscitation using tissue oxygen monitoring. *J Trauma* 1994;36:852–858.
37. Drucker W, Pearce F, Glass-Heidenreich L, et al. Subcutaneous tissue oxygen pressure: a reliable index of peripheral perfusion in humans after injury. *J Trauma* 1996;40(Suppl):S116–S122.
38. Knudson MM, Bermudez KM, Doyle CA, et al. Use of tissue oxygen tension measurements during resuscitation from hemorrhagic shock. *J Trauma* 1997;42:608–614.
39. Ikossi DG, Knudson MM, Morabito DJ, et al. Continuous muscle tissue oxygenation in critically injured patients: a prospective observational study. *J Trauma* 2006;61:780–790.
40. Taylor RW, Manganaro L, O'Brien J, et al. Impact of allogenic packed red blood cell transfusion on nosocomial infection rates in the critically ill patient. *Crit Care Med* 2002;30(10):2249–2254.
41. Gazmuri RJ, Shakeri SA. Blood transfusion and the risk of nosocomial infection: an underreported complication? *Crit Care Med* 2002;30(10): 2389–2391.
42. McCrossan L, Masterson G. Blood transfusion in critical illness. *Br J Anaesth* 2002;88(1):6–9.
43. Steffes CP, Bender JS, Levison MA. Blood transfusion and oxygen consumption in surgical sepsis. *Crit Care Med* 1991;19(4):512–517.
44. Marik PE, Sibbald WJ. Effect of stored-blood transfusion on oxygen delivery in patients with sepsis. *JAMA* 1993;269(23):3024–3029.
45. Lorente JA, Landin L, De Pablo R, et al. Effects of blood transfusion on oxygen transport variables in severe sepsis. *Crit Care Med* 1993;21(9): 1312–1318.
46. Conrad SA, Dietrich KA, Hebert CA, et al. Effect of red cell transfusion on oxygen consumption following fluid resuscitation in septic shock. *Circ Shock* 1990;31(4):419–429.
47. Blumberg N, Heal JM. Immunomodulation by blood transfusion: an evolving scientific and clinical challenge. *Am J Med* 1996;101(3):299–308.
48. Watkins TR, Rubenfeld GD, Martin TR, et al. Effects of leukoreduced blood on acute lung injury after trauma: a randomized controlled trial. *Crit Care Med* 2008;36:1493–1499.
49. Hebert PC, Wells G, Blajchman MA, et al. A multicenter, randomized, controlled clinical trial of transfusion requirements in critical care. Transfusion Requirements in Critical Care Investigators, Canadian Critical Care Trials Group. *N Engl J Med* 1999;340(6):409–417.
50. Contreras M, Ala FA, Greaves M, et al. Guidelines for the use of fresh frozen plasma. British Committee for Standards in Haematology, Working Party of the Blood Transfusion Task Force. *Transfus Med* 1992; 2(1):57–63.
51. Tranbaugh RF, Lewis FR. Crystalloid versus colloid for fluid resuscitation of hypovolemic patients. *Adv Shock Res* 1983;9:203–216.
52. Boldt J. The good, the bad, and the ugly: should we completely banish human albumin from our intensive care units? *Anesth Analg* 2000; 91(4):887–895.
53. Waters LM, Christensen MA, Sato RM. Hetastarch: an alternative colloid in burn shock management. *J Emerg Nurs* 1990;16(4):279–287.
54. Powers KA, Kapus A, Khadaroo RG, et al. Twenty-five percent albumin prevents lung injury following shock/resuscitation. *Crit Care Med* 2003;31(9):2355–2363.
55. Ferguson ND, Stewart TE, Etchells EE. Human albumin administration in critically ill patients. *Intensive Care Med* 1999;25(3):323–325.
56. Schierhout G, Roberts I. Fluid resuscitation with colloid or crystalloid solutions in critically ill patients: a systematic review of randomised trials. *BMJ* 1998;316(7136):961–964.
57. Cochrane Injuries Group Albumin Reviewers. Human albumin administration in critically ill patients: systematic review of randomised controlled trials. *BMJ* 1998;317(7153):235–240.
58. The SAFE Study Investigators. A comparison of albumin and saline for fluid resuscitation in the intensive care unit. *N Engl J Med* 2004;350: 2247–2256.
59. Waters JH, Gottlieb A, Schoenwald P, et al. Normal saline versus lactated Ringer's solution for intraoperative fluid management in patients undergoing abdominal aortic aneurysm repair: an outcome study. *Anesth Analg* 2001;93(4):817–822.
60. Rocha-e-Silva M, Negraes GA, Soares AM, et al. Hypertonic resuscitation from severe hemorrhagic shock: patterns of regional circulation. *Circ Shock* 1986;19(2):165–175.
61. Gemma M, Cozzi S, Piccoli S, et al. Hypertonic saline fluid therapy following brain stem trauma. *J Neurosurg Anesthesiol* 1996;8(2):137–141.
62. Young WF, Rosenwasser RH, Vasthare US, et al. Preservation of postcompression spinal cord function by infusion of hypertonic saline. *J Neurosurg Anesthesiol* 1994;6(2):122–127.
63. Vassar MJ, Perry CA, Gannaway WL, et al. 7.5% sodium chloride/dextran for resuscitation of trauma patients undergoing helicopter transport. *Arch Surg* 1991;126(9):1065–1072.
64. Mattox KL, Maningas PA, Moore EE, et al. Prehospital hypertonic saline/dextran infusion for post-traumatic hypotension. The U. S. A. Multicenter Trial. *Ann Surg* 1991;213(5):482–491.
65. Junger WG, Coimbra R, Liu FC, et al. Hypertonic saline resuscitation: a tool to modulate immune function in trauma patients? *Shock* 1997;8(4): 235–241.
66. Coimbra R, Hoyt DB, Junger WG, et al. Hypertonic saline resuscitation decreases susceptibility to sepsis after hemorrhagic shock. *J Trauma* 1997;42(4):602–606; discussion 606–607.
67. Arbabi S, Rosengart MR, Garcia I, et al. Hypertonic saline solution induces prostacyclin production by increasing cyclooxygenase-2 expression. *Surgery* 2000;128(2):198–205.
68. Cuschieri J, Gourlay D, Garcia I, et al. Hypertonic preconditioning inhibits macrophage responsiveness to endotoxin. *J Immunol* 2002; 168(3):1389–1396.
69. *New analysis of halted trial of hypertonic saline for patients in traumatic shock.* Barclay L; 2009. Available at: http://www.medscape.com/viewarticle/590647. Accessed May 07, 2009.
70. Pruitt BA Jr. Does hypertonic burn resuscitation make a difference? *Crit Care Med* 2000;28(1):277–278.
71. Koustova E, Stanton K, Gushchin V, et al. Effects of lactated Ringer's solutions on human leukocytes. *J Trauma* 2002;52(5):872–878.
72. Koustova E, Rhee P, Hancock T, et al. Ketone and pyruvate Ringer's solutions decrease pulmonary apoptosis in a rat model of severe hemorrhagic shock and resuscitation. *Surgery* 2003;134(2):267–274.
73. Veech RL, Fowler RC. Cerebral dysfunction and respiratory alkalosis during peritoneal dialysis with D-lactate-containing dialysis fluids. *Am J Med* 1987;82(3):572–574.

CHAPTER

17

Fluid and Electrolyte Abnormalities

Bradley D. Freeman

INTRODUCTION

Intravenous fluid therapy is integral to the practice of surgery. For many patients, such as those undergoing minor procedures or requiring parenteral hydration for only brief periods, intravenous fluid prescription is uncomplicated. In contrast, for patients who have undergone complex operations, sustained major trauma, or possess significant comorbidities, meticulous attention to fluid therapy is essential to avoid serious electrolyte disturbance and other adverse sequelae. Further, because of the substantial range of acquisition costs of currently available intravenous fluid preparations, coupled with an environment increasingly focused on cost containment, economic considerations are becoming a greater part of surgical decision-making in this area. A comprehensive discussion of fluid and electrolyte management is beyond the scope of this text. Rather, the purpose of this chapter is to focus on basic aspects of fluid management, discuss potential complications and electrolyte derangements associated with commonly used intravenous fluids, and review recent literature examining the relative risks and benefits of selected therapies. The ultimate goal of this analysis is to promote an approach to intravenous fluid management that is evidence-based and cost-effective.

Fluid compartments

Knowledge of body fluid compartment distribution is essential both for understanding the physiological changes that occur following surgery or injury, and to guide intravenous fluid use. Total body water equals roughly 60% of lean body weight, is slightly higher in men, is most concentrated in skeletal muscle, and declines with age. Total body water can be divided into two major compartments: an intracellular fluid compartment, comprising 60% of the total body water compartment (or 40% of lean body weight), and an extracellular fluid compartment, comprising 40% of the total body water compartment (or 20% of lean body weight). The extracellular fluid space is further subdivided into an intravascular compartment (equaling roughly 10% of total body water or 25% of the extracellular fluid space) and an extravascular or interstitial compartment (roughly 30% of the total body water or 75% of the extracellular fluid space). Surgeons speak frequently of "third space" fluid losses or "fluid third spacing." The third fluid space is extracellular fluid that is neither intravascular nor interstitial and is not immediately physiologically connected to these compartments. This third fluid space represents a patient's nonspecific response to acute insult, from surgery, infection, or trauma. The magnitude and duration of third space fluid accumulation is directly proportional to the degree of the inciting insult and the time required for its resolution. Third space fluid accumulation must be taken into account when prescribing intravenous fluids either for maintenance therapy or for resuscitation.

Crystalloids

Types of Crystalloid Solutions

Commonly used intravenous fluids are derived from two categories, crystalloids and colloids. Crystalloids contain sodium as their osmotically active particle and distribute throughout the extracellular space, such that 25% to 30% of the infused volume remains in the intravascular compartment (1). The predominant effect of crystalloid administration is to expand the interstitial, not the intravascular, space (2). While a variety of crystalloid solutions are available, the prototypes are 0.9% NaCl (normal saline) and lactated Ringer's solution. Normal saline contains Na^+ and Cl^- at concentrations slightly greater than those found in plasma; lactated Ringer's solution contains these constituents as well as K^+, Ca^{2+}, and a HCO_3^- source at near physiologic levels. With minor exceptions, 0.9% NaCl and lactated Ringer's solution can be used interchangeably, and few complications are specifically associated with these formulations. Lactated Ringer's solution should not be used in patients with hyperkalemia. Further, the Ca^{2+} present in lactated Ringer's can bind certain drugs, diminishing bioavailability, as well as chelate citrate present in packed red blood cells, promoting coagulation (2). For this reason, lactated Ringer's solution is contraindicated as a diluent for blood (2). The lactate present in lactated Ringer's solution does not interfere with serum lactate measurements (1). Most commonly used crystalloid solutions are derivatives

Bradley D. Freeman: Department of Surgery, Washington University School of Medicine St. Louis, MO.

of either lactated Ringers solution or 0.9% NaCl (e.g., D_5/0.45% NaCl, D_5/lactated Ringer's, etc.).

Dextrose is a common additive to crystalloids. The original intent of incorporating dextrose into intravenous fluids was to provide a source of nonprotein calories, thus potentially diminishing protein catabolism. A 5% dextrose solution provides approximately 170 kcal/L. While the clinical benefit of this protein sparing effect is unproven, the use of dextrose-containing fluids is essential in the perioperative management of fasting diabetics to decrease the likelihood of ketosis (3). These solutions are likewise useful as a source free water replacement in patients unable to tolerate oral hydration. Solutions containing only 5% dextrose are not effective volume expanders (e.g., only 10% of the infused volume remains within the intravascular space) (1). There are some potentially adverse effects of dextrose solutions. Dextrose adds an additional osmotic load to crystalloid solutions. In situations in which glucose utilization is impaired, such as critical illness, the infused glucose may accumulate and create an osmotic effect that can promote dehydration (2). Further, dextrose infusions may theoretically result in increased CO_2 and lactate production (4,5). This is of uncertain clinical importance in most surgical patients.

Indications for Crystalloid Solution Use

Crystalloids are used in several situations, perhaps most commonly as a maintenance fluid. Maintenance fluids must replace the approximately 75 mEq of Na^+ lost daily and provide approximately 40 to 50 mEq/d of K^+ (6). Because of the large body stores and limited daily losses of Ca^{2+} and Mg^{2+}, maintenance replacement of these elements is unnecessary in patients that require a short course of intravenous therapy (6). For a patient with intact renal and cardiopulmonary function, a common maintenance fluid prescription is Dextrose 5%/0.45% NaCl with supplemental KCl (20 mEq/L) or D5LR infused at 1 to 2 mL/kg/hr. The presence of acute or chronic organ dysfunction frequently requires modification of the volume or composition of fluid infused. For most general surgical patients requiring short courses of intravenous therapy, such as those awaiting resolution of postoperative ileus, it is not necessary to determine serum electrolyte concentrations on a frequent (e.g., daily) basis.

Historically, liberal approaches to fluid volume infusion have been utilized empirically in the perioperative period to counteract the effects of fasting, third space fluid shifts, and other factors that might result in intravascular volume depletion (7). Such an approach has been challenged recently by studies suggesting a relationship between the volume of fluid infused in this context and clinically important outcomes. In a small prospective trial, Lobo et al. randomized patients to receive either standard fluid therapy (defined as volume exceeding 3 L/d and sodium load of 154 mEq/d or greater) or fluid restriction (fluid volume not exceeding 2 L/d and sodium load not exceeding 77 mEq/d) following elective colon surgery (8). Gastric emptying, studied on the fourth postoperative day, was significantly delayed in patients receiving standard fluid therapy, compared with that in patients managed with fluid restriction. Likewise, patients receiving standard fluid therapy had slower resolution of ileus and longer hospital stays. The mechanism underlying these findings is unclear but attributed to the possible development of bowel wall edema secondary to hypoalbuminemia or sodium excess. Similarly, in a prospective multicenter study, patients undergoing elective colon resection and randomized to a restricted intravenous fluid regimen designed to maintain preoperative body weight experienced significantly fewer cardiopulmonary and tissue-healing complications than patients assigned to the usual fluid management (9). In contrast, MacKay et al. demonstrated no difference in the length of hospital stay comparing patients receiving restricted and liberal fluid regimens (10). These conflicting results may reflect variability in the patients studied as well as differences in trial design and treatment regimens. Based on available evidence, it is not possible to make recommendations n what constitutes optimal intravenous fluid use in this context.

A second indication for crystalloid use is as **replacement** therapy in individuals with either pre-existing or ongoing fluid losses or electrolyte disturbances. The nature or source of fluid loss may lead to predictable electrolyte abnormalities and dictate the composition of the intravenous fluid to be used. While a detailed discussion of all the conceivable electrolyte abnormalities occurring in general surgical patients is beyond the scope of this chapter, two commonly encountered scenarios merit mention. The most common electrolyte abnormality observed in general surgical patients is hypokalemic, hypochloremic metabolic alkalosis resulting from loss of gastric secretions via nasogastric tubes. This electrolyte abnormality is a chloride responsive alkalosis; accordingly, its correction requires administration of a Cl^- source in addition to supplemental K^+ (e.g., normal saline with supplemental KCl). For patients who have substantial nasogastric losses (>1 L/d), serial electrolytes should be determined daily and this abnormality should be anticipated and corrected accordingly. A second electrolyte disturbance frequently encountered in surgical practice is metabolic acidosis secondary to high HCO_3^- loss, such as occurs in the presence of proximal small bowel enterocutaneous fistula. Lactated Ringer's solution, because it contains a HCO_3^- source, is the appropriate replacement fluid in this setting.

A third indication for crystalloid use is **resuscitation.** Crystalloids are appropriate as a first line treatment of shock, regardless of etiology, and have the advantages of being inexpensive, readily available, and reaction free. Excessive crystalloid administration may result in peripheral and pulmonary edema, which may occur before intravascular volume is completely restored. Indicators of adequate resuscitation, such as central venous pressure, pulmonary capillary wedge pressure, or end organ function, should guide the volume of crystalloid administered,

negatively, that effect is small (e.g., less than a 10% difference in mortality), and would require a study enrolling nearly 6,000 patients to demonstrate (19). In the absence of unequivocal clinical evidence and given the costs of most colloid preparations relative to crystalloids, it is difficult to recommend their routine use as resuscitation fluids. These agents are licensed and approved for a variety of indications; whether they are beneficial in these settings is not convincingly demonstrated.

Hypertonic saline

Hypertonic saline is a very efficient volume expander. For each milliliter of hypertonic saline infused, approximately 7 mL of free water is drawn into the extracellular space (1). The intravascular hypertonic benefit dissipates within 15 minutes as a result of equilibration between the intravascular and interstitial compartments. To achieve a more sustained effect, hypertonic saline is typically co-infused with a colloid (most clinical trials have used Dextran 70). Hypertonic saline infusion may theoretically be of benefit in patients following head trauma. By increasing systemic blood pressure, hypertonic saline improves cerebral blood flow. Unlike other crystalloids, hypertonicity antagonizes the development of cerebral edema and intracranial hypertension, and may result in improvement of cerebral perfusion pressure (23). There have been several prospective, randomized evaluations to determine the feasibility of hypertonic saline as a prehospital resuscitation strategy. None of these studies showed a convincing benefit of hypertonic saline use (24–26). Similar findings were reported in a secondary data analysis that involved 17 trials enrolling 869 patients (23). (Fig. 17.1) Given that the trials analyzed were small, included heterogeneous patient populations, and were of variable quality, the possibility that hypertonic saline might be of benefit could not be excluded (23). A large multicenter trial comparing prehospital resuscitation using hypertonic saline with isotonic solution in severely injured patients is ongoing (27). In the absence of results from definitive studies, hypertonic saline cannot be recommended for routine use.

CONCLUSION

Despite a history dating back over 150 years, intravenous fluid therapy continues to be an area of debate and investigation (28). This chapter has attempted an evidence-based approach to guide prescription of representative commercially available intravenous fluids. With the exceptions noted, the predominantly used crystalloid solutions (e.g., lactated Ringer's solution or 0.9% NaCl) and their respective derivatives may be used interchangeably for maintenance therapy and as resuscitation fluids. Use of these agents as replacement fluids should be individualized to the clinical situation. The bulk of clinical evidence does not suggest that the use of colloid solutions provides benefit over that of crystalloids as a resuscitation strategy. However, given the heterogeneity of the studies published to date, with respect to both populations of patients enrolled and quality, colloid resuscitation may be of benefit in selected circumstances and cannot be excluded as otherwise. Finally, as evidenced by recent *in vitro* investigations of hypertonic saline suggesting modulatory effects on inflammation and microcirculation (29–31), future uses of intravenous fluids may possess therapeutic value beyond volume and electrolyte replenishment.

REFERENCES

1. Rainey TG, Read CA. Pharmacology of colloids and crystalloids. In: Chernow B, ed. *The pharmacological approach to the critically ill patient*. Baltimore: Williams & Wilkins; 1994:272–290.
2. Marino PL. Colloid and crystalloid resuscitation. In: Marino PL, ed. *The ICU book*. Baltimore: Williams & Wilkins; 1998:228–241.
3. Jonasson O. Surgical aspects of diabetes mellitus. In: Sabiston DC, Lyerly HK, eds. *Textbook of surgery*. Philadelphia: W.B. Saunders Co.; 1997:176–185.
4. Degoute CS, Ray MJ, Manchon M, et al. Intraoperative glucose infusion and blood lactate: endocrine and metabolic relationships during abdominal aortic surgery. *Anesthesiology* 1989;71:355–361.
5. Talpers SS, Romberger DJ, Bunce SB, et al. Nutritionally associated increased carbon dioxide production. *Chest* 1992;102(2):551–555.
6. O' Flaherty D, Giesecke AH. Crystalloid fluid therapy. In: Nimmo WS, Rombotham DJ, Smith G, eds. *Anaesthesia*. London: Blackwell Scientific Publications; 1994:554–567.
7. Jacob M, Chappell D, Rehm M. Clinical update: perioperative fluid management. *Lancet* 2007;369:1984–1986.
8. Lobo DN, Bostock KA, Neal KR, et al. Effect of salt and water balance on recovery of gastrointestinal function after elective colonic resection: a randomized controlled trial. *Lancet* 2002;359:1812–1818.
9. Brandstrup B, Tonnesen H, Beier-Hogersen R, et al. Effects of intravenous fluid restriction on postoperative complications: comparison of two perioperative fluid regimens. *Ann Surg* 2003;238:641–648.
10. MacKay G, Fearon K, McConnachie A, et al. Randomized clinical trial of the effect of postoperative intravenous fluid restriction on recovery after elective colorectal surgery. *Br J Surg* 2006;93:1469–1474.
11. Freeman BD, Natanson C. Hypotension, shock, and multiple organ failure. In: Wachter RM, Goldman L, Hollander H, eds. *Hospital medicine*. Baltimore: Lippincott Williams & Wilkins; 2000:123–132.
12. Wilkes MM, Navickis RJ. Patient survival after human albumin administration. *Ann Intern Med* 2001;135:149–164.
13. Ratner LE, Smith GW. Intraoperative fluid management. *Surg Clin North Am* 1993;73(2):229–241.
14. Brunkhorst FM, Engel C, Bloos F, et al. Intensive insulin therapy and pentastarch resuscitation in severe sepsis. *N Engl J Med* 2008;358(2): 125–139.
15. Goldwasser P, Feldman J. Association of serum albumin and mortality risk. *J Clin Epidemiol* 1997;50:693–703.
16. Cochrane Injuries Group Albumin Reviewers. Human albumin administration in critically ill patients: systematic review of randomized controlled trials. *Br Med J* 1998;317:235–240.
17. Roberts I, Edwards P, McLelland B. More on albumin. Use of human albumin in UK fell substantially when systematic review was published. *Br Med J* 1999;318:1214–1215.
18. Choi PTL, Yip G, Quinonez LG, et al. Crystalloids vs. colloids in fluid resuscitation: a systematic review. *Crit Care Med* 1999;27(1):200–210.
19. Cook DJ, Guyatt G. Colloid use for fluid resuscitation: evidence and spin. *Ann Intern Med* 2001;135(3):205–208.
20. The Albumin Reviewers (Alderson P, Bunn F, Li Wan Po A, et al.). Human albumin solution for resuscitation and volume expansion in critically ill patients. *Cochrane Database Syst Rev* 2004; (4): CD001208. DOI: 10.1002/14651858.CD001208.pub2.
21. Perel P, Roberts IG. Colloids versus crystalloids for fluid resuscitation in critically ill patients. *Cochrane Database Syst Rev* 2007; (4): CD000567. DOI: 10.1002/14651858.CD000567.pub3.

22. Freeman BD, Gerstenberger EP, Banks S, et al. Using secondary data in statistical analysis. In: Gallin JI, ed. *Principles and practice of clinical research*. San Diego, CA: Academic Press; 2002:251–257.
23. Bunn F, Roberts I, Tasker R, et al. Hypertonic versus isotonic crystalloid for fluid resuscitation in critically ill patients. *Cochrane Database Syst Rev* 2004; (3): CD002045. DOI: 10.1002/14651858.CD002045. pub2.
24. Mattox KL, Maningas PA, Moore EE, et al. Prehospital hypertonic saline/dextran infusion for post-traumatic hypotension. *Ann Surg* 1991; 213(5):482–491.
25. Vassar MJ, Fischer RP, O'Brien PE, et al. A multicenter trial of resuscitation of injured patients with 7.5% sodium chloride. *Arch Surg* 1993;128: 1003–1013.
26. Wade CE, Kramer GC, Grady JJ, et al. Efficacy of hypertonic 7.5% saline and 6% dextran-70 in treating trauma: a meta-analysis of controlled clinical trials. *Surgery* 1997;122:609–616.
27. Brasel KJ, Bulger E, Cook AJ, et al. Hypertonic resuscitation: design and implementation of a pre-hospital intervention trial. *J Am Coll Surg* 2008;206(2):220–232.
28. Cosnett JE. The origins of intravenous fluid therapy. *Lancet* 1989; 333(8641):768–771.
29. Gushchin V, Alam HB, Rhee P, et al. cDNA profiling in leukocytes exposed to hypertonic resuscitation fluids. *J Am Coll Surg* 2003;197(3): 426–432.
30. Shields CJ, O'Sullivan AW, Wang JH, et al. Hypertonic saline enhances host response to bacterial challenge by augmenting receptor-independent neutrophil intracellular superoxide formation. *Ann Surg* 2003; 238(2):249–257.
31. Pascual JL, Khwaja KA, Chaudhury P, et al. Hypertonic saline and the microcirculation. *J Trauma* 2003;54(5, Suppl):S133–S140.

CHAPTER

18

Acute Renal Failure

Robert E. Southard and Craig M. Coopersmith

DEFINITION AND EPIDEMIOLOGY

Acute renal failure (ARF) develops in 2% to 7% of hospitalized patients, an incidence that has remained stable for the last 25 years. Surgery is a common cause of ARF and accounts for 20% to 50% of all hospital-acquired cases, making it the second most common cause of hospital-acquired ARF. ARF is associated with markedly worse outcomes after surgery, with patients requiring dialysis in the postoperative period having mortalities greater than 50% (1). Additionally, postoperative ARF increases both the length and cost of hospitalization (2). However, if patients with ARF survive, they are likely to recover renal function prior to discharge. This has been demonstrated by a recent multicenter study showing that only 14% of intensive care unit (ICU) patients with ARF required renal replacement therapy (RRT) at discharge (3).

Although ARF is a commonly encountered complication, there has historically been no well-accepted definition of it. Various studies have used absolute or relative increases in serum creatinine or blood urea nitrogen, decreases in creatinine clearance, and need for RRT as definitions of ARF. This variability in definition made clinical studies difficult to interpret. For instance, it has previously been estimated that ARF develops in 1% to 25% of ICU patients with mortality rates ranging from 15% to 60% (4). Based on this, the Acute Dialysis Quality Initiative Group developed the RIFLE criteria as a consensus definition and classification scheme for acute kidney injury (AKI) (5). The RIFLE criteria (risk, injury, failure, loss, end-stage kidney disease) define AKI using five components. The first three grade the severity of AKI based on changes in either serum creatinine criteria or urine output criteria (Table 18.1). The final two components of the RIFLE criteria involve clinical outcomes. "Loss" is defined as persistent AKI with complete loss of renal function for a period greater than 4 weeks, while end-stage kidney disease indicates permanent renal failure. Although they are likely to be updated in the future as biomarkers replace creatinine and urine output, the RIFLE criteria are a significant improvement over past definitions of ARF. Since their initial description, the RIFLE criteria have been validated in numerous studies and allow clinicians and researchers to use a uniform classification system to define their patients.

Robert E. Southard: Washington University in St. Louis School of Medicine, Department of Surgery.

Craig M. Coopersmith: Emory University School of Medicine, Department of Surgery.

RISK FACTORS

Multiple risk factors contribute to the development of ARF in the postoperative setting, of which the most important is pre-existing renal dysfunction (Table 18.2). Diabetics have been reported to have a 7% incidence of ARF following general surgical procedures, which increases to 20% to 30% in diabetic patients with concomitant infection, peripheral vascular disease, and/or peripheral neuropathy (1). Diabetics also have a ten-fold greater risk of deteriorating renal function in the presence of hypovolemia. Patients with pre-existing renal insufficiency and diabetes mellitus are particularly susceptible to toxic reactions to radiocontrast dye.

The elderly are also especially susceptible to ARF due to the aging kidney's loss of functional reserve and inability to withstand acute insults, as well as the fact that older patients typically have more comorbidities. Since glomerular filtration rate (GFR) decreases with age, elderly patients are more susceptible to volume depletion secondary to the inability of an aged kidney to conserve salt and maximally concentrate urine. Sepsis also increases the risk of ARF in the perioperative setting. The incidence of ARF is 16% in septic surgical intensive care unit (SICU) patients, compared to 1% to 7% in nonseptic ICU patients (6). ARF usually occurs 3 days after the onset of sepsis and is associated with an increase in both morbidity and mortality.

One under-recognized risk factor for perioperative ARF is elevated intra-abdominal pressure. Elevated intra-abdominal pressure can lead to abdominal compartment syndrome, which may cause ARF in addition to a number of other life-threatening abnormalities. Either acute or chronic factors can contribute to elevated intra-abdominal pressure, but the devastating effects of abdominal compartment syndrome are more commonly seen when elevations in intra-abdominal pressure are acute (7). This can occur in a wide range of perioperative settings, and abdominal pressures should be measured when this is suspected. When a patient's intra-abdominal pressure is greater than 20 mm Hg and new onset organ failure is documented, abdominal

Table 18.1 Acute kidney injury network staging of acute kidney injury

	Serum Creatinine (Cr) Criteria	Urine Output Criteria
Risk	Cr increase of ≥0.3 mg/dL or 150%–200% above baseline	<0.5 mL/kg/h for 6 hours
Injury	Cr increase 200%–300% above baseline	<0.5 mL/kg/h for 12 hours
Failure	Cr increase >300% or Cr >4.0 mg/dL	<0.3 mL/kg/h for 24 hours or anuria for 12 hours

decompression should be performed emergently as a lifesaving measure (7).

Although intraoperative injury to the renal collecting system cannot always be avoided, its incidence can be minimized with careful preoperative planning and intraoperative technique. Any patient whose ureters are expected to be difficult to identify during laparotomy should have ureteral stents placed preoperatively. Intraoperative identification of the ureters must also be performed during any case where dissection and/or electrocautery could result in their inadvertent division. Finally, the type of operation performed correlates to risk of postoperative ARF. Procedures that are associated with higher rates of perioperative ARF are cardiac, thoracoabdominal aortic, emergent abdominal aortic, liver transplant, and biliary procedures (1).

DIAGNOSIS AND CLASSIFICATION

An accurate assessment of the etiology of ARF is crucial to prevent further worsening of renal function and to treat reversible causes. A thorough history (including recent medications and exposure to radiocontrast dye), physical examination, and proper diagnostic testing will lead to the best clinical management of patients. Initial laboratory measurements should include a basic metabolic profile, measurement of urine electrolytes including calculation of a fractional excretion of sodium (FENa), urinalysis, and measurement of urine osmolality. It should be noted that the results of most of these tests are altered in critical illness and may therefore be of less utility in the ICU setting. In addition, electrolyte concentrations in urine are affected by diuretics and spillage of glucose into the urine; therefore, urine electrolyte studies are unreliable in patients who have recently received diuretics or those with hyperglycemia.

Table 18.2 Risk factors for development of postoperative acute renal failure

Pre-existing renal dysfunction
Age
Left ventricular dysfunction (ejection fraction <35%, cardiac index <1.7 L/min/m^2)
Hypertension
Peripheral vascular disease
Diabetes mellitus
Jaundice
Increased intra-abdominal pressure
Chronic obstructive pulmonary disease
Cirrhosis
Sepsis
Use of nephrotoxic drugs or agents
Procedure type Cardiac Thoracoabdominal aortic Emergency abdominal aortic Liver transplant Surgery for biliary obstruction

ARF may be classified by etiology or the amount of urine produced per day. For diagnostic and therapeutic purposes, ARF is divided into prerenal (12% to 60% of cases), intrarenal (20% to 80% of cases), and postrenal (1% to 10% of cases) causes. Patients who have prerenal ARF typically have a FENa of less than 1%, urine osmolality greater than 500 mOsm/kg, or urine sodium concentration less than 20 mEq/L. Prerenal ARF is most commonly encountered in the setting of hypovolemia. Ensuring adequate volume status with a fluid challenge and invasive monitoring, if necessary, is an important part of the therapy of postoperative patients with oliguria or increasing serum creatinine levels. When recognized early, prerenal ARF is readily correctable with fluid resuscitation.

Patients with acute tubular necrosis (ATN), the predominant intrarenal cause of ARF, typically have a FENa of greater than 2%, urine osmolality less than 400 mOsm/kg and urine sodium concentration greater than 20 mEq/L. As opposed to patients with prerenal ARF (who may have no findings or have occasional hyaline casts on urinalysis), patients with ATN will generally exhibit renal tubular epithelial cells and granular casts on microscopic analysis.

ATN is precipitated by ischemia of the nephron, which can be due to either decreased renal blood flow and oxygen delivery or to increased oxygen utilization caused by nephrotoxins. Rapid identification and reversal of renal ischemia is the most important method of prevention of ATN. Intraoperative renal ischemia may be unavoidable, but should be minimized as much as possible. It must be noted that prolonged prerenal ARF, if uncorrected, ultimately leads to intrarenal ATN.

Patients with postrenal ARF typically also have a FENa of greater than 2% and urine osmolality less than 400 mOsm/kg. Postrenal ARF occurs when the ureters, bladder or urethra are injured or occluded. It is important to recognize ARF arising from obstruction of the collecting system because this condition is often completely reversible.

The most common cause of ureteral damage is iatrogenic injury. Obstruction or injury of the ureter should be suspected in any patients with ARF after any procedure during which the ureter is at risk. Ureteral injury most commonly occurs during procedures involving the distal colon and rectum or gynecologic procedures, but any procedure involving retroperitoneal or pelvic dissection can result in ureteral injury. A renal ultrasound may be a useful diagnostic study when ureteral obstruction is suspected as a cause of ARF. Preoperative ureteral stent placement is commonly recommended in situations where injury to the ureter is possible, although there is no prospective data to support this practice.

Urethral obstruction is another cause of postrenal ARF. Gross hematuria, benign prostatic hypertrophy, and urinary catheter obstruction can lead to outflow obstruction from the bladder, resulting in ARF if not treated in a timely fashion. The development of oliguria should prompt placement of a Foley catheter. If there is already a catheter in place, the catheter should be flushed to ensure it is draining properly.

Patients with ARF can also be subdivided into those with nonoliguric (urine output >400 mL/d), oliguric (urine output <400 mL/d), and anuric renal failure (urine output <50 mL/d). Patients with nonoliguric renal failure have a better prognosis, although there is no evidence that "converting" oliguric ARF to nonoliguric ARF with diuretics improves outcomes.

PREVENTION

Since ARF significantly worsens prognosis, prevention of ARF and/or minimizing progression of the disease is of utmost importance. However, despite decades of research in how to prevent ARF, very few interventions have been reproducibly successful.

Optimizing fluid status

The single most important measure to prevent perioperative ARF is maintenance of adequate intravascular volume. Depending on the clinical situation, this may range from aggressive fluid administration with isotonic crystalloids or colloids, to keeping the patient on maintenance fluids to balance their insensible losses. When the patient has an adequate cardiac function, euvolemia ensures sufficient renal blood flow, reduces vasoconstrictive stimuli, and improves urine flow. In contrast, prolonged renal hypoperfusion and prerenal ARF can lead to ATN and ultimately complete renal failure.

It is essential to determine whether the cause of renal insufficiency is prerenal hypoperfusion or an intrinsic event, because prerenal ARF is completely reversible if renal perfusion and glomerular filtration pressure are restored rapidly. Assessment of intravascular volume status is based upon physical examination, urine output, laboratory values, and, potentially, invasive monitoring. Depending upon the severity of hypovolemia, the patient may present along a spectrum from subtle signs to cardiovascular collapse. The simplest method to examine volume status is measurement of urine output. A hydrated patient without a Foley catheter in place should void at least once every eight hours and make 0.5 mL/kg/h (280 mL per shift in a 70 kg person). If urine output appears inadequate, placement of a Foley catheter will aid in monitoring urine volume. Two common clinical scenarios that result in seemingly adequate urine output despite intravascular hypovolemia are hyperglycemia (an obligate osmotic diuresis can begin with glucose levels greater than 180 mg/dL) and recent diuretic administration. Patients with elevated blood glucose or those who receive diuretics intraoperatively therefore require special attention to their volume status since they can become markedly intravascularly depleted and yet still appear to have adequate urine output.

Oliguria in the postoperative period usually reflects hypovolemia. In addition to maintenance fluids and replacement of blood loss, intraoperative insensible losses may be estimated to be 1 to 3 mL/kg/h for a small incision, 3 to 7 mL/kg/h for a medium incision and 9 to 11 mL/kg/h for a large incision. While adequate fluid resuscitation should be performed intraoperatively by the anesthesiologist, the surgeon must verify each patient's fluid balance in the immediate postoperative period and administer additional fluid if necessary. Nearly all patients with oliguria in the perioperative period are able to tolerate two boluses of 500 mL of isotonic crystalloid solution or a single bolus of 500 mL of a colloid. Special care should be given to patients with a severely decreased left ventricular ejection fraction, those who are dependent on high dose diuretic preoperatively, and those whose operations would not be expected to result in postoperative hypovolemia.

For patients who do not respond to initial fluid boluses, the physician must decide whether to administer additional fluid boluses or obtain additional monitoring. No universal guidelines can dictate what constitutes a "reasonable" amount of fluid administration before pursuing additional monitoring. However, patients with larger incisions and longer operations may require more fluid than average surgical patients, and younger patients generally tolerate fluid overload better than older ones. For patients in whom additional information is needed to estimate intravascular volume, central venous pressure (CVP) provides a useful reflection of right heart filling pressures. This is relevant because while hypovolemia should be avoided, the injudicious use of fluids should likewise be avoided. For example, a recent study of fluid management in patients with acute respiratory distress syndrome demonstrated a strong trend toward decreased risk of ARF requiring dialysis in patients treated with a conservative fluid management strategy (less fluid at a given CVP) than those with a liberal fluid management strategy (8).

In cases where the CVP is a poor estimate of left heart filling volumes (as occurs with significant valvular disease or pulmonary hypertension), a pulmonary artery catheter or esophageal Doppler may be useful. However, there is a paucity of convincing evidence that these devices prevent renal failure or improve outcomes. In the unusual event that renal blood flow is limited by a poor cardiac output, inotropic agents may be necessary as adjuvants to proper fluid administration.

Blood pressure

Another important factor in the maintenance of renal perfusion is mean arterial pressure. While autoregulation of renal blood flow may be impaired at mean arterial pressures less than 75 mm Hg, two studies have shown no further improvement in urine output with mean arterial pressures greater than 65 mm Hg (9,10). While this means that most patients with possible renal hypoperfusion should have their mean arterial pressure kept above 65 mm Hg, in elderly patients and patients with pre-existing hypertension, autoregulation of renal blood flow is frequently impaired, and these patients may benefit from higher arterial pressures (11).

Avoidance of nephrotoxins

The use of nephrotoxins should be minimized or altogether avoided if possible. Once a patient develops ARF, a prompt review of the patient's recent medications should be undertaken to discontinue agents if safe alternatives exist. The nephrotoxins most commonly encountered in the surgical patient include radiocontrast dye (discussed below), nonsteroidal anti-inflammatory drugs (NSAIDs), cyclosporine, aminoglycosides, and amphotericin B. Once a patient develops ARF, the renal clearance of many drugs will also be decreased, occasionally resulting in nephrotoxic levels of a drug in plasma. Vancomycin is the most commonly encountered drug in this category and should be avoided in evolving renal failure if possible; otherwise trough levels should be followed closely.

Contrast induced acute kidney injury

Contrast induced acute kidney injury (CI-AKI) accounts for 10% of ARF in hospitalized patients. Although nephropathy induced by radiocontrast dye is uncommon in patients with normal renal function, its incidence increases to 5% in patients with mild renal insufficiency and 50% in those with severe renal dysfunction and diabetes. CI-AKI is frequently defined as an increase in serum creatinine of at least 0.5 mg/dL or 25% above the baseline. While transient increases in serum creatinine are common, the need for RRT after contrast administration is low. The incidence of CI-AKI is highest for noncoronary angiography and lowest for CT scans using intra venous (IV) contrast (12).

The most effective therapy to prevent CI-AKI is administration of IV fluid around the time of contrast administration. Another commonly used therapy employs sodium bicarbonate. There have been around 20 studies published on the use of sodium bicarbonate to prevent CI-AKI (half of these have been only in abstract form) with widely varying results. Two recent meta-analyses on the use of sodium bicarbonate demonstrate that the therapy has statistical significance in preventing CI-AKI but has no effect on need for RRT or mortality (13,14). Based on these results as well as the low quality and heterogeneity of many of the studies, one meta-analysis concluded that "only a limited recommendation can be made in favour" of using sodium bicarbonate for CI-AKI prophylaxis. If this strategy is used, the sodium bicarbonate solution is prepared by injecting 154 mmol of sodium bicarbonate into 1 liter of 5% dextrose in water and administering it at a rate of 3 mL/kg/h for 1 hour prior to contrast administration, and then at 1 mL/kg/h for 6 hours after the procedure.

N-acetylcysteine (NAC) is another widely studied therapy to prevent CI-AKI. NAC is thought to act as a free radical scavenger and ameliorate ischemia-reperfusion injury. NAC is usually administered as 600 mg dosed orally twice daily with at least one dose prior to the procedure and continued for at least 1 day afterward. Over 25 studies on the utility of NAC have yielded conflicting results. The two most recent meta-analyses (published in 2008 and 2009) demonstrate a benefit of NAC in preventing CI-AKI (15,16); however, no benefit was seen in a 2007 meta-analysis (17). Like sodium bicarbonate, NAC has not been shown to prevent the need for RRT or decrease mortality. NAC is also similar to sodium bicarbonate in that both therapies are inexpensive and carry little risk. It is of note that preoperative use of NAC has also been studied in over 1,000 patients to determine whether it can prevent ARF in patients undergoing major surgery who do not receive radiocontrast. NAC has no effect on either CI-AKI or mortality in this setting and is therefore not recommended for this usage (18). Multiple other agents including fenoldopam, dopamine, furosemide, mannitol, and theophylline have been studied to determine whether they prevent CI-AKI (15). None of these have been proven to be beneficial. Additionally, furosemide has been shown to increase serum creatinine after IV contrast administration so should not be used in this setting.

Diuretics

The rationale for using diuretics to prevent ARF is based on the observation that nonoliguric renal failure has a better prognosis than oliguric renal failure. However, multiple randomized trials have failed to show improvement with diuretic use. In a trial randomizing 126 patients undergoing cardiac surgery to furosemide, dopamine, or placebo, patients who received furosemide had higher rates of ARF and higher serum creatinine than those who received either dopamine or placebo (19). Similarly, a large retrospective study of 552 patients demonstrated that patients who received diuretics early in the evolution of ARF were less likely to recover renal function than those who did not receive diuretics (20). Thus, while diuretics may play a role in helping the physician manage fluid status (to treat pulmonary edema, for example), they should not be used as a method of preventing ARF.

Dopaminergic agonists

Low-dose ("renal dose," 1 to 3 μg/kg/min) dopamine has been studied for over 30 years and is still widely used by many practitioners. Although numerous theoretical benefits of low dose dopamine exist, it is an ineffective agent in preventing ARF. While low-dose dopamine is frequently successful in improving urinary output, it does not alter mortality, the need for dialysis, or the onset of ARF. Both a prospective randomized trial on this agent in patients with the systemic inflammatory response syndrome and oliguria (21) as well as a recent meta-analysis of 24 studies involving over 1,000 patients demonstrate this (22). Because low-dose dopamine may worsen splanchnic oxygenation, impair GI function, impair endocrine and immunologic systems, and blunt ventilatory drive while not preventing ARF, dialysis, or mortality, this strategy should not be used in clinical practice.

Fenoldopam is a dopamine analogue that is specific for the dopamine-1 receptors. Fenoldopam theoretically increases renal blood flow without the vasoconstrictive effect that may limit the usefulness of dopamine. Although no large randomized trials have demonstrated a mortality benefit with fenoldopam, a recent meta-analysis of more than 1,000 patients in 13 trials concludes that fenoldopam decreases the need for RRT and mortality in patients undergoing cardiovascular surgery (23). Although its routine use cannot be recommended for the prevention of ARF at this time, a large clinical trial to definitively study the effects of fenoldopam following surgery is warranted.

Other pharmacologic therapies

Multiple other therapies have been tried for the prevention of postoperative ARF with limited evidence of their benefit. Calcium channel blockers may provide some benefit in renal transplant patients but their use for other indications has not been proven to be beneficial. Other therapies with potential benefit but limited clinical evidence for efficacy include pentoxifylline, theophylline, anaritide, and nesiritide (synthetic atrial- and brain-type natriuretic peptides, respectively.)

Treatment

The treatment of ARF depends on the etiology. Prerenal ARF typically responds to increased renal perfusion, and postrenal ARF is treated by relieving the obstruction of the collecting system. However, once a patient has developed ATN, there are no therapies proven to hasten the return of renal function, and care is generally supportive. Maintenance of renal perfusion is important as injury to the renal tubules extends in the first 24 hours after the onset of ATN due to inflammation and vascular congestion. Avoidance of nephrotoxins in this period is imperative.

Ultimately, ARF either responds to conservative therapy or progresses to the point that patients require RRT. Indications for dialysis are listed in Table 18.3. Although these indications are generally accepted, there is no absolute threshold for any of these indications that requires initiation of RRT; thus, the timing of initiation of RRT is clinician dependent. However, a recent observational study in 54 ICUs demonstrated that initiation of RRT "late" (defined as >5 days after admission) was associated with a longer duration of RRT, hospital stay, and dialysis dependence (24). This is consistent with a study of 69 patients who developed ARF after cardiac surgery, in which patients randomized to receive RRT for oliguria received dialysis earlier than those who received it based upon serum creatinine or potassium had significantly lower mortality (25)

Table 18.3 Indications for renal replacement therapy
Volume overload
Electrolyte abnormalities (e.g., hyperkalemia)
Acidosis
Symptomatic uremia (e.g., encephalopathy, pericarditis)
Acute poisoning

There are several modalities of RRT, including intermittent hemodialysis, sustained low-efficiency daily dialysis, and continuous venovenous hemodialysis. While hemodynamically unstable patients may not tolerate intermittent hemodialysis, there are no differences in clinical outcomes with intermittent hemodialysis or continuous venovenous hemodialysis in the hemodynamically stable patient. Additionally, a recent prospective randomized trial of 1,124 ICU patients demonstrated that as long as dialysis is adequate, intensive dialysis does not improve outcome (mortality, renal recovery) when compared to less-intensive dialysis (26).

Temporary dialysis in perioperative patients with ARF is typically initiated through a large bore, double lumen central venous catheter. The preferred site is the right internal jugular vein, which yields consistent flow rates and is technically simple. The femoral veins may also be used for access, but long term presence of femoral venous access predisposes the patient to infection. The left subclavian vein often gives acceptable flow rates, but large bore catheters at this site may lead to thrombosis and stenosis of the vein, complicating long term access in the upper extremity if permanent RRT is required. This is one of the few instances in which the internal jugular vein is preferred over the subclavian vein for vascular access, secondary to the increased risk of infection in catheters placed in the internal jugular vein.

Complications of dialysis catheters are similar to those seen with the placement of any central venous catheter. Immediate complications include pneumothorax, arterial cannulation, bleeding, and air embolism. A common delayed complication is catheter-related bloodstream infection. Catheter-related bloodstream infection is manifested by fever, leukocytosis, and hypotension in severe cases, and although this complication can occur at any time, the risk of infection increases the longer the vascular access device is in place. If no other source of infection is apparent, the catheter should be removed, and two sets of blood cultures should be drawn. The patient should also be started on broad-spectrum antibiotics until culture results are known. The decision to remove or keep a dialysis catheter in a septic patient with another possible source of infection must be made on an individual basis. Another frequent complication of dialysis access is thrombosis of the vessel into which the catheter has been placed. Thrombosis is frequently clinically silent but can have significant implications for long-term dialysis access if a patient's renal failure does not resolve.

Patients with chronic renal failure should be dialyzed through their previously placed arteriovenous fistula (or, much less commonly, their peritoneal dialysis catheter). While surgery at another site should not impact continuation of dialysis *per se*, perioperative hypotension increases the risk of thrombosis of a previously patent fistula and should be avoided if possible.

One cause of renal failure that occurs disproportionately in the trauma surgery population is rhabdomyolysis. Rhabdomyolysis results from the destruction of skeletal muscle, most commonly from crush injuries. Other situations in which surgical patients develop rhabdomyolysis include compartment syndrome, ischemia-reperfusion of skeletal muscle, and muscle destruction from positioning during long surgical procedures or in the ICU. Rhabdomyolysis is associated with myoglobinuria. The excretion of myoglobin by the kidneys may lead to tubular obstruction and direct injury to the nephron by myoglobin.

The treatment of ARF due to rhabdomyolysis, as with that for other forms of ARF, is supportive, with special emphasis placed on maintenance of intravascular volume. Because renal damage results from the mechanical obstruction of tubules by myoglobin, there are theoretical advantages to enforcing diuresis (with adequate intravascular volume). Mannitol, an osmotic diuretic that does not enter cells and is freely filtered and not reabsorbed by the tubules, not only flushes necrotic tubular debris from nephrons but also has free radical scavenging properties. The evidence supporting mannitol is based upon experimental animal studies and retrospective clinical studies, and there is no clear evidence demonstrating its efficacy in preventing and/or treating ARF in rhabdomyolysis. Maintaining an alkaline (pH >6.5) urine has also been advocated in the treatment of rhabdomyolysis to decrease the toxicity of myoglobin to renal tubules. There is no clear evidence in patients to determine the efficacy of alkalinizing the urine.

A retrospective review of 2,083 trauma patients demonstrated no difference in mortality or need for RRT in patients treated with mannitol and bicarbonate; however, a trend toward better outcomes was noted in patients with the highest creatine kinase levels (>30,000 IU/L.) (27)

SUMMARY

ARF is a potentially life-threatening complication of surgery that portends a negative outcome. Patients with preexisting renal insufficiency are at the highest risk of ARF. Patients displaying evidence of ARF, such as oliguria or increasing serum creatinine, should be rapidly evaluated. Untreated prerenal and postrenal ARF may lead to ATN and prolonged renal failure. These conditions must be identified and treated as soon as possible. Optimizing fluid status and avoiding nephrotoxins are the only clearly beneficial methods of preventing ATN. Once a patient develops ATN, there are no proven therapeutic interventions to hasten its reversal. Specific situations such as rhabdomyolysis, contrast administration, and abdominal compartment syndrome are potentially treatable or preventable causes of ARF and should be identified rapidly. Once a patient develops indications, RRT should be started. Except in the hemodynamically unstable patient, there is no evidence supporting preference of one mode of RRT over another.

REFERENCES

1. Carmichael P, Carmichael AR. Acute renal failure in the surgical setting. *ANZ J Surg* 2003;73(3):144–153.
2. Dasta JF, Kane-Gill SL, Durtschi AJ, et al. Costs and outcomes of acute kidney injury (AKI) following cardiac surgery. *Nephrol Dial Transplant* 2008;23(6):1970–1974.
3. Uchino S, Kellum JA, Bellomo R, et al. Acute renal failure in critically ill patients: a multinational, multicenter study. *JAMA* 2005;294(7): 813–818.
4. Kellum JA, Bellomo R, Ronco C. Definition and classification of acute kidney injury. *Nephron Clin Pract* 2008;109(4):c182–c187.
5. Bellomo R, Ronco C, Kellum JA, et al. Acute renal failure – definition, outcome measures, animal models, fluid therapy and information technology needs: the Second International Consensus Conference of the Acute Dialysis Quality Initiative (ADQI) Group. *Crit Care* 2004;8(4): R204–R212.
6. Hoste EA, Lameire NH, Vanholder RC, et al. Acute renal failure in patients with sepsis in a surgical ICU: predictive factors, incidence, comorbidity, and outcome. *J Am Soc Nephrol* 2003;14(4):1022–1030.
7. Cheatham ML. Abdominal compartment syndrome. *Curr Opin Crit Care* 2009;15(2):154–162.
8. Wiedemann HP, Wheeler AP, Bernard GR, et al. Comparison of two fluid-management strategies in acute lung injury. *N Engl J Med* 2006; 354(24):2564–2575.
9. Bourgoin A, Leone M, Delmas A, et al. Increasing mean arterial pressure in patients with septic shock: effects on oxygen variables and renal function. *Crit Care Med* 2005;33(4):780–786.
10. LeDoux D, Astiz ME, Carpati CM, et al. Effects of perfusion pressure on tissue perfusion in septic shock. *Crit Care Med* 2000;28(8):2729–2732.
11. Inscho EW. Lewis K. Dahl memorial lecture. Mysteries of renal autoregulation. *Hypertension* 2009;53(2):299–306.
12. Weisbord SD, Mor MK, Resnick AL, et al. Prevention, incidence, and outcomes of contrast-induced acute kidney injury. *Arch Intern Med* 2008;168(12):1325–1332.

13. Hoste EA, De Waele JJ, Gevaert SA, et al. Sodium bicarbonate for prevention of contrast-induced acute kidney injury: a systematic review and meta-analysis. *Nephrol Dial Transplant* 2009;25(3):747–758.
14. Navaneethan SD, Singh S, Appasamy S, et al. Sodium bicarbonate therapy for prevention of contrast-induced nephropathy: a systematic review and meta-analysis. *Am J Kidney Dis* 2009;53(4):617–627.
15. Kelly AM, Dwamena B, Cronin P, et al. Meta-analysis: effectiveness of drugs for preventing contrast-induced nephropathy. *Ann Intern Med* 2008;148(4):284–294.
16. Trivedi H, Daram S, Szabo A, et al. High-dose N-acetylcysteine for the prevention of contrast-induced nephropathy. *Am J Med* 2009;122(9):874–815.
17. Gonzales DA, Norsworthy KJ, Kern SJ, et al. A meta-analysis of N-acetylcysteine in contrast-induced nephrotoxicity: unsupervised clustering to resolve heterogeneity. *BMC Med* 2007;5:32.
18. Ho KM, Morgan DJ. Meta-analysis of N-acetylcysteine to prevent acute renal failure after major surgery. *Am J Kidney Dis* 2009;53(1):33–40.
19. Lassnigg A, Donner E, Grubhofer G, et al. Lack of renoprotective effects of dopamine and furosemide during cardiac surgery. *J Am Soc Nephrol* 2000;11(1):97–104.
20. Mehta RL, Pascual MT, Soroko S, et al. Diuretics, mortality, and nonrecovery of renal function in acute renal failure. *JAMA* 2002;288(20): 2547–2553.
21. Bellomo R, Chapman M, Finfer S, et al. Low-dose dopamine in patients with early renal dysfunction: a placebo-controlled randomised trial. Australian and New Zealand Intensive Care Society (ANZICS) Clinical Trials Group. *Lancet* 2000;356(9248):2139–2143.
22. Kellum JA, Decker M. Use of dopamine in acute renal failure: a meta-analysis. *Crit Care Med* 2001;29(8):1526–1531.
23. Landoni G, Biondi-Zoccai GG, Marino G, et al. Fenoldopam reduces the need for renal replacement therapy and in-hospital death in cardiovascular surgery: a meta-analysis. *J Cardiothorac Vasc Anesth* 2008; 22(1):27–33.
24. Bagshaw SM, Uchino S, Bellomo R, et al. Timing of renal replacement therapy and clinical outcomes in critically ill patients with severe acute kidney injury. *J Crit Care* 2009;24(1):129–140.
25. Demirkilic U, Kuralay E, Yenicesu M, et al. Timing of replacement therapy for acute renal failure after cardiac surgery. *J Card Surg* 2004; 19(1):17–20.
26. Palevsky PM, Zhang JH, O'Connor TZ, et al. Intensity of renal support in critically ill patients with acute kidney injury. *N Engl J Med* 2008; 359(1):7–20.
27. Brown CV, Rhee P, Chan L, et al. Preventing renal failure in patients with rhabdomyolysis: do bicarbonate and mannitol make a difference? *J Trauma* 2004;56(6):1191–1196.

CHAPTER 19

Pulmonary Complications

Mark R. Hemmila

INTRODUCTION

The fire of life is maintained by the oxidation of metabolic substrates and the production of carbon dioxide. This creates the kinetic energy that sustains all bodily functions. As a vital organ, the lungs serve a dual role in allowing the absorption of oxygen gas into the body and the excretion of carbon dioxide to the atmosphere. For surgical patients undergoing elective or emergent operation, safe airway management and maintenance of optimal pulmonary function are paramount to successful perioperative care. Pulmonary complications can occur on multiple levels and at varying rates of clinical urgency. The successful clinician lives by the rule that "chance favors the prepared mind" and is ever vigilant for compromise in a patient's pulmonary function.

Pulmonary complications span a wide range of different etiologies but have a similar result in that they affect either oxygenation or ventilation of the patient. The following is a discussion of risk for pulmonary complications, diagnosis, and management of life-threatening pulmonary problems. The pathogenesis, clinical presentation, prevention, and treatment of severe pulmonary insufficiency will be covered. Basic management of mechanical ventilation in the surgical patient with acute lung injury (ALI) will also be described, along with novel strategies to manage patients with severe acute respiratory distress syndrome (ARDS).

PREOPERATIVE PULMONARY FUNCTION

Risk factors for pulmonary complications

Preoperative assessment of respiratory status and identification of high-risk patients is of critical importance in preventing pulmonary complications in surgery patients. Several potential factors increase the risk of developing pulmonary complications during or following surgery, as outlined in Table 19.1. A respiratory complication is defined as any pulmonary abnormality that produces identifiable disease or dysfunction that is clinically significant and impairs a patient's clinical course (1–4). Important examples of clinically significant pulmonary complications include atelectasis, pneumonia, respiratory failure with prolonged mechanical ventilation, exacerbation of underlying chronic lung disease, and bronchospasm (4). Patient-related risk factors that increase the risk of postoperative pulmonary complications are older age, male gender, smoking, congestive heart failure, metabolic abnormalities, and chronic obstructive pulmonary disease (COPD) (4,5). Procedure related factors which increase risk are higher American Society of Anesthesiologists (ASA) classification, emergency operation, and more complex operation (work relative value units) (5). Certain types of surgery, such as thoracic and upper abdominal procedures, are associated with a reduction in functional residual capacity (FRC) (6). Diaphragmatic dysfunction, postoperative pain, and splinting are factors contributing to this loss in FRC. Loss of FRC places the patient at risk for atelectasis, pneumonia, transpulmonary shunting, and impaired gas exchange due to ventilation/perfusion mismatch.

Smoking is a known and repeatedly demonstrated risk factor for postoperative pulmonary complications. Smoking increases the relative risk of pulmonary complications among all patients who smoke as compared to nonsmokers by an odds ratio (OR) of 1.1 to 4.3 (5–9). This increased risk among smokers extends to those without chronic lung disease (7). In a prospective study of 200 patients who underwent coronary artery bypass surgery, there was a lower risk of pulmonary complications in patients who stopped smoking at least 8 weeks prior to surgery than in current smokers (15% vs. 33%) (10). Ironically, patients who ceased smoking less than 8 weeks before surgery had an increased risk of pulmonary complications compared to current smokers (57% vs. 33%). Patients who stopped smoking for more than 6 months had rates similar to those who never smoked (11% vs. 12%).

General health status is an excellent determinant of overall fitness for surgical intervention and is an important predictor of pulmonary risk. The Goldman cardiac risk index can predict pulmonary as well as cardiac complications (11–13). The commonly used ASA classification, which evaluates overall risk of perioperative mortality, has been shown to be an effective predictor of postoperative respiratory complications (5,14,15). An ASA class of 3 or greater places the patient at a 2.9-fold to 4.9-fold increased

Mark R. Hemmila: Trauma Burn Center, University of Michigan Medical School, University of Michigan Health System, Ann Arbor, MI 48109.

Table 19.1 Risk factors for developing postoperative pulmonary complications

Definite risk factors
Age ≥40 years
Male gender
Chronic obstructive lung disease
Congestive heart failure
Current smoking history
Cessation of smoking less than 8 weeks prior to surgery
Poor general health status, defined as ASA class >2
Serum albumin ≤3.5 gm/dL
Serum creatinine ≥1.5 mg/dL
Emergency surgery
Type of operation (upper abdominal, thoracic, aortic, mouth/palate)
Complexity of operation
Surgery lasting greater than three hours
Use of pancuronium as a neuromuscular blocker
Probable risk factors
General anesthesia
Obstructive sleep apnea
$Paco_2$ >45 mm Hg
Abnormal chest x-ray
Current upper respiratory tract infection

Modified from Smetana GW. Evaluation of preoperative pulmonary risk. UpToDate 17.1. Available online at: http://www.utdol.com. Accessed May 20, 2009, with permission.

Table 19.2 Postoperative respiratory failure risk index

Preoperative Predictor	Point Value
Type of surgery	
Abdominal aortic aneurysm	27
Thoracic	21
Neurosurgery, upper abdominal, or peripheral vascular	14
Neck	11
Emergency surgery	11
Albumin (<3 g/dL)	9
Blood urea nitrogen (>30 mg/dL)	8
Partially or fully dependent functional status	7
History of chronic obstructive pulmonary disease	6
Age (years)	
≥70	6
60–69	4

Class	Point Total	Predicted Probability of Pulmonary Failure
1	≤10	0.5%
2	11–19	2.2%
3	20–27	5.0%
4	28–40	11.6%
5	>40	30.5%

Adapted from Arozullah AM, Daley J, Henderson WG, et al. Multifactorial risk index for predicting postoperative respiratory failure in men after major noncardiac surgery. *Ann Surg* 2000;232:250, with permission.

risk for pulmonary complications from general or vascular surgery (5). Poor exercise tolerance is a strong identifier of patients at risk for pulmonary complications. For patients over 65, the inability to complete 2 minutes of stationary bicycle exercise, sufficient to raise the heart rate to greater than 99 beats/minute, was the strongest predictor of pulmonary complications in a multivariate analysis of patients undergoing abdominal or noncardiac thoracic surgery (13).

The National Surgical Quality Improvement Program (NSQIP) is a multi-institutional study that has prospectively collected data on surgical outcomes and comorbidities. The program relates this data to observed versus expected morbidity and mortality ratios using risk adjusted indices. A multifactorial risk index model for predicting postoperative respiratory failure in men after major noncardiac surgery was created from this study (Table 19.2) (16). A more robust model now exists which applies to men and woman undergoing general or vascular surgery and utilizes 28 predictive variables (5). Risk factor scores are assigned for the 28 covariates and summation of the individual covariate scores results in the final risk factor score. Patients with a risk factor score <8 (Low) have a predicted risk of respiratory failure of 0.2 %, those with a score between 8 and 12 (Medium) have a risk of 1.0%, and patients with a score >12 (High) have a 6.5% risk of respiratory failure. Operation type identified with current procedural terminology (CPT) coding, operative complexity, need for emergent surgery, and preoperative ASA classification continue to be among the most important determinants of respiratory failure risk.

Chronic lung disease is the most important patient-related risk factor for postoperative pulmonary complications. Unadjusted relative risks of postoperative complications for patients with COPD range from 2.7 to 6.0 (4,17). Patients with severe COPD are up to six times more likely to have a postoperative pulmonary complication than patients without COPD (17). In a case control study of 164 patients undergoing abdominal surgery, patients with abnormal findings on lung examination consistent with COPD had an OR of 5.8 for pulmonary complications (12). Medical treatment of patients with symptomatic COPD should be optimized prior to elective general surgery. The use of bronchodilators, physical therapy, antibiotics, smoking cessation, and in selected cases systemic corticosteroids can reduce the risk of postoperative complications in patients with COPD (4). Patients with COPD have an increased risk for pulmonary complications, but there is no exact level of impaired pulmonary function below which all surgery is contraindicated. In a study of 12 very high-risk surgical patients who all had an FEV1 of <1 L, only three of 15 surgeries were associated with postoperative complications, and there were no deaths in these patients (18).

Age and obesity are two common risk factors that have been assumed to be associated with increased risk for pulmonary complications. However, when data are analyzed to account for coexisting medical conditions, both of these risk factors are not always independently predictive of increased pulmonary risk. The risk of surgical mortality is fairly similar for all age groups when stratified by ASA class (19). A multivariate analysis for postoperative respiratory failure from the Patient Safety in Surgery Study identified age ≥40 years as a risk factor (5). Patients aged 40 to 65 had an OR of 1.7, and patients aged >65 had an OR of 2.1 for pulmonary complications when compared with patients <40 years of age.

A review of ten published series of bariatric surgery patients showed a 4% incidence of pneumonia and postoperative atelectasis, which is similar to the general population (20). Prospective studies show that a body mass index >25 kg/m^2 is an independent risk factor for postoperative pulmonary complications (9,21). Published discrepancies exist because the literature does not always distinguish between obesity and comorbid conditions associated with obesity that can contribute to increased pulmonary risk. A large review of six studies with 4,526 patients showed that the risk for pulmonary complications was identical for obese and nonobese patients undergoing abdominal or thoracic surgery (4). Compared with normal weight patients, the morbidly obese patients (body mass index ≥35 kg/m^2) have a higher risk of postoperative pulmonary embolism which can result in mortality (22,23). However, in patients undergoing colectomy for cancer, the risk of pneumonia was not increased in the morbidly obese when adjustments were made for other comorbidities using NSQIP data (23). In summary, the increase in risk for pulmonary complications from age or obesity is small and is probably more directly related to preexisting comorbidities associated with these two conditions.

Preoperative assessment

Patient history and physical examination are the classic starting points for evaluating preoperative pulmonary risk. Identification of findings in the patient history, such as exercise intolerance, dyspnea on exertion, wheezing, cigarette smoking, cough, and sputum production, might indicate a need for more detailed evaluation of pulmonary function. Physical examination should focus on detecting hypoventilation in weak or debilitated patients and hyperinflation in patients with chronic pulmonary disease. Wheezing, rales, or rhonchi on auscultation should trigger further examination. Physical evidence of cardiac insufficiency, obesity, cyanosis, tobacco use, and poor oral hygiene should be considered a relative indication for pulmonary function assessment.

A chest x-ray is part of the complete evaluation of any patient with abnormalities discovered on history or physical examination. Chest x-ray should also be routine for any patient scheduled to undergo thoracotomy. Performance of a maximal respiratory inhalation and exhalation maneuver in the clinic can be revealing. The ability to climb two flights of stairs at a constant pace without dyspnea is a reasonable screening tool for detecting patients with respiratory, cardiac, or joint disease. Some patients might be too obese, weak, sedentary, or debilitated to complete this test. Inability to succeed at this test should prompt further investigation into overall fitness for elective operation, and corrective measures might need to be instituted.

Much confusion and debate exists over the benefit of preoperative pulmonary function testing (PFT). Often these tests confirm what is already clinically evident based on history and physical examination without adding substantially to the clinical estimate of pulmonary risk. A subset of patients with reversible pulmonary disease on spirometry might benefit from aggressive correction with bronchodilators and anti-inflammatory medications. A 2006 American College of Physicians (ACP) consensus statement on preoperative strategies to reduce perioperative pulmonary complications for patients undergoing noncardiothoracic surgery offered the recommendation that preoperative PFTs or chest radiography may be appropriate in patients with a previous diagnosis of COPD or asthma (24). However, preoperative spirometry and chest radiography should not be used routinely for predicting risk for postoperative pulmonary complications. The following is an objective approach to spirometry recommended by Smetana (6) and based on recent literature:

- Obtain PFTs for patients with COPD or asthma if clinical evaluation cannot determine whether the patient is at his or her best baseline and that bronchoconstriction is optimally reduced. Testing might identify patients who will benefit from more aggressive perioperative medical management and conditioning.
- Obtain PFTs for patients with dyspnea or exercise intolerance that is unexplained after clinical evaluation.
- PFTs should not be ordered routinely prior to abdominal surgery or other high risk surgeries.
- PFTs should not be used as the primary factor to deny surgery.

A preoperative arterial blood gas analysis identifies patients with hypercapnia. No data suggest that carbon dioxide retention increases pulmonary risk beyond that already established on the basis of clinical risk factors recognized on history and physical examination. Patients with a $Pa{CO_2}$ of >45 mm Hg usually have severe COPD, which is an already identified risk factor associated with a potential sixfold increase in risk for pulmonary complications. Preoperative arterial blood gas values serve primarily as a baseline for postoperative comparison and for decisions about postoperative ventilation rather than as a screening test for adequacy of pulmonary function (25). The ACP recommends preoperative arterial blood gas analysis in the following patients (26):

- Patients scheduled to undergo coronary artery bypass surgery or upper abdominal surgery with a history of tobacco use or dyspnea.
- All patients undergoing formal lung resection.

As with PFTs, preoperative arterial blood gas analysis alone cannot be the basis to identify high risk patients or to deny surgery.

ACUTE PULMONARY COMPROMISE

In the awake, alert, and conversive patient, patency and protection of the airway is a given. During major operations the airway is usually orotracheally intubated with a cuffed tube that provides a secure conduit for flow of respiratory gases. Many surgical patients are at risk for acute pulmonary compromise during the immediate perioperative period. A surgical patient can experience acute compromise in his or her respiratory status for several reasons.

Loss of airway

Patients who have undergone neck operations such as parathyroidectomy, thyroidectomy, or carotid endarterectomy are at risk for postoperative airway compromise. Hoarseness and stridor in the first 48 hours after operation can be caused by vocal cord edema from intubation, possible recurrent laryngeal nerve injury, or wound hematoma. Symptoms of hypoxia such as restlessness, irritability, and somnolence all might occur in the postoperative patient for a variety of reasons but should heighten suspicion for a respiratory problem as part of the differential diagnosis. Prompt physical examination of the patient helps to establish the etiology and severity of airway compromise. Pulse oximetry should be performed on all patients with respiratory difficulties. Patients with obvious neck swelling and compromise due to wound hematoma should have their wounds opened immediately, and appropriate clinical measures should be taken, including evacuation, reestablishment of hemostasis, endotracheal intubation, and possible tracheostomy. The latter can be performed at the bedside if necessary (27).

Vocal cord edema can be distinguished from recurrent laryngeal nerve injury by indirect laryngoscopy using a flexible fiberoptic nasopharyngoscope. Mild to moderate vocal cord edema can be managed with humidification of the inspired air and close airway monitoring. More severe cases might require treatment with steroids such as dexamethasone 10 mg IV every 6 to 12 hours or even tracheostomy performed in the operating room. The use of steroids is controversial and has only been proven beneficial in prospective randomized clinical trials of neonates and children under 5 years old who were administered dexamethasone 0.25 to 0.5 mg per kg IV prior to planned extubation (28,29). Dexamethasone treated patients had fewer episodes of stridor and reintubation compared to the control group who did not get steroids. However, when a dangerous degree of airway compromise has developed, as evidenced by nasal flaring, subcostal retraction, and use of accessory muscles, the patient should be prepared for immediate tracheostomy. Oral tracheal intubation might be extremely difficult or impossible in this situation and should be attempted only once, if at all, prior to tracheostomy.

Table 19.3 Signs and symptoms of laryngeal nerve injury

	Voice	Glottic Closure	Airway
Recurrent			
Unilateral	Weak	Weak	Good
Bilateral	Normal	Adequate	Poor
External branch, superior recurrent			
Unilateral	Lowered	Weakened	Good
Bilateral	Lowered	Loss of reflex	Good
Combined injury			
Unilateral	Weak	Poor	Good
Bilateral	Weak	Weak	Adequate

Adapted from Newsome HH Jr. Complications of thyroid surgery. In: Greenfield LG, ed. *Complications in surgery and trauma*, 2nd ed. Philadelphia: J.B. Lippincott Company; 1990:654, with permission.

Damage to the recurrent laryngeal nerve can lead to acute airway compromise. Clinical evidence of a unilateral recurrent laryngeal injury is suggested by a weak, whispery voice (Table 19.3). Voice changes might also be accompanied by difficulty with complete glottic closure during coughing or Valsalva maneuver. Inability to close the glottis might be exacerbated with combined injury to the external branch of the superior laryngeal nerve and the recurrent laryngeal nerve. In isolated recurrent laryngeal nerve injury, the intact external branch of the superior laryngeal nerve innervates the cricothyroid muscle to maintain full adduction of the ipsilateral vocal cord. When the superior laryngeal nerve is also damaged, full adduction and glottic closure is not possible, and the vocal cord is paralyzed in the intermediate position, away from the midline. In most instances of isolated recurrent laryngeal nerve injury, the contralateral vocal cord will move across the midline over a few weeks time to abut the paralyzed cord. This produces a relatively normal voice. Therefore, it is imperative to exclude occult recurrent laryngeal nerve injury by performing indirect laryngoscopy prior to neck operation in any patient who has had previous neck surgery, regardless of the quality of the patient's voice (27).

If both recurrent laryngeal nerves are rendered nonfunctional, the vocal cords will become paralyzed in the fully adducted position. This might lead to acute respiratory compromise. The patient will experience difficulty with inspiration, and severe stridor is usually evident. Paradoxically, the voice might be normal during this crisis as the vocal cords are apposed in the midline. Immediate treatment of bilateral recurrent laryngeal nerve injury involves reintubation or tracheostomy. Some patients will have a temporary loss of function that recovers over the next few weeks (27).

Tension pneumothorax

Tension pneumothorax occurs when air enters the potential space between the parietal and visceral pleura of the chest and becomes trapped. The affected lung collapses and subsequently mediastinal shift occurs. Shift in the mediastinum leads to kinking of the superior and inferior vena cava with concomitant impairment in venous return and cardiac output. Ventilation of the contralateral lung is also diminished, and high peak airway pressures can be observed. Common causes of tension pneumothorax include traumatic injury, spontaneous rupture of a pneumocele, laparoscopy with operation at the esophageal hiatus, and mechanical ventilation with positive end-expiratory pressure (PEEP) (30).

Diagnosis of a tension pneumothorax requires timely clinical assessment. Signs and symptoms that are consistent with tension pneumothorax include the following: severe respiratory distress, hypotension, unilateral absence of breath sounds, neck vein distention, tracheal deviation, chest wall crepitus, and cyanosis. Waiting for a confirmatory chest x-ray in the setting of a tension pneumothorax will most certainly result in a fatal outcome. Treatment is based on the clinical examination. The pleural space should be decompressed with a large bore angiocatheter (12 to 14G) inserted through the chest wall into the second intercostal space in the midclavicular line. This will convert the tension pneumothorax to a simple pneumothorax. Chest decompression should be immediately followed by insertion of a thoracostomy tube to re-expand the collapsed lung. Patients who are not intubated and undergo bilateral needle thoracostomies require immediate or simultaneous airway intubation and positive-pressure ventilation.

SMOKE INHALATION AND BURNS

Fires in confined spaces can have devastating consequences, as evidenced by the mass casualty event resulting in approximately 100 deaths at a West Warwick, RI nightclub in the winter of 2003. Most deaths from a fire scene are due to smoke inhalation injury rather than from cutaneous burns and associated complications (31,32). The presence of inhalation injury in association with a burn increases the overall mortality rate and often results in significant pulmonary complications (33). In a patient with a >40% total body surface area burn, the presence of inhalation injury increases mortality from 3% to 27%. The same patient has over 95% mortality if he or she is older than 60.

Smoke inhalation

Smoke inhalation leads to injury by four mechanisms: direct thermal injury to the airways, hypoxia, exposure of the bronchopulmonary system to toxins, and pulmonary absorption of systemic toxins. Smoke tends to be dry and therefore has a low specific heat even at high temperatures. Thermal injuries tend to be limited to the airway above the glottis, including the nasopharynx, oropharynx, and larynx (34). Thermal injuries to the lower respiratory tract are unusual and occur in situations in which the smoke contains superheated particles or steam (35). Injury to the upper airway mucosa from heat produces erythema, ulceration, and edema. Heat damage to the pharynx can cause edema severe enough to lead to obstruction of the airway. Upper airway edema usually occurs during the first 24 hours after thermal injury, but it can be delayed in unresuscitated patients until fluid administration is under way. When present, edema usually resolves in 2 to 5 days (36). Diagnosis depends on the history and surveillance physical examination for signs and symptoms of smoke exposure. Symptoms such as dyspnea, stridor, and cyanosis should prompt early control of the airway by endotracheal intubation. Securing of the endotracheal tube in a burn patient is of paramount importance as a dislodged tube might be impossible to replace because of upper airway edema.

Hypoxia is primarily a result of consumption of oxygen by the fire that drives down the FIO_2 of the ambient air that the victim breathes. Severe hypoxia leads to a critical reduction in the level of oxygen delivery to the organs beyond which the body cannot compensate, eventually resulting in death by asphyxiation. Hypoxemia can potentiate the toxicity of inhaled carbon monoxide and hydrogen cyanide (37). Hypoxemia can also result in an increase in respiratory rate and minute ventilation, thereby markedly increasing the amount of smoke subsequently inhaled and worsening exposure to systemic and bronchopulmonary toxins (34).

Small particles and toxic gases in smoke can reach the distal airways and alveoli. These compounds result in an acute inflammatory reaction initially mediated by neutrophils (37). Symptoms might include persistent coughing, bronchorrhea, dyspnea, and wheezing. Physiologic changes triggered by the inflammatory cascade can result in worsened ventilation/perfusion (V/Q) matching and increased susceptibility to pulmonary infections. Severe cases can progress to ARDS. Bronchoscopy in these patients will reveal erythema, edema, and ulcerations of the airways, often in conjunction with carbonaceous sputum (34).

Carbon monoxide poisoning

Carbon monoxide gas in smoke can be systemically absorbed across the lung and have potentially fatal consequences. Carbon monoxide binds to hemoglobin with an affinity 200 times greater than oxygen (31). If a sufficient amount of circulating hemoglobin is bound to carbon monoxide, tissue hypoxia and cell death will occur. The most immediate threat is to oxygen-sensitive organs such as the brain. Carboxyhemoglobin (HbCO) levels of 40% to

60% cause obtundation and loss of consciousness. Levels of 20% to 40% cause central nervous system dysfunction of varying degrees. Interestingly, HbCO levels of 5% to 10% are found in smokers and in people in urban areas who are exposed to heavy traffic, but these levels of carbon monoxide absorption are rarely symptomatic (31).

The diagnosis of carbon monoxide poisoning is based on compatible history and physical examination. Symptoms and signs are relatively nonspecific and can include headache, nausea, malaise, altered cognition, dyspnea, angina, seizures, cardiac arrhythmias, congestive heart failure, and coma (38). Elevated HbCO levels might cause a cherry-red appearance of the skin. This physical finding is present in only half of patients with severe carbon monoxide poisoning (31). In carbon monoxide poisoning the blood's oxygen content is reduced, but the amount of oxygen dissolved in the plasma is unaffected by the hemoglobin-bound carbon monoxide. Arterial blood gas analysis will appear normal except for the HbCO level, which requires a cooximeter for measurement. HbCO levels correlate poorly with the extent of poisoning (Table 19.4), and do not predict delayed neurologic sequelae. Neurologic deficits, particularly loss of consciousness, worsen prognosis (39).

Placing the patient with carbon monoxide poisoning on 100% oxygen reduces the half life of carbon monoxide in the blood from 4 hours for patients on room air to 1 hour. All patients with elevated HbCO levels should receive 100% oxygen until levels of <10% are reached. Given limited availability and the absence of proven benefit within the medical literature, hyperbaric oxygen (HBO) is considered optional. Transfer to a burn center should not usually be delayed in favor of HBO treatment for carbon monoxide poisoning (38).

All patients with suspected carbon monoxide poisoning or inhalational injury should initially receive humidified 100% oxygen by face mask. Additional evidence must be sought on history and physical examination to confirm suspected inhalational injury. Confinement to fire in a closed space, breathing of large quantities of smoke or noxious fumes, singed facial hair, facial burns, perioral soot, carbonaceous sputum, hoarseness, stridor, and impaired consciousness are all signs and symptoms that might warrant further investigation into the possibility of inhalational injury and trigger potential intervention. An arterial blood gas analysis should be performed and cooximetry obtained to evaluate the level of HbCO in the bloodstream. Patients with a high suspicion for inhalation injury or evidence of severe carbon monoxide poisoning should undergo elective orotracheal intubation to secure the airway. In equivocal cases, the use of flexible fiberoptic nasopharyngeal endoscopy might reveal upper airway erythema and soft tissue edema that can progress to airway compromise if left untreated.

If severe injury to the tracheobronchial tree has occurred, the necrotic epithelium of the airways will begin sloughing around postinjury day 3 to 4 (37,40). This increase in secretions places the patient at risk for airway compromise from obstruction, development of atelectasis, and onset of bacterial pneumonia. Impairment of pulmonary host defense mechanisms, such as mucociliary clearance, function of alveolar macrophages, and recruitment of polymorphonuclear leukocytes can also increase the risk for pneumonia (41). Management of the patient in this clinical phase is largely supportive and involves chest physical therapy, postural drainage, and bronchoscopy, if necessary, to control secretions. Antibiotics should only be used empirically when bacterial pneumonia is suspected and continued only subsequent to confirmatory sputum or quantitative bronchoalveolar lavage culture.

Use of heparin and N-acetylcysteine in combination is based on scavenging of the oxygen free radicals produced when alveolar macrophages are activated by chemicals in smoke or compounds in the arachidonic cascade (32). A retrospective study showed that use of nebulized heparin and N-acetylcysteine to be effective in decreasing mortality, reducing the reintubation rate, and lowering the rate of atelectasis in pediatric patients with inhalation injury (42). The Shriners Hospital for Children in Galveston, TX, utilizes a treatment regimen consisting of 5,000 to 10,000 units of heparin in 3 mL normal saline nebulized every 4 hours, alternating with 3 to 5 mL of 20% *N*-acetylcysteine for 7 days.

Table **19.4** **Signs and symptoms of carbon monoxide poisoning**

Level of Carboxyhemoglobin (%HbCO)	Signs and Symptoms
<20	None, headache, confusion
20–40	Disorientation, fatigue, nausea, visual disturbances
40–60	Hallucination, combativeness, coma, shock
>60	Death

Adapted from Demling RH. Burn care in the immediate resuscitation period. In: Wilmore DW, Cheung LY, Harken AH, et al, eds. *ACS surgery: principles and practice*, 2003 ed. New York, NY: WebMD Inc; 2003:52, with permission.

ASPIRATION PNEUMONIA

Aspiration pneumonia is a pulmonary complication that occurs following abnormal entry of fluid, particulate matter, or gastrointestinal (GI) secretions into the respiratory tract. Two physiologic requirements are usually necessary to produce aspiration pneumonia. First, there must be a compromise in the normal upper airway defenses that protect the distal respiratory tree from exposure to noxious substances. This can consist of loss of glottic closure, inhibition of cough reflex, and failure of clearance mechanisms, all of which are commonly found in the obtunded or anesthetized patient. Second, an inoculation of the lower airways with deleterious fluid or particulate matter must occur. This inoculum can be detrimental to pulmonary function from direct toxic

Table 19.5 Conditions that predispose to aspiration pneumonia

Reduced consciousness
Diminished cough reflex
Compromised glottic closure
Neurologic insult
Dysphagia
Disorders of the upper GI tract
Esophageal disease
Surgery of upper airway or esophagus
Gastroesophageal reflux
Mechanical disruption of glottic closure or esophageal sphincter
Endotracheal intubation
Bronchoscopy
Upper endoscopy
Nasoenteric intubation
Other
Pharyngeal anesthesia
Protracted vomiting
Recumbent position

effect, stimulation of an inflammatory process due to a large bacterial bolus, or creation of airway obstruction from a sufficient volume of particulate matter (43).

Aspiration pneumonia should be distinguished from pneumonia itself. Community acquired or nosocomial pneumonia commonly occurs following small volume aspiration of microorganisms found in the oral cavity or nasopharynx. The organisms that typically produce pneumonia, such as *Staphylococcus aureus*, *Streptococcus pneumoniae*, *Haemophilus influenzae*, and Gram-negative bacilli, are all considered virulent bacteria, and only a small inoculum is required. Aspiration pneumonia is a term reserved for pulmonary infection and/or pneumonitis caused by altered clearance mechanisms of less virulent, primarily anaerobic bacteria that constitute the normal flora of a patient susceptible to aspiration. Conditions found in surgical patients that predispose them to aspiration pneumonia are listed in Table 19.5.

Chemical pneumonitis

Aspiration of gastric and oropharyngeal contents can lead to pulmonary complications from three mechanisms: chemical pneumonitis, bacterial infection, and mechanical obstruction. The aspiration of 1 to 3 mL/kg of gastric contents with a pH $\leq$2.5 leads to rapid pneumonitis characterized by atelectasis, peribronchial hemorrhage, pulmonary edema, and damage to bronchial epithelial cells (44–46). An intense inflammatory response occurs, and within 4 hours the alveoli are filled with marginated polymorphonuclear leukocytes and fibrin. The lung parenchyma eventually becomes grossly edematous and hemorrhagic with loss of alveoli and consolidation. Patients usually follow one of three scenarios after aspiration of gastric contents: (a) rapid progressive respiratory failure resulting in death within 24 hours (12%), (b) prompt resolution over 4 to 5 days (62%), or (c) initial improvement followed by development of nosocomial bacterial pneumonia (26%) (47).

The diagnosis of chemical pneumonitis following aspiration is presumptive and is based on clinical suspicion and features such as abrupt onset of severe respiratory symptoms with significant dyspnea, low-grade fever, cyanosis, diffuse crackles on auscultation, severe hypoxemia, and infiltrates on chest x-ray involving dependent lung segments. Treatment is largely supportive and centers on the provision of oxygen, protection of the airway, and tracheal suctioning. The acid material is rapidly neutralized in the lung, and damage is already well established by the time a physician or other healthcare professional becomes aware of the aspiration event. Animal studies have demonstrated therapeutic benefit from positive-pressure ventilation, intravenous administration of high molecular weight colloids, and infusion of sodium nitroprusside into the pulmonary artery (48–51). The usefulness of mechanical ventilation to support a patient with acute respiratory failure is obvious. However, recommendations on the use of the latter two therapies in the treatment of human patients with aspiration remain indeterminate. The immediate use of corticosteroids to treat chemical pneumonitis following gastric aspiration is unsupported (52).

Bacterial pneumonia

Bacterial pneumonia following aspiration is usually caused by organisms that commonly reside in the upper airways or stomach. These bacteria are less virulent and are primarily anaerobes that reside in the gingival creases. Compared to community-acquired pneumonia, onset is quite slow, with patients manifesting cough, fever, purulent sputum, and dyspnea evolving over a period of several days or weeks rather than hours (43). The absence of rigors is characteristic of nonpyogenic pneumonia since patients with aspiration pneumonia from anaerobes almost never have shaking chills. Many patients with aspiration pneumonia do not present acutely with infection. Instead, they present late with complications characterized by suppuration and necrosis within the lung (53–55). Lung abscesses, necrotizing pneumonia, or empyema all represent delayed presentations of untreated aspiration pneumonia.

Antibiotics are the most important component of treatment for aspiration pneumonia associated with bacterial infection. Based on transthoracic culture data, a switch has been made from Clindamycin to Piperacillin/Tazobactam as the currently the preferred drug for aspiration pneumonia with or without lung abscess (56). This change is based upon a surprising frequency of the bacteria *Klebsiella pneumoniae* found in these aspirates (57). Alternative regimens include Ceftriaxone plus Metronidazole or Moxifloxacin (56). When nosocomial pneumonia is suspected, companion aerobic bacteria, particularly Gram-negative bacilli or *Staphylococcus aureus*, are more important than anaerobes. Therapy should therefore be directed at these virulent organisms.

Mechanical obstruction

Aspiration can flood the lung with fluid and particulate matter. These materials might not be intrinsically toxic to the lung, but they can cause acute airway obstruction. Fluids that can be aspirated that are not toxic to the lung are saline, barium, most ingested fluids, including water, and gastric contents with a pH >2.5. Patients who are at risk for mechanical obstruction are those who cannot protect their airways or cough secondary to neurologic deficit or impaired consciousness. The obvious treatment is tracheal suctioning and prevention. The most important preemptive measure in hospitalized patients is to keep the patient in the semiupright or upright position (58–60).

Solid objects such as peanuts, vegetable particles, small parts, and teeth can become aspirated and lodged in the airway (43). Foreign body aspiration is more common among young children, and plant products are problematic because they cannot be visualized on chest x-ray. For large objects that become lodged in the larynx or trachea, sudden respiratory distress with cyanosis, stridor, and aphonia can ensue. Treatment consists of the Heimlich maneuver with firm rapid pressure applied to the upper abdomen in an attempt to force the diaphragm upward, generating enough pressure to dislodge the particle. Smaller particles will become lodged in the more distal portions of the tracheal-bronchial tree. These patients present with cough, and chest x-ray demonstrates atelectasis or obstructive emphysema with cardiac shift and elevated diaphragm. Unilateral wheezing might be appreciated if there is partial obstruction. The primary intervention is therapeutic rigid or fiberoptic bronchoscopy performed to remove the obstructive element (61).

NOSOCOMIAL PNEUMONIA

Nosocomial pneumonia is defined as pneumonia occurring 48 hours after admission to the hospital and excluding any infection that is present or incubating at the time of admission (62). Ventilator-associated pneumonia is a specific form of nosocomial pneumonia that refers to the development of bacterial pneumonia in patients with acute respiratory failure who have been receiving mechanical ventilation for more than 48 to 72 hours (62). Patients in the surgical intensive care unit (ICU) have higher rates of nosocomial pneumonia than in the medical ICU (63). Data from the National Nosocomial Infection Surveillance system shows that the four types of ICUs with the highest incidence of ventilator-associated pneumonia all care for surgical patients: burn, neurosurgical, trauma, and surgical ICUs, in decreasing order of incidence (64).

Risk factors, etiology, and prevention

The leading risk factor for nosocomial pneumonia is mechanical ventilation. Endotracheal intubation increases the risk of nosocomial pneumonia between 6-fold and 21-fold (65,66). Other significant risk factors for nosocomial pneumonia identified on multivariate analysis include the following: age >70 years, chronic lung disease, depressed consciousness, large volume aspiration, thoracic surgery, frequent ventilator circuit changes, presence of intracranial pressure monitor, presence of nasogastric tube, H-2 blocker or antacid therapy, transport from the ICU to diagnostic or therapeutic procedures, previous exposure to antibiotics, reintubation, hospitalization during the fall or winter, and mechanical ventilation for ARDS (66). Increased gastric pH may play a significant role in elevating the risk for nosocomial pneumonia. A randomized controlled trial compared three strategies of stress ulcer prophylaxis (Ranitidine, antacid, and Sucralfate) (67). The incidence of ventilator-associated pneumonia was significantly lower with Sucralfate (5%) than with antacids (16%) and Ranitidine (21%). Supine positioning can predispose patients to microaspiration and development of nosocomial pneumonia. A randomized trial of positioning in 90 intubated patients was terminated early when interim analysis revealed a significantly lower incidence of nosocomial pneumonia in the semirecumbent versus supine patients (5% vs. 23%) (60).

Preventive measures for which there is now support in the literature include avoidance of acid-blocking medications in patients not at high risk of developing a stress ulcer or stress gastritis, selective decontamination of the GI tract, decontamination of the oropharynx, and patient positioning with the head-of-bed at ≥30 to 45 degrees (62,66). Two other potential preventive measures are subglottic drainage and silver-coated endotracheal tubes. These two items require special equipment and replacing of the existing endotracheal that hinders their widespread acceptance; however, the evidence for these two modalities to reduce the frequency of ventilator-associated pneumonia exists. Daily interruption of sedative infusions and evaluation of patient's mental status as well as physiologic suitability for extubation is associated with a reduction in complications associated with mechanical ventilation, one of which is ventilator-associated pneumonia (62,68). Avoidance of unnecessary use of chemical paralytic agents is also recommended as they suppress the patient's ability to cough and clear secretions (62). Use of haloperidol to manage agitation in mechanically ventilated patients has been shown to result in significantly lower hospital mortality when compared to patients who did not receive haloperidol (21% vs. 36%) (69).

Nosocomial pneumonias are caused by a wide-spectrum of bacterial pathogens. They are frequently polymicrobial in origin and are rarely due to viral or fungal microbes in an immunocompetent patient (62). Common microbial pathogens identified on culture include Gram-negative bacilli such as *Pseudomonas aeruginosa*, *Escherichia coli*, *Klebsiella pneumoniae*, *Enterobacter* species, and *Acinetobacter* species (62,70). Infections due to Gram-positive organisms include *Staphylococcus aureus* and in particular methicillin-resistant S. *aureus* (MRSA) as well as and *Streptococcus* species. Each separate ICU has its own intrinsic flora and might have other virulent bacterial organisms that are high in prevalence for nosocomial pneumonia. It is therefore of critical importance to know the offending pathogens in the ICU in which one practices when choosing empiric antibiotic therapy for patients with suspected nosocomial pneumonia.

Diagnosis and treatment

Accurate diagnosis of pneumonia remains elusive. Clinical signs and symptoms suggestive of pneumonia include new or progressive infiltrate on chest x-ray, fever, white blood cell (WBC) count greater than 10,000 per mm^3, purulent sputum, and increasing oxygen requirements (71). Presence of positive findings for three or more of these signs and symptoms should trigger the obtaining of a sputum sample for Gram stain and confirmatory bacterial culture followed by empiric administration of antibiotics. Tracheal aspirate, protected specimen brush, or bronchoalveolar lavage can be used to obtain sputum samples for culture. Quantitative bronchoscopic specimens are more accurate in confirming the diagnosis but have the disadvantage of being time-consuming and expensive. A prospective randomized clinical study evaluated whether an invasive test using protected brush specimens or bronchoalveolar lavage was superior to clinical criteria in 431 patients with suspicion of ventilator-associated pneumonia (72). Patients who underwent invasive testing had a significantly lower 14-day mortality rate (16% vs. 26%). This survival advantage remained at day 28 and was also associated with an increase in antibiotic-free days as well as a lower mean number of antibiotics administered. Operator variability and differences between ICUs make it difficult to universally replicate and apply these results. Also, the threshold for a positive quantitative bronchoalveolar lavage culture varies between 10^4 and 10^5 cfu/mL in published studies. However, there is a definite trend in the literature toward utilizing bronchoalveolar lavage to improve the accuracy of pneumonia diagnosis and to decrease pneumonia treatment costs through the reduction of false-positive cultures (71,73–75).

Because definitive diagnosis is difficult, many patients are incorrectly suspected of having pneumonia. This error can lead to overtreatment from empiric antibiotic therapy with all of its risks for superinfection and antibiotic toxicity. Conversely, it has been established that inadequate antibiotic therapy significantly affects mortality from infections and is an important independent predictor of hospital mortality with an OR of 4.3 (76,77). Inadequate initial antibiotic selection is associated with a significant increase in ventilator-associated pneumonia mortality (37% vs. 15%) compared to adequate initial therapy (78). The choice of proper antibiotic treatment for nosocomial pneumonia should be guided by recent antibiotic therapy, the indigenous bacterial flora of the hospital and ICU, the presence of underlying diseases, the type of patient (e.g., trauma, burn, general surgery), and the available culture data. The type of patient impacts heavily on the organism that is the most likely culprit for nosocomial pneumonia—for example, trauma patients: aspiration, oral flora type organisms; burn patients: *Staphylococcus aureus*; general surgery patients: virulent Gram-negative bacilli. In the absence of positive microbial culture data, patients with three of the five clinical signs and symptoms of pneumonia should be placed on empiric antibiotic therapy and a lower respiratory tract sample for culture promptly obtained.

Four questions are vital in choosing the appropriate empiric antibiotic therapy for each individual hospital, ICU, and patient (79):

- Is the patient at risk for methicillin-resistant *Staphylococcus aureus* (MRSA)?
- Is *Acinetobacter baumannii* a problem in the institution?
- Is the patient at risk for *Pseudomonas aeruginosa* infection?
- Is the patient at risk for multidrug resistance Gram-negative organisms?

At a bare minimum, the empiric antibiotic regimen chosen should have activity against *Enterobacter* species, *Klebsiella* species, *E. coli*, *Proteus* species, *Serratia marcescens*, *Haemophilus influenzae*, methicillin-sensitive *Staphylococcus aureus*, and *Streptococcus pneumoniae* (62). Patients who have aspirated, who have underlying medical conditions such as recent abdominal surgery, coma, head trauma, diabetes mellitus, renal failure, or COPD, are being treated with steroids or antibiotics, or who have a prolonged ICU stay might require additional coverage for anaerobes, MRSA, and Legionella. Coverage for *Pseudomonas aeruginosa* and multidrug resistant Gram-negative bacilli such as *Acinetobacter baumannii* should also be considered in critically ill patients receiving antibiotics prior to the onset of pneumonia and in institutions in which these bacteria are common pathogens.

If MRSA is a frequent nosocomial pathogen in the institution, Vancomycin or Linezolid will be a necessary first choice for empiric *Staphylococcal* coverage, but it should be discontinued if MRSA is not isolated on culture. The literature supports empiric monotherapy with third-generation cephalosporins with antipseudomonal activity, but caution is suggested as monotherapy has been associated with the development of resistant strains in documented cases of *Pseudomonas aeruginosa* infection (80). Combination therapy is associated with a survival benefit compared to monotherapy in patients with pseudomonal pneumonia and bacteremia (81).

A current empiric antibiotic strategy for nosocomial pneumonia employed in our surgical, trauma, and burn ICU follows:

- Intubated patients suspected of having nosocomial pneumonia are identified by having three of five clinical criteria for pneumonia (new or progressive infiltrate on chest x-ray, fever, elevated WBC count >10,000/mm^3, purulent sputum, and increasing oxygen requirements).
- Perform quantitative bronchoalveolar lavage.

- Initiate empiric antibiotic therapy with one of the following antibiotic combinations based on patients medical comorbidities:
  - If >4 days on the mechanical ventilator or patient has been hospitalized, start Vancomycin, Piperacillin/Tazobactam, and Tobramycin. If aminoglycoside contraindicated replace with Levofloxacin.
  - If <4 days on the mechanical ventilator, consider monotherapy for aspiration-type organisms with Ceftriaxone, Ampicillin/Sulbactam, or Piperacillin/Tazobactam.
- If the quantitative bronchoalveolar lavage culture results are $>10^4$ cfu/mL, continue antibiotics and tailor coverage based on organism and sensitivities.
- If the quantitative bronchoalveolar lavage culture results are $<10^4$ cfu/mL, discontinue antibiotic therapy.

The American Thoracic Society (ATS)/Infectious Diseases Society of America guidelines for the management of ventilator-associated or hospital-acquired pneumonia are also an excellent resource for guidance of empiric antibiotic therapy and can be accessed through the ATS web site at www.thoracic.org/sections/publications/statements/index.html.

Previously, experts have recommended long courses (14 to 21 days) of antibiotic treatment for nosocomial pneumonia. Recent prospective randomized studies on this subject have begun to challenge this dogma. In a large European study of 401 patients diagnosed with ventilator-associated pneumonia by quantitative bronchoalveolar lavage culture, 197 patients were randomly assigned to receive 8 days of antibiotic therapy, and 204 to receive 15 days of antibiotic treatment (82). Primary outcome measures were mortality, recurrence of pneumonia, and antibiotic-free days. Patients treated for 8 days had no excess mortality (18.8% vs. 17.2%). It has been our practice to treat chromosomally mediated resistance-prone bacteria such as *Acinetobacter* species, *Pseudomonas aeruginosa*, *Enterobacter* species, *Serratia* species, and *Citrobacter* species for a minimum of 10 days. *Pseudomonas aeruginosa*, *Enterobacter* species, and *Acinetobacter* species are known to be highly resistant and therefore commonly receive double coverage with two antibiotics. However, there is not conclusive evidence to support combination therapy for nosocomial pneumonia due to these Gram-negative pathogens. A large randomized clinical trial suggests that monotherapy of ventilator-associated pneumonia is as effective as combination therapy with there being no difference in 28-day mortality between groups (83). For pneumonia as a result of resistant *Staphylococcus aureus*, *Pseudomonas aeruginosa*, or *Acinetobacter* species repeat quantitative bronchoalveolar lavage culture is performed at 6 days and if lavage culture results are $>10^4$ cfu/mL, antibiotics are continued to complete a full 15 day course of treatment. Patients suspected of having anaerobic bacterial pneumonia should also be placed on Clindamycin or Flagyl empirically. The selection of empiric antibiotic therapy must take into account patient data and should be institution-specific.

ACUTE RESPIRATORY DISTRESS SYNDROME

ARDS refers to patients with acute and progressive respiratory disease of a noncardiac nature, in association with diffuse, bilateral pulmonary infiltrates demonstrated on chest x-rays, and with hypoxemia (84). ALI and its more severe form, known as ARDS, are clinical syndromes pathologically characterized by acute and persistent pulmonary inflammation with increased vascular permeability. In 1994, the American-European Consensus Conference on ARDS established written clinical definitions of ALI and ARDS, which are listed in Table 19.6 (85). In recent years, significant advances in understanding of the pathophysiology of ARDS and lung injury have been made, leading to prospective randomized clinical trials and attempts to improve therapy on the basis of scientific knowledge. Despite these recent advances, the mortality from severe ARDS remains high—between 40% and 50% in both adults and children (86,87).

The pathophysiology of ARDS is complex but can be summarized as massive capillary leak that is the result of an excessive inflammatory response in the host's lung tissue. ARDS has a rapid onset over 4 to 48 hours and can persist for days to weeks. ARDS progresses through four distinct clinical phases. Phase one is the initial prodrome that is characterized by dyspnea, tachypnea, and a respiratory alkalosis with a normal PaO_2. This phase is driven by inflammatory mediators and activation of inflammatory cells such as alveolar macrophages. Phase two is marked by the onset of lung injury in the first 24 hours. This results in the clinical findings of hypoxemia and radiographic evidence of scattered pulmonary infiltrates bilaterally. During this time, increased pulmonary capillary permeability leads to interstitial edema, neutrophil margination, and an interstitial inflammatory response. This process ultimately causes a severe loss of alveolar units in the patient. The third phase results in progressive lung injury. Injury is evidenced by increased shunt fraction and severe hypoxemia. The pulmonary parenchyma undergoes microvascular thrombosis, redistribution of pulmonary blood flow, and increasing

Table 19.6 Definition of acute lung injury and acute respiratory distress syndrome (ARDS) (75)

Acute lung injury
Acute onset of pulmonary failure
PaO_2/FiO_2 Ratio <300 mm Hg[a]
Bilateral infiltrates on chest x-ray
Pulmonary capillary wedge pressure <18 mm Hg
Acute respiratory distress syndrome
All of criteria for acute lung injury
PaO_2/FiO_2 Ratio <200 mm Hg[a]

[a]Regardless of the level of positive end-expiratory pressure (PEEP).
Adapted from Bernard GR, Artigas A, Brigham KL, et al. The consensus committee report of the American-European consensus conference on ARDS: definitions, mechanisms, relevant outcomes and clinical trial coordination. *Intensive Care Med* 1994;20:225–232, with permission.

edema of the alveolar capillary membranes. During the fourth and final phase, the inflammatory response switches from acute to chronic and is associated with ongoing inflammation and pulmonary fibrosis. Macrophages and progressive interstitial fibrosis that can become irreversible dominates the inflammatory response (88,89).

Basic scientific advances have improved our understanding of the pathophysiology of ARDS, and therapeutic options are emerging to treat the excessive inflammatory response of early ARDS and the irreversible fibroproliferative response of late ARDS (88). Identification of risk factors for ARDS has allowed early implementation of alternative ventilator strategies to reduce iatrogenic lung injury and exacerbation of pulmonary failure in surgical patients at increased risk. Treatment of ARDS is focused on eliminating the inciting source, utilizing protective ventilator strategies to minimize ventilator-induced lung injury, avoidance of additional organ failure, and provision of adequate nutrition. Failing all other therapies, extracorporeal life support (ECLS) may be employed in rare circumstances for severe ARDS patients.

The diagnosis of ARDS is based on findings of acute onset of severe hypoxemia (PaO_2 <200 mm Hg) and bilateral infiltrates on chest x-ray (Fig. 19.1) in the absence of pulmonary edema. In some clinical situations, it might

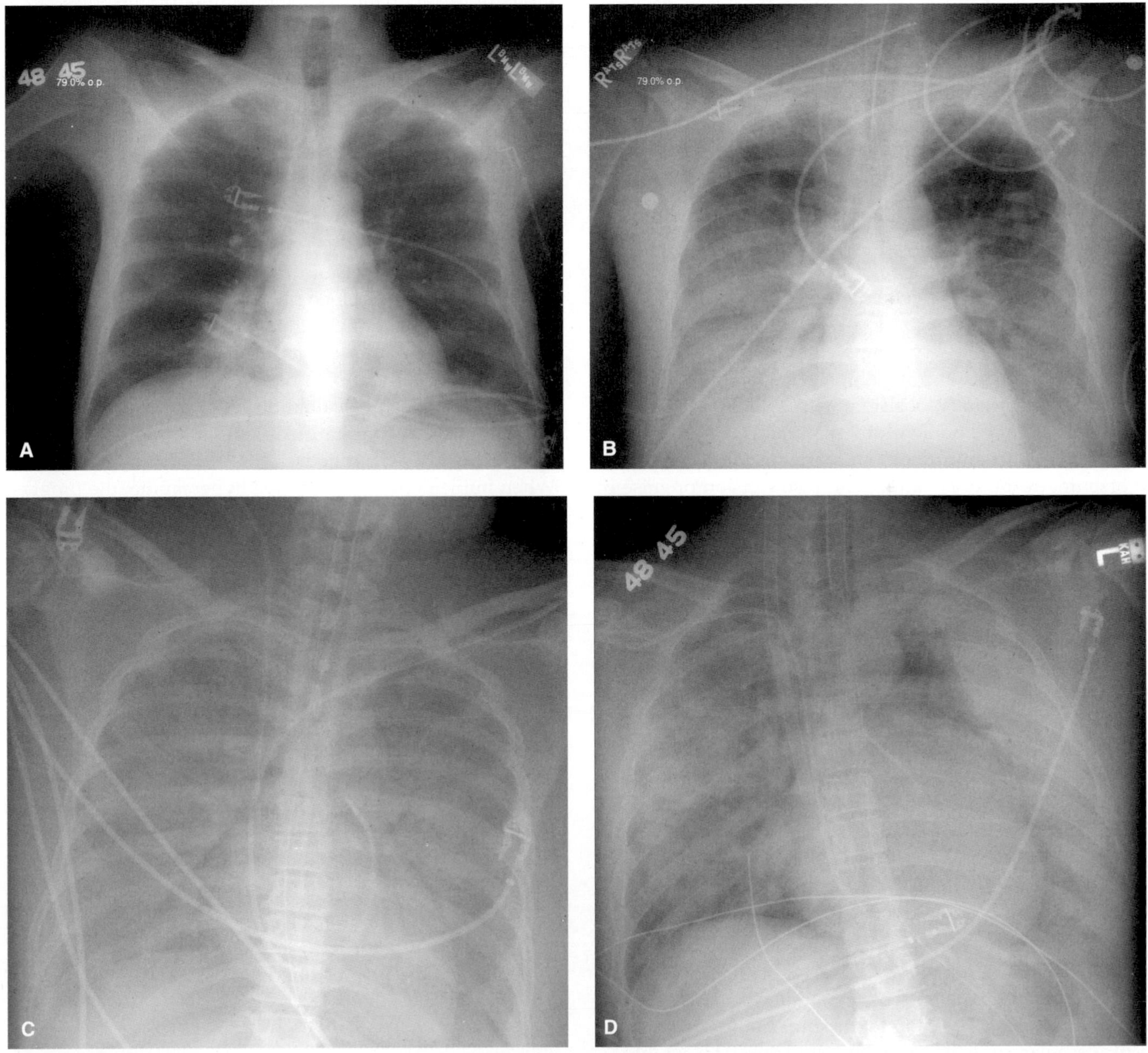

FIGURE 19.1. Common radiologic features of acute respiratory distress syndrome (ARDS). All chest x-rays are portable anteroposterior projection. **A:** 40-year-old man with diabetic ketoacidosis and right lower lobe infiltrate from streptococcal pneumonia. **B:** Same man 1 day later with severe bilateral blossoming of pulmonary infiltrates. **C:** 49-year-old woman with staphylococcal sepsis and bilateral ground glass pulmonary infiltrates. Note the presence of air bronchograms. **D:** 36-year-old man with blastomycosis pneumonia and dense patchy infiltrates bilaterally. This patient required extracorporeal life support for 16 days and was discharged to rehabilitation on hospital day 32.

become necessary to place a Swan-Ganz catheter into the pulmonary artery to verify that the pulmonary capillary wedge pressure (PCWP) is <18 mm Hg in order to rule out pulmonary edema as the etiology of acute respiratory failure. The presence of a PCWP <18 mm Hg favors ALI or ARDS over hemodynamic pulmonary edema. However, an elevated PCWP does not exclude ARDS. If pulmonary infiltrates on chest x-ray and hypoxemia do not improve within 24 to 48 hours following normalization of PCWP, ALI or ARDS has most likely occurred simultaneously with hemodynamic pulmonary edema (90).

Low tidal volume ventilation and permissive hypercapnia

Management of mechanical ventilation for patients with ARDS involves understanding how to minimize and prevent ventilator-induced lung injury. Webb and Tierney (91) first demonstrated ventilator-induced lung injury in animals in 1974, when they revealed the detrimental effects of ventilation at a peak inspiratory pressure of 45 cm H_2O in rats. Subsequently, investigators have documented an increase in pulmonary edema and histopathology in rats ventilated at a peak inspiratory pressure of 45 cm H_2O for only 5 to 20 minutes (92). Healthy sheep, when mechanically ventilated at a peak inspiratory pressure as low as 30 to 40 cm H_2O, showed an increase in wet-to-dry lung weight, deterioration in gas exchange, an increase in the surface tension of lung lavage fluid, and lung lesions consistent with ARDS (93).

The use of high tidal volumes (V_T) and/or high ventilator pressures in an attempt to ventilate the patient with worsening respiratory failure can result in compromise of cardiopulmonary function and the development of ventilator induced lung injury. There is evidence that alveolar stretch induced by large inspired V_Ts plays a significant role in the development of ventilator-induced lung injury through the incitement of an exaggerated alveolar inflammatory response which is associated with systemic inflammation as well (94). In ARDS, large proportions of the lung alveoli become consolidated and are not available for gas exchange. The resulting available lung units are small in number and give the patient a functional lung that is analogous to a "baby lung" in size. Attempting to force adult magnitude V_T breaths into this "baby lung" can result in overdistention of the remaining open alveoli and high distending pressures. This alveolar overinflation can exacerbate existing lung injury leading to microvascular injury and worsening pulmonary edema (95).

Using a low-V_T (6 mL/kg) approach to mechanical ventilation in animals with *Pseudomonas aeruginosa* induced ALI resulted in enhanced oxygenation, increased arterial blood pH, increased blood pressure, and a decrease in extravascular lung water when compared to a high-V_T group (15 mL/kg) (96). The ARDS Network trial conclusively demonstrated the clinical value of a low-V_T versus high-V_T approach in the mechanical ventilatory support of patients with severe respiratory failure (86). This trial was a multicenter, randomized, controlled study that compared a V_T of 6 mL/kg ideal body weight (and plateau pressure <30 cm H_2O) with a V_T of 12 mL/kg ideal body weight (and plateau pressure <50 cm H_2O). The trial showed a significantly lower mortality, 31% versus 40%, in the low-V_T group. The number of ventilator-free days in the first 28 days was significantly higher in the group treated with lower V_Ts (12 vs. 10) as was the number of days without failure of nonpulmonary organs or systems (15 vs. 12). In patients with ALI and ARDS, high levels of plasma interleukin-6 and -8 are associated with increased morbidity and mortality. Lower V_T ventilation in the ARDS Network prospective randomized trial was also associated with a more rapid attenuation of the inflammatory response (97).

Mechanical ventilatory strategies to reduce V_Ts and alveolar overdistension can result in inadequate lung ventilation. Permissive hypercapnia is a consequence of a ventilator strategy that accepts deliberate hypoventilation in an effort to reduce pulmonary overdistention and high transalveolar pressures within the compliant noncollapsed lung in patients with ARDS. This technique induces the side effect of hypercarbia and respiratory acidosis which are managed medically. The V_T is gradually reduced to allow a progressive rise in the $Paco_2$ to levels as high as 120 mm Hg while the blood pH is maintained above 7.1 to 7.2 by the intravenous administration of buffer solutions (98).

Mortality in adults was reduced to 26% compared to the expected mortality of 53% based on an Acute Physiology and Chronic Health Evaluation (APACHE) II score when low-volume, pressure-limited ventilation with permissive hypercapnia was applied to patients with ARDS (99). When implementing permissive hypercapnia, the progressive rise in $Paco_2$ should not exceed 10 mm Hg/hour and only rarely should the maximum level exceed 80 to 100 mm Hg. Patients might require heavy sedation and even chemical paralysis to overcome the hypercapnic respiratory drive and avoid discomfort. Potential deleterious effects of hypercapnia include elevation in intracranial pressure in patients with brain injury, mild hypertension, increased cardiac output, and increased pulmonary vascular resistance (88). A secondary analysis of the ARDS Network low V_T multicenter trial (n = 861) documented that hypercapnic acidosis was associated with a reduced 28-day mortality (adjusted odds ratio 0.14, 95% CI 0.03–0.70) in the 12 mL/kg predicted body weight V_T group after controlling for comorbidities and severity of lung injury, but no difference was identified in the 6 mL/kg V_T group (100). These results are consistent with a protective effect of hypercapnic acidosis against ventilator-induced lung injury that was not found when the further ongoing injury was reduced by 6 mL/kg predicted body weight V_Ts.

Pressure control and inverse ratio ventilation

Conventional ventilation involves volume cycling with V_Ts in the 10 to 15 mL/kg range. An alternative mode of ventilation used in ARDS patients is pressure control ventilation. In this mode the target peak and plateau airway pressure is kept <30 to 35 cm H_2O by feedback servo regulation of the ventilator flow rate. The pressure versus time curve for a breath in pressure control ventilation resembles a square wave in which a uniform pressure is generated throughout the inspiratory cycle. This results in noticeably smaller V_Ts (4 to 8 mL/kg) with each breath and possible hypercapnia, especially in stiff noncompliant lungs. The V_T generated will vary considerably with changes in compliance, and rapid decreases in compliance can lead to inadequate ventilation. Use of pressure control ventilation allows tight control of airway pressures, minimization of barotrauma, and enhanced recruitment of collapsed alveoli throughout the inspiratory cycle.

The normal inspiratory to expiratory ratio is 1:3 or 1:4. By lengthening the time of the inspiratory phase, one increases the time available for gas exchange and potentially inflates collapsed alveoli. In some instances, it is necessary to invert this ratio so that more time is spent during inspiration than expiration—so-called inverse ratio ventilation. Inverse ratio ventilation allows for less time for recruited alveoli to collapse during expiration. As long as there is adequate time for CO_2 clearance, mean airway pressure is monitored, and the patient is appropriately sedated to overcome the unnatural breathing pattern provided by this mode of ventilation, it can be a safe and effective way of increasing oxygenation and recruiting FRC in severe respiratory failure. Pressure control ventilation and pressure control-inverse ratio ventilation are standard techniques used in neonatal mechanical ventilation.

Open lung approach

One of the more common means of recruiting collapsed alveoli and increasing FRC is to use PEEP. By not allowing all the pressure in the lung to escape during expiration, alveoli that are unstable and prone to collapse cannot do so. This technique can be thought of as holding the lung partially open so that the next breath is not starting from total collapse in a noncompliant lung. The optimal level of PEEP to use in ARDS patients is difficult to determine, but evidence is emerging to suggest that optimal recruitment and maintenance of lung volume occurs when PEEP is set at a value that matches or exceeds the lower inflection point (P_{flex}) on the inspiratory static pressure-volume curve (101). A single breath compliance curve with V_T plotted against static airway pressure will demonstrate two inflection points. The lower one represents the theoretical critical opening pressure of most alveoli available for recruitment, and the upper point represents the loss of elastic properties of the lung secondary to overdistension (88).

The combination of PEEP to recruit FRC and pressure control ventilation to minimize barotrauma has been termed the "open lung" approach (102,103). This strategy involves maintaining the PEEP above the lower inflection point of the pressure-volume curve, keeping the V_T ≤6 mL/kg, avoiding high plateau airway pressures >30 to 35 cm H_2O, utilizing permissive hypercapnia, and the stepwise use of pressure-limited modes of ventilation (102). A study of this strategy showed an improved survival at 28 days (62% vs. 29%), a higher rate of weaning from mechanical ventilation, and a lower rate of barotrauma in the patient group that received the protective lung strategy or "open lung" approach compared to controls (103). There was, however, no difference in the in-hospital mortality for these patients. The low 28-day survival in the control group has raised questions about this trial's validity. In the National Institutes of Health (NIH) ARDS Network trial of low V_Ts (6 mL/kg) compared to traditional V_Ts (12 mL/kg) for mechanical ventilation in ARDS, mortality was significantly lower in the group treated with lower V_Ts than in the group with traditional V_Ts (31% vs. 40%) (86). The mean plateau pressures were 25 ± 6 and 33 ± 8 cm H_2O, respectively. A reduction of 25% in the mortality of these patients with lower V_Ts offers strong evidence for a protective lung strategy approach to mechanical ventilation in patients with ARDS.

Based on the ARDS Network trials and others detailing the "open lung" approach, most clinicians today avoid high plateau pressures, use low-V_Ts, and apply appropriate levels of PEEP to encourage lung recruitment and avoid cyclical atelectasis. However, the extent to which V_Ts and inspiratory airway pressures should be reduced to optimize clinical outcomes is a controversial topic. A recent study examined all patients with plateau pressures in the ARDS Network lower V_T trial (104). Figure 19.2 demonstrates the relationship of mortality versus P_{plat} for all patients and shows decreasing mortality as Day 1 P_{plat} declines from high to low levels. It does not reveal a safe P_{plat} threshold within the range of Day 1 P_{plat} levels measured in patients with ALI/ARDS. Bivariate analysis also demonstrated that lower P_{plat} quartiles were associated with reduced mortality when compared with higher P_{plat} quartiles.

In the French led "Express trial," use of an approach to set PEEP at a level to reach a plateau pressure of 28 to 30 cm H_2O (increased recruitment strategy) did not reduce mortality, but did improve lung function, reduced the duration of mechanical ventilation, and the duration of organ failure when compared to patients assigned to a moderate PEEP strategy (5–9 cm H_2O, minimal distension strategy) (105). An "open lung" approach that compared target V_Ts of 6 mL/kg, plateau pressure ≤30 cm H_2O, and conventional levels of PEEP with an experimental strategy of target V_Ts of 6 mL/kg, plateau pressure ≤40 cm H_2O, recruitment maneuvers, and higher levels of PEEP showed no difference in mortality rate (36% vs. 40%) (106). This open lung approach did result in apparent improvements within the secondary endpoints of hypoxemia and use of rescue therapies. In conclusion, one should use a volume or pressure support ventilator mode that keeps the V_T near 6 mL/kg, limits the plateau pressure to as low a level as possible to maintain ventilation, and makes appropriate use of PEEP to recruit FRC.

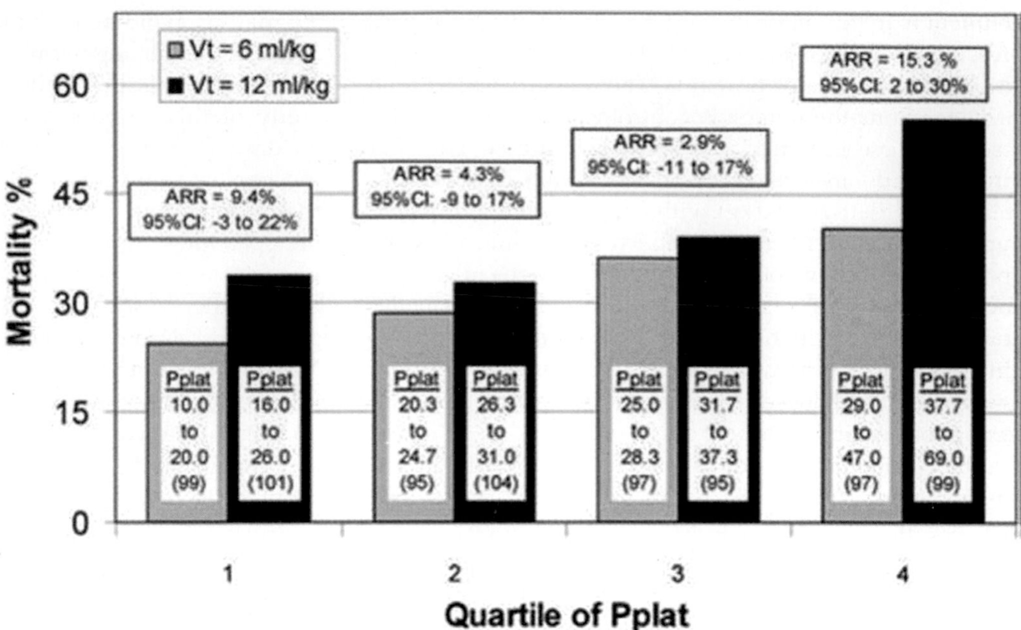

FIGURE 19.2. Mortality difference by quartile of Day 1 P_{plat}. The range of P_{plat} levels in cm H_2O and the number of patients (n) is detailed in each bar of the graph. ARR, absolute risk reduction; CI, confidence interval. (From Hager DN, Krishnan JA, Hayden DL, et al. Tidal volume reduction in patients with acute lung injury when plateau pressures are not high. *Am J Respir Crit Care Med* 2005;172:1241–1245, with permission.)

Airway pressure release ventilation

Airway pressure release ventilation (APRV) is a pressure limited, time-cycled mode of mechanical ventilation that allows a patient unrestricted spontaneous breathing during the application of continuous positive airway pressure (P-High, P_H) (Fig. 19.3). It is an alternative approach to open-lung ventilation. Although recruitment maneuvers may be effective in improving gas exchange and compliance, these effects may not be sustained and may require repeated maneuvers. APRV may be viewed as a nearly continuous recruitment maneuver with P_H providing 80% to 95% of the cycle time creating a stabilized "open lung" while facilitating spontaneous breathing. The ventilator

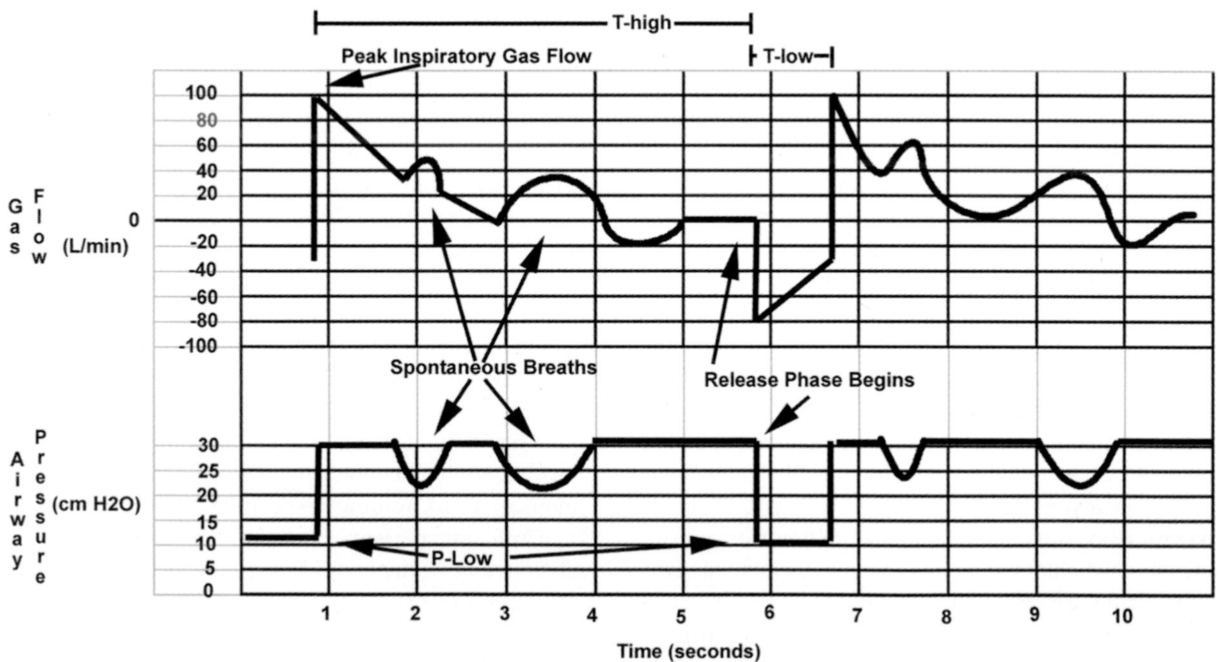

FIGURE 19.3. Example of gas flow and airway pressure for airway pressure release ventilation or BiLevel ventilation mode. This mode maintains a high airway pressure (P_{high}) with intermittent release periods to a low pressure analogous to positive end-expiratory pressure (P_{low}). Patients who are not chemically paralyzed can take spontaneous breaths during the T_{high} phase that allow additional pressure support. The clinician sets the high and low pressure settings, number of breaths, and the release time (T_{low}). This mode provides increased inspiratory time to allow for gas exchange and alveolar recruitment, avoidance of alveolar derecruitment, and the ability to improve hemodynamics by allowing the patient to breathe spontaneously.

maintains a high-pressure setting (P_H) for the bulk of the respiratory cycle which is followed by a periodic release to a low-pressure setting (P_L) analogous to PEEP. Patients (who are not receiving neuromuscular blockade) can spontaneously breathe on top of this form of continuous positive airway pressure, which is periodically lowered to allow ventilation and CO_2 clearance. The spontaneous breathing allowed during APRV can decrease intrathoracic pressure as inspiration by the patient results in periodic cycles of negative pressure from diaphragm and chest wall excursion. APRV is no different than pressure-controlled inverse ratio mechanical ventilation in patients receiving neuromuscular blockade. To date, an adequately designed and powered study to demonstrate a reduction in mortality or ventilator days with APRV compared with optimal lung protective conventional ventilation has not yet been performed.

Prone positioning

Patient positioning can have a sometimes dramatic effect on oxygenation and ventilation in severe ARDS. Changing patient position to prone or steep lateral decubitus positions can improve the distribution of perfusion to ventilated lung regions leading to improvement in oxygenation (107,108). Prone positioning in ARDS patients can improve oxygenation in 60% to 70% of patients (109). A multicenter randomized trial of conventional treatment versus placing patients in a prone position for 6 or more hours daily for 10 days was conducted on patients with ALI or ARDS (109). The mortality rate did not differ for the prone versus conventional positioning group at any point during the study, with up to 6 months follow-up. The mean increase in the PaO_2 to FIO_2 ratio was greater in the prone than supine group (63 ± 67 vs. 45 ± 68). There was no difference between the two groups in the incidence of complications related to positioning. The mean PaO_2 of 85 to 88 mm Hg and mean PaO_2/FIO_2 ratio of 125 to 129 are still quite high for patients with severe ARDS, and therefore these patients might not have been likely to benefit considerably by the prone intervention in terms of mortality.

Prone positioning is labor-intensive and complicated. The main risks are extubation and pressure sores. However, a trained and dedicated nursing staff that is aware of potential benefits in critically ill patients with severe pulmonary failure can safely perform the technique. Prone positioning is a crucial rescue tool for keeping patients with severe respiratory failure off ECLS and for lung recruitment in patients on ECLS. Prone positioning is not used until PaO_2 and PaO_2/FIO_2 ratio are significantly below 100. The technique involves alternating prone with supine positioning every 6 hours using appropriate cushioning of the dependent portions of the body. Patients will often experience an initial worsening in respiratory status with each change in position, but this passes quickly in the first 15 to 30 minutes to eventual improvement in oxygenation and ventilation, with 70% of the overall improvement occurring in the first hour of pronation (109). Prone positioning, although not associated with a significant survival advantage, may serve a role as rescue therapy for patients with ARDS and refractory life-threatening hypoxemia.

Corticosteroids

Prior studies have suggested a benefit for the use of corticosteroids in refractory disease, or the late, fibroproliferative stage of ARDS (88). The mechanism of action for the steroid effect on the fibroproliferative response seems to involve modulation of macrophage and fibroblast activity that can lead to irreversible pulmonary fibrosis. In a randomized clinical trial of steroid administration in late ARDS, there were 24 patients enrolled in the study; 16 were treated with methylprednisolone and eight were randomized to placebo (110). Four of the eight control patients crossed over to the steroid arm for failure to improve. The dose administered was 2 mg/kg/day in divided doses, starting 7 days after the diagnosis of ARDS and continuing for 32 days total. There were significant reductions in lung injury and organ failure scores and an improvement in the PaO_2/FIO_2 ratio. Hospital associated mortality was 12% for the treatment group and 62% for the control group; however, only four patients remained in the placebo group because of patient crossover during the study.

Within the multicenter trial from the ARDS Clinical Trials Network, a sub-trial randomized patients with ARDS of at least 7 days duration to receive either methylprednisolone or placebo in a double-blind manner (111). Methylprednisolone therapy was associated with increased ventilator-free and shock-free days, improved oxygenation, and improved pulmonary compliance during the first 28 days. However, compared with placebo, methylprednisolone was associated with no difference in overall mortality and a significant increase in 60- and 180-day mortality rates for patients enrolled at least 14 days after the onset of ARDS. These results do not support the routine use of methylprednisolone for persistent ARDS.

Extracorporeal life support

In patients who have acute and severe respiratory failure who are failing all advanced modes of mechanical ventilation the use of ECLS is an option. The technique of ECLS for patients with severe ARDS involves a veno-venous or veno-arterial life support circuit with an oxygenator to temporarily take over the function of the lung to provide oxygenation and ventilation. While on ECLS, mechanical ventilator settings are adjusted to minimize ventilator-induced lung injury and to maximize the recruitment of FRC.

Use of ECLS for severe ARDS in neonates is of proven benefit (112,113), but for adult patients the technique remains controversial. Although ECLS has failed to demonstrate a conclusive survival advantage for adults in previous prospective randomized clinical trials, considerable

Table 19.7 Outcome in acute respiratory distress syndrome (ARDS) with extracorporeal life support (ECLS) in adults

		Severe ARDS Survival	
Author	**Year**	**Conventional Rx (%)**	**ECLS Rx (%)**
Zapol	1979	8	10
Gattinoni	1986	—	49
Brunet	1993	—	50
Morris	1994	42	33
Macha	1996	—	39
Kolla	1997	—	54
Peek	1997	—	66
Lewandowski	1997	—	55
Ullrich	1999	—	62
Hemmila	2004	—	52
ELSO Registry	2004	—	53

Modified from Bartlett RH. Extracorporeal life support in the management of severe respiratory failure. *Clin Chest Med* 2000;21:555–561, with permission.

data support its ability to salvage severe ARDS patients failing all other means of respiratory support (Table 19.7). The recently concluded CESAR trial (Conventional ventilation or ECMO for severe adult respiratory failure) demonstrated a survival/absence of severe disability benefit at 6 months in favor of the ECLS group. Data published in *Lancet* from the adult CESAR trial showed survival without disability at 6 months was 47% in the conventional mechanical ventilation group and 63% in the ECLS group (Odds Ratio 0.69, 95% CI 0.05–0.97, $p = 0.03$) (114).

The University of Michigan experience with ECLS has yielded survival to hospital discharge rates of 85% in neonates, 74% in children, and 52% in adults with severe ARDS (115). The treatment program for adults involves an algorithm that aims to normalize body physiology, aggressively recruit FRC, and minimize barotrauma (Table 19.8). This algorithm used in 141 patients with respiratory failure referred for consideration of ECLS yielded a survival rate of 62% in patients with severe ARDS (median initial PaO_2/FIO_2 ratio of 66) (116). Referral to an ECLS center should occur early if there is a suspected need for this technology. This will allow safe transport of the patient and avoidance of the "crash on" with all of its inherent complications.

The primary circumstance for use of ECLS in patients with severe respiratory failure is when, after optimal ventilator and medical management, the risk of dying from ARDS is considered to be >80% (Table 19.9). This requirement translates to an alveoli-arterial oxygen gradient >600 mm Hg or a PaO_2/FIO_2 ratio of <70 on 100% oxygen. Patients should also have a transpulmonary shunt fraction >30% despite maximal conventional therapy. Adult patients are typically cannulated percutaneously with large 21 to 23 Fr catheters for drainage and infusion

Table 19.8 Algorithm for treatment of severe acute respiratory distress syndrome (ARDS)

Mechanical ventilator
- Pressure control mode
- Limit PIP to 30–35 cm H_2O
- Best PEEP
- Titrate FIO_2 for SaO_2 >90 and SvO_2 >70
- Inverse I:E ratio

Monitors
- Continuous cardiac output Swan-Ganz catheter
- Arterial line

Treatments
- Prone positioning
- Transfuse to Hct 35–40
- Diuresis to dry weight (Furosemide drip or CVVH)
- Chemical sedation and paralysis
- Full nutrition

of blood. Anticoagulation is necessary and is titrated as measured by whole blood activated clotting time. ECLS allows for a decreasing of mechanical ventilator settings to nondamaging "rest" levels while maintaining FRC recruitment measures. Once native lung function has improved, the patient is trialed off of ECLS at moderate ventilator settings that allow for potential increases in therapy—for example, FIO_2 0.5 to 0.6. If the trial off of ECLS is successful, the cannulas are removed and recovery continues.

In a series of 255 adult patients who were placed on ECLS for severe ARDS refractory to all other treatment, 67% were weaned off ECLS and 52% survived to hospital discharge (117). Multivariate analysis identified the following pre-ECLS variables as significant independent predictors of survival: (a) age, (b) gender, (c) arterial blood pH ≤7.10, (d) PaO_2/FIO_2 ratio, and (e) days of mechanical ventilation. None of the patients who survived required permanent mechanical ventilation or supplemental oxygen therapy. Patients who can be successfully decannulated from ECLS have a 77% chance of being discharged from the hospital alive and going on to complete recovery.

Table 19.9 Adult extracorporeal life support (ECLS) criteria

Indications	**Contraindications**

• Duration of ventilation
  • <5–7 days, 7–10 days only if ventilated with high pressures for <7 days
• Compliance
  • <0.5 mL/cm H_2O/kg
• Oxygenation
  • PaO_2/FiO_2 <100
  • Shunt >30%
	• Prolonged conventional mechanical ventilation
	• Poor neurologic status
	• Incurable disease
	• Age >70 years
	• Pulmonary artery pressures >2/3 systemic blood pressure
	• Unresolved surgical issues

REFERENCES

1. Kroenke K, Lawrence VA, Theroux JF, et al. Operative risk in patients with severe obstructive pulmonary disease. *Arch Intern Med* 1992;152: 967–971.
2. Pedersen T, Eliasen K, Henriksen E. A prospective study of risk factors and cardiopulmonary complications associated with anaesthesia and surgery: risk indicators of cardiopulmonary morbidity. *Acta Anaesthesiol Scand* 1990;34:144–155.
3. Gracey DR, Divertie MB, Didier EP. Preoperative pulmonary preparation of patients with chronic obstructive pulmonary disease: a prospective study. *Chest* 1979;76:123–129.
4. Smetana GW. Preoperative pulmonary evaluation. *N Engl J Med* 1999; 340:937–944.
5. Johnson RG, Arozullah AM, Neumayer L, et al. Multivariable predictors of postoperative respiratory failure after general and vascular surgery: results from the patient safety in surgery study. *J Am Coll Surg* 2007;204:1188–1198.
6. Smetana GW. Evaluation of preoperative pulmonary risk. UpToDate 17.1. Available at: http://www.utdol.com. Accessed May 20, 2009.
7. Wightman JA. A prospective survey of the incidence of postoperative pulmonary complications. *Br J Surg* 1968;55:85–91.
8. Morton HJV. Tobacco smoking and pulmonary complications after surgery. *Lancet* 1944;1:368–370.
9. Brooks-Brunn JA. Predictors of postoperative pulmonary complications following abdominal surgery. *Chest* 1997;111:564–571.
10. Warner MA, Offord KP, Warner ME, et al. Role of preoperative cessation of smoking and other factors in postoperative pulmonary complications: a blinded prospective study of coronary artery bypass patients. *Mayo Clin Proc* 1989;64:609–616.
11. Goldman L, Caldera DL, Nussbaum SR, et al. Multifactorial index of cardiac risk in noncardiac surgical procedures. *N Engl J Med* 1977; 297:845–850.
12. Lawrence VA, Dhanda R, Hilsenbeck SG, et al. Risk of pulmonary complications after elective abdominal surgery. *Chest* 1996;110: 744–750.
13. Gerson MC, Hurst JM, Hertzberg VS, et al. Prediction of cardiac and pulmonary complications related to elective abdominal and noncardiac thoracic surgery in geriatric patients. *Am J Med* 1990;88:101–107.
14. Wong D, Weber EC, Schell MJ, et al. Factors associated with postoperative pulmonary complications in patients with severe chronic obstructive pulmonary disease. *Anesth Analg* 1995;80:276–284.
15. Warner DO, Warner MA, Barnes RD, et al. Perioperative respiratory complications in patients with asthma. *Anesthesiology* 1996;85:460–467.
16. Arozullah AM, Daley J, Henderson WG, et al. Multifactorial risk index for predicting postoperative respiratory failure in men after major noncardiac surgery. *Ann Surg* 2000;232:242–253.
17. Kroenke K, Lawrence VA, Theroux JF, et al. Postoperative complications after thoracic and major abdominal surgery in patients with and without obstructive lung disease. *Chest* 1993;104:1445–1451.
18. Milledge JS, Nunn JF. Criteria of fitness for anaesthesia in patients with chronic obstructive lung disease. *Br Med J* 1975;3:670–673.
19. Thomas DR, Ritchie CS. Preoperative assessment of older adults. *J Am Geriatr Soc* 1995;43:811–821.
20. Pasulka PS, Bistian BR, Benotti PN, et al. The risks of surgery in obese patients. *Ann Intern Med* 1986;104:540–546.
21. Hall JC, Tarala MD, Hall JL, et al. A multivariate analysis of the risk of pulmonary complications after laparotomy. *Chest* 1991;99:923–927.
22. Morino M, Toppino M, Forestieri P, et al. Mortality after bariatric surgery: analysis of 13871 morbidly obese patients from a national registry. *Ann Surg* 2007;246:1002–1009.
23. Merkow RP, Bilimoria KY, McCarter MD, et al. Effect of body mass index on short-term outcomes after colectomy for cancer. *J Am Coll Surg* 2009;208:53–61.
24. Qaseem A, Snow V, Fitterman N, et al. Risk assessment for and strategies to reduce perioperative pulmonary complications for patients undergoing noncardiothoracic surgery: a guideline from the American College of Physicians. *Ann Intern Med* 2006;144:575–580.
25. Bartlett RH, Rich PB. Pulmonary insufficiency. In: Wilmore DW, Cheung LY, Harken AH, et al, eds. *ACS Surgery: principles and practice*, 2003 ed. New York, NY: WebMD Inc; 2003:1047–1057.
26. Zibrak JD. Preoperative pulmonary function testing. American College of Physicians. *Ann Intern Med* 1990;112:793–794.
27. Newsome HH Jr. Complications of thyroid surgery. In: Greenfield LG, ed. *Complications in surgery and trauma*, 2nd ed. Philadelphia, PA: J.B. Lippincott Company; 1990:649–659.
28. Couser RJ, Ferrara TB, Falde B, et al. Effectiveness of dexamethasone in preventing extubation failure in preterm infants at increased risk for airway edema. *J Pediatr* 1992;121:591–596.
29. Anene O, Meert KL, Uy H, et al. Dexamethasone for the prevention of postextubation airway obstruction: a prospective, randomized, double-blind, placebo-controlled trial. *Crit Care Med* 1996;24:1666–1669.
30. Pryor JP, Schwab CW, Peitzman AB. Thoracic injury. In: Peitzman AB, Rhodes M, Schwab CW, et al, eds. *The trauma manual*, 2nd ed. Philadelphia: Lippincott Williams & Wilkins; 2002:203–223.
31. Airway management and smoke inhalation injury. In: *Advanced burn life support course: provider's manual*. 2003:25–31.
32. Mlcak RP, Suman OE, Herndon DN. Respiratory management of inhalational injury. *Burns* 2007;33:2–13.
33. Ryan CM, Schoenfeld DA, Thorpe WP, et al. Objective estimates of the probability of death from burn injuries. *N Engl J Med* 1998;338: 362–366.
34. Haponik EF, Crapo RO, Herndon DN, et al. Smoke inhalation. *Am Rev Respir Dis* 1988;138:1060–1063.
35. Weiss SM, Lakshiminarayan S. Acute inhalation injury. *Clin Chest Med* 1994;15:103–116.
36. Heimbach DM, Waeckerle JF. Inhalation injuries. *Ann Emerg Med* 1988;17:1316–1320.
37. Demling R. Smoke inhalation injury. *New Horiz* 1993;1:422–484.
38. Mandel J, Hales CA. Smoke inhalation. UpToDate 17.1. Available at: http://www.utdol.com. Accessed May 22, 2009.
39. Seger D, Welch L. Carbon monoxide controversies: Neuropsychologic testing, mechanisms of toxicity, and hyperbaric oxygen. *Ann Emerg Med* 1994;24:242–248.
40. Demling RH. Smoke inhalation injury. In: Shoemaker WC, Ayres SM, Genvik A, et al, eds. *Textbook of critical care*, 3rd ed. Philadelphia: W.B. Saunders Company; 1995:1506–1516.
41. Herlihy JP, Vermeulen PM, Joseph PM, et al. Impaired alveolar macrophage function in smoke inhalation injury. *J Cell Physiol* 1995; 163:1–8.
42. Desai MH, Mlcak R, Richardson J, et al. Reduction in mortality in pediatric patients with aerosolized heparin/N-acetylcysteine therapy. *J Burn Care Rehabil* 1998;19:210–212.
43. Bartlett JG. Aspiration pneumonia. UpToDate 17.1. Available at: http://www.utdol.com. Accessed May 26, 2009.
44. Greenfield LJ, Singleton RP, McCaffree DR, et al. Pulmonary effects of experimental graded aspiration of hydrochloric acid. *Ann Surg* 1969; 170:74–86.
45. Fisk RL, Symes JF, Aldrige LL, et al. The pathophysiology and experimental therapy of acid pneumonitis in ex vivo lungs. *Chest* 1970;57: 364–370.
46. Cameron JL, Caldini P, Toung JK, et al. Aspiration pneumonia: physiologic data following experimental aspiration. *Surgery* 1973;72:238–245.
47. Bynum LJ, Pierce AK. Pulmonary aspiration of gastric contents. *Am Rev Respir Dis* 1976;114:1129–1136.
48. Broe PJ, Toung TJ, Permutt S, et al. Aspiration pneumonia: treatment with pulmonary vasodilators. *Surgery* 1983;94:95–99.
49. Cameron JL, Sebor J, Anderson PR, et al. Aspiration pneumonia: results of treatment by positive-pressure ventilation in dogs. *J Surg Res* 1968;8:447–457.
50. Peitzman AB, Shires GT III, Illner HK, et al. Pulmonary acid injury: effects of positive end-expiratory pressure and crystalloid vs. colloid fluid resuscitation. *Arch Surg* 1982;117:662–668.
51. Toung TJ, Cameron JL, Kimera T, et al. Aspiration pneumonia: treatment with osmotically active agents. *Surgery* 1981;89:588–593.
52. Wolfe JE, Bone RC, Ruth WE. Effects of corticosteroids in the treatment of patients with gastric aspiration. *Am J Med* 1977;63:719–722.
53. Bartlett JG. Anaerobic bacterial infections of the lung and pleural space. *Clin Infect Dis* 1993;4:S248–S255.
54. Finegold SM. Aspiration pneumonia. *Rev Infect Dis* 1991;13(Suppl 9): S737–S742.
55. Bartlett JG. Anaerobic bacterial pneumonitis. *Am Rev Respir Dis* 1979; 119:19–23.
56. Gilbert DN, Moellering RC Jr, Eliopoulos GM, et al, eds. *The Sanford guide to antimicrobial therapy*, 38th ed. Sperryville, VA: Antimicrobial Therapy, Inc.; 2008.
57. Wang JL, Chen KY, Fang CT, et al. Changing bacteriology of adult community-acquired lung abscess in Taiwan: *Klebsiella pneumoniae* versus anaerobes. *CID* 2005;40:915–925.
58. Torres A, Serra-Batlles J, Ros E, et al. Pulmonary aspiration of gastric contents in patients receiving mechanical ventilation: the effect of body position. *Ann Intern Med* 1992;116:540–543.

59. Orozco-Levi M, Torres A, Ferrer M, et al. Semirecumbent position protects from pulmonary aspiration but not completely from gastroesophageal reflux in mechanically ventilated patients. *Am J Respir Crit Care Med* 1995;152:1387–1390.
60. Drakulovic M, Torres A, Bauer TT, et al. Supine body position as a risk factor for nosocomial pneumonia in mechanically ventilated patients: a randomized trial. *Lancet* 1999;354:1851–1858.
61. Zavala DC, Rhodes ML. Foreign body removal: a new role for the fiberoptic bronchoscope. *Ann Otol Rhinol Laryngol* 1975;84:650–656.
62. American Thoracic Society, Infectious Diseases Society of America. Guidelines for the management of adults with hospital-acquired, ventilator-associated, and healthcare-associated pneumonia. *Am J Respir Crit Care Med* 2005;171:388–416.
63. Cunnion KM, Weber DJ, Broadhead WE, et al. Risk factors for nosocomial pneumonia: comparing adult critical-care populations. *Am J Respir Crit Care Med* 1996;153:158–162.
64. National Nosocomial Infections Surveillance (NNIS) report, data summary from October 1986-April 1997, issued May 1997. A report from the NNIS System. *Am J Infect Control* 1997;25:477–487.
65. Tablan OC, Anderson LJ, Arden NH, et al. Guideline for prevention of nosocomial pneumonia. Centers for Disease Control and Prevention. *Respir Care* 1994;39:1191–1198.
66. File TM Jr. Risk factors and prevention of hospital-acquired, ventilator-associated, and healthcare-associated pneumonia in adults. UpToDate 17.1. Available at: http://www.utdol.com. Accessed May 27, 2009.
67. Prod'hom G, Leuenberger P, Koerfer J, et al. Nosocomial pneumonia in mechanically ventilated patients receiving antacid, ranitidine, or sucralfate. *Ann Intern Med* 1994;120:653–662.
68. Schweickert WD, Gehlbach BK, Pohlman AS, et al. Daily interruption of sedative infusions and complications of critical illness in mechanically ventilated patients. *Crit Care Med* 2004;32:1272–1276.
69. Milbrandt EB, Kersten A, Kong L, et al. Haloperidol use is associated with lower hospital mortality in mechanically ventilated patients. *Crit Care Med* 2005;33:226–229.
70. File TM Jr. Epidemiology, pathogenesis, and microbiology of hospital-acquired, ventilator-associated, and healthcare-associated pneumonia in adults. UpToDate 17.1. Available at: http://www.utdol.com. Accessed May 27, 2009.
71. Wahl WL, Franklin GA, Brandt MM, et al. Does bronchoalveolar lavage enhance our ability to treat ventilator-associated pneumonia in a trauma-burn intensive care unit? *J Trauma* 2003;54:633–639.
72. Fagon JY, Chastre J, Wolff M, et al. Invasive and noninvasive strategies for management of suspected ventilator-associated pneumonia. A randomized trial. *Ann Intern Med* 2000;132:621–630.
73. Croce MA, Fabian TC, Schurr MJ, et al. Using bronchoalveolar lavage to distinguish nosocomial pneumonia from systemic inflammatory response syndrome: a prospective analysis. *J Trauma* 1995;39:1134–1140.
74. Croce MA, Fabian TC, Wadde-Smith L, et al. Utility of Gram's stain and efficacy of quantitative culture for posttraumatic pneumonia. *Ann Surg* 1998;227:743–751.
75. Minei JP, Nathens AB, West M, et al. Guidelines for prevention, diagnosis, and treatment of ventilator-associated pneumonia (VAP) in the trauma patient. *J Trauma* 2006;60:1106–1113.
76. Meduri GU, Johanson WG Jr. International consensus conference: clinical investigation of ventilator-associated pneumonia. Introduction. *Chest* 1992;102:551S–552S.
77. Kollef MH, Sherman G, Ward S, et al. Inadequate antimicrobial treatment of infections: a risk factor for hospital mortality among critically ill patients. *Chest* 1999;115:462–474.
78. Rello J, Gallego M, Mariscal D, et al. The value of routine microbial investigation in ventilator-associated pneumonia. *Am J Respir Crit Care Med* 1997;156:196–200.
79. Rello J, Diaz E. Pneumonia in the intensive care unit. *Crit Care Med* 2003;31:2544–2551.
80. Galil K, Zaleznik DF. Nosocomial pneumonia. UpToDate 11.3. Available at: http://www.utdol.com. Accessed February 17, 2003.
81. Hilf M, Yu VL, Sharp J, et al. Antibiotic therapy for pseudomonas aeruginosa bacteremia: outcome correlations in a prospective study of 200 patients. *Am J Med* 1989;87:540–546.
82. Chastre J, Wolff M, Fagon JY. Comparison of 8 vs 15 days of antibiotic therapy for ventilator-associated pneumonia in adults: a randomized trial. *JAMA* 2003;290:2588–2598.
83. Heyland DK, Dodek P, Muscedere J, et al. Canadian Critical Care Trials Group. Randomized trial of combination versus monotherapy for the empiric treatment of suspected ventilator-associated pneumonia. *Crit Care Med* 2008;36:737–744.
84. Hemmila MR, Hirschl RB. Advances in ventilatory support of the pediatric surgical patient. *Curr Opin Pediatr* 1999;11:241–248.
85. Bernard GR, Artigas A, Brigham KL, et al. The Consensus Committee Report of the American-European Consensus Conference on ARDS: definitions, mechanisms, relevant outcomes and clinical trial coordination. *Intensive Care Med* 1994;20:225–232.
86. Brower RG, Morris A, Schoenfeld D, et al. The Acute Respiratory Distress Syndrome Network. Ventilation with lower tidal volumes as compared with traditional tidal volumes for acute lung injury and the acute respiratory distress syndrome. *N Engl J Med* 2000;342: 1301–1308.
87. Beaufils F, Mercier JC, Farnoux C, et al. Acute respiratory distress syndrome in children. *Curr Opin Pediatr* 1997;9:207–212.
88. Bulger EM, Jurkovich GJ, Gentilello LM, et al. Current clinical options for the treatment and management of acute respiratory distress syndrome. *J Trauma* 2000;48: 562–572.
89. Demling RH. Pulmonary dysfunction. In: Wilmore DW, Cheung LY, Harken AH, et al, eds. *ACS Surgery principles and practice 2003*. New York, NY: WebMD Inc; 2003:1433–1453.
90. Hansen-Flaschen J, Siegel MD. Acute respiratory distress syndrome: definition; epidemiology; diagnosis; and etiology. UpToDate 17.1. Available at: http://www.utdol.com. Accessed May 27, 2009.
91. Webb HH, Tierney DF. Experimental pulmonary edema due to intermittent positive pressure ventilation with high inflation pressures. Protection by positive end-expiratory pressure. *Am Rev of Resp Dis* 1974;110:556–565.
92. Dreyfuss D, Basset G, Soler P, et al. Intermittent positive-pressure hyperventilation with high inflation pressures produces pulmonary microvascular injury in rats. *Am Rev of Resp Dis* 1985;132:880–884.
93. Tsuno K, Prato P, Kolobow T. Acute lung injury from mechanical ventilation at moderately high airway pressures. *J Appl Physiol* 1990;69: 956–961.
94. Ranieri VM, Suter PM, Tortorella C, et al. Effect of mechanical ventilation on inflammatory mediators in patients with acute respiratory distress syndrome: a randomized, controlled trial. *JAMA* 1999;282;54–61.
95. Kolobow T, Moretti MP, Fumagalli R, et al. Severe impairment in lung function induced by high peak airway pressure during mechanical ventilation. An experimental study. *Am Rev Respir Dis* 1987;135: 312–315.
96. Savel RH, Yao EC, Gropper MA. Protective effects of low tidal volume ventilation in a rabbit model of *Pseudomonas aeruginosa*-induced acute lung injury. *Crit Care Med* 2001;29:392–398.
97. Parsons PE, Eisner MD, Thompson BT, et al. Lower tidal volume ventilation and plasma cytokine markers of inflammation in patients with acute lung injury. *Crit Care Med* 2005;33:1–6.
98. Hickling KG, Henderson SJ, Jackson R. Low mortality associated with low volume pressure limited ventilation with permissive hypercapnia in severe adult respiratory distress syndrome. *Intensive Care Med* 1990;16:372–377.
99. Hickling KG, Walsh J, Henderson S, et al. Low mortality rate in adult respiratory distress syndrome using low-volume, pressure-limited ventilation with permissive hypercapnia: a prospective study. *Crit Care Med* 1994;22:1568–1578.
100. Kregenow DA, Rubenfeld GD, Hudson LD, et al. Hypercapnic acidosis and mortality in acute lung injury. *Crit Care Med* 2006;34:229–231.
101. Artigas A, Bernard GR, Carlet J, et al. The American-European Consensus Conference on ARDS, part 2: ventilatory, pharmacologic, supportive therapy, study design strategies and issues related to recovery and remodeling. *Intensive Care Med* 1998;24:378–398.
102. Amato MB, Barbas CS, Medieros DM, et al. Beneficial effects of the "open lung approach" with low distending pressures in acute respiratory distress syndrome: a prospective randomized study on mechanical ventilation. *Am J Respir Crit Care Med* 1995;152:1835–1846.
103. Amato MB, Barbas CS, Medieros DM, et al. Effect of a protective-ventilation strategy on mortality in the acute respiratory distress syndrome. *N Engl J Med* 1998;338:347–354.
104. Hager DN, Krishnan JA, Hayden DL, et al. Tidal volume reduction in patients with acute lung injury when plateau pressures are not high. *Am J Respir Crit Care Med* 2005;172:1241–1245.
105. Mercat A, Richard JM, Vielle B, et al. Positive end-expiratory pressure setting in adults with acute lung injury and acute respiratory distress syndrome. *JAMA* 2008;299:646–655.
106. Meade MO, Cook DJ, Guyatt GH, et al. Ventilation strategy using low tidal volumes, recruitment maneuvers, and high positive end-

expiratory pressure for acute lung injury and acute respiratory distress syndrome. *JAMA* 2008;299:637–645.

107. Piehl MA, Brown RS. Use of extreme position changes in acute respiratory failure. *Crit Care Med* 1976;4:13–14.
108. Douglas WW, Rehder K, Beynen FM, et al. Improved oxygenation in patients with acute respiratory failure: the prone position. *Am Rev Respir Dis* 1977;115:559–566.
109. Gattinoni L, Tognoni G, Pesenti A, et al. Effect of prone positioning on the survival of patients with acute respiratory failure. *N Engl J Med* 2001;345:568–573.
110. Meduri GU, Headley AS, Golden E, et al. Effect of prolonged methylprednisolone therapy in unresolving acute respiratory distress syndrome. *JAMA* 1998;280:159–165.
111. Steinberg KP, Hudson LD, Goodman RB. National Heart, Lung, and Blood Institute Acute Respiratory Distress Syndrome (ARDS) Clinical Trials Network. Efficacy and safety of corticosteroids for persistent acute respiratory distress syndrome. *N Engl J Med* 2006;354:1671–1684.
112. Bartlett RH, Roloff DW, Cornell RG, et al. Extracorporeal circulation in neonatal respiratory failure: a prospective randomized study. *Pediatrics* 1985;76:479–487.
113. UK Collaborative ECMO Trial Group. UK collaborative randomized trial of neonatal extracorporeal membrane oxygenation. *Lancet* 1996; 348:75–82.
114. Peek GJ, Mugford M, Tiruvoipati R, Wilson A, Allen E, Thalanany MM, Hibbert CL, Truesdale A, Clemens F Cooper N, Firmin RK, Elbourne D; CESAR trial collaboration. Efficacy and economic assessment of conventional ventilatory support versus extracorporeal membrane oxygenation for severe adult respiratory failure (CESAR): a multicentre randomised controlled trial. *Lancet* 2009;374: 1351–1363.
115. Extracorporeal Life Support Organization. *Annual ECMO Registry Report*. 2003.
116. Rich PB, Awad SS, Kolla S, et al. An approach to the treatment of severe adult respiratory failure. *J Crit Care* 1998;13:26–36.
117. Hemmila MR, Rowe SA, Boules TN, et al. Extracorporeal life support for severe acute respiratory distress syndrome in adults. *Ann Surg* 2004;240:595–607.

CHAPTER

20

Abnormalities in Coagulation

Alvin H. Schmaier

INTRODUCTION

Bleeding or thrombosis is a serious complication associated with elective or emergent surgery. When approaching the proposed surgical patient, a few critical items should be obtained to exclude the possibility of abnormal bleeding and increased risk for thrombosis arising independent of complications during the procedure. This chapter aims (a) to provide a concise and thorough approach to assessing bleeding risk in the prospective surgical patient; (b) to provide a practical and thorough differential diagnosis of causes of surgical bleeding and thrombosis; and (c) to suggest general and specific means to manage various bleeding states and prevent postoperative thrombosis in surgical patients.

ASSESSING RISK FOR BLEEDING IN PROSPECTIVE SURGICAL PATIENTS

Bleeding or thrombosis is the ill consequence of a loss in the delicate balance between hemostasis (clot formation), fibrinolysis (clot lysis), and anticoagulation (regulation) of the various plasma proteins and cells in the intravascular compartment. For 40 years, the blood coagulation system has been represented as a cascade of proteolytic reactions leading to clot formation (1). This concept really describes blood coagulation that occurs in a test tube and not physiologic hemostasis. A current hypothesis is that the blood coagulation, fibrinolysis, and anticoagulant systems are an interacting group of proteins that amplify the activation and inhibition of each other (Fig. 20.1) (2,3). In physiologic hemostasis, the initiating event is factor VIIa-tissue factor (TF-VIIa) activating factor IX to factor IXa. This pathway occurs because a protein called tissue factor pathway inhibitor (TFPI) blocks the direct physiologic activation of factor X by TF-VIIa (2). Factor IXa (IXa) in the presence of factor VIIIa (VIIIa) activates factor X to factor Xa (Xa) which in the presence of factor Va (Va) activates prothrombin (II) to thrombin (IIa) (Fig. 20.1). A little thrombin proteolyzes fibrinogen to make a fibrin clot. However, this same thrombin also activates factor XI to factor XIa (XIa) to amplify more thrombin activation through factors IXa and VIIIa and, subsequently, factors Xa and Va (Fig. 20.1). Inhibitors to each of the coagulation and fibrinolysis enzymes additionally regulate this system. Under physiologic circumstances, factor XIIa is not an activator of factor XI to initiate coagulation reactions to prevent bleeding. In disease or injury such as that seen after platelet thrombus, sepsis, trauma, and cardiopulmonary bypass (CPB), factor XIIa forms by autoactivation on polysomes, ribonucleic acid (RNA), aggregated protein, and exposed collagen to activate factor XI, increasing thrombin formation as well (Fig. 20.1). In these circumstances factor XII contributes to the extent of thrombus formation in injured vessels and intravascular coagulation (4–6).

Although there is a present-day elegant understanding of physiologic hemostasis, the clinician needs to make management decisions based upon clinical tests. The current means to diagnosis of a bleeding risk in the prospective surgery patient is still by history and simple laboratory tests (Table 20.1) (7). Prospectively, thrombosis risk in a patient cannot be assessed by any laboratory testing; it requires assessment of the patient's past medical history, ambulatory ability, and the nature of the proposed surgery. The physician should ask if there have been prior surgeries, injuries, or tooth extractions, and, if so, whether there has been abnormal bleeding requiring additional care, transfusions, or revisits to the physician or hospital, for either the patient or an immediate family member. Similarly, these questions should be asked concerning any bleeding history of an immediate family member. Furthermore, the surgeon needs to take a thorough medication history. The common use of aspirin and other platelet inhibitors (e.g., clopidogrel, serotonin release inhibitor antidepressants, and vitamin E) that interfere with platelet function needs to be recorded. A positive answer to any one of these questions puts the patient into a higher bleeding risk category. Alternatively, thrombosis risk is assessed by prior history and the ambulatory nature of the patient. As will be discussed below, the nature of the surgical procedure contributes to the risk for thrombosis.

The clinical laboratory provides useful information to assess bleeding risk in a patient preparing for surgery. There is controversy regarding the cost-effective approach to assess bleeding risk. The activated partial thromboplastin time (APTT) is the most global screening assay for a

Alvin H. Schmaier: Case Western Reserve University, 2103 Cornell, WRB 2-130, Cleveland, OH 44106-7284

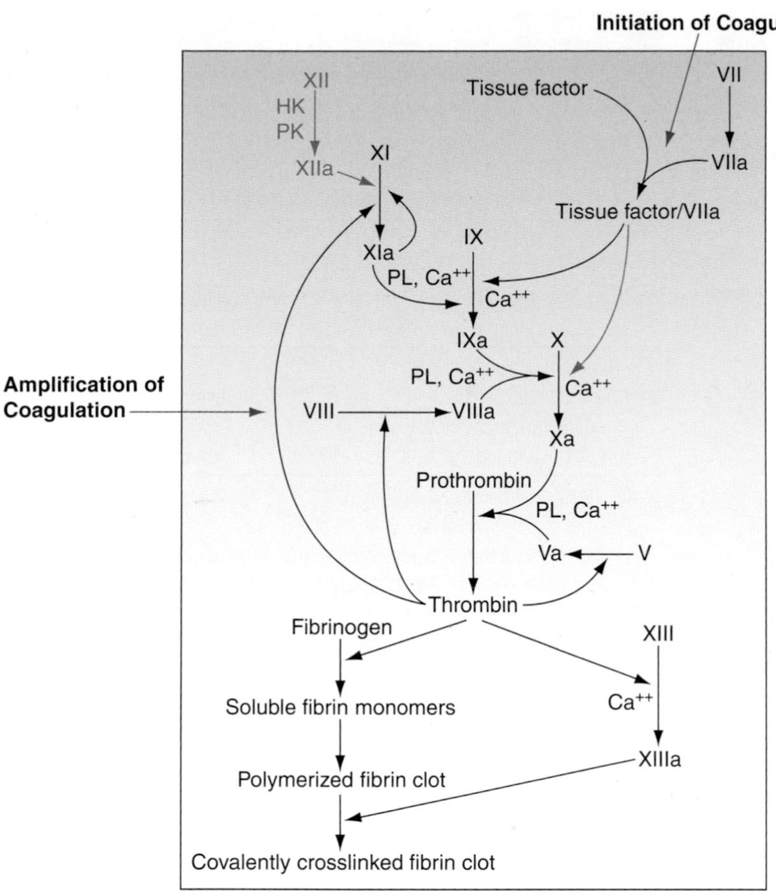

FIGURE 20.1. Physiologic hemostasis. Physiologic hemostasis is initiated by tissue factor-factor VIIa (TF-VIIa) activating factor IX. The plasma protein tissue factor pathway inhibitor (TFPI) blocks factor VIIa-TF from directly activating factor X. Factor IXa in the presence of factor VIIIa (IXa + VIIIa) activates factor X to factor Xa. Factor Xa in the presence of factor Va (Xa + Va) then activates prothrombin to thrombin (IIa). Formed thrombin (IIa) can clot fibrinogen to make fibrin. Thrombin also activates factor XIII to covalently crosslink the fibrin clot making it insoluble. If the need to generate thrombin is great, the initially formed thrombin will also activate factor XI to factor XIa (XIa). Formed factor XIa then amplifies factor IX activation leading to amplified thrombin formation (IIa).

coagulation protein defect, but it will not pick up the rare (1/500,000 to 1/1,000,000) patient with factor VII deficiency. Alternatively, the prothrombin time (PT), if abnormal, is probably a better predictor of bleeding at the time of surgery than the APTT, if abnormal. The bleeding time, which is not used much anymore, has been shown not to predict abnormal surgical bleeding. However, a patient who has a bleeding disorder, but who is on no medications and has a normal APTT and PT, may have von Willebrand disease or a platelet function disorder. These platelet function disorders may be diagnosed by bleeding time or a newer assay that has become widely available, the platelet function analyzer (PFA-100). Use of these latter tests requires that the patient being studied is on no interfering medication. The bleeding time and the PFA-100 are not analogous. The PFA-100 measures platelet activation induced by two agonists under high shear. It does not make a diagnosis of a bleeding disorder. Its result, like that of the bleeding time test, is only either "normal" or "abnormal." In my practice, which is hemostasis and thrombosis consultation, I use neither the bleeding time nor PFA-100 when I suspect a bleeding disorder by history in a patient with a normal APTT and PT. I prefer to obtain the specific assays for von Willebrand disease and platelet function defects. Making a specific diagnosis as to the bleeding state is essential because prophylactic therapies for von Willebrand disease or a platelet function defect, respectively, are quite different. The following is a description of what the tests measure. The decision to use all or a portion of these tests for screening to determine risk for bleeding has to rest in the hands of the clinician, based on the history of the patient.

The APTT and PT screening tests measure specific portions of the coagulation protein system (Fig. 20.2, Table 20.2). Knowing the results of these assays provides major diagnostic power to predict the potential cause of bleeding in a prospective surgical patient. The differential diagnosis of an isolated prolonged APTT is dependent upon whether the patient has a bleeding history or not. If there is a bleeding history, factor VIII (VIII) deficiency is nine times more common than factor IX (IX) deficiency. Both occur almost exclusively in males since they are sex-linked. These

Table 20.1 Presurgical variables to assess bleeding and clotting risk

History
Patient history of bleeding at surgery, trauma, tooth extractions
Family history of bleeding at surgery, trauma, tooth extractions
Medication history: antiplatelet agents, NIADS, anticoagulants
:
Complete blood count including platelet count
Activated partial thromboplastin time
Prothrombin time

NIADS, nonsteroidal anti-inflammatory drugs.

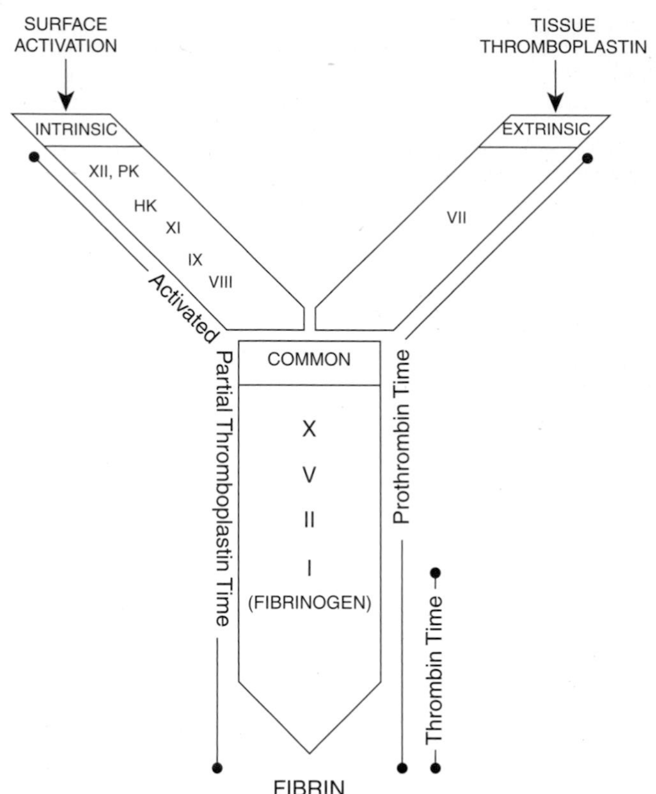

FIGURE 20.2. Description of common coagulation blood tests and what proteins these tests measure. The activated partial thromboplastin time (APTT) measures the functional integrity of all of the proteins of the so-called intrinsic (INTRINSIC) and common (COMMON) pathways of the coagulation system. These proteins include factor XII (XII), prekallikrein (PK), high molecular weight kininogen (HK), factors XI, IX, VIII, X, V, II (thrombin), and I (fibrinogen). The prothrombin time (PT) measures the functional integrity of the proteins of the so-called extrinsic (EXTRINSIC) pathway [Factor VII (VII)] and the proteins of the common pathway. The thrombin clotting time only measures the functional integrity of fibrinogen.

Table 20.2 Differential diagnosis of abnormal screening tests for bleeding disorders

Abnormal activated partial thromboplastin time (APTT) alone
Associated with bleeding: VIII, IX, XI defects
Not associated with bleeding: XII, prekallikrein (PK), high molecular weight kininogen (HK), lupus anticoagulants
Abnormal prothrombin time (PT) alone
VII defects
Mild defects in fibrinogen, factors II, X, or V can sometime appear as slight prolongations of the PT alone, before the APTT lengthens
Combined abnormal APTT and PT
Medical conditions: anticoagulants, DIC, liver disease, vitamin K deficiency, massive transfusion
Rarely dysfibrinogenemias, factors X, V, and II defects
Long bleeding time or PFA-100
Normal platelet count: von Willebrand disease or a platelet function defect (congenital or acquired—usually medication)
Low platelet count (<100,000/μl); low hematocrit (<20%) will give an abnormal PFA-100 result

individuals have a life-long bleeding history. Spontaneous inhibitors to VIII arise in patients who are elderly, postpartum, have a connective tissue disorder, or have a B cell malignancy. Factor XI (XI) deficiency is much less common and 50% of the patients are individuals who are Jewish with an Eastern European background. Alternatively, if there is no bleeding history, but the APTT alone is prolonged, the most likely cause for the prolonged APTT will be a lupus anticoagulant. A lupus anticoagulant is not a bleeding risk; paradoxically, it is a thrombosis risk. Other causes of long APTT that are not associated with bleeding include factor XII (XII), prekallikrein, or high molecular weight kininogen (HK) deficiencies (Fig. 20.2, Table 20.2). These last three protein defects are quite rare, and most physicians will never see a patient with these defects.

An isolated abnormal PT is commonly associated with a factor VII (VII) deficiency. This disorder is quite uncommon, but is associated with abnormal bleeding at the time of surgery. Depending upon the sensitivity of the thromboplastin in the PT reagent, an isolated abnormal PT can also occur with a dysfibrinogenemia or factor X, V, and II deficiencies.

When both the APTT and PT are prolonged, the physician needs to consider a number of medical conditions. These kinds of defects are most likely with inpatients. The most common causes of combined prolonged APTT and PT are the following: anticoagulation, disseminated intravascular coagulation (DIC), liver disease, vitamin K deficiency, and massive transfusions. Each of these entities will be discussed in more detail in the next section of this chapter. Once these medical conditions are excluded, only rare coagulation protein defects or deficiencies should be considered. The most common cause of an abnormal coagulation protein defect giving a prolonged PT and APTT is an abnormal fibrinogen (dysfibrinogenemia). Dysfibrinogenemias are most commonly seen in patients with liver disease, from any cause. Much less common would be deficiency or inhibitors to factors X, V, and II (prothrombin). True deficiencies of each of these three proteins are probably incompatible with normal fetal gestation and parturition. The extremely rare patient who appears to be fully deficient in these proteins actually has a small amount of the protein of interest being produced. More commonly, antibodies to factors V that arise spontaneously or after topical thrombin use from a previous surgery and antibodies to factor II and X arising in patients with systemic lupus erythematosus anticoagulants and malignancy may be seen. Acquired factor X deficiency also arises in patients with amyloidosis.

A bleeding patient with a normal PT, APTT, and platelet count may have von Willebrand disease or, less commonly, a true platelet function defect (ratio 9:1, von Willebrand disease : platelet function defect not induced by medication). Patients with von Willebrand disease and platelet function defects suffer from easy bruisability of soft tissues. Specialized testing is required to make the diagnosis of a deficiency or defect in the von Willebrand factor or a platelet function defect. Finally, all patients with a reduction in their platelet count so that it is below 100,000/μl are at increased risk of bleeding at the time of surgery. The platelet count should never be overlooked in the preoperative evaluation. Thus, all preoperative patients should have a PT, APTT, and platelet count. If there is a strong bleeding history and these tests are normal, the patient should be referred to a hematologist for a specific evaluation for von Willebrand disease or a platelet function defect.

DETERMINING THE DIAGNOSIS OF A BLEEDING SURGICAL PATIENT IN THE OPERATING ROOM OR RECOVERY ROOM

One of the most challenging aspects of consultative medicine is the emergency telephone call to see to the bleeding patient in the operating room (OR) or recovery room. It is the job of the hemostasis consultant to be certain that the cause of bleeding is not due to some medical factor(s) that can be corrected by means other than additional surgery. Although their problems may be acute, the approach to these patients is the same as that for assessing risk for bleeding in the preoperative evaluation. The first issue is the documentation of the preoperative variables examined prior to surgery. For example, patients with a long medication list could be on anticoagulants and/or antiplatelet agents (e.g., low-molecular-weight heparin, warfarin, aspirin, clopidogrel [Plavix®], vitamin E, serotonin release inhibitor antidepressants) that do not necessarily prolong screening coagulation tests but increase a patient's risk of bleeding at the time of surgery or postoperatively. Thus, the surgeon needs to be aware of prior medication history and its possible role in surgical bleeding. After the medications are reviewed, the assessment for other specific acquired bleeding states proceeds. As mentioned above, acquired bleeding states are usually due to anticoagulation, DIC, liver disease, vitamin K deficiency, or massive transfusion (Table 20.3) (8,9). Each of these conditions is associated with a prolonged PT and APTT.

Table 20.3 Acquired surgical bleeding

Anticoagulation
Antifibrin agents
Unfractionated heparin (standard heparin)
Low-molecular-weight heparin
Fondaparinux
Warfarin
Direct thrombin inhibitors: hirudin (Refludan, Leperudin), argatroban, bivalirudin (Angiomax)
Antiplatelet agents
Aspirin
Clopidogrel
Glycoprotein IIb/IIIa antagonists [Abciximab (ReoPro), tirofiban (Aggrastat), eptifibatide (Integrilin)
Disseminated intravascular coagulation—acute
Liver disease
Vitamin K deficiency
Massive transfusion

Anticoagulation

Anticoagulant and antiplatelet agents suffuse medical practice today, allowing for interventional procedures as well as preventing thrombosis. Some of these agents do not prolong the blood coagulation times and their presence in the patient would thus not be recognized unless appreciated upon a careful review of a patient's medication list. The surgeon needs to be aware of these agents and their pharmacokinetics in preparing the patient for surgery. In this section, only currently approved drugs will be discussed (Table 20.3). In general, anticoagulants can be classified into two groups: antifibrin agents and antiplatelet agents. Antifibrin agents can be subclassified into nonspecific inhibitors and specific inhibitors. The nonspecific anticoagulants consist of unfractionated heparin and warfarin. These agents at their usual therapeutic dose prolong the PT and APTT. Unfractionated heparin (standard heparin) has a short half-life (1 to 2 hours) allowing for normalization of bleeding risk within 4 hours after its infusion is stopped. With the exception of CPB surgery usage, patients on unfractionated heparin need only be delayed 4 hours once stopping the drug before commencing with the procedure. Individuals on unfractionated heparin who start to bleed only need red blood cell (RBC) and plasma support (see the discussion below on the effect of massive transfusion) for the duration of time they are at risk. Usually, sufficient amounts of the drug are metabolized within hours to remove the need for additional therapy. Protamine sulfate is almost never needed to correct abnormal bleeding in an individual on heparin.

Warfarin therapy, however, presents different challenges. Normally, it takes at least 5 days to fully anticoagulate someone on warfarin. The delay in anticoagulating someone on warfarin is the result of the fact that the drug needs to inhibit and alter the synthesis of four coagulation protein zymogens (proenzymes factors II, VII, IX, X) before its anticoagulation effect is achieved. Since these targets have variable half-lives (4 hours to 5 days), it takes at least 5 days before a full anticoagulation effect is achieved. Thus, the patient on warfarin at the time of surgery also needs a minimum of 5 days to correct its anticoagulation effect. Patients on warfarin should have this medication stopped at least 1 week before having elective surgery. Current practice is to continue to anticoagulate the patient with low-molecular-weight heparin up to 24 hours before the time of operation to prevent thrombosis (10). Postoperatively, the patient will need to be treated with at least 5 days of parenteral low-molecular-weight heparin if the risk of early anticoagulation is warranted by the risk of thrombosis until the reinstituted warfarin therapy can become effective as an anticoagulant again. It is appropriate to start anticoagulation in high-risk patients 12 to 24 h after surgery (10). If surgery is emergent within 24 h and the patient is on warfarin, there are a few options. In general, a patient fully anticoagulated on warfarin has only about 5% to 15% normal activity of coagulation factors II, VII, IX, and X. Further, the remaining 85% to 95% of these factors is synthesized abnormally, and thus acts as a coagulation protein inhibitor, potentiating the risk to bleed. Since normal hemostasis requires normal coagulation factor levels to be at least 50%, these patients would require at least 50% or more of their plasma volume to be replaced. In a 70 kg person, plasma volume is 60% of blood volume (~7% of body weight) or ~3 liters plasma (or 12 units of fresh frozen plasma [FFP] [1 Unit FFP ~250 mL]). If 50% of the plasma volume needs to be given to the patient to correct their hemostatic defect, the patient would require 1.5 liters of FFP over a very short period of time. Most patients and blood banks cannot tolerate a replacement prescription like this. Thus, surgery should be avoided at all costs in a patient fully anticoagulated with warfarin. However, if truly life saving therapy is needed in such a patient (e.g., intracerebral hemorrhage in a patient on warfarin), there are a few options. One would be to consider whole body plasma exchange by plasmapheresis. Another would be to acutely replace the patient with a vitamin K coagulation factor concentrate, if available (11). Third, would be acute replacement with recombinant factor VIIa (rFVIIa) (12,13). Abnormal bleeding in all locations other than the central nervous system (CNS) in patients on warfarin is corrected with a single dose of rFVIIa at 20 to 40 μg/kg as a single intravenous (IV) infusion along with 2 units FFP (12). More rFVIIa is not better. Too much rFVIIa that costs $1.00/μg has been reported to be associated with myocardial infarction or stroke. It has a 3-hour half-life. A second dose is occasionally helpful. If more than two doses are needed to stop bleeding, a structural etiology needs to be looked for. If there is bleeding within the skull, that is, a closed space, a single IV dose of rFVIIa at 90 μg/kg with 2 units FFP is appropriate to reverse intracerebral hemorrhage in a patient on warfarin (13).

In addition to the above nonspecific anticoagulants, several antifibrin agents are specifically directed to coagulation factors Xa and thrombin (IIa). All the low-molecular-weight heparins and fondaparinux are mostly directed to factor Xa and not thrombin. At doses that are therapeutic for the treatment for deep venous thrombosis, these agents may, in various individuals, only slightly prolong the screening tests of the PT and APTT. Therefore, these assays cannot be used to exclude the possibility that these agents are present in the patient. Although the PT and APTT are not markedly prolonged, the risk of bleeding in patients treated with low-molecular-weight heparin or fondaparinux is similar to that for those on unfractionated heparin. If hemorrhage occurs, there is no immediate antidote, although rFVIIa infusion could be used in cases of serious bleeding (See below). Low-molecular-weight heparins have slightly longer half-lives (2 to 4.5 hours) than unfractionated heparin; the half-life depends upon the preparation. However, these agents accumulate, and after chronic therapy, it will take up to 24 hours to completely eliminate them. Fondaparinux has an 18-hour half-life, so if bleeding occurs while on this agent, support has to be given for a longer period of time. Both low-molecular-weight heparin and fondaparinux are excreted renally. Therefore, patients with renal dysfunction have longer clearance times. Also, both agents are stored in adipose tissue, allowing for anticoagulant accumulation in obese patients. These factors are associated with abnormal bleeding as result of higher drug levels than anticipated.

The direct thrombin inhibitors, hirudin, argatroban, and bivalirudin, are antifibrin agents that interact specifically with the thrombin active site, exosite I, or both. All will prolong the screening tests for coagulation disorders. If renal and liver functions are normal, hirudin or bivalirudin and argatroban are eliminated in 0.5 to 2 hours, respectively. Thus, if a patient is on these drugs, only a short time must pass before the patient can go to surgery. Further, support for abnormal bleeding will be for a short time. Alternatively, renal dysfunction and failure delay the clearance of hirudin, making this recombinant, foreign protein impossible to eliminate. In cases of severe renal failure, even with a normal blood urea nitrogen and creatinine on continuous venovenous hemofiltration (CVVH), hirudin can become virtually impossible to eliminate. Great care is essential when choosing to use this drug in dynamic clinical situations. I generally do not use hirudin in my practice.

In addition to the above list of antifibrin agents, antiplatelet agents are increasingly being used in clinical medicine (Table 20.3). These agents do not influence the PT and APTT, but will prolong the bleeding time or PFA-100. Aspirin, a platelet cyclo-oxygenase I and II inhibitor, has become ubiquitous in the management of coronary artery disease. A single 80 mg tablet of aspirin interferes with platelet function for all platelets present at the instant when the agent was taken. Thus, after aspirin administration, the patient's platelet function will not become normal until at least half of the entire platelet pool has been resynthesized (10 to 14 days). Patients taking aspirin may require platelet transfusions in planned or emergent operations. Clopidogrel (Plavix®) is a platelet ADP $P2Y_{12}$ receptor antagonist. It is also an irreversible platelet inhibitor. Patients on clopidogrel should stop taking the agent before elective surgery. Vitamin E is a protein kinase C inhibitor that interferes with platelet function. Some patients on vitamin E will also have abnormal bleeding at the time of surgery. Serotonin release inhibitor antidepressants are commonly used and all produce an acquired platelet storage pool disorder that increases bleeding risk. Last, the glycoprotein IIb/IIIa ($\alpha_{2b}\beta_3$ integrin) antagonists are used to inhibit platelets in the acute coronary syndrome. Although tirofiban or eptifibatide is rapidly excreted when its infusion is stopped, the monoclonal antibody glycoprotein IIb/IIIa antagonist, abciximab, can remain in the circulation system for 15 days, with the potential to cause hemorrhage.

Disseminated intravascular coagulation

DIC is a clinicopathologic condition that arises in patients due to sepsis, malignancy, obstetrical complications at the time of surgery, and massive tissue injury. In the surgery patient, DIC is usually not a preoperative variable, except with obstetrical catastrophes or after major brain trauma. Rather, it is a complication that occurs during surgery or in the postoperative period. DIC during surgery occurs in a number of conditions. Surgery for prostate cancer and into the brain have been associated with acute DIC. In circulatory arrest operations on the arch of the aorta or main pulmonary arteries, DIC is a frequent complication due to the chilling of the patient to 19°C followed by tissue rewarming. Abruptio placenta and placenta previa are associated with acute hemorrhagic DIC, whereas retained dead fetus is associated with a DIC that is not hemorrhagic, but prothrombotic. DIC also occurs in the postoperative period due to sepsis. DIC with sepsis is most commonly seen with gram negative infections, but can occur with gram positive infections and, in the immunosuppressed patient, with fungemia.

The diagnosis of DIC is through the presence of certain abnormal clinical test results in an appropriate clinical setting. Finding a prolonged PT and APTT with a reduced fibrinogen and platelet count usually points to DIC in the hospitalized patient until proven otherwise (14). The diagnosis of DIC is made by a confirmatory test that shows the simultaneous presence of thrombin and plasmin formation. Currently, the D-dimer assay is the confirmatory test that, if positive, shows that both thrombin and plasmin have been formed. The D-dimer measures plasmin-cleaved, insoluble, cross-linked fibrin that originally arose from thrombin cleavage of fibrinogen. D-dimer assays are characteristic for DIC, but not pathognomonic. D-dimer assays can be positive in individuals with resolving large vessel thrombosis and soft tissue hematomas, which can also occur in surgery patients (15).

Management of DIC first starts with recognition of the syndrome and treatment of the underlying disease. Treatment of abruptio placenta, placenta previa, or retained dead fetus is removal of the inciting etiology by surgical means. DIC associated with sepsis is first treated with removal of the inciting infectious focus with antibiotics or, if appropriate, through surgical means. Once the inciting cause is appreciated and any specific therapy applied, general medical therapy can be provided for the DIC. Most cases of DIC associated with surgery are hemorrhagic coagulopathies resulting in consumption of coagulation factors and platelets. Thus, therapy should be directed towards replacement of missing coagulation factors or platelets, or both. Each platelet transfusion is bathed in fresh plasma. Therefore, platelet infusion also provides some plasma replacement and additional replacement with FFP may not be necessary. The purpose of FFP replacement is not only to replace the consumed coagulation proteins, but also provide plasma protease inhibitors, for example, antithrombin, α_2-antiplasmin, C1 esterase inhibitor, and so on, that reduce the degree of active proteolytic reactions occurring in the plasma. If the fibrinogen levels are low, that is, <150 mg/dL, specific replacement with cryoprecipitate or a recently approved purified fibrinogen concentrate is also indicated. The entire purpose of therapy in these patients is to support the patient so that the underlying condition can be brought under control. Anticoagulant therapy has little role in most of these patients, except in individuals with acryl cyanosis and digital ischemia where small doses of heparin (4 to 5 U/kg constant infusion without a bolus), may ameliorate the prothrombotic nature of the inciting etiology. Heparin usage (unfractionated heparin or low-molecular-weight heparin) should only be used if there is an endpoint in a limited disease state that needs to be achieved.

Liver disease

It is important that surgeons know if a proposed patient has liver disease. In addition to the anesthesia risk, most coagulation proteins and inhibitors are made in the liver. Thus, these patients have increased risk of bleeding. Patients with serious liver disease will have prolonged PT and APTT. Not only are the synthesis of these proteins reduced, but those proteins made are often abnormal in structure, functioning as inhibitors to normal coagulation proteins. As in patients on warfarin, replacement therapy with FFP is not completely feasible because too much replacement is usually needed. Also, since this is dependent upon the half-life of the protein (e.g., factor VII is only 3 to 4 hours), it is not practical to keep up with replacement needs over long periods (i.e., >12 to 24 hours). In addition to reduction in synthesis of coagulation proteins and inhibitors in patients with liver disease, liver disease itself results in abnormal anatomy such as portal hypertension that increases patients' risk of bleeding from esophageal varices, gastritis, and hemorrhoids. Furthermore, portal hypertension results in hypersplenism, thrombocytopenia, and granulocytopenia. In general, prekallikrein is one of the first proteins to decrease in liver disease; fibrinogen is one of the last proteins to decrease in liver disease. Abnormal fibrinogens (dysfibrinogenemias) are very common in patients with liver disease. All the vitamin K dependent proteins (factors II, VII, IX, and X, proteins C, S, and Z) decrease in liver disease. Factors VIII and V also decrease at late end-stage liver disease. Moreover, antithrombin and other serpin plasma protein inhibitors decrease in liver disease. Thus, these patients have reduced procoagulants and anticoagulants, adjusting the baseline for hemostasis at a level other than that seen in normal people.

Preoperative management of patients with liver disease requires thought with regard to a number of variables. All these patients should be given vitamin K to ensure that they are not deficient. The nature and duration of surgery also needs to be considered. If it is a short procedure, replacement coverage with FFP may be sufficient. However, its duration may be too short to be effective. If a patient is mostly deficient in fibrinogen (i.e., <100 mg/dL) or the fibrinogen functions abnormally, cryoprecipitate or newly approved fibrinogen concentrate infusion may be sufficient to correct the defect. Alternatively, if the patient has a decrease in all factors and is thrombocytopenic, the most global means to treat such a patient is with platelet transfusions, aiming to keep the platelet count greater than 100,000/μL throughout the operative procedure and during the first 24 hours post operation, subsequently tapering off slowly. Finally, if all fails, rFVIIa infusion at 40 to 60 μg/kg as a single IV bolus acutely can be used to get a bleeding diathesis under control. Again, rFVIIa therapy is to be used with caution and not repetitively.

Vitamin K deficiency

Vitamin K, a lipid soluble vitamin, is provided by dietary intake of leafy green vegetables and by synthesis of intestinal flora. The body has 1 month stores. Vitamin K deficiency is mostly seen in the very ill surgical patient on antibiotics who has subsisted on parenteral nutrition. Not infrequently, IV fluids are not supplemented with vitamin K. After 4 to 6 weeks of parenteral nutrition and antibiotic treatment, the patient becomes vitamin K deficient. Vitamin K deficiency can also be seen in patients who have anatomic bypass of the small intestine, malabsorption, biliary tract obstruction, and, rarely, reduced dietary intake. For example, alcoholics are often vitamin K deficient. Warfarin also interferes with two enzymes necessary for vitamin K utilization. Vitamin K has a critical role in the γ-carboxylation reaction of glutamic acid residues, γ-carboxyglutamic acid, of the so-called vitamin K-dependent coagulation proteins, factors II, VII, IX, and X and proteins C, S, and Z. This reaction on certain amino acids on the amino terminus of these proteins is critical for these proteins to bind to cells and phospholipids so that they can participate in physiologic coagulation reactions. Vitamin K is usually replaced by oral therapy. However, if necessary, parenteral replacement can be given. Intramuscular rather than IV is the preferred, safe route of administration.

Massive transfusion

Bleeding complications from massive transfusions themselves occur as result of the amount of anticoagulant being poured into the patient by substantial transfusion within a short period of time. Sixteen percent of the volume of each unit of packed RBCs, platelets, and FFP consists of acid-citrate-dextrose anticoagulant. This anticoagulant chelates plasma divalent cations such as calcium, magnesium, and zinc, such that they cannot participate in the blood protein coagulation reactions. If in a 24-hour period, 1.5 times the patient's blood volume is transfused, the accumulation of the citrate anticoagulant can be massive, producing anticoagulation itself and an acquired coagulopathy. For example, in the 70 kg man, 7% of body weight or 4.9 kg or liters are the blood volume. If this individual received 1.5 times his blood volume, he was transfused 7.35 liters of blood products of which 1176 mL was anticoagulant alone. Thus, the anticoagulant volume and dilution of his endogenous plasma from all the transfusions conspire to lead to an anticoagulated state. Such a situation occurs in the OR when there is vigorous RBC replacement. In most circumstances, this problem can be avoided by linking 1 unit of FFP to every 4 to 6 units of RBC transfusion. In addition, one ampule of calcium should be administered for every four to six units of transfused RBCs and 1 unit of FFP to overcome the anticoagulant effect of the sodium citrate.

Managing massive bleeding

There are times in the OR when bleeding occurs and appropriate therapy has been instituted, but the surgeon still believes that hemostasis has not been achieved in a sufficiently timely manner. In these critical situations, an immediate, short-term means to get a handle on the hemorrhage is the use of IV infusion of rFVIIa (16,17). Recombinant FVIIa infusion directly activates IX and/or X to lead to thrombin formation. In essence, its infusion makes a patient prothrombotic. However, life-threatening bleeding in the OR may require its use to get control of a situation. Although the literature provides a wide range of dosing that can be used, our experience tells us that a more conservative dosage from 40 to 60 μg/kg rFVIIa is often sufficient to achieve hemostasis safely in most patients with an acute hemorrhage, not immediately controllable by more traditional means. rFVIIa therapy works best in individuals who have been replenished with coagulation proteins in FFP.

ASSESSING RISK AND PREVENTION FOR THROMBOSIS IN THE SURGICAL PATIENT

Although bleeding in any patient is dramatic and anxiety provoking, thrombosis is a silent cause of more morbidity and mortality. More surgical patients die of thrombotic complications resultant from surgery than bleeding. It is incumbent upon the physician to be knowledgeable about the risks for thrombosis that occur in the surgical patient. The best treatment for thrombosis is thrombosis prevention. In general, venous thrombosis occurs in areas of low flow and consists of an initial platelet thrombus followed by an accumulation of red cells in a fibrin mesh. Alternatively, arterial thrombus is mostly platelet-rich, occurring in areas of high blood flow. Both venous and arterial thromboses have known risk factors (18).

Arterial thrombosis

It is beyond the scope of this chapter to fully discuss the risk factors for myocardial infarction and stroke. To date, no fundamental cohesive hypothesis has been formulated to understand a common pathway for increased arterial thrombosis. Both hypertension and atherosclerosis are associated with it, but "how" has not been precisely defined. However, we do know of certain protein risk factors that contribute to arterial thrombosis. In particular, elevation of homocysteine and antiphospholipid antibodies contribute to risk of both arterial and venous thrombosis. Each will be discussed in the section below on venous thrombosis. Another factor for increased risk for arterial thrombosis is the elevation of lipoprotein(a) [Lp(a)]. Lp(a) consists of low density lipoprotein (LDL) and apolipoprotein(a). Apolipoprotein(a) has 98% sequence identity to kringle 4 of plasminogen, the portion of plasminogen that binds to cells and phospholipids, the place where clinically significant thrombolysis occurs. Therefore, Lp(a) is both atherogenic and prothrombotic.

Venous thrombosis

Risk factors for venous thrombosis in the surgical patient are numerous. After 2 weeks of bed rest, there is 20% likelihood of thrombosis in a 20-year-old individual, but 60% likelihood of thrombosis in a 60-year-old patient. Obesity is a risk factor for venous thrombosis in 55% of patients. A preoperative ambulatory patient has a lower risk of thrombosis than a bed-ridden individual. Further, a patient with a stroke is more likely to have thrombosis in the paretic limb than in the nonparetic limb. The surgical patient with cardiac disease is more thrombus prone than if there was no cardiac disease. Women on oral contraceptives put on bed rest will have an greater risk of thrombosis than if they were not on contraceptives. Surgery itself promotes thrombosis. The degree of risk depends on the nature of the surgery and the amount of time the patient is under anesthesia. For example, orthopedic surgery (hip, knee) is associated with actual flexing and occlusion of the femoral and popliteal veins, respectively. The incidence of deep venous thrombosis is 35% to 40% and 50%, respectively. In abdominothoracic surgery, the risk of thrombosis is 14% to 35%. In urologic surgery, the risk of a deep venous thrombosis is 7% for a transurethral resection, but 35% for a suprapubic prostatectomy. Similarly, in gynecologic surgery, a vaginal hysterectomy has a 7% risk of thrombosis but a total abdominal hysterectomy, 27%. Last, surgical patients with malignancy have a higher risk of thrombosis as result of their malignancy itself. This risk can manifest itself years before the clinical presentation of the cancer.

In addition to these situation causes for thrombosis, there are now a number of recognized protein defects that increase the risk of thrombosis in surgical patients (Table 20.4). The importance of recognizing these conditions preoperatively is that in the affected patient special attention to thrombosis risk at the time of surgery and postoperatively may temper the risk. By far, the most common molecular defect associated with thrombosis is the factor V Leiden nucleotide polymorphism (20% to 60% of patients with venous thromboembolism, VTE) (G to A mutation at base pair 1691 of coagulation factor V) that results in a protein that is resistant to activated protein C inactivation (i.e., activated protein C resistance) (19,20). The factor V Leiden defect is the most common inherited cause of thrombosis in western populations, approaching 20% of unselected cases and 60% of cases with family histories (21). Further, it is associated with other prothrombotic risk factors. Factor V Leiden is considered a low risk factor for thrombosis. However, when combined with other risk factors or when individuals with the defect are put in high risk for thrombosis situations, it can summate with the other entities increasing thrombosis risk. Some data suggest that patients with the factor V Leiden defect may have early graft closure after coronary artery bypass surgery.

Table **20.4** **Protein basis for increased thrombosis risk**

Table 20.4 Protein basis for increased thrombosis risk
Factor V Leiden (20%–60%)[a] (activated protein C resistance) (sevenfold increased risk for VTE)
Elevated homocysteine (10%)
Prothrombin 20210 (6%) (threefold increased risk for VTE)
Protein C deficiency or defect (<5%) (75% risk for VTE)[b]
Protein S deficiency or defect (3%–4%) (74% risk for VTE)[b]
Dysfibrinogenemias (1%–3%)
Antithrombin (<1%) (50% risk for VTE)[b]

[a]The parenthesis indicates the frequency in patients with VTE.
[b]High risk for VTE.
VTE, venous thromboembolism.

Homocysteine (~10%) is the next most common entity associated with increased risk for thrombosis. Homocysteine levels of 11 or greater are a risk factor for cardiovascular disease. Elevated homocysteine injuries endothelium, producing free radicals, and thus interferes with thromboprotective mechanism on vascular endothelium and promotes atherosclerosis. Patients who have elevations in homocysteine should be treated with oral folate. The third most common risk factor for increased thrombosis risk is a gene mutation in prothrombin, prothrombin 20210 (~6%). This polymorphism in the 3′ untranslated region of the prothrombin gene produces increased amounts of a normal prothrombin, thus tipping the balance towards a prothrombotic state. Like factor V Leiden, both elevations of homocysteine and the prothrombin 20210 mutation are weak isolated risk factors for thrombosis. However, with surgery, their importance summates.

More serious, but less common, protein defects associated with thrombosis are protein C (<5%) and S (3% to 4%) deficiencies (Table 20.4). These protein defects interfere with the major anticoagulant function of the protein C and S systems. Patients with these protein defects and a history of thrombosis may require life-long anticoagulation since they have a 75% risk of having venous thromboembolism. Abnormal fibrinogens (dysfibrinogens) are a heterogeneous group of disorders, some of which carry an increased risk of thrombosis. Antithrombin deficiency or defects give a very serious prothrombotic risk with a 50% likelihood of having venous thromboembolism. Fortunately, these patients are quite rare and constitute less than 1% of all patients seen with thrombosis. Recognition of this defect in a patient with thrombosis requires life-long anticoagulation.

Table **20.5** Medical/hematologic conditions associated with increased risk for thrombosis
Disseminated intravascular coagulation
Heparin-induced thrombocytopenia and thrombosis syndrome
Antiphospholipid syndrome
Thrombotic thrombocytopenic purpura
Hemolytic-uremic syndrome
Myeloproliferative disorders

In addition to the molecular/protein defects that increase a patient's risk o thrombosis, certain medical conditions are also associated with thrombosis. The surgeon needs to be aware of these conditions as well so that special precautions can be made to protect these patients from thrombosis at the time of elective or emergent surgery (Table 20.5). As mentioned above, DIC can be associated with thrombosis. If DIC is seen in a patient with malignancy, special effort is necessary to prevent venous thrombosis that can occur in these individuals. Best prevention for thrombosis in the cancer patient is prophylaxis with low-molecular-weight heparin (22). Another medical condition predisposing to thrombosis is heparin-induced thrombocytopenia and thrombosis syndrome (HITTS). This entity is most commonly seen in patients who have had CPB. A very high percentage of patients after CPB will have antibodies that are positive to heparin. Also, about 1% and 2.5% of patients who get deep venous thrombosis prophylaxis with low-molecular-weight heparin or unfractionated heparin, respectively, will develop HITTS anywhere from 3 to 14 days after completion of therapy. Any patient who presents with new thrombosis postoperatively and who received prophylactic heparin therapy has to be considered to have HITTS until proven otherwise. When recognized, these patients are treated with withdrawal of the heparin and anticoagulation with an alternative anticoagulant such as argatroban or bivalirudin.

Antiphospholipid antibody syndrome is another entity that increases thrombosis risk in surgical patients. These patients can have both arterial and venous thrombosis. The condition is recognized by evidence of antiphospholipid antibodies as determined by measuring antibodies to anticardiolipin or β_2-glycoprotein I and studies for lupus anticoagulants, such as the confirmatory test for the dilute Russell's viper venom time (dRVVT). The diagnosis of antiphospholipid antibody syndrome is made by any one of these 3 assays that are positive for a minimum of 3 months when tested twice. Antiphospholipid antibodies interfere with the anticoagulant nature of annexin II, preventing it from getting to endothelial cell membranes to reduce thrombin formation. Patients with antiphospholipid antibodies are prone to thrombosis and, thus, care needs to be taken to prevent it from occurring. The rare hematologic conditions of thrombotic thrombocytopenic purpura (TTP), a deficiency or antibody to the von Willebrand factor cleaving enzyme, ADAMTS13 (a disintegrin and metalloproteases with a thrombospondin-1-like domain), and hemolytic uremic syndrome (HUS), due to Shiga toxin from *Escherichia coli* 0157:H7, present with severe thrombocytopenia and a microangiopathic hemolytic anemia. Usually, these patients are excluded from surgical intervention. Last, myeloproliferative disorder such as polycythemia vera and essential thrombocytosis are conditions with elevated platelet counts and a high increased risk for thrombosis. A majority of these individuals have a polymorphism in JAK2V617F resulting in constitutive overproduction of RBCs and/or platelets. Prior to surgery, efforts should be made to reduce the elevated platelet or RBC counts as well as provide generous prophylaxis for thrombosis since these patients have a 30% to 40% risk for VTE.

Therapy for thrombosis and its prevention

The best therapy in the patient at increased risk for thrombosis is its prevention. In trial of 4,121 patients undergoing major surgical procedures, the use of low dose unfractionated heparin resulted in a reduction of deep venous thrombosis to only 7.7% of patients versus 24.6% of patients in the untreated control group (23). This landmark study in 1975 established the need for deep vein thrombosis (DVT) prophylaxis in the surgical patient. This study was repeated with low-molecular-weight heparin showing the same as unfractionated heparin (24). In the United States, Medicare recognized that this well-documented treatment was underutilized. It instituted a policy of no hospital reimbursement for management costs of a postoperative venous thrombosis or pulmonary embolism if the patient had not previously received prophylactic anticoagulation. It is beyond the scope of this chapter to discuss the pros and cons of subcutaneous heparin or low-molecular-weight heparin versus compression stockings to prevent postoperative DVT in surgical patients. Both approaches have merit. In preparation for surgery, the patient on anticoagulants should have their oral anticoagulant, warfarin, stopped 5 to 7 days before surgery (10). In its place, subcutaneous low-molecular-weight heparin should be administered up to 24 hours prior to surgery (10). Likewise, as soon as the surgeon determines that the risk for postoperative bleeding has passed, usually 12 to 24 hours postoperatively, subcutaneous low-molecular-weight heparin should be started on the patient with increased thrombosis risk (10). If DVT arises in the postoperative patient, therapy should proceed based upon current treatment protocols for all DVT patients (25). The use of vena cava umbrellas should be reserved for the rare patient who cannot tolerate full anticoagulation (e.g., active gastrointestinal or GI bleed) in the postoperative period. In the patients who require vena cava umbrellas, requests for removable filters should preferentially be made since the presence of the umbrella itself will require life-long anticoagulation (10).

SUMMARY

Evaluation of the surgery patient for bleeding and thrombosis risk follows from the same kind of evaluation of any patient for bleeding and thrombosis. Current diagnostic tools are good for assessing bleeding risk; thrombosis risk, on the other hand, requires a good knowledge of the patient's history as well as the nature of the surgical situation the patient will be in. Much information is available to guide the surgeon in diagnosis and therapy. As in all situations, attention to history and simple laboratory assays makes a difference in providing care to our patients.

REFERENCES

1. Davies E, Ratnoff OD. Waterfall sequence for intrinsic blood coagulation. *Science* 1964;145:1310–1320.
2. Schmaier AH. Principles of hemostasis. In: Schmaier AH, Petruzzelli LM, eds. *Hematology for the medical student*, 1st ed. Baltimore: Lippincott, Williams & Wilkins; 2003:71–77.
3. Gailani D, Broze GJ. Factor XI activation in a revised model of blood coagulation. *Science* 1991;253:909–912.
4. Smith SA, Mutch NJ, Baskar D, et al. Polyphosphate modulates blood coagulation and fibrinolysis. *Proc Natl Acad Sci U S A* 2006;103:903–908.
5. Kannemeier C, Shibamiya A, Nakazawa F, et al. Extracellular RNA constitutes a natural procoagulant cofactor in blood coagulation. *Proc Natl Acad Sci U S A* 2007;104:6388–6393.
6. Maas C, Govers-Riemslag JW, Bouma B, et al. Misfolded protein activate factor XII in humans, leading to kallikrein formation without initiating coagulation. *J Clin Invest* 2008;118:3208–3212.
7. Schmaier AH. Laboratory evaluation of hemostatic and thrombotic disorders. In: Hoffman R, Benz EJ, Shattil SJ, et al. eds. *Hematology basic principles and practice*, 5th ed. Philadelphia: Churchill Livingstone Elsevier; 2009:1877–1884.
8. Schmaier AH. Acquired disorders of blood coagulation. In: Humes HD, ed. *Kelley's textbook of internal medicine*, 4th ed. Philadelphia: Lippincott, Williams & Wilkins; 2000:1718–1723.
9. Schmaier AH. Acquired bleeding disorder. In: Schmaier AH, Petruzzelli LM, eds. *Hematology for the medical student*, 1st ed. Philadelphia: Lippincott, Williams & Wilkins; 2003:99–104.
10. Hirsh J, Gordon G, Albers GW, et al. Executive summary: American College of Chest Physicians evidence-based clinical practice guidelines (8th Edition). *Chest* 2008;133:71–109.
11. Boulis NM, Bobek MP, Schmaier AH, et al. Use of factor IX complex in warfarin-related intracranial hemorrhage. *Neurosurgery* 1999;45: 1113–1118.
12. Deveras RAE, Kessler CM. Reversal of warfarin-induced excessive anticoagulation with recombinant human factor VIIa concentrate. *Ann Intern Med* 2002;137:884–888.
13. Lin J, Hanigan WC, Tarantino M, et al. The use of recombinant activated factor VII to reverse warfarin-induced anticoagulation in patients with hemorrhage in the central nervous system: preliminary findings. *J Neurosurg* 2003;98:737–740.
14. Colman RW, Robboy SJ, Minna JD. Disseminated intravascular coagulation (DIC): an approach. *Am J Med* 1972;52:679–689.
15. Rectenwald JE, Myers DD, Hawley AE, et al. D-dimer, P-selectin and microparticles: novel markers to predict deep venous thrombosis. *Thromb Haemost* 2005;94:1312–1317.
16. Midathada MV, Mehta P, Waner M, et al. Recombinant factor VIIa in the treatment of bleeding. *Am J Clin Pathol* 2004;121:124–137.
17. Bijsterveld NR, Moons AH, Boekholdt M, et al. Ability of recombinant factor VIIa to reverse the anticoagulant effect of the pentasaccharide Fondaparinux in healthy volunteers. *Circulation* 2002;106: 2550–2554.
18. Schmaier AH. Evaluation of thrombosis. In: Schmaier AH, Petruzzelli LM, eds. *Hematology for the medical student*, 1st ed. Philadelphia: Lippincott, Williams & Wilkins; 2003:121–126.
19. Svensson PJ, Dahlback B. Resistance to activated protein C as a basis for venous thrombosis. *N Engl J Med* 1994;330:517–522.
20. Greengard JS, Eichinger S, Griffin JH, et al. Brief report: variability of thrombosis among homozygous siblings with resistance to activated protein C due to an Arg-Gln mutation in the gene for factor V. *N Engl J Med* 1994;331:1559–1562.
21. Bavikatty NR, Killeen AA, Akel N, et al. Association of the prothrombin G20210 A mutation with Factor V Leiden in a midwestern American population. *Am J Clin Pathol* 2000;114:272–275.
22. Lee AY, Levine MN, Baker RI, et al. Randomized comparison of low molecular-weight heparin versus oral anticoagulant therapy for the prevention of recurrent venous thromboembolism in patients with recurrent venous thromboembolism in patients with cancer. *N Engl J Med* 2003;349:146–153.
23. Kakkar VV, Corrigan TP, Fossard DP, et al; An International Multicentre Trial Group. Prevention of fatal postoperative pulmonary embolism by low doses of heparin. *Lancet* 1975;II:46–51.
24. Kakkar VV, Boeckl O, Boneu B, et al. Efficacy and safety of a low-molecular-weight heparin and standard unfractionated heparin for prophylaxis of postoperative venous thromboembolism: European multicenter trial. *World J Surg* 1997;21:2–9.
25. Bates SM, Ginsberg JS. Treatment of deep-vein thrombosis. *N Engl J Med* 2004;351:268–277.

CHAPTER

21

Complications of Nutritional Support

Imad F. Btaiche, Eiichi Miyasaka, and Daniel H. Teitelbaum

Nutritional support can be provided by intravenous (parenteral) or gastrointestinal (enteral) delivery of nutrients. In general, enteral nutrition is less complicated and preferable. However, the development of parenteral nutrition (PN) within the last four decades has allowed critical nutritional support for many patients.

PARENTERAL NUTRITION

PN is the administration of complete and balanced nutrition via the intravenous route to support anabolism and weight maintenance or gain when the gastrointestinal tract cannot or should not be used. Adequate nutrition is essential for patient recovery, and PN is a life-saving therapy in patients with intestinal failure. Conversely, a lack of adequate nutrition may lead to a decline in wound healing and possibly an increase in perioperative complications. However, PN can be associated with many complications, including metabolic, infectious, and technical. Aside from the delivery of PN, good nutritional care requires careful assessment of the patient's nutritional status and a determination of which patients should, or should not, receive PN.

Indications for parenteral nutrition in surgical patients

PN is indicated when the gastrointestinal tract cannot be fully used. This includes patients with significant peritonitis, lack of adequate intestinal length, or a malabsorptive state. Additionally, patients with specific gastrointestinal disorders, including intractable diarrhea, protracted vomiting, enterocolitis, motility disorders, inflammatory bowel disease, enteric fistulae with high output, and bowel obstruction may require parenteral feedings for a prolonged length of time.

Indications for Preoperative Nutrition

In adults, provision of enteral feedings preoperatively for 2 to 3 weeks may reduce postoperative wound infections, anastomotic leakage, hepatic and renal failure, and length of hospital stay (1). Data for PN support is much less clear. The first definitive study to approach this question was the Veteran's Administration (VA) cooperative study, which examined a large number of malnourished patients who required major abdominal or thoracic operations (2). Patients were randomized to preoperative PN (along with a short course of postoperative PN) versus surgery without any PN. Surprisingly, those patients who received PN had higher rates of infectious complications, including pneumonias, urinary tract infections, and wound infections. The only patients with proven benefit from perioperative PN were the ones with severe malnutrition. A meta-analysis of patients receiving PN in the perioperative period showed that PN was associated with a 10% increase in the absolute rate of postoperative complications (3). This finding was confirmed by a more recent meta-analysis of critically ill adults, which demonstrated only a marginal benefit of preoperative PN in mildly or moderately malnourished patients (4). A benefit of preoperative PN was noted only in those patients who were severely undernourished. The European Society of Parenteral and Enteral Nutrition (5) guidelines define severe undernutrition to exist when one of the following criteria are present: weight loss >10% to 15% within 6 months, body mass index (BMI) <18 kg/m^2, subjective global assessment (SGA) Grade C (See section below, visible somatic muscle wasting), or serum albumin <3 g/dL (with no evidence of hepatic or renal dysfunction) (5). The cause of these increased infections has not been definitively determined. However, these studies have had a dramatic effect in reducing the aggressive use of PN in surgical patients, confining the preoperative use to those patients with severe malnutrition.

Indications for Postoperative Nutrition

Use of aggressive postoperative nutritional support is even more controversial (6). In adults, the provision of enteral nutrients may reduce the rate of sepsis and may lower costs. However, enteral intolerance can limit the ability to achieve complete nutritional support (7). These data suggest that, when indicated, postoperative nutrition should be started early, utilizing a combination of PN and enteral nutrition until the gastrointestinal tract fully recovers. The effect of PN on postoperative healing is also unclear, as many studies are contradictory. Because results in the area

Imad F. Btaiche: Department of Pharmacology, University of Michigan Health Systems **Eiichi Miyasaka:** Section of Pediatric Surgery, C.S. Mott Children's Hospital, University of Michigan **Daniel H. Teitelbaum:** Section of Pediatric Surgery, C.S. Mott Children's Hospital, University of Michigan, Ann Arbor, MI 48109-5245

of postoperative nutritional support are not clear, aggressive postoperative feedings are recommended only in those patients who can receive enteral nutrition without complication. Postoperative PN should be restricted to those patients who will not start enteral nutrition for at least 5 to 7 days and when PN therapy is expected for at least 7 days (8,9). In malnourished adult patients when enteral nutrition is not possible, PN should be started 5 to 7 days before elective surgery and continued postoperatively until adequate oral or enteral feeding can be achieved (9).

NUTRITIONAL ASSESSMENT AND MONITORING

As stated earlier, many patients who require operative intervention suffer from malnutrition due either to a variety of feeding disorders or to the underlying disease for which they will need surgery. Nutritional assessment is a critical aspect of the initial evaluation of all surgical patients, and the incidence of malnutrition in surgical patients has been well documented in several reviews. In one review by Mullen et al., 95% of all surgical patients had one abnormal nutritional parameter and 35% had three indicators of malnutrition (10). In addition to adults, pediatric surgical patients may also be at risk for malnutrition. Cameron et al. showed that the prevalence of chronic malnutrition was similarly high at 65%, and the incidence increased to 80% in cardiac surgical infants (11). Clearly, recognizing and categorizing the severity of the malnourished state is the best way to determine which patient will require perioperative nutrition support. Recognition and correction of malnutrition prior to elective surgery may eliminate or reduce the rates of surgical morbidity and mortality. Although a significantly malnourished patient can easily be identified, patients with mild to moderate malnutrition are frequently difficult to identify. Classically, indicators of malnutrition have relied on biochemical and physical parameters. These have included measurements of albumin and morphometric measurements, including triceps skin fold and forearm circumferences. Hypoalbuminemia has long been considered an index of protein depletion and has been shown to be associated with an increased rate of postoperative mortality (12). Unfortunately, low serum albumin levels are not a good indicator of nutritional status and may lead to incorrect classification of the nutritional status (13). Serum prealbumin levels may offer the advantage of a shorter half-life as compared to albumin (about 2 days vs. 20 days, respectively) and thus respond more quickly to nutritional changes. Similar to albumin, prealbumin is a negative acute phase protein and its sensitivity and specificity is affected by stress and other diseases (14). It is reasonable, however, to measure serum prealbumin levels once weekly and follow their trend as a marker of adequate anabolism and nutritional repletion in response to nutrition support. A more reliable modality to define malnutrition is the use of a baseline SGA. Such an assessment is easy to obtain and has a high degree of reliability with regard to the determination of degree of malnutrition (15). An SGA consists of a history and physical examination and should include an evaluation of weight loss (10% for severe malnutrition), anorexia, or vomiting, as well as physical evidence of muscle wasting. Patients at particular risk for malnutrition include those with large open wounds with the concomitant loss of protein and increased metabolic needs, extensive burns, blunt trauma, and sepsis.

MALNUTRITION

Kwashiorkor and marasmus

Classically, malnutrition has been divided into two basic forms, protein-calorie malnutrition, or marasmus, and protein deficiency, or kwashiorkor (Table 21.1). Although these conditions are most prevalent in third-world countries, they may also be manifested in hospitalized patients. The most common clinical example of a marasmic patient is one who has been consuming an inadequate diet for a period of several weeks to months. A common example would be an elderly individual who receives little supportive care, often one with a depressed mental condition. Such a patient, if

Table **21.1** Comparison of marasmus and kwashiorkor

Disease	Clinical Setting	Time to Develop	Clinical Features	Laboratory	Clinical Course	Mortality
Marasmus	↓ Calorie intake	Months or years	Starved appearance, weight <80% of UBW, TSF <3 mm, MAMC <15 cm	Possible normal albumin and transferrin	Reasonably preserved responsiveness to short-term stress	Low, unless related to underlying disease
Kwashiorkor	↓ Protein intake during stress	Weeks	Well-nourished appearance, easy hair pluckability, edema	Low albumin and transferrin decubitus ulcers, skin breakdown	Poor wound healing	High

UBW, usual body weight; TSF, triceps skin fold; MAMC, midarm muscle circumference.

From Khalidi N, Btaiche IF, Kovacevich DS, eds. *The parenteral and enteral nutrition manual*, 8th ed. Ann Arbor, MI: The University of Michigan Hospitals and Health Centers; 2003.

admitted and deprived of any nutritional support, will begin to utilize the remaining somatic muscle to support gluconeogenesis (formation of glucose from noncarbohydrate sources). In this case, the patient will develop a mixed picture of an acute kwashiorkor state over a baseline state of marasmus. The outcome of such patients is notoriously poor (16). Common settings in which such conditions can occur or be aggravated are in the septic, severely burned, or multiple trauma patients. These patients may lose as much as 30 g of nitrogen/day, the equivalent of 2.5 lb of wet muscle weight loss daily. Along with this loss of muscle mass will be a number of adverse complications which directly affect the outcome for surgical patients.

Complications of malnutrition

Impaired healing can result from severe states of malnutrition and potentially lead to disruption of intestinal anastomoses as well as wound dehiscence and infection. Previous studies have shown decreased tensile strength of intestinal anastomoses in malnourished rats, which could be prevented by PN repletion. An effort should be made, when possible, to minimize impaired wound healing by preoperatively nutritionally repleting patients who are *severely* undernourished and by preventing postoperative starvation. Zinc, vitamin C (ascorbic acid), and vitamin A deficiencies may also lead to impaired wound healing and should be corrected. Malnutrition may also lead to an increased risk of respiratory difficulties, such as atelectasis and pneumonia, secondary to decreased strength of respiratory muscles and the inability to cough. The lack of muscle strength probably decreases the patient's forced vital capacity and tidal volume and, therefore, prolongs the need for intubation and mechanical ventilation with their associated complications of pneumothorax, baro-trauma, tracheal stenosis, and sepsis. Early and, if possible, preoperative nutrition support is indicated in the malnourished patient. In critically ill patients with a functional gastrointestinal tract, enteral nutrition should be started early, within 24 to 48 hours of admission to the intensive care unit (ICU), and then advanced to the nutritional goal over the next 48 to 72 hours as patients are hemodynamically stabilized. Early enteral nutrition in critically ill patients has been shown to reduce infectious complications (9). Several investigators have found a marked increase in septic complications in malnourished patients (17). Undernutrition alone results in depressed T-lymphocyte numbers and function (18). Impaired leukocyte function could increase the risk of pneumonia. Recent studies suggest that severe malnutrition can cause breakdown of the intestinal mucosal barrier to bacteria with bacterial translocation from the gut lumen to the portal venous system (19,20). Neutropenia has also been noted with copper deficiency, and impaired neutrophil chemotaxis and phagocytosis have also been found with phosphate deficiency. Impaired body defenses will increase the risk of pneumonia, wound infections, and intracavitary abscesses.

Efficacy of correcting malnutrition

It is important to note that although pneumonia and respiratory failure are the major causes of death for persons who are starved, there is little evidence that nutritional repletion improves pulmonary function and prevents pneumonia (21). One of the best controlled studies to suggest that early nutritional support may help surgical patients is by Sandstrom et al. (22). In this study, patients were randomized to receive postoperative PN versus intravenous dextrose. Patients who did not initiate enteral intake prior to 14 days and who were randomized to receive only dextrose had a 10-fold higher mortality and a two-fold higher rate of sepsis. However, those patients who received PN and were overfed actually had a worse outcome. Thus, judicious use of perioperative nutrition is critical. In fact, based on meta-analyses, correction of malnutrition is indicated only for severely malnourished surgical patients (23). Overly aggressive use of PN may lead to a much higher incidence of complications. In fact, a meta-analysis of the routine use of postoperative PN support suggests that PN is associated with a 10% increase in complications (3). Although PN has numerous associated complications, enteral nutrition is associated with several complications as well. In a detailed meta-analysis comparing enteral nutrition and PN, no advantage was noted other than that the cost of enteral nutrition was ten times lower (24).

METABOLIC COMPLICATIONS OF PARENTERAL NUTRITION

Just as malnutrition may lead to a number of problems with perioperative morbidity, use of PN may be equally or more deleterious. Thus, use of PN requires an extensive understanding of indications of PN, knowledge of proper prescribing, and careful monitoring.

Hyperglycemia

Hyperglycemia is the most common complication associated with PN. Dextrose infusion rate and the patient's underlying conditions determine carbohydrate tolerance. Dextrose oxidation is reduced under stress, such as in critically ill and surgical patients (25). Predisposing factors to hyperglycemia also include sepsis, multiorgan failure, diabetes, acute pancreatitis, and drug therapy that alters glucose metabolism (e.g., corticosteroids, tacrolimus, catecholamine vasopressors).

Stress-induced hyperglycemia is the result of increased endogenous glucose production in response to increased release of counter-regulatory hormones and cytokines that stimulate glycogenolysis and gluconeogenesis. In stressed patients, elevated insulin levels fail, however, to suppress gluconeogenesis or to increase cellular glucose uptake, which results in hyperglycemia. In a small study group ($n = 5$) of low stress postoperative adult patients, dextrose infusion rates up to 7 mg/kg/min were tolerated (26).

Table **21.2** **Consequences of overfeeding**

Source of Overfeeding	Consequences
Total calories	Hepatic steatosis; cholestasis; respiratory decompensation
Dextrose	Hyperglycemia; hypertriglyceridemia; hepatic steatosis; hypercapnia; increased infection risk
Lipid emulsions	Hyperlipidemia; hypertriglyceridemia; hepatic steatosis

However, data from hypermetabolic adult burn patients showed a maximum tolerable glucose infusion rate of 5 mg/kg/min (27). Even lower rates ≤4 mg/kg/min in stressed adult patients are better tolerated. In a retrospective review of 102 nondiabetic adult patients who received PN, hyperglycemia occurred in 49% of patients with dextrose infusion rates >5 mg/kg/min, and 11% of patients developed hyperglycemia with dextrose infusion rates between 4.1 and 5 mg/kg/min. None of the patients who received dextrose infusions ≤4 mg/kg/min had hyperglycemia (28).

Hyperglycemia, if left untreated, can result in serious complications, including fluid and electrolyte imbalances, hyperglycemic hyperosmolar nonketotic coma, and increased infectious risk (see Table 21.2). *In vitro* and animal studies have shown that hyperglycemia can impair neutrophil chemotaxis and adhesion, reduce phagocytosis, and inhibit complement fixation (29,30). Poorly controlled diabetics have shown impaired polymorphonuclear leucocyte function (31) and reduced bactericidal activity (32), with phagocytic function improving with glycemic control (33). Notably, hyperglycemia has been shown to increase the risk for nosocomial and wound infections in surgical diabetic patients (34,35).

Hyperglycemia has been defined as serum glucose concentrations >200 mg/dL (36), and serum glucose concentrations of 150 to 200 mg/dL have been long considered acceptable in stressed patients (37). However, recent data from surgical intensive care patients show that tighter glucose control may be more beneficial in reducing patient morbidity and mortality (38). Van den Berghe et al. conducted a prospective, randomized, controlled study to evaluate the outcomes of intensive and conventional insulin therapy in 1,548 adult surgical ICU patients. Patients were randomized to receive intensive insulin therapy with a goal of serum glucose concentrations of 80 to 110 mg/dL or a conventional insulin therapy to maintain serum glucose concentrations between 180 and 200 mg/dL when serum glucose levels were exceeding 220 mg/dL. Study results showed that patients in the intensive insulin group had a 43% reduction in mortality, a 46% reduction in sepsis, and a 35% reduction in need for prolonged antibiotic therapy, as compared to the conventional insulin treatment group. Patients in the intensive insulin group also had reduced acute renal failure and ventilator dependency. Benefits of intensive insulin therapy on reducing mortality were notable in the long-stay ICU patients (>5 days) (38). A follow-up multivariate logistic regression analysis of results showed that benefits derived from intensive insulin therapy were the result of normoglycemia rather than the insulin dose. Also, a direct correlation was found between blood glucose concentrations and hospital mortality. In the long-stay patients the cumulative hospital mortality was 15% in patients with mean blood glucose concentrations <110 mg/dL, about 27% in those with mean blood glucose concentrations between 110 and 150 mg/dL, and 40% in patients with mean blood glucose concentrations >150 mg/dL (39). These data suggest that even small reductions in blood glucose may have a significant effect on improving patient outcomes. However, the benefits of tight glucose control that were derived from the Van den Berghe study were not replicated in the Normoglycemia in Intensive Care Evaluation—Survival Using Glucose Algorithm Regulation (NICE-SUGAR) study. The NICE-SUGAR study was a large, multicenter, prospective, parallel group, unblinded, randomized, controlled study of 6,104 medical and surgical adult patients admitted to the ICUs of 42 international hospitals. Patients were enrolled in the study if they were expected to require at least 3 days of ICU stay. Patients were randomized to an intensive glucose control group with a goal of serum glucose concentrations of 81 to 108 mg/dL or a conventional group with a goal of serum glucose concentrations of 180 mg/dL or less. Study results showed a significantly higher 90-day mortality rate (primary endpoint) in the intensive glucose control group as compared with the conventional group (27.5% vs. 24.9%, respectively). Further, there was no benefit from intensive glucose control on secondary and tertiary endpoints including days on mechanical ventilation, renal replacement therapy, length of ICU stay, blood transfusions, or bloodstream infections. Severe hypoglycemia, defined as blood glucose concentrations of 40 mg/dL or less, was reported in 6.8% of patients in the intensive insulin group as compared with 0.5% in the conventional group ($p < 0.001$), without any reported permanent sequelae. Although the available results of the NICE-SUGAR study would prompt the adoption of a moderate target for serum glucose concentrations between 144 and 180 mg/dL in critically ill patients, more data from subgroup analyses might provide an explanation of the study findings and of any differences in group effects, especially with the heterogeneous population of critically ill patients (40). Thus far, lower degrees of tight glucose control are now applied to most ICU groups. The American Society for Parenteral and Enteral Nutrition (ASPEN) and Society for Critical Care Medicine (SCCM) 2009 Critical Care Guidelines suggest a range of serum glucose concentrations between 110 and 150 mg/dL as appropriate (9).

In order to avoid hyperglycemia and allow physiologic adaptation to dextrose infusion, dextrose infusion rate in adult PN patients should be started at ≤2 mg/kg/min as a continuous infusion. The rate can thereafter be advanced to the goal over the next few days, based on caloric needs and glucose tolerance to a maximum of 4 mg/kg/min. The dextrose infusion rate should be kept at ≤2 mg/kg/min in patients requiring insulin until glucose control is achieved. A dextrose infusion rate of approximately 2 mg/kg/min is mostly sufficient to suppress gluconeogenesis for a maximal body protein sparing effect. In obese patients (body mass index (BMI), ≥30) the dextrose infusion rate should be calculated based on the adjusted ideal body weight since adipose tissue is not a highly metabolically active tissue (41). Caloric distribution in PN is best maintained at 50% to 60% from dextrose, 20% to 30% from lipids, and 10% to 20% from proteins. If hyperglycemia occurs, a portion of the dextrose may be substituted with lipids until glucose control is achieved without exceeding 60% of the total daily calories from lipids (42).

If a patient is receiving PN, 70% of the average sliding scale insulin dose used can be added to the PN solution and the insulin dose can be adjusted thereafter. However, the normal serum glucose target between 80 and 110 mg/dL proposed by the Van den Berghe et al. study necessitates the use of an insulin drip for the control of severe hyperglycemia (38). This allows titration of the insulin dose based on serum glucose concentrations and provides a safe and effective method of glycemic control, although the practice of intensive insulin therapy has also been associated with increased incidence of hypoglycemia (38,43). Such tight control of glucose should be confined to the ICU setting. Although exogenous insulin increases cellular glucose uptake and normalizes blood glucose levels, insulin does not increase glucose oxidation. As such, little benefit is derived from excessive dextrose infusion at a rate that exceeds the body's glucose oxidative capacity. Instead, excess dextrose is converted to fat, which results in hypertriglyceridemia and fatty liver (hepatic steatosis).

In order that they are provided with adequate calories and not overfed, critically ill patients should ideally have their energy expenditure measured using indirect calorimetry on an average of two to three times weekly instead of relying on caloric estimates (44). Data from indirect calorimetric measurements should be interpreted in relation to specific patient factors. Matching caloric intake to energy expenditure is not always possible. In fact, attempting to adjust the carbohydrate and lipid calories to match the high-energy expenditure during severe hypermetabolism would likely result in intolerance and metabolic complications. In select patients, heavier sedation, better pain control, or wound treatment may be of benefit in reducing energy expenditure. Studies have shown that the use of the β-adrenergic blocker propranolol in burn (45) and head injury (46) patients may attenuate hypermetabolism and possibly reduce catabolism. This therapy, in an ICU setting, may have tremendous benefit and improve outcomes in a number of patients.

Hypoglycemia

Although such symptoms of hypoglycemia as diaphoresis, confusion, and agitation have been reported when PN is abruptly terminated, hypoglycemia is rarely observed in adults; it is more common in children. In a randomized controlled study by Nirula et al., 21 adult patients receiving PN for >24 hours who were started on a clear liquid diet were randomized to abrupt cessation or gradual tapering of PN. No significant difference in nadir glucose levels were seen, and changes in hypoglycemic symptom assessment scores were similar (47). However, a study of children younger than 3 years by Bedorf et al. reported that 55% (6 of 11) developed hypoglycemia (serum glucose concentration <40 mg/dL) within 120 minutes of abrupt discontinuation of PN (48). It should also be noted that 2 out of 10 patients whose PN was gradually tapered off developed hypoglycemia. In adult patients, gradual tapering of PN appears unnecessary; however, weaning children from PN should be done with much greater caution, and capillary blood glucose levels should be monitored at least once within 1 or 2 hours after PN is discontinued.

Hyperlipidemia

Hyperlipidemia in patients receiving PN usually manifests as increased serum triglyceride levels, although other alterations in the plasma lipid profile may also occur. Hypertriglyceridemia associated with PN is mainly the result of excessive fat synthesis from dextrose overfeeding, of excessive lipid infusion, or of impaired lipid clearance (49). Severe hypertriglyceridemia (serum triglyceride concentrations >1,000 mg/dL) may precipitate acute pancreatitis (50).

Dextrose overfeeding (see Table 21.2), not excess lipid infusion, is the main cause of hypertriglyceridemia in patients receiving PN. One-third of glucose is normally converted to fat during lipogenesis. However, the amount of fat generated can be higher with dextrose overfeeding, with formed fat being deposited in the liver or transported from the liver as triglyceride-rich very low-density lipoproteins (VLDLs) (51). In patients receiving PN, several factors cause reduction in lipid emulsion clearance, including sepsis, multiorgan failure (52), obesity, diabetes (53), liver disease (54), renal failure (55), pancreatitis (56), and medications that alter fat metabolism (e.g., cyclosporine, sirolimus, corticosteroids). Propofol, a sedative agent formulated in a 10% lipid emulsion that is commonly used in the ICU, can also cause a dose-dependent elevation in serum triglyceride concentrations (57).

Intravenous lipid emulsions currently marketed in the United States are composed of long-chain triglycerides (LCTs). LCT-based lipid emulsions are available in 10%, 20%, and 30% emulsions that provide 1.1, 2, and 3 kcal/mL, respectively. Following infusion, the lipoprotein lipase (LPL) enzyme hydrolyzes lipid particles in the bloodstream to release fatty acids. The liver lipase enzyme metabolizes lipid remnants in the liver to generate VLDLs and low-density lipoproteins (LDLs). Normally, about 80% of lipids are cleared in 1 hour. However, lipid emulsion clearance is reduced in critically ill patients as a result of stress-induced reduction in LPL activity (58).

The differences in the phospholipid-to-triglyceride (PL/TG) ratio in the various lipid emulsion formulations are the basis for clearance differences between the lipid formulations. The PL/TG ratio of the 10% and 20% lipid emulsions is 0.12 and 0.06, respectively, and of the 30% lipid emulsion 0.06 (30% Liposyn III®) or 0.04 (30% Intralipid®). An excess of phospholipids in the 10% emulsion is believed to result in the formation of abnormal lipoprotein X particles. Lipoprotein X is a large particle made predominantly from phospholipids and cholesterol and has a long half-life of 2 to 4 days (59). The lipoprotein X particles that appear in the blood of patients with the infusion of the 10% lipid emulsions are believed to cause hyperlipidemia by competing for metabolism with the infused lipid emulsion particles (60). A 5-day infusion of the 10% emulsion to postoperative trauma patients resulted in increased plasma phospholipids and cholesterol levels. Although this was not observed with the infusion of the 20% lipid emulsion (61), others have made such observations (62–64). Although the difference has not been shown to alter the clinical course of patients, higher concentrations of lipid emulsions may be less desirable in critically ill surgical patients (65). There are concerns about the possible immunosuppressive effects of the soy-based ω-6 long-chain fatty acid formulations and their proinflammatory characteristics (9). The 30% lipid emulsion is FDA-approved for infusion in total nutrient admixtures (TNA; admixture of amino acids, dextrose, and lipid emulsions in one solution) and is most advantageous in patients with fluid restriction, due to its higher caloric concentration.

In acutely ill patients receiving PN, serum triglyceride concentrations should be monitored at the baseline once the lipid goal is achieved and then once weekly thereafter. If hypertriglyceridemia occurs, dextrose overfeeding should be ruled out first and the dextrose load should be reduced if needed. Reducing the lipid dose may be necessary if hypertriglyceridemia does not improve following the reduction of the dextrose amount. Lipid emulsions should preferably be infused continuously over 24 hours to improve their clearance (66).

Another possible etiology of hypertriglyceridemia is carnitine deficiency; carnitine is essential for the transport of fatty acids into the mitochondria where they undergo oxidation. This state is particularly prevalent in premature patients. Daily lipid infusion should be withheld when the patient's serum is lipemic or when serum triglyceride concentrations are >400 mg/dL. In such cases, the lipid emulsion dose should be given only two to three times weekly. In order to prevent essential fatty acid deficiency, linoleic acid should provide 3% to 4% of daily caloric intake. Practically, providing 500 mL once weekly or 250 mL twice weekly of the 20% lipid emulsion is sufficient to prevent essential fatty acid deficiency in adults.

Fatty acid deficiency is extremely uncommon as long as some supplementation of the PN contains lipids. Nevertheless, withdrawal of lipids will be manifested in skin changes, anemia, thrombocytopenia, and fatty liver.

Respiratory decompensation

Hypercapnia in PN patients can be the result of excess total calories and carbohydrate overfeeding with a subsequent excess production of carbon dioxide (CO_2). The respiratory quotient ($RQ = VCO_2/VO_2$) for carbohydrate, protein, and fat is 1, 0.8, and 0.7, respectively, with carbohydrate oxidation generating the most CO_2 production. Normally, energy-mixed substrates yield an RQ around 0.85 (67). An RQ >1 indicates overfeeding and lipogenesis (68). Dextrose infusion rates >4 mg/kg/min in critically-ill patients may cause an increase in RQ that is >1 (69).

The increased respiratory workload associated with the generation of excess CO_2 production may exacerbate or result in acute respiratory acidosis, respiratory insufficiency, and prolongation of ventilator dependence (70). These deleterious effects may occur within hours of dextrose overfeeding, especially in cachectic patients and those with limited pulmonary reserves (71). In PN patients, keeping dextrose infusion rates ≤4 mg/kg/min and reducing the total caloric delivery will result in lower CO_2 production (66). Although an RQ >1 may reflect excess carbohydrate feeding, an RQ <1 does not exclude overfeeding. This is the case for hypermetabolic patients for whom oxygen consumption and minute ventilation increase with increased CO_2 production (72).

Refeeding syndrome

Refeeding syndrome describes the fluid and electrolyte disturbances, vitamin deficiencies, and glucose intolerance that occur in severely malnourished patients upon rapid initiation of feeding (oral, enteral, or parenteral). Metabolic derangements of the refeeding syndrome can result in cardiac, pulmonary, renal, and neuromuscular complications that can be reflective of severe electrolyte depletion and/or the state of starvation or severe malnutrition. Patients at high risk for refeeding syndrome include those with chronic starvation, significant weight loss, chronic alcoholism, anorexia nervosa, wasting diseases, and malabsorption syndromes (73,74).

Hypophosphatemia, hypokalemia, and hypomagnesemia (see section below) are the three most common and potentially severe electrolyte disturbances that may occur during the refeeding syndrome. Potassium, magnesium, and organic phosphates are primarily intracellular ions and are cofactors in macronutrients metabolism. As a result of significant weight loss, the total body stores of these electrolytes become depleted. Serum concentrations may appear normal at first due to their extracellular shift to maintain homeostasis. As a result of anabolism and increased insulin secretion in response to feeding initiation following starvation, these electrolytes are redistributed intracellularly, resulting in decreased serum concentrations (75). With rapid initiation of carbohydrate feeding, insulin secretion is stimulated and shifts phosphorus and potassium intracellularly. Phosphorus demands are also increased for the synthesis of high-energy phosphates such as adenosine triphosphate (ATP), 2,3-diphosphoglycerate (2,3-DGP), and glycerol-3-phosphate dehydrogenase (G-3PD). With limited phosphorus availability in starved patients, the increased phosphorus demand results in severe hypophosphatemia (76,77). A key to preventing the refeeding syndrome is to first identify patients at highest risk. Once identified, nutrient delivery, especially of carbohydrates, should be started at low amounts and then advanced slowly to the caloric goal over 3 to 5 days. Frequent serum electrolyte monitoring (serum phosphorus, potassium, and magnesium initially monitored one to two times daily) with adequate supplementation of phosphate, potassium, and magnesium before and during feeding is usually necessary to replenish electrolyte stores and maintain normal serum electrolyte levels. Providing additional vitamin supplementation to cachectic patients especially with thiamine 100 mg/day and folic acid 1 mg/day is recommended during the first 5 to 7 days of initiating nutrition support (78).

Electrolyte abnormalities

These issues occur more commonly with PN. Deficiency or excess of any of the electrolytes may happen—the most frequent problems are with sodium, potassium, phosphorus, and magnesium.

Sodium

By far the most common problem encountered is hyponatremia, typically resulting from the administration of hypotonic solutions and to a lesser extent from renal or gastrointestinal sodium losses. Hypotonic PN solutions and excess free water given enterally may lead to lower serum sodium. If serum sodium levels drop below 120 mmol/L, neurologic symptoms can occur; it is imperative to correct the sodium deficiency over a period of time to avoid central pontine myelinolysis (79). A minimum dose of sodium is 1 mEq/kg/d, and in general, most patients can receive 2 to 3 mEq/kg/d. Preventing hyponatremia and other common electrolyte aberrancies is possible with daily laboratory monitoring when starting PN and adjusting nutrient delivery as needed. When a steady state is reached, laboratory parameters can be checked less frequently, three times a week, and then weekly to monthly in chronic PN patients. In the event of any significant change in the PN composition or clinical situations, such as excess emesis and diarrhea, serum sodium levels should be checked more frequently.

Conversely, hypernatremia is the result of dehydration due to inadequate free water intake (either enteral or parenteral) or excess water losses (emesis, stoma output, diarrhea, sweating). Again, neurologic symptoms may occur, especially when serum sodium levels exceeds 160 mmol/L. In this case, the free water deficit is calculated and replaced over a 24- to 48-hour period to prevent complications (79,80). Serum sodium levels should be corrected upward or downward at no faster than 12 mmol/L. The formula for replenishing free water is

$$\text{Free water deficit } (L) \simeq 0.6 \times \text{body weight (kg)} \times [1 - (140/\text{serum sodium})]$$

Potassium

Hypokalemia can occur when there are excess potassium losses or inadequate intake. Potassium is essential in electrical conduction and has a profound effect on muscle function, including that of cardiac muscles. Severe hypokalemia can cause cardiac, neuromuscular, gastrointestinal, metabolic, and renal dysfunction. Hypokalemia may contribute to postoperative ileus in surgical patients, and maintaining normal serum potassium levels postoperatively is essential to restoring intestinal motility. As a patient on PN becomes anabolic and begins to synthesize new proteins, an obligatory requirement exists for intracellular potassium utilization. Intravenous potassium is typically administered in PN at 2 to 4 mEq/kg/d in infants and small children, and 40 mEq/L/d in older children and adults. Higher potassium doses may be required in the early phase of refeeding; the need can be determined by monitoring the patient's serum potassium levels. Replacement may be more rapid when central venous access is available. Continuous electrocardiogram (EKG) monitoring is advised when higher doses are used such as when exceeding potassium infusion of 20 mEq/h in adults. One may anticipate excess potassium losses with emesis and diarrhea or when the patient is treated with loop and thiazide diuretics. In these cases, prophylactic potassium supplementation should be provided to avoid hypokalemia, and serum potassium levels should be monitored more frequently.

Hyperkalemia occurs less frequently and may be due to an error in PN compounding. Patients receiving PN may have an elevated serum potassium level if they are not significantly anabolic and are unable to fully utilize the administered potassium. Other causes of hyperkalemia include decreased renal function, metabolic acidosis, tissue necrosis, and sepsis. Potassium intake should be reduced or withheld in PN and all other sources until hyperkalemia resolves.

Phosphate and Magnesium

Magnesium and phosphate, as well as potassium, are required during an anabolic state and during protein synthesis. Phosphate and magnesium abnormalities are usually noted shortly after initiation of nutritional support. This is due to a rapid production of ATP from depleted stores, which uses up the available phosphate store and shifts it intracellularly (see the section above, titled "Refeeding Syndrome"). It is important to be cognizant of this phenomenon and check serum phosphorus levels frequently after starting enteral or PN in a severely malnourished patient. Severe hypophosphatemia has resulted in respiratory, neuromuscular, and hematologic complications, and even death in cachectic patients following nutritional initiation without adequate phosphorus supplementation (75,81). Hypophosphatemia can also manifest as paresthesia, weakness, and convulsions within a few days of PN initiation (82). Typically, every 1,000 kcal requires about 10 to 15 mmol of phosphates for adequate metabolism.

Conditions leading to hypokalemia may also cause hypomagnesemia (e.g., renal losses and anabolic state), and successful correction of hypokalemia depends on normalizing serum magnesium levels. Hypomagnesemia may cause functional ileus, hyperreflexia, seizures, and cardiac and neuromuscular dysfunction. Typically, an adult PN formulation is supplemented with 1 to 2 g (8 to 16 mEq) of magnesium sulfate daily, in the absence of severe magnesium losses (renal or intestinal) or deficiency.

Acid-base disturbances

Acid-base disturbances in adult patients receiving PN are primarily related to the underlying patient conditions rather than to the PN components. However, excess acetate in PN can lead to metabolic alkalosis (83), and excess chloride can cause metabolic acidosis (84). Acid-base disorders are managed primarily by correcting the underlying problem. However, altering the chloride-to-acetate ratio in PN may be useful in correcting minor acid-base abnormalities. Acetate is converted *in vivo* at a one-to-one molar ratio to bicarbonate. As such, diarrhea and enterocutaneous fistula losses resulting in a bicarbonate deficit can be adjusted by increasing the acetate sources (as sodium or potassium) in PN. Conversely, in patients with high gastric suctioning, increasing the chloride salts (such as sodium or potassium) in PN can compensate for loss of gastric hydrochloric acid.

Vitamins and trace elements

Vitamin deficiencies, especially of water-soluble vitamins, occur in malnourished patients. Dextrose infusion increases thiamine demands since thiamine is a cofactor in the intermediate carbohydrate metabolism. Thiamine deficiency has resulted in Wernicke encephalopathy (85) and lactic acidosis (86). PN supplementation with at least the five trace elements (zinc, selenium, copper, manganese, chromium) is critical, as a number of trace element deficiencies may occur especially in PN-dependent patients with intestinal fluid losses (zinc and selenium lost in diarrhea, enterocutaneous fistulas, short bowel syndrome; see Tables 21.3 and 21.4).

Liver complications

A transient elevation of liver enzymes is common within 1 to 2 weeks of PN initiation, but liver enzymes will return to normal following PN cessation (87). However, prolonged PN can lead to more severe liver toxicities, including steatosis, steatohepatitis, cholestasis, and cholelithiasis.

Hepatic steatosis describes fat accumulation in hepatocytes when liver lipid accumulation exceeds its removal (88). Steatohepatitis describes an advanced stage of severe hepatic inflammation that can rapidly progress to liver fibrosis and cirrhosis (89). Patients with hepatic steatosis are usually asymptomatic, and liver enzymes correlate poorly with the degree of fatty infiltration (90). Steatosis should be ruled out when hepatomegaly, malaise, and abdominal discomfort occur. Although hepatic steatosis in PN patients is primarily the result of dextrose overfeeding (91), other factors, such as lipid overfeeding (92), and deficiencies of carnitine (93), choline (87), and essential fatty acids, may also contribute (94).

Excess calories and imbalance in the carbohydrate-to-lipid ratio in PN can lead to hepatic steatosis (95). Patients who receive dextrose infusions have a much greater tendency (53%) to develop hepatic steatosis compared to only 17% of those who receive a mixed lipid and dextrose solution (30% and 70% of nonprotein calories from lipids and dextrose, respectively) (96). Also, patients who received lipid-free PN developed fatty liver, possibly as a result of essential fatty acid deficiency, and steatosis resolved following lipid supplementation (97). In rare instances of fat overfeeding, fat overload syndrome characterized by hypertriglyceridemia, fatty liver, hepatosplenomegaly, coagulopathy, fever, and multiorgan dysfunction have been described (98).

Avoiding carbohydrate and total calorie overfeeding and providing balanced PN are essential to prevent hepatic steatosis. Up to one-third of total calories can be provided from lipids, carbohydrates should provide no more than 60% of total calories, and the remaining calories should come from proteins.

Carnitine deficiency has been proposed as a cause of hepatic steatosis. Carnitine is an amine that transports LCTs into the mitochondria for oxidation and is not a normal supplement of PN. Carnitine deficiency has been proposed to cause liver fat accumulation (99). However, carnitine deficiency is primarily described in premature infants and is extremely rare in adults. The role of carnitine in enhancing fat clearance and preventing hepatic steatosis remains questionable. The correlation between plasma and tissue carnitine levels is uncertain; patients may have normal plasma carnitine levels and still develop hypertriglyceridemia.

The role of choline deficiency in hepatic steatosis is also unclear. Choline is a quaternary amine that is ubiquitous in diet. It is also derived *in vivo* from methionine metabolism. Deficiency of phosphatidylcholine, a byproduct of choline and a component of lipoprotein synthesis, has been proposed to cause abnormal lipoprotein production and to promote triglyceride accumulation in the liver (100). Although methionine is provided from amino acids in PN, choline deficiency may still occur as intravenous methionine is metabolized differently than it is with enteral

Table 21.3 Requirements and clinical characteristics of some generally recognized micronutrients

Nutrient	Adult Dietary Reference Intakes (DRIs) and Recommended Dietary Allowances (RDAs)[a]	Signs of Deficiency	Laboratory Assay	Adult Dose for Oral Supplementation to Treat Deficiency	Daily Maintenance Requirements for Parenteral Supplementation
Iron	8–18 mg/d (DRIs)	Pallor, fatigue, microcytic anemia	Iron/TIBC ratio, ferritin	2–3 mg/kg/d elemental iron, in 2 to 3 divided doses	1–1.2 mg
Iodine	150 μg/day (RDAs)	Goiter, hypothyroidism	Urine iodine	150–300 μg potassium iodide 400 μg (di-iodotyrosine for endemic goiter)	100 μg
Zinc	8–11 mg/d (RDAs)	Acrodermatitis enteropathica, growth retardation, hair loss, delayed wound healing	Serum and urine zinc	2.5–15 mg/d elemental zinc	2.5–5 mg
Copper	900 μg/d (RDAs)	Hypochromic anemia not responsive to iron, neutropenia, steely hair	Serum copper, ceruloplasmin	2–3 mg/d elemental copper (cupric sulfate)	0.3–0.5 mg
Manganese	1.8–2.3 mg/d (DRIs)	Scaly dermatitis, retarded hair and nail growth, increased prothrombin time (PT) not responsive to vitamin K, hypercalcemia, hyperphosphatemia	Urinary *N*-methyl nicotinamide	2–5 mg/d elemental manganese	0.2–0.3 mg
Chromium	20–35 μg/d (DRIs)	Neuropathy, high free fatty acids, glucose intolerance not responsive to insulin	Glucose tolerance test	200 μg/d	10–15 μg
Selenium	55 μg/d (DRIs)	Cardiomyopathy, muscle pain, weakness, macrocytosis, skin and hair depigmentation, glucose intolerance	Serum selenium, glutathione peroxidase activity	70 μg/d	20–60 μg

[a]Based on the Food and Nutrition Board, Institute of Medicine—National Academy of Sciences, DRIs are reference values that are quantitative estimates of nutrient intakes to be used for planning and assessing diets of healthy people. RDAs are set to meet the needs of almost all (97%–98%) individuals in a group. From Btaiche IF, Khalidi N, Kovacevich DS, eds. *The parenteral and enteral nutrition manual*, 8th ed. Ann Arbor, MI: The University of Michigan Hospitals and Health Centers; 2009.
Food and Nutrition Board, Institute of Medicine-National Academy of Sciences: www.iom.edu.
Daily Requirements for Parenteral Supplementation from ESPEN Guidelines on Parenteral Nutrition: Surgery.

Table 21.4 Vitamin deficiencies/toxicities with clinical characteristics

Vitamin	Deficiency	Toxicity
A	Dry skin, hyperkeratosis, dry conjunctiva	Hepatomegaly, muscle pain, malaise, ophthalmoplegia, fever, icterus, rash, pseudotumor cerebri
B_1 (thiamine)	Beriberi, encephalopathy, heart failure, confusion, decreased tendon reflexes, acidosis	None
B_2 (riboflavin)	Angular stomatitis, cheilosis, atrophy of lingual papillae, glossitis, magenta tongue	Photohemolysis in premature infants
B_6 (pyridoxine)	Personality changes, irritability, depression, filiform hypertrophy of lingual papillae, aphthous stomatitis, nasolabial seborrhea, forehead rash	Sensory neuropathy, degeneration of sensory root Ganglia
B_{12}	Megaloblastic anemia, neurologic symptoms, sore tongue, weakness, neuropsychiatric manifestations	None
K	Elevated prothrombin time	None

administration (101). Limited data are available about the effects of choline supplementation on reversing steatosis in PN patients (102). A pilot study of home PN patients with hepatic steatosis showed that intravenous choline chloride supplementation at 2 g/day in PN for up to 24 weeks was safe and effective in reducing the degree of hepatic steatosis (103). More research, however, is needed to clarify the role of choline in liver disease and before routine choline supplementation to PN can be recommended.

PN-associated cholelithiasis is the result of decreased gallbladder contractility during fasting. In the absence of oral intake or enteral stimulation, there is decreased secretion of cholecystokinin (CCK), a peptide hormone secreted by the duodenum in response to meals to induce gallbladder contractility (104). Fasting PN patients have been observed to have a distended gallbladder and absence of gallbladder contractions, a finding not observed in enterally fed patients (105). As a result of bile stasis, bile accumulation in the biliary tract facilitates cholesterol gallstone formation (106) and calcium bilirubinate precipitation in the form of sludge (107). Biliary sludge, gallstones, and hyperviscous and tenacious bile were recovered during gallbladder surgery to relieve refractory cholestasis in PN-dependent patients (108,109). Patients with short bowel syndrome are especially at increased risk for cholelithiasis and biliary sludge (110). This is due to impaired bile flow, disrupted bile enterohepatic cycling, and canalicular accumulation of toxic bile acids, such as lithocholic acid (111). Although use of cholecystokinin-octapeptide has been suggested in patients receiving a prolonged course of PN, results have been mixed at best (112,113), and a recent study has failed to show efficacy in preventing cholelithiasis in neonates (114).

PN-associated cholestasis (PNAC) occurs primarily in infancy and is less common in older children and adults (115,116). Factors predisposing to PNAC include duration of PN, prematurity, overfeeding, short bowel, bowel rest, and sepsis (117,118). More recently, PNAC has been described in a number of adult patients on long-term PN (119). The etiology of PNAC is unknown. Bowel rest leads to increased intestinal permeability, alteration in gut hormone secretion, reduction in bile flow, decreased bile salt excretion, bacterial overgrowth, bacterial and endotoxin translocation from the gut, and impaired intestinal immunologic mechanisms (120,121). All these factors may contribute to the development of PNAC. Most recently, a derangement in the expression of bile canalicular transport proteins has been shown in a rodent model of PN (122–124). These transport proteins are responsible for the production of bile within the canalicular space, and a loss of this function may well be a major mechanism in the development of PNAC. Liver function tests in patients with PNAC may show increased serum liver transaminases, alkaline phosphatase, bilirubin, and gamma glutamyl transferase concentrations (125). However, a rise in serum conjugated bilirubin concentration >2 mg/dL is considered the most commonly accepted marker of cholestasis. Jaundice occurs with advanced cholestasis (126).

PNAC is reversible if PN is discontinued before irreversible liver damage occurs. Because of the detrimental effects of bowel rest, early initiation of enteral or oral feedings and weaning PN is the best way to prevent PNAC. In addition, it is essential to avoid overfeeding, use balanced sources of calories, cycle PN, and avoid and promptly treat sepsis.

Pharmacologic measures have been used to prevent PNAC, improve bile flow, provide symptomatic relief of cholestasis, and reduce the toxic insults to the liver. Unfortunately, there is little evidence showing definitive efficacy. Ursodeoxycholic acid has been shown to improve bile flow and reduce the clinical signs and symptoms of cholestasis; however, a prospective study in infants (the group most prone to PNAC) failed to demonstrate drug efficacy (127). Cholecystokinin-octapeptide (sincalide) was used in infants to induce gallbladder contraction and improve bile flow (128). In a recently performed controlled trial, however, use of cholecystokinin was not shown to be effective in preventing PNAC (129). Treatment of bacterial overgrowth with oral antibiotics (e.g., metronidazole, gentamicin, neomycin) during prolonged bowel rest may be beneficial in reducing bacterial translocation across the intestinal wall and possibly prevent their potential hepatotoxic effects (130).

The lipid composition within total PN (TPN) has been garnering more attention as a potential contributing factor to the development of PN associated liver disease (PNALD). Traditional lipid emulsions contain mainly omega-6 polyunsaturated fatty acids (sometimes referred to as n-6 PUFA) derived from soy or safflower oils. These n-6 PUFAs have been associated with proinflammatory activity (3,23,131). Some researchers have suggested that the accumulation of n-6 PUFA as well as other products found in commercial products, including phytosterols, contribute to the development of PNAC (4,132). The use of alternative fatty acids, such as medium chain triglycerides, olive oil, or omega-3 fatty acids have been proposed as potential methods for treatment of PNALD. Three small case series report a dramatic improvement in PNALD in patients treated with omega-3 fish oil based lipids (6–8). In addition to these effects, several studies comparing fish oil supplemented TPN to standard soy-based TPN, found shorter postoperative hospital stay (10), decreased severe infectious complications (10), and decreased mortality (11) associated with the former. A larger study showed a trend towards decreased hospital length of stay in the fish oil group, but this did not reach statistical significance (12).

Olive oil or medium chain triglyceride-based lipid formulations have also been examined in smaller, short-term clinical trials. While results indicate that these formulations are safe to administer, there are conflicting findings as to whether there is a real clinical benefit in terms of reduced infectious complication rate or shorter hospital stay. At this point, more research is needed to clarify the mechanism of action of these various lipid formulations and their clinical effects.

Short bowel syndrome patients with end-stage liver disease may benefit from combined liver and bowel transplantation. Early referral of short bowel syndrome patients at high risk for liver complications for bowel transplantation may possibly become a viable life-saving option before irreversible liver damage occurs (133).

COMPLICATIONS OF NUTRITION SUPPORT DELIVERY

Delivery systems depend on the route of nutritional support—parenteral or enteral. In addition, there are a limited number of broad categories of these delivery problems, including mechanical, infectious, and thrombotic complications for the intravenous route, and mechanical and infectious for the enteral route (Tables 21.5 and 21.6).

Parenteral nutrition

Mechanical

Although PN can be delivered via the peripheral route, it has several limitations, including osmolarity-induced thrombosis and phlebitis, which limits the concentration of dextrose to 10% in adolescents and adults and 12.5% in infants and small children, thus limiting the total number of calories via this route. PN via central vein infusion is thus preferred. Central venous access is usually obtained via a percutaneous route to the internal jugular or subclavian or the common femoral veins. More commonly, access may be obtained by peripherally inserted central catheters (PICC) (134). Needle injury to the vein or an adjacent artery is rare but does occur, especially in unskilled hands (135). Malposition of the catheter can lead to problems as well. This includes cardiac injury, pericardial effusion and tamponade, and arrhythmias. Additionally, if the catheter is not located centrally, these hypertonic solutions can result in thrombotic complications. Malpositioning occurs frequently with subclavian access with the catheter tip ending in the ipsilateral jugular vein or the contralateral innominate. Therefore, it is mandatory to check the catheter position radiographically before usage—either with fluoroscopy or static images. Pneumothorax occurs in 1% to 2% of cases of central venous catheter insertion; this usually occurs when obtaining subclavian access and less commonly with the internal jugular vein. This is due to transgression of the pleural space and puncture of lung apex (136). Another complication of malpositioning is the pinch-off syndrome (137,138). In this condition, a catheter placed into the subclavian vein is pinched between the first rib and clavicle due to it being inserted too medially. It may manifest itself as catheter occlusion depending on body position or as the inability to aspirate blood. If clinically suspected, it should be confirmed by chest radiography and removed with insertion of a more laterally placed device. Failure to replace such a line may lead to catheter disruption and embolus of the distal end. The details of proper central venous access insertion are beyond the scope of this section, but Table 21.5 contains a list of the potential complications.

Table 21.5 Potential complications of central venous access
Pneumothorax
Hemothorax
Subclavian artery/vein injury
Cardiac injury/arrhythmias
Carotid artery injury
Catheter malposition
Catheter embolism
Thromboembolism
Thoracic duct injury
Lung injury
Nerve injury
Air embolism

Infectious

Infectious complication rates associated with PN range from 7% to 27% (139). If proper sterile and aseptic techniques are not used while obtaining central venous access, acute catheter infections can occur. It is vital to perform placement with gown, gloves, and mask. This is especially true when performing tunneled catheter access for prolonged nutritional support. Care must be taken when accessing these catheters as well. Use of central venous catheters (CVC) for multiple drugs and blood draws, as well as PN, has been shown to increase infectious complications (140,141). In fact, when a formal protocol for catheter insertion and care is instituted, a dramatic reduction in catheter infections can be seen. In one prospective study, the rate of catheter infections declined from 11.3/1,000 catheter days to 1.6/1,000 catheter days over the 4-year period in which these methods were used (142). It appears that multiple central venous lumens may predispose patients to a higher risk of infection, but this association is not proven (143). PICCs did not have a significantly lower incidence of infection; however, PICCs have been associated with higher rates of thrombophlebitis (144).

Catheter infections may occur from one of three sources: the insertion site, the hub, or seeded via the bloodstream. The hub has often been considered the most common source of CVC infections, and great care must be used to protect this site when gaining access to these catheters (145). Infections secondary to bacteria from around the entrance site include skin contaminants such as staphylococci or streptococci (146). These organisms can colonize the fibrin sleeve that develops around the catheter tip and start proliferating. Other infections are a result of seeding from other foci, such as bacterial translocation, and may be Gram-negative or enteric in nature (147). One of the most common sources of

Table 21.6 Potential complications of enteral feeding and preventive interventions

Complication	Possible Reasons	Suggested Treatment
Gastrointestinal		
Diarrhea (6–8 loose, watery stools per day)	Osmotic overload	• Review medications for hypertonic elixirs, sorbitol-containing oral liquid medications, and antacids • Dilute elixirs and change to nonsorbitol-containing oral liquid medications • Provide continuous feeding rather than bolus • May require judicious use of antidiarrheal medication
	Lactose intolerance	• Change formula to lactose-free • Monitor lactose intake if also taking oral diet
	Contaminated formula	• Change bag and tubing every 24 hours
	Nervous tension	• Promote restful environment
	Bacterial overgrowth; oral medications	• Review oral medications, especially for antibiotics and H_2 receptor antagonists for possible side effects
	Intestinal infection	• Rule out and treat *Clostridium difficile* infection
	Low residue feedings	• Use of fiber-enriched formula may be helpful
Nausea	Volume overload	• Decrease total volume/flow rate
Vomiting	Obstruction, delayed gastric emptying, drug-induced	• Rule out obstruction • Evaluate medication profile
Cramping	Intolerance due to rapid administration	• Decrease total volume/flow rate
Delayed gastric emptying	Diabetes, gastric surgery, trauma, sepsis	• Check gastric residuals every 4 hours and return up to 200 mL into the stomach • If residuals >200 mL, hold tube feeding for 1 hour and recheck • May also consider small bowel feeding
Constipation	Insufficient fluid intake	• Increase fluid intake
	Decreased bowel mobility	• Increase physical activity as tolerated
	Low residue feedings	• Use of fiber-enriched formula may be helpful
Metabolic		
Altered glucose, electrolyte, LFTs, and renal function tests	Excess or insufficient administration; prolonged administration of tube feeding containing low sodium; excessive free water	• Monitor glucose, especially in diabetics and in elderly • Sudden glucose intolerance may indicate sepsis • Measure electrolytes and input and outputs • Weigh regularly • Reassess appropriateness of feeding formula • Reduce free water requirements
Dehydration	Insufficient free water	• Increase fluid intake • Administer additional free water each day based on body weight • Monitor input and output
	Diarrhea	• See gastrointestinal complications
	Hyperglycemia	• Monitor glucose, especially in elderly and diabetic patients
Overhydration	Excess fluid administration; renal failure	• Decrease volume of fluid administered • Monitor input and output • Reassess appropriateness of feeding formula; switch to a calorie dense formula
Mechanical		
Dislodged tube	Confused patient	• Restrain patient, bridle tube, place decoy tube, or place permanent feeding tube
Obstructed tube	Inadequate flushing	• Flush tubes with 5–30 mL every 4 hours, after checking gastric residuals, medication administration, and stopping feeding
	Incompatible medications	• Administer medication individually; do not add medications to feeding bag
	Tablets	• Crush medications well or use liquid forms • Have patient take tablet orally, if possible • Suggested treatment: instill in tube a mixture of one crushed tablet of Viokase® with one crushed tablet of sodium bicarbonate dissolved in 5 mL of warm water; clamp tube for 5–10 minutes, then gently flush tube
Aspiration	Rapid administration of feeding	• Decrease administration flow rate • Check gastric residuals every 4 hours • Hold tube feeding if gastric residual volume >200 mL on two successive checks, hold feeding for 1 hour and recheck residuals
	Incorrect patient position	• Raise head of bed at least 30 to 45 degree during continuous feeding and 1 hour after and during bolus feedings
	Tube malposition	• Confirm placement with low upright chest x-ray • Be aware that a feeding tube can come into the pharynx with coughing or other activity; if in doubt, check by aspiration, insufflation, or x-ray

From Btaiche IF, Khalidi N, Kovacevich DS, eds. *The parenteral and enteral nutrition manual*, 9th ed. Ann Arbor, MI: The University of Michigan Hospitals and Health Centers; 2009.

CVC infections is the hub itself. In one study, the majority of CVC infections were due to an infected hub, with negative skin cultures (145). Although tunneling of the catheter was initially thought to reduce the rate of CVC infections, this does not appear to reduce infection rates (148).

Fungal infections are dreaded problems, as they are associated with higher mortality, especially in immunocompromised adults (149). In general, a positive fungal culture will require catheter removal as they are otherwise recalcitrant to therapy (150). Attempts to clear a fungal infection are only occasionally successful and often result in death. For most bacterial infections, if the patient is clinically not in septic shock, treating through the catheter with antibiotics is appropriate (151,152). This applies to silastic catheters; temporary polyvinyl chloride lines, however, must be removed. In general, bacterial infections will clear from a silastic catheter 80% to 90% after the first infection and less frequently with subsequent infections (153). Lack of clearance requires removal of the catheter. Treatment failure is much more frequently seen in the presence of abscess, immunocompromised status, and the organisms *Pseudomonas aeruginosa* and *Candida albicans*. Data from a series of pediatric patients with short bowel syndrome suggest that these populations are at highest risk for catheter infections (154,155). Patients who manifest with a catheter infection along the subcutaneous track require catheter removal, as antibiotics are generally ineffective in these cases.

The usual workup of a patient on PN who develops an acute, unexplained fever should include a blood culture. The clinical practice guidelines for the diagnosis and management of intravascular catheter-related infection by the Infectious Diseases Society of America recommend that paired blood samples are drawn from the suspected catheter and a peripheral vein for culture. If a blood sample cannot be drawn from a peripheral vein, then two blood samples should be drawn from different catheter lumens. A definitive diagnosis of catheter-related blood stream infection (CRBSI) should be based on the finding of the same organism that grows from at least one percutaneous blood culture and from a catheter tip culture; alternatively, two blood samples should be drawn one from the catheter hub and from a peripheral vein, so that, when cultured, they meet the CRBSI criteria for quantitative blood cultures or differential time to positivity (156). Empiric antibiotic therapy may be used if the patient appears septic. Most fevers are due to some other source; however, if fever persists, a catheter change over a wire (for temporary lines) with a quantitative or semiquantitative culture of the catheter tip should be performed. Newer catheters that are impregnated with antibiotics may reduce the incidence of infections (157).

Recent data have shown tremendous benefit in prevention of central venous line infections with the use of ethanol lock therapy (158). A retrospective study showed that use of a 70% ethanol lock therapy was able to both treat over 80% of central venous line infections in a pediatric hematology oncology setting. A more recent paper has shown that this approach can also be used to prevent the development of such infections (159).

Thrombotic

Chronic indwelling central catheters are associated with development of thrombi. These may present acutely with ipsilateral limb swelling and inability to infuse solutions. Fortunately, they rarely lead to a pulmonary embolism. Treatment by catheter removal and replacement in an alternate site is usually sufficient. Unfortunately, in patients with long-term dependence on PN, this may lead to loss of access sites and, with no access, loss of nutrition. Some advocate the use of anticoagulation therapy in low doses (e.g., warfarin or urokinase) to prevent these complications, with some success (160,161); however, there is no evidence to support the routine use of anticoagulation to prevent CVC-associated venous thrombosis (5). The catheter itself may also become occluded due to thrombosis. Such problems may be treated with intracatheter lytic therapy. Catheters that have been in place for longer periods of time may also suffer occlusion from calcium deposits or lipid deposits, which may respond to dilute infusion of hydrochloric acid or ethanol (162).

Enteral nutrition

Like parenteral administration, enteral delivery of nutrition is associated with a wide number of complications (Table 21.6).

Mechanical

Enteral nutritional support is usually obtained by some form of access to the gastrointestinal tract. For relatively short-term support, temporary tubes via the nose or mouth are used. These tubes can irritate and damage the mucosa of the nasal passage, causing rhinorrhea, epistaxis, and a blockage of the sinuses, leading to sinusitis. A well-described source of fevers of unknown origin in a patient with a long-standing nasoenteric tube is maxillary sinusitis. This is best treated by removal of the tube, nasal decongestant sprays, and occasional drainage of the sinus. Occasionally, if the feeding tube is not secured appropriately, the cartilage of the anterior nares may be damaged. Inflammation around the eustachian tubes in the nasopharynx may lead to otitis media. To avoid these problems, the newer enteral feeding tubes are smaller and less rigid; however, these smaller tubes may carry an increased risk of being positioned in the tracheobronchial tree, especially in an obtunded or sedated patient (163). To identify this problem before damage occurs, it is necessary to obtain radiologic confirmation of the tube position prior to initiating feeds. Auscultatory confirmation alone, though a helpful adjunct, is not adequate.

In certain patients with gastric emptying problems or reflux, postpyloric tubes are used. These are placed via the nares and have weighted tips that allow them to be carried past the pylorus into the duodenum with peristaltic action

(164). These tubes must be marked after confirming placement as they may be dislodged. Occasional complications noted with these tubes have been damage to the esophagus or stomach with gastritis and perforations. These occur more often with the more rigid tubes. Acute gastric distention may also occur, especially in patients receiving nasogastric bolus feeding or with gastroparesis. This can lead to vomiting and aspiration (see the next section) as well as perforation of the stomach. Additionally, acute distention of the stomach may cause hypotension from a vagal response. To avoid this, the stomach should be aspirated periodically to ensure that it is emptying. Occasionally, medications may be required to enhance gastric motility or a change to a postpyloric tube may be called for.

Long-term enteral access is usually obtained surgically. Access can be either to the stomach or to the jejunum, depending on the patient's specific needs. Technical complications from the operation may occur. These tubes may also be malpositioned and dislodged, requiring replacement. In the past 20 years most enteral feeding tubes have been placed using minimally invasive techniques [percutaneous endoscopic gastrostomy (PEG) or laparoscopic] (165,166). Early dislodgement of a PEG may cause the stomach to pull away from the abdominal wall and lead to peritonitis (165). After 3 months the stomach is generally well adhered to the abdominal wall. When these tubes become dislodged, especially in children, the access hole shrinks fairly rapidly, often within a few hours. The caregivers and patients must be instructed to take immediate action to replace the tube if this occurs.

Infectious

Aspiration is the most feared complication from enteral nutrition (167). This can result from either a primary tube malposition in the tracheobronchial tree or from reflux/emesis. Aspiration of stomach contents may be particularly harmful as the acid leads to severe pneumonitis and a capillary leak into the alveoli, causing the adult respiratory distress syndrome (ARDS). Although enteral feedings are clearly less expensive than PN, complications in the two groups are not dissimilar. In a recent meta-analysis examining complications by these two routes, complication rates were the same in both groups (24). Although postpyloric feedings have been advocated in the early postoperative period (7), this may not have as great an advantage as initially perceived. In fact, the incidence of aspiration does not significantly differ for patients in relation to whether they are receiving postgastric or intragastric feedings (168,169). In cases where gastric acid secretion has been controlled with histamine receptor blocking drugs or proton pump inhibitors, the stomach contents become colonized with Gram-negative bacteria; aspiration of this would potentially lead to a bacterial pneumonia. These complications significantly prolong hospital and intensive care stays, may lead to mortality, and certainly lead to increased health care costs. Thus, taking precautions to avoid them should be part of routine and protocol driven care.

As mentioned previously, sinusitis and otitis media can occur in patients with nasal tubes. Sinusitis is more common and is seen almost universally with these tubes. It may present as unexplained fevers in patients or with nasal discharge. Using smaller caliber tubes has decreased but not eliminated this problem. A computerized tomography (CT) scan of the head is frequently used to make this diagnosis. Treatment consists of moving the tube to the other side and employing nasal sprays and antibiotics. If longer term nutritional support is deemed necessary, consideration should be given to surgical access.

SUMMARY

Advances in nutritional science over the last four decades have improved the care of countless patients. The management of nutrition can have complications, however, in the provision of too much or too little of any nutrient or supplement, as well as mechanical or infectious complications of the delivery mechanism. Knowledge of these complications is critical to proper planning and patient management.

REFERENCES

1. Kudsk K, Croce M, Favian T, et al. Enteral versus parenteral feeding. Effects on septic morbidity after blunt and penetrating abdominal trauma. *Ann Surg* 1992;215(5):503–511.
2. Buzby G. Perioperative total parenteral nutrition in surgical patients. The Veterans Affairs Total Parenteral Nutrition Cooperative Study Group. *N Engl J Med* 1991;325(8):525–532.
3. Klein S, Kinney J, Jeejeebhoy K, et al. Nutrition support in clinical practice: review of published data and recommendations for future research directions. *JPEN J Parenter Enteral Nutr* 1997;21:133–156.
4. Heyland DK, MacDonald S, Keefe L, et al. Total parenteral nutrition in the critically ill patient: a meta-analysis. *JAMA* 1998;280(23):2013–2019.
5. Braga M, Ljungqvist O, Soeters P, et al. ESPEN guidelines on parenteral nutrition: surgery. *Clin Nutr* 2009;28(4):378–386.
6. Minard G, Kudsk KA. Postoperative nutrition in surgery for major trauma. *Curr Opin Clin Nutr Metab Care* 1998;1(1):35–39.
7. Boulanger BR, Brennemann FD, Rizoli SB, et al. Insertion of a transpyloric feeding tube during laparotomy in the critically injured: rationale and plea for routine use. *Injury* 1995;26(3):177–180.
8. August D, Teitelbaum DH. Guidelines for the use of parenteral and enteral nutrition in adult and pediatric Patients. *JPEN J Parenter Enteral Nutr* 2002;26(1):1SA–137SA.
9. McClave SA, Martindale RG, Vanek VW. Guidelines for the provision and assessment of nutrition support therapy in the adult critically ill patient: Society of Critical Care Medicine (SCCM) and American Society for Parenteral and Enteral Nutrition (ASPEN). *JPEN J Parenter Enteral Nutr* 2009;33:277–316.
10. Mullen JL, Buzby GP, Waldman MT. Prediction of operative morbidity and mortality by preoperative nutritional assessment. *Surg Forum* 1979;30:80.
11. Cameron JW, Rosenthal A, Olson AD. Malnutrition in hospitalized children with congenital heart disease. *Arch Pediatr Adolesc Med* 1995; 149(10):1098–1102.
12. Merritt RJ, Blackburn GL. Nutritional assessment and metabolic response to illness of the hospitalized child. In: Suskind RM, ed. *Textbook of Pediatric Nutrition*. New York: Raven Press; 1981:285–307.
13. Baker J, Detsky A, Wesson D. Nutritional assessment: A comparison of clinical judgement and objective measurements. *N Engl J Med* 1982; 306:969–972.
14. Ingenbleek Y, Young VR. Significance of transthyretin in protein metabolism. *Clin Chem Lab Med* 2002;40:1281–1291.
15. Detsky JM, Baker JP, O'Rourke K, et al. Perioperative parenteral nutrition: A meta-analysis. *Ann Intern Med* 1987;107:195–203.

16. Bistrian BR. Nutritional assessment and therapy of protein–calorie malnutrition in the hospital. *J Am Diet Assoc* 1977;71(4):393–397.
17. Bistrian BR. Interaction of nutrition and infection in the hospital setting. *Am J Clin Nutr* 1977;30(8):1228–1235.
18. Keenan RA, Moldawer LL, Yang RD, et al. An altered response by peripheral leukocytes to synthesize or release leukocyte endogenous mediator in critically ill, protein-malnourished patients. *J Lab Clin Med* 1982;100(6):844–857.
19. Reynolds JV, O'Farrelly C, Feighery C, et al. Impaired gut barrier function in malnourished patients. *Br J Surg* 1996;83(9):1288–1291.
20. Wiren M, Soderholm JD, Lindgren J, et al. Effects of starvation and bowel resection on paracellular permeability in rat small-bowel mucosa in vitro. *Scand J Gastroenterol* 1999;34(2):156–162.
21. Torosian MH. Perioperative nutrition support for patients undergoing gastrointestinal surgery: critical analysis and recommendations. *World J Surg* 1999;23(6):565–569.
22. Sandstrom R, Drott C, Hyltander A, et al. The effect of postoperative intravenous feeding (TPN) on outcome following major surgery evaluated in a randomized study. *Ann Surg* 1993;217(2):185–195.
23. Group TVATPNCS. Perioperative total parenteral nutrition in surgical patients. *N Engl J Med* 1991;325(No. 8):525–532.
24. Braunschweig C, Levy P, Sheean P, et al. Enteral compared with parenteral nutrition: A meta-analysis. *Am J Clin Nutr* 2001;74(4):534–542.
25. Bjerke HS, Shabot MM. Glucose intolerance in critically ill surgical patients: relationship to total parenteral nutrition and severity of illness. *Am Surg* 1992;58:728–731.
26. Wolfe RR, O'Donnell TF, Stone MD, et al. Investigation of factors determining the optimal glucose infusion rate in total parenteral nutrition. *Metabolism* 1980;29:892–900.
27. Burke JF, Wolfe RR, Mullany CJ, et al. Glucose requirements following burn injury. *Ann Surg* 1979;190:274–285.
28. Rosmarin DK, Wardlaw GM, Mirtallo J. Hyperglycemia associated with high, continuous infusion rates of total parenteral nutrition dextrose. *Nutr Clin Pract* 1996;11:151–156.
29. Hostetter MK. Perspectives in diabetes: handicaps to host defense: effects of hyperglycemia on C3 and Candida albicans. *Diabetes* 1990;39: 271–275.
30. Van Oss CJ, Border JR. Influence of intermittent hyperglycemic glucose levels on the phagocytosis of microorganisms by human granulocytes in vitro. *Immunol Commun* 1978;7:669–676.
31. Kjersem H, Hilsted J, Madsbad S, et al. Polymorphonuclear leucocyte dysfunction during short term metabolic changes from normo- to hyperglycemia in type 1 (insulin dependent) diabetic patients. *Infection* 1988;16:215–221.
32. Rayfield EJ, Ault MJ, Keusch GT, et al. Infection and diabetes: the case for glucose control. *Am J Med* 1982;72:439–450.
33. Bagdade JD, Nielson KL, Bulger RJ. Reversible abnormalities in phagocytic function in poorly controlled diabetic patients. *Am J Med Sci* 1972;263:451–456.
34. Furnay AP, Zerr KJ, Grunkemeier GL, et al. Continuous intravenous insulin infusion reduces the incidence of deep sternal wound infection in diabetic patients after cardiac surgical procedures. *Ann Thorac Surg* 1999;67:352–362.
35. Pomposelli JJ, Baxter JK, Babineau TJ, et al. Early postoperative glucose control predicts nosocomial infection rate in diabetic patients. *JPEN J Parenter Enteral Nutr* 1998;22:77–81.
36. McCowen KC, Malhotra A, Bistrian BR. Stress-induced hyperglycemia. *Crit Care Clin* 2001;17:107–124.
37. Golden SH, Peart-Vigilance C, Kao WH, et al. Perioperative glycemic control and the risk of infectious complications in a cohort of adults with diabetes. *Diabetes Care* 1999;22:1408–1414.
38. Van den Berghe G, Wouters PJ, Weekers F, et al. Intensive insulin therapy in the critically ill patients. *N Engl J Med* 2001;345(19):1359–1367.
39. Van Den Berghe G, Wouters PJ, Bouillon R, et al. Outcome benefit of intensive insulin therapy in the critically ill: insulin dose versus glycemic control. *Crit Care Med* 2003;31:359–366.
40. Finfer S, Chittock DR, Su SY, et al. The NICE-SUGAR Study Investigators. Intensive versus conventional glucose control in critically ill patients. *N Engl J Med* 2009;360:1283–1297.
41. Amato P, Keating KP, Quercia RA, et al. Formulaic methods of estimating caloric requirements in mechanically ventilated obese patients: a reappraisal. *Nutr Clin Pract* 1995;10:229.
42. Btaiche IF, Khalidi N. Metabolic complications of parenteral nutrition in adults, part 1. *Am J Health Syst Pharm* 2004;61:1938–1949.
43. Brown G, Dodek P. Intravenous insulin nomogram improves blood glucose control in the critically ill. *Crit Care Med* 2001;29:1714–1719.
44. Hunter DC, Jaksic T, Lewis D, et al. Resting energy expenditure in the critically ill: estimations versus measurements. *Br J Surg* 1988;75(9): 875–878.
45. Herndon DN, Hart DW, Wolf SE, et al. Reversal of catabolism by betablockade after severe burns. *N Engl J Med* 2001;345:1223–1229.
46. Chiolero RL, Breitenstein E, Thorin D, et al. Effects of propranolol on resting metabolic rate after severe head injury. *Crit Care Med* 1989;17: 328–334.
47. Nirula R, Yamada K, Waxman K. The effect of abrupt cessation of total parenteral nutrition on serum glucose: a randomized trial. *Am Surg* 2000;66(9):866–869.
48. Bendorf K, Friesen CA, Roberts CC. Glucose response to discontinuation of parenteral nutrition in patients less than 3 years of age. *JPEN J Parenter Enteral Nutr* 1996;20(2):120–122.
49. Jeejeebhoy KN, Anderson GH, Nakhooda AF, et al. Metabolic studies in total parenteral nutrition with lipid in man. Comparison with glucose. *J Clin Invest* 1976;57:125–136.
50. Cameron JL, Capuzzi DM, Zuidema GD, et al. Acute pancreatitis with hyperlipemia: evidence of persistence defect in lipid metabolism. *Am J Med* 1974;56:482–487.
51. Aarsland A, Chinkes D, Wolfe RR. Hepatic and whole-body fat synthesis in humans during carbohydrate overfeeding. *Am J Clin Nutr* 1997;65:1774–1782.
52. Samra JS, Summers LK, Frayn KN. Sepsis and fat metabolism. *Br J Surg* 1996;83:1186–1196.
53. Garber AJ, Vinik A, Creeps SR. Detection and management of lipid disorders in diabetic patients. *Diabetes Care* 1992;15:1068–1073.
54. Muscaritoli M, Cangiano C, Cascino A, et al. Exogenous lipid clearance in compensated liver cirrohsis. *JPEN J Parenter Enteral Nutr* 1986;10:599–603.
55. Attman PO, Samuellson O, Alaupovic P. Diagnosis and classification of dyslipidemia in renal disease. *Blood Purif* 1996;14:49–57.
56. Carmen JL. Lipid abnormalities and acute pancreatitis. *Hosp Pract* 1977;12:95–101.
57. Eddleston JM, Shelly MP. The effect on serum lipid concentrations of a prolonged infusion of propofol. Hypertriglyceridaemia associated with propofol administration. *Intensive Care Med* 1991;17:424–426.
58. Tsuguhiko T, Mashima Y, Yamamori H, et al. Intravenous intralipid 10% vs 20% hyperlipidemia and increase in lipoprotein X in humans. *Nutrition* 1992;8:155–160.
59. Messing B, Peynet J, Poupon J, et al. Effect of fat-emulsion phospholipids on serum lipoprotein profile during 1 mo of cyclic total parenteral nutrition. *Am J Clin Nutr* 1990;52:1094–1100.
60. Carpentier YA. Intravascular metabolism of fat emulsions. *Clin Nutr* 1989;8:115–125.
61. Roulet M, Wiesel PH, Pilet M, et al. Effects of intravenously infused egg phospholipids on lipid and lipoprotein metabolism in postoperative trauma. *JPEN J Parenter Enteral Nutr* 1993;17:107–112.
62. Haumont D, Richelle M, Deckelbaum RJ, et al. Effect of liposomal content of lipid emulsions on plasma lipid concentrations in low birth weight infants receiving parenteral nutrition. *J Pediatr* 1992;121: 759–763.
63. Kalfarentzos F, Kokkinis K, Leukaditi K, et al. Comparison between two fat emulsions: Intralipid 30 cent vs intralipid 10 cent in critically ill patients. *Clin Nutr* 1998;17:31–34.
64. Nordenstrom J, Thorne A. Comparative studies on a new concentrated fat emulsion: Intralipid 30% vs. 20%. *Clin Nutr* 1993;12:160–167.
65. Druml W, Fischer M, Ratheiser K, et al. Use of intravenous lipids in critically ill patients with sepsis without and with hepatic failure. *JPEN J Parenter Enteral Nutr* 1998;22:217–223.
66. Abbott WC, Grakauskas AM, Bistrian BR, et al. Metabolic and respiratory effects of continuous and discontinuous lipid infusions. Occurrence in excess of resting energy expenditure. *Arch Surg* 1984;119: 1367–1371.
67. Ireton-Jones CS, Turner WWJ. The use of respiratory quotient to determine the efficacy of nutrition support regimens. *J Am Diet Assoc* 1987;87:180–183.
68. Elia M, Livesey G. Theory and validity of indirect calorimetry during net lipid synthesis. *Am J Clin Nutr* 1988;47:591–607.
69. Guenst JM, Nelson LD. Predictors of total parenteral nutrition-induced lipogenesis. *Chest* 1994;105:553–559.
70. Covelli HD, Black JW, Olsen MS, et al. Respiratory failure precipitated by high carbohydrate loads. *Ann Intern Med* 1981;95:579–581.
71. Aguilaniu B, Goldstein-Shapses S, Pajon A, et al. Muscle protein degradation is severely malnourished patients with COPD subject to short-term TPN. *JPEN J Parenter Enteral Nutr* 1992;16:248–254.

72. Rodriguez JL, Askanazi J, Weissman C, et al. Ventilatory and metabolic effects of glucose infusions. *Chest* 1985;88:512–518.
73. Brooks MJ, Melnik G. The refeeding syndrome: an approach to understanding its complications and preventing its occurrence. *Pharmacotherapy* 1995;15:713–726.
74. Solomon SM, Kirby DF. The refeeding syndrome: a review. *JPEN J Parenter Enteral Nutr* 1990;14:90–97.
75. Nesbakken R, Reinlie S. Magnesium and phosphorus: the electrolytes of energy metabolism. *Acta Anaesthesiol Scand* 1985;29:60–64.
76. Lichtman MA, Miller DR, Cohen J, et al. Reduced red cell glycolysis, 2, 3 diphosphoglycerate and adenosine triphosphate concentration, and increased hemoglobin-oxygen affinity caused by hypophosphatemia. *Ann Intern Med* 1971;74:562–568.
77. O'Connor LR, Wheeler WS, Bethune JE. Effect of hypophosphatemia on myocardial performance in man. *N Engl J Med* 1977;297:901–903.
78. Kraft MD, Btaiche IF, Sacks GS. Review of the refeeding syndrome. *Nutr Clin Pract* 2005;20:625–633.
79. Luckey A, Parsa C. Fluid and electrolytes in the aged. *Arch Surg* 2003; 138:1055–1060.
80. Beaty L, Pemberton D. *Treatment of water, electrolyte, and acid-base disorders in the surgical patient*. New York: McGraw-Hill Companies; 1994.
81. Weinsier RL, Krumdieck CL. Death resulting from overzealous total parenteral nutrition: the refeeding syndrome revisited. *Am J Clin Nutr* 1980;34:393–399.
82. Silvis SE, Paragas PD. Paresthesias, weakness, seizures, and hypophosphatemia in patients receiving hyperalimentation. *Gastroenterology* 1972;62:513–520.
83. Eliahou HE, Feng PH, Weinberg U, et al. Acetate and bicarbonate in the correction of uraemic acidosis. *Br Med J* 1970;4:399–401.
84. Richards CE, Drayton M, Jenkins H, et al. Effect of different chloride infusion rates on plasma base excess during neonatal parenteral nutrition. *Acta Paediatrica* 1993;82:678–682.
85. Baughman FA, Papp JP. Wernike's encephalopathy with intravenous hyperalimentation: remarks on similarities between Wernike's encephalopathy and the phosphate depletion syndrome. *Mt Sinai J Med* 1976;43:48–52.
86. Kitamura K, Takahashi T, Tanaka H, et al. Two cases of thiamine deficiency-induced lactic acidosis during total parenteral nutrition. *Tohoku J Exp Med* 1993;171:129–133.
87. Sheldon GF, Petersen SR, Snaders R. Hepatic dysfunction during hyperalimentation. *Arch Surg* 1978;113(4):504–508.
88. Zamir O, Nussbaum MS, Bhadra S, et al. Effect of enteral feeding on hepatic steatosis induced by total parenteral nutrition. *JPEN J Parenter Enteral Nutr* 1994;18:20–25.
89. Powell EE, Cooksley WGE, Hanson R, et al. The natural history of nonalcoholic steatohepatitis: a follow-up study of forty-two patients for up to 21 years. *Hepatology* 1990;11:74–80.
90. Sax HC, Bower RH. Hepatic complications of total parenteral nutrition. *JPEN J Parenter Enteral Nutr* 1988;12(No. 6):615–618.
91. Lowry SF, Brennan MF. Abnormal liver function during parenteral nutrition: relation to infusion excess. *J Surg Res* 1979;26:300–307.
92. Nussbaum MS, Fischer JE. Pathogenesis of hepatic steatosis during total parenteral nutrition. *Surg Annu* 1991;23(Pt 2):1–11.
93. Palombo JD, Schnure F, Bistrian BR, et al. Improvement of liver function tests by administration of L-carnitine to a carnitine-deficient patient receiving home parenteral nutrition: a case report. *JPEN J Parenter Enteral Nutr* 1987;11:88–92.
94. Richardson TJ, Sgoutas D. Essential fatty acid deficiency in four adult patients during total parenteral nutrition. *Am J Clin Nutr* 1975;28:258–263.
95. Campos AC, Oler A, Meguid MM, et al. Liver biochemical and histological changes with graded amounts of total parenteral nutrition. *Arch Surg* 1990;125:447–450.
96. Zagara G, Locati L. Role of total parenteral nutrition in determining liver insufficiency in patients with cranial injuries. Glucose vs glucose + lipids. *Minerva Anestesiol* 1989;55(12):509–512.
97. Reif S, Tano M, Oliverio R, et al. Total parenteral nutrition-induced steatosis: reversal by parenteral lipid infusions. *JPEN J Parenter Enteral Nutr* 1991;15:102–104.
98. Heyman MB, Storch S, Ament ME. The fat overload syndrome. Report of a case and literature review. *Am J Dis Child* 1981;135:628–630.
99. Tao RC, Peck GK, Yoshimura NN. Effect of carnitine on liver fat and nitrogen balance in intravenously fed growing rats. *J Nutr* 1981;111: 171–177.
100. Yao ZM, Vance DE. The active synthesis of phosphatidylcholine is required for very low density lipoprotein secretion from rat hepatocytes. *J Biol Chem* 1988;263:2998–3004.
101. Buchman AL. Choline deficiency during parenteral nutrition in humans. *Nutr Clin Pract* 2003;18:353–358.
102. Buchman AL, Dubin M, Jenden D, et al. Lecithin increases plasma free choline and decreases hepatic steatosis in long-term parenteral nutrition patients. *Gastroenterology* 1992;102(4 pt 1):1363–1370.
103. Buchman AL, Ament M, Sohel M, et al. Choline deficiency causes reversible hepatic abnormalities in patients receiving parenteral nutrition: proof of a human choline requirement: a placebo-controlled trial. *JPEN J Parenter Enteral Nutr* 2001;25:260–268.
104. Roslyn JJ, DenBesten L, Pitt HA, et al. Resident research award. Effects of cholecystokinin on gallbladder stasis and cholesterol gallstone formation. *J Surg Res* 1981;30(3):200–204.
105. Jawaheer G, Pierro A, Lloyd DA, et al. Gall bladder contractility in neonates: effects of parenteral and enteral feeding [published erratum appears in *Arch Dis Child Fetal Neonatal Ed* 1995;73(3):F198]. *Arch Dis Child Fetal Neonatal Ed* 1995;72(3):F200–F202.
106. Gurll NJ, Meyer PD, DenBesten L. The effect of cholesterol crystals on gallbladder function in cholelithiasis. *Surg Forum* 1977;28:412–413.
107. Allen B, Bernhoft R, Blanckaert N, et al. Sludge is calcium bilirubinate associated with bile stasis. *Am J Surg* 1981;141:51–56.
108. Cooper A, Ross AJ, O'Neill JA Jr, et al. Resolution of intractable cholestasis associated with total parenteral nutrition following biliary irrigation. *J Pediatr Surg* 1985;20(6):772–774.
109. Rintala R, Lindahl H, Pohjavuori M, et al. Surgical treatment of intractable cholestasis associated with total parenteral nutrition in premature infants. *J Pediatr Surg* 1993;28(5):716–719.
110. Caniano DA, Starr J, Ginn-Pease ME. Extensive short-bowel syndrome in neonates: Outcome in the 1980s. *Surgery* 1989;105:119–124.
111. Hofmann AF. Defective biliary secretion during total parenteral nutrition: probable mechanisms and possible solutions. *J Pediatr Gastroenterol Nutr* 1995;20(4):376–390.
112. Sitzmann JV, Pitt HA, Steinborn PA, et al. Cholecystokinin prevents parenteral nutrition induced biliary sludge in humans. *Surg Gynecol Obstet* 1990;170(1):25–31.
113. Teitelbaum DH, Han-Markey T, Drongowski RA, et al. Use of cholecystokinin to prevent the development of parenteral nutrition-associated cholestasis. *JPEN J Parenter Enteral Nutr* 1997;21(2):100–103.
114. Tsai S, Strouse P, Drongowski R, et al. Use of cholecystokinin-octapeptide to prevent TPN-associated gallstone disease. *J Pediatr Surg* 2005; 40(1):263–267.
115. Beath SV, Davies P, Papadopoulou A, et al. Parenteral nutrition-related cholestasis in postsurgical neonates: multivariate analysis of risk factors. *J Pediatr Surg* 1996;31(4):604–606.
116. Teitelbaum DH, Tracy T. Parenteral nutrition-associated cholestasis. *Semin Pediatr Surg* 2001;10(2):72–80.
117. Btaiche IF, Khalidi N. Parenteral nutrition-associated liver complications in children. *Pharmacotherapy* 2002;22:188–211.
118. Teitelbaum DH. Parenteral nutrition-associated cholestasis. *Curr Opin Pediatr* 1997;9:270–275.
119. Cavicchi M, Beau P, Crenn P, et al. Prevalence of liver disease and contributing factors in patients receiving home parenteral nutrition for permanent intestinal failure. *Ann Intern Med* 2000;132(7):525–532.
120. Kiristioglu I, Antony P, Fan Y, et al. Total parenteral nutrition-associated changes in mouse intestinal intraepithelial lymphocytes. *Dig Dis Sci* 2002;47(5):1147–1157.
121. Yang H, Finaly R, Teitelbaum DH. Alteration in epithelial permeability and ion transport in a mouse model of total parenteral nutrition. *Crit Care Med* 2003;31(4):1118–1125.
122. Tazuke Y, Drongowski RA, Btaiche I, et al. Effects of lipid administration on liver apoptotic signals in a mouse model of total parenteral nutrition (TPN). *Pediatr Surg Int* 2004;20(4):224–228.
123. Tazuke Y, Kiristioglu I, Heidelberger KP, et al. Hepatic P-glycoprotein changes with total parenteral nutrition administration [see comment]. *JPEN J Parenter Enteral Nutr* 2004;28(1):1–6.
124. Tazuke Y, Teitelbaum D. Alteration of canalicular transporters in a mouse model of total parenteral nutrition. *J Pediatr Gastroenterol Nutr* 2009;48(2):193–202.
125. Beale E, Nelson R, Bucciarelli R, et al. Intrahepatic cholestasis associated with parenteral nutrition in premature infants. *Pediatric* 1979;64: 342–347.
126. Vileisis RA, Inwood RJ, Hunt CE. Prospective controlled study of parenteral nutrition-associated cholestatic jaundice: effect of protein intake. *J Pediatr* 1980;96(5):893–897.
127. Heubi JE, Wiechmann DA, Creutzinger V, et al. Tauroursodeoxycholic acid (TUDCA) in the prevention of total parenteral nutrition-associated liver disease.[see comment]. *J Pediatr* 2002;141(2):237–242.

128. Teitelbaum DH, Han-Markey T, Drongowski RA, et al. Use of cholecystokinin to prevent the development of parenteral nutrition-associated cholestasis. *JPEN J Parenter Enteral Nutr* 1997;21(2):100–103.
129. Teitelbaum DH, Tracy TF Jr, Aouthmany MM, et al. Use of cholecystokinin-octapeptide for the prevention of parenteral nutrition-associated cholestasis. *Pediatrics* 2005;115(5):1332–1340.
130. Capron JP, Gineston JL, Herve MA, et al. Metronidazole in prevention of cholestasis associated with total parenteral nutrition. *Lancet* 1983;1(8322):446–447.
131. Kudsk K, Croce M, Fabian T. Enteral versus parenteral feeding: effects on septic morbidity after blunt and penetrating abdominal trauma. *Ann Surg* 1992;215:503–513.
132. Iyer K, Spitz L, Clayton P. New insight into mechanisms of parenteral nutrition—associated cholestasis: role of plant sterols. *J Pediatr Surg* 1998;33(1):1–6.
133. Teitelbaum D, Drongowski R, Spivak D. Rapid development of hyperbilirubinemia in infants with the short bowel syndrome as a correlate to mortality: Possible indication for early small bowel transplantation. *Transplant Proc* 1996;28(5):2677–2678.
134. Correia M, Guimaraes J, de Mattos L, et al. Peripheral parenteral nutrition: an option for patients with an indication for short-term parenteral nutrition. *Nutr Hosp* 2004;19(1):14–18.
135. Foley MJ. Radiologic placement of long-term central venous peripheral access system ports (PAS Port): results in 150 patients. *J Vasc Interv Radiol* 1995;6(2):255–262.
136. Domino K, Bowdle T, Posner K. Injuries and liability related to central vascular catheters: a closed claims analysis. *Anesthesiology* 2004;100(6):1411–1418.
137. Andris DA, Krzywda EA, Schulte W, et al. Pinch-off syndrome: a rare etiology for central venous catheter occlusion. *JPEN J Parenter Enteral Nutr* 1994;18(6):531–533.
138. Hinke DH, Zandt-Stastny DA, Goodman LR, et al. Pinch-off syndrome: a complication of implantable subclavian venous access devices. *Radiology* 1990;177(2):353–356.
139. Lane R, Matthay M. Central line infections. *Curr Opin Crit Care* 2002;8:441–448.
140. Faubion WC, Wesley JR, Khalidi N, et al. Total parenteral nutrition catheter sepsis: impact of the team approach. *JPEN J Parenter Enteral Nutr* 1986;10(6):642–645.
141. Reed CR, Sessler CN, Glauser FL, et al. Central venous catheter infections: concepts and controversies. *Intensive Care Med* 1995;21(2):177–183.
142. Berenholtz S, Pronovost P, Lipsett P, et al. Eliminating catheter-related bloodstream infections in the intensive care unit. *Crit Care Med* 2004;32(10):2014–2020.
143. Dezfulian C, Lavelle J, Nallamothu B, et al. Rates of infection for single-lumen versus multilumen central venous catheters: A meta-analysis. *Crit Care Med* 2003;31(9):2385–2390.
144. Cowl C, Weinstock J, Al-Jurf A. Complications and cost associated with parenteral nutrition delivered to hospitalized patients through either subclavian or peripherally-inserted central catheters. *Clin Nutr* 2000;19:237–243.
145. Sitges-Serra A, Puig P, Linares J, et al. Hub colonization as the initial step in an outbreak of catheter-related sepsis due to coagulase negative staphylococci during parenteral nutrition. *JPEN J Parenter Enteral Nutr* 1984;8(6):668–672.
146. King DR, Komer M, Hoffman J, et al. Broviac catheter sepsis: the natural history of an iatrogenic infection. *J Pediatr Surg* 1985;20(6):728–733.
147. Kurkchubasche AG, Smith SD, Rowe MI. Catheter sepsis in short-bowel syndrome. *Arch Surg* 1992;127:21–25.
148. Sitges-Serra A, Linares J. Tunnels do not protect against venous-catheter-related sepsis [letter]. *Lancet* 1984;1(8374):459–460.
149. Lecciones JA, Lee JW, Navano EE, et al. Vascular catheter associated fungemia: Analysis of 155 episodes. *Clin Infect Dis* 1992;14:875.
150. Widmer AF. Management of catheter-related bacteremia and fungemia in patients on total parenteral nutrition. *Nutrition* 1997;13(4, Suppl):18S–25S.
151. Mermel LA. Prevention of catheter-related infections. *Ann Intern Med* 2000;132:391–402.
152. O'Grady NP, Alexander M, Dellinger EP, et al. Guidelines for the prevention of intravascular catheter-related infections. Centers for Disease Control and Prevention. *MMWR Morb Mortal Wkly Rep* 2002;51(RR-10):1–29.
153. Krzywda EA, Andris DA, Edmiston CE. Catheter infections: diagnosis, etiology, treatment and prevention. *Nutr Clin Pract* 1999;14:178.
154. Coran AG, Spivak D, Teitelbaum DH. An analysis of the morbidity and mortality of short-bowel syndrome in the pediatric age group. *Eur J Pediatr Surg* 1999;9(4):228–230.
155. Johnson PR, Decker MD, Edwards KM, et al. Frequency of Broviac catheter infections in pediatric oncology patients. *J Infect Dis* 1986;154(4):570–578.
156. Mermel LA, Allon M, Bouza E, et al. Clinical practice guidelines for the diagnosis and management of intravascular catheter-related infection: 2009 update by the Infectious Diseases Society of America. *Clin Infect Dis* 2009;49:1–45.
157. Attar A, Messing B. Evidence-based prevention of catheter infection during parenteral nutrition.[see comment]. *Curr Opin Clin Nutr Metab Care* 2001;4(3):211–218.
158. Onland W, Shin C, Fustar S, et al. Ethanol-lock technique for persistent bacteremia of long-term intravascular devices in pediatric patients. *Arch Pediatr Adolesc Med* 2006;160(10):1049–1053.
159. Mouw E, Chessman K, Lesher A, et al. Use of an ethanol lock to prevent catheter-related infections in children with short bowel syndrome. *J Pediatr Surg* 2008;43(6):1025–1029.
160. Andrew M, Marzinotto V, Pencharz P, et al. A cross-sectional study of catheter-related thrombosis in children receiving total parenteral nutrition at home. *J Pediatr* 1995;126(3):358–363.
161. Klerk C, Smorenburg S, Buller H. Thrombosis prophylaxis in patient populations with a central venous catheter: a systematic review. *Arch Intern Med* 2003;163(16):1913–1921.
162. Werlin SL, Lausten T, Jessen S, et al. Treatment of central venous catheter occlusions with ethanol and hydrochloric acid. *JPEN J Parenter Enteral Nutr* 1995;19(5):416–418.
163. Dwolatzky T, Berezovski S, Friedmann R. A prospective comparison of the use of nasogastric and percutaneous endoscopic gastrostomy tubes for long-term enteral feeding in older people. *Clin Nutr* 2001;20(6):535–540.
164. Boulton-Jones J, Lewis J, Jobling J, et al. Experience of post-pyloric feeding in seriously ill patients in clinical practice. *Clin Nutr* 2004;23:35–41.
165. Ganga UR, Ryan JJ, Schafer LW. Indications, complications, and long-term results of percutaneous endoscopic gastrostomy: a retrospective study. *S D J Med* 1994;47(5):149–152.
166. Gauderer ML, Ponsky JL, Izant RJ Jr. Gastrostomy without laparotomy: A percutaneous endoscopic technique. *J Pediatr Surg* 1980;15:872–875.
167. Metheny NA, Eisenberg P, Spies M. Aspiration pneumonia in patients fed through nasoenteral tubes. *Heart Lung* 1986;15(3):256–261.
168. Spain DA, DeWeese RC, Reynolds MA, et al. Transpyloric passage of feeding tubes in patients with head injuries does not decrease complications. *J Trauma* 1995;39(6):1100–1102.
169. Strong R, Condon S, Soling M, et al. Equal aspiration rates from postpylorus and intragastric-placed small bore nasoenteric feeding tubes: A randomized prospective study. *JPEN J Parenter Enteral Nutr* 1992;16:59–63.

CHAPTER

22

Complications of Immunosuppression

Niraj M. Desai and Christina L. Klein

INTRODUCTION

Modern advances in medical therapy have resulted in a large number of individuals with a compromised immune system. The cause of immunodeficiency may be intentional (immunosuppression administration to patients with organ transplants or with autoimmune disease), the unintended consequence of a particular therapy (chemotherapy for cancer), or the result of a disease state (large burns or acquired immunodeficiency syndrome [AIDS]). As a result of the increasing number of patients receiving immunosuppressive agents, the diagnosis, treatment, and prevention of immunosuppression related complications has become commonplace. This chapter first reviews immunosuppressive medications and their specific side effects. Commonly occurring complications of immunosuppression are then reviewed from the perspective of the consulting surgeon. A thorough understanding of these complications is essential when providing care to these complex patients.

IMMUNOSUPPRESSIVE AGENTS

Over the past five decades, several classes of immunosuppressive agents have been discovered, with many new compounds becoming part of routine clinical use. These medications are primarily used for the prevention and treatment of rejection and have allowed for an impressive improvement in the survival of solid organ transplant recipients. In addition, immunosuppressive medications have been used increasingly for the treatment of autoimmune diseases. Immunosuppressive agents are often used in at high doses for a short time period as induction therapy, for the treatment of rejection, or the treatment of an autoimmune flare. They are also used on a chronic basis in lower doses as maintenance therapy. The available medications can be classified into five major categories: corticosteroids, calcineurin inhibitors (CNIs), mammalian target of rapamycin (mTOR) inhibitors, antiproliferative agents, and antibodies. The immunosuppressive medications and their common side effects are summarized in Table 22.1 (1). The activation of T cells and the inhibitory sites of action for commonly used immunosuppressive agents are shown in Figure 22.1 (2).

Corticosteroids

Corticosteroids were first used clinically in 1949 and, since that time, have been used for a variety of indications including allergies, autoimmune diseases, arthritis, asthma, cancer therapies, neurosurgery, organ transplantation, and numerous others. Steroids are the most commonly prescribed immunosuppressive medication due to their efficacy in a variety of diseases, long-standing experience with their use, and low cost. They are usually used in high doses when therapy is initiated or for the rapid treatment of immune activation (asthma exacerbation, organ rejection). Dosing is often then tapered to a maintenance dose or completely discontinued. Dexamethasone, prednisone, prednisolone, and methylprednisolone are examples of commonly used steroids.

Corticosteroids have a variety of effects on the immune system. Most importantly, they inhibit the production of several cytokines by T cells and antigen presenting cells (APCs), including IL-1, IL-2, IL-3, IL-6, tumor necrosis factor-alpha, and interferon-gamma. Steroids initially enter the cell and bind to intracellular receptors. The steroid-receptor complex then enters the nucleus and binds to sequences of deoxyribonucleic acid (DNA) on the promoter region of cytokine genes called glucocorticoid response elements, and thereby block the transcription of those cytokines. In addition, steroids inhibit the action of nuclear factor-kappa B, another key element in the cytokine response (3,4). Given the effect on multiple cytokines, steroids inhibit T cell activation at several stages. Additional immunosuppressive effects of steroids include inhibition of monocyte migration and suppression of chemokine production.

Given the ubiquitous nature of glucocorticoid receptors in most human cells, corticosteroids are associated with adverse effects on a variety of tissues. Transient side effects can occur with short term use of high-dose steroids, such as hypertension and diabetes mellitus. However, severe complications occur with long-term use, even when steroids are taken at low maintenance doses. The metabolic side effects of steroids are hypertension, diabetes, hyperlipidemia, sodium

Niraj M. Desai: Department of Surgery, The Johns Hopkins University School of Medicine, Baltimore, MD 21205.

Christina L. Klein: Department of Surgery, Washington University School of Medicine, St. Louis, MO 63110.

Table **22.1** **Summary of immunosuppressive medication side effects**

Medication	Side Effects
Corticosteroids	Hypertension, glucose intolerance, hyperlipidemia, fluid retention, protein wasting, adipose weight gain, cataracts, glaucoma, peptic ulcers, pancreatitis, osteoporosis, osteonecrosis, mood disturbances, psychosis, acne, delayed wound healing
Cyclosporine	Hypertension, glucose intolerance, hyperlipidemia, nephrotoxicity, electrolyte disturbances, neurotoxicity, gingival hyperplasia, hirsutism
Tacrolimus	Hypertension, glucose intolerance, hyperlipidemia, nephrotoxicity, electrolyte disturbances, neurotoxicity, alopecia
Sirolimus	Hyperlipidemia, anemia, leukopenia, thrombocytopenia, mouth sores, gastrointestinal disturbances, lymphedema, impaired wound healing, pneumonitis
Azathioprine	Leukopenia, thrombocytopenia, gastrointestinal disturbances, pancreatitis
Mycophenolate mofetil/ mycophenolic acid	Leukopenia, thrombocytopenia, gastrointestinal disturbances
Antithymocyte globulin	Fever, chills, rash, leukopenia, thrombocytopenia, allergic reactions
Intravenous immune globulin	Fever, chills, rash, aseptic meningitis, acute renal dysfunction, hypersensitivity reaction
Muromonab-CD3 (OKT3)	Fever, chills, rigors, headache, myalgia, hypertension, flash pulmonary edema, aseptic meningitis, hypersensitivity reaction
Basiliximab/daclizumab	Hypersensitivity reaction (rare)
Alemtuzumab	Fever, rash, nausea, shortness of breath, chest discomfort, hypersensitivity reaction
Rituximab	Fever, rash, nausea, shortness of breath, chest discomfort, hypersensitivity reaction

Adapted from Hardinger KL, Koch MJ, Brennan DC. Current and future immunosuppressive strategies in renal transplantation. *Pharmacotherapy* 2004; 24:1159–1176, with permission.

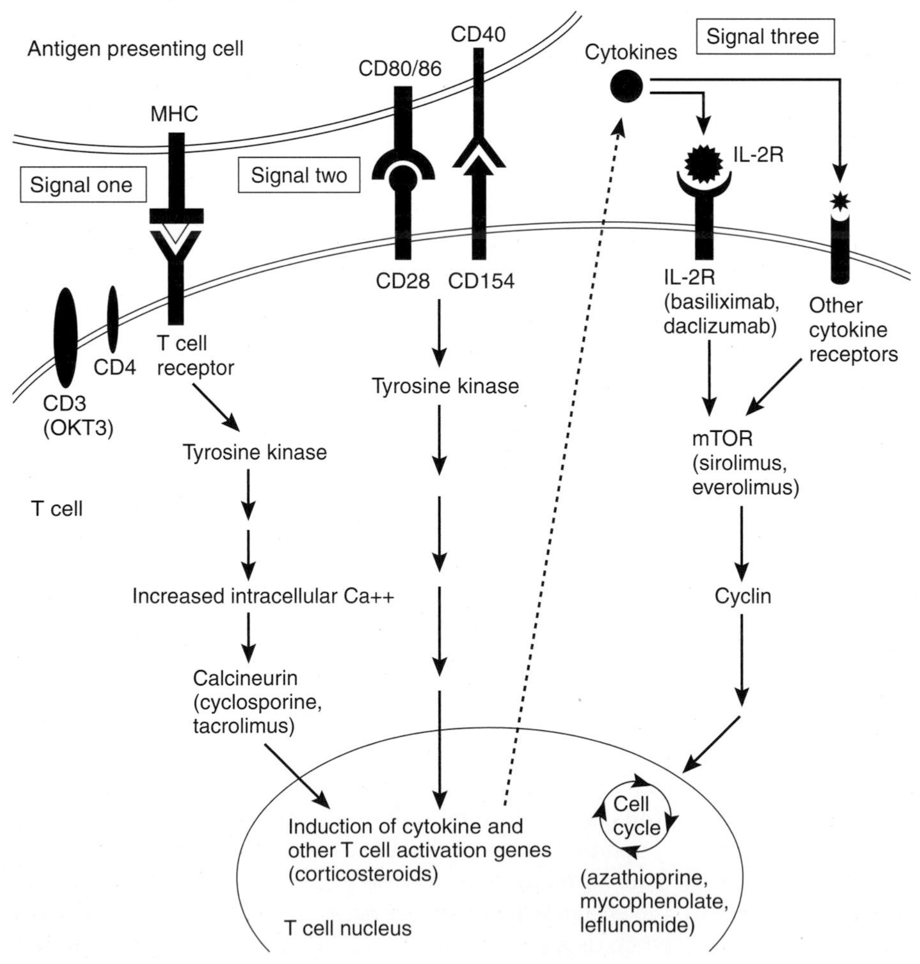

FIGURE 22.1. Signaling pathways involved in T cell activation. Sites of inhibition by commonly used immunosuppressive medications are indicated in parentheses. (From Helderman JH, Goral S. Transplantation immunobiology. In: Danovitch GM, ed. *Handbook of kidney transplantation*, 3rd ed. Philadelphia, PA: Lippincott Williams & Wilkins; 2001:17–38, with permission.)

and fluid retention, protein wasting, growth retardation, and adipose weight gain. Gastrointestinal (GI) side effects include gastritis, duodenal ulcers, and pancreatitis. The ocular complications are glaucoma and cataracts. Osteoporosis often affects vertebral bodies of the spine, while osteonecrosis often affects the femoral head. Psychiatric effects such as mood disturbances and psychosis, cosmetic side effects including acne and the development of Cushingoid features, and delayed wound healing are all observed with steroids (1,3–5). This broad range of side effects associated with chronic steroid use, along with the development of more specific immunosuppressive medications, has led to efforts to minimize or completely avoid the use of steroids (6,7). However, for the majority of patients with organ transplants and with autoimmune disease, steroids remain a cornerstone of immunosuppressive therapy.

Calcineurin inhibitors

The currently available CNIs are cyclosporine and tacrolimus (formerly known as FK-506). Both agents inhibit the activation and proliferation of T lymphocytes by suppressing the production of the cytokines interleukin-2 (IL-2), IL-4, interferon-gamma, and tumor necrosis factor-alpha by T lymphocytes. The agents are biochemically distinct – cyclosporine is an 11 amino acid cyclic polypeptide produced by the fungal species *Tolypocladium inflatum Gams* and tacrolimus is a macrolide antibiotic produced by the fungus *Streptomyces tsukubaensis*. Both agents have distinct cytoplasmic binding proteins (immunophilins), with cyclosporine binding to cyclophilin and tacrolimus binding to FKBP-12. However, in both cases, the drug-immunophilin complex binds calcineurin, and thus inhibits its ability to upregulate the activity of certain nuclear regulatory proteins (1,4). Both agents have a relatively narrow therapeutic window and close monitoring of drug levels is necessary to achieve a balance between efficacy and toxicity.

The original oil-based oral cyclosporine formulation depends upon bile for absorption and has erratic absorption patterns. In contrast, cyclosporine modified (also known as cyclosporine microemulsion), depends less on bile for absorption and exhibits increased bioavailability and more consistent absorption. In terms of dosing, the two cyclosporine formulations are not considered interchangeable. Appropriate drug levels can sometimes be maintained with a lower relative dose of cyclosporine modified, and monitoring of levels is mandatory if the patient is changed to an alternate formulation. Intravenous cyclosporine (nonmodified) is rarely used; however when necessary, approximately one-third of the total oral daily dose is administered intravenously either over 2 to 6 hours or by 24 hour continuous infusion. Tacrolimus does not depend upon bile for absorption and has excellent oral bioavailability. Due to its ready absorption, tacrolimus very rarely needs to be given intravenously with therapeutic levels achievable in almost any patient via either an oral or sublingual route, even after major abdominal surgery (1). Rather than administering intravenous cyclosporine, it is preferable to convert a patient from cyclosporine to oral tacrolimus if absorption of drug is a concern in the postoperative setting. In contrast to cyclosporine, where administration with food tends to increase bioavailability, administration of tacrolimus with food can decrease the rate and extent of absorption.

Table 22.2 Medication interactions for cytochrome P450 IIIa substrates—cyclosporine, tacrolimus, and sirolimus

Increased Immunosuppressant Levels	Decreased Immunosuppressant Levels
Ketoconazole	Rifampin
Fluconazole	Rifabutin
Itraconazole	Phenytoin
Voriconazole	Phenobarbital
Erythromycin	Carbamazepine
Clarithromycin	St. John's wort
Diltiazem	Isoniazid
Verapamil	
Cimetidine	
Danazol	
Grapefruit juice	
Nefazodone	
Fluvoxamine	
Amiodarone	

Adapted from Hardinger KL, Koch MJ, Brennan DC. Current and future immunosuppressive strategies in renal transplantation. *Pharmacotherapy* 2004;24:1159–1176, with permission.

Oral cyclosporine and tacrolimus are usually given twice daily. They are both metabolized in the liver by the cytochrome P450 IIIA (CYP3 A) pathway and are excreted in the bile. Potential drug interactions are important to recognize, and vigilance in monitoring drug levels is required when any agent is added or adjusted that induces or inhibits CYP3 A levels (Table 22.2) (1). There is only minimal renal excretion of either drug and neither is significantly affected by dialysis. Cyclosporine and tacrolimus levels have traditionally been measured as morning trough levels; however an increasing trend has been to measure the cyclosporine level 2 hours after oral dosing (C_2 level). The appropriate therapeutic levels depend on the type of organ transplant, the length of time since transplantation, and other factors (8).

CNIs are associated with numerous toxicities. Nephrotoxicity is a critical side effect that is dose dependent and results from vasoconstriction of the afferent arteriole, resulting in a "prerenal" type of renal dysfunction. In addition, long term use of CNIs can lead to the development of interstitial fibrosis due to the production of profibrotic cytokines (4,9,10). Concomitant administration of CNIs with other nephrotoxic medications, such as aminoglycosides, amphotericin B deoxycholate, and nonsteroidal anti-inflammatory drugs, should be avoided. Intravenous contrast should be used cautiously, taking specific measures, such as hydration, administration of N-acetylcysteine or sodium bicarbonate, and possible adjustment of the CNI dose, to protect the kidneys. Another major side effect that often results in the development of frank diabetes is glucose intolerance. The incidence of post-transplant diabetes is higher in those receiving tacrolimus compared to those on cyclosporine (11). The development of diabetes may be mild and require only diet control, or it may be more severe and require an oral agent or insulin to treat.

Other common side effects of CNIs include hypertension, electrolyte abnormalities, hyperlipidemia, and neurotoxicity. Hypertension, although seen with both cyclosporine and tacrolimus, is often more severe with cyclosporine. This side effect is due to both renal and peripheral vasoconstriction. Electrolyte abnormalities on CNIs include hyperkalemia due to impaired renal excretion of potassium, and hypomagnesemia due to wasting of magnesium in the urine (4). Hyperlipidemia is more often seen with cyclosporine than with tacrolimus. Neurologic side effects are more often associated with tacrolimus, and may be mild, such as tremor or headache, or may be severe, such as seizures and posterior reversible encephalopathy syndrome. Two common cosmetic side effects that are specific to cyclosporine are gingival hyperplasia and hirsutism, while alopecia is sometimes seen with tacrolimus (1). While the cosmetic side effects of cyclosporine may seem minor compared to the pathophysiologic ones mentioned above, they are important to the patient and can result in medication noncompliance and graft loss. Due to a more favorable side effect profile, tacrolimus has become the preferred CNI for most solid organ transplant recipients, and is almost exclusively used in pediatric patients. Generic preparations of both cyclosporine and tacrolimus are available and in common use. It is recommended that frequent monitoring of levels be performed when a patient is changed from branded to generic product (or vice versa) to ensure that the intended therapeutic range is maintained.

Mammalian target of rapamycin inhibitors

Sirolimus and everolimus are mTOR inhibitors. Sirolimus is a macrocyclic antibiotic produced by the bacteria *Streptomyces hygroscopicus*, and everolimus is the 2-hydroxyethyl derivative of sirolimus. The mTOR inhibitors also bind to FKBP-12 in the cytoplasm of cells (like tacrolimus); however, the mechanism of action is quite different. The drug/FKBP-12 complex inhibits mTOR, a key regulatory protein kinase that controls cytokine-dependant cell proliferation (1). Like the CNIs, the mTOR inhibitors require monitoring of drug levels to achieve proper therapeutic efficacy.

Both sirolimus and everolimus are available in oral form only and are readily absorbed. The half-life of sirolimus is 60 hours, allowing for once daily dosing, while the half-life of everolimus is 28 hours and typical dosing is twice daily. Both drugs are metabolized in the liver and counter transported to the gut lumen leading to elimination in the feces. The CYP3 A pathway is involved in drug metabolism; thus, recognizing potential drug interactions is important (Table 22.2) (1).

A major distinction between mTOR inhibitors and the CNIs is the lack of renal toxicity from vasoconstriction from using the former. However, significant proteinuria has been observed in some individuals with the use of mTOR inhibitors; thus, they also have nephrotoxic potential. When combined with a CNI, mTOR inhibitors appear to actually increase the renal toxicity associated with the CNI (4). This effect is probably most pronounced with cyclosporine, but is also seen with tacrolimus. Given this potential renal toxicity, the combined use of a CNI and an mTOR inhibitor on a chronic basis is avoided.

Another important toxicity of mTOR inhibitors is hyperlipidemia (hypercholesterolemia and hypertriglyceridemia) affecting upwards of 50% of patients (4). In most instances, the lipid abnormalities can be managed by placing the patient on either a HMG-CoA reductase inhibitor ("statin") or a fibrate depending on the specific lipid abnormality. A unique and interesting side effect of mTOR inhibitors is the development of painful mouth sores that are associated with high drug levels and generally resolve with dose reduction. The mTOR inhibitors can also cause hematologic abnormalities such as leukopenia, thrombocytopenia, and anemia that may require dose reduction or changing immunosuppression. Lymphedema is an increasingly recognized complication of mTOR inhibitors and can present any time after initiation (1). Impaired wound healing is an important side effect from the surgeon's perspective that is discussed later in this chapter.

Antiproliferative agents

A variety of antiproliferative agents are used for immunosuppression. These agents work by inhibiting DNA synthesis and therefore cell proliferation. Azathioprine, mycophenolate mofetil (MMF), and mycophenolate sodium are used in transplant recipients as part of maintenance immunosuppression, and in patients with autoimmune diseases. Other commonly used antiproliferative agents include cyclophosphamide and methotrexate for treatment of cancer and immune-mediated diseases.

Azathioprine is a purine analog that inhibits lymphocyte and myelocyte proliferation. It is typically administered orally as part of a maintenance immunosuppression regimen, although intravenous dosing at one-half the oral dose is occasionally necessary. Azathioprine should be avoided, or the dosing reduced significantly, if administered with allopurinol or febuxostat, since xanthine oxidase is necessary for the conversion of azathioprine to inactive metabolites. The major side effect observed is hematological, with a reversible, dose-dependent leukopenia and anemia most commonly observed. In addition, hepatotoxicity and acute pancreatitis are rarely seen in patients on azathioprine, with both conditions being reversible with timely cessation of therapy (1,4).

MMF and mycophenolate sodium both become mycophenolic acid (MPA) *in vivo*. A product of several *Penicillium* species, MPA affects DNA replication by noncompetitive reversible inhibition of inosine monophosphate dehydrogenase, an important enzyme for *de novo* guanosine synthesis. Because lymphocytes depend upon *de novo* guanosine synthesis, MPA has a more selective cytostatic effect on lymphocytes compared to other cell types that have a salvage pathway. Both drugs are primarily administered orally in two divided doses, although an intravenous form of MMF can be given at the same dosing regimen. The major side effects of both MMF and mycophenolate sodium are related to the GI tract and are generally dose-dependent. Nausea, diarrhea, and bloating are often seen, while esophagitis and gastritis are uncommon and may be related to invasive cytomegalovirus (CMV) disease. Evaluation of MMF-related GI distress often includes colonoscopy and mucosal biopsy, and a spectrum of histologic changes is described (12,13). Hematological side effects including anemia, leukopenia, and thrombocytopenia are also fairly common and usually improve by temporary medication discontinuation and resumption at lower doses once counts recover (1,4).

Antibodies

Antibodies are often administered for induction therapy in the critical early period after transplantation to decrease the risk of acute rejection and to allow for lower overall intensity of maintenance immunosuppression. They are also used for the treatment of steroid resistant acute rejection. Antibody therapies can be divided into the polyclonal preparations that have a broad range of antibody specificities, and the monoclonal preparations that target a single specific molecule to evoke their mechanism of action.

Rabbit-derived and horse-derived polyclonal antithymocyte globulin preparations are currently available. They both contain a variety of antibodies against many lymphocyte surface antigens—these antibodies bind to the surface of the lymphocyte, cause depletion, and thus interfere with cell-mediated and humoral immune responses (1,14). This depletion occurs by both complement-dependent cell lysis and by macrophage phagocytosis. The side effects of this medication include infusion related ones such as fever, chills, headache, and rarely anaphylaxis. In addition, severe lymphocyte depletion and thrombocytopenia may occur, which can limit the ability to safely administer successive doses (4). Lymphocyte counts remain abnormally low for several months in most patients and may persist for several years in some (15). Thus, it is important to remember that recipients of antithymocyte globulin may develop complications related to persistent lymphopenia weeks, months, or even years after treatment.

Intravenous immune globulins (IVIGs) are also polyclonal antibody preparations that are commonly used to treat autoimmune and inflammatory diseases, and are increasingly being used in organ transplant recipients. IVIG is prepared by pooling immunoglobin G (IgG) antibody from thousands of normal volunteers. It has complex immunoregulatory properties, but is not immunosuppressive and therefore does not lead to the associated complications (16). As with antithymocyte globulin, infusion-related side effects are observed. When IVIG is used in high doses, self-resolving aseptic meningitis can develop. The high osmotic load of the medication can cause tubular injury that may lead to acute renal dysfunction (4). Renal dysfunction associated with IVIG administration has most commonly been reported in the setting of rapid administration and the use of products stabilized with sucrose.

Currently there are several monoclonal antibodies available that target the T lymphocyte. In contrast to polyclonal antibodies, each of these agents has a specific target on the T lymphocyte that the antibody binds to and on which it exerts its mechanism of action. The oldest of these agents is muromonab-CD3 (OKT3), a mouse monoclonal antibody against the human T cell surface molecule CD3. OKT3 leads to the rapid depletion of T cells and blocks the action of activated cytotoxic T cells. Severe side effects with initial administration are fairly common due to a cytokine release syndrome that occurs. Fever, chills, rigors, headache, and muscle pain are commonly observed in patients receiving OKT3, especially with the first few doses. In patients that are fluid overloaded, "flash" pulmonary edema can occur and should be closely monitored for. Volume status should be optimized prior to administering this agent. An aseptic meningitis picture has also been observed in patients receiving OKT3 (4). Basiliximab is a monoclonal antibody that targets the IL-2 receptor that is used for induction therapy only. This antibody blocks the IL-2 receptor on T cells, preventing activation and proliferation, but does not lead to depletion and an associated cytokine storm (1).

Antibody preparations approved for use in hematology, oncology, and autoimmunity are being used "off-label" in transplant. Alemtuzumab is an anti-CD52 antibody that depletes T and B lymphocytes and monocytes. It has been used for both induction therapy and for the treatment of rejection (1). A prolonged depletion in the white blood cell count can occur, with many patients still having abnormally low counts 6 to 12 months after receiving alemtuzumab (17). Rituximab is a monoclonal antibody directed against the CD20 marker on B cells and is used for prophylaxis and treatment against antibody-mediated immunity (1). Its use in kidney transplantation has increased due to the growing number of transplants performed in sensitized and ABO-incompatible recipients. Both alemtuzumab and rituximab have infusion-related side effects such as fever, rash, nausea, shortness of breath, chest discomfort, and allergic reactions. Eculizumab, a humanized monoclonal antibody specific for complement component C5a, inhibits membrane attack complex formation and is approved for use in paroxysmal nocturnal hemoglobinuria. This agent is under investigation in kidney transplant recipients for desensitization protocols and treatment of antibody mediated rejection (18).

Medications in development

The greater understanding of immune activation at the cellular level has allowed for the development of several new biologics, including fusion proteins and small molecules. The fusion proteins combine a receptor targeting a ligand of interest with the Fc portion of an IgG molecule. They target the "immune synapse" between the APC and the T lymphocyte (Fig. 22.1). The fusion protein LEA29Y (Belatacept), which strongly binds to CD80 and CD86 on APCs and interrupts T cell activation, has completed phase III clinical trials in renal transplant recipients and is under governmental review. Alefacept, a fusion protein that binds to CD2 on T lymphocytes, also inhibits T cell activation. It is approved for use in psoriasis and ongoing clinical trials are being conducted in transplant patients. Early clinical experience with a monoclonal antibody against CD154 demonstrated major thrombotic events, including myocardial infarction and stroke; thus, any new agent will be carefully scrutinized for safety and efficacy prior to receiving approval for use in patients (19).

Small molecule immunosuppressive drug development also continues with numerous agents being studied. Janus kinase 3 (JAK3) is an important intracellular signaling protein involved in cytokine mediated T cell proliferation (20). Phase II clinical trials using a JAK3 inhibitor (CP-690550) in renal transplant patients have demonstrated promising results compared to standard CNI-based regimens. Potential adverse effects include increased rates of CMV disease and BK virus nephropathy, as well as anemia (18). Protein kinase C (PKC) mediates signalling downstream of the T-cell receptor, and PKC inhibitors are being studied in transplant. Phase II trials involving tacrolimus withdrawal in renal transplant patients receiving a PKC inhibitor (AEB071) were halted due to an increased incidence of acute rejection. However, PKC inhibitors are still under investigation as adjunctive therapy in both CNI and mTOR based regimens (18).

Bortezomib, a proteosome inhibitor approved for the treatment of multiple myeloma, is being investigated off-label in kidney transplant desensitization protocols and for treatment of antibody mediated rejection (21). It directly targets the mature plasma cell, unlike other therapies currently used for prevention and treatment of antibody mediated rejection.

COMMON PROBLEMS ASSOCIATED WITH IMMUNOSUPPRESSION

The complications that occur due to immunosuppression can affect any part of the body and are wide ranging in their scope. Many of them are related to the previously mentioned side effects of a particular immunosuppressive agent; however, additional complications occur that are the result of combination therapy with multiple agents or a consequence of the global immunosuppressed state of the patient. This section will cover whole body and organ system based problems associated with immunosuppression, especially as they pertain to the consulting surgeon involved in the care of these patients.

Infection

The majority of the morbidity and mortality from immunosuppression was once primarily due to infection. These infectious complications not only resulted from common pathogens seen in nonimmunosuppressed patients, but often were caused by opportunistic agents that attacked the immune deficient host primarily. With experience, clinicians developed effective prophylactic strategies against the more commonly seen infections. This experience, coupled with the development of more T cell specific agents, decreased the overall incidence of infectious complications. Despite these advances, infectious complications remain a major concern when caring for immunosuppressed individuals.

The variety of pathogens that have been observed in immunosuppressed patients far exceeds what is seen in the "normal" host, with many of these opportunistic pathogens only being observed in these individuals. Bacterial infections are often resistant to routinely used antibiotics because of previous patient exposure to these agents or colonization of the patient with resistant bacteria during prolonged hospital stays. Vancomycin resistant *Enterococcus* (VRE), methicillin-resistant *Staphylococcus aureus* (MRSA), and extended-spectrum beta-lactamase producing *Escherichia coli* and *Klebsiella* species are examples. Cystic fibrosis patients awaiting lung transplantation can become colonized with *Pseudomonas aeruginosa*, *Stenotrophomonas maltophilia*, or *Burkholderia cepacia* that are resistant to beta lactams, aminoglycosides, and fluoroquinolones, leading to high morbidity and mortality after transplantation (22). Mycobacterial infection with either *Mycobacterium tuberculosis* or atypical mycobacterium occurs far more frequently in immunosuppressed patients, but is still rare in developed countries (22).

Viral infections are often the consequence of reactivation of latent infections once the patient has become immunosuppressed. In organ transplant recipients, an extremely problematic viral infection was CMV until prophylaxis with antiviral therapy became routine. CMV disease can occur as a viral syndrome with fever, malaise, leukopenia, and thrombocytopenia, and it can also present as a tissue invasive disease causing pneumonitis, hepatitis, retinitis, or GI tract disease (22). Other viral diseases due to Epstein-Barr, herpes simplex, human herpesvirus-6 and -7, varicella zoster, respiratory syncytial, influenza, parvovirus, and adenovirus are all described (22).

Invasive fungal infections are considered the most difficult to treat infections in immunosuppressed patients. *Pneumocystis jiroveci* (formerly known as *Pneumocystis carinii*) causes a pneumonia that is characterized by hypoxemia and dyspnea that is disproportional to physical exam and radiographic findings. This disease was the initial defining illness in 63% of AIDS patients in 1987 and affected up to 15% of transplant recipients (22,23). Fortunately, effective prophylaxis strategies have reduced these rates considerably. *Candida* species can cause mucocutaneous infection, esophagitis, pyelonephritis, candidemia, endocarditis, brain abscess, sinusitis, empyema, peritonitis, and wound infection. *Aspergillus* species most commonly cause lung and upper respiratory tract infections, including sinusitis, tracheobronchitis, necrotizing pneumonia, and empyema. Disseminated disease with brain abscess formation can occur as can fungal ball formation in preexisting cavities. This organism is especially problematic for lung transplant recipients (22,24). *Cryptococcus neoformans* most commonly causes central nervous system disease and pulmonary disease. In organ transplant recipients, there is a typical timeline for occurrence of the more common fungal infections—*Candida* in the first few weeks after transplantation, *Aspergillus* and *Pneumocystis* in the first 1 to 6 months after transplantation, and *Cryptococcus* after 6 months (22). Of course, these times can vary based upon environmental factors and the overall degree of immunosuppression in the individual patient.

Malignancy

Malignancy has been considered a greater problem in those receiving immunosuppression compared to the general population, with the absolute increase in risk depending on the amount of immunosuppression used and the type of malignancy (25–27). The majority of the studies regarding malignancy and immunosuppression are based upon transplant recipients, although the findings should be applicable to all immunosuppressed patients. In kidney transplant recipients, the risk of developing cancers of the colon, lung, prostate, stomach, esophagus, pancreas, ovary, and breast are approximately two-fold greater than for the general population for the first 3 years following transplantation. Testicular and bladder cancers are increased three-fold, and leukemia, hepatobiliary cancers, cervical and vulvovaginal cancers are increased approximately five-fold (28). Thus, prevention strategies and screening methods for these common cancers are likely to be even more relevant for immunosuppressed individuals.

Skin cancer is the most common malignancy in patients on immunosuppressive therapy, causing serious morbidity and potential mortality. Several studies have shown that the incidence of skin cancers in transplant patients is between 40% and 80% after 20 years of immunosuppressive therapy. Compared to the general population, melanoma occurs two to four times more often, squamous-cell carcinoma occurs 65 to 250 times more frequently, and basal-cell carcinoma occurs 10 times more often (29). As a result, the number of squamous-cell skin cancers exceeds the number of basal-cell skin cancers in transplant recipients—the opposite of the general population. The key risk factor for development is ultraviolet light exposure, and patients on immunosuppression should be counseled regarding prevention strategies and careful skin exams to aid early detection.

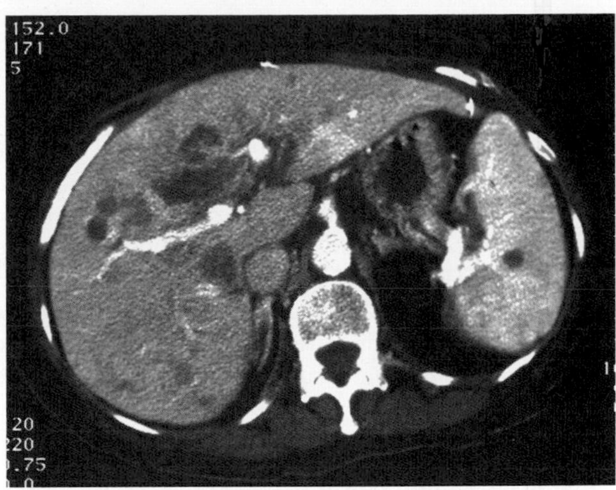

FIGURE 22.2. Abdominal CT scan demonstrating cancer metastases to the liver and spleen of unknown primary origin in a recipient 4 months after kidney transplantation. A CT scan 3 months earlier was normal.

Treatment of solid organ and skin cancers in patients on immunosuppressive therapy should follow established guidelines for that particular cancer. When possible, surgical resection with adequate margins should be performed to control the primary site of disease. Additional chemotherapy should be administered when indicated. Even with an aggressive approach to cancer treatment, the development of recurrences and distant metastases is common on immunosuppressive therapy. If possible, consideration should be given to immunosuppression reduction or withdrawal. Regardless of whether immunosuppressive therapy can be reduced, frequent monitoring for the development of recurrence and metastases should be performed since the propensity for rapid tumor spread in these patients is well documented (Fig. 22.2).

Two cancers that occur in the general population but are observed at much higher rates in immunosuppressed individuals deserve additional mention. Post-transplant lymphoproliferative disease (PTLD) represents a variety of B lymphocyte disorders ranging from mild polyclonal hyperplasia to malignant monoclonal lymphoma. In the majority of instances, the disease appears related to Epstein-Barr virus (EBV) mediated transformation of B cells. The incidence is estimated between 1% and 10% of transplant recipients (30). In one series of 500 liver transplant recipients, 2.4% developed PTLD at a mean of 19.5 months after transplantation (31). Patients may present with fever, fatigue, weight loss, a high EBV viral load, and lymphadenopathy—either by physical exam or by imaging study. Patients can also present with solid organ masses, skin lesions, central nervous system symptoms, and tonsil enlargement, especially in children. Biopsy is sometimes required to confirm the diagnosis, help determine the severity of the disease, and determine therapy. Treatment for milder forms is usually by immunosuppression reduction and antiviral therapy, while more malignant variants require chemotherapy and immunotherapy with anti-CD20 monoclonal antibody (32). Surgical resection or radiation for disease localized to a single lesion has also been reported.

Kaposi's sarcoma is characterized by multiple angiomatous lesions. There is an 80- to 500-fold increased incidence in immunosuppressed patients, and human herpesvirus 8 (HHV-8) has a causal role. Most patients with Kaposi's sarcoma have mucosal or skin lesions, with most skin lesions occurring on the legs. Patients with visceral disease usually present with lesions in the lungs, GI tract, or lymph nodes (29). Immunosuppression reduction is first-line therapy for Kaposi's sarcoma, often resulting in disease regression, with chemotherapy being reserved for persistent disease.

Impaired wound healing

Impaired wound healing has been recognized to be a consequence of corticosteroid therapy since its introduction. Several studies have documented that steroid administration before or at the time of surgery impairs wound healing as measured by tensile strength. Histologic studies have shown that steroids interfere with the migration of monocytes and macrophages into the wound, thus reducing the inflammatory phase of wound healing and reducing the number of fibroblasts in the wound. Studies with corticosteroids have demonstrated a two-fold to five-fold increase in wound healing complications compared to control subjects not receiving steroids (5).

More recently, mTOR inhibitors have been documented to lead to impaired wound healing. This impairment is related to the antiproliferative effects of the drug on many different cell types. From the transplantation literature, it has been demonstrated that sirolimus causes a five-fold increased incidence of wound infections, lymphoceles, and hernias in kidney recipients, and an increased incidence of bronchial anastomosis dehiscence in lung recipients (33,34). Other anecdotal reports describe decreased wound healing in transplant patients on sirolimus undergoing other procedures. Consideration should be given to temporarily substituting an mTOR inhibitor with a CNI at the time of an operative procedure, or much earlier in the setting of elective surgery. The use of additional closure methods such as retention sutures should be considered when operating on patients receiving an mTOR inhibitor. Other than steroids and mTOR inhibitors, the other immunosuppressive medications do not significantly inhibit wound healing. However, the consequences of wound infections can be severe and thus vigilant observation for the development of wound complications is recommended.

Cardiovascular disease

Cardiovascular disease in patients on immunosuppression is frequently observed, but the exact contribution of immunosuppressive agents to cardiovascular complications is difficult to assess since preexisting disease often carries its own risk of cardiovascular complications (35). For example, renal failure patients have a 10 to 20 times higher mortality from cardiovascular events than the general population (36). However, several studies have demonstrated that kidney transplantation reduces this mortality risk when compared with ongoing dialysis; thus, the potential harm caused by immunosuppressive therapy is overshadowed by the benefit of transplantation (37,38). Within the population of immunosuppressed patients, differences in cardiovascular mortality have been observed between groups of patients on different immunosuppressive medications, implying a contributory role of these medications to cardiovascular complications. Perhaps the best way to assess the influence of immunosuppressive agents on cardiovascular complications is by examining their impact on the risk factors of cardiovascular disease (36).

Many of the immunosuppressive agents negatively impact cardiovascular risk factors, such as diabetes, hypertension, and hyperlipidemia. As mentioned previously, corticosteroids, tacrolimus, and cyclosporine all cause diabetes, hypertension, and hyperlipidemia to varying degrees. In addition, sirolimus and everolimus also cause hyperlipidemia to a greater extent than any of the other immunosuppressive agents (1,4,36). Modification of risk factors through diet and exercise is encouraged in patients on immunosuppressive medications. In addition, the aggressive treatment of these risk factors with pharmacologic agents is widely practiced. It is important to remember that patients on longstanding immunosuppression will often have cardiac disease, either as a result of native disease or the result of these medications. Thus, noninvasive stress testing is recommended prior to major elective procedures in this patient population.

Gastrointestinal disease

Serious and often life threatening complications involving the entire GI tract have been reported in association with immunosuppressive therapy. Mucosal ulceration leading to bleeding or perforation has been reported with the esophagus, stomach, small intestine, and colon. In addition, biliary tract disease and pancreatitis have also been frequently observed. The most commonly observed problems are gastroduodenal ulcers and colon perforations. Historically, the initial culprit was corticosteroids, with numerous reports documenting GI complications in 10% to 30% of patients on steroids, and a high associated mortality (5,39). As additional immunosuppressive agents were introduced, reduced doses of corticosteroids have been used and the incidence of GI complications has decreased. In addition, the availability of histamine receptor antagonists and proton pump inhibitors has allowed for routine prophylaxis against gastroduodenal ulcer disease and reduced the incidence of upper GI complications dramatically (40).

The highest rate of GI complications appears to occur in recipients of heart and lung transplants. In one report, a 20% rate of GI complications was observed within 30 days following cardiac transplantation, including perforated duodenal ulcer, pancreatitis, colonic pneumatosis, cholecystitis, appendicitis, and colonic necrosis. Most of these patients underwent successful surgical intervention with over 90% surviving with normal GI function (41). Another report documented a 40% rate of major GI complications following lung transplantation, with 18% requiring an operative procedure and the remainder being managed with endoscopic intervention or medications. Most of these GI complications occurred within the first month after lung transplantation (42). A more recent analysis of renal transplant recipients documented a 10% rate of severe GI complications following transplantation, with the most common problems being gastroduodenal ulcers, colonic diverticulitis, and pancreatitis (43).

Diagnosis of GI complications in immunosuppressed individuals is often difficult because systemic signs such as abdominal pain, fever, and leukocytosis are often minimal or absent despite significant disease. Abdominal distension and hypoactive bowel sounds may be the only signs of an abdominal catastrophe. A high index of suspicion is required to diagnose these GI complications, with frequent abdominal exams and the liberal use of diagnostic studies being helpful. Plain radiographs, computed tomography scans, contrast studies, selective arteriography, and upper and lower endoscopy have all been reported to be helpful in making the diagnosis in these patients. Once the diagnosis of a major GI complication is made, immediate and aggressive intervention is required to optimize patient outcomes. When operative therapy is necessary, most experienced surgeons advocate a conservative approach in terms of performing the simplest procedure that controls the problem at hand. When small bowel resection is necessary, intestinal continuity can usually be restored safely. However, when large bowel resection is necessary, diversion is preferred over an anastomosis due to the risk of breakdown and the development of further complications. Meticulous surgical care can lead to successful outcomes in patients with major immunosuppression related GI complications.

CMV is a common human pathogen that can lead to significant disease in immunosuppressed individuals, as described elsewhere in this chapter. The systemic signs and symptoms of CMV disease include fever, malaise, lethargy, and leukopenia. CMV disease of the GI tract is characterized by mucosal ulcerations, erosions, and hemorrhage that can affect the esophagus, stomach, small bowel, and colon. Lesions in these sites can lead to intestinal tract bleeding or perforation. The diagnosis of CMV disease in the intestinal tract is often made by the presence of GI symptoms in the setting of a high viral load detected by polymerase chain reaction (44). However, significant GI tract CMV disease may be present in the absence of symptoms, and investigation with endoscopy and biopsy is recommended when CMV disease is suspected (45). Treatment of GI tract CMV disease is with systemic antiviral therapy, and in severe cases, CMV immune globulin is also administered. In some situations, patients may present with perforation, and require surgical intervention, albeit with a high morbidity and mortality.

Chronic renal insufficiency and failure

Renal insufficiency and renal failure are relatively common problems that develop in patients that receive long-term immunosuppressive therapy (10). Although this is primarily a consequence of CNI therapy, other complications of immunosuppression such as hypertension, diabetes, and dyslipidemia all contribute to the development of chronic kidney disease. The prolonged use of cyclosporine or tacrolimus leads to tubular atrophy, interstitial fibrosis, and arteriole hyalinosis in the kidney (46). This development of renal failure is most pronounced in recipients of nonrenal solid organ transplants, primarily due to the dependence on cyclosporine or tacrolimus to prevent rejection and thereby prolong graft and patient survival. Preexisting renal disease from chronic hypoperfusion often contributes as well, particularly in heart and liver recipients. The cumulative incidence of chronic renal failure in the United States at 5 years following transplantation is 10.9% for heart, 21.3% for intestine, 18.1% for liver, and 15.8% for lung recipients (Fig. 22.3) (47).

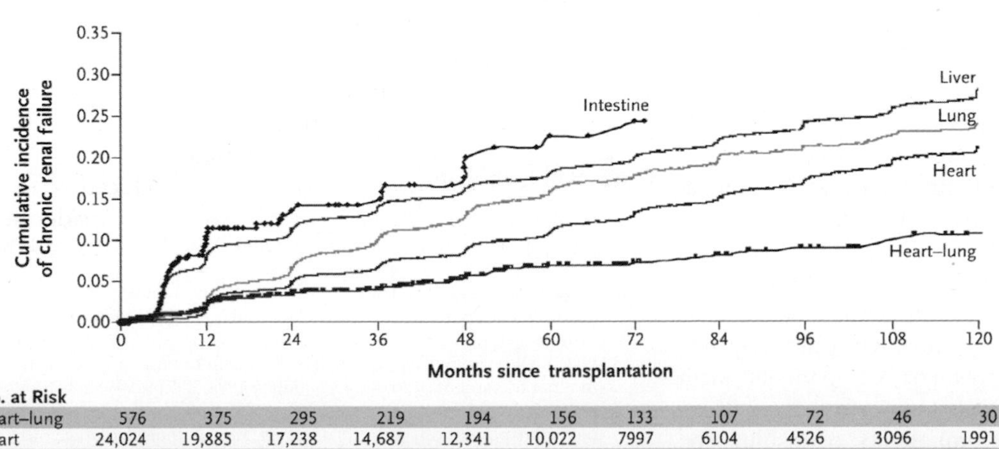

No. at Risk

	0	12	24	36	48	60	72	84	96	108	120
Heart–lung	576	375	295	219	194	156	133	107	72	46	30
Heart	24,024	19,885	17,238	14,687	12,341	10,022	7997	6104	4526	3096	1991
Intestine	228	152	110	84	57	33	23	13	8	5	5
Liver	36,849	28,495	24,041	19,508	15,724	12,564	9844	7345	5292	3614	2261
Lung	7,643	5,633	4,316	3,184	2,327	1,629	1136	745	468	258	133

FIGURE 22.3. Cumulative incidence of chronic renal failure in recipients of nonrenal solid organ transplants in the United States. (From Ojo AO, Held PJ, Port FK, et al. Chronic renal failure after transplantation of a nonrenal organ. *N Engl J Med* 2003;349:931–940, with permission.)

Although the majority of patients on CNI therapy do not develop chronic renal failure, most have some degree of impaired renal function (48). Patients on CNIs have a mean glomerular filtration rate that is approximately 40% less than that of comparable patients not on CNIs, with this difference being a result of reduced renal blood flow and therefore reduced ultrafiltration (9,46,49). Impaired renal function may or may not be fully reflected in the plasma creatinine, and it may require calculation or measurement of the creatinine clearance to appreciate the degree of renal dysfunction present. When caring for these patients, it is important to prevent intravascular volume depletion because hypovolemia further exacerbates the chronic effects of CNI on renal function. It is also recommended that the use of nephrotoxic medications be avoided and interventions that can further disturb renal function (i.e., intravenous contrast) be minimized in patients receiving CNIs.

The management of dialysis access in immunosuppressed patients is often quite complicated. The preferred long-term access is an arterial-venous fistula because infectious complications are often severe in these patients and are much more likely to occur with artificial grafts, peritoneal dialysis catheters, and hemodialysis catheters. The ideal therapy for the recipient of a nonrenal solid organ transplant with renal failure is renal transplantation since the patient is already receiving immunosuppressive therapy. This is an increasingly common scenario with reports indicating good outcomes (50).

Endocrine abnormalities

Diabetes mellitus is the most common endocrine abnormality in patients on immunosuppression and is largely due to the use of steroids and CNIs. The diabetes is primarily due to insulin resistance, although it may also result from diminished insulin release. Risk factors for diabetes include African-American race, family history of diabetes, obesity, hepatitis C, and older age. The contribution of steroids to diabetes is dose related—the majority of individuals receiving high doses of steroids in the immediate period following transplantation demonstrate impairment in glucose tolerance; however, as the dose is reduced, most patients return to near normal glucose levels. Since CNIs are most commonly used in conjunction with corticosteroids, their contribution to inducing diabetes is difficult to assess. It is generally accepted that both cyclosporine and tacrolimus can cause diabetes and that the risk is greater with tacrolimus. One analysis of renal transplant recipients demonstrated that 18% of patients receiving tacrolimus had developed diabetes by two years after transplantation compared to 8% of those receiving cyclosporine (11). Targeting lower therapeutic CNI levels as well as minimization of steroid dosing will often improve glycemic control (51). Management of patients with immunosuppression induced diabetes is similar to others and includes diet and exercise, oral agents, or insulin. The general goal is to maintain a hemoglobin A1c below 7% and to monitor and prevent diabetes related complications.

Adrenal insufficiency has been a major concern in patients receiving chronic glucocorticoid therapy, since an early report of death due to adrenal atrophy in a patient receiving steroids undergoing an operation (52). Thus, for many years these patients received additional large doses of steroids at the time of stress. However, more recent studies have documented the safety of avoiding "stress steroids" in patients receiving maintenance prednisone therapy of 5 to 10 mg/day (53,54). "Stress steroids" should not routinely be given in the perioperative setting to patients on chronic steroid therapy, since their administration increases the risk of infection, delays wound healing and often significantly increases blood glucose levels. When minor or moderate stress is expected, steroids should be continued at maintenance doses and the patient should be observed for signs of adrenal insufficiency, such as hypotension, myalgia, arthralgia, ileus, fever, hyponatremia, and eosinophilia. If signs of adrenal insufficiency develop, then a 24- to 48-hour course of "stress steroids" should be given. When a major stressor occurs in a patient on chronic steroid therapy, such as major multiorgan trauma or a ruptured aortic aneurysm, most clinicians agree that adrenal insufficiency should be investigated and administration of "stress steroids" should be considered.

SUMMARY

The complications of immunosuppression remain a challenging problem for patients and their healthcare providers. While numerous individuals have suffered due to immunodeficiency disease states, there is little doubt that the lives of others have been extended and enhanced by the availability of various medications that allow for the control of autoimmunity, transplant rejection, and cancer. The hope for both groups of patients is based on the growing number of therapeutic agents combined with the increased understanding of the human immune system. It is to be hoped that there will soon be a day when the negative consequences of immunodeficiency will be prevented. Until then, a thorough understanding of the complications associated with immunosuppression combined with an aggressive approach to diagnosis and treatment will generally lead to optimal outcomes.

REFERENCES

1. Hardinger KL, Koch MJ, Brennan DC. Current and future immunosuppressive strategies in renal transplantation. *Pharmacotherapy* 2004;24(9):1159–1176.
2. Helderman J, Goral S. Transplantation immunobiology. In: *Handbook of kidney transplantation,* 3rd ed. Philadelphia, PA: Lippincott Williams & Wilkins, 2001:17–38.
3. Hricik DE, Almawi WY, Strom TB. Trends in the use of glucocorticoids in renal transplantation. *Transplantation* 1994;57(7):979–989.
4. Danovitch G. Immunosuppressive medications and protocols for kidney transplantation. In: *Handbook of kidney transplantation,* 4th ed. Philadelphia, PA: Lippincott Williams & Wilkins, 2005:72–134.
5. Diethelm AG. Surgical management of complications of steroid therapy. *Ann Surg* 1977;185(3):251–263.

6. Matas AJ, Kandaswamy R, Humar A, et al. Long-term immunosuppression, without maintenance prednisone, after kidney transplantation. *Ann Surg* 2004;240(3):510–516; discussion 516–517.
7. Woodle ES, First MR, Pirsch J, et al. A prospective, randomized, double-blind, placebo controlled, multicenter trial comparing early (7 day) corticosteroid cessation versus long-term, low-dose corticosteroid therapy. *Ann Surg* 2008;248(4):564–577.
8. Nashan B, Cole E, Levy G, et al. Clinical validation studies of Neoral C(2) monitoring: a review. *Transplantation* 2002;73(Suppl 9):S3–S11.
9. Myers BD, Ross J, Newton L, et al. Cyclosporine-associated chronic nephropathy. *N Engl J Med* 1984;311(11):699–705.
10. Bennett WM, DeMattos A, Meyer MM, et al. Chronic cyclosporine nephropathy: the Achilles' heel of immunosuppressive therapy. *Kidney Int* 1996;50(4):1089–1100.
11. Woodward RS, Schnitzler MA, Baty J, et al. Incidence and cost of new onset diabetes mellitus among U.S. wait-listed and transplanted renal allograft recipients. *Am J Transplant* 2003;3(5):590–598.
12. Selbst MK, Ahrens WA, Robert ME, et al. Spectrum of histologic changes in colonic biopsies in patients treated with mycophenolate mofetil. *Mod Pathol* 2009;22(6):737–743.
13. Papadimitriou JC, Cangro CB, Lustberg A, et al. Histologic features of mycophenolate mofetil-related colitis: a graft-versus-host disease-like pattern. *Int J Surg Pathol* 2003;11(4):295–302.
14. Gaber AO, First MR, Tesi RJ, et al. Results of the double-blind, randomized, multicenter, phase III clinical trial of Thymoglobulin versus Atgam in the treatment of acute graft rejection episodes after renal transplantation. *Transplantation* 1998;66(1):29–37.
15. Brennan DC, Flavin K, Lowell JA, et al. A randomized, double-blinded comparison of Thymoglobulin versus Atgam for induction immunosuppressive therapy in adult renal transplant recipients. *Transplantation* 1999;67(7):1011–1018.
16. Kazatchkine MD, Kaveri SV. Immunomodulation of autoimmune and inflammatory diseases with intravenous immune globulin. *N Engl J Med* 2001;345(10):747–755.
17. Calne R, Moffatt SD, Friend PJ, et al. Campath IH allows low-dose cyclosporine monotherapy in 31 cadaveric renal allograft recipients. *Transplantation* 1999;68(10):1613–1616.
18. Vincenti F, Kirk AD. What's next in the pipeline. *Am J Transplant* 2008;8(10):1972–1981.
19. Vincenti F. What's in the pipeline? New immunosuppressive drugs in transplantation. *Am J Transplant* 2002;2(10):898–903.
20. Nashan B. Review of T-cell activation: impact of Janus kinase 3 inhibition. *Transplantation* 2003;75(11):1783–1785.
21. Everly MJ, Everly JJ, Susskind B, et al. Bortezomib provides effective therapy for antibody- and cell-mediated acute rejection. *Transplantation* 2008;86(12):1754–1761.
22. Green M, Avery R, Preiksaitis J. Guidelines for the prevention and management of infectious complications of solid organ transplantation. *Am J Transplant* 2004;10S:6–166.
23. Morris A, Lundgren JD, Masur H, et al. Current epidemiology of Pneumocystis pneumonia. *Emerg Infect Dis* 2004;10(10):1713–1720.
24. Patterson TF, Kirkpatrick WR, White M, et al. Invasive aspergillosis. Disease spectrum, treatment practices, and outcomes. I3 Aspergillus Study Group. *Medicine (Baltimore)* 2000;79(4):250–260.
25. Trofe J, Beebe TM, Buell JF, et al. Posttransplant malignancy. *Prog Transplant* 2004;14(3):193–200.
26. Penn I. The effect of immunosuppression on pre-existing cancers. *Transplantation* 1993;55(4):742–747.
27. Feng S, Buell JF, Chari RS, et al. Tumors and transplantation: The 2003 Third Annual ASTS State-of-the-Art Winter Symposium. *Am J Transplant* 2003;3(12):1481–1487.
28. Kasiske BL, Snyder JJ, Gilbertson DT, et al. Cancer after kidney transplantation in the United States. *Am J Transplant* 2004;4(6): 905–913.
29. Euvrard S, Kanitakis J, Claudy A. Skin cancers after organ transplantation. *N Engl J Med* 2003;348(17):1681–1691.
30. Green M. Management of Epstein-Barr virus-induced post-transplant lymphoproliferative disease in recipients of solid organ transplantation. *Am J Transplant* 2001;1(2):103–108.
31. Norin S, Kimby E, Ericzon BG, et al. Posttransplant lymphoma–a single-center experience of 500 liver transplantations. *Med Oncol* 2004;21(3): 273–284.
32. Verschuuren EA, Stevens SJ, van Imhoff GW, et al. Treatment of post-transplant lymphoproliferative disease with rituximab: the remission, the relapse, and the complication. *Transplantation* 2002;73(1):100–104.
33. Dean PG, Lund WJ, Larson TS, et al. Wound-healing complications after kidney transplantation: a prospective, randomized comparison of sirolimus and tacrolimus. *Transplantation* 2004;77(10):1555–1561.
34. Groetzner J, Kur F, Spelsberg F, et al. Airway anastomosis complications in de novo lung transplantation with sirolimus-based immunosuppression. *J Heart Lung Transplant* 2004;23(5):632–638.
35. Kasiske BL, Chakkera HA, Roel J. Explained and unexplained ischemic heart disease risk after renal transplantation. *J Am Soc Nephrol* 2000; 11(9):1735–1743.
36. Boots JM, Christiaans MH, van Hooff JP. Effect of immunosuppressive agents on long-term survival of renal transplant recipients: focus on the cardiovascular risk. *Drugs* 2004;64(18):2047–2073.
37. Wolfe RA, Ashby VB, Milford EL, et al. Comparison of mortality in all patients on dialysis, patients on dialysis awaiting transplantation, and recipients of a first cadaveric transplant. *N Engl J Med* 1999;341(23): 1725–1730.
38. Ojo AO, Hanson JA, Meier-Kriesche H, et al. Survival in recipients of marginal cadaveric donor kidneys compared with other recipients and wait-listed transplant candidates. *J Am Soc Nephrol* 2001;12(3):589–597.
39. Penn I, Groth CG, Brettshneider L, et al. Surgically correctable intra-abdominal complications before and after renal homotransplantation. *Ann Surg* 1968;168(5):865–870.
40. Troppmann C, Papalois BE, Chiou A, et al. Incidence, complications, treatment, and outcome of ulcers of the upper gastrointestinal tract after renal transplantation during the cyclosporine era. *J Am Coll Surg* 1995;180(4):433–443.
41. DiSesa VJ, Kirkman RL, Tilney NL, et al. Management of general surgical complications following cardiac transplantation. *Arch Surg* 1989; 124(5):539–541.
42. Lubetkin EI, Lipson DA, Palevsky HI, et al. GI complications after orthotopic lung transplantation. *Am J Gastroenterol* 1996;91(11):2382–2390.
43. Sarkio S, Halme L, Kyllonen L, et al. Severe gastrointestinal complications after 1,515 adult kidney transplantations. *Transpl Int* 2004;17(9):505–510.
44. Goodgame RW. Gastrointestinal cytomegalovirus disease. *Ann Intern Med* 1993;119(9):924–935.
45. Mayoral JL, Loeffler CM, Fasola CG, et al. Diagnosis and treatment of cytomegalovirus disease in transplant patients based on gastrointestinal tract manifestations. *Arch Surg* 1991;126(2):202–206.
46. Young EW, Ellis CN, Messana JM, et al. A prospective study of renal structure and function in psoriasis patients treated with cyclosporin. *Kidney Int* 1994;46(4):1216–1222.
47. Ojo AO, Held PJ, Port FK, et al. Chronic renal failure after transplantation of a nonrenal organ. *N Engl J Med* 2003;349(10):931–940.
48. Avitzur Y, De Luca E, Cantos M, et al. Health status ten years after pediatric liver transplantation–looking beyond the graft. *Transplantation* 2004;78(4):566–573.
49. Hollander AA, van Saase JL, Kootte AM, et al. Beneficial effects of conversion from cyclosporin to azathioprine after kidney transplantation. *Lancet* 1995;345(8950):610–614.
50. Coopersmith CM, Brennan DC, Miller B, et al. Renal transplantation following previous heart, liver, and lung transplantation: an 8-year single-center experience. *Surgery* 2001;130(3):457–462.
51. Gaston RS, Chandrakantan A. Diabetes mellitus after kidney transplantation. *Am J Transplant* 2003;3(5):512–513.
52. Fraser CG, Preuss FS, Bigford WD. Adrenal atrophy and irreversible shock associated with cortisone therapy. *J Am Med Assoc* 1952;149(17): 1542–1543.
53. Bromberg JS, Alfrey EJ, Barker CF, et al. Adrenal suppression and steroid supplementation in renal transplant recipients. *Transplantation* 1991;51(2):385–390.
54. Bromberg JS, Baliga P, Cofer JB, et al. Stress steroids are not required for patients receiving a renal allograft and undergoing operation. *J Am Coll Surg* 1995;180(5):532–536.

PART

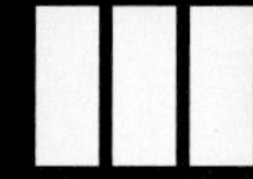

Complications of Thoracic Surgery

CHAPTER

23

Complications of Intubation, Tracheotomy, and Tracheal Surgery

Kevin Fung and Norman D. Hogikyan

INTRODUCTION

The development of orotracheal intubation for the administration of anesthesia by William Macewen in 1878 was one of the most important advances in the history of surgery. With the passage of time, however, acute and chronic complications of intubation have become evident. Tracheotomy is currently indicated in patients for prolonged ventilation in order to avoid long-term complications of intubation. Benefits attributed to tracheotomy include enhanced patient comfort, improved pulmonary toilet, decreased ventilator-associated pneumonia, and accelerated ventilator weaning, although strong supportive evidence is lacking (1). Although some view tracheotomy as a routine procedure, the potential complications are significant and can be devastating. As a consequence of prolonged intubation, acquired laryngotracheal stenosis can occur and is the most common indication for tracheal resection. An understanding of the complications of procedures involving the airway, including intubation, tracheotomy, and tracheal surgery, is important for all surgeons.

Terminology

The terms "vocal cord" and "vocal fold" are used in various ways in the literature. Although both terms refer to the same anatomical structures, vocal fold is the more correct contemporary term and will be used throughout the chapter.

INTUBATION

The surgeon should employ current techniques to achieve airway control during administration of general anesthesia and their associated complications. Injury can occur to any part of the upper aerodigestive tract as a consequence of the intubation event itself or as a consequence of the endotracheal tube residing in the airway. Injuries are classified according to anatomic location as well as timing—acute (i.e., complications during the intubation event) versus chronic (i.e., complications while the patient is intubated) (2,3). Pertinent risk factors for these injuries are summarized in Table 23.1.

Kevin Fung and Norman D. Hogikyan: University of Western Ontario, London, Ontario, Canada 800

Nasal complications

Nasotracheal intubation is indicated for surgical procedures involving the oral cavity when endotracheal intubation is expected to be prolonged and when there is a contraindication to orotracheal intubation.

Acute Epistaxis

Epistaxis can occur as a result of injury to nasal mucosa during nasotracheal intubation. Injury can occur at the level of the septum (Kiesselbach plexus), lateral nasal wall (branches of internal maxillary artery), nasal turbinates, or nasopharyngeal mucosa. Treatment consists of direct pressure, anterior nasal pack, topical decongestion, or otolaryngologic consultation for cauterization or posterior nasal pack if persistent and profuse. The following preventive measures are suggested.

1. Preoperative recognition and correction of bleeding disorders
2. Preoperative recognition of abnormal anatomy (i.e., deviated nasal septum, septal spur, nasal polyps, enlarged adenoids)
3. Adequate topical decongestion (i.e., pseudoephedrine, oxymetazoline, cocaine)
4. Use of an appropriate size tube (i.e., internal diameter 6.5 mm for men and 6.0 mm for women) (4)
5. Judicious use of lubrication and heat to prepare the tube
6. Proper technique (i.e., angulation of the tube in an inferior and posterior direction along the nasal floor)

Traditionally, it has been believed that in the presence of a midline nasal septum, the right nostril should be used for nasotracheal intubation because endotracheal tubes have a bevel on the tip such that the flat side faces to the left. A recent prospective study randomized nostril side in 128 patients undergoing nasotracheal intubation and found no difference in the incidence of epistaxis or the difficulty of intubation (4).

Chronic Sinusitis

The ostiomeatal complex represents the final common pathway of paranasal sinus drainage. Its patency ensures proper ventilation, aeration, mucociliary clearance, and prevention of effusion and infection. In response to the presence of an endotracheal tube in the nasal cavity, edema and inflammation of the lateral nasal wall mucosa can lead to obstruction

Table 23.1 Risk factors for intubation complications

Patient factors
Unfavorable anatomy—short, thick neck
Abnormal anatomy—facial skeletal abnormality, trismus
Preexisting anatomic conditions—loose dentition, nasal septal deviation, cervical spine abnormalities
Preexisting medical conditions—gastroesophageal reflux disease (GERD), diabetes, coagulopathy
Tube factors
Tube too large
Cuff pressure too high
Coexisting nasogastric (NG) tube
Technical factors
Forceful intubation
Poor visualization of larynx
Numerous intubation attempts

of the ostiomeatal complex, thereby resulting in effusion and infection within the paranasal sinuses. Obstruction is less common than previously thought. A study of nasotracheally intubated patients demonstrated sinus effusion on ultrasound within 3 days of intubation in 31% of patients (5). No patients developed sinusitis and all effusions resolved with removal of the tube. Longer-term intubation is associated with a higher incidence of sinusitis. At risk are immunocompromised patients and head injury patients with blood in the sinuses. Clinical manifestations of sinusitis include purulent rhinorrhea, fever, facial pain, and unilateral facial swelling. Pus obtained from the ostiomeatal complex with endoscopic guidance should be sent for culture and sensitivity. Computerized tomography (CT) can demonstrate effusion, but not all effusions represent true bacterial sinusitis. Sinusitis is not an important source of sepsis unless purulent sinusitis exists (2). Treatment involves removal of the tube if possible, a 3-day course of topical decongestant (i.e., pseudoephedrine, oxymetazoline, cocaine), and culture-directed antibiotics, including coverage for anaerobes and *Staphylococcus aureus*. Occasionally, antral lavage is necessary in refractory cases.

Nasal Alar Necrosis

Within hours, pressure necrosis can occur from the nasotracheal tube or its securing ties. This rare complication has been reported in isolated case reports in the literature (6,7). Surgical correction of this devastating cosmetic problem is extremely difficult. Prevention consists of proper cushioning between the nose, the tube, and securing ties.

Oral cavity and oropharyngeal complications

Acute Dental Injury

Injury to dentition is a relatively common complication of intubation, with a reported incidence of 1 in 150 to 1 in 1,500 intubations (8). This is an avoidable complication. Preventive measures include preoperative recognition of poor dentition or loose teeth and the use of a tooth guard during intubation. Injuries may include dental fracture, avulsion, and partial root avulsion. It is important to ensure that an avulsed tooth is recovered in order to prevent aspiration. Once the tooth is recovered, it should be placed in saline and a dental consultation should be obtained to consider reimplantation (3). In the case of a partial fracture, dental restoration can be considered. In the case of a partial avulsion, the tooth can be splinted or wired to an adjacent tooth.

Lip Injury

The upper lip can be lacerated if it is caught between the laryngoscope blade and the upper teeth. Likewise, the lower lip can be injured as the laryngoscope or the endotracheal tube drags the lip down across the lower teeth. Superficial injuries can be treated conservatively with topical antibiotic ointment, and deeper lacerations can be primarily closed with attention to accurate approximation of the vermillion border.

Temporomandibular Joint Injury

The temporomandibular joint can be dislocated as a consequence of forceful intubation or difficult intubation. At risk are patients with facial skeletal abnormalities. Clinically, the mandible is found to be locked in open position. The mechanism involves disruption of the ligamentous attachment of the temporomandibular disc to the condyle and subsequent displacement of the disc in the anteromedial direction due to the pull of the lateral pterygoid muscle. Immediate manual reduction under anesthesia with muscle relaxation is recommended. Postoperatively, the patient should be on a soft diet for 2 weeks.

Mucosal Injury

Injury to the mucosa of the oral cavity or oropharynx can be superficial, deep, or full-thickness. Risk factors include unfavorable anatomy (i.e., short, thick neck), limited neck extension, and trismus. Injury can manifest as laceration, hematoma, infection, or perforation. Superficial lacerations are treated conservatively while full-thickness lacerations are closed primarily. In the event of hematoma, antibiotics should be administered to prevent infection. Infection outside the pharynx can lead to abscess formation in the retropharyngeal or parapharyngeal spaces and can spread via tissue planes to the mediastinum. Neck abscess should be drained surgically. Perforation can be treated conservatively with nothing by mouth (NPO) and antibiotics if isolated, but should be repaired via an external cervical approach with closed suction drainage if large. Definitive airway management with prolonged intubation or tracheotomy may be necessary. It is important to note that positive pressure ventilation in the presence of pharyngeal injury can lead to subcutaneous emphysema, pneumomediastinum, or pneumothorax. These complications are discussed in the section on complications of tracheotomy.

Acute laryngeal complications

Mucosal Injury

Mucosal injury to the larynx can be superficial, deep, or transmural. Superficial mucosal injury heals spontaneously within days. Minor mucosal injury can result in troublesome bleeding into the airway (3), and attempts at suctioning can precipitate laryngeal edema. Superficial mucosal injury can also lead to vocal fold hematoma, which resolves spontaneously and does not require intervention except for voice rest. Vocal fold hematoma is more commonly left-sided because of right-handed intubators. Deep mucosal injury can result in cartilage exposure with subsequent chondritis. Symptoms include pain, dysphonia, and odynophagia. Patients with severe edema are treated with steroids and antibiotics (9). Airway obstruction requires definitive airway management. Transmural laryngeal injuries should undergo surgical repair via an open, laryngofissure approach. Laryngotracheal separation can occur from intubation in the setting of acute laryngeal trauma. Awake tracheotomy is the preferred method of airway control in this scenario.

Laryngospasm

Inadequate anesthesia on induction can lead to laryngospasm as a response to noxious stimuli anywhere in the body or stimulation of the airway. Aspiration of gastric contents may be an inciting event. Laryngospasm can also occur following extubation. The mechanism of airway obstruction is adduction of the true and false vocal folds, foreshortening of the larynx, pressing the preepiglottic soft tissues against the upper surface of the vocal folds, and complete closure of the larynx (10). Because there is no air movement through the larynx, there is no stridor despite obvious respiratory effort. Management consists of immediate removal of the noxious stimulus, proper positioning (i.e., head extended on a flexed neck) and positive pressure bag and mask ventilation. Lightening the anesthetic may restore tone to vocal fold abductors, thus enabling easier ventilation. If ventilation is not possible, a short-acting muscle relaxant such as succinylcholine should be administered, followed by maintenance of ventilation via a mask or endotracheal intubation if necessary. Prevention consists of adequate anesthesia on induction, avoidance of unnecessary stimuli while the patient is lightly anesthetized, and application of topical lidocaine on the vocal folds following endoscopic laryngeal surgery.

Arytenoid Dislocation/Subluxation

The paired arytenoids are irregular pyramidal-shaped cartilages situated on the cricoid cartilage. The base of the arytenoid cartilage is concave and articulates with the cricoid via the cricoarytenoid joint. This synovial joint allows rotation and translation, which are fundamental movements for proper vocal fold function. Inappropriately forceful or blind intubation can result in arytenoid dislocation or subluxation. Overall, however, this is a very uncommon complication. Clinical features include hoarseness after extubation, odynophagia, weak cough, and dysphagia. Diagnosis is made by bedside awake flexible laryngoscopy, revealing an immobile vocal fold, and the injured arytenoid cartilage is tipped anteriorly and medially (i.e., intubation injury) or posteriorly and laterally (i.e., extubation injury). One would also expect to see contractile activity in vocal fold musculature with phonation on stroboscopic evaluation (11). Definitive diagnosis is made by direct laryngoscopy with palpation of the joint. Laryngeal electromyography (EMG) and CT scan may also be helpful (11). The most important differential diagnosis to rule out is vocal fold paralysis from recurrent laryngeal nerve (RLN) injury. In this case, the joint would be freely mobile, and treatment is discussed in the section on complications of tracheal surgery. Voice therapy for dysphonia associated with suspected arytenoid dislocation or subluxation may be helpful in some patients (11), although manual endoscopic reduction is indicated as the definitive treatment (12).

Recurrent Laryngeal Nerve Injury

The RLN typically enters the larynx between the cricoid and thyroid cartilages near their articulation and travels a short distance submucosally. A cuffed endotracheal tube might compress the nerve in this region. Patients may develop vocal fold paralysis. Vocal fold paralysis can be an acute injury or can occur as a consequence of long-term intubation and inappropriately high cuff pressure. Patients complain of hoarseness and dysphagia postextubation. Principles of diagnosis and management of RLN injury are discussed in the section on tracheal surgery.

Chronic laryngeal complications

Laryngeal injury is common following prolonged intubation. After 10 days of intubation, the incidence of erythema and vocal fold ulceration is 94% and 67%, respectively, and most resolve within 8 weeks (13). The mechanism is straightforward: The posterior position of the endotracheal tube in the airway leads to compression of the mucosa overlying the cricoid cartilage, medial aspect of the arytenoid cartilages, interarytenoid region, and subglottis, leading to ischemic necrosis when the force of compression exceeds mucosal capillary perfusion pressure [i.e., >25 mm Hg (14)]. Following prolonged periods of intubation, granulation and fibrosis can result. Contributing factors include presence of a nasogastric (NG) tube, gastroesophageal reflux disease (GERD), diabetes, systemic vascular disease, and multiple intubation attempts (3).

Laryngotracheal Stenosis

Acquired postintubation stenosis is traditionally classified as glottic, subglottic, and tracheal. The incidence following prolonged intubation has been found to be 4% after 5 to 10 days and 14% beyond 10 days (15). Patients are initially asymptomatic but will develop symptoms weeks to months later. Symptoms may include decreased exercise tolerance, dysphonia, stridor, or dyspnea.

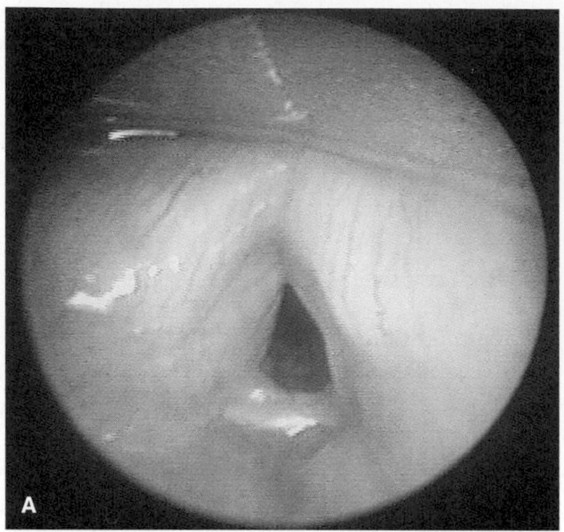

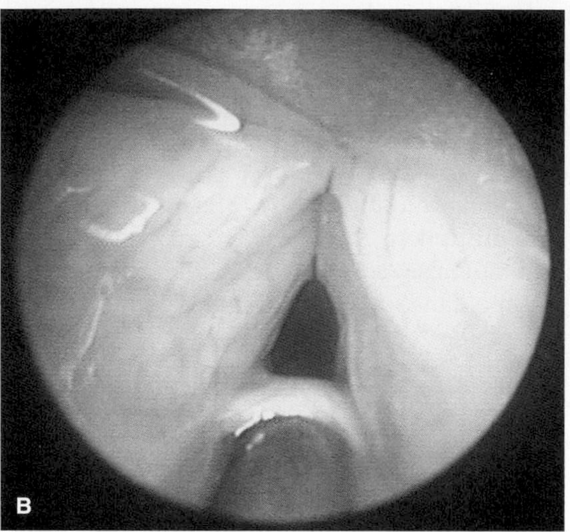

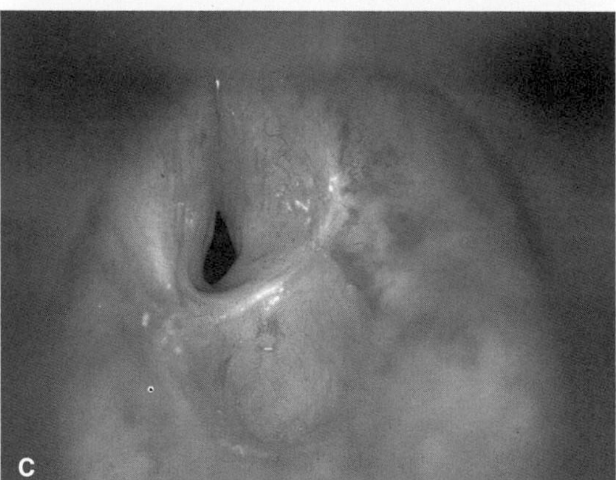

FIGURE 23.1. Two different extremes of posterior glottic stenosis. A relatively simple interarytenoid scar band (**A**) with demonstration of mucosalized tract posterior to scar band by passage of suction tip (**B**). Severe stenosis with dense posterior commissure scarring (**C**). Definitive surgical management depends on the location and extent of disease.

Accurate awake flexible endoscopic examination is important to determine laryngeal function and extent of glottic involvement. If there is combined laryngeal and tracheal damage, the larynx should be addressed first (16). Stenosis at the level of glottic larynx is typically posterior, at the level of the posterior vocal folds, vocal processes of the arytenoid cartilages, and interarytenoid region. A classification system for posterior glottic stenosis has been defined that ranges from a relatively simple interarytenoid scar band (Figs. 23.1A and B) to dense posterior commissure scarring involving both cricoarytenoid joints (Fig. 23.1C) (17). Subglottic stenosis occurs at the level of the cricoid cartilage, the narrowest portion of the airway (Fig. 23.2). Because stenoses can occur simultaneously from the larynx to the trachea, it is imperative to endoscopically assess the entire upper respiratory tract prior to surgical intervention. Awake endoscopy in the outpatient clinic is the optimum way to assess vocal fold mobility, while operative laryngoscopy and bronchoscopy under general anesthesia is often employed to determine the level and degree of injury, staging, and to confirm the diagnosis. Endoscopy of the subglottic larynx and trachea using topical anesthesia in the outpatient clinic has also been described as an alternative to operative endoscopy (18). CT scan with fine (2 mm) cuts through the larynx and upper trachea is useful to further delineate the extent of stenosis for diagnosis and surgical planning. Imaging studies, including chest x-ray and lateral neck x-ray, as well as pulmonary function studies, such as flow-volume loops, are imprecise.

Patients without a critical degree of airway compromise can be managed in the elective setting. Initial airway management in the setting of acute respiratory distress includes temporizing measures such as elevation of the head of the bed, cool humidified air, nebulized racemic epinephrine, corticosteroids, and heliox (i.e., a mixture of oxygen and helium that is low in density and flows more efficiently through a constricted airway). Critical airway stenosis that precludes the possibility of intubation is managed with immediate tracheotomy. If critical stenosis is not immediately present, the patient should be transferred to the operating room with an experienced anesthesiologist, otolaryngologist, and operating room staff. Available equipment should include a tracheotomy set, laryngoscope, dilators, rigid bronchoscopes, and endotracheal tubes of various sizes. The bronchoscope can be used to establish an airway rapidly and to dilate the stenotic segment if necessary. If a tracheotomy is performed, it should be done through the area of maximal tracheal damage in

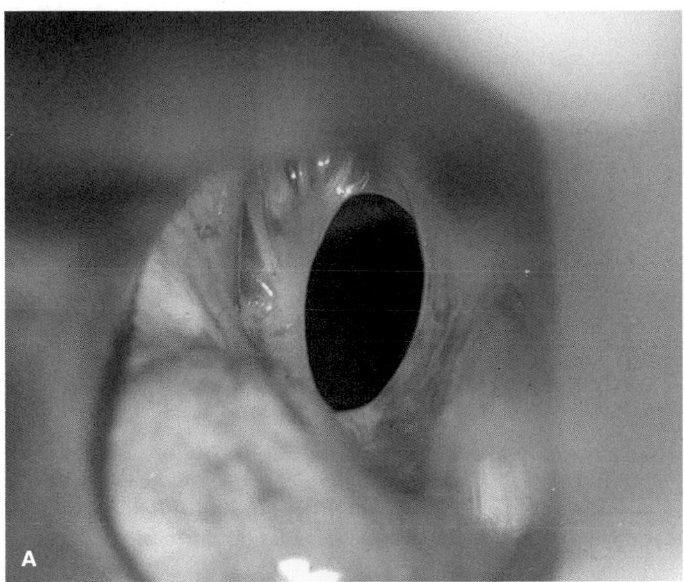

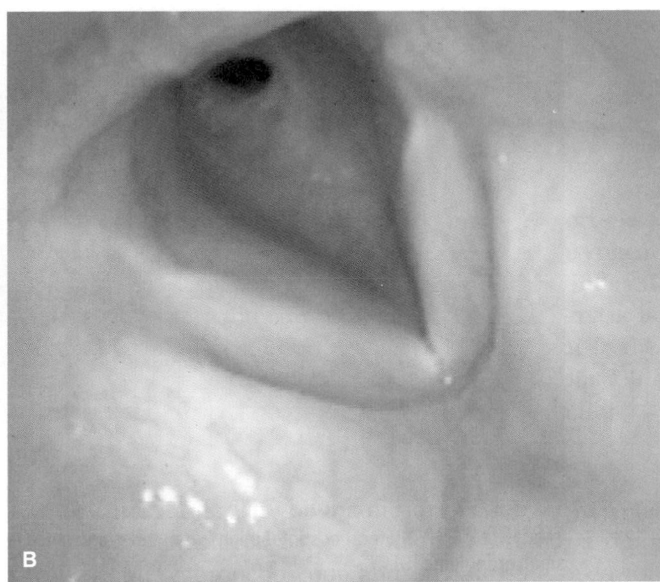

FIGURE 23.2. **A**: Mild short-segment subglottic stenosis. **B**: Severe subglottic stenosis.

order to preserve length for subsequent reconstruction (19). A T-tube can be used to stent the stenotic segment while awaiting surgery.

Glottic stenosis. Posterior glottic stenosis is often a challenging clinical problem. Options for posterior glottic stenosis include directed treatment at the area of stenosis itself, such as simple excision of a scar band, scar excision with endoscopic postcricoid advancement flap (20), open placement of a posterior cartilage graft, or open scar excision via laryngofissure with mucosal graft and postoperative stenting with either a Montgomery T-tube or a solid laryngeal stent for 6 to 8 weeks. Alternatively, enhancement of the airway can be accomplished by reduction or release of glottic tissue that may or may not be directly involved with the scar. This includes procedures such as arytenoidectomy or posterior cordotomy.

Subglottic stenosis. If the stenotic segment is $<$10 mm long, treatment can include endoscopic approaches, such as CO_2 laser excision with a microtrap door mucosal flap or radial incisions followed by dilation. Additionally, topical mitomycin-C is believed to be a useful adjunct for limiting restenosis (21). When an endoscopic approach is unfavorable, external approaches are warranted, such as cricoid division with cartilage graft or cricotracheal resection and primary thyrotracheal anastomosis.

Tracheal Stenosis

Treatment depends on the length of the stenotic segment, whether the stenosis is circumferential or not, and whether it is thin (membranous) or thick (fibrotic). Thin, short-segment stenosis can be managed with endoscopic dilation and CO_2 laser excision. Long-segment stenosis is best managed externally with segmental resection and primary end-to-end anastomosis. The details of tracheal resection for postintubation tracheal stenosis are discussed elsewhere (22). Basic principles include:

1. Accurate preoperative endoscopic evaluation of the anatomy of the stenotic segment
2. Preservation of tracheal blood supply
3. Tension-free anastomosis, which may require one or a combination of various described tracheal mobilization techniques (23)—finger dissection in the pretracheal plane, suprahyoid release, infrahyoid release, hilar release, reimplantation of left mainstem bronchus, and neck flexion
4. Careful patient selection (i.e., no mechanical ventilation, optimization of medical conditions)

Vocal process granuloma

Postintubation laryngeal granulomas arise at the medial aspect of the arytenoids, where there is greatest mechanical compression from the endotracheal tube. Terms in the literature used to describe this disease entity include "contact ulcer," "contact granuloma," and "vocal process granuloma."

Patients present with hoarseness after extubation, globus sensation (i.e., sensation of a lump in the throat), or laryngeal pain. Awake laryngoscopy is diagnostic (Figs. 23.3A and B). Typical endoscopic findings include proliferative tissue appearing pale gray to red in color, polypoid, nodular, or ulcerated in shape, and a posterior location. Biopsy should be considered if the appearance is not typical or there is no history of recent intubation.

Thinking of these lesions as wounds rather than as mass lesions helps to guide treatment. Medical treatment includes proton pump inhibitors and antireflux behavior, based on the premise that subclinical reflux can irritate the posterior glottis and delay healing of the granuloma (24). Voice therapy may

anterior jugular veins anteriorly, the innominate artery inferiorly, the lung apices inferolaterally, and the esophagus posteriorly.

Recurrent Laryngeal Nerve Injury

The RLN is in the tracheoesophageal groove and therefore should never be injured if dissection is precisely midline. This complication is usually identified when there is dysphonia after plugging the tracheostomy tube or decannulation and is verified with indirect laryngoscopy. Management of RLN injury is discussed in the section on complications of tracheal surgery.

Esophageal Injury

Transmural injury to the posterior wall of the trachea can extend into the esophagus. Management consists of prompt airway stabilization followed by surgical repair. TEF can also be a long-term complication of tracheotomy and is discussed later in this section.

Hemorrhage

Minor hemorrhage can be life-threatening if it interferes with the airway. Bleeding usually originates from the edges of the thyroid isthmus if this structure is divided during the procedure. Depending on surgeon preference, the thyroid isthmus can be divided sharply and suture ligated, carefully divided with monopolar cautery, or left intact. Whatever the technique chosen, it is advisable to check hemostasis at this site prior to incision of the trachea in order to avoid bleeding into the airway and to decrease risk of airway fire associated with the use of cautery in proximity to an open airway (32).

Major hemorrhage from great vessels is life-threatening. Bleeding from the innominate artery is discussed in the section on tracheoinnominate artery fistula (TIF). Bleeding from the internal jugular vein or common carotid artery is managed with recognition of the injury, proximal and distal vascular control, and repair or ligation by a surgeon with appropriate expertise.

Airway Fire

Supplemental oxygen may be present in the airway, originating from the ventilator through the endotracheal tube or from mask ventilation if an awake tracheotomy is performed under local anesthesia. In either scenario, the surgeon should be aware that an electrical arc from electrocautery, in the presence of supplemental oxygen, can result in airway fire. Airway fire is a devastating but rare complication that has been reported in the literature (32,33). Combustion is easily avoidable with proper precautions. There should be open communication between the anesthesiologist and the surgeon, particularly at the time of surgical entry into the airway. Electrocautery should not be used in the presence of an oxygen-enriched environment and potentially combustible material. In the event of airway fire, supplemental oxygen should be immediately discontinued. All potentially flammable material should be removed from the patient, including the endotracheal tube and surgical drapes. Direct laryngoscopy and rigid bronchoscopy with saline lavage should be performed to extinguish the fire, to re-establish airway control, and to assess damage.

Early postoperative complications

The early postoperative period, beginning in the recovery room, is the setting for several important treatable complications. These can be thought of as problems with the tracheotomy tube, problems associated with air outside the tracheobronchial tree, and other problems.

Tube Problems

Cannula obstruction. The tracheotomy tube itself can be obstructed by blood, secretions, or mucus. This problem is manifested clinically by decreased bilateral breath sounds and hypoxia. Cannula obstruction is easily managed with suction or removal and cleaning of the inner cannula. Prevention of obstruction is achieved by meticulous tracheostomy care, including humidified air and frequent suctioning after instillation of 1 to 2 cc of sterile saline (3).

Accidental decannulation. When accidental decannulation occurs, it is important for the surgical staff to replace the tube using the proper introducer and to confirm placement by verifying good ventilation or with flexible endoscopy through the tube. A tube that is blindly placed by well-meaning paramedical personnel can result in false passage. Prevention of decannulation is achieved by securing the tracheostomy tube to the patient with suture and tracheostomy ties. Anticipation is paramount in cases in which recannulation may be difficult, such as in obese patients with abundant cervical subcutaneous tissue, in difficult tracheotomies, and in pediatric cases. In such cases, the surgeon can consider placement of guide sutures to assist with recannulation. Nonabsorbable sutures can be placed around adjacent tracheal rings, brought out of the wound on either side of the tracheostomy tube, and taped to the skin. In the event of decannulation, manual tension of these sutures would bring the airway to the skin to permit easy recannulation. The Björk flap is an inferiorly based flap of anterior tracheal wall at the tracheostoma that is sutured to the overlying subcutaneous tissue; it is another useful technique in cases with the potential for difficult recannulation (34).

False passage. Consequences of the tracheotomy tube being in the subcutaneous tissue between the skin and the trachea include subcutaneous emphysema, pneumomediastinum, pneumothorax, and hypoventilation (i.e., loss of airway). This problem may occur with initial tube placement or by retraction of the distal end of the tube with patient movement or tube manipulation. Management consists of prompt recognition, re-establishment of the airway, and treatment of the complication. In the early postoperative period, the tracheotomy tract is not well formed, and therefore, recannulation should be performed with appropriate lighting, patient positioning, and equipment.

Air outside the tracheobronchial tree. As a consequence of the surgery itself, positive pressure ventilation into a false passage, or injury to pleura, air can dissect into various tissue planes, resulting in subcutaneous emphysema, pneumomediastinum, or pneumothorax. These complications are uncommon (incidence of 0.34%) (31). They share similar mechanisms—excessive dissection of tissue planes, cannula blockage, assisted ventilation with excessive pressure (35), excessive coughing against a mechanical ventilator, rupture of subpleural bleb, and discrepancy between size of tracheal opening and size of cannula. Prevention consists of avoiding unnecessary paratracheal dissection, creating an opening into the trachea that is similar in size to that of the cannula, and avoiding tight closure of the tracheotomy site. We do not close the surgical wound around the cannula.

Subcutaneous emphysema. This complication is heralded by the presence of neck swelling and crepitus. One must first exclude pneumomediastinum and pneumothorax. Management includes removal of skin sutures, replacement of cannula with one of a larger size, insertion of a cuffed tube, adequate sedation, and ventilation of the patient.

Pneumomediastinum and pneumothorax. Management includes observation, chest tube placement, adequate sedation, or reduction in positive end-expiratory pressure (PEEP).

Other problems. In patients with chronic upper airway obstruction, tracheotomy results in immediate relief of obstruction but can also result in postobstructive pulmonary edema. This is treated by mechanical ventilation with PEEP and appropriate diuresis.

Late postoperative complications

Long-term complications of tracheotomy include stenosis and fistulae. These problems are typically related to direct pressure necrosis at the cuff site (36). Initial mucosal ulceration leads to cartilage exposure, infection, and necrosis. A fibrotic stricture or full-thickness posterior perforation into the esophagus or anterior perforation into the innominate artery can occur (19). Tracheostomy tube cuffs should be kept between 20 and 25 mm Hg because pressures above 25 mm Hg have been shown to occlude submucosal tracheal capillaries (14). Since the advent of high volume, low-pressure cuffs, and specially designed tracheotomy tubes for unusual neck anatomy, these complications have decreased.

Tracheal Stenosis

This section will focus on tracheal stenosis as it relates to tracheotomy. The diagnosis and management of tracheal stenosis following intubation are discussed in the section on complications of intubation.

Fortunately, tracheal stenosis following tracheotomy is a rare complication. One study of 2,000 tracheotomies demonstrated the incidence of tracheal stenosis to be 0.5% (37). Technical factors in tracheotomy contributing to development of tracheal stenosis include excessively large opening into the trachea, neglected infection or chondritis, and excessive traction or movement of the tracheotomy tube. Some authors also cite specific tracheostoma techniques (i.e., inferiorly based Björk flap, excision of window, and H-shaped window) as risk factors for development of tracheal stenosis (38). Tracheal stenosis following tracheotomy can be classified anatomically into suprastomal (subglottic), stomal, and infrastomal. Some patients present early, with granulation tissue at the tip of the cannula. Granulation occurs as a result of friction of the tip against the tracheal mucosa. Most patients present following decannulation. Complaints include shortness of breath, exertional dyspnea, cough, or biphasic stridor and respiratory distress if severe. Symptoms may be exacerbated with a viral respiratory illness and may mimic bronchitis, asthma, or pneumonia.

Fistulae

Erosion of the tracheotomy tube into an adjacent structure is a dreaded, potentially life-threatening, and preventable complication. The tube can erode anteriorly into the innominate artery (TIF) and posteriorly into the esophagus (TEF), and decannulation can result in persistent tracheocutaneous fistula if the wound does not heal completely. Mechanisms include a tracheotomy that is too low (i.e., below the third tracheal ring), a cuff that is inflated too high, and local wound healing problems (i.e., infection, irradiation, and tube movement during mechanical ventilation).

Tracheoesophageal Fistula

The incidence of this uncommon but highly morbid complication is 0.5% (39). TEF is life-threatening because of contamination of the airway and interference with nutrition. TEF is commonly associated with tracheal stenosis since it shares a common pathophysiology. Patients present with a dramatic increase in tracheal secretions, resembling enteral feedings. Coughing may follow oral swallowing. Gastric distension may occur secondary to ventilated air into the stomach. Initial diagnosis is made with endoscopy through the stoma and can be confirmed with methylene blue dye swallow and observation of dye in the trachea. Barium swallow is diagnostic. If the patient is ventilated, a low-pressure cuffed endotracheal tube should be advanced below the fistula site and a gastrostomy performed for gastric drainage and a jejunostomy for enteral nutrition (39). There is evidence that TEFs do not close spontaneously (19). Therefore, management is surgical. Principles of surgical management include multilayered repair with interposition of muscle between the esophagus and trachea.

Tracheoinnominate Artery Fistula

TIF is a rare, often fatal complication that occurs when a tracheostomy tube erodes anteriorly into the posterior wall of the innominate artery. TIF can also occur as a consequence of tracheal resection and tracheal stenting. The incidence is reported to be 0.3% following tracheotomy, and most occur

Cricothyroidotomy

In 1921, Chevalier Jackson published a landmark paper condemning cricothyroidotomy (57). He stated that "high tracheotomy should never be done" because of the high observed rate of laryngeal stenosis (57). This doctrine remained unchallenged until 1976, when Brantigan and Grow published study of a large series of cardiothoracic surgery patients who underwent cricothyroidotomy for elective airway management (58). Cricothyroidotomy is appropriate in the emergency airway situation because it is rapid and can be life-saving. The controversies are (i) whether cricothyroidotomy should be converted to formal tracheostomy for long-term airway management and (ii) whether elective cricothyroidotomy should be performed.

Jackson reviewed 200 cases of chronic laryngeal stenosis and found that 158 cases were due to "high tracheotomy" (57). Not all cases were true cricothyroidotomies, as most involved division of the cricoid cartilage and 32 cases were performed through the cricothyroid membrane *and* thyroid cartilage. Many patients had an underlying inflammatory disorder of the larynx that may have predisposed them to the development of stenosis. Jackson reasoned that the subglottis is the narrowest segment of the airway and that the subglottic mucosa is intolerant to trauma. He therefore advocated "low tracheotomy" below the second tracheal ring in order to prevent laryngeal stenosis. Brantigan and Grow challenged this doctrine in their review of 655 thoracic surgery patients who underwent elective cricothyroidotomy. They observed no cases of chronic subglottic stenosis but found five cases of chronic tracheal stenosis at the cuff site, all requiring tracheal resection. They cite absence of cross-contamination of median sternotomy wounds, simplicity, and safety as the basis of their recommendation that routine elective cricothyroidotomy is appropriate. However, follow-up was limited (i.e., obtained in many cases with telephone calls to patients or referring physicians) and data on vocal quality was lacking. Subsequently, several studies demonstrated variable rates of subglottic stenosis, ranging from 1% to 48%. A meta-analysis of 875 patients who underwent cricothyroidotomy revealed a 4% overall incidence of subglottic stenosis. The authors demonstrated that if patients with contraindications to cricothyroidotomy are excluded, this incidence drops to 1% (59). Contraindications include prolonged endotracheal intubation at 7 days or greater (59), coexisting laryngeal infection (57,60), and upper airway difficulties after endotracheal intubation. Other risk factors for subglottic stenosis following elective cricothyroidotomy include prolonged cannulation beyond 30 days (61) and patients under the age of 18 (59,62). This seemingly low incidence of subglottic stenosis contrasts with a 0.5% incidence of tracheal stenosis following tracheotomy (37). Subglottic stenosis is significantly more difficult to manage than tracheal stenosis and should therefore be prevented whenever possible.

The effect of cricothyroidotomy on voice has been neglected in much of the early, nonotolaryngologic literature on cricothyroidotomy complications. Several studies have documented a high incidence of voice disturbance following cricothyroidotomy, ranging from 40% to 75% (60,63,64). The mechanism involves (i) scarring of the cricothyroid membrane, which limits the pivoting of the thyroid cartilage on the cricoid cartilage that is necessary to increase length and tension of the vocal folds, and (ii) glottic scarring, as a consequence of the close proximity (10 mm) of the true vocal folds with the upper limit of the cricothyroid membrane (59).

In summary, subglottic stenosis can occur following cricothyroidotomy, even in carefully selected patients, and vocal dysfunction is a common complication that is difficult to manage. We conclude that (i) cricothyroidotomy is indicated in the emergency airway setting, (ii) emergency cricothyroidotomy should be expeditiously converted to a formal tracheotomy in an elective setting in order to limit vocal dysfunction and prevent subglottic stenosis, and (iii) elective cricothyroidotomy for long-term airway management *may* be indicated in cases in which it is crucial to maintain separation between the cervical wound and the median sternotomy wound and is contraindicated in patients who have been intubated for 7 days or longer, patients with coexisting laryngeal pathology, occupational and professional voice users, and patients under the age of 18 (59).

TRACHEAL SURGERY

Indications for tracheal resection include primary tracheal tumors, tumors invading the trachea, and stenosis. The most common indication for tracheal resection and reconstruction is postintubation tracheal stenosis (45); therefore, most complications of tracheal surgery can be avoided by prevention of tracheal stenosis. Prevention is achieved by atraumatic intubation technique, proper selection of endotracheal tube, proper inflation of a low-pressure cuff, and avoidance of long-term endotracheal intubation. However, when tracheal resection is indicated, the surgeon must be aware of potential adverse outcomes, their management, and their prevention. Tracheal resection and primary anastomosis are highly successful. A recent series of 23 cases of acquired upper airway stenosis treated with segmental resection and primary reanastomosis had a decannulation rate of 96% (65). The complication rate of tracheal surgery has been found to increase as the anastomotic level rises (45).

Intraoperative complications

Recurrent Laryngeal Nerve Injury

Given its proximity to the trachea, the RLN is prone to injury during tracheal surgery. This is particularly true in the upper cervical trachea and near the laryngotracheal junction. Meticulous surgical technique and knowledge of pertinent anatomy are the most important safeguards to lessen the likelihood of injury.

The primary clinical manifestations of unilateral RLN injury are a paralyzed vocal fold and dysphonia (66). Some patients will also have dysphagia and signs of aspiration. Airway compromise, usually with stridor due to bilateral vocal fold paralysis, is the hallmark of bilateral RLN injury.

Treatment options for unilateral RLN injury include the nonsurgical alternatives of observation or voice therapy. Surgical treatment options include vocal fold medialization with injection laryngoplasty or laryngeal framework surgery, or laryngeal reinnervation (67). The ideal treatment option, that is able to restore physiologic movements, is not yet at hand.

Expectant management is appropriate in circumstances where the paralysis may be temporary, such as a neurapraxia due to traction injury or when the symptom severity does not mandate treatment. When observing for possible spontaneous recovery, a period of 6 months to 1 year is generally advocated.

Voice therapy by a speech pathologist should be considered to help ameliorate symptoms during a period when spontaneous recovery is possible, in poor surgical candidates, or for patients whose symptoms are toward the less severe side of the spectrum. Vocal therapy may also be employed as an adjunctive treatment either preoperatively or postoperatively in surgically treated patients.

Although surgical medialization of a paralyzed vocal fold does not restore normal dynamic laryngeal physiology, it is typically a very effective geometrical solution for incomplete glottic closure (Fig. 23.5). Medialization allows the contralateral, normal vocal fold to make better contact with the paralyzed vocal fold during phonation and deglutition.

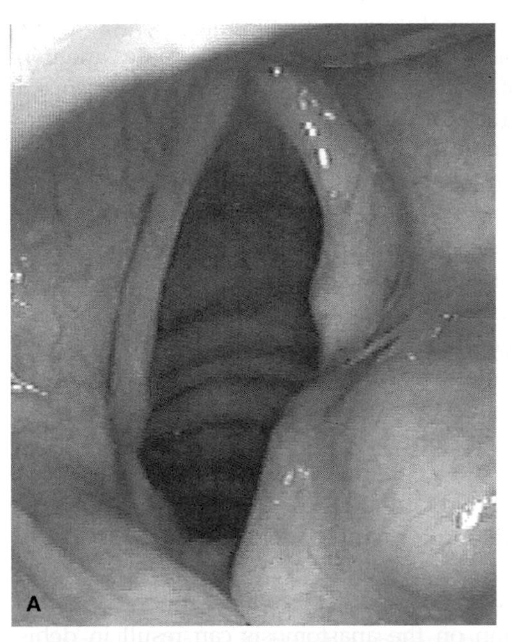

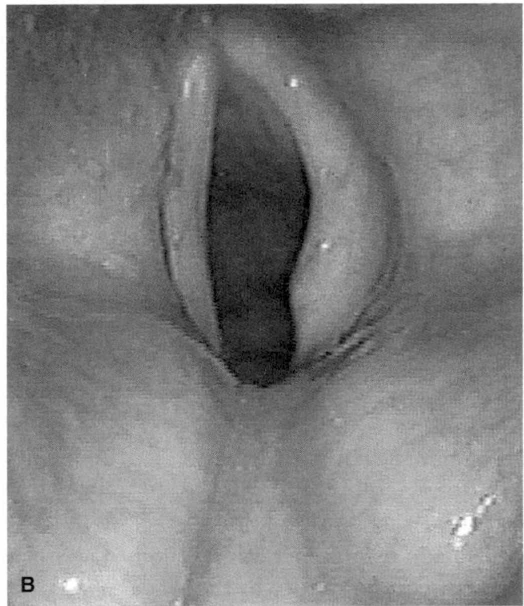

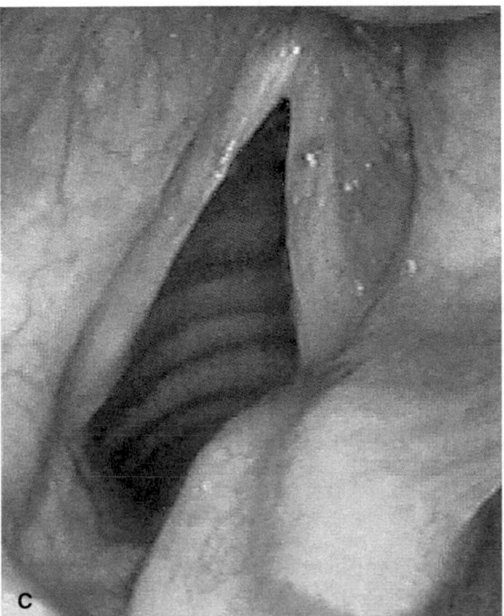

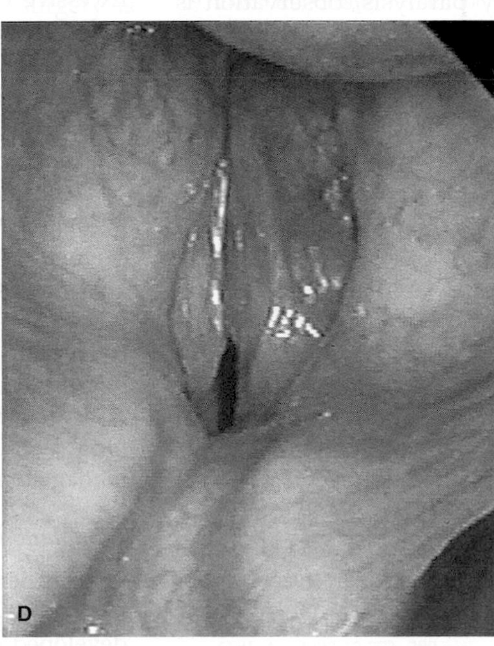

FIGURE 23.5. Patient with unilateral vocal fold paralysis due to right recurrent laryngeal nerve (RLN) injury during inspiration (**A**) and phonation (**B**) prior to laryngeal framework surgery with type-I thyroplasty. Same patient during inspiration (**C**) and phonation (**D**) postsurgical medialization of the paralyzed vocal fold.

40. Grillo HC, Donahue DM, Mathisen DJ, et al. Postintubation tracheal stenosis: treatment and results. *J Thorac Cardiovasc Surg* 1995;109:486–493.
41. Grillo HC, Mathisen DJ. Cervical exenteration. *Ann Thorac Surg* 1990;49: 401–408.
42. Jones JW, Reynolds M, Hewitt RL, et al. Tracheo-innominate artery erosion: successful surgical management of a devastating complication. *Ann Surg* 1976;184:194–204.
43. Allan JS, Wright C. Tracheoinnominate fistula: diagnosis and management. *Chest Surg Clin N Orth Am* 2003;13:331–341.
44. Utley JR, Singer MM, Roe BB, et al. Definitive management of innominate artery hemorrhage complicating tracheostomy. *JAMA* 1972;220: 577–579.
45. Lanuti M, Mathisen DJ. Management of complications of tracheal surgery. *Chest Surg Clin N Orth Am* 2003;13:385–397.
46. Lawson DW, Grillo HC. Closure of persistent tracheal stomas. *Surg Gynecol Obstet* 1970;130:995–996.
47. Bishop JB, Bostwick J, Nahai F. Persistent tracheostomy stoma. *Am J Surg* 1980;140:709–710.
48. Carr MM, Poje CP, Kingston L, et al. Complications in pediatric tracheostomies. *Laryngoscope* 2001;111:1925–1928.
49. Kremer B, Botos-Kremer A, Eckel HE, et al. Indications, complications and surgical techniques for pediatric tracheostomies—an update. *J Pediatr Surg* 2002;37:1556–1562.
50. Rodgers BM, Rooks JJ, Talbert JL. Pediatric tracheostomy: long-term evaluation. *J Pediatr Surg* 1979;14(14):258–263.
51. Carron JD, Derkay CS, Strope GL, et al. Pediatric tracheotomies: changing indications and outcomes. *Laryngoscope* 2000;110: 1099–1104.
52. Toye FJ, Weinstein JD. A percutaneous tracheotomy device. *Surgery* 1969;65:384–389.
53. Ciaglia P, Firsching R, Syniec C. Elective percutaneous dilatational tracheostomy: a new simple bedside procedure: preliminary report. *Chest* 1985;87:715–719.
54. Sharpe MD, Parnes LS, Drover JW. Translaryngeal tracheostomy: experience of 340 cases. *Laryngoscope* 2003;113(3):530–536.
55. Oliver ER, Gist A, Gillespie MB. Percutaneous versus surgical tracheotomy: an updated meta-analysis. *Laryngoscope* 2007;117(9): 1570–5.
56. Anderson HL, Bartlett RH. Elective tracheotomy for mechanical ventilation by the percutaneous technique. *Clin Chest Med* 1991;12(3):555–560.
57. Jackson C. High tracheotomy and other errors—the chief causes of chronic laryngeal stenosis. *Surg Gynecol Obstet* 1921;32:392–398.
58. Brantigan CO, Grow JB. Cricothyroidotomy: elective use in respiratory problems requiring tracheotomy. *J Thorac Cardiovasc Surg* 1976;71: 72–80.
59. Burkey B, Esclamado R, Morganroth M. The role of cricothyroidotomy in airway management. *Clin Chest Med* 1991;12(3): 561–571.
60. Cole RR, Aguilar EA. Cricothyroidotomy versus tracheotomy: an otolaryngologist's perspective. *Laryngoscope* 1988;98:131–135.
61. Kuriloff DB, Setzen M, Portnoy W, et al. Laryngotracheal injury following cricothyroidotomy. *Laryngoscope* 1989;99:125–130.
62. Sise MJ, Shackford SR, Cruickshank JC, et al. Cricothyroidotomy for long-term tracheal access: a prospective analysis of morbidity and mortality in 76 patients. *Ann Surg* 1984;200(1):13–17.
63. Gleeson MJ, Pearson FG, Armistead S, et al. Voice changes following cricothyroidotomy. *J Laryngol Otol* 1984;98:1015–1019.
64. Holst M, Hertegard S, Persson A. Vocal dysfunction following cricothyroidotomy: a prospective study. *Laryngoscope* 1990;100:749–755.
65. Wolf M, Shapira Y, Talmi YP, et al. Laryngotracheal anastomosis: primary and revised procedures. *Laryngoscope* 2001;111:622–627.
66. Hoff PT, Hogikyan ND. Unilateral vocal fold paralysis. *Curr Opin Otolaryngol Head Neck Surg* 1996;4:176–181.
67. Zeitels SM, Casiano RR, Gardner GM, et al. Management of common voice problems: committee report. *Otolaryngol Head Neck Surg* 2002;126: 333–348.
68. Isshiki N, Morita H, Okamura H, et al. Thyroplasty as a new phonosurgical technique. *Acta Otolaryngol (Stockh)* 1974;78:451–457.
69. Lundy D, Casiano RR, Xue JW, et al. Thyroplasty type I: short versus long-term results. *Otolaryngol Head Neck Surg* 2000;122: 533–536.
70. Hogikyan ND, Wodchis WP, Terrell JE, et al. Voice-related quality of life (V-RQOL) following type I thyroplasty for unilateral vocal fold paralysis. *J Voice* 2000;14:378–386.
71. Crumley RL. Update: ansa cervicalis to recurrent laryngeal nerve anastomoses for unilateral laryngeal paralysis. *Laryngoscope* 1991;101: 384–387.
72. Olson D, Goding GS, Michael DD. Acoustic and perceptual evaluation of laryngeal reinnervation by ansa cervicalis. *Laryngoscope* 1998;108: 1767–1772.
73. Flint PW, Shiotani A, O'Malley BW. IGF-I gene transfer into denervated rat laryngeal muscle. *Arch Otolaryngol Head Neck Surg* 1999;125:274–279.
74. Rubin AD, Mobley B, Hogikyan ND, et al. Delivery of an adenoviral vector to the crushed recurrent laryngeal nerve. *Laryngoscope* 2003;113: 985–989.
75. Hillel AD, Benninger M, Blitzer A, et al. Evaluation and management of bilateral vocal cord immobility. *Otolaryngol Head Neck Surg* 1999;121: 760–765.
76. Cunningham M, Eavey RD, Vlahakes GJ, et al. Slide tracheoplasty for long-segment tracheal stenosis. *Arch Otolaryngol Head Neck Surg* 1998; 124(1):98–103.

CHAPTER

24

Complications of Esophageal Surgery

Andrew C. Chang and Mark D. Iannettoni

ANATOMIC AND PHYSIOLOGIC CONSIDERATIONS

Many of the complications of esophageal surgery are related directly to the unique features of esophageal anatomy and physiology. Detailed knowledge and thorough understanding of these characteristics are essential for the surgeon to identify potential pitfalls of esophageal surgery and avert complications before they occur. A unique feature of esophageal anatomy is its unusually fatty submucosa, which allows greater mobility of the overlying squamous mucosa. In performing a manual esophageal anastomosis, every suture should transfix the mucosal edge, which at times can retract more than 1 cm from the cut esophageal margin (Fig. 24.1). The esophagus is also unique in the gastrointestinal tract because it lacks a serosal layer. The soft and often tenuous muscle holds sutures poorly and cannot be relied upon to maintain a fundoplication, for example, unless the associated submucosa is included by the esophageal stitch.

The esophagus is nourished by four to six paired aortic-esophageal arteries as well as collateral circulation from the inferior thyroid, intercostals, bronchial, inferior phrenic, and left gastric arteries. Although the segmental "poor" blood supply of the esophagus has frequently been incriminated as the cause of anastomotic disruption, the submucosal collateral circulation of the esophagus is extensive. Even after the cardia has been divided and the intrathoracic esophagus mobilized completely out of the chest, the distal end of the esophagus maintains good arterial bleeding so long as the inferior thyroid arteries remain intact. Poor technique, not poor blood supply, is the more likely explanation for the complication of esophageal anastomotic disruption. Finally, parasympathetic innervation of the esophagus is supplied by the vagus nerves, and the recurrent laryngeal supplies the upper portion of the esophagus. Recurrent laryngeal nerve injury during esophageal surgery can result in one of the most devastating complications, cricopharyngeal muscle dysfunction with subsequent incapacitating cervical dysphagia and aspiration pneumonia (1). Similarly, injury to the vagal nerve trunks in operations on the distal esophagus may produce neurogenic dysphagia or gastric atony and pylorospasm, which are very troublesome complications after esophageal surgery.

Physiologic considerations influence other complications following surgery of the esophagus. The pathophysiology of gastroesophageal reflux and secondary reflux esophagitis directly influences the results of antireflux surgery and hence the complication of recurrent reflux. For example, it has been demonstrated that the incidence of recurrent reflux in patients undergoing the standard Belsey Mark IV transthoracic hiatal hernia repair in the presence of esophagitis or a stricture is between 25% and 75% (2,3). In the presence of the intramural inflammation and esophageal shortening that may accompany reflux esophagitis, the esophageal sutures of the Belsey repair may not be reliable, and tension on the repair to reduce the requisite 3 to 5 cm of distal esophagus below the diaphragm sets the stage for recurrence of the hernia (Fig. 24.2). These same considerations apply to the Nissen fundoplication and the Hill posterior gastropexy, which also aim to restore an intra-abdominal segment of distal esophagus and require esophageal or periesophageal sutures. To avert the complication of disruption of the repair due to the need to suture inflamed esophagus and tension on the repair, the esophagus-lengthening Collis gastroplasty can be combined with a fundoplication (4–6). The gastroplasty tube functions as a new distal esophagus and provides healthy, resilient tissue, i.e., the gastric wall, around which to perform the fundoplication. Furthermore, the additional "esophageal length" provided by the gastroplasty tube reduces tension on the repair (Fig. 24.3). The presence of reflux esophagitis and a peptic stricture also complicates an antireflux procedure if the stricture is perforated during attempted dilation.

An intrathoracic esophagogastric anastomotic leak, perhaps the most dreaded complication of esophageal surgery, owes its morbidity in part to associated gastroesophageal reflux. An intrathoracic esophagogastric anastomosis is associated almost invariably with the development of reflux esophagitis, compared with a cervical esophagogastric anastomosis, which is rarely associated with clinically significant reflux. Although it has been argued that with

Andrew C. Chang: University of Michigan Medical Center, Ann Arbor, MI 48109.

Mark D. Iannettoni: University of Iowa Hospitals and Clinics, Iowa City, IA 52242.

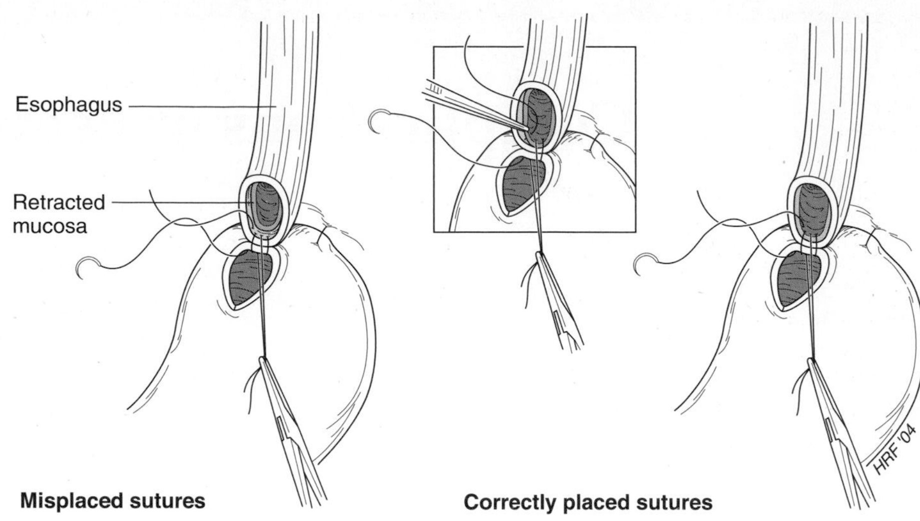

FIGURE 24.1. Misplacement of the esophagogastric anastomotic suture. The relatively great mobility of the esophageal mucosa over the fatty submucosa permits the cut mucosal edge to retract proximally. Unless care is taken to identify the mucosa and properly transfix it with each suture, mucosal apposition will not occur and an anastomotic disruption will follow. (Reproduced with permission from Orringer MB. Complications of esophageal surgery and trauma. In: Greenfield LJ, ed. *Complications in surgery and trauma,* 2nd ed. Philadelphia, PA: J.B. Lippincott; 1990:303.)

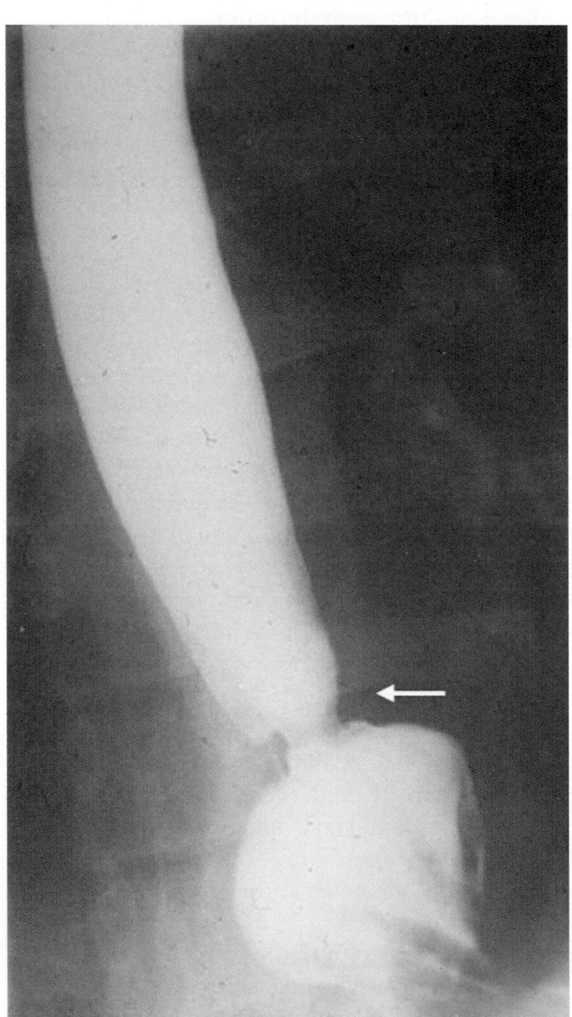

FIGURE 24.2. A sliding hiatus hernia with a peptic stricture at the esophagogastric junction (*arrow*). Standard antireflux operation (Hill, Belsey, or Nissen) require reduction below the diaphragm not only of the esophagogastric junction but also the distal 3 to 5 cm of esophagus. The relative shortening associated with the distal esophagitis in this patient prevented a tension-free standard repair. (Reproduced with permission from Orringer MB. Complications of esophageal surgery and trauma. In: Greenfield LJ, ed. *Complications in surgery and trauma,* 2nd ed. Philadelphia, PA: J.B. Lippincott; 1990:305.)

appropriate attention to detail, an intrathoracic esophagogastric anastomosis can be performed reliably and with an exceedingly low morbidity rate (7), the potential for an anastomotic leak and secondary mediastinitis cannot be eliminated totally, and this fact perhaps more than anything else has influenced our current "defensive posture" that the best esophagogastric anastomosis is a cervical anastomosis, with which the consequence of a leak is a salivary fistula and not life-threatening mediastinitis and sepsis.

Gastroesophageal reflux after esophageal resection and an esophagogastric anastomosis may be responsible for life-threatening aspiration of gastric contents into the tracheobronchial tree in the early postoperative period. For this reason, initial decompression of the intrathoracic stomach with a nasogastric tube and placement of the patient in a 45° head-up position are important. Similarly, because of the potential for regurgitation and aspiration after eating, patients who have a fresh esophagogastric anastomosis should not be permitted to undergo postural drainage as part of their postoperative pulmonary physiotherapy within 1 to 2 hours of mealtime.

The potential pulmonary complications, primarily aspiration pneumonia, resulting from esophageal obstruction due to a variety of causes cannot be overestimated. Particularly in the patient with a megaesophagus of advanced achalasia, the risk of massive regurgitation and aspiration on induction of general anesthesia is enormous. Awareness of this possibility dictates the need for nasogastric tube esophageal decompression and emptying in these patients before a rapid sequence induction of general anesthesia and endotracheal intubation.

ESOPHAGEAL PERFORATION

Perforation of the thoracic esophagus, with resultant mediastinitis, poses a devastating threat. Regardless of the cause of perforation (Table 24.1), delay in recognition and definitive management increases concomitant mortality and

Table 24.1 Causes of esophageal perforation

Instrumental
Endoscopy
Direct injury
Transesophageal echocardiography
Injury occurring during removal of a foreign body
Dilatation
Intubation (esophageal, endotracheal)
Catheter-based radiofrequency ablation for atrial fibrillation
Noninstrumental
Barogenic trauma
Postemetic
Blunt chest or abdominal trauma
Other (e.g., labor, convulsion, defecation)
Penetrating neck, chest or abdominal trauma
Postoperative
Anastomotic disruption
Devascularization following pulmonary resection, vagotomy or repair of hiatal hernia
Injury following ingestion of caustic agent
Erosion by adjacent infection with resultant fistula involving the tracheobronchial tree, pericardium, pleural cavity or aorta
Pathologic
Severe reflux esophagitis
Candidal, herpetic and opportunistic infection

morbidity. Repair of an acute esophageal tear in an otherwise normal esophagus within 6 to 8 hours carries a risk of morbidity that 1is essentially the same as that imposed by elective esophagotomy and primary esophageal closure. If operative intervention is delayed beyond this early period, local inflammation greatly jeopardizes primary healing of the esophageal tear and mortality rises dramatically (8–10).

Esophageal instrumentation accounts for the large majority of iatrogenic perforation, with the cricopharyngeal area most commonly injured (Fig. 24.4). Perforation of the mid and distal esophagus is most likely to occur following biopsy or dilatation (Fig. 24.5). There has been increasing awareness of esophageal necrosis and atrioesophageal fistula due to thermal injury sustained during catheter-based radiofrequency ablation for atrial fibrillation, with incidence ranging from 0.03% to 0.5% and possibly higher (11). Spontaneous perforation usually occurs following straining (Boerhaave's syndrome) with rupture involving the left posterior aspect of the distal esophagus (12).

DIAGNOSIS

Patients with esophageal perforation typically present with pain, directly referring to the site of perforation. The presence of mediastinal air or hydropneumothorax on chest radiograph in a patient suspected of having a perforation is confirmatory. However, a normal chest radiograph does not exclude the possibility of esophageal perforation. Not every esophageal tear is a full-thickness disruption. For example, pneumatic dilatation of the esophagus for achalasia may result in a tear of the distal esophageal mucosa and submucosa. Air insufflation through a flexible esophagoscope may result in mediastinal, cervical or subcutaneous air, exaggerating the extent of injury. Following esophagoscopy or esophageal operation, postoperative pain or fever should be considered a result of esophageal perforation until proven otherwise. Contrast esophagogram should be performed immediately in order to limit any further delay in establishing proper drainage and/or definitive repair. Water-soluble contrast esophagogram, followed by dilute barium, best identifies the site of perforation (Fig. 24.6), whether the perforation communicates with either the pleural or peritoneal cavities, or is confined to the mediastinum.

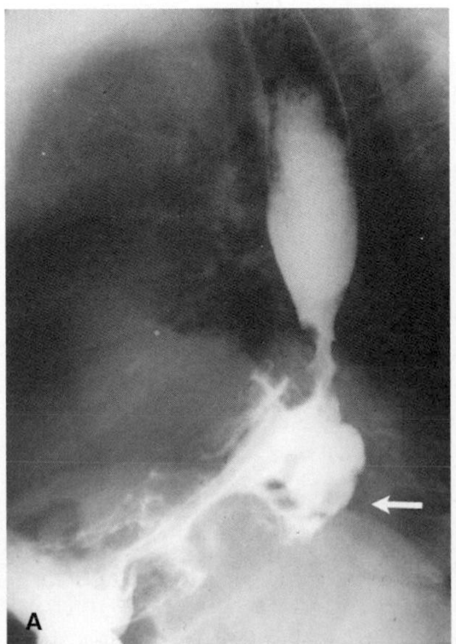

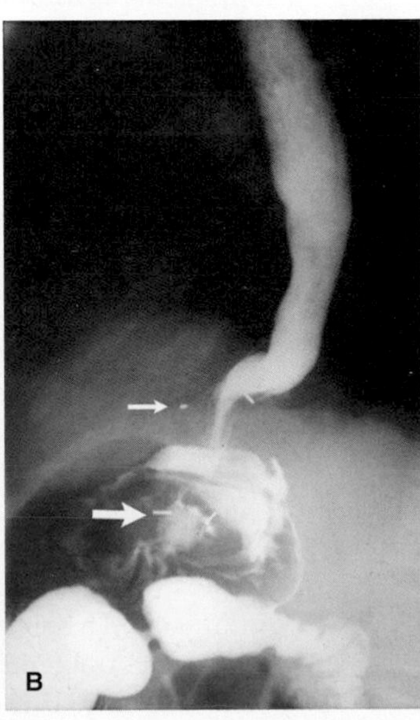

FIGURE 24.3. **A:** This lateral view from a preoperative esophagogram show a large, sliding hiatus hernia with half of the stomach above the left hemidiaphragm (*arrow*), a proximal stricture, and esophageal dilatation from the obstruction. **B:** Postoperative appearance of the reconstructed distal esophagus following intraoperative dilatation of the stricture and a Collis gastroplasty-Nissen fundoplication. The horizontal gastric folds in the fundoplication around the distal 5 to 7 cm of the functional esophagus can be seen. Also visible are the titanium clips (*small arrow*) marking the diaphragmatic hiatus and those at the new esophagogastric junction (*large arrow*). There is no evidence of esophageal stenosis, and the dilation proximal to the obstruction has resolved. (Reproduced with permission from Orringer MB. Complications of esophageal surgery and trauma. In: Greenfield LJ, ed. *Complications in surgery and trauma,* 2nd ed. Philadelphia; PA. J.B. Lippincott; 1990:308.)

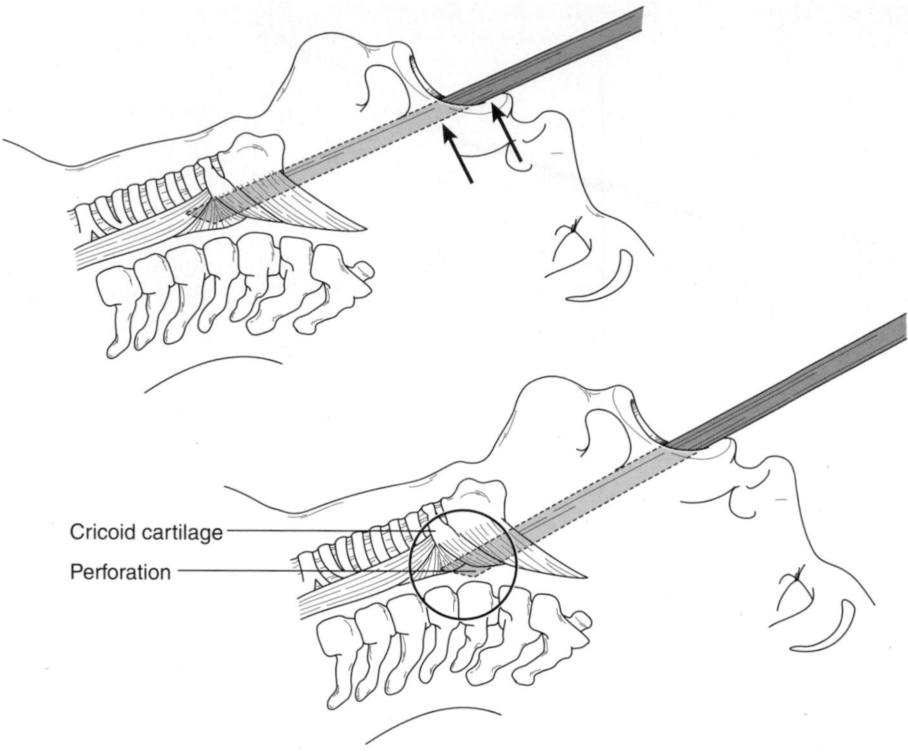

FIGURE 24.4. The mechanism of endoscopic cervical esophageal perforation. In performing rigid esophagoscopy, it is essential that a gentle, steady, lifting force (*arrow*) be exerted to displace forward the larynx and cricoid cartilage. Failure to overcome the natural pull of the upper esophageal sphincter against the cricoid cartilage results in a typical posterior perforation (*inset*). (Reproduced with permission from Orringer MB. Complications of esophageal surgery and trauma. In: Greenfield LJ, ed. *Complications in surgery and trauma,* 2nd ed. Philadelphia, PA. J.B. Lippincott; 1990:309.)

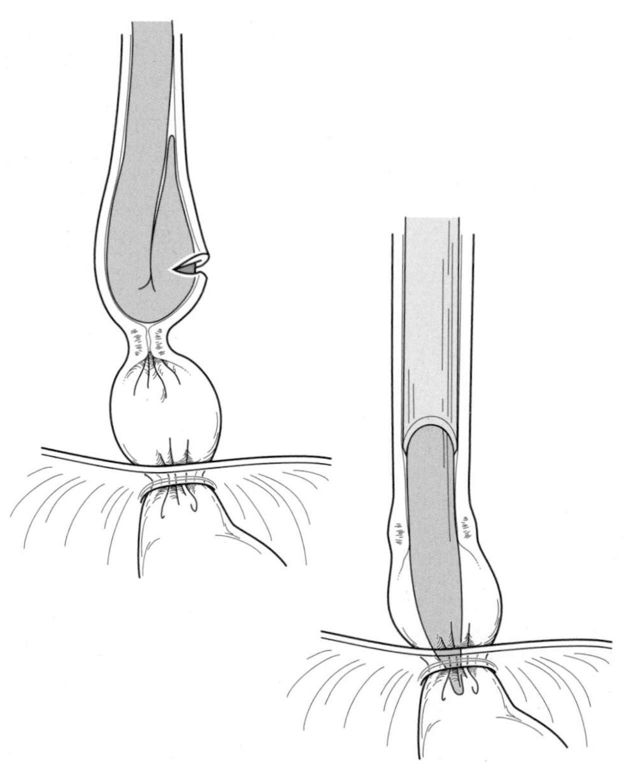

FIGURE 24.5. Esophageal perforation during an attempt at blind passage of a dilator through a tight stricture. (*Left*) The dilator has curled proximal to the stenosis, and as the bougie is advanced, disruption of the esophagus may occur. (*Right*) Using a special-order, large esophagoscope that will accommodate up to a 50-French dilator, the stricture can be visualized directly for dilatation. (Reproduced with permission from Orringer MB. Complications of esophageal surgery and trauma. In: Greenfield LJ, ed. *Complications in Surgery and Trauma,* 2nd ed. Philadelphia, PA. J.B. Lippincott; 1990:310.)

TREATMENT

Once the diagnosis of esophageal perforation is established, oral intake by the patient should cease. Aggressive intravenous fluid resuscitation, facilitated by using either a central venous pressure catheter or pulmonary artery catheter, is indicated if there is hypovolemia associated with intrathoracic perforation. Broad-spectrum antibiotic coverage is initiated. The presence of carious teeth increases the morbidity risk of esophageal injury owing to the virulence of swallowed oral bacteria. Thus, oral hygiene cannot be neglected in the patient with an esophageal perforation.

There is controversy about the best method of treatment of patients with esophageal perforations. Nonoperative "conservative" therapy is successful in some patients with esophageal perforation, primarily those with pre-existing periesophageal and mediastinal fibrosis that contains the injury. Thus, for the esophageal disruption in which contrast material extends only a few millimeters from the esophageal lumen and the patient is doing well clinically, antibiotic therapy, chest tube drainage as indicated and observation may suffice (13–15). More frequently, successful outcome following esophageal perforation requires surgical intervention (Fig. 24.7).

Perforation of the cervical and upper thoracic esophagus is approached through an oblique cervical incision that parallels the anterior border of the left sternocleidomastoid muscle. The sternocleidomastoid muscle and carotid sheath are retracted laterally, and the trachea and thyroid gland medially. If the perforation can be identified, it is

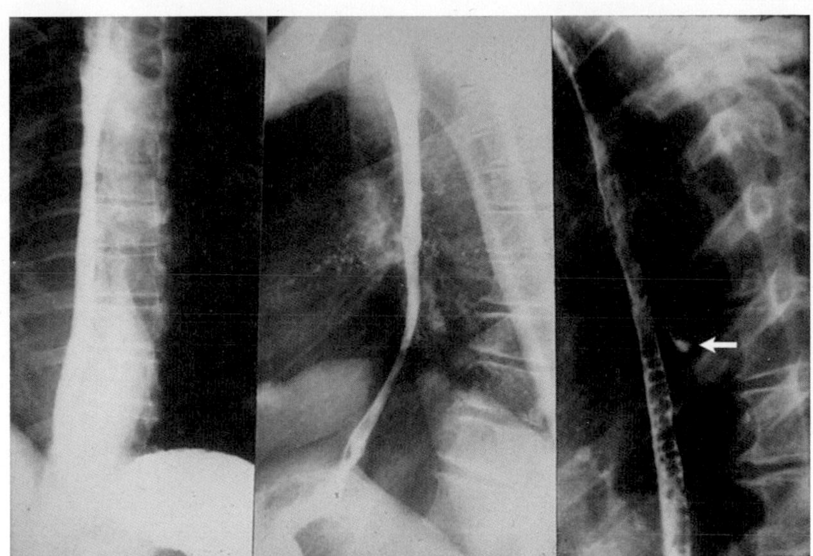

FIGURE 24.6. Posteroanterior (*left*) and lateral (*center*) views from Gastrografin (meglumine diatrizoate) esophagogram in a patient with acute caustic injury that was incorrectly dilated prematurely within 10 days of caustic ingestion. There was still acute inflammation in this esophagus, and the patient had fever and chest pain following dilation. Despite the negative Gastrografin swallow, dilute barium was administered (*right*), and a perforation (*arrow*) of the midesophagus was demonstrated. (Reproduced with permission from Orringer MB. Complications of esophageal surgery and trauma. In: Greenfield LJ, ed. *Complications in surgery and trauma,* 2nd ed. Philadelphia, PA: J.B. Lippincott; 1990:312.)

closed with absorbable polyglycolic acid sutures. If the injury cannot be visualized adequately for repair, the retroesophageal prevertebral space is dissected bluntly with the finger and the superior mediastinum is drained with two 1-inch Penrose drains brought out through the neck wound. Esophageal perforations to the level of the tracheal bifurcation can generally be treated successful

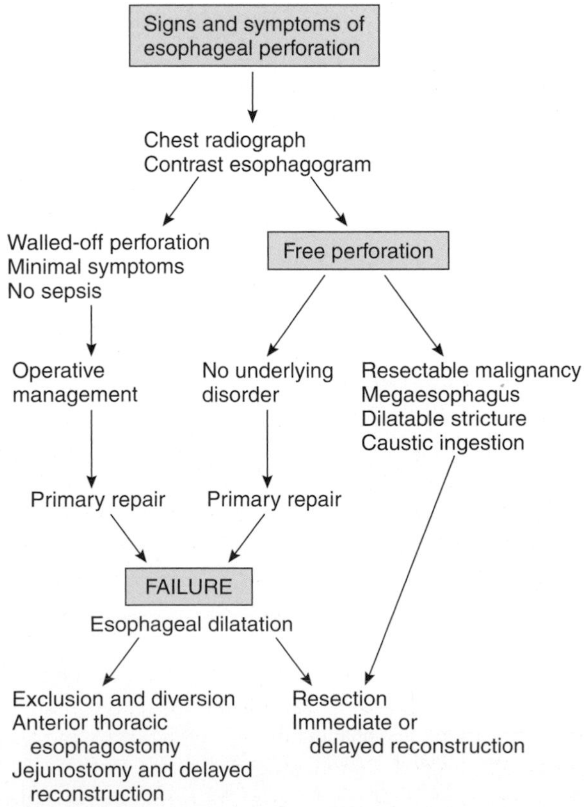

Signs and symptoms of esophageal perforation

Chest radiograph
Contrast esophagogram

Walled-off perforation
Minimal symptoms
No sepsis

Free perforation

Operative management

No underlying disorder

Resectable malignancy
Megaesophagus
Dilatable stricture
Caustic ingestion

Primary repair

Primary repair

FAILURE
Esophageal dilatation

Exclusion and diversion
Anterior thoracic esophagostomy
Jejunostomy and delayed reconstruction

Resection
Immediate or delayed reconstruction

FIGURE 24.7. Treatment algorithm for esophageal perforation.

with such a cervical approach. Midthoracic esophageal perforations must be approached through a right thoracotomy and those of the distal third of the esophagus are approached through a left thoracotomy.

Traditional surgical dogma teaches that esophageal perforations beyond 6 to 12 hours in duration are virtually impossible to repair primarily, the pouting inflamed mucosa at the edge of the tear holding sutures poorly. Isolated reports, however, have emphasized that even after marked delay in repair, successful closure of the esophageal injury may be possible (8,16). Several groups have found that the majority of esophageal tears can in fact be repaired successfully using meticulous surgical technique that includes identification of adjacent submucosa by dissecting away the overlying muscle, defining the limits of the mucosal tear (Fig. 24.8), reapproximation of the disrupted mucosa and submucosa with a surgical stapler (Auto Suture Endo-GIA II Stapler, U.S. Surgical Corporation, Auto Suture Company Division, Norwalk, CT) (17), and reapproximation of the muscle over the staple suture line (Fig. 24.9). The esophageal repair should be performed with an esophageal bougie in place, to limit excessive narrowing of the lumen. Limited esophagomyotomy performed 180° opposite the site of injury may permit enough advancement of adjacent esophageal wall for adequate repair of the perforation (18). In patients with chronic mediastinitis and pleural reaction, the adjacent mediastinal pleura is thickened and provides an excellent flap with which to reinforce the esophageal suture line. Alternatively, if there is not sufficient parietal pleural thickening to provide adequate support for the suture line, reinforcement with either a pedicled intercostal muscle flap, omentum, pericardium, visceral pleura, or diaphragm can be carried out (19,20). The mediastinal pleura must be opened from the apex of the chest to the diaphragm to permit wide drainage of the mediastinum. After copious irrigation of the mediastinum and pleural

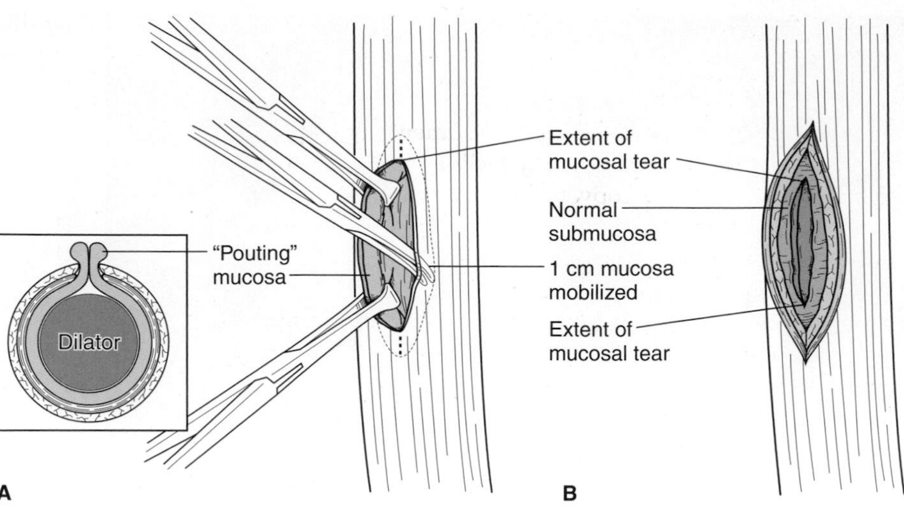

FIGURE 24.8. Technique of primary repair of esophageal perforation. Mucosa at the site of the tear (*inset*) is grasped with Allis clamps **(A)**, and the adjacent esophageal muscle is mobilized around the entire tear until 1 cm of normal submucosa is exposed around the defect **(B)**. (Reproduced with permission from Whyte RI, Iannettoni MD, Orringer MB. Intrathoracic perforation: the merit of primary repair. *J Thorac Cardiovasc Surg* 1995;109:140–146.)

cavity and decortication of any acute fibrinous exudate that may have formed over the lung, a large-bore chest tube is left near the esophageal suture line so that if disruption occurs, the result will be an esophagopleural cutaneous fistula.

In treating an esophageal perforation, associated esophageal pathology cannot be ignored. Thus, a perforation proximal to a carcinoma or a caustic or reflux stricture may necessitate an emergent esophagectomy with either primary or delayed esophageal reconstruction. Patients who present with esophageal perforation and a long-standing history of reflux stricture are more likely to develop postoperative dysphagia requiring repeated esophageal dilatation. In this subset of patients, consideration should be given for primary esophagectomy, if their physiologic status at the time of operation permits (21). Alternatively, if it is possible to dilate a benign stricture intraoperatively to relieve the distal obstruction, closure of a proximal esophageal perforation may be successful. A subsequent disruption of the esophageal closure may still eventually heal if dilation of the associated stricture is continued. A perforated pulsion diverticulum of the esophagus may be resected within several hours of the injury. The associated obstruction must be dealt with and the neuromotor esophageal dysfunction responsible for formation of the pouch relieved by performing a concomitant esophagomyotomy.

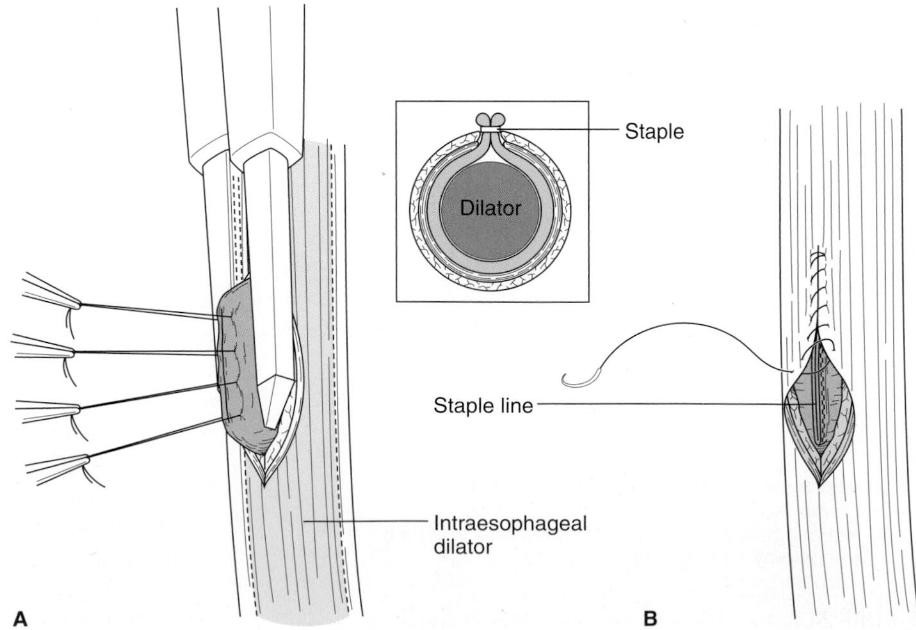

FIGURE 24.9. Technique of primary repair of esophageal perforation. Traction sutures placed along the inflamed mucosal edge of the tear elevate the submucosa so that an EndoGIA-II cartridge can be applied and deployed. The esophageal lumen is maintained by passage of an intraesophageal dilator **(A)** (*inset*). The staple line is covered by approximating the adjacent muscle with a running absorbable suture **(B)**. (Reproduced with permission from Whyte RI, Iannettoni MD, Orringer MB. Intrathoracic perforation: the merit of primary repair. *J Thorac Cardiovasc Surg* 1995;109:140–146.)

PROCEDURAL COMPLICATIONS

Esophagoscopy

Technologic advances in the development of flexible fiberoptic instruments have greatly facilitated the performance of esophagogastroscopy, particularly with the advent of endoscopic ultrasound. Furthermore, there has been a concomitant increase in the number of these studies being performed on an outpatient basis. The consequences of esophageal disruption, however, have not changed. Perforation occurs in as many as 0.8% of all patients during flexible upper endoscopy, with rates as high as 4% for those patients undergoing esophageal dilatation (22). Perforation following rigid esophagoscopy can occur in as many as 5% of patients following therapeutic procedures (e.g., biopsy, dilation, or removal of foreign body) and 1.5% of patients following rigid esophagoscopy alone (23).

1. Adequate preoperative and intraoperative sedation and anesthesia are mandatory. In some patients, general anesthesia is the only means of creating acceptable conditions for performance of esophagoscopy for both the patient and the surgeon.
2. Esophagoscopy should not be carried out unless a prior barium esophagogram has been performed and reviewed by the endoscopist, particularly if the patient presents with symptoms of dysphagia or esophageal obstruction. The barium swallow provides information about preexisting pathology and its expected location. For example, a Zenker diverticulum identified with contrast esophagogram should be expected to be encountered at the level of the upper esophageal sphincter, approximately 15 cm from the upper incisors. A midesophageal carcinoma at the level of the tracheal bifurcation is encountered approximately 25 cm from the upper incisors. An epiphrenic diverticulum located proximal to the esophagogastric junction is encountered before the esophagoscope reaches a point 40 cm from the upper incisors. Perforation of a cervical esophageal diverticulum or a midesophageal stricture cannot be justified because the endoscopist was unaware of these lesions as a prior barium swallow examination had been neither obtained nor personally reviewed.
3. Failure to introduce the rigid esophagoscope properly through the upper esophageal sphincter may result in a perforation. The cricopharyngeus muscle originates from the cricoid cartilage, and the natural "pull" of this muscle against the cartilage will result in a posterior perforation unless the larynx is "lifted" anteriorly as the esophagoscope is advanced.
4. The esophagoscope should not be advanced unless the lumen is visible.
5. As the esophagoscope is advanced, adjustment must be made for the natural course of the esophagus. Because the distal esophagus courses anteriorly and to the left as it joins the stomach, particularly when performing rigid endoscopy, the instrument must be angled toward the right side of the patient's mouth and the occiput of the head lowered as the esophagoscope is advanced into the distal esophagus.
6. The initial dilatation of a tight esophageal stricture is frequently painful, and patients must be adequately sedated and anesthetized, minimizing patient discomfort and allowing the surgeon to concentrate on the visual field. When a rigid esophagoscope is used for this initial evaluation, flexible gum-tipped Jackson bougies are inserted through the stricture under direct vision, and the pliability and extent of the stenosis are assessed (Fig. 24.10). With a

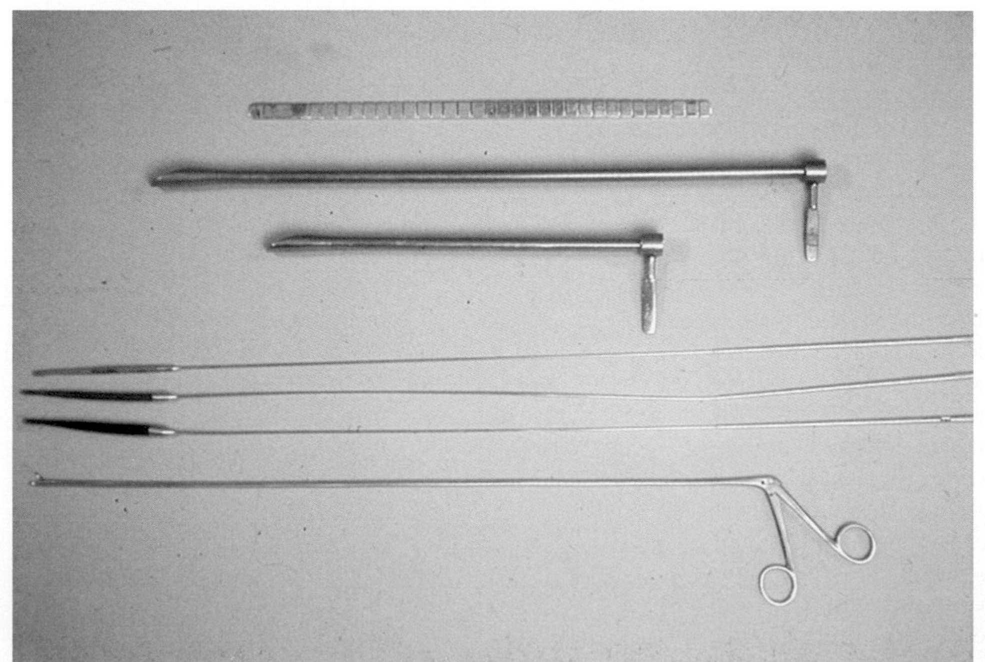

FIGURE 24.10. The instruments required for evaluating an esophageal stricture. Precisely measured localization of the stricture (in centimeters from the incisor teeth) and adequate biopsies and brushings from the stricture must be obtained. The gum-tipped Jackson dilators, gently manipulated through the stenosis, permit evaluation of the extent and pliability of the obstruction. The 26-French dilator is the largest one that will pass through the standard 45-cm rigid esophagoscope. (Reproduced with permission from Orringer MB. Complications of esophageal surgery and trauma. In: Greenfield LJ, ed. *Complications in surgery and trauma,* 2nd ed. Philadelphia, PA: J.B. Lippincott; 1990:309.)

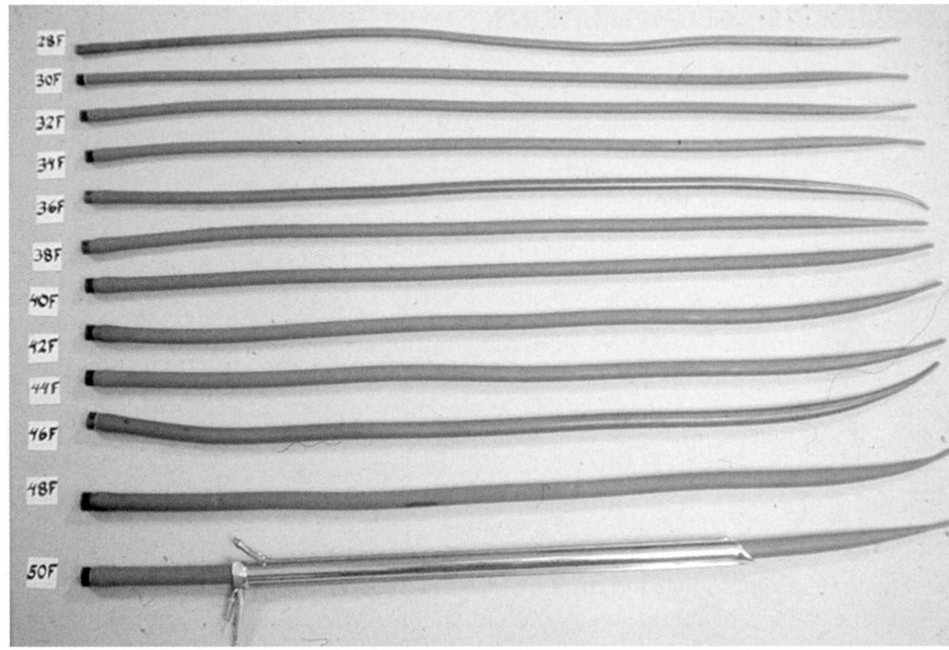

FIGURE 24.11. Tapered Hurst-Maloney esophageal dilators and a 45-cm Pilling esophagoscope, which accommodates up to a 50-French bougie, thus permitting progressive dilatation of severe peptic strictures under direct vision. (Reproduced with permission from Orringer, MB. Complications of esophageal surgery and trauma. In: Greenfield LJ, ed. *Complications in surgery and trauma*, 2nd ed. Philadelphia, PA: J.B. Lippincott; 1990:311.)

mild "soft" stenosis, dilation by advancing the esophagoscope through the stenosis might be possible. With more firm, high-grade strictures, it is safer to pass progressively larger dilators through the narrowing. This can be accomplished using the Savary-Gilliard guidewire and dilating system, with fluoroscopic guidance, or with the Maloney tapered esophageal dilators (Fig. 24.11). The latter instruments are our preference for repeated outpatient dilatations of esophageal strictures, requiring none of the sedation or anesthesia necessary when endoscopic balloon dilatations are performed.

Hiatal hernia repair

Hiatal herniorrhaphy, although conceptually quite simple, can result in a number of serious complications (Table 24.2). Acute esophageal perforation can occur when concomitant esophagoscopy is performed during an antireflux operation or when a distal esophageal stricture is disrupted during intraoperative dilatation. A delayed perforation, usually within 1 week of surgery, can occur when esophageal sutures placed too deeply during the repair result in local mural necrosis.

Acute esophageal tears recognized before the incision should be approached transthoracically and repaired, and the esophageal suture line reinforced with either the fundoplication if the tear is in the distal esophagus, or with pedicled anterior mediastinal fat or a pedicled intercostal muscle flap for a more proximal tear. When an intercostal muscle pedicle is used to reinforce an esophageal suture line, it should be sutured to the esophagus as an onlay patch, not placed circumferentially around the esophagus; regeneration of bone or cartilage from the perichondrium or periosteum mobilized with the flap may result in a late obstructing ring around the esophagus. When a reflux stricture is perforated during attempted dilation at the time of a planned antireflux operation, unless the involved tissues are relatively healthy and amenable to repair, esophageal resection is generally a better option. Although most reflux strictures can be dilated, and many regress after an antireflux

Table 24.2 Complications of hiatal herniorrhaphy

Intraoperative Complications
Perforation
Vagus nerve injury
Hemorrhage
Splenic laceration
Short gastric vessel
Postoperative Complications
Perforation
Stricture
Suture placement
Dysphagia
Mechanical
Tight hiatal closure
Excessive fundoplication
Inadequate gastroplasty
Edema
Gastric atony, pylorospasm
Early anatomic recurrence
Crural repair disruption
Functional
Postvagotomy diarrhea
Ileus
Cardiac tamponade
Chylothorax
Pleural effusion
Incisional pain

Modified from Patel HJ, Tan BT, Yee J, et al. A twenty-five year experience with open primary transthoracic repair of paraesophageal hiatal hernia. *J Thorac Cardiovasc Surg* 2004;127:843–849.

procedure has been carried out, disruption of a stricture during attempted dilation is one of the definitions of an "undilatable" stricture that justifies esophageal resection. Our preference in this situation is to proceed with a transthoracic esophagectomy and then reposition the patient supine and carry out a cervical esophagogastric anastomosis. Several additional options for the treatment of a disrupted distal stricture are available. Unfortunately, none is without its associated morbidity. The Thal fundic patch esophagoplasty utilizes adjacent gastric fundus to "patch" the opened narrowed esophagus. This procedure not only relies on the healing of the opened, inflamed distal esophagus to which the stomach is sutured but also requires the addition of an intrathoracic fundoplication (Thal-Woodward procedure) to control gastroesophageal reflux, in effect, creation of a man-made paraesophageal hiatal hernia. The incidence of suture line disruption and mechanical complications associated with this operation condemn its use. For the same reason, we oppose use of an intrathoracic fundoplication (without a Thal procedure) to control reflux. The complications of such an approach outweigh its benefits.

Gastric ulceration may complicate 3% to 10% of fundoplications and may occur both in supradiaphragmatic fundic wraps and in intra-abdominal fundoplications. In the former, one is dealing with a complication of an iatrogenic paraesophageal hiatal hernia, and operative repair is generally indicated. In the latter, ulceration may be due to relative ischemia in the wrap, and treatment with H_2-receptor blockers, proton pump inhibitors, or cytoprotective agents may suffice. The development of fever, chest pain, or respiratory distress during the first week after a hiatal hernia operation mandates a contrast study. If a distal esophageal perforation is diagnosed, treatment usually involves reoperation. The site of the perforation is identified intraoperatively, at times by insufflating air through a nasogastric tube. A leak from an intra-abdominal fundoplication suture may be closed and reinforced with adjacent omentum. If the leak is in the chest, pedicled anterior mediastinal fat, intercostal muscle, or pleura is used to reinforce the closure using a transthoracic approach. A jejunostomy feeding tube should be placed to allow nutritional support and unimpeded ambulation in case the repair is unsuccessful and an esophageal fistula ensues. Either a large-bore chest tube should be left near the thoracic esophageal repair or a drain should be placed near the transabdominally repaired fundoplication to ensure external drainage of a recurrent fistula.

Low retrosternal dysphagia after an antireflux operation may have one of several causes: (a) distal esophageal edema after intraoperative manipulation; (b) distal esophageal motor dysfunction due to manipulation of the vagus nerves; (c) obstruction due to too tight a fundoplication; (d) or obstruction from excessive closure of the hiatus. Performance of the fundoplication over at least a 54 French intraesophageal dilator minimizes the likelihood of this latter complication. Dysphagia after truncal vagotomy has been recognized for more than 40 years, and it is apparent that neuromotor esophageal dysfunction may follow manipulation of the vagus nerves at the level of the distal esophagus. This complication after antireflux surgery is more likely with a transthoracic than with a transabdominal repair because identification and displacement of the main vagal trunks are more routine with the former approach. Such patients have dysphagia immediately after the antireflux procedure. On barium swallow examination, the distal esophagus is tapered and empties poorly, resembling the picture of achalasia or esophageal spasm. Reassurance and maintenance of a soft diet for several days usually constitute adequate therapy, although passage of an esophageal dilator is at times required for relief. This problem typically subsides spontaneously, but occasionally reoperation, takedown of the repair, and at times, even esophageal resection may be needed.

Another complication of intraoperative vagus nerve injury occurring during a hiatal hernia repair is impaired gastric motility or pylorospasm resulting in delayed gastric emptying and secondary gastric dilation. This complication has direct implications for the long-term success of the hiatal hernia repair because sustained gastric dilation in combination with a competent distal esophageal sphincter mechanism may eventually result in disruption of the esophageal sutures used to construct the fundoplication and failure of the repair. When the patient who has undergone an antireflux operation develops gastric dilation immediately after operation, a 7- to 10-day trial of gastric decompression with a nasogastric tube is indicated. At times, an anticholinergic (e.g., atropine 0.4 mg either per os or intramuscularly every 4 to 6 hours) may relieve the associated pylorospasm. This problem should not be permitted to persist indefinitely, and it is best to perform an early gastric drainage procedure (pyloromyotomy or pyloroplasty) than to risk recurrent gastroesophageal reflux. Finally, vagal nerve injury may result in varying degrees of "dumping syndrome" (e.g., postprandial diarrhea, cramping, abdominal pain, nausea, diaphoresis, palpitations). This problem generally subsides within a few months, but at times long-term management with antidiarrheal medication and dietary restriction may be required.

Chylothorax following an antireflux procedure may result from injury to the thoracic duct, which passes from the abdomen through the aortic hiatus and then courses in the lower chest anterior to the spine between the esophagus and the aorta. Injury may occur during mobilization of the cardia or during placement of the crural sutures. This complication is heralded by prolonged chest tube drainage after a transthoracic repair, and the true cause of this serosanguineous drainage may not become apparent until the patient's diet is liberalized and its fat content increases. If chylothorax is present, the oral administration of 60 to 90 mL of cream for 4 to 6 hours will cause the chest tube drainage to become opalescent and milky chyle. The diagnosis can also be established by staining the fluid with Sudan R, which stains the globules of fat. Determination of the cholesterol and triglyceride levels in the fluid is usually not necessary. A cholesterol/triglyceride ratio of less than 1 is characteristic of a chylous effusion, whereas nonchylous effusions have a ratio of greater than 1. In most cases, a chylothorax following a hiatal hernia repair can be managed nonoperatively by administering a low-residue elemental diet and maintaining prolonged chest tube suction. If the output of chyle remains significant (>400 to 600 mL per consecutive 8-hour periods) after 7 to 10 days of this treatment, then reoperation with identification and ligation of the injured thoracic duct is indicated.

Acute postoperative hemorrhage after an antireflux operation is most often the result of bleeding from an unsecured divided short gastric vessel along the high greater curvature of the stomach. This possibility should always be borne in mind as the short gastric vessels are divided and ligated before performing a fundoplication. Hemorrhage from these vessels may be a particularly treacherous complication following a transthoracic hiatal hernia repair because the resulting hypovolemic shock may be attributed to other causes (e.g., myocardial infarction) when there is minimal chest tube drainage and the chest roentgenogram shows no hemothorax. Abdominal exploration, evacuation of the blood, and ligation of the bleeding vessel is the proper course of therapy. Splenic injury also occurs in a small percentage of patients undergoing antireflux surgery, particularly in reoperations. The incidence of splenic injury is slightly higher with transabdominal as compared with transthoracic antireflux operations, particularly in obese patients. Rarely, postoperative hemorrhage manifests as a pericardial effusion causing tamponade and cardiopulmonary collapse (24). This may arise by avulsion of an epicardial vessel occurring during esophageal mobilization for repair of a large hiatal hernia. Rapid diagnosis by surface echocardiogram followed by sternotomy, relief of tamponade, and repair of the bleeding vessel is indicated (25).

Before the patient's discharge from the hospital after an antireflux operation, a routine barium swallow examination should be performed to document the postoperative appearance of the reconstructed esophagogastric junction. At times, this contrast study may reveal a "silent" localized extravasation of contrast material at the site of one of the fundoplication sutures that was placed too deeply. If the patient is asymptomatic and the "leak" is very small, no therapy may be required because the supporting fundoplication has prevented a more major disruption. A far more disconcerting radiographic finding on the "routine" postoperative barium swallow obtained prior to discharge is the asymptomatic migration of the fundoplication or gastric fundus into the chest as a result of disruption of the posterior crural repair (Fig. 24.12). This iatrogenic paraesophageal hiatal hernia is subject to the same mechanical complications of paraesophageal herniation in the patient who has had no surgery. Reoperation is necessary to reduce the fundoplication back into the abdomen and to replace the posterior crural sutures if they have pulled through the crural muscle (or to narrow the hiatus further if they have not), before postoperative adhesions form between the herniated stomach and adjacent tissues, making any subsequent repair more difficult. It may be difficult to tell the asymptomatic patient recovering from an antireflux operation that reoperation is necessary, but conservative management of this problem is ill-advised.

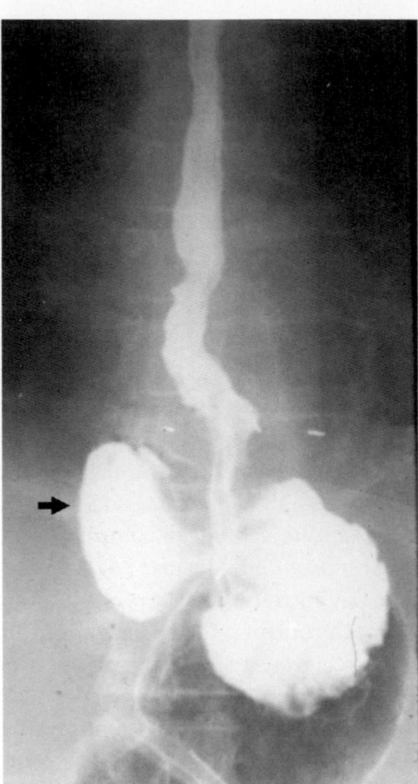

FIGURE 24.12. An esophagogram taken 1 week after a combined Collis gastroplasty-Nissen fundoplication. A portion of the fundoplication (*arrow*) has slipped into the chest through the diaphragmatic hiatus because of disruption of the posterior crural sutures. Although this patient was asymptomatic, reoperation and reduction of the herniated fundus below the diaphragm were carried out to prevent the potential complications of this "paraesophageal" hernia. (Reproduced with permission from Orringer, MB. Complications of esophageal surgery and trauma. In: Greenfield LJ, ed. *Complications in surgery and trauma,* 2nd ed. Philadelphia, PA: J.B. Lippincott; 1990:316.)

Controversy remains regarding the role of surgical therapy for patients with complications of gastroesophageal reflux disease, particularly Barrett's esophagus. Both symptoms and requirement for antisecretory medications decrease significantly following antireflux operation (26). However, no long-term data are available regarding regression of Barrett's esophagus, regarded as a precursor lesion to esophageal adenocarcinoma. Currently, patients with Barrett's esophagus undergoing hiatal herniorrhaphy should continue routine surveillance esophagoscopy with biopsies in order to screen for the progression from metaplasia to dysplasia and esophageal adenocarcinoma (27).

Laparoscopic antireflux/hiatal hernia surgery

Since 1991, when the first reports of laparoscopic antireflux surgery were published, minimally-invasive surgical approaches to the diaphragmatic esophageal hiatus have been used with increasing frequency. Although mortality rates for laparoscopic fundoplication have been low (0% to

1.4%), early morbidity rates were acceptable, and conversion rates to the open procedure were from 0% to 14%, so the learning curve for this operation is substantial (28,29).

As operator experience increases, laparoscopic antireflux operations or hiatal hernia repairs can be accomplished safely in obese patients, those with intra-abdominal adhesions from prior surgery, or in those with an unusually large left hepatic lobe. These factors remain indications for open transthoracic hiatal hernia repair. Perforations of the distal esophagus or gastric fundus have been reported during laparoscopic fundoplication. Blind dissection posterior to the esophagus should be avoided to prevent this complication. When recognized at the time of, or soon after operation, laparoscopic repair is feasible, but repair may also warrant conversion to an open procedure.

Early postoperative dysphagia may result from an overly tight fundoplication, which is more likely to occur with minimally invasive procedures in which tactile sensation is not used to assess the tightness of the wrap. Performance of the fundoplication over at least a size 54 French Maloney dilator minimizes the likelihood of this complication. Postoperative dysphagia due to fibrotic stenosis of the muscular esophageal hiatus, attributed to a diathermy injury during the esophageal dissection, has also been reported and treated with laparoscopic hiatal division. Persistent dysphagia after a laparoscopic fundoplication, refractory to dilatation therapy, may necessitate reoperation, takedown of the wrap, and construction of a looser fundoplication. The author's approach for such reoperative procedures is a transthoracic approach, generally with a combined esophageal lengthening Collis gastroplasty and Nissen fundoplication. Additional complications of laparoscopic fundoplication include pneumothorax or pneumomediastinum from CO_2 tracking into the chest during the operation, incisional hernia at a port site, and herniation of the fundoplication through the diaphragmatic hiatus (particularly when the crura were not closed at the time of the original operation).

As enthusiasm for laparoscopic fundoplication has grown, this approach has also been used to repair large paraesophageal hiatal hernias, which are often associated with an attenuated, abnormally wide esophageal hiatus. In 1983, Pearson et al. emphasized that esophageal shortening is common in these patients, most of whom have combined sliding and paraesophageal hiatus hernias, and the authors used the combined Collis gastroplasty-fundoplication operation liberally in this group (30,31). With the laparoscopic approach, one cannot assess the degree of tension on the distal esophagus that results from reduction of the esophagogastric junction below the diaphragm, because, again, direct manual palpation of the esophagus is not possible. Furthermore, with the diaphragm pushed abnormally upward by CO_2 insufflation of the abdomen, a false sense of ease of reduction of the esophagogastric junction into the abdomen may occur. Although several groups have developed minimally-invasive techniques for combined Collis gastroplasty and fundoplication, with acceptable early and intermediate-term results (29,32), our group believes that most large combined sliding and paraesophageal hiatal hernias should be approached through the chest with an open operation, generally a combined Collis gastroplasty and Nissen fundoplication. The increasing number of fundoplications that have "slipped" through the hiatus into the chest after laparoscopic repair likely reflect, at least in part, a lack of recognition by the original surgeon that there was unacceptable tension on the repair. Recurrent herniation of an intact or a partially disrupted fundoplication is the most common reason for failure of laparoscopic fundoplications. Body habitus is another important but often overlooked factor in recurrence after laparoscopic (or any) antireflux operation; obesity is present in a significant number of patients who experience disruption of repairs.

Another laparoscopic technique for the repair of paraesophageal hiatal hernias is the use of prosthetic mesh to repair the diaphragmatic defect. This is an ill-conceived operation because the constant diaphragmatic motion against the adjacent esophagus at the hiatus may result in esophageal or gastric erosion and perforation (33) as late as 9 years following operation (34). This approach is mentioned only to condemn its use.

Esophageal resection and visceral esophageal substitution

In almost every large series of patients undergoing a traditional esophageal resection and substitution with either stomach or intestine, the leading causes of death are (a) respiratory insufficiency associated with the physiologic insult of a combined thoracic and abdominal operation and (b) sepsis from mediastinitis resulting from disruption of an intrathoracic anastomosis. As a result, our group has adopted a general policy of performing no intrathoracic esophageal anastomoses and prefers a cervical esophagogastric anastomosis instead. A cervical esophagogastric anastomotic leak generally represents little more morbidity than a salivary fistula, and spontaneous closure with local wound care is the rule. The authors and associates reported a dramatic reduction in the incidence of postoperative cervical esophagogastric anastomotic leak to less than 3% with a side-to-side stapled cervical esophagogastric anastomosis (35) constructed with the Auto Suture Endo-GIA II Stapler (U.S. Surgical Corporation, Auto Suture Company Division, Norwalk, CT). The authors have also found that a transhiatal esophagectomy without thoracotomy and a cervical esophagogastric anastomosis is applicable in most patients requiring esophageal resection and reconstruction for both benign and malignant disease. This procedure minimizes the operative insult to the patient by avoiding a thoracotomy. The incidence of postoperative pulmonary complications is thereby reduced, and the possibility of mediastinitis resulting from an intrathoracic leak is virtually eliminated.

The authors recommend a No. 14 French rubber catheter feeding jejunostomy tube secured in place with a Witzel maneuver, not a "needle catheter" jejunostomy, in every patient undergoing esophagectomy and esophageal reconstruction. The jejunostomy tube is regarded as an "insurance policy" if anastomotic disruption necessitates an alternate means of nourishment. If use of the tube is not required postoperatively, it is removed after several weeks. Alternatively, if an anastomotic leak occurs, a feeding jejunostomy tube is safer and more effective in providing calories than intravenous hyperalimentation.

Anastomotic leak

After completion of a cervical esophageal anastomosis, the neck wound is closed loosely with only four or five 4-0 sutures over a 1/4-in Penrose drain placed adjacent to the anastomosis. If an anastomotic leak does occur, the neck wound is opened at the bedside in its entirety, and gentle wound packing with gauze is initiated. The size of the leak can be estimated by having the patient drink water and evaluating the amount that escapes from the neck wound with a disposable bedside suction catheter. In general, within several days of opening the wound, the drainage diminishes considerably, and the patient may resume oral intake while maintaining steady gentle pressure over the wound to occlude the fistula. Passage of tapered Maloney dilators (generally, Nos. 40 and 46 French) at the bedside during the first week after drainage of the cervical fistula ensures that no element of obstruction from either local edema or spasm contributes to continued drainage of the fistula (36). More than 98% of cervical esophagogastric anastomotic leaks are small and respond to the open drainage and packing as described. A small proportion, however, are associated with catastrophic complications: major gastric tip necrosis necessitating takedown of the anastomosis, construction of cervical esophagostomy and resection of nonviable stomach, vertebral body osteomyelitis, epidural abscess with resultant paraplegia, pulmonary microabscesses from an internal jugular vein abscess, and tracheoesophagogastric anastomotic fistula (37).

Early disruption of an intrathoracic esophageal anastomosis occurring within the first 10 critical days after operation is characterized by the signs and symptoms of mediastinitis. Symptoms, including fever, chest pain, tachycardia, tachypnea, respiratory distress, peripheral cyanosis, vasoconstriction, hypotension, and shock, when associated with a chest roentgenogram that demonstrates hydrothorax or pneumothorax, leave little question about the diagnosis. Diagnosis should be documented with a contrast study. In an otherwise asymptomatic patient found to have a small (<1 cm) contained anastomotic leak on a routine postoperative barium swallow, observation alone may be sufficient. In most cases, however, anastomotic disruption warrants immediate re-exploration, irrigation of the chest and mediastinum, repair of the fistula, if possible, and chest tube drainage. A localized anastomotic leak with viable adjacent tissue may be amenable to direct suture repair. A pedicled flap of anterior mediastinal fat, intercostal muscle flap, pleura, or omentum should be mobilized to reinforce the repair. Decompression of the esophageal substitute with a nasogastric tube, placement of a jejunostomy tube for nutritional support, and appropriate antibiotics complete the therapy. Following removal of the chest tubes, a barium swallow examination should be performed 10 days following reoperation to be certain that healing has occurred. If disruption of the anastomosis recurs, a controlled esophagopleural cutaneous fistula should be established. Rib resection with placement of a large-bore drainage tube adjacent to the fistula may be required to ensure that all drainage from the esophageal leak can flow freely out of the chest. Gastric contents that are aspirated through the nasogastric tube can be returned to the alimentary tract through the jejunostomy tube to minimize electrolyte imbalance and to simplify fluid and electrolyte replacement.

During re-exploration of the chest for a disrupted esophageal anastomosis, extensive local necrosis of the tissue with a major anastomotic dehiscence mandates reversal of the anastomosis, resection of nonviable stomach, and replacement of the remaining stomach into the abdomen. Only nonviable distal esophagus should be resected. However, a diverting lateral cervical esophagostomy with oversewing of the divided proximal intrathoracic esophagus should not be attempted. Disruption of the intrathoracic esophageal suture line is not only likely, but if subsequent reconstruction is possible, management of the remaining segment of intrathoracic esophagus presents a considerable technical problem. The best alternative is to mobilize the esophagus circumferentially well into the neck through the thoracic incision. After the thoracotomy is closed, formal end esophagostomy, with the patient returned to the supine position, should be performed. As indicated earlier, the submucosal collateral circulation of the esophagus is excellent, and most of the length of the thoracic esophagus will remain viable so long as at least one inferior thyroid artery remains intact. Therefore, after delivering the divided thoracic esophagus out of the neck incision, the maximum length of remaining esophagus should be preserved to facilitate later reconstruction. This is achieved by developing a subcutaneous tunnel anteriorly to the left clavicle onto the chest wall, in order to construct an anterior thoracic esophagostomy. An esophagostomy stoma placed on the relatively flat upper anterior chest wall is much more easily cared for by the patient because a stomal appliance is more readily adapted to this location than to the usual site of a standard cervical esophagostomy (Fig. 24.13). A feeding jejunostomy is, of course, required until later esophageal reconstruction can be performed.

When colon or jejunum has been used to replace the esophagus and necrosis of the graft is documented at re-exploration for an anastomotic leak, there is similarly little recourse but to remove the nonviable graft and insert a feeding tube. If the patient survives the sequelae of the mediastinal sepsis, later reconstruction can be considered.

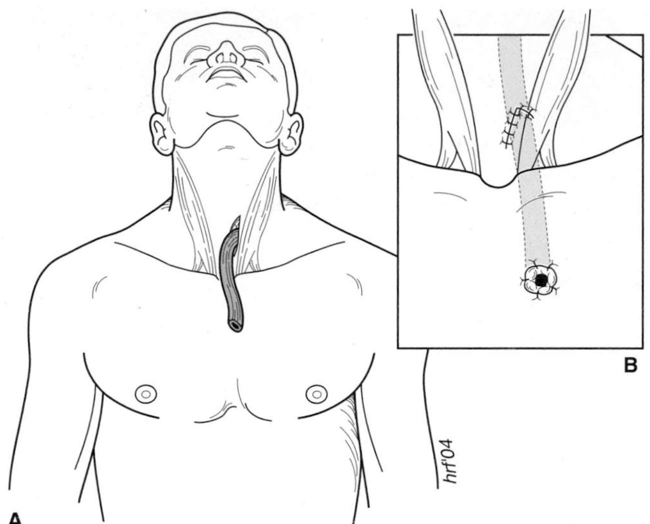

FIGURE 24.13. Construction of an anterior thoracic esophagostomy instead of a traditional end-cervical esophagostomy. **A:** The mobilized thoracic esophagus is placed on the anterior chest wall so that the location of the stoma can be determined. **B:** All viable remaining esophagus is preserved and tunneled subcutaneously, and an end anterior thoracic esophagostomy is constructed. Stomal appliances are readily applied to the flat surface of the anterior chest, and when performing a later colon interposition, 7 to 12 cm of esophagus is available for the reconstruction. (Reproduced with permission from Orringer, MB. Complications of esophageal surgery and trauma. In: Greenfield LJ, ed. *Complications in surgery and trauma,* 2nd ed. Philadelphia, PA: J.B. Lippincott; 1990:317.)

Anastomotic stricture

Although the management of a cervical anastomotic leak is generally straightforward and seldom associated with death, the long-term sequelae of a cervical leak are far from inconsequential. As many as 50% of cervical esophagogastric anastomotic leaks result in an anastomotic stricture as healing occurs, and this represents an unsatisfactory outcome of an operation that is intended to provide comfortable swallowing. The implications are similar in patients who survive an intrathoracic esophageal anastomotic leak. Our group has previously reported in over 2000 transhiatal esophagectomy patients at the University of Michigan an anastomotic leak rate averaging 12%, with nearly half of these patients developing subsequent anastomotic strictures (38), consistent with reports in the literature for the incidence of both anastomotic leak from 5% to 26%, and stenosis from 10% to 31% (39–42). Without question, the prevention of an anastomotic leak is the key to a successful functional outcome in these patients. In our initial experience with side-to-side stapled cervical esophagogastric anastomosis, which has been associated with an anastomotic leak rate of less than 3%, we observed a dramatic reduction in the need for late postoperative anastomotic dilatations (35).

In the patient who has experienced an esophageal anastomotic leak, early passage of a No. 46 French or larger dilator within 1 week of drainage is carried out to maintain a satisfactory lumen and to prevent late high-grade stenosis. A cervical fistula generally heals within 7 to 10 days of external drainage. When the patient returns for follow-up within 2 weeks of discharge, a No. 46 French or larger Maloney dilator is passed through the anastomosis. If the patient has no dysphagia and there is no resistance to passage of the dilator, the need for subsequent dilatations is dictated by the return of cervical dysphagia. In patients with anastomotic narrowing that prevents the free passage of a No. 46 French or larger Maloney dilator, a more aggressive program of esophageal dilatation is undertaken. With an early program of weekly dilatations, anastomotic healing in a patent configuration is often achieved. Patients whose anastomotic stricture produces resistance as the dilator is passed may need more frequent dilatations. In this situation, over several weeks, the patient is taught to pass a No. 46 or 48 French dilator with the assistance of a family member or friend. Once facility with passage of the dilator is achieved, the patient is issued a dilator with instructions to pass it daily for 1 week, then every other day for 1 week, and then at increasingly longer intervals until the longest duration between dilatations without the recurrence of dysphagia can be established. With this aggressive initial program of dilatation, long-term comfortable swallowing with little or no need for subsequent dilatations is generally achieved (43). Few patients require anastomotic revision. Occasionally, endoscopic injection of steroids into a refractory anastomotic scar facilitates the management of this problem (44,45).

Pulmonary complications

Respiratory insufficiency after esophageal resection and reconstruction is exceedingly common and is associated with a mortality rate of up to 40% (46,47). Patients with esophageal squamous cell cancer, particularly those treated with preoperative chemoradiation, may have a greater risk for postoperative pulmonary morbidity, including pleural effusion, pneumonia and respiratory insufficiency following esophagectomy (48). A vital part of minimizing postoperative pulmonary complications after esophageal resection and reconstruction is rigorous preoperative pulmonary physiotherapy. The authors insist on total abstinence from cigarette smoking for a minimum of 2 weeks before esophagectomy. Home use of an incentive inspirometer and instruction in deep-breathing exercises are also begun 2 weeks preoperatively. This investment of time and energy in improving the patient's preoperative respiratory status is repeatedly rewarded by a lower incidence of postoperative pulmonary complications after esophageal resection and reconstruction. Postoperatively, patients are extubated immediately after operation and resume pulmonary physiotherapy as early as possible. Adequate postoperative analgesia, particularly epidural anesthesia, is of great value in minimizing postoperative pulmonary problems.

One of the most disastrous complications after esophageal resection is the development of a fistula between the tracheobronchial tree and either the esophagus or esophageal substitute, generally at the anastomotic site. Among 207 patients with malignant esophagorespiratory fistulas treated at the Memorial Sloan-Kettering Cancer Center in New York, Burt at al. reported that 13 patients developed their fistulas after resections for esophageal carcinoma (49). Once a fistula between the airway and adjacent alimentary tract develops, there are few options other than to prevent continued contamination of the respiratory tree by identifying and dividing the fistula and repairing the airway, generally a major undertaking in a desperately ill patient.

Gastric outlet obstruction

The need for a routine gastric drainage procedure following the vagotomy that inevitably accompanies esophagectomy has been debated. It has been shown, for example, that most patients who undergo an esophagectomy and esophagogastric anastomosis without a concomitant drainage procedure do not develop difficulty with gastric outlet obstruction (50,51). However, in a prospective trial in which 200 patients undergoing esophageal resection were randomized to receive either a pyloroplasty or no gastric drainage procedure, gastric emptying was found to be four times longer in those who did not have a pyloroplasty (52). Adverse postprandial symptoms were less in those who had a drainage procedure, and there was no morbidity from the pyloroplasty. For the occasional patient who does develop significant gastric outlet obstruction after esophageal resection (Fig. 24.14), the outcome may be disastrous aspiration pneumonia and impaired nutrition due to inability to eat. Further, reoperation to perform a drainage procedure may be very difficult after the stomach has been mobilized into the chest. For these reasons, the authors advocate performance of a gastric drainage procedure in every patient undergoing esophagectomy and esophageal reconstruction, preferring a Ramstedt-type extramucosal pyloromyotomy, which avoids the intra-abdominal suture line of a pyloroplasty. After performing the pyloromyotomy, silver clip markers placed at the level of the pylorus aid in interpreting subsequent radio logic studies used to evaluate gastric emptying. In more than 1,500 such pyloromyotomy performed during esophageal bypass or replacement with stomach, our group has experienced one leak postoperatively. This leak resulted in fatal peritonitis. Intrathoracic gastric outlet obstruction may also result from failure to enlarge the diaphragmatic hiatus adequately before mobilizing the stomach into the chest. The diaphragmatic hiatus should accommodate at least three fingers comfortably alongside the mobilized stomach to prevent this complication.

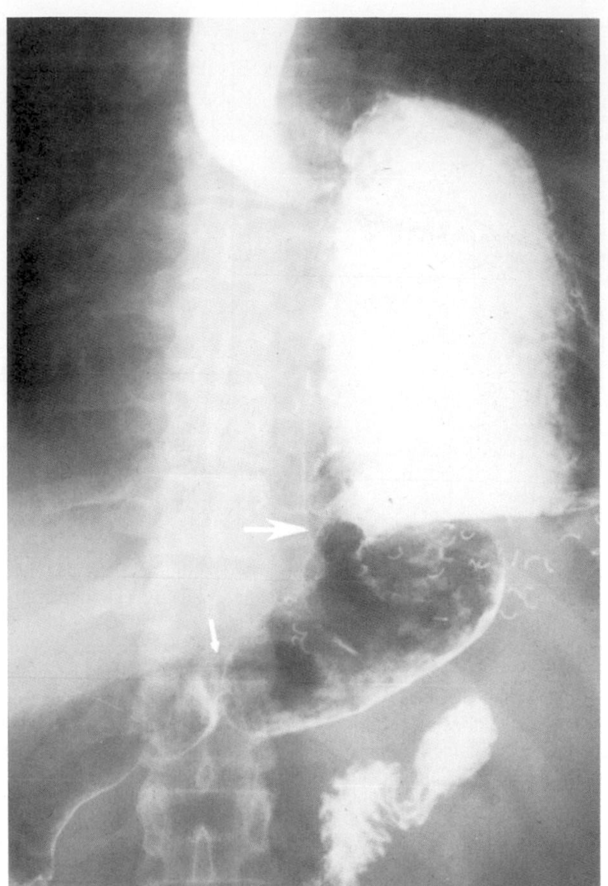

FIGURE 24.14. A barium study of a patient with regurgitation and dilatation of the intrathoracic stomach following esophagectomy for distal-third carcinoma. This complication was the result of two technical errors: failure to enlarge the diaphragmatic hiatus sufficiently, with resultant relative obstruction at the diaphragmatic hiatus (*large arrow*), and failure to perform a gastric drainage procedure, with resultant pyloric obstruction (*small arrow*). (Reproduced with permission from Orringer MB. Complications of esophageal surgery and trauma. In: Greenfield LJ, ed. *Complications in surgery and trauma*, 2nd ed. Philadelphia, PA: J.B. Lippincott; 1990:318.)

Diaphragmatic hiatus obstruction or herniation

Not only must the hiatus be enlarged sufficiently to prevent the esophageal substitute from becoming obstructed at the level of the diaphragm, but the esophageal replacement, whether stomach or intestine, should also be carefully sutured to the edge of the diaphragmatic hiatus to prevent subsequent herniation of abdominal viscera through the hiatus and into the chest (Fig. 24.15). As our group and others have observed, this complication may occur acutely within the first several days of operation or years after the esophagectomy (53,54). Such a hernia may be an asymptomatic finding on a postoperative chest roentgenogram on which intestinal gas is seen above the level of the hiatus, or the patient may present with vague left upper quadrant abdominal or lower thoracic discomfort, nausea, and vomiting as is the case with chronic traumatic diaphragmatic hernias. Because the risk of incarceration and strangulation of the herniated viscera is substantial, reduction of the hernia is advised. Herniation of intestine through the diaphragmatic hiatus following esophagectomy can generally be repaired transabdominally. In the case of chronic traumatic diaphragmatic hernias, the opening in the diaphragm is relatively

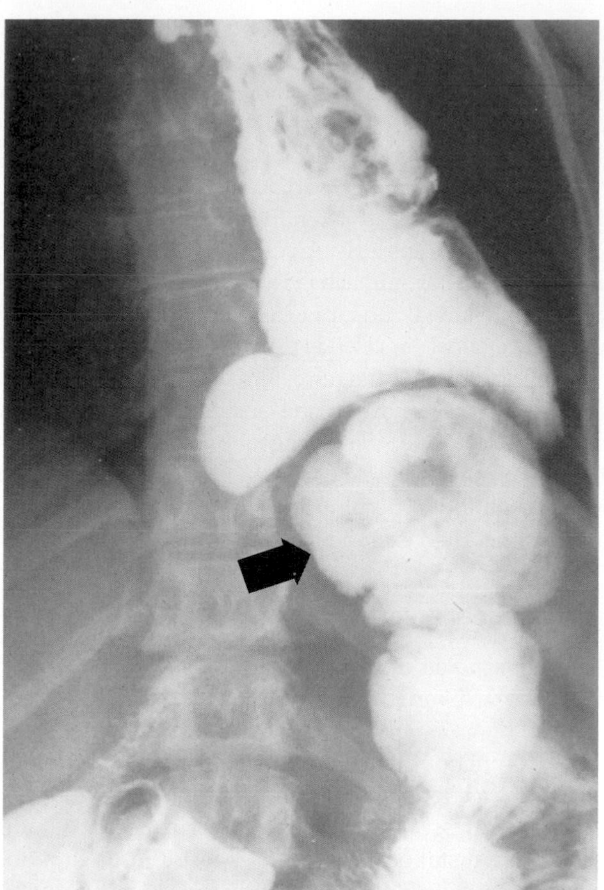

FIGURE 24.15. Herniation of the splenic flexure of the colon (*large arrow*) through the diaphragmatic hiatus following esophageal replacement with stomach for a caustic stricture. No sutures had been placed between the intrathoracic stomach (*small arrow*) and the edge of the diaphragmatic hiatus to prevent this complication. (Reproduced with permission from Orringer MB. Complications of esophageal surgery and trauma. In: Greenfield LJ, ed. *Complications in surgery and trauma,* 2nd ed. Philadelphia, PA: J.B. Lippincott; 1990:318.)

small and the herniated viscera may become adherent to adjacent intrathoracic structures requiring a transthoracic approach for reduction. The majority of herniations of intestine alongside the intrathoracic stomach, on the other hand, occur through a relatively patulous hiatus. Reduction of the hernia and narrowing of the hiatus are readily achieved through the abdomen. As is the case with other complications that follow esophageal surgery, this situation can also generally be prevented. When the esophageal substitute has been brought through the diaphragmatic hiatus and the anastomosis has been completed, several heavy diaphragmatic crural sutures should be used to narrow the hiatus so that it admits three fingers alongside the stomach or colon. Then a few interrupted sutures between the edge of the diaphragmatic hiatus and the visceral esophageal substitute should be used to limit the migration of other intra-abdominal viscera through the hiatus into the chest. Finally, the divided triangular ligament of the mobilized liver should be sutured to the edge of the hiatus to provide one additional barrier to herniation at this site.

Chylothorax

Owing to the proximity of the thoracic duct and the esophagus, chylothorax following esophagectomy is a recognized complication. Ligation of the divided periesophageal tissues at the time of esophagectomy minimizes this complication. Compared with the relatively healthy patient who sustains a chylothorax after aortic surgery, however, this complication occurring in the debilitated patient with esophageal obstruction is not well tolerated, with reported mortality as high as 50% (55,56). Patients with chronic esophageal obstruction are already nutritionally depleted. Further loss of protein-rich chyle is not well tolerated. Only a few days should be expended trying to treat this complication nonoperatively. With aggressive operative intervention and direct ligation of the point of thoracic duct injury, patient salvage is the rule (57). Thoracic duct ligation at the point where the thoracic duct emerges through the diaphragmatic hiatus can be accomplished either by right posterolateral thoracotomy or VATS techniques.

Pancreatitis

Postoperative pancreatitis may occur following esophagectomy due to pancreatic injury during performance of either the Kocher maneuver or gastric mobilization. The possibility should be suspected in patients who develop unexplained fever, respiratory distress, or prolonged ileus after esophagectomy. The diagnosis is confirmed by determining serum amylase and lipase levels. Standard treatment of pancreatitis with nasogastric tube decompression of the gastrointestinal tract and intravenous fluids is usually sufficient, although progression to fatal hemorrhagic pancreatitis may occur.

Splenic injury

Injury to the spleen may occur during esophagectomy, particularly during mobilization of the stomach for esophageal replacement. Careful avoidance of undue traction on the short gastric vessels during gastric mobilization and early division of adhesions between the stomach and the spleen on opening the abdomen minimize this complication. Routine splenectomy as part of the "cancer operation" for esophageal carcinoma is not advocated because splenectomy is associated with a well-documented increased morbidity of its own.

Peripheral atheroembolism

Thromboembolic sequelae after transhiatal esophagectomy have been reported in two patients and attributed to inadvertent dislodgement of debris from the diseased aorta in the process of mobilizing the esophagus through the diaphragmatic hiatus (58). This complication has not been encountered by our group in a combined experience with more than 2,000 transhiatal esophagectomies.

Complications of substernal esophageal replacement

Several unique complications of esophageal replacement are related to retrosternal placement of the esophageal substitute. The most obvious is potential obstruction at the level of the retrosternal neohiatus due to failure to create an adequate opening. When creating a retrosternal tunnel, it is our practice to dilate this space until the entire hand and forearm can be inserted retrosternally, ensuring sufficient room for either the stomach or the colon. Compression and obstruction of the retrosternal esophageal substitute at the superior opening into the anterior mediastinum is a function of the posterior prominence of the clavicular head, which narrows the anterior thoracic inlet. For this reason, when performing a retrosternal interposition of stomach or colon, which requires relocation of the cervical esophagus anteriorly from its usual position to the left and posterior to the trachea, the medial third of the clavicle, the adjacent manubrium, and usually the medial first rib as well should be resected to ensure an adequate opening into the anterior mediastinum.

Complications of bypassing or excluding the native esophagus

Management of the diseased native esophagus is controversial when performing retrosternal replacement of the esophagus. An esophagus that is severely strictured from a caustic injury, for example, may simply be left in the posterior mediastinum and bypassed with a retrosternal colon. The potential complications arising from the residual diseased esophagus, however, mandate that it be removed whenever possible. The small but definite increased risk of late development of carcinoma in the caustic strictured esophagus is a less compelling reason to resect it than the potential for subsequent reflux esophagitis. A caustic injury may destroy the lower esophageal sphincter mechanism owing to subsequent fibrosis, and such a patient undergoing substernal colon interposition may develop reflux symptoms and severe esophagitis in the native esophagus.

Although substernal bypass of the excluded esophagus with either stomach or colon has been used for treatment of both benign and malignant disease, the complications from such an approach are appreciable. The excluded esophagus may become a giant posterior mediastinal mucocele that causes respiratory distress due to tracheobronchial compression. Of more immediate concern in the postoperative period is the incidence of disruption of the distal end of the excluded esophagus with resultant left subphrenic abscess. When esophageal replacement is necessary for benign disease, the authors advocate resection of the esophagus. It is always preferable to place the esophageal substitute in the posterior mediastinum in the original esophageal bed because (a) this is the shortest distance between the neck and the abdominal cavity; (b) if subsequent anastomotic dilation is required, it is far safer and more direct to perform it when one does not have to negotiate the anterior angulation of the cervical esophagus that has been anastomosed to a retrosternal graft; and (c) the incidence of postoperative cervical anastomotic leak is lower. In the original esophageal bed in the neck, the anastomosis is buttressed by adjacent tissues: the spine posteriorly, the carotid sheath laterally, the trachea medially, and the strap muscles anteriorly. An esophageal anastomosis to a retrosternal colon or stomach is basically subcutaneous in the neck and is relatively unsupported. Coughing or a Valsalva maneuver against a closed upper esophageal sphincter results in distention of the retrosternal esophageal substitute with increased pressure on the anastomosis and a higher anastomotic leak rate. If esophageal bypass is performed in patients with unresectable esophageal carcinoma, the distal esophagus should be decompressed into a Roux-en-Y limb or jejunum rather than excluded (59,60).

Esophageal diverticulectomy

Pulsion diverticula of the esophagus, whether oropharyngeal (Zenker diverticulum) or intrathoracic, result from associated distal esophageal obstruction, most often neuromotor dysfunction. Thus, if the underlying neuromotor abnormality responsible for the formation of the diverticulum is not addressed at the time of diverticulectomy, failure to relieve the distal obstruction may result in disruption of the suture line (Fig. 24.16). Following resection of a diverticulum, the esophagus should be insufflated with air through an indwelling nasogastric tube positioned within the esophagus, and an air leak should be looked for by immersing the pouting esophageal submucosa in saline solution (Fig. 24.17). The most opportune time to treat such a pinhole leak is at the time of operation, and a single 5-0 monofilament stitch may avert a great deal of postoperative morbidity. Alternatively, if a cervical esophageal leak occurs after diverticulectomy and esophagomyotomy, the neck wound must be opened, irrigated, and drained, as described earlier for the treatment of cervical anastomotic disruption. Nutrition may be maintained with either nasogastric feedings or total parenteral support. Broad-spectrum antibiotics are administered. With an adequate esophagomyotomy that has relieved the distal obstruction, the incidence of leak from a diverticulectomy suture line should be exceedingly low (61). If a cervical salivary fistula does occur, however, spontaneous closure within 7 to 10 days should be expected. If an intrathoracic esophageal suture line leak occurs within several days of diverticulectomy, immediate re-exploration of the chest with closure of the fistula and reinforcement with anterior mediastinal fat, adjacent pleura, intercostal muscle, or omentum is indicated.

Esophagomyotomy for achalasia or esophageal spasm

The megaesophagus of achalasia may contain 1 to 2 liters of stagnant intraesophageal contents. Induction of general

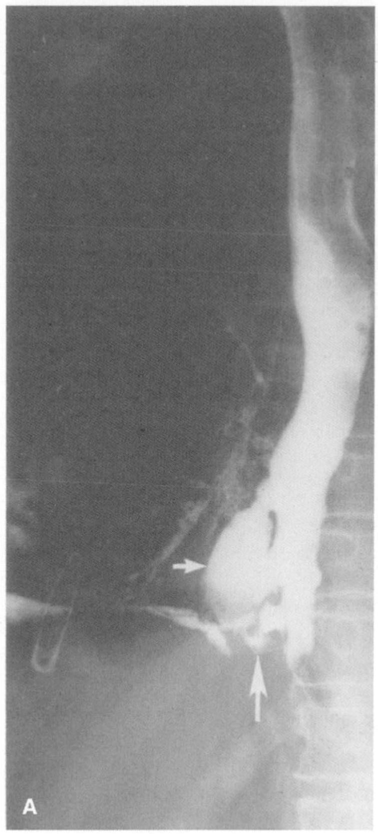

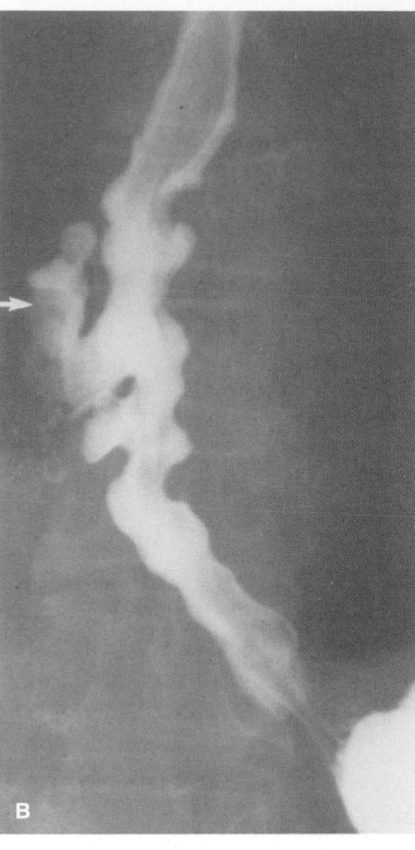

FIGURE 24.16. **A:** This esophagogram shows an esophagopleural cutaneous fistula (*large arrow*) and a recurrent esophageal diverticulum (*small arrow*) in a patient who had undergone prior resection of the diverticulum *without* an esophagomyotomy. **B:** The patient's underlying esophageal neuromotor problem is evident in this view from the same study, showing a typical corkscrew esophagus. The relative obstruction secondary to intermittent spasm distal to the esophageal suture line had not been relieved when the diverticulum was resected; hence disruption of the suture line with fistula formation and recurrence of the diverticulum (*arrow*) followed. (Reproduced with permission from Orringer MB. Complications of esophageal surgery and trauma. In: Greenfield LJ, ed. *Complications in surgery and trauma,* 2nd ed. Philadelphia, PA: J.B. Lippincott; 1990:320.)

anesthesia in such a patient represents the most dangerous part of the operation. Because a nasogastric tube interferes with deep breathing and adequate clearing of pulmonary secretions, one should not use an intraesophageal nasogastric tube preoperatively to decompress the dilated esophagus. Rather, the patient is restricted to a clear liquid diet for 2 days before the operation, and then immediately before induction of general anesthesia, with the patient in a sitting position, a nasogastric tube is passed, and the esophagus is aspirated and evacuated. Rapid-sequence induction of anesthesia is then carried out while constant pressure is maintained on the cricoid cartilage to prevent regurgitation of esophageal contents into the pharynx until the endotracheal tube balloon is inflated. Once the airway is protected,

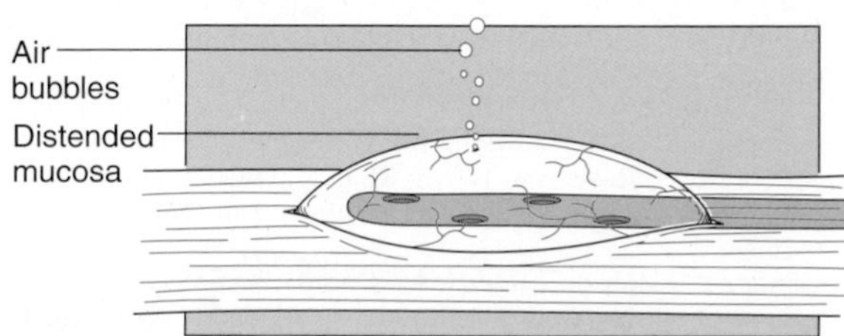

FIGURE 24.17. Testing for inadvertent esophageal perforation following esophagomyotomy. The esophageal mucosa is distended by insufflating air down an intraesophageal nasogastric tube. Air bubbles escaping from the esophagus submerged under saline indicate a perforation. (Reproduced with permission from Orringer MB. Complications of esophageal surgery and trauma. In: Greenfield LJ, ed. *Complications in surgery and trauma,* 2nd ed. Philadelphia, PA: J.B. Lippincott; 1990:322.)

rigid esophagoscopy is carried out, and the esophagus is evacuated and irrigated.

After completion of the esophagomyotomy for either achalasia or esophageal spasm, integrity of the esophageal mucosa is documented by insufflating air into the esophagus through an indwelling intraesophageal nasogastric tube. As described earlier, identification and closure of an inadvertent esophageal injury at this point is far simpler than when the perforation is detected hours to days after operation. Patients with achalasia are frequently referred for operation following failed pneumatic dilatation or, more recently, unsuccessful intrasphincteric injection of botulinum toxin. These previous endoscopic interventions may increase the difficulty in identifying tissue planes prior to successful esophagomyotomy. In particular, patients who have previously undergone botulinum toxin injection, and obtained some relief of achalasia symptoms, are more likely to have periesophageal fibrosis resulting in a greater risk, as high as 50%, for esophageal perforation during esophagomyotomy and less palliation of their symptoms following operation. Periesophageal fibrosis was less prevalent among patients who had previously been treated by pneumatic dilatation and did not appear to affect surgical outcomes following esophagomyotomy (62,63).

Regardless of the approach used, potential complications exist and may require reoperation in 10% to 15% of patients following esophagomyotomy. If a complete distal esophagomyotomy is not performed and the obstruction relieved, dysphagia and regurgitation will continue in the immediate postoperative period and reoperation may be necessary (64). Alternatively, if the esophagomyotomy is carried onto the stomach to ensure adequate relief of the esophageal obstruction, the uncoordinated lower esophageal sphincter may be converted to an incompetent one, with ensuing long-term complications of reflux esophagitis. Furthermore, "long" esophagomyotomy, over 5 cm with extension onto the stomach, has been associated with "diverticularization" of the mucosa in long-term follow-up (65,66).

Controversy exists about the need for a concomitant antireflux procedure with the distal esophagomyotomy, which may render the lower esophageal sphincter incompetent (67–69). With a few notable exceptions, the majority of esophageal surgeons now advocate partial fundoplication to prevent the subsequent development of gastroesophageal reflux following esophagomyotomy for achalasia (70). A Belsey-type partial fundoplication has been recommended when esophagomyotomy is approached transthoracically, whereas Toupet (posterior) or Dor (anterior) fundoplication is typically recommended following transabdominal esophagomyotomy. When performing a fundoplication to ensure lower esophageal sphincter competence in an atonic esophagus, care must be exercised to avoid subsequent obstruction due to an overaggressive fundoplication.

Among the more difficult problems of surgery for achalasia is the development of recurrent dysphagia and regurgitation due to esophageal obstruction occurring 1 or more years after a previous esophagomyotomy. Although esophagomyotomy has become the standard surgical approach to patients with achalasia, in those with a tortuous megaesophagus and a supradiaphragmatic pouch of esophagus, delayed esophageal emptying may occur even after a satisfactory esophagomyotomy. Furthermore, the patient who has undergone a previous esophagomyotomy and has recurrent symptoms has only a 40% to 70% chance of experiencing a good result from a "redo" esophagomyotomy (71,72). Finally, esophagomyotomy remains a palliative operation for patients with esophageal motor disorders involving the body of the esophagus and lower esophageal sphincter. Patients with achalasia remain at risk for the development of esophageal squamous cell carcinoma, and should undergo routine surveillance upper endoscopy following esophagomyotomy. In patients with either recurrent or persistent symptoms of achalasia with or without associated reflux esophagitis, esophagectomy may provide the best option, eliminating the esophageal obstruction as well as the potential for late development of carcinoma (73). Several groups have suggested that the presence of megaesophagus does not preclude successful esophagomyotomy (74,75), particularly if the long axis of the esophagus remains near-vertical (75). In contrast, others have shown that duration of symptoms, sigmoidal esophagus (megaesophagus), and diminished lower esophageal sphincter pressures appear to be factors predictive of worse outcomes following esophagomyotomy (76), and these factors should be taken into consideration in determining whether patients should undergo esophagomyotomy or primary esophagectomy.

REFERENCES

1. Henderson RD, Boszko A, Van Nostrand AW, et al. Pharyngoesophageal dysphagia and recurrent laryngeal nerve palsy. *J Thorac Cardiovasc Surg* 1974;68:507–512.
2. Salama FD, Lamont G. Long-term results of the Belsey Mark IV antireflux operation in relation to the severity of esophagitis. *J Thorac Cardiovasc Surg* 1990;100:517–519.
3. Orringer MB, Skinner DB, Belsey RH. Long-term results of the Mark IV operation for hiatal hernia and analyses of recurrences and their treatment. *J Thorac Cardiovasc Surg* 1972;63:25–33.
4. Pearson FG, Langer B, Henderson RD. Gastroplasty and Belsey hiatus hernia repair. An operation for the management of peptic stricture with acquired short esophagus. *J Thorac Cardiovasc Surg* 1971;61: 50–63.
5. Orringer MB, Orringer JS, Dabich L, et al. Combined Collis gastroplasty–fundoplication operations for scleroderma reflux esophagitis. *Surgery* 1981;90:624–630.
6. Pearson FG. Hiatus hernia and gastroesophageal reflux: indications for surgery and selection of operation. *Sem Thorac Cardiovasc Surg* 1997;9: 163–168.
7. Lam TC, Fok M, Cheng SW, et al. Anastomotic complications after esophagectomy for cancer. A comparison of neck and chest anastomoses. *J Thorac Cardiovasc Surg* 1992;104:395–400.
8. Michel L, Grillo HC, Malt RA. Esophageal perforation. *Ann Thorac Surg* 1982;33:203–210.
9. White RK, Morris DM. Diagnosis and management of esophageal perforations. *Am Surg* 1992;58:112–119.
10. Bufkin BL, Miller JI Jr, Mansour KA. Esophageal perforation: emphasis on management. *Ann Thorac Surg* 1996;61:1447–1451.
11. Bahnson TD. Strategies to minimize the risk of esophageal injury during catheter ablation for atrial fibrillation. *Pacing Clin Electrophysiol.* 2009;32:248–260.
12. Zwischenberger JB, Savage C, Bidani A. Surgical aspects of esophageal disease: perforation and caustic injury. *Am J Resp Crit Care Med* 2002;165: 1037–1040.
13. Cameron JL, Kieffer RF, Hendrix TR, et al. Selective nonoperative management of contained intrathoracic esophageal disruptions. *Ann Thorac Surg.* 1979;27:404–408.
14. Andersen OS, Giustra PE. Nonoperative management of contained esophageal perforation. *Arch Surg* 1981;116:1214–1217.
15. Michel L, Grillo HC, Malt RA. Operative and nonoperative management of esophageal perforations. *Ann Surg* 1981;194:57–63.
16. Flynn AE, Verrier ED, Way LW, et al. Esophageal perforation. *Arch Surg* 1989;124:1211–1214.
17. Whyte RI, Iannettoni MD, Orringer MB. Intrathoracic esophageal perforation: the merit of primary repair. *J Thorac Cardiovasc Surg* 1995;109: 140–146.
18. Orringer MB. Complications of esophageal surgery and trauma. In: Greenfield LJ, ed. *Complications in surgery and trauma* Philadelphia, PA: J.B. Lippincott; 1990:313.
19. Gouge TH, Depan HJ, Spencer FC. Experience with the Grillo pleural wrap procedure in 18 patients with perforation of the thoracic esophagus. *Ann Surg* 1989;209:612–617.
20. Wright CD, Mathisen DJ, Wain JC, et al. Reinforced primary repair of thoracic esophageal perforation. *Ann Thorac Surg* 1995;60:245–248.
21. Iannettoni MD, Vlessis AA, Whyte RI, et al. Functional outcome after surgical treatment of esophageal perforation. *Ann Thorac Surg* 1997;64: 1606–1609.
22. Hernandez L, Jacobson J, Harris M. Comparison among the perforation rates of Maloney, balloon, and savary dilation of esophageal strictures. *Gastrointest Endosc* 2000;51:460–462.
23. Kubba H, Spinou E, Brown D. Is same-day discharge suitable following rigid esophagoscopy? Findings in a series of 655 cases. *Ear Nose Throat J* 2003;82:33–36.
24. Puchakayala MR, Abbey K, Haft J, et al. Delayed pericardial tamponade following transthoracic hiatal hernia repair. *J Cardiothorac Vasc Anesth* 2006;20:245–246.

25. Patel HJ, Tan BB, Yee J, et al. A twenty-five year experience with open primary transthoracic repair of paraesophageal hiatal hernia. *J Thorac Cardiovasc Surg* 2004;127:843–849.
26. Khaitan L, Ray WA, Holzman MD, et al. Health care utilization after medical and surgical therapy for gastroesophageal reflux disease: a population-based study, 1996 to 2000. *Arch Surg* 2003;138:1356–1361.
27. Bowers SP, Mattar SG, Smith CD, et al. Clinical and histologic follow-up after antireflux surgery for Barrett's esophagus. *J Gastrointest Surg* 2002;6:532–539.
28. Watson DI, Baigrie RJ, Jamieson GG. A learning curve for laparoscopic fundoplication. Definable, avoidable, or a waste of time? *Ann Surg* 1996;224:198–203.
29. Nason KS, Luketich JD, Qureshi I, et al. Laparoscopic repair of giant paraesophageal hernia results in long-term patient satisfaction and a durable repair. *J Gastrointest Surg* 2008;12:2066–2075.
30. Pearson FG, Cooper JD, Ilves R, et al. Massive hiatal hernia with incarceration: a report of 53 cases. *Ann Thorac Surg* 1983;35:45–51.
31. Maziak DE, Todd TR, Pearson FG. Massive hiatus hernia: evaluation and surgical management. *J Thorac Cardiovasc Surg* 1998;115:53–60.
32. Johnson AB, Oddsdottir M, Hunter JG. Laparoscopic Collis gastroplasty and Nissen fundoplication. A new technique for the management of esophageal foreshortening. *Surg Endosc* 1998;12:1055–1060.
33. Tatum R, Shalhub S, Oelschlager B, et al. Complications of PTFE mesh at the diaphragmatic hiatus. *J Gastrointest Surg* 2008;12:953–957.
34. Stadlhuber R, Sherif A, Mittal S, et al. Mesh complications after prosthetic reinforcement of hiatal closure: a 28-case series. *Surg Endosc* 2009;23:1219–1226.
35. Orringer MB, Marshall B, Iannettoni MD. Eliminating the cervical esophagogastric anastomotic leak with a side-to-side stapled anastomosis. *J Thorac Cardiovasc Surg* 2000;119:277–288.
36. Orringer M, Lemmer J. Early dilation in the treatment of esophageal disruption. *Ann Thorac Surg* 1986;42:536–539.
37. Iannettoni MD, Whyte RI, Orringer MB. Catastrophic complications of the cervical esophagogastric anastomosis. *J Thorac Cardiovasc Surg* 1995;110:1493–1500.
38. Orringer MB, Marshall B, Chang AC, et al. Two thousand transhiatal esophagectomies: changing trends, lessons learned. *Ann Surg* 2007;246:363–372.
39. Dewar L, Gelfand G, Finley RJ, et al. Factors affecting cervical anastomotic leak and stricture formation following esophagogastrectomy and gastric tube interposition. *Am J Surg* 1992;163:484–489.
40. Vigneswaran WT, Trastek VF, Pairolero PC, et al. Transhiatal esophagectomy for carcinoma of the esophagus. *Ann Thorac Surg* 1993;56:838–844.
41. Gandhi SK, Naunheim KS. Complications of transhiatal esophagectomy. *Chest Surg Clin N Am* 1997;7:601–610.
42. Rice TW. Anastomotic stricture complicating esophagectomy. *Thorac Surg Clin* 2006;16:63–73.
43. Chang AC, Orringer MB. Management of the cervical esophagogastric anastomotic stricture. *Sem Thorac Cardiovasc Surg* 2007;19:66–71.
44. Kirsch M, Blue M, Desai RK, et al. Intralesional steroid injections for peptic esophageal strictures. *Gastrointest Endosc* 1991;37:180–182.
45. Lee M, Kubik C, Polhamus C, et al. Preliminary experience with endoscopic intralesional steroid injection therapy for refractory upper gastrointestinal strictures. *Gastrointest Endosc* 1995;41:598–601.
46. Law SY, Fok M, Cheng SW, et al. A comparison of outcome after resection for squamous cell carcinomas and adenocarcinomas of the esophagus and cardia. *Surg Gyn Obstet* 1992;175:107–112.
47. Gillinov AM, Heitmiller RF. Strategies to reduce pulmonary complications after transhiatal esophagectomy. *Dis Esoph* 1998;11:43–47.
48. Doty JR, Salazar JD, Forastiere AA, et al. Postesophagectomy morbidity, mortality, and length of hospital stay after preoperative chemoradiation therapy. *Ann Thorac Surg* 2002;74:227–231.
49. Burt M, Diehl W, Martini N, et al. Malignant esophagorespiratory fistula: management options and survival. *Ann Thorac Surg* 1991;52:1222–1228.
50. Urschel JD, Blewett CJ, Young JE, et al. Pyloric drainage (pyloroplasty) or no drainage in gastric reconstruction after esophagectomy: a meta-analysis of randomized controlled trials. *Dig Surg* 2002;19:160–164.
51. Ludwig DJ, Thirlby RC, Low DE. A prospective evaluation of dietary status and symptoms after near-total esophagectomy without gastric emptying procedure. *Am J Surg* 2001;181:454–458.
52. Fok M, Cheng SW, Wong J. Pyloroplasty versus no drainage in gastric replacement of the esophagus. *Am J Surg* 1991;162:447–452.
53. Katariya K, Harvey JC, Pina E, et al. Complications of transhiatal esophagectomy. *J Surg Oncol* 1994;57:157–163.
54. Heitmiller RF, Gillinov AM, Jones B. Transhiatal herniation of colon after esophagectomy and gastric pull-up. *Ann Thorac Surg* 1997;63:554–556.
55. Merigliano S, Molena D, Ruol A, et al. Chylothorax complicating esophagectomy for cancer: A plea for early thoracic duct ligation. *J Thorac Cardiovasc Surg* 2000;119:453–457.
56. Wemyss-Holden SA, Launois B, Maddern GJ. Management of thoracic duct injuries after oesophagectomy. *Br J Surg* 2001;88:1442–1448.
57. Orringer MB, Bluett M, Deeb GM. Aggressive treatment of chylothorax complicating transhiatal esophagectomy without thoracotomy. *Surgery* 1988;104:720–726.
58. Magee MJ, Landreneau RJ, Keenan RJ, et al. Peripheral atheroembolism from the aorta complicating transhiatal esophagectomy. *Am Surg* 1994;60:634–637.
59. Kirschner M. Ein neues verfahren der oesophagus plastik. *Arch Klin Chir* 1920;114:606–663.
60. Meunier B, Stasik C, Raoul J-L, et al. Gastric bypass for malignant esophagotracheal fistula: a series of 21 cases. *Eur J Cardiothorac Surg* 1998;13:184–189.
61. Varghese TK Jr, Marshall B, Chang AC, et al. Surgical treatment of epiphrenic diverticula: a 30-year experience. *Ann Thorac Surg* 2007;84:1801–1809.
62. Patti MG, Feo CV, Arcerito M, et al. Effects of previous treatment on results of laparoscopic Heller myotomy for achalasia. *Dig Dis Sci* 1999;44:2270–2276.
63. Wiechmann RJ, Ferguson MK, Naunheim KS, et al. Video-assisted surgical management of achalasia of the esophagus. *J Thorac Cardiovasc Surg* 1999;118:916–923.
64. Patti MG, Molena D, Fisichella PM, et al. Laparoscopic Heller myotomy and Dor fundoplication for achalasia: analysis of successes and failures. *Arch Surg* 2001;136:870–877.
65. Chen LQ, Chughtai T, Sideris L, et al. Long-term effects of myotomy and partial fundoplication for esophageal achalasia. *Dis Esoph* 2002;15:171–179.
66. Ellis FH Jr. Failure after esophagomyotomy for esophageal motor disorders. Causes, prevention, and management. *Chest Surg Clin N Am* 1997;7:477–487.
67. Richards WO, Sharp KW, Holzman MD. An antireflux procedure should not routinely be added to a Heller myotomy. *J Gastrointest Surg* 2001;5:13–16.
68. Peters JH. An antireflux procedure is critical to the long-term outcome of esophageal myotomy for achalasia. *J Gastrointest Surg* 2001;5:17–20.
69. Lyass S, Thoman D, Steiner JP, et al. Current status of an antireflux procedure in laparoscopic Heller myotomy: outcomes of laparoscopic fundoplication for gastroesophageal reflux disease and paraesophageal hernia. *Surg Endosc* 2003;17:554–558.
70. Ellis FH Jr, Watkins E Jr, Gibb SP, et al. Ten to 20-year clinical results after short esophagomyotomy without an antireflux procedure (modified Heller operation) for esophageal achalasia. *Eur J Cardiothorac Surg* 1992;6:86–89.
71. Gorecki PJ, Hinder RA, Libbey JS, et al. Redo laparoscopic surgery for achalasia. *Surg Endosc* 2002;16:772–776.
72. Ellis FH Jr, Crozier RE, Gibb SP. Reoperative achalasia surgery. *J Thorac Cardiovasc Surg* 1986;92:859–865.
73. Devaney EJ, Lannettoni MD, Orringer MB, et al. Esophagectomy for achalasia: patient selection and clinical experience. *Ann Thorac Surg* 2001;72:854–858.
74. Patti MG, Pellegrini CA, Horgan S, et al. Minimally invasive surgery for achalasia: an 8-year experience with 168 patients. *Ann Surg* 1999;230:587–593.
75. Eldaif SM, Mutrie CJ, Rutledge WC, et al. The risk of esophageal resection after esophagomyotomy for achalasia. *Ann Thorac Surg* 2009;87:1558–1563.
76. Schuchert MJ, Luketich JD, Landreneau RJ, et al. Minimally-invasive esophagomyotomy in 200 consecutive patients: factors influencing postoperative outcomes. *Ann Thorac Surg* 2008;85:1729–1734.

CHAPTER

25

Complications of Pulmonary and Chest Wall Surgery

Christina H. Wei and Jessica S. Donington

INTRODUCTION

Thoracic surgery outcomes are dependent on many factors including patient's cardiopulmonary health, smoking status, primary thoracic pathology, extent of resection, anesthetics, and quality of pre- and postoperative care. When complications arise, early and prompt recognition is important. The majority of pulmonary and chest wall resections are related to the treatment of non-small cell lung cancer (NSCLC). This is a tobacco associated malignancy and therefore a significant proportion of patients undergoing resection have other tobacco related comorbidities including coronary artery disease, hypertension, peripheral vascular disease, chronic obstructive lung disease (COPD). It is also a disease of the elderly with the median age of diagnosis at 67 (1). These factors contribute to a relatively frail surgical population.

SURGERY FOR LUNG CANCER

Surgery remains the primary form of treatment for patients with early stage NSCLC (1). This includes tumors limited to the lung and intrapulmonary lymph nodes, but also encompasses tumors that extend into the chest wall and select tumors that involve mediastinal lymph nodes. Lobectomy via video assisted thoracoscopic surgery (VATS) or standard posterior lateral thoracotomy, with mediastinal lymph node dissection is the current standard of care for medically fit patients with early stage NSCLC. Over the past decade, there has been a meaningful reduction in the morbidity and mortality associated with pulmonary resections. This is attributed to improved patient selection, advances in anesthesia care and surgical technology, and improved postoperative care. The American College of Surgeons Oncology Group (ACOSOG) recently published operative morbidity and mortality results of Z0030, a phase III trial, which compared systematic mediastinal lymph node sampling to complete mediastinal lymph node dissection in clinical stage I and II NSCLC patients undergoing surgical resection (2). The trial randomized 1,023 patients from 102 different institutions, and its morbidity and mortality data represent a modern benchmark for patients undergoing major pulmonary resection in the United States and Canada. Overall mortality in the series was 1.4%, with no increase in mortality with more extensive resections, although the trial was not designed to detect that difference (Table 25.1). One or more complications occurred in 38% of patients, with atrial arrhythmias seen in 14%, prolonged chest tube duration in 11%, and persistent air leaks in 8% being most common (Table 25.2). Other contemporary series from Strand et al. (3) and Licker et al. (4) report similar mortality to the ACOSOG trial at 4.4% and 2.9% respectively. A series from Dominguez-Ventura et al. (5) looking exclusively at surgical outcome in octogenarians reported mortality of 6.3% and overall morbidity of 48%. A history of chronic heart failure or myocardial infarction (MI) was an indicator of increased mortality, and the greatest increase in morbidity compared to a younger population was in the rate of atrial arrhythmias (21%).

INTRAOPERATIVE COMPLICATIONS

Intraoperative hemorrhage

Massive intraoperative hemorrhage is usually the result of injury to a pulmonary artery or vein branch sustained during dissection. The pulmonary arteries are thin walled and prone to injury during traction or manipulation. The wall of pulmonary veins is more resilient and can better withstand surgical manipulation. Inflammatory changes to the surrounding soft tissue resulting from neoadjuvant chemotherapy, radiation therapy, or chronic infection can render dissection more difficult. Expeditious control of bleeding is crucial and can usually be accomplished with application of pressure to the bleeding site. The surgeon should be cognizant of the patient's hemodynamic status during this time. Mode of repair is dependent on the size and location of injury. The fragile nature of the pulmonary artery often mandates proximal hilar control to assure tension free repair.

Ventilatory complications

Intraoperative ventilatory complication can be a result of multiple causes. Ventilation circuitry should be assessed and appropriate placement and position of the endotracheal tube

Christina H. Wei, Jessica S. Donington: NYU School of Medicine, Department of Cardiothoracic Surgery, New York, NY 10016.

Table **25.1** **Operative mortality following lung cancer resections**

			Mortality				
Study	**Year**	***N***	**Overall (%)**	**Pneumonectomy (%)**	**Bilobectomy (%)**	**Lobectomy (%)**	**Sublobar (%)**
Strand	2007	4,395	4.4	8.6	7.3	2.5	2.2
Allen	2006	1,023	1.37	0	5	1	3
Dominguez-Ventura	2006	379	6.3	8	14.3	5	8.4
Rostad	2006	3,224	8.0	11.6	N/R	5.3	N/R
Licker	1999	634	3.2	7.9	3	1.2	2.7
Romano	1992	12,439	5.0	11.6	N/R	3.9	3.7
Wada	1988	7,099	1.3	3.2	N/R	1.2	0.8
Ginsberg	1983	2,220	3.7	6.2	N/R	2.9	1.4
Weiss	1974	547	12.4	17	N/R	10	0

confirmed. Double lumen endotracheal tubes (DLETT) are frequently used during pulmonary resections and greatly facilitate surgery by providing lung collapse and a quiet surgical field but require more precise positioning than standard single lumen tubes. If the DLETT is advanced too far, it occludes the take off of left upper lobe orifice, resulting in hypoxia and hypoventilation during right-sided resections. Withdrawal of the tube can relieve the obstruction. The DLETT can also be placed too proximally, resulting in poor lung isolation or occlusion of the right main stem bronchus by the herniated bronchial cuff. This can be prevented by bronchoscopic confirmation of tube position after the patient is placed in the decubitus position. Patients with pre-existing emphysema are at risk of ventilator-associated pneumothorax. Pneumothorax can occur in the contralateral lung during surgery while the patient is on positive pressure ventilation. This typically results in an acute increase in the airway pressure, hypotension, loss of rhythmic movement of mediastinum, or bulging mediastinum. This problem can be alleviated by opening into the contralateral pleural space through the mediastinum.

POSTOPERATIVE COMPLICATIONS

Postoperative bleeding

Etiology and Risk Factors

Substantial postoperative bleeding following pulmonary resections is rare. Inadequate intraoperative hemostasis is the most common reason for postoperative bleeding (6). According to a National Veterans Affairs Surgical Quality Improvement Program, which analyzed outcomes after

Table **25.2** **Operative morbidity following lung cancer resections**

	Study		
Complication	**Licker (1999)** *n* **= 634**	**Dominguez-Ventura (2006)** *n* **= 379**	**Allen (2006)** *n* **= 1,023**
One or more complication	N/R	48	38
Air leaks >7 days (%)	N/R	7	7.6
Chest tube >7 days (%)	N/R	N/R	11.5
Chylothorax (%)	N/R	1.0	1.3
Hemorrhage (%)	0.6	1.0	2.4
Myocardial infarction (%)	2.4	4.0	0.9
Empyema	N/R	1.0	1.1
Recurrent nerve injury (%)	N/R	2.0	0.7
Arrhythmia (%)	N/R	21.0	14.4
Respiratory failure (%)	1.3	6.0	5.5
Broncho-pleural fistula (%)	N/R	N/R	0.5
Pneumonia (%)	0.8	4.0	2.5

3,516 lung resections, significant postoperative bleeding, defined as requiring ≥4 units transfusion, occurred in 3% of patients (7). Factors associated with postoperative bleeding include a history of antiplatelet or anticoagulation therapy and neoadjuvant radiation or chemotherapy (8).

Clinical Presentation

Presentation can range from obvious to occult. The common thresholds for reoperation for postoperative bleeding include a chest tube output of 1,000 mL in 1 hour or 200 mL/hour for 2 to 4 hours. However, low chest tube output does not exclude active bleeding since the chest tube can clot. In occult cases, patients remain hemodynamically stable but bleed slowly into the thorax with retained blood that evolves into clotted hemothorax.

Management and Prevention

Hemodynamic stabilization and reversal of coagulopathy are the initial management steps, followed by a decision for re-exploration. The goals at re-exploration are controlling ongoing blood loss and evacuation of retained hemothorax. Sources of bleeding include mediastinal, bronchial, intercostal, and hilar vessels, or along lung parenchymal staple lines in the lung. In many cases, no specific site of bleeding is identified at re-exploration.

Thromboembolism

Etiology and Risk Factors

Venous thromboembolism is a relatively rare but potentially devastating complication of pulmonary surgery. Thoracic surgical procedures are considered a moderate risk for the development of deep venous thrombosis (DVT) due to the increased perioperative hypercoagulable state. The classic Virchow's triad of stasis (from anesthetics), hypercoagulability (associated with tobacco use, malignancy, and age), and endothelial injury (from surgery) are present in most thoracic surgery patients. The incidence of thromboembolism in patients undergoing pulmonary resection is between 7% and 14% for DVT and up to 5% for pulmonary embolism (PE) (9–11).

Clinical Presentation

PE presents with sudden respiratory distress, hypotension, tachycardia, syncope, or circulatory arrest (9). Ambulation in the early postoperative period should be monitored since many symptomatic cases of PE occur during patients' first walking attempt.

Diagnosis and Prevention

Diagnosis of PE is most commonly made by contrast computed tomography (CT) of the chest performed with specific PE protocols. Once diagnosed, patients are typically placed on anticoagulation therapy. Thrombolytic therapy is not an option in the early postoperative period. Thromboembolectomy is an option for only a very select group of hemodynamically unstable patients with large central clots. Prophylaxis includes the use of mechanical means with compression hose and intermittent compression devices and pharmacological means with low dose heparin. The prophylaxis should be started prior to the induction of anesthesia and continued throughout the hospital course.

Cardiac arrhythmia

Etiology and Risk Factors

Cardiac arrhythmia, specifically atrial fibrillation (AF), is by far the most common cardiac complication after thoracic surgery, with an incidence of 4% after wedge resection, 10% to 20% following lobectomy, and 40% after pneumonectomy (12,13). The incidence of AF after lobectomy does not differ for open and VATS approaches (14). The peak onset of AF is 2 to 3 days post surgery. Patients who develop perioperative AF are at increased risk for stroke. The risk of stroke related to postoperative AF is 1.9% (15). The only consistent independent preoperative risk factor for development of atrial arrhythmia is age greater than 60 (12). Other predictors include male gender, history of AF, and prolonged P wave on a 12-lead electrocardiogram (ECG). Another interesting predictor is a twofold increase in white count on the first postoperative day, which is most likely a reflection of increased adrenergic activation post surgery (16). Other arrhythmias are much less frequently encountered. The incidence of sustained ventricular tachycardia is <1.6% and the incidence of bradyarrhythmias requiring treatment is <0.4% (12).

Treatment and Prevention

There are four key treatment issues with regard to postoperative AF: (a) control of ventricular response, (b) conversion to normal sinus rhythm, (c) prevention of thromboembolic events, and (d) prophylaxis (17). In patients with postoperative AF without structural heart disease, who are hemodynamically stable, rate-controlling agents such as β-blockers or calcium channel blockers are recommended. Rhythm control agents such as amiodarone show no overt advantage over rate control agents (18). For hemodynamically unstable patients, cardioversion is recommended to quickly achieve stability. Once arrhythmia resolves, the rate or rhythm control agent is continued for 8-week treatment. With appropriate pharmacologic intervention, approximately 85% of these cases will resolve before hospital discharge. In cases of persistent AF, about 98% will revert back to sinus rhythm within two months of surgery (18). Contraindications of commonly prescribed antiarrhythmic agents exist and vary according to individual medical history. Cardiology consultation is recommended in complex cases.

Another important aspect of AF treatment is prevention of thromboembolism. The potential for the development of thromboembolic events usually occur within 24 to 48 hours of new-onset AF; hence, prompt restoration of sinus rhythm is crucial and anticoagulation should be considered for arrhythmias that persist for greater than 24 hours.

Available evidence for perioperative prophylaxis to prevent cardiac arrhythmias indicates that a number of antiarrhythmic drugs have varying degrees of efficacy. The current American College of Chest Physician guidelines recommend using selective β-blockers for AF risk reduction (17). In cases where β-blockers are contraindicated, amiodarone is recommended. There is apprehension about the use of amiodarone for prophylaxis because of the small risk of acute respiratory distress syndrome (ARDS) (19).

Cardiac ischemia

Etiology and Risk Factors

The risk of developing cardiac ischemia related to thoracic surgery varies according to the patient's underlying cardiac performance. The risk of developing transient ischemic ECG changes is 3.8% (20,21), ranging from 0.13% in patients with no prior cardiac history to between 2.8% and 21% in patients with prior history of cardiac infarction (21,22). The mortality associated with postoperative ischemic event ranges between 2.3% and 70% (21,22). The onset of MI is usually on postoperative day 2 or 3. Abnormal exercise tolerance test and intraoperative hypotension are the strongest predictors for postoperative ischemic events (20).

Cardiopulmonary Risk Stratification

Intrathoracic surgery is considered an intermediate cardiac risk procedure (23). The American College of Cardiology and the American Heart Association have published a guideline on perioperative cardiopulmonary risk assessment (24), which reports increased perioperative cardiovascular complications in patients with active cardiac symptoms or cardiac ischemia induced by low-level exercise.

Postoperative respiratory complications

Respiratory complications occur in 10% to 20% of patients after lung resection and are a leading cause of mortality. In a prospective study of 956 patients undergoing resection for NSCLC, the 30-day mortality was 12.5% higher in patients who developed postoperative pulmonary complications than in those who did not (25). Pulmonary complications encompass several entities, including atelectasis, pneumonia, aspiration, and ARDS. The three most frequently reported predictors for pulmonary complications are low forced expired volume in 1 second (FEV_1), low diffusing capacity of lung for carbon monoxide (DLCO), and low predicted postoperative DLCO (26–29). Other risk factors include undergoing pneumonectomy, neoadjuvant chemotherapy, and poor exercise tolerance.

Pulmonary Risk Stratification

All patients being considered for lung resection should have spirometry testing. If the FEV_1 is >80% predicted or >2 L, and there is no evidence of dyspnea on exertion or interstitial lung disease, the patient is suitable for pneumonectomy. Lobectomy is typically feasible if the FEV_1 is >60% predicted or >1.5 L. Patients who do not fulfill these criteria may be at an increased risk for perioperative death and pulmonary complications. In patients with poor cardiopulmonary reserves, such as those who walk <25 shuttles on two shuttle walks or less than one flight of stairs, are at increased risk for perioperative death and cardiopulmonary complications with standard lung resection, and should be counseled about nonstandard surgery or nonoperative options (30).

Aspiration

The risk of aspiration increases when the airway is not protected, typically due to decreased mental status secondary to comorbid condition (stroke, dementia) or oversedation. Narcotic medications increase the risk of aspiration by decreasing gastrointestinal motility, which can lead to vomiting, and oversedation with lack of airway protection. Preventative measures include elevating the head of the bed, use of epidurals to decrease narcotic requirement, and attention to gastrointestinal symptoms including abdominal distension, nausea, or constipation. Treatment for aspiration includes bronchoscopy with washing to remove debris and collect cultures, supplemental oxygen, aggressive pulmonary physiotherapy, and antibiotics directed by cultures.

Sputum Retention

Inability to breathe deeply or cough due to pain or oversedation leads to increased postoperative sputum retention. Stagnation of secretions can result in bronchial plugging, atelectasis, lobar collapse, pneumonia, and respiratory failure. Current smokers, patients with COPD, stroke patients, and those without regional analgesia are at increased risk for sputum retention (31). The value of prophylactic smoking cessation immediately prior to surgery is debated, but those who continue to smoke within 1 month of pneumonectomy are at increased risk of developing postoperative pneumonia and ARDS (32).

Postoperative Pneumonia

Postoperative pneumonia is a significant cause of morbidity and mortality after major thoracic procedures, with an incidence of between 5.3% and 25% (7,33,34). Postoperative pneumonia increases mortality by up to 26.3% after pulmonary resection (35). Risk factors associated with the development of postoperative pneumonia include preoperative respiratory infection, sputum retention, a current smoking habit, poor mental status, poor pain control, COPD, immunodeficiency, and postoperative ventilator support. Pneumonias typically occur in early postoperative course, accompanied by fever, elevated white blood cell count, and persistent infiltrate on chest radiograph, but may be difficult to diagnose because these are nonspecific findings early after lung resection. The most common causative organisms are gram-negative rods, *Streptococcus pneumonia*, and *Staphylococcus aureus* (33,35). Broad-spectrum antibiotics should be initiated in cases of suspected pneumonia and adjusted on the basis of culture result. Prophylactic measures to decrease pneumonia include smoking cessation, good pain control with epidural catheter, chest physiotherapy, incentive spirometry, and early ambulation. The routine use of prophylactic antibiotics is not recommended.

Postresection pulmonary edema

Etiology and Risk Factors

Pulmonary edema is a disastrous complication following pulmonary resection. It is identified using several terms including: noncardiogenic pulmonary edema, acute lung injury (ALI), ARDS, and postpneumonectomy pulmonary edema. The syndrome is characterized by acute onset, fluffy infiltrates on chest radiograph, pulmonary capillary wedge pressure <18 mm Hg, and PAO2/FIO2 <300 mm Hg for ALI and <200 mm Hg for ARDS. The mortality rate for post resection pulmonary edema is reported at 50% to 100%, and correlates with the extent of resection (36,37). The incidence of ARDS following pulmonary resection is between 2.2% and 3.1% and also correlates with the extent of resection (36–38). It complicates 4% to 16% of pneumonectomies, but can also be seen at lower frequencies following lobectomies and VATS resections (36–38).

Although many independent risk factors for ARDS have been identified, the inciting event is often unknown (37–39). The most consistently reported risk factors are low FEV_1, low DLCO, extent of lung resection, and excessive fluid administration (36,37,40–42). In a large prospective study of 1,428 patients undergoing lung resection, Alam et al. found that the odds ratio for developing ALI was 1.17 for every 500 mL incremental increase in perioperative fluid administered (37).

Clinical Presentation

The presentation of postresection pulmonary edema can be subtle in the initial stages with tachypnea and low grade temperature, but quickly progresses to pulmonary edema, refractory hypoxemia, and hypercapnia. One-third of cases will begin within 24 hours of surgery, and most will manifest signs within 3 days of surgery, but onset has been reported as late as 7 days from resection. Once the process is initiated, it progresses with remarkable speed. Radiographic findings typically lag by 24 hours. Differential diagnosis includes iatrogenic fluid overload, cardiogenic pulmonary edema, pulmonary embolus, pneumonia, and aspiration. It is imperative to consider and exclude these etiologies prior to invoking the working diagnosis of postresection pulmonary edema.

Treatment

Optimal treatment remains elusive and is supportive in nature. Therapy should include intubation and mechanical ventilation, diuresis to improve fluid balance, broad-spectrum antibiotics coverage, bronchoscopy to remove any bronchial plugs, and frequent position changes to maximize alveolar recruitment. Steroid therapy is recommended by some but has not been universally used (43). A small series found inhaled nitric oxide useful (44).

Lobar torsion

Etiology and Risk Factors

Lobar torsion is a rare but serious complication after lung resection. The incidence is estimated at 0.1% to 0.3%. Right middle lobe torsion after a right upper lobectomy accounts for 70% of reported cases. Torsion of the bronchovascular pedicle results in strangulation and airway obstruction of the involved lobe. Complete interlobar fissure and absence of parenchymal bridge between contiguous lobes predispose to lobar torsion. Another predisposing factor that promotes lobar motility is atelectasis, and several lobar torsion cases have been reported in the setting of large pleural effusion, pneumothorax, or mass effect from neoplasm (45,46).

Clinical Presentation

Pulmonary torsion typically presents with an abrupt clinical changes in post surgical setting, with acute onset of respiratory distress, acidosis, tachycardia, loss of breath sounds over the affected lung field, loss of air leak, shock, or sepsis. Radiographic signs of torsion include: (a) lobe opacification, (b) change in location of an opacified lobe, (c) hilar displacement, (d) abnormal position of the pulmonary vasculature, (e) lobar air trapping, and (f) bronchial cutoff or distortion (45). A CT scan is the best imaging modality to visualize lobar torsion, but acquisition depends on the patient's hemodynamic stability. Bronchoscopy is diagnostic with the appearance of a distorted or compressed airway with a "fish mouth" appearance.

Treatment and Prevention

Prevention of lobar torsion starts with a careful evaluation of the anatomic lung position prior to chest closure. Staples or sutures are used to fixate a mobile lobe to a nearby lobe (47). If the diagnosis is made postoperatively, immediate re-exploration to restore the blood supply is paramount. Re-exploration should be within 48 hours of the initial surgery to avoid irreversible infarction (48). If viable at re-exploration, the torsed lobe should be fixed in place to prevent recurrent torsion. If frankly gangrenous, or if viability is in doubt, resection is indicated. Broad-spectrum antibiotics should be initiated upon diagnosis.

Bronchial dehiscence/Bronchopleural fistula

Etiology and Risk Factors

Bronchial stump dehiscence is a breakdown of bronchial closure after lung resection that leads to a communication between the bronchus and pleural space, a bronchopleural fistula (BPF). It is a highly morbid event, with incidence estimated at 0.5% to 10% after pulmonary resection and mortality ranging from 25% to 71% (48). Bronchial stump dehiscences are divided into early and late, each with a unique set of risk factors. In general, early dehiscence is secondary to poor surgical techniques. Late dehiscence is usually related to ischemia and patient comorbidities (49). Patient characteristics that predispose to dehiscence include COPD, low FEV_1, malnutrition, diabetes, steroid use, and neoadjuvant therapy. Surgical factors that are associated with increased risk for bronchial dehiscence include right pneumonectomy, residual neoplasm at the bronchial margin, extensive lymph node dissection, blood supplies interruption, stapled versus hand sewn closure, long stump, or tension of the closure (48,50,51). The risk for developing BPF following right pneumonectomy is 13.2%, versus 5% following left pneumonectomy (52). This discrepancy is a due to intrinsic differences in the blood supply and soft tissue coverage. The right main stem bronchus is typically supplied by a single bronchial artery, while the left is supplied by two. The left main stem bronchus is embedded in the richly vascularized mediastinal tissue under the aortic arch, while the right is freely exposed in the pleural space. Positive pressure ventilation in the post operative period subjects the bronchial stump to barotraumas and increases risk of stump dehiscence.

Clinical Presentation

Early bronchial stump dehiscence occurs within the first few days to weeks following resection. Patients present with a large or prolonged air leak or progressive subcutaneous emphysema. Later in the postoperative course, patients may cough copious amount of clear or purulent secretion secondary to drainage of pleural fluid through the stump opening. Hemoptysis may herald an early bronchovascular fistula, where the bronchial stump suture line has eroded into a nearby vascular structure. In late cases of BPF, patients can be minimally symptomatic, but may present with fever, chills, and chronic cough productive of frothy and mucopurulent secretions secondary to pleural space infection. The patients may also develop a preference for sleeping with the surgical side down to prevent leakage of pleural effusion through the stump. Chest radiograph usually demonstrate a fall in the fluid level or development of a new air/fluid level in the ipsilateral pleural space (Fig. 25.1). Bronchoscopy is diagnostic.

Treatment and Prevention

Initial treatment for early BPF is positioning the patient in the reverse Trendelenburg with the surgical side down to minimize drainage and contamination of the contralateral lung. A chest tube should be placed expeditiously to evacuate infected fluid and broad-spectrum antibiotics instituted. Early bronchial stump dehiscence needs to be treated surgically. The thoracic cavity should be explored the pleural space debrided, and the bronchial stump inspected. The stump length should be assessed, and stump resected back if too long. Necrotic of devitalized tissue should be debrided. Stump closure is achieved with interrupted sutures and reinforced with a vascularized pedicle flap of parietal pleural, pericardial fat, serratus anterior, intercostal muscle, or omentum. Small BPF (<5 mm) may be amenable to endoscopic closure with fibrin or acrylic glues with varying degrees of success. Sclerosis of stump dehiscence with ND:YAG laser or submucosal injections has also been reported (53–55).

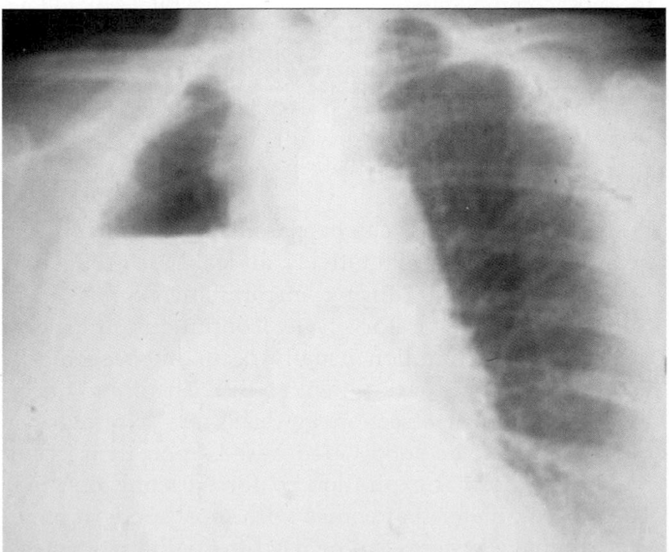

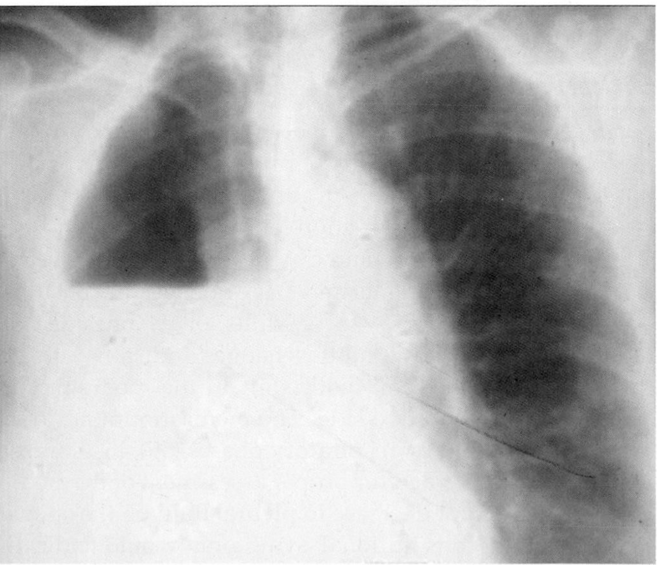

FIGURE 25.1. Chest radiographs from patient who developed a bronchopleural fistula (BPF) two weeks after right pneumonectomy. Radiograph on left is prior to discharge from hospital. The radiograph on right is 10 days later when patient presented with fever, elevated white blood cell count and coughing up copious watery secretions, note the decrease in air fluid level consistent with bronchial dehiscence.

Prevention of BPF starts with mitigating reversible risk factors and optimizing of medical and nutritional status preoperatively. In cases where the patient is immunocompromised, diabetic, on steroids, or has a history of neoadjuvant therapy, additional operative modifications with pedicle flaps to buttress the stump should be considered. Stump ischemia is prevented by avoiding overzealous dissection. The length of the stump should be optimally created so as to avoid stagnation of secretion, and undue tension at the suture line should be avoided. Postoperative positive pressure ventilation should be avoided whenever possible.

Postresection empyema

Etiology and Risk Factors

By definition, postresection empyema is infection of the pleural space after lung resection. Postresection empyema occurs far more commonly after pneumonectomy than after lobectomy or lesser resections. Eighty percent of postpneumonectomy empyema is associated with BPF (50,56,57). The mortality associated with postpneumonectomy empyema is 30% to 40%, but decreases to 5% without BPF (57). A retrospective study from the Mayo Clinic of 713 pneumonectomy patients identified factors associated with increased risk for empyema included: benign indication for surgery, right pneumonectomy, bronchial stump reinforcement, timing of chest tube removal, low FEV_1, low DLCO, low preoperative hemoglobin, and intraoperative and total amount of blood transfusion. The risk of developing empyema is higher following right pneumonectomy than left because of higher risk BPF (56). Early empyema without dehiscence is thought to be caused by a direct contamination of the pleural space during surgery. Late empyema develops as a result of hematogenous dissemination from sources such as dental caries, pneumonia, or appendicitis.

Clinical Presentation

Postresection empyema can occur at any time in the postoperative period. Early empyema is usually diagnosed within 3 months of surgery and represents 60% of cases (58). Late postresection empyema is diagnosed after 3 months of surgery, and can present as late as 40 years after the resection. Patients may have nonspecific constitutional symptoms such as fever, chills, or dyspnea. Chest radiograph may show subtle changes indicative of an early evolving empyema with shift in the mediastinum away from the operative side. The mediastinum position can also be affected by respiratory phases (59); inspiratory films are recommended for proper assessment of the mediastinum. An abrupt decrease in pleural fluid on the operative side with constitutional symptoms would indicate empyema with BPF as outlined above. Patients can present with purulent drainage from the thoracotomy incision via pleurocutaneous fistula, an entity known as empyema necessitatis.

Bronchoscopy should be done to evaluate the bronchial stump and to collect any fluid for bacterial cultures. Thoracentesis is an important step and best done under ultrasound guidance because of the unpredictably of the position of shifted intrathoracic organs after pneumonectomy (58). Broad-spectrum antibiotics should be initiated immediately. The most common causative organisms are *Staphylococcus aureus, Pseudomonas aeruginosa,* or multiple organisms (58,60,61).

Treatment and Prevention

A chest tube without suction should be placed in the infected cavity. Surgical management involves re-exploration of infected space, drainage, washout, debridement, and examination of the bronchial stump. Once a fistula has been ruled out, multiple options are available to clean pleural space, including open packing via Elloesser flap or pleural window, multiple surgical debridements, or placement of antibiotic irrigation system. Once the infection is controlled, and the pleural space is cleaned, it can be reclosed over antibiotic irrigation. There is a paucity of literature on postresection empyema prophylaxis. Two studies looked at intrapleural antibiotic irrigation and reported a reduction in the incidence of empyemas (62,63).

Persistent air leak

Etiology and Risk Factors

Air leak is a condition where air enters into the pleural space through an abnormal communication from the airway or pulmonary parenchyma. Air leaks represent one of the most common complications after pulmonary resection. Most air leaks heal spontaneously, but if a leak lasts for more than 7 days, it is considered persistent. The incidence of persistent air leak ranges between 3% and 25% (2,64–66) and represents the most common reason for prolonged hospital stay following lung resection (66). Risk factors for persistent air leaks include steroid use, malnutrition, diabetes, COPD, low FEV_1, male gender, concomitant pneumothorax, pleural adhesions, upper lobectomy, and bilobectomy (66–68).

Clinical Presentation

Postresection air leaks can be classified qualitatively and quantitatively (68). Qualitatively, air leaks are grouped by whether they occur during inspiration, expiration, or throughout the respiratory cycle. Continuous air leaks or those during inspiration usually occur in mechanically ventilated patients or those with a BPF. The grand majority (98%) of post resection air leaks are expiratory in nature, but can be subdivided based upon their occurrence with normal expiration or forced expiration (68). The air leak meter that comes with most modern pleurevac drainage systems can be used to qualitatively measure the leak. The meters typically contain five to seven chambers, with the first chamber denoting the smallest leak (68). Serial evaluation of air leak severity is important to monitor for improvement trend. As the lung heals, the air leak classification will go from expiratory to occurring with forced expiration only. Cerfolio has demonstrated that patients with large expiratory leaks (extending into the last chambers of the leak monitor) in the immediate postoperative period are at increased risk for persistent air leaks, and may be best managed with early Heimlich valve placement (69).

Treatment and Prevention

The treatment for air leaks is expectant, since almost all eventually heal. Two independent, randomized, prospective studies for air leaks in patients undergoing elective pulmonary resection have reported that early placement of chest tube to water seal leads to shorter duration of leak and decreases the time that the chest tubes remain in place (70,71). The timing of water seal was different in these two studies. In one study, tubes were placed to water seal on postoperative day 2 and in the other, immediately after surgery. A negative pressure intrathoracic environment induced by suction stents opens areas of visceral pleural disruption that impedes healing, and most likely explains the superiority of water seal over suction. A chest x-ray should be obtained within 24 hours of placing a patient with an air leak to water seal to ensure that there is no new or enlarging pneumothorax.

In a patient with a persistent air leak, transition to outpatient chest tube management should be made while the patient is still hospitalized. A 24-hour observation is usually done with the patient's chest tube connected to a Heimlich valve. If the chest x-ray demonstrates no new changes after 24 hours, then the patient can be safely discharged with the Heimlich valve and followed every one to two weeks in the clinic for chest tube removal (69).

Several intraoperative measures have been developed to minimize air leaks. A recent meta-analysis of 16 clinical trials comparing standard closure with or without sealant revealed that surgical sealants reduced postoperative air leaks and time to chest drain removal, but did not reduce the length of postoperative stay (72). Another approach is creation of pleural tent, which involves mobilizing the apical parietal pleura and draping it on to the remaining lung, facilitating pleura-pleura apposition. This is performed after upper lobectomy, and efficacy was reported in a prospectively randomized trial of 200 patients who had undergone elective upper lobectomy (73).

Chylothorax

Etiology and Risk Factors

Chylothorax is the presence of lymphatic fluid in the pleural space and is usually a result of a leak from the thoracic duct or one of its tributaries. Operative injuries are by far the most common cause of chylothorax. The anatomy of the thoracic duct is quite variable with the propensity for multiple mediastinal trunks and crossing levels. In approximately half of the population, it arises from the cisterna chyli and enters the chest through the aortic hiatus. It then ascends along the anterior vertebral column between the azygos vein and the aorta, posterior to the esophagus. It crosses the mediastinum at the level of the carina and travels along the left side of the esophagus until it exits the mediastinum and joins the junction of the left internal jugular and subclavian veins in the neck. The thoracic duct is relatively well protected within the posterior mediastinum but is at risk of injury during complicate cardiac, aortic, esophageal, pulmonary, left cervical, and diaphragmatic operations. During routine resections for NSCLC, the duct is most susceptible to injury during mediastinal lymph node dissection in the subcarinal and subaortic locations (74). The incidence of chylothorax complicating pulmonary resection is less than 1% in most series (75,76), including the recent ACOSOG series (2). Chylothoraces occur at a slightly higher rate following right-sided procedures (75). The thoracic duct is the main conduit for transport of chyle from the intestine and lymphatics from the lower extremities. Large thoracic duct leaks can result in fat depletion, dehydration, hypoproteinemia, loss of fat-soluble vitamins, and immunologic compromise. Chyle is bacteriostatic with an alkaline pH and is an irritant within the pleural space when it leaks.

Clinical Presentation

There are typically 2 to 10 days between the duct injury and the development of a chylothorax. Chylothorax should be suspected when there is rapid or excessive filling of the pleural space following a pneumonectomy or excessive chest tube drainage following lobectomy. Chest tube output >400 mL/day, and especially >700 mL/day, is suggestive of a chyle leak. Chyle is typically milky and nonclotting, but may be clear in the fasting state. Triglyceride concentrations greater than 110 mg/dL, the presence of chylomicrons, or a lymphocyte level in the pleural fluid that is greater than that in the plasma are diagnostic of chylothorax.

Lymphangiography can identify the site and size of the leak in 80% of cases (76,77). It can also differentiate between tributary injury and complete duct transection. Unfortunately, the procedure is technically challenging in centers that do not perform it regularly and uncomfortable for the patient. CT scans are in general not helpful in diagnosis or work up of thoracic duct injuries.

Treatment and Prevention

Initial treatment of a chylothorax is ensuring drainage of the chyle with a chest tube, because chyle is irritating and lung re-expansion can help to seal the leak. Patients should be made NPO (nothing by mouth) and parenteral nutrition started to decrease the chyle flow. Cessation of oral intake inhibits the absorption of fats and markedly diminishes stimulation of secretion into the gastrointestinal tract, decreasing the volume flow through the thoracic duct and reducing fluid, fat, and protein loss from the leak, while increasing the opportunity for the duct to heal. Approximately 50% of injuries will resolve with these conservative measures (76,78). Somatostatin and its analogue octreotide can be used with conservative measures to simultaneously decrease the volume of chyle demonstrated utility in animal studies. There is no standard recommendation for how long to wait for leak closure. Most agree that the maximum observation time is two weeks and earlier intervention for cases where drainage remains >500 mL/day, or in patients with severe nutritional deficits or evidence of clinical deterioration is needed (76,78–80).

Failure of conservative therapy warrants surgical intervention. The primary goal of surgery is to stop the leak. This can be accomplished by identification and direct ligation of the leak or mass by ligation of the duct as it enters the chest at the aortic hiatus. Leak identification is facilitated by preoperative lymphangiography or the administration of enteral fat in the form of cream of olive oil 2 or 3 hours prior to surgery. Tissues around the leak are usually inflamed and require pledgetted sutures for secure closure. Mass ligation involves surrounding and tying all of the tissue between the aorta, esophagus, and azygos vein immediately above the diaphragm typically through the right chest. In cases of right-sided leaks, the approach is straightforward. In left-sided chyle leaks, some controversy exists as to which of the two approaches is more effective and from which side to proceed. Pleurodesis is advocated as complimentary to either procedure. VATS has become an attractive approach for treatment because it provides excellent visualization of mediastinum.

Pleural shunts and percutaneous thoracic duct embolization are alternatives to surgery. Embolization procedures are increasing in use at selective centers with lymphangiography expertise, and are especially useful in cases of multiple bilateral ducts which may escape mass ligation (77).

Nerve injuries

Etiology and Risk Factors

The incidence for nerve injury during thoracic surgery is 1% (81). The risk for injury is influenced by the patient's anatomy, type of procedure, extent of resection, and surgeon's experience. Nerves at risk of injury during pulmonary resection include recurrent laryngeal, phrenic, vagus, and intercostal. The recurrent laryngeal and vagus nerves are at greatest risk during mediastinal surgery, including cervical mediastinoscopy, thymectomy, esophagectomy, thyroid surgery, and tracheostomy. Phrenic nerves are at greatest risk for injury during thymectomy, mediastinal lymph node dissection for NSCLC, pericardiotomy, or intrapericardial pneumonectomy. Intercostal nerves can be injured with an access incision through the chest wall.

Post-thoracotomy pain syndrome is a well recognized complication of thoracotomy with an incidence between 5% and 40% in VATS patients and 9% and 80% in thoracotomy patients (82–87). It is defined as persistent pain along a thoracotomy incision for at least 2 months after the surgery. Intercostal nerve dysfunction and entrapment are thought to be central in the development of this complication (84). Primary hyperalgesia from exaggerated response of local nociceptors to inflammatory mediators, which results in pain hypersensitization, is another explanation for this syndrome (85).

Clinical Presentation

Presentation for nerve injuries depends on the nerve that was injured. Recurrent laryngeal nerve injury leads to ipsilateral vocal cord paralysis, with a brassy or hoarse voice and an increased risk for aspiration. Phrenic nerve injuries result in unilateral diaphragmatic paralysis. Chest x-ray may show elevation of diaphragm, and fluoroscopy can be used to demonstrate paradoxical movement of diaphragm during inspiration. Phrenic nerve conduction studies are available in a few specialized centers. Post-thoracotomy pain syndrome is usually diagnosed at follow up visits with unresolved pain and neuralgia in the distribution of the nerve, usually anterior and inferior to the thoracotomy.

Treatment and Prevention

Treatment of recurrent laryngeal nerve injuries often requires vocal cord medialization to strengthen cough, improve voice quality and decrease the risk for aspiration. Otolaryngologists frequently wait 6 to 12 weeks to differentiate reversible from nonreversible injuries. Treatment for symptomatic phrenic nerve injuries includes diaphragm plication to help decrease the attenuation of the muscle and reduce atelectasis of the adjacent lung. Phrenic nerve pacing typically requires an intact lower motor neuron, and is not applicable to post-thoracotomy injuries. Currently there is no effect treatment to reverse the syndrome, and gabapentin appears to provide the most significant symptomatic relief.

Postpneumonectomy syndrome

Etiology and Risk Factors

Postpneumonectomy syndrome is a rare syndrome defined by a shift of the mediastinal structures into the ipsilateral surgical side secondary to hyperinflation of the residual lung, resulting in rotation and progressive airway obstruction. An understanding of the anatomic changes that occur after pneumonectomy is helpful in understanding this syndrome. The postpneumonectomy space undergoes significant remodeling. It fills with sterile fluid over the first several weeks. The contralateral lung then slowly becomes hyperinflated, and shifts toward the pneumonectomy side. The accumulated fluid in the pneumonectomy is slowly reabsorbed while scar tissue grows to fill the space. After right pneumonectomy, the mediastinum shifts to the right. The heart and great vessels rotate counterclockwise and can result in compression of the left main stem between left pulmonary artery and vertebral column or descending aorta. After left pneumonectomy, the mediastinum shifts to the left, and the heart and great vessels rotate clockwise with the potential to compress the airway between the right pulmonary artery and vertebral column or aorta. The two largest reported cases series are both from Massachusetts General Hospital with a combined number of 29 patients (88,89). In their experience, postpneumonectomy syndrome is more common after right pneumonectomy, occurring in 68% of patients reported. The median time between pneumonectomy and presentation was 7.5 years. Postpneumonectomy syndrome is more likely to develop in infants and young children because of their anatomic plasticity and increased lung compliance.

Clinical Presentation

Patients are typically young and had undergone pneumonectomy in their childhood. Progressive debilitating dyspnea is the hallmark of the syndrome. Dysphagia from displacement of esophagus has also been reported. Patients may also present with positional dyspnea from positional compression of the pulmonary veins (90). The workup includes a pulmonary function test and chest imaging. A CT scan provides the best information on the degree of mediastinal shift and the anatomical details. Other causes of dyspnea should be ruled out, including pulmonary hypertension, congestive heart failure, declining pulmonary reserve, PE, or recurrent cancer.

Treatment and Prevention

No preventive measures are available, but several methods have been devised to surgically correct postpneumonectomy syndrome. The simplest approach is placement of bronchial stents. This typically reserved for older and more debilitated patients because of the risk of stent migration and erosion in younger patients. The more invasive approach involves re-exploration of the pneumonectomy site, lysis of adhesions, and placement of saline prosthesis to anatomically correct the mediastinal shift. This results in an improvement in symptoms in a significant number of patients (88). Successful VATS approaches for the treatment have also been reported (91,92).

Cardiac herniation

Etiology and Risk Factors

Cardiac herniation occurs when the heart migrates through a defect in the pericardium, rotating along its axis and leading to volvulus. It is a rare complication associated with a 40% to 60% mortality rate in recognized cases and 100% in undiagnosed cases (93,94). Herniation of the heart occurs when the pericardium has been opened, as with partial pericardectomy, intrapericardial pneumonectomy, or intrapericardial ligation of pulmonary vessels.

Clinical Presentation

The onset is usually within hours of surgery accompanying alterations in intrathoracic pressure. It can be triggered by applying suction on the chest tube, coughing, or body positional change (21,94). Patients develop hemodynamic instability with elevated central venous pressure suggestive of cardiogenic shock. A high index of suspicion and prompt diagnosis is crucial. Radiographic findings are characteristic and easily recognized. With right cardiac herniation, the heart is displaced to the midline, a globular right cardiac border visible in the right hemithorax (snow cone sign), and if a central line is present, a rotational kink at the level of the right brachiocephalic venous junction. With left cardiac herniation, the entire heart is in the left chest with a cleft between the great vessels and the herniated chambers (93).

Treatment and Prevention

Treatment of symptomatic cardiac herniation requires immediate reoperation to reposition the heart. Prevention of this dreadful complication involves repairing the pericardial defects at the time of resection. All large right-sided pericardial defects must be repaired because of the high risk for developing herniation. The defect may be closed primarily or with a patch of parietal pleural and prosthetic materials (21). Large left-sided defects typically do not require routine closure.

Lung herniation

Etiology and Risk Factors

There is a paucity of literature on lung herniation following thoracotomy (95). Iatrogenic lung hernias, especially intercostals lung hernias, are more frequently reported as a complication of minithoracotomies or VATS. This is probably a result of less meticulous closure of small incisions and the typical lack of closure of intercostal defects during VATS (96,97). Other risk factors associated with lung herniation include steroid use, diabetes, obesity, increased intrathoracic pressure, and lung volume from positive pressure ventilation or emphysema, rib resection, or repeat thoracotomy/thoracostomy (98,99). However, patients who have had large chest wall resections without reconstruction or have gaps in the interspace between paracostal sutures from thoracotomy do not routinely develop hernia (100).

Clinical Presentation

Symptoms related to lung herniation are vague. Patients present with intermittent bulging in the chest wall that may or may not be tender. Careful palpation of the incision site with patient coughing elicits a soft, elastic bulge. Lung herniation can be diagnosed definitively with chest CT.

Treatment and Prevention

Prevention starts with meticulous wound closure, especially at the pericostal level. Medical and nutritional optimizations are important to promote wound healing. Lung hernias, like other hernias, are at risk for incarceration or strangulation, and should be repaired if these signs are present. Numerous repair methods have been reported, including reapproximation of defect with pericostal heavy nylon sutures or wires, coverage with prosthetic material, or coverage with muscle flaps or omentum. VATS techniques have been successfully used to repair lung herniation (96,97,101).

COMPLICATIONS RELATED TO CHEST WALL RESECTION

Malignancy, infection, radiation injury, or any combinations of the three are the most common indication for chest wall resection. Resections for malignancy are performed for primary chest wall malignancies, metastatic spread from distant sites, or for direct extension from NSCLC or breast cancer. The tenets of chest wall resection and reconstruction are (a) removal of all malignant or devitalized tissue, (b) restoration of rigidity to large chest wall defects to prevent flail chest, and (c) healthy soft tissue coverage to seal the pleural space, protect underling organs, and prevent infection. Appropriate planning is required prior to the start of surgery, to ensure that adequate margins are obtained, while necessary muscles and soft tissues needed for reconstruction are preserved.

Flail chest and respiratory complications

Etiology and Risk Factors

Chest wall defects greater than 4 cm or from resection of three or more contiguous ribs have the potential to result in a flail chest with paradoxical movement of the chest wall during respiration, leading to respiratory compromise. Multivariate analysis of complications after chest wall resection identified defect size as the most significant predictor of complication (102). Respiratory complication is the most common complication with an estimated incidence of 11% to 20% (103–105). Respiratory failure is the most common cause of postoperative mortality (102,103).

Clinical Presentation

Patients typically present with respiratory failure in immediate postoperative setting secondary to flail chest. Mechanical ventilation may be required for respiratory insufficiency.

Treatment and Prevention

Intraoperative restoration of chest wall rigidity with prosthetic materials such as, polytetrafluoroethylene (PTFE) patch, methyl methacrylate sandwich, or autologous tissue such as fascia lata reduces this complication. The choice of prosthetic material for chest wall reconstruction mostly depends on surgeon preference.

Wound complications: seroma and wound infection

Etiology and Risk Factors

Wound complications are the second most common postoperative complications associated with chest wall resection, occurring in 7% to 18% of cases (103–105). Fortunately, seroma is more common than wound infection.

Clinical Presentation

A painless soft tissue induration with no erythema is usually a seroma. Aspiration of the induration returns serous fluid. A wound infection may also present with induration, but appear erythematous, is tender to the touch, and has purulent drainage from the surgical site and constitutional symptoms.

Treatment and Prevention

The management of seroma is conservative since the risk of infection is low. Seromas typically respond to repeated drainage. In contrast, wound infection is a dreaded complication in the setting of chest wall resection because the potential to spread to intrathoracic space. Early management involves antibiotics therapy and removal of infected prosthesis. Infection frequently results in significant induration and fibrosis of underling tissue and therefore removal of prosthetics does not typically result in flail chest. Musculocutaneous or omentum flap with skin graft can be used for reconstruction when infection is controlled. Prosthetic materials should not be used in an infectious setting.

Vacuum-assisted closure (VAC) technology has proven to be a very effective tool in the management of complex chest wall wounds. Subatmospheric pressure dressings are now commercially available as the VAC device (KCI, San Antonio, TX) (106). Vacuum-assisted closure devices accelerate wound healing by maintaining an optimal environment with subatmospheric pressure at approximately 125 mm Hg with an alternating cycle of 5 minutes of suction followed by 2 minutes off suction. Subatmospheric pressure also alters the cytoskeleton of the cells in the wound bed, and triggers a cascade of intracellular signals that increase cell division and subsequent formation of granulation tissue (107). These effects make the VAC device an extremely versatile tool in the wound healing armamentarium.

Scapula entrapment

Etiology and Risk Factors

Posterior defects on the superior aspect of the chest wall usually do not need closure because of coverage by scapula. However, if the defect extends past the fourth rib the scapula tips can get trapped in the defect during movement.

Clinical Presentation

Patient presents with pain and inability to move their ipsilateral upper extremity or with painful catching with movement.

Treatment and Prevention

Intraoperative reconstruction of large posterior chest wall defects and those that extend beyond the fourth rib should avoid this complication. Re-exploration through the initial thoracotomy and patch reconstruction is warranted when this presents postoperatively, but scarring can make it far more challenging than initial reconstruction.

CONCLUSION

Lung cancer is the leading cause of cancer-related death in the United States. Lung resection with and without chest wall resection presents surgical and postoperative challenges due to the frail nature of the NSCLC population. Rigorous preoperative assessment, meticulous attention to operative technique, and vigilance in postoperative care will continue to advance the practice, decrease complications, and improve outcomes for this common malignancy.

REFERENCES

1. Jemal A, Siegel R, Ward E, et al. Cancer statistics, 2009. *CA Cancer J Clin* 2009;59(4):225–249.
2. Allen MS, Darling GE, Pechet TT, et al. Morbidity and mortality of major pulmonary resections in patients with early-stage lung cancer: initial results of the randomized, prospective ACOSOG Z0030 trial. *Ann Thorac Surg* 2006;81(3):1013–1019; discussion 1019–1020.
3. Strand TE, Rostad H, Damhuis RA, et al. Risk factors for 30-day mortality after resection of lung cancer and prediction of their magnitude. *Thorax* 2007;62(11):991–997.
4. Licker MJ, Widikker I, Robert J, et al. Operative mortality and respiratory complications after lung resection for cancer: impact of chronic obstructive pulmonary disease and time trends. *Ann Thorac Surg* 2006;81(5):1830–1837.
5. Dominguez-Ventura A, Allen MS, Cassivi SD, et al. Lung cancer in octogenarians: factors affecting morbidity and mortality after pulmonary resection. *Ann Thorac Surg* 2006;82(4):1175–1179.
6. Litle VR, Swanson SJ. Postoperative bleeding: coagulopathy, bleeding, hemothorax. *Thorac Surg Clin* 2006;16(3):203–207, v.
7. Harpole DH Jr, DeCamp MM Jr, Daley J, et al. Prognostic models of thirty-day mortality and morbidity after major pulmonary resection. *J Thorac Cardiovasc Surg* 1999;117(5):969–979.
8. Doddoli C, Thomas P, Thirion X, et al. Postoperative complications in relation with induction therapy for lung cancer. *Eur J Cardiothorac Surg* 2001;20(2):385–390.
9. Sakuragi T, Sakao Y, Furukawa K, et al. Successful management of acute pulmonary embolism after surgery for lung cancer. *Eur J Cardiothorac Surg* 2003;24(4):580–587.
10. Patel A, Anraku M, Darling GE, et al. Venous thromboembolism in patients receiving multimodality therapy for thoracic malignancies. *J Thorac Cardiovasc Surg* 2009;138(4):843–848.
11. Ziomek S, Read RC, Tobler HG, et al. Thromboembolism in patients undergoing thoracotomy. *Ann Thorac Surg* 1993;56(2):223–226; discussion 227.
12. Amar D. Prevention and management of perioperative arrhythmias in the thoracic surgical population. *Anesthesiol Clin* 2008;26(2):325–335, vii.
13. De Decker K, Jorens PG, Van Schil P. Cardiac complications after noncardiac thoracic surgery: an evidence-based current review. *Ann Thorac Surg* 2003;75(4):1340–1348.
14. Park BJ, Zhang H, Rusch VW, et al. Video-assisted thoracic surgery does not reduce the incidence of postoperative atrial fibrillation after pulmonary lobectomy. *J Thorac Cardiovasc Surg* 2007;133(3): 775–779.
15. Creswell LL, Schuessler RB, Rosenbloom M, et al. Hazards of postoperative atrial arrhythmias. *Ann Thorac Surg* 1993;56(3):539–549.
16. Amar D, Goenka A, Zhang H, et al. Leukocytosis and increased risk of atrial fibrillation after general thoracic surgery. *Ann Thorac Surg* 2006;82(3):1057–1061.
17. McKeown PP, Gutterman D. Executive summary: American College of Chest Physicians guidelines for the prevention and management of postoperative atrial fibrillation after cardiac surgery. *Chest* 2005;128(2, Suppl):1S–5S.
18. Lee JK, Klein GJ, Krahn AD, et al. Rate-control versus conversion strategy in postoperative atrial fibrillation: a prospective, randomized pilot study. *Am Heart J* 2000;140(6):871–877.
19. Van Mieghem W, Coolen L, Malysse I, et al. Amiodarone and the development of ARDS after lung surgery. *Chest* 1994;105(6):1642–1645.
20. von Knorring J, Lepantalo M, Lindgren L, et al. Cardiac arrhythmias and myocardial ischemia after thoracotomy for lung cancer. *Ann Thorac Surg* 1992;53(4):642–647.
21. Karamichalis JM, Putnam JB Jr, Lambright ES. Cardiovascular complications after lung surgery. *Thorac Surg Clin* 2006;16(3):253–260.
22. Herrington CS, Shumway SJ. Myocardial ischemia and infarction postthoracotomy. *Chest Surg Clin N Am* 1998;8(3):495–502, vii.
23. Fleisher LA, Beckman JA, Brown KA, et al. 2009 ACCF/AHA Focused Update On Perioperative Beta Blockade incorporated into the ACC/AHA 2007 Guidelines on Perioperative Cardiovascular Evaluation and Care for Noncardiac Surgery: a report of the American College of Cardiology Foundation/American Heart Association Task Force on Practice Guidelines. *Circulation* 2009;120(21):e169–e276.
24. Fleisher LA, Bass EB, McKeown P. Methodological approach: American College of Chest Physicians Guidelines for the Prevention and Management of postoperative atrial fibrillation after Cardiac Surgery. *Chest* 2005;128(2, Suppl):17S–23S.
25. Amar D, Munoz D, Shi W, et al. A clinical prediction rule for pulmonary complications after thoracic surgery for primary lung cancer. *Anesth Analg* 2010;110(5):1343–1348.
26. Brunelli A, Refai M, Salati M, et al. Predicted versus observed FEV1 and DLCO after major lung resection: a prospective evaluation at different postoperative periods. *Ann Thorac Surg* 2007;83(3):1134–1139.
27. Brunelli A, Ferguson MK, Rocco G, et al. A scoring system predicting the risk for intensive care unit admission for complications after major lung resection: a multicenter analysis. *Ann Thorac Surg* 2008;86(1):213–218.
28. Ferguson MK, Durkin AE. A comparison of three scoring systems for predicting complications after major lung resection. *Eur J Cardiothorac Surg* 2003;23(1):35–42.
29. Ferguson MK, Gaissert HA, Grab JD, et al. Pulmonary complications after lung resection in the absence of chronic obstructive pulmonary disease: the predictive role of diffusing capacity [published online ahead of print September 26, 2009]. *J Thorac Cardiovasc Surg* 2009;138(6):1297–1302. DOI: 10.1016/j.jtcvs.2009.05.045.
30. Brunelli A, Belardinelli R, Refai M, et al. Peak oxygen consumption during cardiopulmonary exercise test improves risk stratification in candidates to major lung resection [published online ahead of print November 24, 2008]. *Chest* 2009;135(5):1260–1267. DOI: 10.1378/chest.08-2059.
31. Bonde P, McManus K, McAnespie M, et al. Lung surgery: identifying the subgroup at risk for sputum retention. *Eur J Cardiothorac Surg* 2002;22(1):18–22.
32. Vaporciyan AA, Merriman KW, Ece F, et al. Incidence of major pulmonary morbidity after pneumonectomy: association with timing of smoking cessation. *Ann Thorac Surg* 2002;73(2):420–425; discussion 425–426.
33. Schussler O, Alifano M, Dermine H, et al. Postoperative pneumonia after major lung resection. *Am J Respir Crit Care Med* 2006;173(10): 1161–1169.
34. Duque JL, Ramos G, Castrodeza J, et al. Early complications in surgical treatment of lung cancer: a prospective, multicenter study. Grupo Cooperativo de Carcinoma Broncogenico de la Sociedad Espanola de Neumologia y Cirugia Toracica. *Ann Thorac Surg* 1997;63(4):944–950.
35. Radu DM, Jaureguy F, Seguin A, et al. Postoperative pneumonia after major pulmonary resections: an unsolved problem in thoracic surgery. *Ann Thorac Surg* 2007;84(5):1669–1673.
36. Dulu A, Pastores SM, Park B, et al. Prevalence and mortality of acute lung injury and ARDS after lung resection. *Chest* 2006;130(1):73–78.
37. Alam N, Park BJ, Wilton A, et al. Incidence and risk factors for lung injury after lung cancer resection. *Ann Thorac Surg* 2007;84(4): 1085–1091; discussion 1091.
38. Ruffini E, Parola A, Papalia E, et al. Frequency and mortality of acute lung injury and acute respiratory distress syndrome after pulmonary resection for bronchogenic carcinoma. *Eur J Cardiothorac Surg* 2001;20(1): 30–36, discussion 36–37.
39. Roberts JR. Postoperative respiratory failure. *Thorac Surg Clin* 2006;16(3):235–241, vi.
40. Kutlu CA, Williams EA, Evans TW, et al. Acute lung injury and acute respiratory distress syndrome after pulmonary resection. *Ann Thorac Surg* 2000;69(2):376–380.
41. Licker M, de Perrot M, Hohn L, et al. Perioperative mortality and major cardio-pulmonary complications after lung surgery for non-small cell carcinoma. *Eur J Cardiothorac Surg* 1999;15(3):314–319.
42. Parquin F, Marchal M, Mehiri S, et al. Post-pneumonectomy pulmonary edema: analysis and risk factors. *Eur J Cardiothorac Surg* 1996;10(11):929–932; discussion 933.
43. Steinberg KP, Hudson LD, Goodman RB, et al. Efficacy and safety of corticosteroids for persistent acute respiratory distress syndrome. *N Engl J Med* 2006;354(16):1671–1684.

44. Mathisen DJ, Kuo EY, Hahn C, et al. Inhaled nitric oxide for adult respiratory distress syndrome after pulmonary resection. *Ann Thorac Surg* 1998;66(6):1894–1902.
45. Felson B. Lung torsion: radiographic findings in nine cases. *Radiology* 1987;162(3):631–638.
46. Ohde Y, Nakagawa K, Okumura T, et al. Spontaneous pulmonary torsion secondary to pseudo-Meigs' syndrome. *Interact Cardiovasc Thorac Surg* 2005;4(1):59–60.
47. Higashiyama M, Takami K, Higaki N, et al. Pulmonary middle lobe fixation using TachoComb in patients undergoing right upper lobectomy with complete oblique fissure. *Interact Cardiovasc Thorac Surg* 2004;3(1):107–109.
48. Farkas EA, Detterbeck FC. Airway complications after pulmonary resection. *Thorac Surg Clin* 2006;16(3):243–251.
49. Jichen QV, Chen G, Jiang G, et al. Risk factor comparison and clinical analysis of early and late bronchopleural fistula after non-small cell lung cancer surgery. *Ann Thorac Surg* 2009;88(5):1589–1593.
50. Abbas Ael S, Deschamps C. Postpneumonectomy empyema. *Curr Opin Pulm Med* 2002;8(4):327–333.
51. Liberman M, Cassivi SD. Bronchial stump dehiscence: update on prevention and management. *Semin Thorac Cardiovasc Surg* 2007;19(4): 366–373.
52. Darling GE, Abdurahman A, Yi QL, et al. Risk of a right pneumonectomy: role of bronchopleural fistula. *Ann Thorac Surg* 2005;79(2): 433–437.
53. Kanno R, Suzuki H, Fujiu K, et al. Endoscopic closure of bronchopleural fistula after pneumonectomy by submucosal injection of polidocanol. *Jpn J Thorac Cardiovasc Surg* 2002;50(1):30–33.
54. Kiriyama M, Fujii Y, Yamakawa Y, et al. Endobronchial neodymium: yttrium-aluminum garnet laser for noninvasive closure of small proximal bronchopleural fistula after lung resection. *Ann Thorac Surg* 2002;73(3):945–948; discussion 948–949.
55. Wang KP, Schaeffer L, Heitmiller R, et al. Nd:YAG laser closure of a bronchopleural fistula. *Monaldi Arch Chest Dis* 1993;48(4): 301–303.
56. Deschamps C, Bernard A, Nichols FC III, et al. Empyema and bronchopleural fistula after pneumonectomy: factors affecting incidence. *Ann Thorac Surg* 2001;72(1):243–247; discussion 248.
57. Gharagozloo F, Margolis M, Facktor M, et al. Postpneumonectomy and postlobectomy empyema. *Thorac Surg Clin* 2006;16(3):215–222.
58. Kopec SE, Irwin RS, Umali-Torres CB, et al. The postpneumonectomy state. *Chest* 1998;114(4):1158–1184.
59. Wechsler RJ, Goodman LR. Mediastinal position and air-fluid height after pneumonectomy: the effect of the respiratory cycle. *AJR Am J Roentgenol* 1985;145(6):1173–1176.
60. Pairolero PC, Arnold PG, Trastek VF, et al. Postpneumonectomy empyema. The role of intrathoracic muscle transposition. *J Thorac Cardiovasc Surg* 1990;99(6):958–966; discussion 966–958.
61. Zumbro GL Jr, Treasure R, Geiger JP, et al. Empyema after pneumonectomy. *Ann Thorac Surg* 1973;15(6):615–621.
62. Miller JD, Nemni J, Simone C, et al. Prophylactic intracavitary (pneumonectomy space) antibiotic instillation: a comparative study. *Ann Thorac Cardiovasc Surg* 2001;7(1):14–16.
63. Goldstraw P. Prophylaxis of postpneumonectomy empyema. *Thorax* 1980;35(2):107–110.
64. Stolz AJ, Schutzner J, Lischke R, et al. Predictors of prolonged air leak following pulmonary lobectomy. *Eur J Cardiothorac Surg* 2005;27(2): 334–336.
65. Isowa N, Hasegawa S, Bando T, et al. Preoperative risk factors for prolonged air leak following lobectomy or segmentectomy for primary lung cancer. *Eur J Cardiothorac Surg* 2002;21(5):951.
66. Abolhoda A, Liu D, Brooks A, et al. Prolonged air leak following radical upper lobectomy: an analysis of incidence and possible risk factors. *Chest* 1998;113(6):1507–1510.
67. Brunelli A, Fianchini A, Al Refai M, et al. Internal comparative audit in a thoracic surgery unit using the physiological and operative severity score for the enumeration of mortality and morbidity (POSSUM). *Eur J Cardiothorac Surg* 2001;19(6):924–928.
68. Cerfolio RJ. Recent advances in the treatment of air leaks. *Curr Opin Pulm Med* 2005;11(4):319–323.
69. Cerfolio RJ, Bass CS, Pask AH, et al. Predictors and treatment of persistent air leaks. *Ann Thorac Surg* 2002;73(6):1727–1730; discussion 1730–1721.
70. Cerfolio RJ, Bass C, Katholi CR. Prospective randomized trial compares suction versus water seal for air leaks. *Ann Thorac Surg* 2001; 71(5):1613–1617.
71. Marshall MB, Deeb ME, Bleier JI, et al. Suction vs water seal after pulmonary resection: a randomized prospective study. *Chest* 2002; 121(3):831–835.
72. Belda-Sanchis J, Serra-Mitjans M, Iglesias Sentis M, et al. Surgical sealant for preventing air leaks after pulmonary resections in patients with lung cancer. *Cochrane Database Syst Rev* 2010;(1):CD003051.
73. Brunelli A, Al Refai M, Monteverde M, et al. Pleural tent after upper lobectomy: a randomized study of efficacy and duration of effect. *Ann Thorac Surg* 2002;74(6):1958–1962.
74. Haniuda M, Nishimura H, Kobayashi O, et al. Management of chylothorax after pulmonary resection. *J Am Coll Surg* 1995;180(5): 537–540.
75. Le Pimpec-Barthes F, D'Attellis N, Dujon A, et al. Chylothorax complicating pulmonary resection. *Ann Thorac Surg* 2002;73(6):1714–1719.
76. Cerfolio RJ, Allen MS, Deschamps C, et al. Postoperative chylothorax. *J Thorac Cardiovasc Surg* 1996;112(5):1361–1365; discussion 1365–1366.
77. Cope C, Salem R, Kaiser LR. Management of chylothorax by percutaneous catheterization and embolization of the thoracic duct: prospective trial. *J Vasc Interv Radiol* 1999;10(9):1248–1254.
78. Shimizu K, Yoshida J, Nishimura M, et al. Treatment strategy for chylothorax after pulmonary resection and lymph node dissection for lung cancer. *J Thorac Cardiovasc Surg* 2002;124(3):499–502.
79. Guillem P, Papachristos I, Peillon C, et al. Etilefrine use in the management of post-operative chyle leaks in thoracic surgery. *Interact Cardiovasc Thorac Surg* 2004;3(1):156–160.
80. Patterson GA, Todd TR, Delarue NC, et al. Supradiaphragmatic ligation of the thoracic duct in intractable chylous fistula. *Ann Thorac Surg* 1981;32(1):44–49.
81. Krasna MJ, Forti G. Nerve injury: injury to the recurrent laryngeal, phrenic, vagus, long thoracic, and sympathetic nerves during thoracic surgery. *Thorac Surg Clin* 2006;16(3):267–275, vi.
82. Gotoda Y, Kambara N, Sakai T, et al. The morbidity, time course and predictive factors for persistent post-thoracotomy pain. *Eur J Pain* 2001;5(1):89–96.
83. Allama AM. Intercostal muscle flap for decreasing pain after thoracotomy: a prospective randomized trial. *Ann Thorac Surg* 2010;89(1): 195–199.
84. Maguire MF, Latter JA, Mahajan R, et al. A study exploring the role of intercostal nerve damage in chronic pain after thoracic surgery. *Eur J Cardiothorac Surg* 2006;29(6):873–879.
85. Koehler RP, Keenan RJ. Management of postthoracotomy pain: acute and chronic. *Thorac Surg Clin* 2006;16(3):287–297.
86. Perttunen K, Tasmuth T, Kalso E. Chronic pain after thoracic surgery: a follow-up study. *Acta Anaesthesiol Scand* 1999;43(5):563–567.
87. Dajczman E, Gordon A, Kreisman H, et al. Long-term postthoracotomy pain. *Chest* 1991;99(2):270–274.
88. Shen KR, Wain JC, Wright CD, et al. Postpneumonectomy syndrome: surgical management and long-term results. *J Thorac Cardiovasc Surg* 2008;135(6):1210–1216; discussion 1216–1219.
89. Grillo HC, Shepard JA, Mathisen DJ, et al. Postpneumonectomy syndrome: diagnosis, management, and results. *Ann Thorac Surg* 1992;54(4): 638–650; discussion 650–631.
90. Partington SL, Graham A, Weeks SG. Pulmonary vein stenosis following left pneumonectomy: a variant contributor to postpneumonectomy syndrome. *Chest* 2010;137(1):205–206.
91. Ng T, Ryder BA, Maziak DE, et al. Thoracoscopic approach for the treatment of postpneumonectomy syndrome. *Ann Thorac Surg* 2009; 88(3):1015–1018.
92. Reed MF, Lewis JD. Thoracoscopic mediastinal repositioning for postpneumonectomy syndrome. *J Thorac Cardiovasc Surg* 2007;133(1): 264–265.
93. Mehanna MJ, Israel GM, Katigbak M, et al. Cardiac herniation after right pneumonectomy: case report and review of the literature. *J Thorac Imaging* 2007;22(3):280–282.
94. Rodenwaldt J, Lembcke AE, Wiese TH, et al. Postoperative dislocation of the heart after pneumonectomy. *Circulation* 2002;105(7):e49–e50.
95. DiMarco AF, Oca O, Renston JP. Lung herniation. A cause of chronic chest pain following thoracotomy. *Chest* 1995;107(3):877–879.
96. Berry MF, Friedberg J. Chest wall/diaphragmatic complications. *Thorac Surg Clin* 2006;16(3):277–285, vii.
97. Weissberg D, Refaely Y. Hernia of the lung. *Ann Thorac Surg* 2002;74(6):1963–1966.
98. Van Den Broeck S, Van Rompaey V, Ortmanns P, et al. Intercostal lung herniation after repeat thoracotomy. *Minerva Chir* 2008;63(4):307–310.
99. Moncada R, Vade A, Gimenez C, et al. Congenital and acquired lung hernias. *J Thorac Imaging* 1996;11(1):75–82.

100. Temes RT, Talbot WA, Green DP, et al. Herniation of the lung after video-assisted thoracic surgery. *Ann Thorac Surg* 2001;72(2):606–607.
101. Santini M, Fiorello A, Vicidomini G, et al. Pulmonary hernia secondary to limited access for mitral valve surgery and repaired by video thoracoscopic surgery. *Interact Cardiovasc Thorac Surg* 2009;8(1): 111–113.
102. Weyant MJ, Bains MS, Venkatraman E, et al. Results of chest wall resection and reconstruction with and without rigid prosthesis. *Ann Thorac Surg* 2006;81(1):279–285.
103. Lans TE, van der Pol C, Wouters MW, et al. Complications in wound healing after chest wall resection in cancer patients; a multivariate analysis of 220 patients. *J Thorac Oncol* 2009;4(5):639–643.
104. Mansour KA, Thourani VH, Losken A, et al. Chest wall resections and reconstruction: a 25-year experience. *Ann Thorac Surg* 2002;73(6): 1720–1725; discussion 1725–1726.
105. Deschamps C, Tirnaksiz BM, Darbandi R, et al. Early and long-term results of prosthetic chest wall reconstruction. *J Thorac Cardiovasc Surg* 1999;117(3):588–591; discussion 591–582.
106. Welvaart WN, Oosterhuis JW, Paul MA. Negative pressure dressing for radiation-associated wound dehiscence after posterolateral thoracotomy. *Interact Cardiovasc Thorac Surg* 2009;8(5):558–559.
107. Saxena V, Hwang CW, Huang S, et al. Vacuum-assisted closure: microdeformations of wounds and cell proliferation. *Plast Reconstr Surg* 2004;114(5):1086–1096; discussion 1097–1088.

Table 26.1 Inflammatory mediators and mechanisms of injury during cardiopulmonary bypass

Mediator	Effects
Complement: anaphylatoxins C3a, C4a, C5a	Increased vascular permeability Histamine release from mast cells and basophils Smooth muscle contraction Leukocyte migration Cytokine release Neutrophils and mast cell enzyme release C3a-caused platelet aggregation C5a-caused neutrophil aggregation and adherence to endothelium
Cytokines: TNF-α, IL-6, IL-8, IL-10	Altered myocardial contractility Chemoattraction of neutrophils IL-10 may be protective
Arachidonic acid metabolites	Thromboxane A_2-caused vasoconstriction, platelet aggregation Prostaglandins (E_1, E_2, I_2)-caused vasodilatation, platelet antiaggregant Leukotriene-caused chemoattractant, increased vascular permeability
Clotting and fibrinolytic systems/ kallikrein–bradykinin system	Bradykinin leads to vasodilatation, smooth muscle contraction Increased vascular permeability Kallikrein activates plasminogen to plasmin Endothelial cells facilitate plasminogen activation
Endotoxin (intestinal mucosa)	Activation of complement Increased release of cytokines

TNF, tumor necrosis factor.

of the plasma enzyme systems and formed elements of blood (1). This reaction is called the whole body inflammatory response or cascade. The magnitude of the inflammatory response has been demonstrated to adversely influence clinical outcome following CPB (14). Reduced levels of reactive mediators have been demonstrated with off-pump bypass surgery, but it is unclear how this reduction translates to clinical benefit (15–17). Activation of multiple mediators by CPB ultimately leads to tissue damage and organ injury. These mediators, their sites of origin, and the mechanisms of injury are summarized in Table 26.1 (1,9,18).

Risk factors

Length of CPB is key in the degree of inflammatory reaction invoked and is correlated with mediator and cytokine levels.

Prevention

Strategies to limit the inflammatory response to CPB include leukocyte filtration, ultrafiltration, heparin-bonded circuits, anticytokine antibodies, and steroids (1,19–22). These methods have typically targeted only one specific portion of this complicated process and therefore have not consistently benefited patient outcome. Large, prospective randomized clinical trials are needed to establish the clinical benefit of many of these strategies (18,23).

PROTAMINE REACTION

Protamine is utilized to reverse the systemic anticoagulation effects of heparin following cessation of CPB. During protamine administration, patients may experience a range of reactions from hypotension to a severe catastrophic reaction. A severe protamine reaction leads to massive pulmonary vasoconstriction, systemic hypotension, and right heart failure.

Previous exposure to protamine, fish allergy, diabetes mellitus, and exposure to protamine-containing insulin have been implicated as risk factors for protamine reaction. Previous exposure is the most important predictor (24–27).

Hypotension may be avoided by the slow administration of protamine and by the administration of vasopressors. The often fatal idiosyncratic reaction that includes hypotension, bronchospasm, pulmonary vasoconstriction, and right heart failure is typically refractory to medical therapy and often requires reheparinization and reinstitution of CPB for hemodynamic support. Therapy may then include pulmonary vasodilators, systemic vasoconstriction, steroids, antihistamines, and aminophylline (28).

HEPARIN-INDUCED THROMBOCYTOPENIA

Heparin is required to prevent thrombosis of the CPB circuit. Heparin-induced thrombocytopenia results from the production of immunoglobulin G antibodies that recognize platelet factor 4 when bound to heparin (29). This reaction leads to platelet activation and to activation of the coagulation cascade. Patients develop thrombosis which may lead to limb amputation and death. The presence of antibody is associated with a significant increase in morbidity and mortality (30,31).

Heparin exposure is essential for the development of heparin-induced thrombocytopenia. Unfractionated heparin from porcine intestinal mucosa is preferred over heparin obtained from bovine lung due to its reduced risk of antibody formation (29). Prevention of heparin-induced thrombocytopenia may be facilitated by the limited use of heparin to only surgical procedures requiring its use and reliance on other alternatives for preoperative and postoperative antithrombotic prophylaxis and therapy (32).

The diagnosis of heparin-induced thrombocytopenia must be considered when thrombocytopenia occurs following CPB. If the diagnosis is suspected, *all* heparin should be immediately discontinued. Administration of thrombin inhibitors is essential in the prevention of thrombotic complications related to heparin-induced thrombocytopenia. Direct thrombin inhibitors lepirudin, bivalirudin, or argatroban are recommended, with the choice depending on renal and hepatic function (29).

HEMATOLOGIC COMPLICATIONS

The interaction of blood with air and with the nonendothelial surface of the CPB circuit results in a myriad of effects on the hematologic system. Postoperative bleeding requiring return to the operating room occurs in up to 5% of patients (9). The most dreaded hematologic complication is clotting of the oxygenator or the CPB circuit. The most common complication pertaining to hemostasis is due to qualitative and quantitative platelet defects. Platelets are diluted and destroyed during CPB and are often defective due to preoperative medications such as aspirin, dipyridamole, and clopidogrel.

A variety of events contribute to the hematologic complications following CPB. Coagulation factors are hemodiluted by the pump prime. The fibrinolytic system is activated following contact of factor XII with the circuit and by stimulation of endothelial cells. Thrombin is generated by the coagulation cascade. A systemic dose of heparin is administered to prevent thrombosis of the circuit. Cardiotomy and vent suctions result in turbulence and shear stress of the blood elements, while platelet aggregation leads to impaired function. Platelet function is further inhibited by hypothermia (1,9,33). Heparin resistance is due to antithrombin III depletion preoperatively by heparin therapy, resulting in the need for increased doses of heparin to achieve adequate activated clotting time levels for CPB as well as the need for antithrombin III repletion. Heparin rebound is defined as persistence of active, unmetabolized heparin following the administration and complete metabolism of protamine. Both heparin resistance and rebound may contribute to postoperative bleeding (1,34).

Table 26.2 Treatment of bleeding following cardiopulmonary bypass

Correct abnormal laboratory values: Platelet transfusion Cryoprecipitate administration Fresh frozen plasma administration Additional protamine
Correct hypothermia: Use a blood product warmer for massive transfusions Warm the patient with a topical warming device
Avoid systemic hypertension that places tension on suture lines
Administer supplemental protamine dose to treat heparin rebound
Avoid hemodilution and support blood volume and hemodynamics with packed red blood cell transfusion when appropriate
Increase positive end-expiratory pressure on ventilator
Consider desmopressin or epsilon-aminocaproic acid
Maintain a high suspicion of tamponade if cardiac output decreases, chest tube output decreases, and CVP increases
Surgical exploration if bleeding remains excessive

CVP, central venous pressure.

Risk factors

Factors that result in an increased risk of bleeding following CPB include redo surgery, surgery requiring hypothermia below 27°C, preoperative use of aspirin or anticoagulants, significant liver disease or congestion, end stage renal disease, and congenital or acquired coagulation protein deficiency (1,9,35,36). Prolonged CPB time is also a risk factor for postoperative hematologic complications (37).

Prevention

Multiple strategies may be employed to prevent hematologic complications following CPB. The antifibrinolytics epsilon-aminocaproic acid and tranexamic acid may be used to reduce mediastinal blood loss and transfusion requirements (35). Maintenance of a hematocrit level >22% during CPB will significantly reduce the incidence of postoperative bleeding and morbidity and may improve long-term survival (38). Controlled, gentle cardiotomy suction decreases shear forces and preserves platelets (36). Repletion of antithrombin III by the administration of fresh frozen plasma corrects heparin resistance. Additional doses of protamine are effective in treating heparin rebound. The treatment of bleeding following CPB begins with the investigation of causative factors. A management strategy is summarized in Table 26.2 (39).

ENDOCRINE COMPLICATIONS

Pain, stress, hypothermia, hemodilution, and the contact of blood with a nonendothelial surface lead to physiologic responses during CPB. Multiple changes are noted in endogenous hormone levels despite their relative lack of physiologic control during CPB. Hemodilution results in a decrease in total and ionized calcium, parathyroid hormone, T_3, and T_4 (9,40). Hyperglycemia is noted during CPB secondary to decreased insulin secretion, decreased peripheral glucose utilization secondary to hypothermia, and elevated levels of circulating cortisol and epinephrine (9,33,41). Increased levels of norepinephrine, aldosterone, renin, angiotensin, and vasopressin are noted. There is an increase in free fatty acids and lipid metabolism. Decreased levels of atrial natriuretic factor and adrenocorticotropin hormone are noted during CPB (33,41).

Many of the hormonal changes noted are inevitable during CPB and are limited only by the length of CPB. Increasing the depth of anesthesia during CPB or providing pulsatile perfusion may blunt some hormonal responses. The significance of hormonal responses on ultimate outcome is unknown (41).

FLUID BALANCE AND RENAL COMPLICATIONS

During CPB the intravascular volume of the body is removed, hemodiluted, and then returned. The normal physiologic responses to intravascular volume change are eliminated during CPB as central venous pressure is artificially controlled. The adult patient may gain 1 to 15 lb (up to 6.8 kg) following CPB; the amount of weight gained increases with the length of CPB (33). Fluid accumulation occurs mainly in the extracellular, extravascular interstitial space (42). Renal impairment is observed in 12% of patients following CPB, and the incidence of renal failure requiring hemodialysis is approximately 1% to 5% (9,43). Renal failure following CPB results in an eightfold increase in morbidity and mortality. Mortality rates increase 20-fold in patients who require hemodialysis (43,44).

Renal insufficiency may be attributed to a combination of hemodilution, low perfusion pressure and decreased renal blood flow on CPB, hypothermia, microembolization, circulating hormones (renin, aldosterone, vasopressin, and angiotensin II) that cause renal vasoconstriction, injury secondary to inflammatory mediators, and hemolysis (1,9). Despite the beneficial effects of increased blood flow secondary to decreased viscosity, the hemodilution of CPB results in fluid retention as a decrease in plasma colloid osmotic pressure leads to increased capillary permeability and vasodilatation (33,42). Hypothermia reduces glomerular filtration, renal blood flow, and osmolar clearance (42). Aldosterone and vasopressin promote conservation of sodium and water and renal vasoconstriction (42). Hemolysis results in hemoglobin cast formation in renal tubules (33,42).

Risk factors

Factors that are predictive of postoperative fluid accumulation include obesity, female sex, diabetes mellitus, emergency surgery, advanced age, congestive heart failure, and preoperative anemia (33,42). Risk factors associated with renal dysfunction following CPB include preoperative renal dysfunction, age >70 years, diabetes mellitus, blood transfusion, previous cardiac surgery, congestive heart failure, use of IABP, unstable angina, low cardiac output, emergency surgery, and duration of CPB (9,45–47).

Prevention

Strategies to prevent renal failure focus upon the prevention of oliguria by maximizing cardiac output and utilizing diuretic therapy, the limitation of CPB time, maintenance of an alkaline urine if hemolysis is ongoing, and the avoidance of nephrotoxic drugs or dyes. Consideration should be given to delaying surgery following the administration of nephrotoxic agents such as cardiac catheterization.

Strategies to manage renal injury are based on the maintenance of fluid and electrolyte balance and the use of hemodialysis when indicated. Hemodilution with a crystalloid prime solution and hyperglycemia provide modest diuresis in most patients following CPB. Fluid losses should be repleted and preload maximized. Often the most important strategy in the postoperative period is the improvement of cardiac output with resulting improved renal perfusion.

CENTRAL NERVOUS SYSTEM COMPLICATIONS

Significant neurologic injury is the most disabling of all complications relating to CPB. Central nervous system (CNS) injury ranges from minor cognitive deficit to overt stroke. Injury may include delirium, encephalopathy, confusion, agitation, disorientation, drowsiness, decreased alertness, memory deficit, seizure, or other neuropsychiatric disturbances (48).

Neurologic deficits are often difficult to quantify and categorize. Many studies have underestimated the number of patients with deficits because findings may be subtle and difficult to document (49,50). The incidence of stroke following CPB ranges from 1% to 7% (51,52). The incidence of encephalopathy is as high as 7% (53), and up to 53% of patients undergoing cardiac surgery experience postoperative cognitive deficits (54,55). Neurologic injury is particularly devastating because it significantly increases mortality, length of hospital stay, and cost of hospitalization and requires inpatient and outpatient rehabilitation (49,53).

Neurologic injury is attributed to global or regional hypoperfusion, hemorrhage, or embolic phenomenon. Global hypoperfusion is particularly important in patients with hypertension who require a higher mean arterial pressure during CPB to provide adequate blood flow to the brain. The presence of significant carotid artery disease increases this risk, particularly in the region of the brain at risk.

The number of cerebral emboli detected during CPB has been correlated with the degree of neurologic deficit postoperatively (56). Embolic phenomena may occur as a result of cannulation of the aorta, clamping the aorta, intracardiac debris or clot, or gaseous or particulate matter from the cardiotomy suction and the CPB machine (33,57). Air emboli may result from the reversal or kinking of pump or vent lines, the vortexing of air entering an empty venous reservoir, air entry around vent lines, an intravenous infusion line in a patient with a patent foramen ovale or septal defect, the clotting or detachment of the oxygenator, inadequate deairing of open cardiac chambers, a break in the integrity of the arterial line, and the introduction of air bubbles in solution into the internal mammary artery graft lumen (58).

Microembolization may include gas, lipid particles, atheroma, calcific debris, bone marrow, glove powder, aggregates of blood cells or fibrin, or particles of silicone or polyvinyl chloride tubing (9,59). Using transcranial Doppler ultrasonography, CPB has been demonstrated to significantly increase the number of microemboli compared to the use of off-pump coronary artery bypass techniques (60–62). The number of microemboli has been demonstrated to increase significantly with perfusionist manipulations such as injection of drugs into the CPB circuit or the acquisition of blood samples from the circuit (63).

Table 26.4 Strategies to minimize neurologic injury during cardiopulmonary bypass

Address symptomatic carotid artery stenosis preoperatively
Image ascending aorta using epiaortic ultrasound probe to guide cannulation site
Plan "no touch" technique for calcified aorta
Minimize frequency of aortic cross clamping
Careful deairing maneuvers: vent aorta and use Trendelenburg position when removing cross clamp
Maintain adequate mean arterial pressure
Minimize cardiotomy suction
Perform careful and thorough debridement and irrigation of intracardiac debris
Minimize cardiopulmonary bypass and deep hypothermic circulatory arrest time
Consider retrograde cerebral perfusion during circulatory arrest
Adhere to cooling and warming guidelines to prevent air precipitation

Risk factors

Risk factors for stroke in patients undergoing CPB are summarized in Table 26.3 (49,64,65). Technical strategies may be employed to reduce neurologic injury during CPB (Table 26.4). Prior to cannulation, care should be given to the site of cannulation and the placement of the aortic cross clamp in the patient with the calcified aorta.

Prevention

Alternatives in the case of the severely calcified aorta include femoral artery cannulation, axillary artery cannulation, cold fibrillatory arrest for the placement of proximal coronary artery anastomoses or for the replacement of a mitral valve, the use of off-pump coronary artery bypass techniques with placement of proximal anastomoses on internal mammary artery grafts, replacement of the entire ascending aorta, and the placement of proximal anastomoses on the descending aorta. Other strategies include the use of a higher perfusion pressure during CPB (66). A management strategy for the treatment of massive air embolism during CPB is summarized in Table 26.5 (67).

Two different blood gas management techniques may be used during CPB. Hypothermia results in an elevation of the pH. Using the pH stat method, carbon dioxide is added to the CPB circuit to correct the alkalotic pH to 7.4. Using the α stat method, the numerical pH result is corrected to account for hypothermia and no carbon dioxide is added. Carbon

Table 26.3 Risk factors for stroke following cardiopulmonary bypass

Preoperative	Intraoperative
Age	Atherosclerosis of the ascending aorta
Peripheral vascular disease (especially carotid artery disease)	Duration of cardiopulmonary bypass Return to cardiopulmonary bypass after separation
Renal insufficiency or failure	
Diabetes mellitus	Use of IABP
Previous stroke	Presence of left ventricular thrombus
Urgent or emergency surgery	Severe valvular calcification
Ejection fraction <40%	Repeated manipulation of the aorta
Recent myocardial infarction	
Hypertension	

IABP, intra-aortic balloon pump.

Table 26.5 Management of massive air embolus during cardiopulmonary bypass

Stop the pump immediately
Clamp both arterial and venous lines
Place the patient into deep Trendelenburg position
Ventilate with 100% oxygen
Remove the aortic cannula to deair the aorta
Place the arterial cannula in the SVC for retrograde cerebral perfusion, clamp the SVC proximally, and cool the patient
Compress the heart manually
Compress the carotid arteries manually
Once the aorta is deaired, replace the aortic cannula and resume CPB at a high pressure
Turn off any nitrous gas
Consider the administration of steroids and mannitol

CPB, cardiopulmonary bypass; SVC, superior vena cava.

dioxide added when using the pH stat method results in arteriolar dilatation in the brain. Despite increased blood flow to the brain with the pH stat method, cerebral autoregulation of blood flow is lost (68). The use of α stat blood gas management during hypothermia maintains cerebral blood flow autoregulation and improves myocardial functional recovery when compared to pH stat management (1,68).

The use of off-pump coronary artery bypass technique provides fewer microemboli to the brain and allows for a "no touch" aorta technique (60). Large, randomized prospective trials will be necessary to determine whether this approach significantly reduces the incidence of neurologic injury. Treatment following CPB and CNS injury includes neurologic consultation, supportive care, aggressive physical and occupational therapy, the limitation of cerebral edema when appropriate, and the correction of any contributing metabolic derangements.

GASTROINTESTINAL COMPLICATIONS

The incidence of gastrointestinal complications following CPB is approximately 1% (69). Gastrointestinal complications of CPB are often subtle and difficult to detect because patients are sedated. Diagnosis often requires transportation of the critically ill patient to various radiology departments.

Intraoperative monitoring of splanchnic perfusion is not routinely performed. Injury to the small and large bowel, gallbladder, liver, and pancreas during CPB results from regional malperfusion secondary to hypoperfusion, vasoactive substances, cytotoxins, and microemboli. Angiotensin II release results in splanchnic vasoconstriction that may be harmful in patients with arteriosclerosis of the splanchnic vessels (70,71). Reduced gastrointestinal blood flow combined with systemic anticoagulation may cause gastrointestinal bleeding, gastritis, cholecystitis, ischemic small or large bowel, hepatic damage, and pancreatitis. Relative hypoperfusion is particularly detrimental to the liver and pancreas due to the lack of intrinsic autoregulation mechanisms during CPB (72).

Approximately 10% to 20% of patients will manifest mild jaundice secondary to blood transfusion, hemolysis, and liver injury (1). Hepatic injury can also occur during manual compression of the liver to augment venous return or to fill venous cannulas with blood prior to initiation of CPB. Acute pancreatitis occurs in <1% of patients, but 30% of patients will have temporary asymptomatic elevation of serum amylase or lipase (12,73). Mortality is greatly increased when severe gastrointestinal complications occur following CPB, probably the reflection of a generalized low cardiac output state.

Risk factors

Risk factors for gastrointestinal injury following CPB include advanced age, emergency surgery, prolonged duration of CPB, low cardiac output, prolonged use of vasopressors, peripheral vascular disease, and congestive heart failure (12,70). Risks of pancreatitis include previous history of pancreatitis, renal insufficiency, and high-dose calcium administration (12,73).

Prevention

Strategies to decrease gastrointestinal complications include the use of an increased perfusion flow rate rather than peripheral vasoconstrictors for maintaining perfusion pressure on CPB and limitation of bypass time (74). Optimization of cardiac output improves splanchnic perfusion. Manual compression of the liver should not be used to augment venous return. The management of gastrointestinal complication focuses on prompt recognition and treatment, which often requires further surgery.

REFERENCES

1. Edmunds LH, ed. *Cardiac surgery in the adult*. New York: McGraw-Hill; 1997.
2. Hammermeister KE, Burchfiel C, Johnson R, et al. Identification of patients at greatest risk for developing major complications at cardiac surgery. *Circulation* 1990;82(Suppl 5):IV380–IV389.
3. Parolari A, Alamanni F, Cannata A, et al. Off-pump vs. on-pump coronary artery bypass: meta-analysis of currently available randomized trials. *Ann Thorac Surg* 2003;76:37–40.
4. Braunwald E, Kloner RA. The stunned myocardium: prolonged, postischemic ventricular dysfunction. *Circulation* 1982;66:1146–1149.
5. Menasche P. Strategies to improve myocardial protection during extracorporeal circulation. *Shock* 2001;16(Suppl 1):20–23.
6. Jain U. Myocardial ischemia after cardiopulmonary bypass. *J Card Surg* 1995;10(Suppl 4):520–526.
7. Kalman J. Arrhythmias and pacing. In: Buxton B, Frazier OH, Westaby S, eds. *Ischemic heart disease surgical management*. London: Mosby;1999: 87–89.
8. Jayam VKS, Flaker GC, Jones JW. Atrial fibrillation after coronary bypass: etiology and pharmacologic prevention. *Cardiovasc Surg* 2002; 10(4):351–358.
9. Brodie JE, Johnson RB. *The manual of clinical perfusion*, 2nd ed. Augusta, GA: Glendale Medical Corp; 1997.
10. Ng CSH, Wan S, Yim APC, et al. Pulmonary dysfunction after cardiac surgery. *Chest* 2002;121:1269–1277.
11. Sladen RN, Berkowitz DE. Cardiopulmonary bypass and the lung. In: Gravlee GP, Davis RF, Utley JR, eds. *Cardiopulmonary bypass principles and practice*. Baltimore, MD: Williams & Wilkins; 1993:467–487.
12. Cohn LH, Edmunds LH, eds. *Cardiac surgery in the adult*, 2nd ed. New York: McGraw-Hill; 2003.
13. Rady MY, Ryan T, Starr NJ. Early onset of acute pulmonary dysfunction after cardiovascular surgery: risk factors and clinical outcome. *Crit Care Med* 1997;25(11):1831–1839.
14. Holmes JH, Connolly NC, Paull DL, et al. Magnitude of the inflammatory response to cardiopulmonary bypass and its relation to adverse clinical outcomes. *Inflamm Res* 2002;51(12):579–586.
15. Okubo N, Hatori N, Ochi M, et al. Comparison of m-RNA expression for inflammatory mediators in leukocytes between pump and off-pump coronary artery bypass grafting. *Ann Thorac Cardiovasc Surg* 2003;9(1):43–49.
16. Wildhirt SM, Schulze C, Schulz C, et al. Reduction of systemic and cardiac adhesion molecule expression after off-pump versus conventional coronary artery bypass grafting. *Shock* 2001;16(Suppl 1):55–59.
17. Schulze C, Conrad N, Schutz A, et al. Reduced expression of systemic proinflammatory cytokines after off-pump versus conventional coronary artery bypass grafting. *Thorac Cardiovasc Surg* 2000;48(6): 364–369.
18. Wan S, LeClerc JL, Vincent JL. Inflammatory response to cardiopulmonary bypass: mechanisms involved and possible therapeutic strategies. *Chest* 1997;112:676–692.
19. Kaul TK, Fields BL. Leukocyte activation during cardiopulmonary bypass: limitations of the inhibitory mechanisms and strategies. *J Cardiovasc Surg (Torino)* 2000;41(6):849–862.
20. Lei Y, Haider HK, Chusnsheng W, et al. Dose-dependent effect of aprotinin on aggravated pro-inflammatory cytokines in patients with

pulmonary hypertension following cardiopulmonary bypass. *Cardiovasc Drugs Ther* 2003;17(4):343–348.
21. Gott JP, Cooper WA, Schmidt FE, et al. Modifying risk for extracorporeal circulation: trial of four anti-inflammatory strategies. *Ann Thorac Surg* 1998;66(3):747–753.
22. Schmartz D, Tabardel Y, Preiser JC, et al. Does aprotinin influence the inflammatory response to cardiopulmonary bypass in patients? *J Thorac Cardiovasc Surg* 2003;125(1):184–190.
23. Paparella D, Yau TM, Young E. Cardiopulmonary bypass induced inflammation: pathophysiology and treatment. An update. *Eur J Cardiothorac Surg* 2002;21:232–244.
24. Weiler JM, Gellhaus MA, Carter JG, et al. A prospective study of the risk of an immediate adverse reaction to protamine sulfate during cardiopulmonary bypass surgery. *J Allergy Clin Immunol* 1990;85(4):713–719.
25. Brooks JC. Noncardiogenic pulmonary edema immediately following rapid protamine administration. *Ann Pharmacother* 1999;33(9):927–930.
26. Levy JH, Schwieger IM, Zaidan JR, et al. Evaluation of patients at risk for protamine reaction. *J Thorac Cardiovasc Surg* 1989;98(2): 200–204.
27. Comunale ME, Maslow A, Robertson LK, et al. Effect of site of venous protamine administration, previously alleged risk factors, and preoperative use of aspirin on acute protamine-induced pulmonary vasoconstriction. *J Cardiothorac Vasc Anesth* 2003;17(3): 309–313.
28. Hensley FA, Larach DR, Martin DE. Intraoperative anesthetic complications and their management. In: Waldhausen JA, Orringer MB, eds. *Complications in cardiothoracic surgery*. St. Louis, MO: Mosby–Year Book; 1991:12–14.
29. Warkentin TE, Greinacher A. Heparin-induced thrombocytopenia and cardiac surgery. *Ann Thorac Surg* 2003;76:638–648.
30. Greinacher A, Levy JH. HIT happens: Diagnosing and evaluating the patient with heparin-associated thrombocytopenia. *Anesth Analg* 2008;107(2):356–358.
31. Kerendi F, Thourani VH, Puskas JD, et al. Impact of heparin-induced thrombocytopenia on postoperative outcomes after cardiac surgery. *Ann Thorac Surg* 2007;84:1548–1555.
32. Warkentin TE, Kelton JG. Temporal aspects of heparin-induced thrombocytopenia. *N Engl J Med* 2001;344:1286–1292.
33. Buxton B, Frazier OH, Westaby S, eds. *Ischemic heart disease surgical management*. London: Mosby; 1999.
34. Ranucci M. Antithrombin III. A key factor in extracorporeal circulation. *Minerva Anestesiol* 2002;68(5):454–457.
35. Barrons RW, Jahr JS. A review of post-cardiopulmonary bypass bleeding, aminocaproic acid, tranexamic acid, and aprotinin. *Am J Ther* 1996;3(12):821–838.
36. Weerasinghe A, Taylor KM. The platelet in cardiopulmonary bypass. *Ann Thorac Surg* 1998;66:2145–2152.
37. Woodman RC, Harker LA. Bleeding complications associated with cardiopulmonary bypass. *Blood* 1990;76(9):1680–1697.
38. Habib RH, Zacharias A, Schwann TA, et al. Adverse effects of low hematocrit during cardiopulmonary bypass in the adult: should current practice be changed? *J Thorac Cardiovasc Surg* 2003;125(6):1438–1450.
39. Horrow JC. Management of coagulopathy associated with cardiopulmonary bypass. In: Gravlee GP, Davis RF, Utley JR, eds. *Cardiopulmonary bypass principles and practice*. Baltimore, MD: Williams & Wilkins; 1993:436–466.
40. Klemperer JD. Thyroid hormone and cardiac surgery. *Thyroid* 2002;12 (6):517–521.
41. Kennedy DT, Butterworth JF. Endocrine function during and after cardiopulmonary bypass: recent observations. *J Clin Endocrinol Metab* 1994;78(5):997–1002.
42. Utley JR. Renal function and fluid balance with cardiopulmonary bypass. In: Gravlee GP, Davis RF, Utley JR, eds. *Cardiopulmonary bypass principles and practice*. Baltimore, MD: Williams & Wilkins; 1993:488–508.
43. Conlon PJ, Stafford-Smith M, White WD, et al. Acute renal failure following cardiac surgery. *Nephrol Dial Transplant* 1999;14:1158–1162.
44. Rinder CS, Fontes M, Matthew JP, et al. Neutrophil CD11b upregulation during cardiopulmonary bypass is associated with postoperative renal injury. *Ann Thorac Surg* 2003;75(3):899–905.
45. Suen WS, Mok CK, Chiu SW, et al. Risk factors for development of acute renal failure (ARF) requiring dialysis in patients undergoing cardiac surgery. *Angiology* 1998;49(10):789–800.
46. Ranucci M, Pavesi M, Mazza E, et al. Risk factors for renal dysfunction after coronary surgery: the role of cardiopulmonary bypass technique. *Perfusion* 1994;9(5):319–326.
47. Boldt J, Brenner T, Lehmann A. Is kidney function altered by the duration of cardiopulmonary bypass? *Ann Thorac Surg* 2003;73(3):906–912.
48. Taggart DP, Westaby S. Neurological and cognitive disorders after coronary artery bypass grafting. *Curr Opin Cardiol* 2001;16:271–276.
49. Stamou SS, Hill PC, Dangas G. Stroke after coronary artery bypass: incidence, predictors, and clinical outcome. *Stroke* 2001;32:1508–1513.
50. Sotaniemi KA. Long-term neurologic outcome after cardiac operation. *Ann Thorac Surg* 1995;59:1336–1339.
51. John R, Choudhri AF, Weinberg AD, et al. Multicenter review of preoperative risk factors for stroke after coronary artery bypass grafting. *Ann Thorac Surg* 2000;69:30–36.
52. Trehan N, Mishra M, Sharma OP, et al. Further reduction in stroke after off-pump coronary artery bypass grafting: a 10-year experience. *Ann Thorac Surg* 2001;72(3):S1026–S1032.
53. McKhann GM, Grega MA, Borowicz LM, et al. Encephalopathy and stroke after coronary artery bypass grafting. *Arch Neurol* 2002;59: 1422–1428.
54. Newman MF, Kirchner JL, Phillips-Bute B, et al. Longitudinal assessment of neurocognitive function after coronary-artery bypass surgery. *N Engl J Med* 2001;344(6):395–402.
55. Baker RA, Andrew MJ, Knight JL. Evaluation of neurological assessment and outcomes in cardiac surgical patients. *Semin Thorac Cardiovasc Surg* 2001;13(2):149–157.
56. Mark DB, Newman MF. Protecting the brain in coronary artery bypass graft surgery. *JAMA* 2002;287(11):1448–1450.
57. Appelblad M, Engstrom G. Fat contamination of pericardial suction blood and its influence on in vitro capillary-pore flow properties in patients undergoing routine coronary artery bypass grafting. *J Thorac Cardiovasc Surg* 2002;124(2):377–386.
58. Pae WE, Williams DR, Troncelliti EK, et al. Prevention of complications during cardiopulmonary bypass. In: Waldhausen JA, Orringer MB, eds. *Complications in cardiothoracic surgery*. St. Louis, MO: Mosby-Year Book; 1991:39–44.
59. Mills SA. Cerebral injury and cardiac operations. *Ann Thorac Surg* 1993;56(5 Suppl):S86–S91.
60. Bowles J, Lee JD, Dang CR, et al. Coronary artery bypass performed without the use of cardiopulmonary bypass is associated with reduced cerebral microemboli and improved clinical results. *Chest* 2001;119:25–30.
61. Malheiros SM, Massaro AR, Gabbai AA, et al. Is the number of microemboli signals related to neurologic outcome in coronary bypass surgery? *Arq Neuropsiquiatr* 2001;59(1):1–5.
62. Lee JD, Lee SJ, Tsushima WT, et al. Benefits of off-pump bypass on neurologic and clinical morbidity: a prospective randomized trial. *Ann Thorac Surg* 2003;76(1):18–25.
63. Borger MA, Feindel CM. Cerebral emboli during cardiopulmonary bypass: effect of perfusionist interventions and aortic cannulas. *J Extra Corpor Technol* 2002;34(1):29–33.
64. Likosky DS, Leavitt BJ, Marin CAS, et al. Intra- and postoperative predictors of stroke after coronary artery bypass grafting. *Ann Thorac Surg* 2003;76:428–435.
65. Tuman KJ, McCarthy RJ, Rajafi H, et al. Differential effects of advanced age on neurologic and cardiac risks of coronary artery operations. *J Thorac Cardiovasc Surg* 1992;104(6):1510–1517.
66. Gold JP, Charlson ME, Williams-Russo P, et al. Improvement of outcomes after coronary artery bypass. A randomized trial comparing intraoperative high versus low mean arterial pressure. *J Thorac Cardiovasc Surg* 1995;110(5):1302–1311.
67. Mills NL, Morris JM. Air embolism associated with cardiopulmonary bypass. In: Waldhausen JA, Orringer MB, eds. *Complications in cardiothoracic surgery*. St. Louis, MO: Mosby-Year Book; 1991:60–67.
68. Rogers AT, Newman SP, Stump DA, et al. Neurologic effects of cardiopulmonary bypass. In: Gravlee GP, Davis RF, Utley JR, eds. *Cardiopulmonary bypass principles and practice*. Baltimore, MD: Williams & Wilkins; 1993:542–576.
69. Halm MA. Acute gastrointestinal complications after cardiac surgery. *Am J Crit Care* 1996;5(2):109–118.
70. Zacharias A, Schwann TA, Parenteau GL, et al. Predictors of gastrointestinal complications in cardiac surgery. *Tex Heart Inst J* 2000;27: 93–99.
71. Reilly PM, Bulkley GB. Vasoactive mediators and splanchnic perfusion. *Crit Care Med* 1993;21(Suppl 2):S55–S68.
72. Shangraw RE. Metabolic and splanchnic visceral effects of cardiopulmonary bypass. In: Gravke GP, Davis RF, Utley JR, eds. *Cardiopulmonary bypass principles and practice*. Baltimore, MD: Williams & Wilkins; 1993: 509–541.
73. Fernandez-del Castillo C, Harringer W, Warshaw AL, et al. Risk factors for pancreatic cellular injury after cardiopulmonary bypass. *N Engl J Med* 1991;325(6):382–387.
74. Plestis KA, Gold JP. Importance of blood pressure regulation in maintaining adequate tissue perfusion during cardiopulmonary bypass. *Semin Thorac Cardiovasc Surg* 2001;13(2): 170–175.

CHAPTER

27

Complications of Surgical Coronary Revascularization

Spencer J. Melby, Traves D. Crabtree, and Marc R. Moon

INTRODUCTION

Despite advances in percutaneous techniques for coronary revascularization, coronary artery bypass surgery remains an integral component of the treatment regimen for patients with coronary artery disease. Critical analysis of clinical outcomes with subsequent improvements in care, including critical care management and myocardial protection techniques, have significantly improved outcomes related to surgical revascularization. Based on previous comparisons with nonsurgical techniques, current guidelines for coronary artery bypass grafting (CABG) include left main coronary artery stenosis, triple-vessel disease, single- or double-vessel disease that includes left anterior descending stenosis in patients with poor left ventricular (LV) function, and disease refractory to nonsurgical management (1). CABG has better long-term outcomes, especially in patients with diabetes or other high risk comorbidities (2,3).

Continued efforts to decrease morbidity and mortality associated with surgical revascularization have resulted in persistent survival advantage and decreased need for reinterventions relative to nonsurgical revascularization techniques. Based upon randomized controlled trials of patients with stable angina, CABG has been shown to provide a significant survival advantage in moderate to high-risk patients at 5, 7, and 9 years follow-up compared to medical management (4–8). A meta-analysis of randomized trials also demonstrated a significant long-term survival advantage of CABG over percutaneous transluminal coronary angioplasty (PTCA) and a substantial decrease in the number of repeat interventions required following CABG relative to PTCA (9). These differences were most notable in patients with multivessel disease or diabetes. The purported benefits of drug-eluting devices have not been realized in the short or mid term (10). Long-term investigations comparing contemporary coronary stent technology to CABG are currently unavailable but may have an impact on clinical practice in the future.

Spencer J. Melby, Traves D. Crabtree, Marc R. Moon: Washington University School of Medicine, St. Louis, MO 63110.

OVERALL MORBIDITY AND MORTALITY

With regard to monitored outcome variables, coronary revascularization is one of the most scrutinized surgical procedures performed. With the development of the Society of Thoracic Surgeons (STS) database, surveillance of perioperative morbidity and mortality and identification of significant comorbid conditions have allowed for an unprecedented model of quality control on a local, regional, and national basis. The STS database has also permitted the development of risk stratification models that can estimate perioperative mortality and morbidity based on multiple potential risk factors and comorbid conditions. A report from the STS database of 595,222 isolated coronary revascularization procedures performed between 2000 and 2003 demonstrated an overall 30-day operative mortality of 2.54% (11). Risk factors for perioperative death included increasing age, renal dysfunction, emergency surgery, cardiogenic shock, and repeat operations. Perioperative mortality is closely linked to postoperative morbidity, and many of the risk factors identified for mortality correlate with the development of surgery-related complications (12).

One area of study that has received attention recently is maintenance of normoglycemia. Control of hyperglycemia has been demonstrated in multiple studies to decrease the rates of mortality and morbidity, especially in wound infections and occurrences of stroke (13–15). The STS set out practice guidelines concerning blood glucose management during adult cardiac surgery (16). Key points included evidence that poor perioperative glycemic control is associated with increased morbidity and mortality, and that control of blood sugar with a standardized insulin regimen should be utilized to maintain blood glucose levels <180 mg/dL in patients with diabetes. Glycemic control is unnecessary in nondiabetic patients provided that glucose levels remain <180 mg/dL (16). Evidence also exists to show that excessively tight control of glucose levels may increase morbidity and mortality (17).

Table 27.1 summarizes the incidence of several major complications associated with CABG based on a review of the STS database (11). The characteristics of the population undergoing coronary revascularization have changed considerably over the past decade, increasing the complexity of the surgery as well as postoperative care. Review of the STS database demonstrates that from 1990 to 1999, patients

Table 27.1 Incidence of major complications following isolated coronary revascularization (STS Database, 1997–2000)

Complication	Incidence (%)
30-day mortality	2.54
Permanent stroke	1.50
Renal failure requiring dialysis	3.53
Prolonged mechanical ventilation (>48 hr)	7.24
Deep sternal wound infection	0.50
Reoperation for bleeding	6.19
Any major morbidity/mortality	13.83

From DiSesa VJ, O'Brien SM, Welke KF, et al. Contemporary impact of state certificate-of-need regulations for cardiac surgery: an analysis using the Society of Thoracic Surgeons' National Cardiac Surgery Database. *Circulation* 2006;114(20): 2122–2129.

have become significantly older and are more likely to have a history of smoking, diabetes, renal failure, hypertension, stroke, chronic lung disease, worsening heart failure, and multivessel disease. Risk stratification models have also shown that predicted operative risk has risen from 2.6% in 1990 to 3.4% in 1999 while the observed operative mortality has decreased from 3.9% to 3.0% (18). Although advances in surgical and perioperative care have resulted in improvement in clinical outcomes, the increasing complexity of the patients will require continuing efforts to understand and improve outcomes related to CABG.

NEUROLOGIC COMPLICATIONS

One of the most devastating complications following coronary revascularization is the development of stroke. The reported incidence of stroke following CABG is 1.1% to 2.9% with an associated in-hospital mortality of 22% to 24.8% and a 5-year mortality of 56% (18–22). Risk factors for the development of stroke by multivariate analysis include the presence of a calcified aorta, prior stroke, increasing age, carotid artery disease, increasing duration of cardiopulmonary bypass, unstable angina, renal failure, peripheral vascular disease, smoking history, and diabetes mellitus (18,19,22,23). The most significant risk factor among these is the presence of an atherosclerotic ascending aorta, with atheroemboli accounting for the majority of severe ischemic strokes. The presence of mobile plaques in the ascending aorta has been associated with a stroke rate as high as 33.3% following coronary bypass surgery (24,25). Manipulation of the aorta with or without the institution of cardiopulmonary bypass is a significant risk factor for stroke following coronary revascularization (26). Emboli account for >80% of strokes after cardiac surgery with watershed infarcts contributing to the other sources of ischemic events (27).

Preoperative identification of risk factors allows for risk stratification and patient education but may also help to plan the operation in order to decrease the rate of stroke. Patients with symptomatic carotid artery stenosis or critical asymptomatic stenosis diagnosed preoperatively may undergo endarterectomy prior to bypass surgery or at the time of the bypass operation. Preoperative carotid duplex scanning is performed in patients with a history of a transient ischemic attack (TIA), stroke, amaurosis fugax, or in patients with a carotid bruit. Patients with <80% stenosis, corresponding to an internal carotid artery to common carotid artery (IC:CC) velocity ratio <4.0, typically undergo CABG alone. For patients with high-grade carotid stenosis (IC:CC velocity ratio >4.0) carotid endarterectomy is necessary before cardiopulmonary bypass to minimize the risk of stroke. The approach differs depending on the degree of cardiac disease. Timing of endarterectomy for patients with significant but asymptomatic carotid stenosis remains a subject of debate. For patients with unstable angina and preserved LV function, simultaneous carotid endarterectomy and CABG are performed. For patients with stable angina and severe LV dysfunction, carotid endarterectomy is performed 1 to 2 days prior to coronary revascularization. Patients who undergo combined CABG and carotid endarterectomy often have significant hemodynamic fluctuation in the immediate postoperative period due to carotid body manipulation. Although these fluctuations do not affect patients with normal LV function, the occurrence makes patients with poor LV function difficult to manage perioperatively.

The application of transesophageal echocardiography and sensitive epiaortic echocardiography has improved the ability to diagnose and characterize a severely atherosclerotic aorta (28). This diagnosis poses a formidable challenge to the surgeon. The advancement of "no-touch" techniques that avoid manipulation or clamping of the diseased ascending aorta may be used with or without cardiopulmonary bypass (29,30). Application of such techniques has been shown to significantly decrease the incidence of stroke in high-risk patients undergoing coronary revascularization (30). Another option for patients with a severely atherosclerotic aorta involves institution of circulatory arrest and replacement of the ascending aorta to limit the incidence of stroke in this population (31). Recently developed intra-aortic filters may be used in conjunction with the aortic cannula to decrease the embolic load during cardiopulmonary bypass and may play a future role in reducing the rate of stroke (32,33).

Off-pump CABG (OPCAB) has been found to be protective against strokes in several series, including a large retrospective study of patients in the New York State Registry; the adjusted odds ratio for OPCAB versus on-pump was 0.70 (95% confidence interval 0.57 to 0.86) (34). In a retrospective review of 42,477 consecutive, nonemergency, isolated CABG cases in the STS database (over 16,000 patients underwent OPCAB versus over 26,000 patients who underwent conventional on-pump CABG), the stroke rate decreased in patient who underwent OPCAB (odds ratio was 0.65, 95% confidence interval 0.52–0.80, $p < 0.001$) (35).

Areas of controversy with regard to the conduct of the operation and its effect upon neurologic outcome include the use of a single or sequential clamp technique, temperature management strategies during and after bypass, and perioperative management of hyperglycemia.

Unfortunately, there are few treatment options for patients who develop an intraoperative or perioperative stroke. A small number of patients with a thromboembolic etiology may benefit from early (<6 to 8 hours after the event) thrombolytic therapy.

Neurocognitive changes or encephalopathy may occur following bypass surgery. Encephalopathy is present in 3.0% to 6.9% of patients undergoing CABG and is associated with an increased length of stay and mortality relative to patients without encephalopathy (21,36). Significant risk factors for postoperative encephalopathy or neurocognitive changes include increasing age, the presence of a carotid bruit, hypertension, diabetes mellitus, pulmonary disease, excessive alcohol consumption, and history of a previous stroke (21,36). More stringent neuropsychometric tests have estimated that 19% to 26% of patients have persistent cognitive deficits for >2 months following coronary revascularization surgery (37). The etiology of these subtle deficits is incompletely understood, although microembolization may play a role. Although the use of cardiopulmonary bypass has been implicated, studies have failed to identify long-term differences in neurocognitive testing 3 to 12 months post bypass between patients undergoing on-pump revascularization versus off-pump revascularization (38–40).

POSTOPERATIVE ARRHYTHMIAS

Postoperative arrhythmias are a common problem following coronary bypass surgery, with atrial fibrillation accounting for the majority of occurrences. The incidence of postoperative atrial fibrillation following coronary revascularization is 23% to 40%, with even higher rates reported among patients undergoing combined bypass and valve surgery (41–46). The pathophysiology of atrial fibrillation is related to the development of reentrant circuits within the atrium or pulmonary veins. Potential risk factors for atrial fibrillation include advanced age, male gender, chronic obstructive pulmonary disease (COPD), left atrial enlargement, a preoperative history of paroxysmal atrial fibrillation, increasing severity of coronary artery disease, and preoperative digoxin use (42,45,46). Among these, advanced age is the most consistent predictor of postoperative atrial fibrillation. Following coronary revascularization, the incidence of atrial fibrillation is 26% in patients younger than 70 and 45% in patients older than 70 (41).

Atrial fibrillation typically develops between postoperative days 1 and 5 and is often asymptomatic. Some patients develop hypotension or experience shortness of breath, chest pain, palpitations, or confusion with acute onset of atrial fibrillation. Acute hypotension or a low cardiac output state account for most symptoms and are often related to a rapid ventricular response to the atrial rhythm. In these circumstances, urgent treatment to control the ventricular rate is required. In addition to acute symptoms, the development of postoperative atrial fibrillation significantly increases the risk of stroke following coronary revascularization (46,47). The loss of normal atrial contraction results in the development of thrombus within the atrium that serves as a source for emboli. Such thrombus may develop within 48 hours from the onset of fibrillation. The morbidity associated with postoperative atrial fibrillation results in prolonged hospital stay, prolonged intensive care unit (ICU) stay, increased hospital costs, and need for hospital readmission after discharge (41,43,46–48).

Many trials have examined the prevention of postoperative atrial fibrillation by perioperative pharmacotherapy. Prophylactic administration of β-blockers has consistently been shown to decrease postoperative atrial fibrillation in randomized controlled trials, especially in patients who received preoperative β-blockade. Other trials have demonstrated that preoperative administration of amiodarone decreases the rate of postoperative atrial fibrillation after bypass surgery (49,50). Criticisms of amiodarone prophylaxis have included an inability to reproduce these results in subsequent trials using similar regimens of amiodarone and failure of trials to demonstrate a benefit over β-blockers (51,52). A recent meta-analysis of randomized trials suggests that preoperative administration of β-blockers, sotalol, and amiodarone are all effective at preventing postoperative atrial fibrillation in cardiac patients (53). Despite the ability of these agents to decrease the rate of postoperative atrial fibrillation, their prophylactic administration has not resulted in a significant decrease in the length of stay or in overall hospital costs (51,53–55).

A practical limitation of preoperative prophylaxis with β-blockers or amiodarone in patients requiring coronary revascularization is the inability to provide an adequate therapeutic regimen prior to surgery. In most patients, current surgical practice involves CABG within 1 to 2 days of catheterization, making preoperative treatment impractical. Recent randomized trials have demonstrated that immediate postoperative administration of metoprolol or amiodarone significantly decreases the incidence of postoperative atrial fibrillation (54,56). Prophylactic administration of other agents such as digoxin, calcium channel blockers, and magnesium sulfate have shown mixed results (47,57–63).

A novel technique for the prevention of postoperative atrial fibrillation involves biatrial overdrive pacing in the early postoperative period. Pacing wires are placed in both atria intraoperatively and the patient undergoes overdrive pacing for 4 to 5 days postoperatively. Randomized studies have demonstrated a significant reduction in postoperative atrial fibrillation with biatrial pacing (64–67). Although this technique decreases the incidence of atrial fibrillation, these studies have not demonstrated a consistent decrease in hospital length of stay (64–67).

Initial treatment of atrial fibrillation is based on the severity of symptoms. Immediate electrical cardioversion is indicated in the presence of hemodynamic instability, worsening LV dysfunction, or ischemia. Among patients who are relatively asymptomatic, initial management strategies include identification and treatment of underlying abnormalities such as hypoxia, hypovolemia or hypervolemia, hypokalemia, hypomagnesemia, and elimination of chronotropic drugs. Agents used for rate control include metoprolol and diltiazem, which can be given intravenously initially and subsequently as an oral maintenance dose. Although used less frequently, digoxin can be given when other agents are contraindicated. These agents are titrated to a resting ventricular heart rate of 80 to 110 beats per minute, provided that there is an absence of symptoms or hemodynamic compromise.

Rate control with β-blockers or calcium channel blockers may also result in conversion to sinus rhythm. Other antiarrhythmic agents may also be given specifically to convert patients to sinus rhythm. Administration of intravenous amiodarone has been shown to restore sinus rhythm within 24 hours in 77% to 83% of cardiac surgical patients (68–70). Other agents such as propafenone and sotalol have not been as effective as amiodarone for conversion to sinus rhythm (71,72). Side effects of long-term amiodarone administration include pulmonary fibrosis, hepatic toxicity, and hypothyroidism, although these side effects occur infrequently with short-term (≤6 weeks) treatment (73).

Table 27.2 outlines an approach to the management of postoperative atrial fibrillation. In patients who are hemodynamically stable, amiodarone 150 mg is administered intravenously, followed by initiation of oral amiodarone, 400 mg three times a day. If the patient has a controlled heart rate at the onset of atrial fibrillation (≤100 beats per minute), the intravenous loading dose can be eliminated. If the heart rate remains >120 beats per minute, intravenous amiodarone bolus is repeated or metoprolol or diltiazem is administered for rate control. A diltiazem drip may also be used for rate control in this setting. Fortunately, among patients without a preoperative history of atrial arrhythmias, over 98% will return to sinus rhythm within 8 weeks after cardiac surgery (74).

Many patients will convert to sinus rhythm immediately after initiation of treatment. Patients who do not convert within the first 24 to 48 hours are at risk for mural thrombus within the atrium that may serve as a source of emboli. Patients who remain in atrial fibrillation for >24 hours may be started on a low-dose heparin drip at 500 to 800 units per hour. Anticoagulation with heparin followed by Coumadin has been shown to decrease the risk of thromboembolic events in patients with persistent postoperative atrial fibrillation (75,76). In the absence of anticoagulation, attempts at pharmacologic cardioversion with agents such as amiodarone or electrical cardioversion have been associated with a 1% to 7% risk of thromboembolism (77,78). Patients with persistent or recurrent atrial fibrillation are maintained on Coumadin for 4 to 6 weeks postoperatively to minimize the risk of thromboembolic events.

STERNAL WOUND COMPLICATIONS

According to the STS database, the incidence of sternal wound infections in 2006 was 0.3% among isolated coronary artery bypass procedures (79). A previous surveillance of over 2,400 patients demonstrated an overall chest infection rate of 3% among coronary artery bypass patients, with 1.6% superficial infections and 1.4% deep sternal wound infections (80,81). It is expected that this rate will increase due to a trend toward increasing comorbidities and decreasing LV function among patients undergoing bypass surgery. The most common organisms isolated from sternal wound infections are staphylococcal species. The average time from operation to diagnosis of sternal wound infection is 15 to 19 days, with most diagnosed after discharge (82).

Risk factors for the development of sternal wound infections include steroid use, diabetes mellitus, reoperation for bleeding, increasing operative duration, heart failure, increased number of grafts performed, and prolonged mechanical ventilation (80,83). Previous reports have identified the use of bilateral internal mammary arteries as a significant risk factor for the development of deep sternal wound infections (84,85). Most recent studies have demonstrated a similar infection rate with use of bilateral internal mammary arteries versus use of a single internal mammary

Table 27.2 Treatment options for acute management of postoperative atrial fibrillation

Drug	Initial IV Dose	Maintenance Dose
Amiodarone	150 mg bolus ± 0.5 mg/min drip	400 mg p.o. t.i.d. × 5 days (load) followed by 200–400 mg p.o. q.d. for 4–6 weeks
Metoprolol	2.5–5 mg bolus q 5–10 min (max. 3 doses)	12.5–100 mg p.o. b.i.d.
Atenolol	5–10 mg q 5–10 min	25–100 mg p.o. q.d. or b.i.d.[a]
Diltiazem	2.5–5 mg bolus q 10 min ± initiation of IV drip at 5–15 mg/hr	30–90 mg p.o. q.i.d.

[a]Extended release form may be dosed once daily.

artery in nondiabetics (86,87). A purported advantage of use of both internal mammary arteries is a decrease in recurrent angina post-CABG and a decrease in overall cardiac morbidity (86,87). Skeletonization of the internal mammary artery during mobilization rather than creation of a large pedicle may decrease the rate of sternal wound infections (88). Use of bilateral internal mammary arteries with or without skeletonization may still increase the risk of sternal wound complications in high-risk patients such as obese diabetic women, patients with COPD, and in patients undergoing a repeat sternotomy (89,90).

Because diabetes is a significant risk factor for sternal wound infections and because hyperglycemia has a determined effect upon wound healing, investigations of the impact of improved glucose control perioperatively have been performed. Continuous perioperative intravenous infusion of insulin decreased the rate of deep sternal wound infections to 0.8% from 2.0% among patients receiving standard subcutaneous insulin injections ($p = 0.01$) (91). Continuous infusion of insulin has been shown to decrease overall hospital mortality among diabetics undergoing CABG relative to controls (2.5% vs. 5.3%, $p < 0.0001$) (15). One protocol for insulin infusion consists of three regimens—a conservative regimen, a moderate regimen, and an aggressive regimen. The choice of regimen is based on the patient's preoperative insulin dose or oral hypoglycemic agent, recent hemoglobin A1-C level, and most recent preoperative blood glucose level. Depending on the regimen and the blood glucose level, which is monitored every 1 to 2 hours, insulin infusion may range between 0.5 units per hour and 10 units per hour.

Signs and symptoms of chest wound infections include purulent drainage, erythema, sternal instability, fever, and pain. Clinical history and physical examination are frequently diagnostic, although a computed tomography (CT) scan may help delineate the deep extent of the infectious process. Wound cultures should be performed to direct antibiotic therapy. Surgical debridement is invariably necessary. Care must be taken to debride all necrotic sternal tissue or bone and avoid injury to underlying structures, such as the thin-walled right ventricle, which can be adherent to the posterior sternum. Historical management strategies for deep sternal wound infections included sternal wound debridement followed by sternal rewiring using a closed drainage system. However, early coverage of the wound with pectoralis myocutaneous advancement flaps and greater omental transposition into the wound have been associated with a decreased length of stay, mortality, and recurrent infection rate versus the standard approach (92). Coverage of the wound can be performed after adequate debridement of all necrotic or infected tissue, usually within 3 to 5 days. Most patients can be extubated shortly after sternal debridement. After 3 to 5 days of dressing changes, definitive closure of the wound is performed. Patients who present late or have significant sepsis can expect a prolonged ICU and hospital stay and an increased mortality rate.

POSTOPERATIVE MYOCARDIAL ISCHEMIA

Although uncommon after coronary revascularization, myocardial ischemia or infarction (MI) can occur and is frequently difficult to diagnose in the early postoperative period. Postoperative MI is estimated to occur in 1% to 2% of patients undergoing CABG (93). Risk factors for postoperative ischemia include the presence of preoperative unstable angina and increasing bypass time, with a bypass time of >100 minutes associated with a MI rate of 7.7% (93). Off-pump coronary revascularization may be associated with a hypercoagulable state in the early postoperative period requiring aggressive antiplatelet therapy (94,95). Complicated revascularizations, such as those requiring coronary endarterectomy or grafting of small diffusely diseased vessels, may also require aggressive antiplatelet therapy to avoid early graft failure.

The diagnosis of myocardial ischemia in the early postoperative period can be challenging. The presence of Q waves is not associated with significant myocardial tissue damage and is not predictive of early mortality following coronary revascularization (96). Prospective studies have demonstrated that conventional biochemical markers for postoperative infarction, such as CK-MB, troponin T, and troponin I, are unreliable in determining graft occlusion post bypass because there is significant overlap in these values among patients with and without graft occlusion (97). If postoperative infarction or severe ischemia is identified, efforts should be made to evaluate graft function with reexploration or urgent catheterization to identify and correct the cause of ischemia.

Recent evidence supports the use of statin therapy in patients undergoing cardiac surgery. Although no randomized controlled studies have been performed, retrospective reviews have shown that patients receiving lipid-lowering statin medications have decreased adverse cardiac events, including all-cause mortality and stroke in the postoperative period (98–101). Cessation of statin therapy postoperatively has been shown to increase in-hospital mortality in patients who underwent CABG (100). Studies which have separated patients into hyperlipidemic and normolipidemic groups have found that the protective benefit is only found in patients that are hyperlipidemic; therefore use of statin therapy should be targeted to that group (98). Perioperative statin therapy should be given to any hyperlipidemic patient planning to undergo CABG and should not be discontinued in the postoperative period in any patient that is receiving the medication.

COMPLICATIONS OF CONDUIT HARVEST SITES

One of the most frequent sources of complaints following bypass surgery is related to the saphenous vein harvest site. The incidence of leg wound complications following saphenous vein harvesting is 1% to 28%, with variability related to differences in the definition of leg wound complications as well as variations in harvesting techniques (80,82,102–105). Common minor complications include dermatitis, cellulitis, greater saphenous nerve paresthesias, persistent leg swelling, seromas, and lymphoceles. Major leg wound complications requiring additional surgical procedures occur in less than 0.7% of patients, with nonhealing wounds and wound necrosis accounting for the majority (102,106). Risk factors for the development of major leg wound complications include female gender, peripheral vascular disease, and use of an intra-aortic balloon pump (102). These risk factors emphasize the contribution of vasculopathy and peripheral ischemia to the development of complications.

Several techniques are used to harvest the saphenous vein, including a single incision extending over the entire length of the vein, several smaller intermittent incisions with skin bridges, and endoscopic techniques that further limit the extent of incisions. Endoscopic techniques have recently been developed to decrease wound complications associated with standard open techniques. Prospective studies have provided varying results regarding the ability of endoscopic vein harvest techniques to decrease the local wound complication rate compared to standard open techniques (105,107,108). The learning curve, the cost of additional equipment, and the time required for endoscopic harvesting have been limiting factors. The technique does not appear to affect vein quality (109–111). The most important caveats to limiting leg wound complications include identification of at-risk patients and careful handling of tissue with minimization of the dissection necessary to procure the vein.

With improvements in prevention of radial artery spasm and reports of good long-term patency in radial artery grafts, this conduit has been used with increasing frequency for coronary revascularization (112,113). Complications associated with radial artery harvesting have been uncommon, with hand ischemia occurring rarely (114,115). Neurologic complications, including sensation abnormalities of the hand or forearm or decreased thumb strength, have been reported to be as high as 30% among patients in the early postoperative period (116). Longer follow-up has demonstrated that most of these symptoms resolve over time, with donor arm weakness in 0.7% and cutaneous paresthesias in 3.7% of patients 8 weeks postoperatively (116,117). The incidence of neurologic hand complications in one large study ($n = 786$) showed that conventional scalpel and harmonic scalpel techniques had equivalent complication rates (11.2% using the scalpel, 11.0% using the harmonic scalpel, $p > 0.95$) as well as similar resolution rates (9.0% experienced long-term symptoms in both groups). Although long-term discomfort in the hand was low using both techniques, enough patients had neurologic hand symptoms to warrant preoperative discussion of this risk (118).

Risk factors for the development of these complications include diabetes, peripheral vascular disease, smoking history, and elevated serum creatinine levels. Preoperative demonstration of adequate collateral blood supply from the ulnar distribution using an Allen test is adequate for preventing significant ischemic injury with radial artery harvesting. Careful surgical technique with avoidance of injury or traction on the superficial radial nerve may help limit the degree of neurologic injury associated with radial artery harvesting. Newer techniques of endoscopic radial artery harvesting are currently under investigation (119). Good results have been obtained, but risk of neurologic complications must be weighed against improved cosmetic results compared to the open technique (120–122).

COMPLICATIONS RELATED TO HEMOSTASIS

Postoperative bleeding is a significant early complication following CABG. The incidence of reexploration for bleeding is 2% to 4% for isolated coronary revascularization and accounts for the majority of patients requiring reoperation (79,123,124). The most common etiology of bleeding at the time of reoperation is a surgical cause (67%); diffuse bleeding related to coagulopathy accounts for the remaining third (123). Reoperation for bleeding is associated with an inhospital mortality three times higher than for patients not requiring reoperation (124). Reexploration is also associated with a higher rate of postoperative renal failure, prolonged mechanical ventilation, adult respiratory distress syndrome (ARDS), sepsis, atrial arrhythmias, sternal wound infection, and increased length of stay (124,125). Risk factors for reexploration for bleeding include prolonged cardiopulmonary bypass (CPB) time (>150 minutes), older age, smaller body surface area, and increasing number of distal anastomoses (124). Emergent reexploration, occasionally at the bedside, may be necessary in patients who develop postoperative cardiac tamponade. Tamponade occurred in 0.2% of postoperative cardiac patients in 2006; it should be suspected in all patients who develop hypotension or decreased cardiac output (79).

A thorough preoperative history should identify most patients with a bleeding diathesis and allow for diagnostic evaluation and planning. Although aspirin administration has been shown to improve graft patency postoperatively, it is also associated with an increase in postoperative blood loss and transfusion requirements (126–128). Very little can be done to combat this problem preoperatively as almost all patients are on aspirin prior to surgery. Administration of clopidogrel in the preoperative period has also been shown to increase the number of patients requiring reoperation for bleeding, increased red blood cell transfusion, and transfusion of other blood products (129).

Perioperative administration of aprotinin, a protease inhibitor that works to inhibit fibrinolysis, was routinely used postoperatively as it had been shown to decrease the rate of reoperation for bleeding, postoperative chest tube drainage, and requirement for blood transfusions (130–132). Despite its procoagulant effects, aprotinin has been shown to not affect the occurrence of postoperative MI or overall cardiac-related mortality (133). However, data from large scale studies called into question the safety of the medication concerning increased rates of renal failure and death (134,135). Additional studies have refuted those findings, showing no differences in outcomes when adjusting for patient characteristics (136). The subject remains controversial; aprotinin was suspended from the market and is not available for routine use.

Limiting postoperative transfusion requirements is crucial not only because of the need to decrease the morbidity and cost associated with transfusion therapy but also because transfusion of blood products may be an independent predictor of mortality following bypass surgery (137). Other agents that have been shown to decrease bleeding and the requirement for blood transfusions include tranexamic acid and aminocaproic acid (131,138,139). Although these agents may facilitate hemostasis following coronary revascularization, the most important factor is meticulous surgical technique and control of surgical bleeding at the time of operation.

RENAL COMPLICATIONS

There is wide variation in the literature regarding the incidence of postoperative acute renal failure following coronary revascularization. This inconsistency is related to variability in the definition of renal failure, ranging from an isolated increase in serum creatinine to the requirement for dialysis. Acute renal failure, defined as a rise in serum creatinine of at least 1 mg/dL above the baseline, has been reported in 7.9% to 14.9% of patients following revascularization, with an associated mortality of 14% to 21.5% (140,141). According to the STS database (2006), the incidence of acute renal failure requiring dialysis following revascularization is 3.5% (79). Mortality associated with the need for dialysis after coronary bypass surgery has been reported to be as high as 28% (140). Risk factors for the development of renal failure requiring dialysis include elevated preoperative creatinine, increasing duration of cardiopulmonary bypass, cerebrovascular disease, diabetes, advanced age, postoperative hypotension (systolic blood pressure, 90 mm Hg for >1 hour), LV dysfunction, and atherosclerosis of the ascending aorta (140–142). Maintenance of adequate systemic perfusion during and after bypass is the only way to minimize the risk of renal failure following cardiac surgery.

POSTOPERATIVE PULMONARY COMPLICATIONS

Respiratory failure and pulmonary complications are a significant cause of morbidity and mortality among post-CABG patients. Respiratory failure defined as the requirement for mechanical ventilatory support for more than 72 hours occurs in 5.6% of patients undergoing isolated coronary revascularization, with an associated 30-day mortality of 24.3% (143). Preoperative risk factors for prolonged ventilation include unstable angina, COPD, preoperative renal failure, female gender, and age >70 (144). Intraoperative risk factors for respiratory failure include increasing cardiopulmonary bypass time, while postoperative risk factors for respiratory failure include the presence of sepsis, gastrointestinal (GI) bleeding, renal failure, sternal wound infection, postoperative stroke, and reoperation for bleeding (143). The most important intervention to prevent respiratory complications postoperatively is aggressive pulmonary toilet with early ambulation, especially in the elderly.

GASTROINTESTINAL COMPLICATIONS

Although rare, GI complications following coronary revascularization are associated with high morbidity and mortality. GI complications have been reported to occur in 0.7% to 2.1% of patients undergoing coronary revascularization (145–147). The most common complications include GI bleeding, bowel ischemia, and pancreatitis. Other less frequent complications include perforated duodenal ulcer, pseudomembranous colitis, hepatic failure, and cholecystitis. Clostridium difficile associated diarrhea can be a problem in patients, and increasing incidence with increased use of antibiotics has been shown (148). This complication is associated with longer ventilation time as well as both ICU and hospital length of stay. Overall mortality in patients with postoperative GI complications is 34% to 87% (146,147,149). A significant cause of the poor outcomes associated with these complications is that they are often associated with a delay in diagnosis.

One of the most challenging diagnoses to make in the postoperative CABG patient is intestinal ischemia. Mortality for patients developing intestinal ischemia postoperatively is 64% to 80% (146,147,149), and 50% to 90% of cases of postoperative intestinal ischemia are secondary to nonocclusive mesenteric ischemia, with embolic and thrombotic causes accounting for the remainder (149, 150). Early recognition of signs and symptoms is the most essential component in the prevention of the excessive mortality associated with ischemia. The presence of postoperative abdominal pain, bloating, persistent ileus, sepsis, or lower GI bleeding should prompt an early evaluation for ischemia. Unfortunately, many of these patients remain intubated or sedated in the postoperative period, which makes it more difficult to follow the physical examination, thus contributing to a delay in diagnosis. Serum lactate levels may be used as an adjunct to physical exam findings in identifying patients with ischemia; however, it should be noted that serum lactate may be unreliable in identifying patients with early intestinal ischemia and more likely reflects very advanced disease in the setting of high lactate levels. Flexible sigmoidoscopy should be instituted early to identify signs of mucosal ischemia. As with the prevention of renal failure, maintenance of adequate systemic perfusion and cardiac output both intraoperatively and postoperatively allows for better prevention of GI complications.

The cornerstone of treatment involves optimizing perfusion based on the mechanism of ischemia. Vasopressor agents should be discontinued if possible with optimization of the patient's volume status and cardiac function. If necrotic bowel is suspected, prompt surgical intervention is essential, with thromboembolectomy and resection of residual nonviable bowel. Early surgical intervention—defined as performance of laparotomy within 6 hours of the onset of symptoms—has been shown to decrease mortality in patients with postoperative intestinal ischemia (149).

ON-PUMP VERSUS OFF-PUMP CORONARY ARTERY BYPASS SURGERY

A current area of controversy is the impact of off-pump coronary bypass grafting on outcomes in patients requiring revascularization. Although beating-heart coronary revascularization is not a novel concept, newer technology has improved the ability to manipulate the heart while maintaining hemodynamic stability and has improved the ability to stabilize the isolated coronary vessel for performance of distal anastomoses. A central objective of off-pump surgery is to decrease neurologic and neurocognitive complications and to decrease morbidity related to cardiopulmonary bypass. Previous randomized trials comparing outcomes of on-pump and off-pump surgery failed to demonstrate significant differences in postoperative neurologic injury, neurocognitive dysfunction, or overall mortality (38,151–153). More recent studies have shown some improvements in rates of stroke.

Randomized trials with small numbers have shown a decreased level postoperatively of chemical markers of myocardial injury (e.g., troponin I, creatine kinase-MB, myoglobin) in patients undergoing OPCAB versus those who had conventional cardiopulmonary bypass (152,154). The clinical significance of this finding has not been demonstrated directly. Studies have suggested that off-pump surgery may be associated with decreased incidence of postoperative atrial fibrillation, decreased length of hospital stay, and decreased hospital costs versus the use of cardiopulmonary bypass (151–153,155). Other studies have failed to reproduce such benefits (151,153,156–158).

Large retrospective studies have evaluated outcomes comparing on-pump with off-pump CABG. Utilizing the New York State registry, Racz et al. compared 9,135 patients who underwent OPCAB to 59,044 patients who underwent standard CABG with bypass from 1997 to 2000. Their findings showed that in spite of a decrease in stroke rates (1.6% vs. 2.0%, $p = 0.003$) and reoperation for bleeding (1.6% vs. 2.2%, $p < 0.001$), and a shorter length of stay (5 days vs. 6 days, $p < 0.001$) for the OPCAB group, the 3-year survival was better in the conventional on-pump CABG group (89.6% vs. 88.8%, $p = 0.02$) as was the freedom from death or revascularization (84.7% vs. 82.1%, $p > 0.001$). However, these differences in survival and freedom from revascularization disappeared when they analyzed only patients from the most recent 2 years (159).

To evaluate whether the difference in outcome would change after surgeons had gone through the initial technical learning curve of OPCAB, the New York State registry was analyzed further looking at more contemporary patients (2001–2004). More OPCAB surgeries were performed in these latter years; 13,899 patients underwent OPCAB surgery. They were compared to a matched group from 35,941 patients who underwent on-pump CABG (34). There was no difference in three-year survival (90.1% vs. 89.4%, $p = 0.20$); that has been corroborated by other more recent studies (160,161).

Review of the STS database showed a decrease in the risk-adjusted operative mortality from 2.9% with conventional CABG to 2.3% with OPCAB and a decrease in the risk-adjusted major complication rate from 14.2% to 10.6% in 118,140 CABG procedures performed from 1998 to 2000 (162). Results from a more recent large retrospective review of 42,477 patients in the STS database (limited to 63 North American centers which performed at least 100 OPCAB cases/year) in the years 2004–2005 were similar. Multiple logistic regression analysis showed that in the 16,245 patients in the OPCAB group versus the on-pump CABG group the relative risk of death was decreased (RR = 0.83, 95% CI = 0.69–0.98, $p = 0.03$), stroke (RR = 0.65, 95% CI = 0.52–0.80, $p < 0.001$), and MI (RR = 0.67, 95% CI = 0.54–0.84, $p < 0.001$) as well as renal failure, sternal infections, reoperation, atrial fibrillation, and hospital length of stay (35). A group which seems to particularly benefit from the OPCAB technique is the female population: compared to that for on-pump CABG they have shown improved outcomes in death, MI, stroke, renal failure, reoperation rates, postoperative atrial fibrillation, and hospital length of stay (35,163).

One of the purported advantages of off-pump coronary revascularization is the limitation of blood transfusion requirements (152). Off-pump techniques also prove to be very beneficial in patients with a difficult, severely atherosclerotic aorta by allowing for limited or complete avoidance of aortic manipulation (164). Improvements in technology and in individual comfort level with this technique may provide an additional tool for dealing with challenging patients and may have an advantage over on-pump coronary revascularization in selected patients.

SUMMARY

As the use of percutaneous techniques for coronary artery disease becomes more prevalent, the population of patients undergoing CABG has become more complex. Surgical patients are now significantly older and have more comorbidities than historical cohorts. In spite of these factors, improvements in intraoperative and postoperative management and concerted efforts to improve on quality control practices have allowed for improvements in outcomes for patients undergoing coronary revascularization. As acuity continues to rise, it will be even more challenging to deal with the complications associated with surgical coronary revascularization. To meet this challenge, a multidisciplinary approach involving medicine, cardiology, and cardiac surgery will be necessary to improve clinical management and to foster research directed at the treatment of patients with coronary artery disease.

REFERENCES

1. Eagle KA, Guyton RA, Davidoff R, et al. ACC/AHA 2004 Guideline Update for Coronary Artery Bypass Graft Surgery: summary article: a report of the American College of Cardiology/American Heart Association Task Force on Practice Guidelines (Committee to Update the 1999 Guidelines for Coronary Artery Bypass Graft Surgery). *Circulation* 2004;110(9):1168–1176.
2. Niles NW, McGrath PD, Malenka D, et al. Survival of patients with diabetes and multivessel coronary artery disease after surgical or percutaneous coronary revascularization: results of a large regional prospective study. Northern New England Cardiovascular Disease Study Group. *J Am Coll Cardiol* 2001;37(4):1008–1015.
3. Brener SJ, Lytle BW, Casserly IP, et al. Propensity analysis of long-term survival after surgical or percutaneous revascularization in patients with multivessel coronary artery disease and high-risk features. *Circulation* 2004;109(19):2290–2295.
4. Coronary Artery Surgery Study (CASS). A randomized trial of coronary artery bypass surgery. Survival data. *Circulation* 1983;68(5):939–950.
5. Murphy ML, Hultgren HN, Detre K, et al. Treatment of chronic stable angina. A preliminary report of survival data of the randomized Veterans Administration cooperative study. *N Engl J Med* 1977;297(12): 621–627.
6. Varnauskas E. Twelve-year follow-up of survival in the randomized European Coronary Surgery Study. *N Engl J Med* 1988;319(6):332–337.
7. Yusuf S, Zucker D, Peduzzi P, et al. Effect of coronary artery bypass graft surgery on survival: overview of 10-year results from randomised trials by the Coronary Artery Bypass Graft Surgery Trialists Collaboration. *Lancet* 1994;344(8922):563–570.
8. The European Coronary Surgery Study Group. Prospective randomised study of coronary artery bypass surgery in stable angina pectoris. Second interim report. *Lancet* 1980;2(8193):491–495.
9. Hoffman SN, TenBrook JA, Wolf MP, et al. A meta-analysis of randomized controlled trials comparing coronary artery bypass graft with percutaneous transluminal coronary angioplasty: one- to eight-year outcomes. *J Am Coll Cardiol* 2003;41(8):1293–1304.
10. Hannan EL, Racz MJ, Walford G, et al. Long-term outcomes of coronary-artery bypass grafting versus stent implantation. *N Engl J Med* 2005;352(21):2174–2183.
11. DiSesa VJ, O'Brien SM, Welke KF, et al. Contemporary impact of state certificate-of-need regulations for cardiac surgery: an analysis using the Society of Thoracic Surgeons' National Cardiac Surgery Database. *Circulation* 2006;114(20):2122–2129.
12. Prabhakar G, Haan CK, Peterson ED, et al. The risks of moderate and extreme obesity for coronary artery bypass grafting outcomes: a study from the Society of Thoracic Surgeons' database. *Ann Thorac Surg* 2002;74(4):1125–1130; discussion 1130–1131.
13. Lazar HL, Chipkin SR, Fitzgerald CA, et al. Tight glycemic control in diabetic coronary artery bypass graft patients improves perioperative outcomes and decreases recurrent ischemic events. *Circulation* 2004;109(12):1497–1502.
14. van den Berghe G, Wouters P, Weekers F, et al. Intensive insulin therapy in the critically ill patients. *N Engl J Med* 2001;345(19): 1359–1367.
15. Furnary AP, Gao G, Grunkemeier GL, et al. Continuous insulin infusion reduces mortality in patients with diabetes undergoing coronary artery bypass grafting. *J Thorac Cardiovasc Surg* 2003;125(5):1007–1021.
16. Lazar HL, McDonnell M, Chipkin SR, et al. The Society of Thoracic Surgeons practice guideline series: Blood glucose management during adult cardiac surgery. *Ann Thorac Surg* 2009;87(2):663–669.
17. Lipshutz AK, Gropper MA. Perioperative glycemic control: an evidence-based review. *Anesthesiology* 2009;110(2):408–421.
18. Ferguson TB Jr, Hammill BG, Peterson ED, et al. A decade of change–risk profiles and outcomes for isolated coronary artery bypass grafting procedures, 1990–1999: a report from the STS National Database Committee and the Duke Clinical Research Institute. Society of Thoracic Surgeons. *Ann Thorac Surg* 2002;73(2):480–489; discussion 489–490.
19. John R, Choudhri AF, Weinberg AD, et al. Multicenter review of preoperative risk factors for stroke after coronary artery bypass grafting. *Ann Thorac Surg* 2000;69(1):30–35; discussion 35–36.
20. Puskas JD, Winston AD, Wright CE, et al. Stroke after coronary artery operation: incidence, correlates, outcome, and cost. *Ann Thorac Surg* 2000;69(4):1053–1056.
21. McKhann GM, Grega MA, Borowicz LM Jr, et al. Encephalopathy and stroke after coronary artery bypass grafting: incidence, consequences, and prediction. *Arch Neurol* 2002;59(9):1422–1428.
22. Almassi GH, Sommers T, Moritz TE, et al. Stroke in cardiac surgical patients: determinants and outcome. *Ann Thorac Surg* 1999;68(2): 391–397; discussion 397–398.
23. Gardner TJ, Horneffer PJ, Manolio TA, et al. Stroke following coronary artery bypass grafting: a ten-year study. *Ann Thorac Surg* 1985;40(6):574–581.
24. Barbut D, Lo YW, Hartman GS, et al. Aortic atheroma is related to outcome but not numbers of emboli during coronary bypass. *Ann Thorac Surg* 1997;64(2):454–459.
25. Barbut D, Lo YW, Gold JP, et al. Impact of embolization during coronary artery bypass grafting on outcome and length of stay. *Ann Thorac Surg* 1997;63(4):998–1002.
26. Calafiore AM, Di Mauro M, Teodori G, et al. Impact of aortic manipulation on incidence of cerebrovascular accidents after surgical myocardial revascularization. *Ann Thorac Surg* 2002;73(5):1387–1393.
27. Salazar JD, Wityk RJ, Grega MA, et al. Stroke after cardiac surgery: short- and long-term outcomes. *Ann Thorac Surg* 2001;72(4):1195–1201; discussion 1201–1202.
28. Davila-Roman VG, Barzilai B, Wareing TH, et al. Intraoperative ultrasonographic evaluation of the ascending aorta in 100 consecutive patients undergoing cardiac surgery. *Circulation* 1991;84(5 Suppl): III47–III53.
29. Mills NL, Everson CT. Atherosclerosis of the ascending aorta and coronary artery bypass. Pathology, clinical correlates, and operative management. *J Thorac Cardiovasc Surg* 1991;102(4):546–553.
30. Royse AG, Royse CF, Ajani AE, et al. Reduced neuropsychological dysfunction using epiaortic echocardiography and the exclusive Y graft. *Ann Thorac Surg* 2000;69(5):1431–1438.
31. Wareing TH, Davila-Roman VG, Daily BB, et al. Strategy for the reduction of stroke incidence in cardiac surgical patients. *Ann Thorac Surg* 1993;55(6):1400–1407; discussion 1407–1408.
32. Banbury MK, Kouchoukos NT, Allen KB, et al. Emboli capture using the Embol-X intraaortic filter in cardiac surgery: a multicentered randomized trial of 1,289 patients. *Ann Thorac Surg* 2003;76(2):508–515; discussion 515.
33. Harringer W. Capture of particulate emboli during cardiac procedures in which aortic cross-clamp is used. International Council of Emboli Management Study Group. *Ann Thorac Surg* 2000;70(3):1119–1123.
34. Hannan EL, Wu C, Smith CR, et al. Off-pump versus on-pump coronary artery bypass graft surgery: differences in short-term outcomes and in long-term mortality and need for subsequent revascularization. *Circulation* 2007;116(10):1145–1152.
35. Puskas JD, Edwards FH, Pappas PA, et al. Off-pump techniques benefit men and women and narrow the disparity in mortality after coronary bypass grafting. *Ann Thorac Surg* 2007;84(5):1447–1454; discussion 1454–1456.
36. Roach GW, Kanchuger M, Mangano CM, et al. Adverse cerebral outcomes after coronary bypass surgery. Multicenter Study of Perioperative Ischemia Research Group and the Ischemia Research and Education Foundation Investigators. *N Engl J Med* 1996;335(25): 1857–1863.
37. van Dijk D, Keizer AM, Diephuis JC, et al. Neurocognitive dysfunction after coronary artery bypass surgery: a systematic review. *J Thorac Cardiovasc Surg* 2000;120(4):632–639.
38. Van Dijk D, Jansen EW, Hijman R, et al. Cognitive outcome after off-pump and on-pump coronary artery bypass graft surgery: a randomized trial. *JAMA* 2002;287(11):1405–1412.
39. Kilo J, Czerny M, Gorlitzer M, et al. Cardiopulmonary bypass affects cognitive brain function after coronary artery bypass grafting. *Ann Thorac Surg* 2001;72(6):1926–1932.
40. Hernandez F Jr, Brown JR, Likosky DS, et al. Neurocognitive outcomes of off-pump versus on-pump coronary artery bypass: a prospective randomized controlled trial. *Ann Thorac Surg* 2007;84(6): 1897–1903.
41. Aranki SF, Shaw DP, Adams DH, et al. Predictors of atrial fibrillation after coronary artery surgery. Current trends and impact on hospital resources. *Circulation* 1996;94(3):390–397.

42. Borzak S, Tisdale JE, Amin NB, et al. Atrial fibrillation after bypass surgery: does the arrhythmia or the characteristics of the patients prolong hospital stay? *Chest* 1998;113(6):1489–1491.
43. Mathew JP, Parks R, Savino JS, et al. Atrial fibrillation following coronary artery bypass graft surgery: predictors, outcomes, and resource utilization. MultiCenter Study of Perioperative Ischemia Research Group. *JAMA* 1996;276(4):300–306.
44. Shore-Lesserson L, Moskowitz D, Hametz C, et al. Use of intraoperative transesophageal echocardiography to predict atrial fibrillation after coronary artery bypass grafting. *Anesthesiology* 2001;95(3):652–658.
45. Ducceschi V, D'Andrea A, Liccardo B, et al. Perioperative clinical predictors of atrial fibrillation occurrence following coronary artery surgery. *Eur J Cardiothorac Surg* 1999;16(4):435–439.
46. Almassi GH, Schowalter T, Nicolosi AC, et al. Atrial fibrillation after cardiac surgery: a major morbid event? *Ann Surg* 1997;226(4):501–511; discussion 511–513.
47. Creswell LL, Schuessler RB, Rosenbloom M, et al. Hazards of postoperative atrial arrhythmias. *Ann Thorac Surg* 1993;56(3):539–549.
48. Lahey SJ, Campos CT, Jennings B, et al. Hospital readmission after cardiac surgery. Does "fast track" cardiac surgery result in cost saving or cost shifting? *Circulation* 1998;98(19 Suppl):II35–II40.
49. Guarnieri T, Nolan S, Gottlieb SO, et al. Intravenous amiodarone for the prevention of atrial fibrillation after open heart surgery: the Amiodarone Reduction in Coronary Heart (ARCH) trial. *J Am Coll Cardiol* 1999;34(2):343–347.
50. Daoud EG, Strickberger SA, Man KC, et al. Preoperative amiodarone as prophylaxis against atrial fibrillation after heart surgery. *N Engl J Med* 1997;337(25):1785–1791.
51. Dorge H, Schoendube FA, Schoberer M, et al. Intraoperative amiodarone as prophylaxis against atrial fibrillation after coronary operations. *Ann Thorac Surg* 2000;69(5):1358–1362.
52. Redle JD, Khurana S, Marzan R, et al. Prophylactic oral amiodarone compared with placebo for prevention of atrial fibrillation after coronary artery bypass surgery. *Am Heart J* 1999;138(1 Pt 1):144–150.
53. Crystal E, Connolly SJ, Sleik K, et al. Interventions on prevention of postoperative atrial fibrillation in patients undergoing heart surgery: a meta-analysis. *Circulation* 2002;106(1):75–80.
54. Connolly SJ, Cybulsky I, Lamy A, et al. Double-blind, placebo-controlled, randomized trial of prophylactic metoprolol for reduction of hospital length of stay after heart surgery: the Beta-Blocker Length Of Stay (BLOS) study. *Am Heart J* 2003;145(2):226–232.
55. Lee SH, Chang CM, Lu MJ, et al. Intravenous amiodarone for prevention of atrial fibrillation after coronary artery bypass grafting. *Ann Thorac Surg* 2000;70(1):157–161.
56. Yagdi T, Nalbantgil S, Ayik F, et al. Amiodarone reduces the incidence of atrial fibrillation after coronary artery bypass grafting. *J Thorac Cardiovasc Surg* 2003;125(6):1420–1425.
57. Seitelberger R, Hannes W, Gleichauf M, et al. Effects of diltiazem on perioperative ischemia, arrhythmias, and myocardial function in patients undergoing elective coronary bypass grafting. *J Thorac Cardiovasc Surg* 1994;107(3):811–821.
58. Kowey PR, Taylor JE, Rials SJ, et al. Meta-analysis of the effectiveness of prophylactic drug therapy in preventing supraventricular arrhythmia early after coronary artery bypass grafting. *Am J Cardiol* 1992; 69(9):963–965.
59. Podesser B, Schwarzacher S, Zwolfer W, et al. Combined perioperative infusion of nifedipine and metoprolol provides antiischemic and antiarrhythmic protection in patients undergoing elective aortocoronary bypass surgery. *Thorac Cardiovasc Surg* 1993;41(3):173–179.
60. Toraman F, Karabulut EH, Alhan HC, et al. Magnesium infusion dramatically decreases the incidence of atrial fibrillation after coronary artery bypass grafting. *Ann Thorac Surg* 2001;72(4):1256–1261; discussion 1261–1262.
61. Speziale G, Ruvolo G, Fattouch K, et al. Arrhythmia prophylaxis after coronary artery bypass grafting: regimens of magnesium sulfate administration. *Thorac Cardiovasc Surg* 2000;48(1):22–26.
62. Parikka H, Toivonen L, Pellinen T, et al. The influence of intravenous magnesium sulphate on the occurrence of atrial fibrillation after coronary artery by-pass operation. *Eur Heart J* 1993;14(2):251–258.
63. Kaplan M, Kut MS, Icer UA, et al. Intravenous magnesium sulfate prophylaxis for atrial fibrillation after coronary artery bypass surgery. *J Thorac Cardiovasc Surg* 2003;125(2):344–352.
64. Daoud EG, Dabir R, Archambeau M, et al. Randomized, double-blind trial of simultaneous right and left atrial epicardial pacing for prevention of post-open heart surgery atrial fibrillation. *Circulation* 2000; 102(7):761–765.
65. Fan K, Lee KL, Chiu CS, et al. Effects of biatrial pacing in prevention of postoperative atrial fibrillation after coronary artery bypass surgery. *Circulation* 2000;102(7):755–760.
66. Greenberg MD, Katz NM, Iuliano S, et al. Atrial pacing for the prevention of atrial fibrillation after cardiovascular surgery. *J Am Coll Cardiol* 2000;35(6):1416–1422.
67. Levy T, Fotopoulos G, Walker S, et al. Randomized controlled study investigating the effect of biatrial pacing in prevention of atrial fibrillation after coronary artery bypass grafting. *Circulation* 2000;102(12): 1382–1387.
68. Cochrane AD, Siddins M, Rosenfeldt FL, et al. A comparison of amiodarone and digoxin for treatment of supraventricular arrhythmias after cardiac surgery. *Eur J Cardiothorac Surg* 1994;8(4):194–198.
69. Di Biasi P, Scrofani R, Paje A, et al. Intravenous amiodarone vs propafenone for atrial fibrillation and flutter after cardiac operation. *Eur J Cardiothorac Surg* 1995;9(10):587–591.
70. Galve E, Rius T, Ballester R, et al. Intravenous amiodarone in treatment of recent-onset atrial fibrillation: results of a randomized, controlled study. *J Am Coll Cardiol* 1996;27(5):1079–1082.
71. Campbell TJ, Gavaghan TP, Morgan JJ. Intravenous sotalol for the treatment of atrial fibrillation and flutter after cardiopulmonary bypass. Comparison with disopyramide and digoxin in a randomised trial. *Br Heart J* 1985;54(1):86–90.
72. Costeas C, Kassotis J, Blitzer M, et al. Rhythm management in atrial fibrillation–with a primary emphasis on pharmacological therapy: Part 2. *Pacing Clin Electrophysiol* 1998;21(4, Pt 1):742–752.
73. Dimopoulou I, Marathias K, Daganou M, et al. Low-dose amiodarone-related complications after cardiac operations. *J Thorac Cardiovasc Surg* 1997;114(1):31–37.
74. Liebold A, Haisch G, Rosada B, et al. Internal atrial defibrillation – a new treatment of postoperative atrial fibrillation. *Thorac Cardiovasc Surg* 1998;46(6):323–326.
75. Petersen P, Boysen G, Godtfredsen J, et al. Placebo-controlled, randomised trial of warfarin and aspirin for prevention of thromboembolic complications in chronic atrial fibrillation. The Copenhagen AFASAK study. *Lancet* 1989;1(8631):175–179.
76. The Boston Area Anticoagulation Trial for Atrial Fibrillation Investigators. The effect of low-dose warfarin on the risk of stroke in patients with nonrheumatic atrial fibrillation. *N Engl J Med* 1990;323(22): 1505–1511.
77. Arnold AZ, Mick MJ, Mazurek RP, et al. Role of prophylactic anticoagulation for direct current cardioversion in patients with atrial fibrillation or atrial flutter. *J Am Coll Cardiol* 1992;19(4):851–855.
78. Bjerkelund CJ, Orning OM. The efficacy of anticoagulant therapy in preventing embolism related to D.C. electrical conversion of atrial fibrillation. *Am J Cardiol* 1969;23(2):208–216.
79. Society of Thoracic Surgeons. STS NCD Executive Summary Spring 2007. STS Web site. Available at: http:/www.sts.org/sections/stsnationaldatabase/publications/executive/article.html
80. Slaughter MS, Olson MM, Lee JT Jr, et al. A fifteen-year wound surveillance study after coronary artery bypass. *Ann Thorac Surg* 1993;56(5): 1063–1068.
81. Olsen MA, Lock-Buckley P, Hopkins D, et al. The risk factors for deep and superficial chest surgical-site infections after coronary artery bypass graft surgery are different. *J Thorac Cardiovasc Surg* 2002;124(1): 136–145.
82. L'Ecuyer PB, Murphy D, Little JR, et al. The epidemiology of chest and leg wound infections following cardiothoracic surgery. *Clin Infect Dis* 1996;22(3):424–429.
83. Lu JC, Grayson AD, Jha P, et al. Risk factors for sternal wound infection and mid-term survival following coronary artery bypass surgery. *Eur J Cardiothorac Surg* 2003;23(6):943–949.
84. Borger MA, Rao V, Weisel RD, et al. Deep sternal wound infection: risk factors and outcomes. *Ann Thorac Surg* 1998;65(4):1050–1056.
85. The Parisian Mediastinitis Study Group. Risk factors for deep sternal wound infection after sternotomy: a prospective, multicenter study. *J Thorac Cardiovasc Surg* 1996;111(6):1200–1207.
86. Buxton BF, Komeda M, Fuller JA, et al. Bilateral internal thoracic artery grafting may improve outcome of coronary artery surgery. Risk-adjusted survival. *Circulation* 1998;98(19, Suppl):II1–II6.
87. Lev-Ran O, Mohr R, Amir K, et al. Bilateral internal thoracic artery grafting in insulin-treated diabetics: should it be avoided? *Ann Thorac Surg* 2003;75(6):1872–1877.
88. Sofer D, Gurevitch J, Shapira I, et al. Sternal wound infections in patients after coronary artery bypass grafting using bilateral skeletonized internal mammary arteries. *Ann Surg* 1999;229(4):585–590.

89. Pevni D, Mohr R, Lev-Run O, et al. Influence of bilateral skeletonized harvesting on occurrence of deep sternal wound infection in 1,000 consecutive patients undergoing bilateral internal thoracic artery grafting. *Ann Surg* 2003;237(2):277–280.
90. Matsa M, Paz Y, Gurevitch J, et al. Bilateral skeletonized internal thoracic artery grafts in patients with diabetes mellitus. *J Thorac Cardiovasc Surg* 2001;121(4):668–674.
91. Furnary AP, Zerr KJ, Grunkemeier GL, et al. Continuous intravenous insulin infusion reduces the incidence of deep sternal wound infection in diabetic patients after cardiac surgical procedures. *Ann Thorac Surg* 1999;67(2):352–360; discussion 360–362.
92. Brandt C, Alvarez JM. First-line treatment of deep sternal infection by a plastic surgical approach: superior results compared with conventional cardiac surgical orthodoxy. *Plast Reconstr Surg* 2002;109(7): 2231–2237.
93. Iyer VS, Russell WJ, Leppard P, et al. Mortality and myocardial infarction after coronary artery surgery. A review of 12,003 patients. *Med J Aust* 1993;159(3):166–170.
94. Cartier R, Robitaille D. Thrombotic complications in beating heart operations. *J Thorac Cardiovasc Surg* 2001;121(5):920–922.
95. Mariani MA, Gu YJ, Boonstra PW, et al. Procoagulant activity after off-pump coronary operation: is the current anticoagulation adequate? *Ann Thorac Surg* 1999;67(5):1370–1375.
96. Svedjeholm R, Dahlin LG, Lundberg C, et al. Are electrocardiographic Q-wave criteria reliable for diagnosis of perioperative myocardial infarction after coronary surgery? *Eur J Cardiothorac Surg* 1998;13(6): 655–661.
97. Holmvang L, Jurlander B, Rasmussen C, et al. Use of biochemical markers of infarction for diagnosing perioperative myocardial infarction and early graft occlusion after coronary artery bypass surgery. *Chest* 2002;121(1):103–111.
98. Thielmann M, Neuhauser M, Marr A, et al. Lipid-lowering effect of preoperative statin therapy on postoperative major adverse cardiac events after coronary artery bypass surgery. *J Thorac Cardiovasc Surg* 2007;134(5):1143–1149.
99. Pan W, Pintar T, Anton J, et al. Statins are associated with a reduced incidence of perioperative mortality after coronary artery bypass graft surgery. *Circulation* 2004;110(11 Suppl 1):II45–II49.
100. Collard CD, Body SC, Shernan SK, et al. Preoperative statin therapy is associated with reduced cardiac mortality after coronary artery bypass graft surgery. *J Thorac Cardiovasc Surg* 2006;132(2): 392–400.
101. Ouattara A, Benhaoua H, Le Manach Y, et al. Perioperative statin therapy is associated with a significant and dose-dependent reduction of adverse cardiovascular outcomes after coronary artery bypass graft surgery. *J Cardiothorac Vasc Anesth* 2009;23(5):633–638.
102. Paletta CE, Huang DB, Fiore AC, et al. Major leg wound complications after saphenous vein harvest for coronary revascularization. *Ann Thorac Surg* 2000;70(2):492–497.
103. Utley JR, Thomason ME, Wallace DJ, et al. Preoperative correlates of impaired wound healing after saphenous vein excision. *J Thorac Cardiovasc Surg* 1989;98(1):147–149.
104. Garland R, Frizelle FA, Dobbs BR, et al. A retrospective audit of long-term lower limb complications following leg vein harvesting for coronary artery bypass grafting. *Eur J Cardiothorac Surg* 2003;23(6):950–955.
105. Bitondo JM, Daggett WM, Torchiana DF, et al. Endoscopic versus open saphenous vein harvest: a comparison of postoperative wound complications. *Ann Thorac Surg* 2002;73(2):523–528.
106. DeLaria GA, Hunter JA, Goldin MD, et al. Leg wound complications associated with coronary revascularization. *J Thorac Cardiovasc Surg* 1981;81(3):403–407.
107. Puskas JD, Wright CE, Miller PK, et al. A randomized trial of endoscopic versus open saphenous vein harvest in coronary bypass surgery. *Ann Thorac Surg* 1999;68(4):1509–1512.
108. Schurr UP, Lachat ML, Reuthebuch O, et al. Endoscopic saphenous vein harvesting for CABG – a randomized, prospective trial. *Thorac Cardiovasc Surg* 2002;50(3):160–163.
109. Crouch JD, O'Hair DP, Keuler JP, et al. Open versus endoscopic saphenous vein harvesting: wound complications and vein quality. *Ann Thorac Surg* 1999;68(4):1513–1516.
110. Griffith GL, Allen KB, Waller BF, et al. Endoscopic and traditional saphenous vein harvest: a histologic comparison. *Ann Thorac Surg* 2000;69(2):520–523.
111. Meyer DM, Rogers TE, Jessen ME, et al. Histologic evidence of the safety of endoscopic saphenous vein graft preparation. *Ann Thorac Surg* 2000;70(2):487–491.
112. Acar C, Ramsheyi A, Pagny JY, et al. The radial artery for coronary artery bypass grafting: clinical and angiographic results at five years. *J Thorac Cardiovasc Surg* 1998;116(6):981–989.
113. Maniar HS, Barner HB, Bailey MS, et al. Radial artery patency: are aortocoronary conduits superior to composite grafting? *Ann Thorac Surg* 2003;76(5):1498–1503; discussion 1503–1504.
114. Dumanian GA, Segalman K, Mispireta LA, et al. Radial artery use in bypass grafting does not change digital blood flow or hand function. *Ann Thorac Surg* 1998;65(5):1284–1287.
115. Serricchio M, Gaudino M, Tondi P, et al. Hemodynamic and functional consequences of radial artery removal for coronary artery bypass grafting. *Am J Cardiol* 1999;84(11):1353–1356, A8.
116. Denton TA, Trento L, Cohen M, et al. Radial artery harvesting for coronary bypass operations: neurologic complications and their potential mechanisms. *J Thorac Cardiovasc Surg* 2001;121(5):951–956.
117. Budillon AM, Nicolini F, Agostinelli A, et al. Complications after radial artery harvesting for coronary artery bypass grafting: our experience. *Surgery* 2003;133(3):283–287.
118. Moon MR, Barner HB, Bailey MS, et al. Long-term neurologic hand complications after radial artery harvesting using conventional cold and harmonic scalpel techniques. *Ann Thorac Surg* 2004;78(2):535–538; discussion 535–538.
119. Connolly MW, Torrillo LD, Stauder MJ, et al. Endoscopic radial artery harvesting: results of first 300 patients. *Ann Thorac Surg* 2002;74(2): 502–505; discussion 506.
120. Patel AN, Henry AC, Hunnicutt C, et al. Endoscopic radial artery harvesting is better than the open technique. *Ann Thorac Surg* 2004; 78(1):149–153; discussion 149–153.
121. Bleiziffer S, Hettich I, Eisenhauer B, et al. Neurologic sequelae of the donor arm after endoscopic versus conventional radial artery harvesting. *J Thorac Cardiovasc Surg* 2008;136(3):681–687.
122. Kim G, Jeong Y, Cho Y, et al. Endoscopic radial artery harvesting may be the procedure of choice for coronary artery bypass grafting. *Circ J* 2007;71(10):1511–1515.
123. Hall TS, Brevetti GR, Skoultchi AJ, et al. Re-exploration for hemorrhage following open heart surgery differentiation on the causes of bleeding and the impact on patient outcomes. *Ann Thorac Cardiovasc Surg* 2001;7(6):352–357.
124. Dacey LJ, Munoz JJ, Baribeau YR, et al. Reexploration for hemorrhage following coronary artery bypass grafting: incidence and risk factors. Northern New England Cardiovascular Disease Study Group. *Arch Surg* 1998;133(4):442–447.
125. Moulton MJ, Creswell LL, Mackey ME, et al. Reexploration for bleeding is a risk factor for adverse outcomes after cardiac operations. *J Thorac Cardiovasc Surg* 1996;111(5):1037–1046.
126. Verstraete M, Brown BG, Chesebro JH, et al. Evaluation of antiplatelet agents in the prevention of aorto-coronary bypass occlusion. *Eur Heart J* 1986;7(1):4–13.
127. Kallis P, Tooze JA, Talbot S, et al. Pre-operative aspirin decreases platelet aggregation and increases post-operative blood loss–a prospective, randomised, placebo controlled, double-blind clinical trial in 100 patients with chronic stable angina. *Eur J Cardiothorac Surg* 1994;8(8):404–409.
128. Ferraris VA, Ferraris SP, Joseph O, et al. Aspirin and postoperative bleeding after coronary artery bypass grafting. *Ann Surg* 2002;235(6): 820–827.
129. Yende S, Wunderink RG. Effect of clopidogrel on bleeding after coronary artery bypass surgery. *Crit Care Med* 2001;29(12):2271–2275.
130. Murkin JM, Lux J, Shannon NA, et al. Aprotinin significantly decreases bleeding and transfusion requirements in patients receiving aspirin and undergoing cardiac operations. *J Thorac Cardiovasc Surg* 1994;107(2):554–561.
131. Laupacis A, Fergusson D. Drugs to minimize perioperative blood loss in cardiac surgery: meta-analyses using perioperative blood transfusion as the outcome. The International Study of Peri-operative Transfusion (ISPOT) Investigators. *Anesth Analg* 1997;85(6): 1258–1267.
132. Alvarez JM, Jackson LR, Chatwin C, et al. Low-dose postoperative aprotinin reduces mediastinal drainage and blood product use in patients undergoing primary coronary artery bypass grafting who are taking aspirin: a prospective, randomized, double-blind, placebo-controlled trial. *J Thorac Cardiovasc Surg* 2001;122(3):457–463.
133. Alderman EL, Levy JH, Rich JB, et al. Analyses of coronary graft patency after aprotinin use: results from the International Multicenter Aprotinin Graft Patency Experience (IMAGE) trial. *J Thorac Cardiovasc Surg* 1998;116(5):716–730.

134. Shaw AD, Stafford-Smith M, White WD, et al. The effect of aprotinin on outcome after coronary-artery bypass grafting. *N Engl J Med* 2008;358(8):784–793.
135. Schneeweiss S, Seeger JD, Landon J, et al. Aprotinin during coronary-artery bypass grafting and risk of death. *N Engl J Med* 2008;358(8):771–783.
136. Ngaage DL, Cale AR, Cowen ME, et al. Aprotinin in primary cardiac surgery: operative outcome of propensity score-matched study. *Ann Thorac Surg* 2008;86(4):1195–1202.
137. Engoren MC, Habib RH, Zacharias A, et al. Effect of blood transfusion on long-term survival after cardiac operation. *Ann Thorac Surg* 2002;74(4):1180–1186.
138. Mongan PD, Brown RS, Thwaites BK. Tranexamic acid and aprotinin reduce postoperative bleeding and transfusions during primary coronary revascularization. *Anesth Analg* 1998;87(2):258–265.
139. Bernet F, Carrel T, Marbet G, et al. Reduction of blood loss and transfusion requirements after coronary artery bypass grafting: similar efficacy of tranexamic acid and aprotinin in aspirin-treated patients. *J Card Surg* 1999;14(2):92–97.
140. Conlon PJ, Stafford-Smith M, White WD, et al. Acute renal failure following cardiac surgery. *Nephrol Dial Transplant* 1999;14(5):1158–1162.
141. Suen WS, Mok CK, Chiu SW, et al. Risk factors for development of acute renal failure (ARF) requiring dialysis in patients undergoing cardiac surgery. *Angiology* 1998;49(10):789–800.
142. Davila-Roman VG, Kouchoukos NT, Schechtman KB, et al. Atherosclerosis of the ascending aorta is a predictor of renal dysfunction after cardiac operations. *J Thorac Cardiovasc Surg* 1999;117(1):111–116.
143. Canver CC, Chanda J. Intraoperative and postoperative risk factors for respiratory failure after coronary bypass. *Ann Thorac Surg* 2003;75(3):853–857; discussion 857–858.
144. Legare JF, Hirsch GM, Buth KJ, et al. Preoperative prediction of prolonged mechanical ventilation following coronary artery bypass grafting. *Eur J Cardiothorac Surg* 2001;20(5):930–936.
145. Perugini RA, Orr RK, Porter D, et al. Gastrointestinal complications following cardiac surgery. An analysis of 1477 cardiac surgery patients. *Arch Surg* 1997;132(4):352–357.
146. Byhahn C, Strouhal U, Martens S, et al. Incidence of gastrointestinal complications in cardiopulmonary bypass patients. *World J Surg* 2001;25(9):1140–1144.
147. Huddy SP, Joyce WP, Pepper JR. Gastrointestinal complications in 4473 patients who underwent cardiopulmonary bypass surgery. *Br J Surg* 1991;78(3):293–296.
148. Crabtree T, Aitchison D, Meyers BF, et al. Clostridium difficile in cardiac surgery: risk factors and impact on postoperative outcome. *Ann Thorac Surg* 2007;83(4):1396–1402.
149. Ghosh S, Roberts N, Firmin RK, et al. Risk factors for intestinal ischaemia in cardiac surgical patients. *Eur J Cardiothorac Surg* 2002;21(3):411–416.
150. Pinson CW, Alberty RE. General surgical complications after cardiopulmonary bypass surgery. *Am J Surg* 1983;146(1):133–137.
151. Angelini GD, Taylor FC, Reeves BC, et al. Early and midterm outcome after off-pump and on-pump surgery in Beating Heart Against Cardioplegic Arrest Studies (BHACAS 1 and 2): a pooled analysis of two randomised controlled trials. *Lancet* 2002;359(9313):1194–1199.
152. Puskas JD, Williams WH, Duke PG, et al. Off-pump coronary artery bypass grafting provides complete revascularization with reduced myocardial injury, transfusion requirements, and length of stay: a prospective randomized comparison of two hundred unselected patients undergoing off-pump versus conventional coronary artery bypass grafting. *J Thorac Cardiovasc Surg* 2003;125(4):797–808.
153. Nathoe HM, van Dijk D, Jansen EW, et al. A comparison of on-pump and off-pump coronary bypass surgery in low-risk patients. *N Engl J Med* 2003;348(5):394–402.
154. Chowdhury UK, Malik V, Yadav R, et al. Myocardial injury in coronary artery bypass grafting: on-pump versus off-pump comparison by measuring high-sensitivity C-reactive protein, cardiac troponin I, heart-type fatty acid-binding protein, creatine kinase-MB, and myoglobin release. *J Thorac Cardiovasc Surg* 2008;135(5):1110–1119, 1119.e1–e10.
155. Ascione R, Caputo M, Calori G, et al. Predictors of atrial fibrillation after conventional and beating heart coronary surgery: A prospective, randomized study. *Circulation* 2000;102(13):1530–1535.
156. van Dijk D, Nierich AP, Jansen EW, et al. Early outcome after off-pump versus on-pump coronary bypass surgery: results from a randomized study. *Circulation* 2001;104(15):1761–1766.
157. Bull DA, Neumayer LA, Stringham JC, et al. Coronary artery bypass grafting with cardiopulmonary bypass versus off-pump cardiopulmonary bypass grafting: does eliminating the pump reduce morbidity and cost? *Ann Thorac Surg* 2001;71(1):170–173; discussion 173–175.
158. Shennib H, Endo M, Benhamed O, et al. Surgical revascularization in patients with poor left ventricular function: on- or off-pump? *Ann Thorac Surg* 2002;74(4):S1344–S1347.
159. Racz MJ, Hannan EL, Isom OW, et al. A comparison of short- and long-term outcomes after off-pump and on-pump coronary artery bypass graft surgery with sternotomy. *J Am Coll Cardiol* 2004;43(4):557–564.
160. Sabik JF, Blackstone EH, Lytle BW, et al. Equivalent midterm outcomes after off-pump and on-pump coronary surgery. *J Thorac Cardiovasc Surg* 2004;127(1):142–148.
161. Sedrakyan A, Wu AW, Parashar A, et al. Off-pump surgery is associated with reduced occurrence of stroke and other morbidity as compared with traditional coronary artery bypass grafting: a meta-analysis of systematically reviewed trials. *Stroke* 2006;37(11):2759–2769.
162. Cleveland JC Jr, Shroyer AL, Chen AY, et al. Off-pump coronary artery bypass grafting decreases risk-adjusted mortality and morbidity. *Ann Thorac Surg* 2001;72(4):1282–1288; discussion 1288–1289.
163. Puskas JD, Kilgo PD, Kutner M, et al. Off-pump techniques disproportionately benefit women and narrow the gender disparity in outcomes after coronary artery bypass surgery. *Circulation* 2007;116(11 Suppl):I192–I199.
164. Sharony R, Grossi EA, Saunders PC, et al. Propensity case-matched analysis of off-pump coronary artery bypass grafting in patients with atheromatous aortic disease. *J Thorac Cardiovasc Surg* 2004;127(2):406–413.

CHAPTER

28

Complications in Valvular Cardiac Surgery

Gorav Ailawadi

INTRODUCTION

More than 100,000 operations for cardiac valve repair or replacement are performed in the United States, and more than 1 million valve operations are performed worldwide each year. The earliest valve surgery, closed mitral valvotomy, was performed through a thoracotomy without the use of cardiopulmonary bypass. With the advent of the cardiopulmonary bypass circuit, marked improvements have been made in the surgical treatment of patients with valvular heart disease. Improvements in cardiac protection, prosthetic (mechanical and bioprosthetic) heart valves, and valve reconstructive/repair techniques all have contributed to improved outcomes (1,2). In addition, the widespread use of intraoperative transesophageal echocardiography (TEE) and updated guidelines for timing of surgical intervention have further standardized outcomes related to valve surgery (1,2). The recognition of complications related specifically to valvular surgery has led to the greatest improvement in valvular surgery outcomes (Table 28.1).

PROSTHETIC HEART VALVES

The prosthetic valves available today are of two primary categories: bioprosthetic (biologic tissue) and mechanical valves. Tissue valves include porcine (stented and stentless) and pericardial (bovine or equine) valves. In addition to prosthetic valves, allografts (human cadaveric homografts) and autografts (pulmonic valve) can be used in either the aortic or the mitral position (3). The mechanical prostheses include single tilting disc and bileaflet valves.

Bioprosthetic valves

A significant advantage of tissue valves is the avoidance of the need for lifelong anticoagulation. These valves have a very low thromboembolic complication rate; however, risk does exist in patients with atrial fibrillation or with an enlarged left atrium, a history of previous emboli, an atrial clot, or significantly reduced left ventricular (LV) function. These patients should be *considered* for anticoagulation therapy despite having a tissue prosthesis. Structural valve degeneration eventually leading to valve failure is the most important long-term complication of the bioprosthetic valve. The risk of valve failure increases over time, and this rate is accelerated in both younger patients and those on chronic dialysis. The probability of structural failure with currently available porcine and bovine pericardial valves increases beginning at approximately 10 to 12 years after operation. The life expectancy of these valves, with new anticalcification fixation techniques is thought to be in the 15 to 20 year range (4–8).

Mechanical valves

Mechanical valves have the potential for indefinite long-term durability but have increased risk of thromboembolism and the risk of bleeding secondary to the need for anticoagulation (9). Rates of thrombotic complications are low (1% to 3%) when the patients are adequately anticoagulated. However, anticoagulation-related bleeding remains one of the most common causes of valve-related morbidity (1% to 3% per patient-year) and mortality (0.1% to 0.5% per patient-year), as safe, stable, and effective anticoagulation is often difficult to achieve (10). Ongoing trials are underway, evaluating the use of aspirin alone in patients with mechanical valves.

Prosthetic valve endocarditis

Prosthetic heart valves carry an increased risk for the development of endocarditis that can be precipitated by any cause of transient bacteremia. Prosthetic valve endocarditis (PVE) encompasses 15% to 30% of all cases of endocarditis, is reported in 1% to 2% of all valve implants, and is associated with a mortality rate higher than that of native valve endocarditis (11,12). PVE that occurs in the early postoperative period is frequently due to *Staphylococcus epidermidis*, either due to a break in technique in the operating room or from skin contamination. Late-onset PVE is related to bacteremic seeding of the valve. Common portals of entry include dental procedures, operations, gastrointestinal endoscopy, intravenous catheter contamination, intravenous drug abuse, and infections of the skin, lungs, bowel, and the urinary tract.

Gorav Ailawadi: University of Virginia, Charlottesville, VA 22908.

Table 28.1 Complications of valve surgery

General Complications
- Structural valve degeneration
- Anticoagulation-related bleeding
- Mechanical valve thromboembolism
- Prosthetic valve endocarditis
- Paravalvular leak
- Supraventricular arrhythmias
- Heart block
- Low cardiac output
- Debris, fat, or air embolism

Procedure-Specific Complications
Aortic valve complications
- Aortic-ventricular dehiscence
- Mitral leaflet detachment
- Occlusion of coronary artery ostia
- Inadequate myocardial preservation
- Aortic wall dissection or embolization
- Atrioventricular node block

Mitral Valve Replacement Complications
- Atrioventricular groove rupture
- Circumflex artery injury
- Coronary sinus injury
- Posterior myocardial perforation
- Aortic valve cusp entrapment
- Mitral valve prosthesis leaflet entrapment/suture looping
- Ventricular output failure
- Mechanical valve thrombosis
- Late cardiac tamponade

Mitral Valve Repair Complications
- Residual mitral stenosis or regurgitation
- Persistent mitral regurgitation
- Left ventricular (LV) outflow obstruction
- Hemolysis

Tricuspid Valve Complications
- Persistent right ventricular failure
- Complete heart block
- Recurrent or residual tricuspid regurgitation

Transcatheter Aortic Valve Complications
- Vascular injury
- Bleeding from LV apex
- Inappropriate placement of valve
- Rupture of aortic annulus
- Occlusion of coronary artery ostia
- Heart block

Physical examination, microbiological results, laboratory testing, and imaging procedures are all useful to diagnose PVE. The most common presenting symptoms for PVE are fever, fatigue, malaise, and dyspnea. Pyrexia, newly noted heart murmur, and microscopic hematuria are frequent clinical signs. Thirty percent of patients present with septic emboli, which can involve the spleen, kidneys, cerebral vasculature, and coronary system. Blood cultures are the mainstay of diagnosis and are positive for bacteremia in more than 90% of cases. Septic pulmonary emboli from tricuspid valve (TV) endocarditis can produce patchy infiltrates on chest radiograph. Echocardiogram may show a rocking motion of the prosthesis and the presence of vegetations or a new onset of a paravalvular leak. Often TEE is needed to make the diagnosis.

Although carefully selected antimicrobial therapy, specific for the infecting organisms, is important in the care of PVE, it is rare that antimicrobial therapy alone will cure PVE. Most patients require surgical removal of the valve and valve replacement. Indications for acute surgical intervention in PVE include the presence of new-onset congestive heart failure, complete heart block (CHB), or cardiogenic shock. Surgical intervention should not be delayed in the presence of acute infective PVE when congestive heart failure ensues. However, surgical intervention is futile if complications of the infection (such as severe embolic cerebral damage) or other comorbid conditions make the prospect of recovery remote.

Anesthesia, intraoperative monitoring, cardioplegia, and exposure of the valve are similar to other valvular procedures. Excision of the valve and debridement of the annulus and abscesses must be meticulous and extensive. All necrotic and infected tissue must be removed. After local antibiotic irrigation, the annulus and areas of tissue loss can often be reconstructed by using autologous pericardium or aortic homograft (13).

Abscess formation is the most commonly reported PVE manifestation; it occurs in 20% of cases and is most often caused by *S. aureus*. *Enterococcus* species have been reported in 5% to 17% of the cases, and gram-negative rod infections are rare (1% to 9%). Other secondary manifestations of endocarditis include aortic mycotic infections, cardiac conduction defects, sinus of Valsalva aneurysms, and valve thrombosis. Fungal infections occur more frequently in patients with prosthetic valves who are immunocompromised or intravenous drug users. Fungal vegetations, due to their bulky size, can produce valvular stenosis (14–16). *S. aureus* and fungal infections are particularly aggressive and typically should be treated with surgical valve removal and replacement urgently. Other organisms are often virulent, and the timing of surgery is dictated by their clinical presentation.

Postoperative care should include at least 6 weeks of intravenous antibiotics. Hospital mortality is related primarily to ongoing sepsis, multisystem organ failure, or failure to eradicate the local infection followed by recurrent perivalvular leak. Valve replacement in hemodynamically stable patients with PVE has a favorable outcome in 80% to 95% of cases (17). The reinfection rate overall is uncommon and ranges from 1% to 10%.

Paravalvular leak

Paravalvular leak is an uncommon complication with current surgical techniques. The incidence of paravalvular leak for both mechanical and biologic valves is approximately 0% to 1.5% per patient-year of valve life. Paravalvular leak traditionally was considered slightly more common with the bileaflet valve than with the porcine valve because of a less bulky sewing ring (18). Historically, the use of pledgeted sutures to seat the valve was thought to decrease the risk of paravalvular leak. Recently, our group has demonstrated similarly low paravalvular leak rates with a non-pledgeted suture technique (19).

Atrial arrhythmias

Atrial arrhythmias, primarily atrial fibrillation and atrial flutter, occur in 10% to 40% of patients after valve surgery and can contribute to neurologic morbidity. The usual onset is 1 to 3 days after operation, with a peak incidence at 48 hours; however, arrhythmias may occur at any time, including shortly after discharge. Increasing age is the most consistent predisposing factor; other conditions include a history of rheumatic fever, aortic cross-clamp time and cardiopulmonary bypass time, and abrupt stoppage of β-blocking agents. Acidosis, hypokalemia, or hypoxemia may contribute to the onset of the arrhythmia and should be corrected before initiating definitive therapy. Amiodarone is the first-line agent for both rate control and conversion to sinus rhythm in these patients postoperatively (20,21).

COMPLICATIONS OF AORTIC VALVE SURGERY

Complications related to the aortic valve annulus

Calcific degeneration is the most common cause of aortic valve stenosis. Calcification is nearly always present both in the aortic valve leaflets and the aortic annulus at the time of operation, particularly in the elderly patient. The native valve is excised by using scissors, knife, or a rongeur to remove all calcium allowing the prosthetic valve to seat properly in the annulus. Inadequate debridement of the leaflets can predispose to paravalvular leaks as the prosthetic valve may not be opposed to the aortic annulus or may result in debris in the LV cavity or coronary arteries. To avoid any embolism of this debris, copious rinsing is critical; a sponge placed in the ventricle can be helpful (Fig. 28.1).

On the other extreme, vigorous debridement of calcium in the aortic annulus can result in detachment of the anterior mitral leaflet, which is in continuity with the aortic valve annulus posteriorly. This results in an opening from the aortic root into the left atrium. This defect should be repaired with pledgeted sutures through the anterior leaflet of the mitral valve and the aortic valve annulus. These sutures are then used to secure the prosthesis. Similarly, debridement of calcium in the annulus wall can result in a disruption of the ventriculoaortic junction. If unrecognized, this will lead to ventriculoaortic dissociation and profuse arterial bleeding below the level of the valve. When overly aggressive debridement is performed and disruption of the annulus is of concern, pledgeted sutures should be used to repair the annulus to reapproximate the ventricle to the aorta. If the defect is large, a bovine pericardial patch can be used to close the defect before placing the valve sutures.

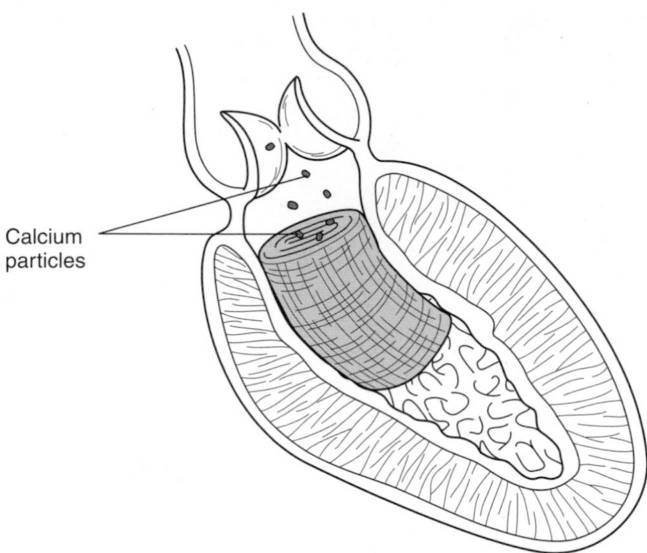

FIGURE 28.1. A sponge placed in the left ventricle during debridement of the aortic or mitral valve annulus can catch the debris. This may prevent small pieces from becoming lodged in the spaces along the wall of the ventricle, only to embolize once contractile cardiac function resumes.

Occlusion of the Coronary Arteries

During aortic valve replacement, the right and left main coronary os are visible. Care must be taken during valve debridement that calcium and debris do not occlude or embolize into the coronary arteries. Importantly, as valve sutures are placed, they should be placed low enough below the os to avoid the prosthetic valve annulus from obstructing the coronary arteries. The commissures of the prosthetic valve should match the native trileaflet aortic valve such that the struts of the prosthetic valve do not obstruct the coronary arteries. Occlusion of the coronary artery manifests are ventricular arrhythmias and low cardiac output. TEE can be used to visualize flow in the coronary ostia. If an occluded coronary artery is discovered, replacement of the valve is usually mandated. Another option is to perform a coronary artery bypass to the affected coronary system with an internal thoracic artery or saphenous vein graft.

Complications related to myocardial preservation

Inadequate myocardial preservation during the aortic valve replacement procedure is the most common cause of postoperative ventricular dysfunction. Most surgeons employ hypothermic cardioplegic preservation during aortic valve replacement. Concomitant coronary artery occlusive disease can result in uneven distribution of the cardioplegia solution. For this reason, most surgeons use retrograde cardioplegia as an adjunct to protection or as the sole method to distribute the cardioplegia. However, retrograde cardioplegia does not distribute adequate doses of cardioplegia to the right coronary system. As such, right heart dysfunction can ensue with inadequate protection of the right heart. This complication can be obviated by administering handheld cardioplegia into the right coronary os after the aorta has been opened to perform the aortic valve replacement. The use of topical cooling solutions around the heart during aortic valve replacement also helps to ensure myocardial preservation, especially of the right ventricle (RV), which is most prone to warming from operative lights. One effective routine is to measure the septal temperature continuously during operation and maintain it at 10°C to monitor the adequacy of myocardial preservation (22). Cardioplegia should be administered at regular intervals of 15 to 20 minutes or on the basis of septal temperature.

Complications related to the aorta and the aortotomy

Either a transverse or an oblique aortotomy is used to provide access to the valve. Patients with bicuspid aortic valve disease have thin and often aneurysmal ascending aortas. In addition, calcification of the ascending aorta frequently accompanies calcific degeneration of the aortic valve, especially in elderly patients. A calcified or even porcelain aorta may preclude safe cannulation of the ascending aorta for cardiopulmonary bypass. In these instances, the risk of aortic injury or stroke is exceedingly high and alternative cannulation sites such as the axillary or femoral artery should be employed. In addition, calcified plaques can fracture when the aortic cross-clamp is applied, causing arterial embolization or later dissection of the aorta. With a severely diseased aorta or porcelain aorta that is too calcified for the safe application of a cross-clamp, the technique of deep hypothermia and circulatory arrest may be a preferable option. Segmental endarterectomy and decalcification are occasionally required to successfully close the aorta. Aortas that are friable or calcified should be closed by using strips of felt to buttress the suture line.

Extreme care must be taken to close the aortotomy as this can be a challenging area to repair should bleeding occur after the cross-clamp is removed. Typically, closure of the aortotomy is performed with a two-layer closure. Taking bites that are too deep can result in excessive tension and tearing of the aorta once systemic pressure is present. Bleeding from the aortotomy can be handled in several different manners. Repair of the aorta can be as simple as placement of additional horizontal mattress pledgeted sutures across the aortotomy to buttress the closure to reclamping the aorta and replacing the aorta. Another option is coverage of the aortotomy with bovine pericardial patch, which can be particular useful if there is concern for placing additional tension on the closure, which repair stitches often do.

One additional mechanism of bleeding from the aortotomy can occur if the aortotomy is placed too low. Bioprosthetic valves have struts at the location of the commissures of the valve that can protrude and abut the aorta. When the aortotomy is placed too low, the strut can abut the suture line and lead to acute or late breakdown of the aortotomy, resulting in major hemorrhage. As such, the aortotomy should be placed at least 2 cm above the annulus of the aortic valve. Newer bioprosthetic valves often have a lower profile with shorter struts such that the risk of this occurring is less frequent. When the aortotomy is placed too low, and there is concern that a strut may erode into the suture line, the aortotomy can be closed with a bovine pericardial patch to decrease the risk the strut will abut the aorta.

Atrioventricular node block

The atrioventricular (AV) node is located in the membranous septum, which is located just below the junction of the right coronary cusp and the noncoronary cusp of the aortic valve. Great care must be taken when placing valve sutures in this location as the AV node may be damaged by placement of deep stitches, overly aggressive debridement, or annular abscess (similar to Fig. 28.2). In most circumstances, AV conduction disturbances at the conclusion of the procedure do not require the placement of permanent pacing electrodes as the majority of temporary AV node dysfunction immediately following aortic valve replacement is transient. Edema from the procedure itself can cause temporary AV conduction block, which resolves within the first postoperative week (23,24). The incidence of pacemaker requirement following aortic valve surgery is on the order of 3% to 5% and is typically not performed until at least a week after surgery.

Paravalvular leak

Paravalvular leak results in aortic insufficiency and can cause hemolysis, cause recurrent symptoms of heart failure, or lead to endocarditis. Most often, paravalvular leaks are created in the operating room during valve insertion. Thus, care must be taken to ensure that sutures (whether placed as simple interrupted or horizontal mattress) have minimal travel between sutures. In addition, deep bites of the annulus and aorta are necessary to ensure the sutures do not pull through. Finally, sizing the valve appropriately and avoiding placing too large a valve given the annulus size will allow the prosthetic valve to seat appropriately in or above the annulus. These maneuvers will minimize the risk of paravalvular leak.

Paravalvular leak is diagnosed by TEE. In addition, a paravalvular leak may be present if there is evidence of pulsatility with the heart beating even when on full cardiopulmonary bypass. This would indicate that blood is regurgitating across the aortic valve and ejecting with each cardiac cycle. Small paravalvular leaks are often related to small gaps between sutures and often resolve after heparin

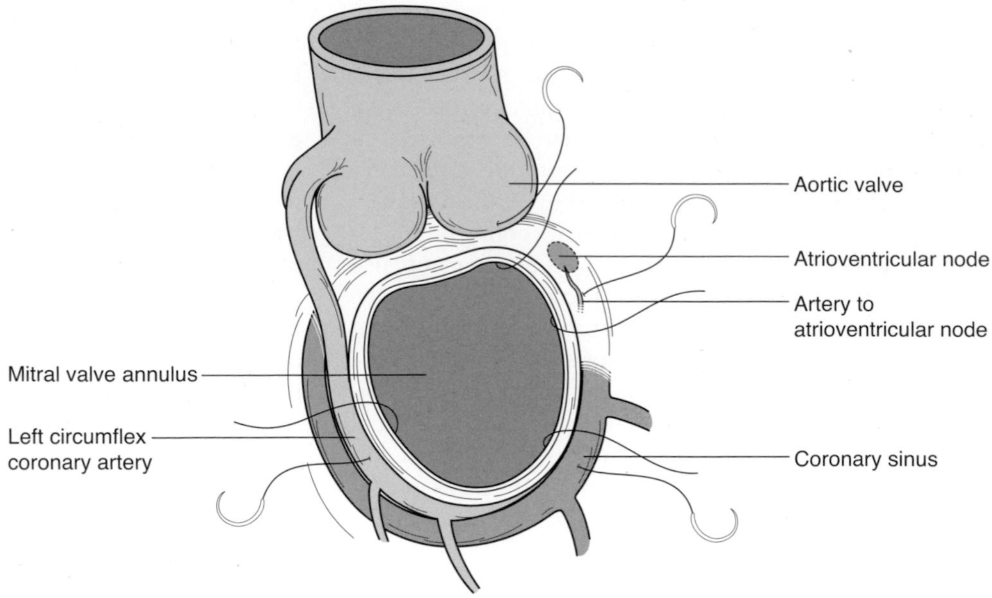

FIGURE 28.2. Suture injuries to structures surrounding the mitral valve annulus. Improper placement of sutures in the annulus can damage the left circumflex artery, aortic valve, atrioventricular node, or coronary sinus.

reversal. Larger paravalvular leaks often require rearresting the heart and repair. This can typically be performed with additional pledgeted sutures placed between the aorta and valve annulus. Often, these are most easily placed from below the valve if a bioprosthetic valve is placed. Mechanical valve paravalvular leaks require placing sutures from the adjacent aorta to the valve sewing ring. If unable to adequately assess or repair the paravalvular leak, removal and reinsertion of the valve may be needed.

COMPLICATIONS OF MITRAL VALVE SURGERY

Injury to the circumflex artery

The anatomy of the mitral valve is such that several major structures lie in near this important valve. The circumflex coronary artery lies in the AV groove along the left side of the valve and can be injured or occluded by placement of the mitral valve sutures too deeply beyond the annulus during valve replacement (Fig. 28.2). This complication presents as decreased cardiac output, poor LV lateral wall motion on intraoperative echocardiogram, or bleeding posteriorly from the heart. Correction requires the reinstitution of cardiopulmonary bypass, removal of the stitch, and, occasionally, a saphenous vein bypass graft to the circumflex coronary. Careful placement of sutures at the junction of the mitral valve annulus and the valve leaflet prevents this complication. Circumflex artery injury is less common during mitral valve repair as the sutures are placed parallel to the valve rather than across the annulus as they are during mitral valve replacement (MVR).

Posterior myocardial perforation

Myocardial rupture is a catastrophic complication of mitral valve surgery. The incidence is rare (0.5% to 2%) and occurs during MVR. This complication is caused by perforation or stretching of the LV by the prosthesis or by a strut. It is manifested as profuse bright-red blood emanating from behind the heart. Because of the potential for this complication, the apex of the heart should not be lifted after MVR is performed. As such, concomitant coronary artery bypass should be performed prior to mitral valve surgery. Treatment requires reinstitution of cardiopulmonary bypass removal of the valve prosthesis. The perforation is located, and repair may be done with the use of Teflon or pericardial strips, both externally and internally. With common techniques of preservation of the posterior mitral leaflet and papillary muscles, this complication is rare.

Atrioventricular groove dissociation

AV dissociation is a dreaded and often fatal complication. This is an extreme form of posterior LV rupture where a portion or the entire posterior left atrium separates from the left ventricle. The risk of this occurrence is greatest in patients with extensive calcification in the posterior mitral annulus and leaflet. This finding is common in elderly patients undergoing mitral valve surgery and is evident by preoperative imaging, including echocardiography and cardiac catheterization. Chest computed tomography without intravenous contrast can be useful in quantifying the degree of posterior mitral annular calcification (also known as *MAC*).

AV dissociation is usually related to vigorous traction or debridement of the posterior leaflet of the valve or to calcium excision in a calcified posterior leaflet. This can cause separation of the AV groove, leading to massive hemorrhage upon separation from cardiopulmonary bypass. This complication is prevented by understanding the pathologic process of calcification of the mitral annulus and avoiding rupture by either placement of traction sutures on the edge of the posterior leaflet or by very careful calcium debridement only in isolated spots. A safer procedure may be to attach the prosthesis to the atrial wall, leaving the entire calcified mass intact. This approach may result in a smaller valve area but a successful operation (25). When this complication occurs, valve prosthesis is removed and the ventricle is reapproximated to the left atrium with felt strips. Often, a pericardial patch is used to cover the defect and the valve sutures are now placed into the pericardial patch. Nevertheless, this complication carries a high mortality.

Embolus

Emboli from the heart can be debris from valve debridement, fat particles, or air. This complication results when there is failure to remove all debris, often from an extensively calcified valve or through technical errors that allow air to remain in the LV outflow tract. Embolism typically occurs on removal of the cross-clamp and resumption of normal cardiac ejection. Prevention is critical and involves copious irrigation of the LV to remove all debris. Air embolism may be prevented by an LV vent, an aortic root aspirating vent, or needle-venting the LV apex. Removal of all air can be confirmed by the intraoperative TEE (26,27).

Entrapment of the noncoronary cusp of the aortic valve

Although rare, this can occur in the area of 10 o'clock to 12 o'clock of the mitral valve, near the anterolateral commissure of the mitral valve. At this point, the commissure is very close to the aortic valve's noncoronary cusp, and this cusp may be entrapped if the mitral valve suture is placed too deeply (Fig. 28.2). This complication may be diagnosed only after the removal of the aortic cross-clamp, when the heart dilates because of severe aortic regurgitation and when aortic insufficiency is observed on TEE. Avoiding excessively deep bites can prevent entrapment. Treatment of entrapment requires reinstitution of cardiopulmonary bypass, re–cross-clamping, removal of the mitral prosthesis, and resuturing the area at this point. In some cases, the aortic root may need to be opened and the aortic valve inspected, repaired, or even replaced.

Leaflet entrapment by retained valvular tissue

Many mechanical valves involve the opening and closing of either single or double leaflets. With these valves, care must be taken that retained native valve structures, chords, or tips of papillary muscles do not interfere with the leaflet action (Fig. 28.3). Tissue retention can produce significant obstruction or regurgitation. Echocardiography is the best way to demonstrate valve malfunction. This complication is prevented by using proper supra-, sub-, or annular suturing technique. To ensure that leaflets open and close without interference at implantation, a cotton-tipped swab or rubber-shod instrument can be used to test the valve. To fix this problem, the mitral valve is removed, and the tissue that prevents opening and closing below the valve should be

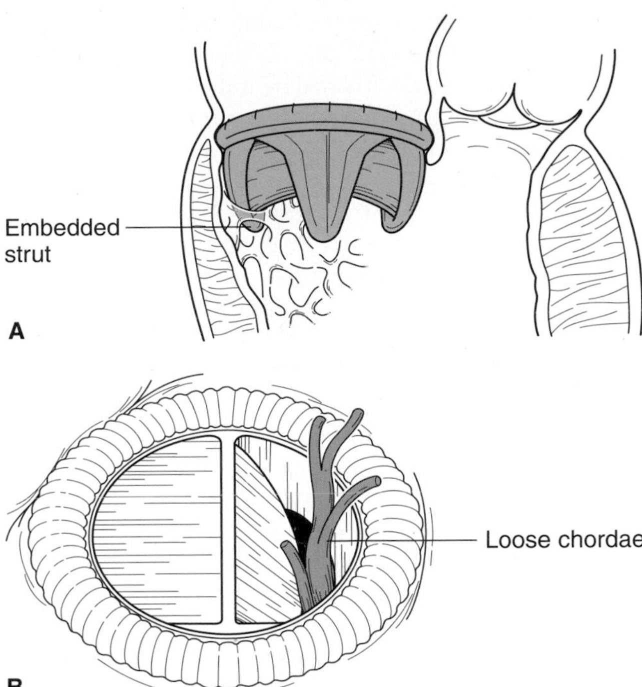

FIGURE 28.3. Dysfunction of prosthetic valves due to interference from periannular structures. **A:** Mitral valve struts can become entrapped along the wall of the ventricle and in the valve remnant, chordae, or papillary muscles. **B:** Remnants of the papillary muscles preventing full closure of the valve.

removed. The valve is then replaced. Often, the placement of sutures in an everting fashion (from atrium to ventricle) allows the valve to seat within the annulus, preventing leaflet tissue from obstructing the mechanical leaflets.

Acute valve dysfunction due to suture looping

This complication causes early bioprosthetic valve dysfunction and severe mitral regurgitation (MR) from immobility of a leaflet. Leaflet looping is preventable by carefully pushing the valve down during insertion or by use of a dental mirror to inspect the valve struts and ensure that no suture is looped over them before the valve sutures are tied down. Failure to do so will result in a large paravalvular leak. Correction of this complication requires removing and reimplanting the valve.

Low cardiac output

Low cardiac output following MVR is a frequent complication that has been documented since this procedure's inception. It has also been one of the most difficult problems to treat because it has many causes. In patients with MR, depression of cardiac performance is common after initial valve replacement. The normally cone-shaped ventricle assumes a spherical shape if there is removal of the papillary muscle-annular continuity. This concept was first promulgated in 1964, and laboratory and clinical studies have substantiated that maintaining papillary muscle-annular continuity is important for the maintenance of normal cardiac output and LV shape. The normal LV geometric relationship can be best maintained by mitral valve repair or, if that is not possible, by preserving the posterior leaflet and papillary muscles with the insertion of a totally intact valve into the mitral apparatus. The prognosis for the patient with low cardiac output from loss of LV geometry is grave and accounts for substantial early and late mortality following MVR (28). Other causes of low cardiac output include inadequate myocardial protection, injury to the circumflex artery, or residual MR.

Paravalvular leak

Paravalvular leak, early or late, producing severe regurgitation may occur in patients whose tissue is friable, in patients with endocarditis, or in patients who have extensive calcification. Patients have a loud holosystolic murmur. The diagnosis is made by echocardiogram and a rise in left atrial pressure with a prominent V wave. Using pledgeted sutures can prevent this complication, particularly when fragile or minimal annular tissue is found. If there is an abscess, a pericardial or Teflon bolster may be necessary to improve the fixation of the valve. Testing the valve prior to closure of the atriotomy with high pressure in the LV (often performed by administering anterograde cardioplegia with retractors in place exposing the mitral valve, rendering the aortic valve incompetent, thus filling the LV with aortic pressure) will often reveal significant paravalvular leaks. These can be repaired with buttressing sutures between the left atrium and valve sewing ring.

Heart Block/Arrhythmias

Atrial fibrillation is associated with mitral valve disease in up to 50% of patients (29). It is not uncommon that these patients develop atrial arrhythmias postoperatively. These can often be treated acutely with β-blockade and antiarrhythmic agents such as amiodarone. Electrical cardioversion can be performed in the operating room or postoperatively if there is hemodynamic compromise.

Heart block can occur with mitral valve surgery and is more common with MVR. Often this is due to edema near the AV node as the sutures are placed near this structure and the heart block is often transient. Rarely, valve sutures are inadvertently placed through the AV node, or the valve prosthesis compresses the node. When heart block persists for more than 7 days, a permanent pacemaker is considered.

Mechanical valve thrombosis

Thrombosis of a mechanical mitral valve can occur late following MVR. The typical presentation is a low cardiac output refractory to all forms of support. Most patients report a recent period with inadequate anticoagulation. The thrombosed mechanical prosthesis has restricted leaflet motion on echocardiography. Since echocardiography can be limited with shadowing from the mechanical valve, definitive diagnosis is made by fluoroscopy. Although immediate operation may be required, thrombolytic therapy is an option if the patient is not moribund. In patients in extremis, insertion of a percutaneous LV assist device such as a TandemHeart (Cardiac Assist, Pittsburgh, Pennsylvania) will allow correction of acidosis and cardiac output and allow for more optimal hemodynamics at the time of reoperation (30). At operation, the prosthesis is inspected and can be reimplanted, or a thrombectomy may be sufficient. If there is an obvious cause for the thrombosis that can be fixed, such as an impinging suture, the clot can be removed and the LV irrigated copiously to ensure complete thrombus removal. If not, the valve should be rereplaced (31). Prior to the operation, the decision must be made with the patient whether a bioprosthetic or mechanical valve should be inserted, on the basis of the patient's ability to take and compliance with anticoagulation.

Late tamponade

Patients who have undergone recent MVR requiring anticoagulation may have late cardiac tamponade. This is due to accumulation of blood in the pericardial space. The diagnosis should be considered in all patients on anticoagulants who have low cardiac output days to weeks after the placement of a mitral valve. It is frequent in patients who have become excessively anticoagulated. Echocardiography is diagnostic for this with great accuracy. The treatment is to reopen the incision and evacuate the fluid collection, which should result in immediate improvement of patients' hemodynamic stability. Directed needle aspiration or subxiphoid pericardial drain placement is also possible but may not be sufficient if the blood is coagulated.

COMPLICATIONS OF MITRAL VALVE REPAIR

Residual mitral stenosis or regurgitation

Mitral valve repair techniques have evolved over the last decades. At highly experienced centers, up to 90% of degenerative/myxomatous valves are able to be repaired. In patients with MR, overaggressive leaflet resection or downsizing of an annuloplasty ring can lead to mitral stenosis. Patients who present with mitral stenosis where mitral valve repair is attempted may have residual mitral stenosis. Diagnosis is made in the operating room by TEE, high left atrial pressure, and low cardiac output following repair (31–33). In this setting, MVR should be considered. Postrepair MR after operation for mitral stenosis is usually the result of an excessive commissurotomy. Significant MR is detected by TEE. Usually, the incisions in the leaflet have missed the fused commissures or a chorda supporting a section of the valve has been inadvertently cut. The aorta must be clamped, cardioplegia reinstituted, and the left atrium reopened. If the MR originates at the commissures, a pledgeted stitch can correct this complication. If regurgitation persists, valve replacement is mandated.

Persistent mitral regurgitation

Residual MR after operation for MR is probably the most vexing of all problems for the mitral repair surgeon. Residual MR almost always results from a lack of understanding of the exact geometry of the underlying pathology and an inability to recreate a functional intraventricular zone of leaflet coaptation. Correction of this residual deficit requires a reconsideration of the valve structure and either re-repair or replacement. The intraoperative TEE is paramount to understanding the pathophysiology of the leaking mitral valve following attempted repair.

Left ventricular outflow tract obstruction or abnormal systolic anterior motion of the anterior leaflet

An often-mentioned complication of mitral valve repair is systolic anterior motion of the anterior leaflet. This occurs when too small an annuloplasty ring is placed during mitral repair in patients with large mitral valves with excessive tissue. This results in the coaptation point between the anterior and posterior leaflets to be pushed anteriorly. The excessively large anterior leaflet then becomes windsocked in the LV outflow tract during systole resulting in an LV outflow track obstruction and significant residual MR. This problem can be diagnosed by an increased left atrial pressure and reduced cardiac output; TEE can confirm the diagnosis. Often, this is a dynamic finding and is associated with hypovolemia and hypercontractility. Discontinuation of pressors and correction of intravascular volume deficit solve this in many cases. Some authors advocate the use of β-blockers. If these maneuvers do not alleviate the obstruction, re-repair of the mitral valve consists of reducing the height of the posterior leaflet, perhaps with a sliding valvuloplasty. As a last resort, MVR is possible. Similarly, a "tilted" placement of a prosthetic mitral valve can obstruct the LV outflow tract (Fig. 28.4). This generally requires repositioning or replacement of the valve.

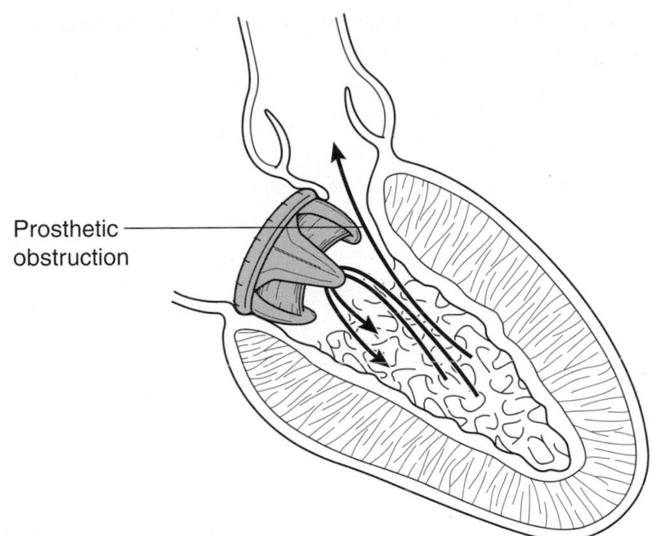

FIGURE 28.4. Obstruction of the left ventricular outflow tract by a prosthetic mitral valve.

Hemolysis

Insertion of an annuloplasty mitral valve ring requires sutures placed around the annulus. If there is dehiscence of a suture, the result is a moving nonsupported ring that can hemolyze red blood cells. Hemolysis may occur also in the absence of dehiscence when a small jet of insignificant MR hits a stitch or the ring itself. One may produce either only a very minor derangement or severe hemolysis with resulting anemia. β-Blockade, to reduce the force of the blood shear, and pentoxifylline, to make the red cells more "pliable," may be a satisfactory therapy. For some patients requiring intermittent transfusion, reoperation is the only choice.

Prosthetic Ring Dehiscence/Endocarditis

Dehiscence of the prosthetic ring is often associated with endocarditis and recurrent MR. When this occurs early following surgery, the cause is usually technical and the annuloplasty sutures were not placed in the true annulus. The other potential mechanism is the use of too small an annuloplasty ring for the given annulus size. This puts excess tension on the mitral annulus and results in ring dehiscence. Careful suture placement in the annulus and sizing of the annuloplasty ring can help decrease this risk. When this occurs, reoperation and repair of the dehiscence, re-repair of the mitral valve, or replacement of the mitral valve is needed.

COMPLICATIONS OF TRICUSPID VALVE SURGERY

Right ventricular failure

The prognosis and complications after TV operation depend less on the valve surgery itself than on the duration of TV disease, particularly tricuspid regurgitation and RV hemodynamic abnormalities. In one series, only 13% of patients with chronic tricuspid regurgitation and severe RV failure had a good outcome, whereas 78% of the patients who had no history of congestive heart failure and less RV dysfunction had a good outcome (34). A recent study suggested that a MELD (model for end-stage liver disease) score of >15 predicts higher mortality during TV surgery due to right heart dysfunction (35). The difficult preoperative decision is whether a patient's tricuspid regurgitation is the result of TV disease or is due to primary RV failure. TV surgery is likely to be curative in the former case but possibly lethal in the latter. Unfortunately, there are no completely reliable preoperative methods to predict recovery of RV systolic function postoperatively. Sound clinical judgment based on a careful examination of the patient over time, along with the response to optimal fluid and electrolyte management, remains the best preoperative indicator. RV failure has become more manageable with the use of vasodilators;

phosphodiesterase inhibitors, such as milrinone; and inhaled nitric oxide (36).

Rhythm disturbances

The most common heart rhythm problem following TV surgery is CHB. The risk of CHB is time-related; the incidence at 5 weeks has been reported to be 5%, but it is 25% by 10 years. The early risk is largely iatrogenic, having to do with suture placement near the AV node, which is at the junction of the anterior and septal leaflets of the TV (37). This can be minimized by judicious placement of valve sutures, particularly near the triangle of Koch. Placing the sutures at the base of the valve leaflet rather than deeper in the annulus ensures the greatest distance from the conduction system. The risk of CHB is greater when tricuspid valve (TV) replacement or annuloplasty is combined with mitral valve procedures than after TV procedures alone, because of swelling on both sides of the AV node or the bundle of His. Heart block appears to occur less frequently after annuloplasty than after replacement of the TV—a difference of 6% versus 24% was observed in one series involving 47 patients. Late CHB is due to scar formation around the prosthetic valve annulus, particularly when a mitral or aortic prosthesis abuts it. CHB usually necessitates a permanent epicardial pacemaker system for the patient.

Recurrent/residual tricuspid regurgitation

Comparative studies of recurrent/residual tricuspid regurgitation after tricuspid annuloplasty are few. One prospective, randomized study compared ring with stitch annuloplasty. At 64 months' follow-up, there was a significantly greater incidence of moderate or severe postoperative tricuspid regurgitation in the DeVega stitch group (38). However, in both groups, control of tricuspid regurgitation was poor, particularly with elevated pulmonary vascular resistance or organic TV disease. Although long-term survival was termed *excellent*, recurrence of at least moderate tricuspid regurgitation occurs in many patients; most do not require reoperation. A very recent study advocated an aggressive approach of TV annuloplasty, even with minor tricuspid regurgitation, if the annulus was dilated. This study showed infrequent recurrent tricuspid regurgitation in the group treated with annuloplasty for less severe dilation (39).

COMPLICATIONS OF TRANSCATHETER AORTIC VALVE REPLACEMENT

Novel methods to replace the aortic valve without the need for sternotomy, arrest of the heart or even cardiopulmonary bypass are widely available in Europe and available in the United States in trials. With these techniques, the native aortic valve is ballooned open but not removed. A stented valve is placed in the aortic annulus either through a transfemoral artery approach or through a transapical approach (through a minithoracotomy on the left chest accessing the LV apex directly).

With these techniques, a host of new complications have been recognized. With the transfemoral approach, vascular injury to the femoral or iliac system is not uncommon as currently available valves require a 18 to 26 F sheath. With the transapical approach, bleeding from the LV apex can be life threatening should the repair sutures not hold. With both approaches, inappropriate placement of the valve can result in severe aortic insufficiency, occlusion of the coronary arteries, or embolization into the left ventricle. Coronary artery occlusion may be treated with emergent percutaneous coronary intervention. If the valve is placed too high, it can sometimes be pulled into the descending aorta, left in place, and a new valve transcatheter valve deployed. Vascular complications can be treated with covered stent grafts if recognized early. Other complications such as embolization of the valve into the left ventricle, severe aortic insufficiency if the valve is not placed properly, or aortic injury usually require open surgical repair.

Injury to the AV node is not uncommon, and depending on the type of valve inserted, upto 25% of patients may require a permanent pacemaker with this approach.

REFERENCES

1. Bonow RO, Carabello B, de Leon AC, et al. ACC/AHA guidelines for the management of patients with valvular heart disease: executive summary. *J Heart Valve Dis* 1998;7:672.
2. Carabello BA, Crawford FA. Medical progress: valvular heart disease. *N Engl J Med* 1997;337:32.
3. Rahimtoola SH. Choice of prosthetic heart valve for adult patients—review article. *J Am Coll Cardiol* 2003;41(6):893–904.
4. Chaitman BR, Bonan R, Lepage G, et al. Hemodynamic evaluation of the Carpentier-Edwards porcine xenograft. *Circulation* 1979;60:1170.
5. Wernly JA, Crawford MH. Choosing a prosthetic heart valve. *Cardiol Clin* 1998;16:491.
6. Edwards TJ, Livesey SA, Simpson IA, et al. Biological valves beyond fifteen years: the Wessex experience. *Ann Thorac Surg* 1995;60:S211.
7. Bernal JM, Rabasa JM, Lopez R, et al. Durability of the Carpentier-Edwards porcine bioprosthesis: role of age and valve position. *Ann Thorac Surg* 1995;60:S248.
8. Doty JR, Flores JH, Millar RC, et al. Aortic valve replacement with Medtronic freestyle bioprosthesis: operative technique and results. *J Card Surg* 1998;13:208.
9. Akins CW. Results with mechanical cardiac valvular prostheses. *Ann Thorac Surg* 1995;60:1836.
10. Hammermeister KE, Henderson WG, Burchfiel CM, et al. Comparison of outcome after valve replacement with a bioprosthesis versus a mechanical prosthesis: initial 5 year results of a randomized trial. *J Am Coll Cardiol* 1987;10:719.
11. Steusse DC, Vlessis AA. Epidemiology of native valve endocarditis. In: Vlessis AA, Bolling SF, eds. *Endocarditis: a multidisciplinary approach.* Armonk, NY: Futura, 1999:77.
12. Vlessis AA, Hovaguimian H, Jaggers J, et al. Infective endocarditis: ten-year review of medical and surgical therapy. *Ann Thorac Surg* 1996; 61:1217.
13. Schwartz CF, Bolling SF. Mitral valve endocarditis. In: Vlessis AA, Bolling SF, eds. *Endocarditis: a multidisciplinary approach.* Armonk, NY: Futura; 1999:263.
14. Husebye DG, Pluth JR, Piehler JM, et al. Reoperation on prosthetic heart valves: an analysis of risk factors in 552 patients. *J Thorac Cardiovasc Surg* 1983;86:543–552.
15. Lytle BW, Cosgrove DM, Taylor PC, et al. Reoperation for valve surgery: perioperative mortality and determinants of risk for 1,000 patients. *Ann Thorac Surg* 1986;42:632–643.

16. Teoh KH, Ivanov J, Weisel RD, et al. Survival and bioprosthetic valve failure. *Circulation* 1989;80(Suppl 1):8–15.
17. David TE, Bos J, Christakis GT, et al. Heart valve operations in patients with active infective endocarditis. *Ann Thorac Surg* 1990;49:701.
18. Lindblom D. Long-term clinical results after aortic valve replacement with the Bjork-Shiley prosthesis. *J Thorac Cardiovasc Surg* 1988;95: 658–667.
19. Lapar DJ, Ailawadi G, Bhamidipati CM, et al. Use of a nonpledgeted suture technique is safe and efficient for aortic valve replacement [published online ahead of print May 18, 2010]. *J Thorac Cardiovasc Surg*. 2011;141(2):388–393.
20. Kalus JS, White CM, Caron MF, et al. Indicators of atrial fibrillation risk in cardiac surgery patients on prophylactic amiodarone. *Ann Thorac Surg* 2004;77(4):1288–1292.
21. Kobayashi J, Kosakai Y, Isobe F, et al. Rationale of the Cox maze procedure for atrial fibrillation during redo mitral valve operations. *J Thorac Cardiovasc Surg* 1996;112:1216.
22. Carr JA, Savage EB. Aortic valve repair for aortic insufficiency in adults: a contemporary review and comparison with replacement techniques—review article. *Eur J Cardiothorac Surg* 2004;25(1):6–15.
23. David TE, Komeda M, Brofman PR. Surgical treatment of aortic root abscess. *Circulation* 1989;80(Suppl 1):269–274.
24. Magovern JA, Pennock JL, Campbell DB, et al. Aortic valve replacement and combined aortic valve replacement and coronary artery bypass grafting: predicting high risk groups. *J Am Coll Cardiol* 1987;9: 38–43.
25. Najafi H, Dye WS, Javid H, et al. Mitral valve replacement: review of seven years' experience—review article. *Am J Cardiol* 1969;24(3): 386–392.
26. Bucerius J, Gummert JF, Borger MA, et al. Stroke after cardiac surgery: a risk factor analysis of 16,184 consecutive adult patients. *Ann Thorac Surg* 2003;75(2):472–478.
27. Jennifer C, O'Brien B, Schneck M. Risk of stroke following valve replacement surgery. *Semin Cerebrovasc Dis Stroke* 2003;3(4):214–218.
28. Fenster MS, Feldman MD. Mitral regurgitation: an overview. *Curr Probl Cardiol* 1995;20:193.
29. Ailawadi G, Swenson BR, Girotti ME, et al. Is mitral valve repair superior to replacement in elderly patients? *Ann Thorac Surg* 2008;86(1):77–85.
30. Solomon H, Lim DS, Ragosta M. Percutaneous ventricular assist device to rescue a patient with profound shock from a thrombosed prosthetic mitral valve. *J Invasive Cardiol* 2008;20(11):E320–E323.
31. David TE, Uden DE, Strauss HD. The importance of the mitral apparatus in left ventricular function after correction of mitral regurgitation. *Circulation* 1983;68:II76.
32. Akins CW, Hilgenberg AD, Buckley MJ, et al. Mitral valve reconstruction versus replacement for degenerative or ischemic mitral regurgitation. *Ann Thorac Surg* 1994;58:668.
33. Roberts WC, McIntosh CL, Wallace RB. Mechanisms of severe mitral regurgitation in mitral valve prolapse determined from analysis of operatively excised valves. *Am Heart J* 1987;113:1316.
34. Bernal JM, Gutiérrez-Morlote J, Llorca J, et al. Tricuspid valve repair: an old disease, a modern experience. *Ann Thorac Surg* 2004;78(6):2069–2074.
35. Ailawadi G, Lapar DJ, Swenson BR, et al. Model for end-stage liver disease predicts mortality for tricuspid valve surgery. *Ann Thorac Surg* 2009;87(5):1460–1467.
36. Thorburn CW, Morgan JJ, Shanahan MX, et al. Long-term results of tricuspid valve replacement and the problem of prosthetic valve thrombosis. *Am J Cardiol* 1983;51:1128–1132.
37. Breyer RH, McClenathan JH, Michaelis LL, et al. Tricuspid regurgitation: a comparison of nonoperative management, tricuspid annuloplasty and tricuspid valve replacement. *J Thorac Cardiovasc Surg* 1976;72: 867–874.
38. Peterffy A, Jonasson R, Henze A. Haemodynamic changes after tricuspid valve surgery: a recatheterization study in forty-five patients. *Scand J Thorac Cardiovasc Surg* 1981;15:161–170.
39. Dreyfus GD, Corbi PJ, John Chan KM, et al. Secondary tricuspid regurgitation or dilatation: which should be the criteria for surgical repair? *Ann Thorac Surg* 2005;79(1):127–132.

CHAPTER

29

Complications of Thoracoscopy

James M. Donahue, Michael A. Smith, and Richard J. Battafarano

BACKGROUND

The use of endoscopy for diagnostic and therapeutic procedures of the chest was introduced in 1910 by the Swedish physician Hans Christian Jacobaeus (1). Over the following decades thoracoscopy developed into a routine procedure for the diagnosis and management of pleural space complications of tuberculosis. As antimicrobial therapy for tuberculosis developed, the use of thoracoscopy waned. Not until the 1990s, with the rapid adoption of minimally invasive laparoscopic techniques, did thoracoscopy become more widely utilized. Today, video-assisted thoracic surgery (VATS) refers to a minimally invasive approach to chest surgery that avoids rib spreading and requires visualization by video technology. Currently, VATS is the standard approach for many diagnostic and therapeutic procedures involving the lung, pleura, esophagus, and mediastinum (Table 29.1). In some ways, the minimally invasive nature of this approach has changed the way in which patients are managed. This is particularly true for biopsies of peripheral pulmonary nodules and densities, which, historically, have been followed with serial imaging studies.

When considering whether to proceed with a VATS approach for a given diagnostic or therapeutic procedure, it is important to consider the advantages and disadvantages as well as contraindications for each individual patient. VATS is often preferable to open procedures because it reduces surgical trauma, decreases pain and postoperative narcotic use, and preserves pulmonary function (2). These factors may allow older patients or patients with significant medical comorbidities who are poor candidates for thoracotomy to undergo diagnostic or therapeutic interventions (3). The appeal of the VATS approach for diagnostic procedures is well-recognized in the thoracic community. More recently, the use of VATS has become increasingly popular for major anatomic pulmonary resections. According to a recent analysis of the Society of Thoracic Surgery (STS) database, 32% of all lobectomies were performed using VATS in 2006 (4).

The disadvantages of VATS include a fairly steep learning curve, the loss of tactile sensation, poor access to and ability to control vital structures in the event of emergent blood loss, and the high cost of specialized equipment. In addition, there are contraindications to thoracoscopy (Table 29.2) that also diminish the prospect of using this approach in certain patients. The technical accomplishment of VATS procedures requires certain conditions in order to be safe and effective. The most important requirement is that the surgeon be able to see the operative field. Therefore, two absolute contraindications to VATS are a fused pleural space from prior surgery or inflammation and an inability to tolerate single lung ventilation secondary to preexisting lung disease or cardiopulmonary instability. In general, resection of tumors >4 cm in diameter is also a contraindication for a VATS approach. Relative contraindications include endobronchial tumors seen on bronchoscopy, obesity, coagulopathy, extensive hilar lymphadenopathy, prior hilar radiation, and chest wall involvement. It is important for surgeons to understand the potential complications associated with the thoracoscopic approach in order to identify the patients most likely to benefit from this minimally invasive technique. If there are no absolute contraindications, many surgeons will begin with the VATS technique and will convert to open thoracotomy if they are unable to proceed safely.

RISK ASSESSMENT

In an effort to avoid complications in the intraoperative and postoperative periods, a preoperative risk assessment must be performed. Many algorithms have been developed to systematically stratify the risk of candidates for chest surgery based upon preoperative data such as age, exercise capacity, spirometric values, and measures of gas exchange and diffusing capacity. No single factor has been proven as being predictive for the development of complications. In an effort to improve predictive ability, various factors have been accounted for in scoring systems. The Cardiopulmonary Risk Index (CPRI) and the Physiological and Operative Severity Score for the Enumeration of Mortality and Morbidity (POSSUM) are general scoring systems that have been used for lung resection with variable predictive ability (5–7). Additional scoring systems specifically developed for lung resection, such as the Predictive Respiratory Quotient (PRQ) (8) and the Predicted Postoperative Product (9), have not gained widespread use.

James M. Donahue, Richard J. Battafarano: Division of General Thoracic Surgery, University of Maryland, Baltimore, MD.

Michael A. Smith: Division of General Thoracic Surgery, Saint Joseph's Hospital and Medical Center, Phoenix, AZ.

Table 29.1 Minimally invasive procedures of the chest

Pulmonary
Wedge resection
Lobectomy
Pneumonectomy
Esophageal
Fundoplication
Myotomy
Leiomyoma resection
Esophagectomy
Cardiac
Pericardial window
Nervous System
Sympathectomy
Other
Thymectomy
Mediastinal mass excision

Most surgeons do not rely completely on a particular scoring system to determine a patient's surgical fitness. However, many of the factors that make up these scoring systems, along with surgical judgment, are used to make the ultimate decision. Some of these factors include patient age, pulmonary function, clinical stage of disease, and the presence of comorbid illnesses. Patients who would normally be considered high risk because of advanced age, poor pulmonary function, and low functional status may actually experience better outcomes with fewer complications using a VATS approach (10,11). However, their risks are still substantial when compared to the general population and should not be underestimated. Another consideration specific to VATS is the clinical stage and location of disease. Central lung lesions are more difficult to deal with than peripheral lesions from both a diagnostic and therapeutic standpoint. The close proximity of central lung lesions to major pulmonary vessels can increase the risk of approaching these using a VATS approach (12). For this reason it is important to set size and location criteria for VATS approaches to lung lesions. Disregarding these criteria will make the patient vulnerable to complications.

Table 29.2 Contraindications to thoracoscopy

Absolute
Fused pleural space
Prior thoracotomy
Severe inflammatory process
Prior pleurodesis
Inability to tolerate single lung ventilation
Prior pneumonectomy
Severe respiratory failure
Hemodynamically unstable patient
Cardiac arrest
Severe trauma
Relative
High risk of incomplete resection or dissemination
Tumor >4 cm
Central pulmonary lesions
Endobronchial tumor
Hilar lymphadenopathy
Prior hilar radiation
Chest wall involvement
Coagulopathy
Obesity

GENERAL COMPLICATIONS

Although the VATS approach may be less traumatic than thoracotomy, the anatomic and physiologic consequences of the operation remain the same. Therefore, all potential complications that may be associated with the open procedure may also be encountered in the same operation performed by VATS. However, there are intraoperative complications that are specific to VATS. In early studies examining the safety of VATS for nonanatomic diagnostic and therapeutic resections, mortality rates ranged from 0.5% to 2.5%, while morbidity rates varied from 4% to 14% (10,13–15). Recent large reviews from individual institutions of excellence examining the use of VATS for major anatomic resections report mortality rates from 0.7% to 1.2% and morbidity rates from 15% to 26% (16–18). A recent report from the American College of Surgeons Oncology Group details the morbidity and mortality following major pulmonary resections in patients with early-stage lung cancer in the Z0030 trial. This prospective, randomized trial was designed to compare lymph node sampling versus mediastinal lymph node dissection in early-stage lung cancer. Because 94% of patients in this study underwent thoracotomy, it serves as an excellent modern benchmark by which to assess results following thoracotomy. In this study, mortality was 1.4%, and morbidity was 38% (19). Finally, an analysis of the STS database using propensity matching to compare a VATS approach versus thoracotomy for patients undergoing lobectomy reported mortality rates of 0.94% in the VATS group and 1.01% in the thoracotomy group. Overall morbidity rates were 26.2% in the VATS group and 34.7% in the thoracotomy group (20).

INTRAOPERATIVE COMPLICATIONS

The initial reservation with minimally invasive surgery in the chest was a concern for safety. However, over the years, it has been shown that minimally invasive chest surgery can be performed for a variety of procedures with safety that is comparable to open thoracotomy. To a great degree, safety depends on good surgical judgment for conversion to open thoracotomy for technical reasons or when an open operation is more appropriate. The most common, immediately life-threatening intraoperative complications of chest surgery are massive hemorrhage, cardiogenic disturbances, and ventilatory problems.

Hemorrhage

Massive intraoperative hemorrhage is the most worrisome complication for surgeons when considering minimally invasive procedures in the chest because of the difficulty in obtaining central control of the pulmonary artery and veins using the VATS technique. Massive hemorrhage in the chest can result from great vessel injury or, more commonly, injury to a pulmonary artery or vein branch sustained during pulmonary dissection. The pulmonary artery and its branches are particularly thin-walled and easily injured during manipulation or traction employed to increase exposure. In contrast, the walls of the pulmonary vein are more resilient and withstand surgical manipulation much better. The risk of a difficult dissection and pulmonary artery injury can be anticipated in patients who have had induction chemotherapy or prior irradiation. In addition, patients with mediastinal granulomatosis or prior silica exposure will have regional bronchopulmonary lymph nodes densely adherent to branch pulmonary arteries. In such cases, it is prudent to begin the surgical dissection by encircling the ipsilateral main pulmonary artery and both pulmonary veins so as to have proximal and distal control in the event of vessel injury. Another reported cause of major intraoperative bleeding is the mechanical failure of vascular staplers, although this is rare (21,22). Some authors recommend the central placement of vascular clamps prior to vessel division to minimize the sequelae of misfiring staplers.

Because the pulmonary circulation is a low-pressure, high-flow system, arterial and venous injury can almost always be immediately controlled with local pressure at the injury site. After local control of the bleeding is obtained, the surgeon, knowing the injury's site and magnitude, must make an immediate decision on what will be required to control the bleeding. In the setting of VATS, the operative view can be lost very quickly. Therefore, attempts to place a vascular clamp to control bleeding should be avoided. In the case of a pulmonary artery injury, this may, in fact, exacerbate the injury. A better alternative to controlling bleeding during VATS is to gain immediate control with a gentle application of pressure using a sponge-stick through the utility incision or a port site. This will give ample time to gain better exposure with an open incision and to repair the injury if needed. Rarely will an injury to the main pulmonary artery, the left atrium medial to the pulmonary vein, or the superior or inferior vena cava require a cardiopulmonary bypass to control the situation for adequate repair.

In addition, injuries to bronchial arteries, parenchymal surfaces, and pleural adhesions, as well as intercostal and internal mammary vessels can also lead to significant intraoperative blood loss if they go unnoticed. It is important to use careful dissection techniques at all times during the operation to avoid injuries to these structures and to control them quickly when they occur. A particular concern during anatomic VATS resections is the failure to correctly recognize vascular or bronchial structures. During open lobectomy, the most common approach involves opening the fissures to obtain control of the pulmonary arterial branches. This approach is generally not performed during the performance of a VATS lobectomy. In the VATS approach, upper lobectomies are generally performed by proceeding with the hilar dissection from anterior to posterior, while lower lobectomies are usually performed from inferior to superior. This may be confusing during the initial experience with the technique. It is essential to correctly identify structures prior to dividing them. This often requires moving the camera to different port sites in order to examine critical structures from different angles.

Intraoperative cardiogenic disturbances

As mentioned previously, adequate visualization is extremely important when using a VATS approach. The insufflation of CO_2 aids in the compression of lung parenchyma and the effacement of subpleural lesions, and it acts as a retractor when combined with changes in the patient's position. Initially, there was reluctance to using CO_2 insufflation because of concern over hemodynamic compromise. Intrapleural CO_2 insufflation has been shown to have adverse hemodynamic consequences in laboratory animal studies (23). However, in the clinical setting, low-pressure (<10 mm Hg) insufflation of CO_2 during thoracoscopy is safe and without significant hemodynamic consequences except for an elevation of central venous pressure (15). The pressures and flow rates should be kept at <10 mm Hg and 2 L/min, respectively, to avoid significant central venous pressures or rapid mediastinal movement. In addition, intrapleural CO_2 insufflation should be initiated only if there are no significant adhesions present to prevent pleural and parenchymal injury.

Patients with preexisting heart disease are at risk for more typical intraoperative cardiogenic disturbances such as ischemia and arrhythmias. It is important to identify these patients from their medical history, physical exam, and preoperative testing to determine the need for preoperative prophylactic measures to avoid cardiac ischemia and to select those who need intraoperative Swan–Ganz catheter monitoring. Of particular note, for patients who have undergone previous CABG using a left internal mammary artery graft, special care must be taken when performing procedures on the left upper lobe so as not to damage the graft. Patients without preexisting cardiac dysfunction can also develop intraoperative arrhythmias due to hypothermia, hypoxemia, hypokalemia, hyperkalemia, hypovolemia, or acidosis. When they occur, these problems must be corrected as soon as possible. Electrical cardioversion may be necessary in the case of hemodynamically significant arrhythmias. However, the arrhythmia may be recalcitrant to electrical cardioversion if the underlying disturbance is not corrected (i.e., hypothermia, hyperkalemia). In addition, manipulation and compression of the heart for exposure can also lead to arrhythmias and ischemia. Often, these maneuvers cannot be completely avoided, but they must be limited in duration and frequency, using close communication between the surgeon and anesthesiologist to help identify the effects on blood pressure and rhythm.

Ventilatory complications

A host of ventilatory problems can put the patient's gas exchange and hemodynamic stability at risk. As ventilation is established through either a double lumen endobronchial tube or a single lumen tube with a bronchial blocking balloon, it is essential for the anesthesiologist, as well as the surgeon, to be confident that proper positioning has been established prior to starting the resection. The surgeon must also be aware of the presentation of tube displacement. High airway pressure and absent CO_2 in the ventilator circuit indicate that the bronchial cuff or bronchial blocking balloon has herniated into the trachea, causing tracheal obstruction. Deflation of the cuff or balloon solves the problem and advancement of the tube or balloon prevents the problem from reoccurring. While conducting a right-sided resection with ventilation only on the left, persistent hypoxemia suggests that the balloon on the left limb of the double lumen tube has advanced too far and has occluded the left upper lobe orifice. This problem is sometimes first detected by the attentive surgeon, who recognizes that the mediastinum's usual ventilatory movement is absent because of the progressive atelectasis of the left upper lobe. Repositioning the tube solves the problem. Communication between the surgeon and anesthesiologist is critical for the successful completion of VATS procedures. Early recognition of a patient not tolerating single lung ventilation is of critical importance to avoid having to inflate the lung on the operative side immediately. This could prove disastrous if it coincides with a critical portion of the hilar dissection and could lead to significant bleeding.

Patients undergoing lung surgery are more susceptible to pneumothorax secondary to barotrauma because of preexisting emphysema from smoking. Pneumothorax can occur at the time of induction and at the onset of positive pressure ventilation or at any point during the actual operation on the contralateral side. The surgeon should be aware of this development since airway pressures will increase, and the rhythmic movement of the mediastinum will be absent. Indeed, the mediastinum will sometimes balloon out toward the operative side, causing an obstruction of the venous return and hemodynamic compromise. Opening the mediastinal pleura easily remedies the problem.

POSTOPERATIVE COMPLICATIONS

General considerations

Several complications can arise after chest surgery. Many can be fatal if not recognized and managed early and aggressively. Paying attention to the details of patient symptoms, clinical exams, and routine chest X-rays, in addition to having a high index of suspicion during the postoperative period will help the clinician to identify complications and manage them effectively. Recent outcome analyses of large series of anatomic VATS resections provide insights into the post-operative complications of these procedures when compared to resections performed via thoracotomy. When interpreting these results, it must be kept in mind that patients in these nonrandomized studies are highly selected and may not represent the general patient population. In this section, we will examine the results and management strategies for three of the most common postoperative complications: prolonged air leaks, pneumonia, and atrial fibrillation. Many thoracic surgical investigators are interested in the differences in the incidence of these complications between open and VATS approaches.

Residual air space and prolonged air leaks

During the normal conduct of VATS or open pulmonary resections, there can be small injuries to the visceral pleura, resulting in air leaks. These small visceral pleural injuries can be minimized with meticulous technique. Normally, these small air leaks resolve with the apposition of pleural surfaces once the lung is reexpanded. A residual air space exists when there is a failure in filling the chest cavity after the reexpansion of the lung. Greater amounts of parenchymal resection increase the risk of residual air space. Thus, bilobectomies and lobectomies have higher rates of residual air space than segmentectomies and wedge resections. Usually the space is noted at the apex after upper lobectomy and at the base near the diaphragm after lower lobectomy. In many patients, residual air space in the absence of a persistent air leak will not be associated with any significant morbidity. The space gradually disappears over several weeks, secondary to the reabsorption of gases within the space, further reexpansion of the lung, shift of the mediastinum to the operative side, and elevation of the ipsilateral hemidiaphragm. When a residual air space is associated with symptoms such as pain, dyspnea, hemoptysis, or fever, a bronchopleural fistula with empyema should be suspected and requires appropriate intervention with thoracostomy tube placement and possible reoperation.

As with open lung resection, prolonged air leak is the most common cause of morbidity and prolonged hospital stay after VATS lung resection. It also increases patient discomfort, cost of care, and the utilization of resources. Prolonged air leak is responsible for approximately 25% of all morbidity after lung resection. An air leak that persists for more than 5 to 7 days after surgery is generally considered a prolonged air leak. As depicted in Table 29.3, the occurrence of a prolonged air leak after VATS lobectomy in the Cedars Sinai series was 5.1%. In the ACOSOG Z0030 trial, the incidence of prolonged air leak after open resection was 7.6%. The incidence of prolonged air leak in other large VATS series ranges from 4% to 7.7% (17,18). In the propensity-matched analysis of the STS database depicted in Table 29.4, prolonged air leak occurred in 7.6% of

Table 29.3 VATS versus thoracotomy: morbidity and mortality comparison from large series of anatomic resections

	VATS (Cedars Sinai)	Thoracotomy (ACOSOG Z0030)
Patients	1,100	1,023
Mortality	0.8	1.4
Reoperation for bleeding	0	1.5
Prolonged air leak	5.1	7.6
Empyema	0.4	1.1
Pneumonia	1.2	2.5
Bronchopleural fistula	0.3	0.5
Atelectasis	0.2	6.4
ARDS	0.1	0.7
Atrial fibrillation	2.9	14.4

ARDS, adult respiratory distress syndrome; VATS, video-assisted thoracic surgery.

patients after VATS lobectomy versus 8.7% of patients in the open lobectomy group (p NS).

The most consistent risk factor for prolonged air leak after anatomic resection is severe obstructive pulmonary disease. Other potential risk factors for prolonged air leak include advanced age, pleural adhesions, preoperative steroid use, and induction chemo/radiation therapy. Preoperative awareness of increased risk for prolonged air leaks should engender extra measures in addition to meticulous technique during the operation to help prevent them. The use of bovine pericardial strips as a buttress along the lung staple line to decrease air leaks was first described for lung volume reduction surgery (24). However, their efficacy for completing fissures during lobectomy and segmentectomy is unclear. Previously, Venuta et al. (25) found that the use of pericardial strips to complete interlobar fissures for pulmonary lobectomy significantly reduced the duration of postoperative air leaks and hospital stay. The use of pericardial buttressing strips has been described in conjunction with the VATS approach (26) and has been shown to lower the prolonged air leak rate after VATS lung volume reduction surgery (27,28).

Other measures to reduce the incidence of prolonged air leaks in high-risk patients are maneuvers that displace the potential residual space to an extrapleural position, thereby making the apposition of pleural surfaces more likely. One common practice is the creation of a pleural tent. In a prospective randomized study of 200 patients undergoing upper lobectomy (29), it was found that pleural tenting reduced the duration of air leaks and hospital costs. Similarly, other randomized and retrospective studies (30,31) showed that pleural tenting following lobectomy shortens the duration of chest tube drainage and hospital costs. The use of pleural tents has also been described with the VATS approach (25). A second way to limit the potential residual pleural air space is to elevate the diaphragm by insufflating air into the peritoneal cavity. Pneumoperitoneum has been described to treat air leaks and residual spaces after lung volume reduction surgery (32). Subsequently, De Giacomo et al. (33) described its use after pulmonary resection. In a prospective randomized study of 16 patients undergoing bilobectomy, Cerfolio et al. showed that intraoperative creation of pneumoperitoneum decreased the incidence of air leaks and shortened hospital stay without increasing morbidity (34).

A third measure that has been used for prolonged air leak is the use of biologic sealants. Prior reports have shown (35,36) that fibrin glue is not effective in reducing the duration of air leaks after lobectomy. However, Fabian et al. (37) showed in a randomized study that fibrin glue reduced the rate of postoperative air leak from 15% to 2% after lung resection. Similarly, Wain et al. (38) found that fibrin glue–treated patients had a mean air leak time of 31 hours while untreated patients had a mean air leak time of 52 hours. Although this difference was significant, there was no reduced time for chest tube removal or earlier hospital discharge. Because thoracoscopic procedures were excluded from both of these sealant trials, further study is needed to determine efficacy, patient selection, and the cost effectiveness of fibrin sealants for preventing prolonged air leak for VATS pulmonary resection.

Despite preventive measures, many patients go on to develop prolonged air leak. Although this is the most common problem thoracic surgeons deal with in the postoperative period, there is no consensus on its management. Most surgeons believe that conversion from suction to water seal is an effective way of encouraging an air leak to seal. Development of a pneumothorax in the setting of an expiratory air leak is uncommon. This is supported by a study by

Table 29.4 VATS versus thoracotomy: morbidity and mortality comparison in propensity-matched analysis of patients undergoing lobectomy in STS database

	VATS	Thoracotomy	*p*-value
Patients	1,281	1,281	–
Mortality	0.9	1.0	NS
Reoperation for bleeding	1.3	0.6	NS
Prolonged air leak	7.6	8.7	NS
Pneumonia	3.0	4.4	NS
Bronchopleural fistula	0.2	0.2	NS
Atelectasis	2.1	3.3	NS
ARDS	0.7	0.8	NS
Reintubation	1.4	3.1	0.0046
Atrial fibrillation	7.3	11.5	0.0004

ARDS, adult respiratory distress syndrome; VATS, video-assisted thoracic surgery.

Cerfolio et al. (39) in which 33 patients with postoperative air leak were randomized to continued suction versus water seal on postoperative day 2. They found that 67% of the patients treated with water seal had air leak resolution by postoperative day 3 versus 7% of the patients who remained on suction. Air leaks that do not resolve on water seal should be placed on a Heimlich valve once the fluid drainage is minimal. The patient can be discharged with the chest tube and Heimlich valve in place as long as there is no new or enlarging pneumothorax apparent on the chest X-ray. Outpatient chest tube management is well-tolerated and desirable for the patient since it avoids prolonged hospitalization. Most air leaks stop after several days, and the chest tube can be removed at that time. As an alternative to discharging patients with chest tubes, chemical pleurodesis can be employed in the management of prolonged postoperative air leak. In a recent retrospective analysis, 41 patients with a prolonged air leak underwent chemical pleurodesis through an indwelling chest tube. Sclerosis was successful in 40 of the 41 patients, with a mean duration of air leak after sclerosis of 2.8 days. Five patients required repeat sclerosis, and one patient developed an empyema (40).

Sputum retention and pneumonia

Poor airway hygiene is a significant life-threatening problem after chest surgery. Acutely, it can cause hypoxia, tachycardia, and hemodynamic embarrassment. Postoperative pain and compromised mental status leading to an inability to breathe deeply or cough are the main factors contributing to the retention of airway secretions. In many cases, postoperative pain leads to increased narcotic use with subsequent compromised mental status and sputum retention. These airway secretions can go on to plug the airways, causing atelectasis, lobar collapse, pneumonia, and respiratory failure. Patients at higher risk for postoperative sputum retention are current smokers; patients with a history of chronic obstructive pulmonary disease, cerebrovascular accident, or ischemic heart disease; and those without regional analgesia (41). In case-controlled studies, the VATS approach has been shown to be associated with less immediate postoperative pain compared to the thoracotomy approach by an objective assessment of analgesic requirements (42,43) and by subjective scales (2). However, one prospective randomized trial comparing VATS lobectomy with thoracotomy showed only a trend toward less narcotic use that was not statistically significant (44). The lack of statistical significance in this study may have been related to small sample sizes and low statistical power. In general, however, it is believed that the VATS approach indeed lowers postoperative pain and the need for analgesia. Diminished pain and a reduced need for narcotic analgesia should lower the risk of sputum retention and poor postoperative airway hygiene.

As depicted in Table 29.3, the occurrence of pneumonia after VATS resection in the Cedars Sinai series was 1.2%. In the Z0030 trial, the incidence of pneumonia after open resection was 2.5%. The incidence of pneumonia in the Duke VATS series was 5% (17). Because pneumonia is a clinical diagnosis, other measures of sputum retention and poor airway hygiene must be analyzed in order to more completely gauge its prevalence. As mentioned above, many patients with significant sputum retention ultimately require bronchoscopy for atelectasis. In the Cedars Sinai series, only 0.2% of patients were reported as experiencing atelectasis, while 6.4% of patients in the Z0030 trial had atelectasis. In the propensity-matched analysis of the STS database depicted in Table 29.4, pneumonia occurred in 3.0% of patients after VATS lobectomy versus 4.4% of patients in the open lobectomy group (p NS). The incidence of patients with atelectasis was 2.1% after VATS lobectomy and 3.3% after thoracotomy (p NS). The incidence of postoperative intubation was significantly different, occurring in 1.4% of patients following VATS lobectomy and 3.1% of patients following thoracotomy ($p = 0.0046$). Although the need for intubation encompasses post-operative complications other than atelectasis and pneumonia, these are major reasons for reintubation following pulmonary resection.

In addition to the surgical approach, there are other measures to reduce the incidence of sputum retention. The most important tactic is smoking cessation prior to surgery. Vaporciyan et al. (45) found in a retrospective analysis of 237 patients undergoing pneumonectomy that patients who continued to smoke within 1 month of the operation were at increased risk for developing pneumonia and adult respiratory distress syndrome (ARDS). Chest physiotherapy, including coughing, early ambulation, incentive spirometry, and percussion with postural drainage, is the standard approach for postoperative prophylaxis and therapy for sputum retention. However, patients with recalcitrant sputum retention may require more invasive measures such as transcricoid saline injection to stimulate coughing. As mentioned above, bronchoscopy may ultimately be required to aspirate secretions and to stimulate a more vigorous cough. Many recommend the liberal use of minitracheostomies in high-risk patients as a form of prophylaxis and treatment. The minitracheostomy tube allows immediate and repeated aspiration of the tracheobronchial tree. It is placed percutaneously through the cricothyroid membrane either at the time of surgery or at the bedside postoperatively. In a prospective randomized trial of 102 high-risk patients, Bonde et al. (46) found that prophylactic use of minitracheostomy significantly lowered the incidence of sputum retention. Similarly, Au et al. (47) reported a decreased need for suction bronchoscopy in patients who had undergone minitracheostomy placement.

Atrial fibrillation

The incidence of atrial fibrillation (AF) following noncardiac thoracic surgery has been documented to range from 10% to 40% (48,49). Although the exact mechanism for the development of AF following noncardiac thoracic surgery is not known, a number of associated clinical features have been described. Major risk factors include advanced age, concomitant lung disease, and extensive hilar dissection (50–52). Although generally transient and self limiting, AF can increase the length of stay and cost of hospitalization. In addition, it is associated with increased 30-day mortality and can lead to embolic events (53).

Following pulmonary resection, meticulous management of fluid balance and electrolyte levels, particularly potassium and magnesium, are imperative to decrease the incidence of AF. In addition to such measures, the ability of numerous agents including β-blockers, calcium channel blockers, digoxin, and amiodarone to provide effective prophylaxis against the development of postoperative AF has been investigated (54). Patients already taking β-blockers or calcium channel blockers pre-operatively should continue on those medications post-operatively. For patients not taking a rate control agent pre-operatively, several prospective randomized trials have demonstrated a statistically significant reduction in the incidence of AF in patients receiving prophylactic calcium channel blockers. In the most recent study, published by Amar and colleagues, the incidence of AF was reduced from 25% to 15% in patients receiving diltiazem prophylaxis (55).

When AF does occur, management decisions must be made quickly. Hemodynamically unstable patients require immediate electrical cardioversion. For stable patients, providers must choose between controlling the rate—generally with beta or calcium channel blockers—and attempting to chemically cardiovert with amiodarone. Approximately 50% of AF episodes will convert to normal sinus rhythm with rate controlling agents alone within 12 hours, so this is generally an appropriate initial strategy (56). β-blockers need to be used with caution in patients with COPD, who represent a large proportion of patients undergoing pulmonary surgery. The use of nonselective β-blockers such as propranolol may induce or worsen bronchospasm. β1-selective blockers such as metoprolol are generally well-tolerated except in patients with severe COPD. Many patients, particularly those with other risk factors for stroke, whose AF persists beyond 48 hours, are started on anticoagulation therapy for 4 to 6 weeks. In order to attempt to avoid this and the attendant bleeding risk, most patients whose AF persists for more than 24 hours should undergo an attempt at chemical cardioversion with amiodarone. This drug is successful in restoring sinus rhythm in up to 86% of postoperative patients (57). As with β-blockers, amiodarone needs to be used with caution in patients who have undergone lung resection because of the risk of pulmonary toxicity. It is generally not recommended for use in patients who have undergone pneumonectomy or who are mechanically ventilated due to an unacceptably high rate of ARDS developing when amiodarone was used as a prophylaxis in pneumonectomy patients (58).

With the decrease in postoperative pain and the presumably lowered adrenergic state following VATS resections, it has been hoped that the incidence of AF would be less than that after thoracotomy. In the Cedars Sinai series, the incidence of AF following VATS resection was 2.9%, while it was 14.4% in the Z0030 trial. In the Duke VATS series, the incidence of AF was 10% (17). In the propensity-matched analysis of the STS database depicted in Table 29.4, AF occurred in 7.3% of patients after VATS lobectomy versus 11.5% of patients in the open lobectomy group (p = 0.0004). An important caveat in interpreting these results is that there may be a higher percentage of peripheral tumors in the VATS group than in the thoracotomy group. As mentioned above, extensive dissection involving the hilum, as is required for central tumors, is associated with an increased incidence of AF.

SUMMARY

The revival of thoracoscopy for the management of diseases of the chest is one of the most important recent advancements in thoracic surgery. With proper judgment and skill, the surgeon can safely apply this approach to a wide variety of cardiothoracic procedures. Although the approach is minimally invasive, the risks for complications must not be overlooked. Anticipation and attention to the details of patient selection, intraoperative technique, and postoperative patient management will help with prevention, early identification, and successful management of complications after thoracoscopy. Recent data from several large series suggest a decrease in the incidence of atrial fibrillation following VATS lung resection compared with thoracotomy. Improvements in the rates of postoperative air leak and pneumonia have been more modest.

REFERENCES

1. Jacobeus HC. Ueber die möglichkeit die zytoskopie bei untersuchung seroser hohlungen anzuwenden. *Munch Med Wochenschr* 1910;57:2090–2092.
2. Demmy TL, Curtis JJ. Minimally invasive lobectomy directed toward frail and high-risk patients: a case-control study. *Ann Thorac Surg* 1999;68:194–200.
3. Lewis RJ, Caccavale RJ, Sisler GE, et al. One hundred consecutive patients undergoing video-assisted thoracic operations. *Ann Thorac Surg* 1992;54:421–426.
4. Boffa DJ, Allen MS, Grab JD, et al. Data from the Society of Thoracic Surgeons General Thoracic Surgery database: the surgical management of primary lung tumors. *J Thorac and Cardiovasc Surg* 2008;135:247–254.
5. Epstein SK, Faling LJ, Daly BD, et al. Predicting complications after pulmonary resection. Preoperative exercise testing vs a multifactorial cardiopulmonary risk index. *Chest* 1993;104:694–700.
6. Melendez JA, Carlon VA. Cardiopulmonary risk index does not predict complications after thoracic surgery. *Chest* 1998;114:69–75.
7. Brunelli A, Fianchini A, Gesuita R, et al. POSSUM scoring system as an instrument of audit in lung resection surgery. Physiological and operative severity score for the enumeration of mortality and morbidity. *Ann Thorac Surg* 1999;67:329–331.
8. Melendez JA, Barrera R. Predictive respiratory complication quotient predicts pulmonary complications in thoracic surgical patients. *Ann Thorac Surg* 1998;66:220–224.
9. Pierce RJ, Copland JM, Sharpe K, et al. Preoperative risk evaluation for lung cancer resection: predicted postoperative product as a predictor of surgical mortality. *Am J Respir Crit Care Med* 1994;150:947–955.
10. DeCamp MM Jr, Jaklitsch MT, Mentzer SJ, et al. The safety and versatility of video-thoracoscopy: a prospective analysis of 895 consecutive cases. *J Am Coll Surg* 1995;181:113–120.

11. Jaklitsch MT, DeCamp MM Jr, Liptay MJ, et al. Video-assisted thoracic surgery in the elderly. A review of 307 cases. *Chest* 1996;110:751–758.
12. Demmy TL, Wagner-Mann CC, James MA, et al. Feasibility of mathematical models to predict success in video-assisted thoracic surgery lung nodule excision. *Am J Surg* 1997;174:20–23.
13. Jancovici R, Lang-Lazdunski L, Pons F, et al. Complications of video-assisted thoracic surgery: a five-year experience. *Ann Thorac Surg* 1996; 61:533–537.
14. Yim AP, Liu HP. Complications and failures of video-assisted thoracic surgery: experience from two centers in Asia. *Ann Thorac Surg* 1996; 61:538–541.
15. Krasna MJ, Deshmukh S, McLaughlin JS. Complications of thoracoscopy. *Ann Thorac Surg* 1996;61(4):1066–1069.
16. McKenna RJ, Houck W, and Fuller CB. Video-assisted thoracic surgery lobectomy: experience with 1100 cases. *Ann Thorac Surg* 2006;81: 421–426.
17. Onaitis MW, Petersen RP, Balderson SS, et al. Thoracoscopic lobectomy is a safe and versatile procedure: experience with 500 consecutive patients. *Ann Surg* 2006;244:420–425.
18. Roviaro G, Varoli F, Vergani C, et al. Video-assisted thoracoscopic major pulmonary resections: technical aspects, personal series of 259 patients, and review of the literature. *Surg Endosc* 2004;18: 1551–1558.
19. Allen MS, Darling GE, Pechet TV, et al. Morbidity and mortality of major pulmonary resections in patients with early-stage lung cancer: initial results of the randomized, prospective ACOSOG Z0030 trial. *Ann Thorac Surg* 2006;81:1013–1020.
20. Paul S, Altorki NK, Sheng S, et al. Thoracoscopic lobectomy is associated with lower morbidity than open lobectomy: a propensity-matched analysis from the STS database. *J Thorac Cardiovasc Surg* 2010;139:366–378.
21. Yim AP, Ho JK. Malfunctioning of vascular staple cutter during thoracoscopic lobectomy. *J Thorac Cardiovasc Surg* 1995;109:1252.
22. Watanabe A, Abe T, Yamauchi A, et al. Reinforcement of a bronchial stump in VATS lobectomy. *Thorac Cardiovasc Surg* 2000;48:242–243.
23. Jones DR, Graeber GM, Tanguilig GG, et al. Effects of insufflation on hemodynamics during thoracoscopy. *Ann Thorac Surg* 1993;55: 1379–1382.
24. Cooper JD. Technique to reduce air leaks after resection of emphysematous lung. *Ann Thorac Surg* 1994;57:1038–1039.
25. Venuta F, Rendina EA, De Giacomo T, et al. Technique to reduce air leaks after pulmonary lobectomy. *Eur J Cardiothorac Surg* 1998;13:361–364.
26. Eugene J, Dajee A, Kayaleh R, et al. Reduction pneumonoplasty for patients with a forced expiratory volume in 1 second of 500 milliliters or less. *Ann Thorac Surg* 1997;63:186–190; discussion 190–192.
27. Hazelrigg SR, Boley TM, Naunheim KS, et al. Effect of bovine pericardial strips on air leak after stapled pulmonary resection. *Ann Thorac Surg* 1997;63:1573–1575.
28. Stammberger U, Klepetko W, Stamatis G, et al. Buttressing the staple line in lung volume reduction surgery: a randomized three-center study. *Ann Thorac Surg* 2000;70:1820–1825.
29. Brunelli A, Al Refai M, Monteverde M, et al. Pleural tent after upper lobectomy: a randomized study of efficacy and duration of effect. *Ann Thorac Surg* 2002;74:1958–1962.
30. Okur E, Kir A, Halezeroglu S, et al. Pleural tenting following upper lobectomies or bilobectomies of the lung to prevent residual air space and prolonged air leak. *Eur J Cardiothorac Surg* 2001;20:1012–1015.
31. Robinson LA, Preksto D. Pleural tenting during upper lobectomy decreases chest tube time and total hospitalization days. *J Thorac Cardiovasc Surg* 1998;115:319–326; discussion 326–327.
32. Handy JR Jr, Judson MA, Zellner JL. Pneumoperitoneum to treat air leaks and spaces after a lung volume reduction operation. *Ann Thorac Surg* 1997;64:1803–1805.
33. De Giacomo T, Rendina EA, Venuta F, et al. Pneumoperitoneum for the management of pleural air space problems associated with major pulmonary resections. *Ann Thorac Surg* 2001;72:1716–1719.
34. Cerfolio RJ, Holman WL, Katholi CR. Pneumoperitoneum after concomitant resection of the right middle and lower lobes (bilobectomy). *Ann Thorac Surg* 2000;70:942–946; discussion 946–947.
35. Fleisher AG, Evans KG, Nelems B, et al. Effect of routine fibrin glue use on the duration of air leaks after lobectomy. *Ann Thorac Surg* 1990;49: 133–134.
36. Wong K, Goldstraw P. Effect of fibrin glue in the reduction of post-thoracotomy alveolar air leak. *Ann Thorac Surg* 1997;64:979–981.
37. Fabian T, Federico JA, Ponn RB. Fibrin glue in pulmonary resection: a prospective, randomized, blinded study. *Ann Thorac Surg* 2003;75: 1587–1592.
38. Wain JC, Kaiser LR, Johnstone DW, et al. Trial of a novel synthetic sealant in preventing air leaks after lung resection. *Ann Thorac Surg* 2001;71:1623–1628; discussion 1628–1629.
39. Cerfolio RJ, Bass C, Katholi CR. Prospective randomized trial compares suction versus water seal for air leaks. *Ann Thorac Surg* 2001;71: 1613–1617.
40. Liberman M, Muzikansky A, Wright CD, et al. Incidence and risk factors of persistent air leak after major pulmonary resection and use of chemical pleurodesis. *Ann Thorac Surg* 2010;89:891–897.
41. Bonde P, McManus K, McAnespie M, et al. Lung surgery: identifying the subgroup at risk for sputum retention. *Eur J Cardiothorac Surg* 2002;22:18–22.
42. Yim AP, Ko KM, Chau WS, et al. Video-assisted thoracoscopic anatomic lung resections. The initial Hong Kong experience. *Chest* 1996;109:13–17.
43. Walker WS, Pugh GC, Craig SR, et al. Continued experience with thoracoscopic major pulmonary resection. *Int Surg* 1996;81:255–258.
44. Kirby TJ, Mack MJ, Landreneau RJ, et al. Lobectomy—video-assisted thoracic surgery versus muscle-sparing thoracotomy. A randomized trial. *J Thorac Cardiovasc Surg* 1995;109(5):997–1001.
45. Vaporciyan AA, Merriman KW, Ece F, et al. Incidence of major pulmonary morbidity after pneumonectomy: association with timing of smoking cessation. *Ann Thorac Surg* 2002;73:420–425; discussion 425–426.
46. Bonde P, Papachristos I, McCraith A, et al. Sputum retention after lung operation: prospective, randomized trial shows superiority of prophylactic minitracheostomy in high-risk patients. *Ann Thorac Surg* 2002; 74:196–202; discussion 202–203.
47. Au J, Walker WS, Inglis D, et al. Percutaneous cricothyroidotomy (minitracheostomy) for bronchial toilet: results of therapeutic and prophylactic use. *Ann Thorac Surg* 1989;48:850–852.
48. Roselli EE, Murthy SC, Rice TW, et al. Atrial fibrillation complicating lung cancer resection. *J Thorac Cardiovasc Surg* 2005;130:438–444.
49. Vaporciyan AA, Correa AM, Rice DC, et al. Risk factors associated with atrial fibrillation after noncardiac thoracic surgery: Analysis of 2588 patients. *J Thorac Cardiovasc Surg* 2004;127:779–786.
50. Asamura H, Naruke T, Tsuchiya R, et al. What are the risk factors for arrhythmias after thoracic operations? A retrospective multivariate analysis of 267 consecutive thoracic operations. *J Thorac Cardiovasc Surg* 1993;106:1104–1110.
51. Krowka MJ, Pairolero PC, Trastek VF, et al. Cardiac dysrhythmia following pneumonectomy. Clinical correlates and prognostic significance. *Chest* 1987;91:490–495.
52. Ciriaco P, Mazzone P, Canneto B, et al. Supraventricular arrhythmia following lung resection for non-small cell lung cancer and its treatment with amiodarone. *Eur J Cardiothorac Surg* 2000;18:12–16.
53. Irshad K, Feldman LS, Chu VF, et al. Causes of increased length of hospitalization on a general thoracic surgery service: a prospective observational study. *Can J Surg* 2002;45:264–268.
54. Sedrakyan A, Treasure T, Browne J, et al. Pharmacologic prophylaxis for postoperative atrial tachyarrhythmia in general thoracic surgery: evidence from randomized clinical trials. *J Thorac Cardiovasc Surg* 2005;129:997–1005.
55. Amar D, Roistacher N, Rusch VW, et al. Effects of diltiazem prophylaxis on the incidence and clinical outcome of atrial arrhythmias after thoracic surgery. *J Thorac Cardiovasc Surg* 2000;120:790–798.
56. Amar D. Postoperative atrial fibrillation. *Heart Dis* 2002;4:117–123.
57. Barbetakis N, Vassiliadis M. Is amiodarone a safe antiarrhythmic to use in supraventricular tachyarrhythmias after lung cancer surgery? *BMC Surg* 2004;4:7.
58. Van Mieghem W, Coolen L, Malysse I, et al. Amiodarone and the development of ARDS after lung surgery. *Chest* 1994;105:164.

PART

IV

Complications of Vascular Surgery

CHAPTER

30

Complications of Arterial Surgery

Gilbert R. Upchurch Jr., Jonathan L. Eliason, John E. Rectenwald, and James C. Stanley

INTRODUCTION

The practice of surgery has evolved significantly over the last 5 to 10 years with all specialties migrating toward minimally invasive approaches. Vascular surgery, in particular, has been affected by this trend with the majority of all arterial lesions now being first treated using endovascular techniques. For example, in the past, aortoiliac occlusive disease (AIOD) was managed primarily by aortobifemoral bypass, whereas presently, this disease process is managed percutaneously with angioplasty and stenting (1). It is predictable that, over time, with endovascular first approaches, the number of open arterial operations performed will decline, thus impacting outcomes and complications as well as the training of future surgeons. In addition to changes in practice patterns, the literature reporting complications has shifted from primarily single institution reports from centers of excellence to large databases or registries with statewide or national samples (2–11). While this shift in reporting allows increased power in analyzing morbidity and mortality through coding across large populations, the details or granularity of specific complications have become less visible in the resulting reports.

Despite these shifts in vascular practice and reporting, many of the life- and organ-threatening complications that occur during open arterial surgery remain the same (12). In the present chapter, specific complications accompanying operations on the extracranial carotid arteries, the aorta, and the lower extremity arteries are highlighted, as these three regions of the vasculature comprise the majority of arterial reconstructions. In addition, studies from large databases will document significant variability in practice across a wide range of complications.

EXTRACRANIAL CAROTID ARTERY

Although carotid artery stenting is being undertaken with increasing frequency (13,14), carotid endarterectomy (CEA) remains one of the most commonly performed peripheral vascular operations in the United States (15). To achieve its primary goal of stroke prevention, CEA must be performed with a low complication rate. The incidence of stroke after CEA varies widely, with established morbidity and mortality standards reported by experienced surgeons as being between 3% and 7% (16,17). This variation in postoperative morbidity and mortality may be secondary to the patients' presenting symptoms, ranging from asymptomatic carotid disease to frank stroke. It may also be influenced by the surgeon's volume of carotid procedures (18). Specific complications (Table 30.1) and complication rates (Table 30.2) from centers of excellence deserve individual comment (19–23).

Early complications

Myocardial Infarction

With the exception of stroke, cardiac complications remain the most common source of mortality after CEA. In an important early study, DeBakey and associates (24) noted the risk of perioperative myocardial infarction to be three times higher in patients who had hypertension or symptomatic carotid artery disease than in those who did not. Myocardial infarction is also the most common cause of late death in patients who have undergone prior CEA. The 10-year survival after CEA when patients with coronary artery disease underwent coronary artery bypass grafting (CABG) prior to CEA was 55%, compared to 32% among those whose coronary artery disease remained uncorrected (25).

Given this increased risk of myocardial infarction following CEA, many have advocated combined CEA and CABG (26,27). While single institutional experiences have reported acceptable results, current recommendations are that combined CEA–CABG be performed only in the setting of symptomatic internal carotid artery (ICA) disease. This subject remains controversial. In contemporary series, with the more frequent use of statins and antiplatelet agents, no evidence-based data exist to establish guidelines (28). A recent study by Brown et al. suggested that stroke and death rates nationally following CEA–CABG were higher than those reported from isolated centers of excellence (29). In that study, the combined CEA–CABG stroke and death rate was 17.7%. Importantly, the diagnosis of stroke in this series was often delayed with most strokes not involving the same hemisphere as the CEA.

Cerebral Ischemia or Infarction

This complication may occur during endarterectomy as a result of internal carotid occlusion and inadequate collateral flow to the brain. The risk of cerebral ischemia is

Gilbert R. Upchurch Jr.: University of Veginia, Charlottesville, VA Jonathan L. Eliason, John E. Rectenwald, and James C. Stanley: University of Michigan, Ann Arbor, MI

Table 30.1 Common early and late complications following carotid endarterectomy

Early
Stroke
Myocardial infarction
Cranial nerve injury
 Vagus nerve (recurrent laryngeal, superior laryngeal)
 Hypoglossal nerve
 Facial nerve (marginal mandibular)
Hemodynamic instability
 Hypotension and bradycardia
 Hypertension
Neck hematoma
Acute internal carotid artery thrombosis
Carotid dissection

Late
Recurrent Carotid Artery Stenosis (neointimal hyperplasia 0–24 months, recurrent atherosclerosis (>24 months)
Pseudoaneurysm (patch infection, suture line failure, arterial wall disruption)

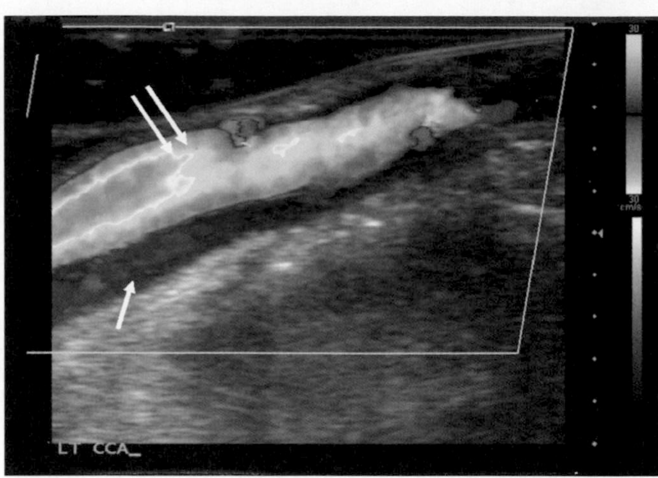

FIGURE 30.1. Intraoperative duplex documenting common carotid artery dissection (*single arrow*) and patent common carotid artery (*double arrow*) that occurred secondary to the insertion of a shunt during carotid endarterectomy (CEA).

greater among patients with contralateral carotid occlusion or prior stroke affecting the ipsilateral hemisphere (30).

A variety of techniques have been used to lessen cerebral ischemia during CEA. One approach is to place an indwelling carotid shunt in all patients. However, many surgeons find the technical performance of this to be more difficult when a shunt is in place and believe that the process of shunt insertion may cause complications, including intimal tears and dissections (Fig. 30.1), embolization of proximal atherosclerotic debris, and air emboli. Use of a shunt is appropriate in those patients who have inadequate cerebral blood flow during carotid artery occlusion. Some surgeons prefer to perform CEA under local or regional anesthesia, and if carotid cross-clamping initiates neurologic dysfunction, then a shunt is inserted (31,32). The use of selective shunting under regional anesthesia appears to offer a reasonable means of recognizing intraoperative cerebral ischemia during carotid clamping. In addition, this approach may reduce cardiovascular complications, such as perioperative blood pressure instability accompanying general anesthesia.

One of the original techniques used for assessing the adequacy of cerebral blood flow in anesthetized patients was the measurement of carotid artery "stump pressure" or "back pressure" after the common and external carotid arteries are clamped. A 20-gauge needle, connected to a pressure transducer, is inserted into the carotid artery distal to the common carotid artery clamp. A mean stump pressure below 25 mm Hg (33) or 50 mm Hg (34) becomes an indication for the placement of a shunt. However, neurologic deficits are known to occur in patients who are operated on under regional anesthesia with stump pressures above these levels (35).

Continuous electroencephalographic (EEG) monitoring during carotid artery occlusion has been proposed to provide a sensitive technique for monitoring the adequacy of cerebral blood flow. Approximately 15% of patients evaluated in this fashion will require shunting during CEA (36). Some patients with stump pressures above 75 mm Hg will develop EEG evidence of cerebral ischemia. In one study, the EEG remained normal in 39 out of 1,009 patients subjected to endarterectomy under local anesthesia who showed obvious cerebral ischemia (37). In 52 other patients in this series, the EEG became abnormal, but the clinical status did not suggest cerebral ischemia. Thus, while EEG

Table 30.2 Early complications following carotid endarterectomy from contemporary, large, single institutional series

Primary Author	Year of Report	Study Period	Carotid Endarterectomies Performed (*N*)	Mortality (%)	Stroke (%)	Cranial Nerve Injury (%)	Postoperative Bleeding (%)
Ballotta	2004	1990–2002	1,150	0.3	0.9	4.5	Not stated
Conrad	2003	1990–1999	1,045	0.9	3.0	2.5	1.7
Darling	2003	1994–1999	3,429	1.1	1.7	0.6	2.3
Ecker	2003	1988–2000	1,000	0.9	1.0	0.7	Not stated
Illig	2003	1993–2000	1,168	0.6	2.7	0.8	2.7

may provide a means of monitoring cerebral perfusion during CEA, it is not consistently reliable.

A second cause of perioperative stroke is the embolization of the thrombus or atheromatous debris from within the diseased carotid artery. This complication may occur during the dissection of the carotid artery, placement or release of a clamp, or from platelet aggregates accumulating at the endarterectomy site during the operation or in the immediate postoperative period. Carotid artery dissection should always be performed with minimal manipulation of the internal carotid artery, using the so-called "no touch technique." Similarly, at the completion of the endarterectomy, the vessel lumen should be carefully irrigated with heparinized saline and all pieces of loose intima or media removed. Perioperative use of aspirin or other antiplatelet agents reduces the deposition of platelets on the surface of the endarterectomized vessel. The use of statins has also been associated with a reduced incidence of stroke following CEA (38).

A third cause of stroke following CEA is acute thrombosis of the internal carotid artery. This complication results most often from subintimal hemorrhage under a loose flap or inadequate control of proximal or distal endarterectomy end points. The completion duplex of the carotid artery has altered the traditional algorithm for the treatment of acute ICA thrombosis since it has been suggested that a normal completion duplex eliminates the need to immediately return the patient to the operating room (39). Intraoperative use of a carotid duplex has recently gained favor over "on-table" cerebral angiography. However, one could not be faulted for an aggressive approach and for returning all patients suspected of carotid thrombosis to the operating room in the setting of acute stroke after CEA.

A final cause of postendarterectomy stroke is intracerebral hemorrhage. This problem typically occurs on the second or third day after carotid endarterectomy, often during a period of severe hypertension (40). Neurologic deficits occurring on the second or third postoperative day should lead to duplex scanning or angiography to ensure the patency of the carotid artery. If a significant carotid artery defect is identified, the patient should be returned to the operating room and the vessel repaired. Computed tomography (CT) or magnetic resonance imaging (MRI) of the brain should be obtained if the carotid artery is normal. The presence of intracerebral hemorrhage carries a poor prognosis, and some have recommended neurosurgical evacuation of the hematoma in selected patients (32).

Cerebral hyperperfusion syndrome is a rare but potentially lethal complication following either CEA or carotid stenting (41). Following the carotid intervention with improved blood flow and pressure, patients with this complication develop a constellation of symptoms, including ipsilateral migraine-like headache, seizure, and transient focal neurologic deficits in the absence of frank cerebral ischemia. While this syndrome is defined by the clinical picture, the diagnosis is confirmed with imaging techniques. The incidence of cerebral hyperperfusion syndrome is reported to be between 0.4% and 14%. A partial list of preoperative and perioperative risk factors for the development of cerebral hyperperfusion syndrome includes long-standing hypertension, diabetes mellitus, increased age, recent contralateral CEA (<3 months), high-grade ipsilateral carotid stenosis with poor collateral flow, contralateral carotid occlusion, and refractory postoperative cerebral hyperperfusion. No specific therapies have been documented to adequately treat patients with cerebral hyperperfusion (41). However, strategies involving the prevention of cerebral edema with head elevation, limiting fluid resuscitation, and aggressively treating hypertension seem justified. As cerebral hyperperfusion syndrome can result in severe brain edema, intracerebral hemorrhage, and death, treatment should be directed toward reducing blood pressure and limiting excessive increases in cerebral perfusion.

Cranial Nerve Injury

Cranial nerve injury is not an uncommon complication following CEA, accompanying as many as 39% of these procedures (42). Certain cranial nerve injuries are not detectable upon casual examination, in that one-third of these injuries produce no clinical symptoms such as hoarseness, difficulty in swallowing, or changes in speech (42,43). The most common injuries involve the recurrent laryngeal nerve with subsequent hoarseness, and the hypoglossal nerve with the resultant tongue deviation toward the side of the injury and difficulty in mastication. Recurrent laryngeal nerve injury is usually a manifestation of injury to the ipsilateral vagus nerve, most often by a retractor or clamps. Other injuries involve the superior laryngeal nerve with a resultant voice fatigue and the marginal mandibular nerve with a drooping of the lower lip. Less commonly injured nerves are the greater auricular nerve, which results in numbness over the lower earlobe, the spinal accessory nerve and the glossopharyngeal nerve with shoulder shrugging and difficulty swollowing respectively.

Many cranial nerve injuries are secondary to traction and usually resolve within 6 months. However, bilateral injuries may be severely disabling or even life-threatening. This is particularly true in the case of bilateral recurrent laryngeal nerve injury. All patients who undergo CEA should be subjected to careful cranial nerve examination before and after operation. In addition, bilateral CEAs should not be performed simultaneously but should be staged following appropriate neurologic examination, including indirect laryngoscopy between operations.

Hematoma

Hematoma after CEA, although rare, may, in part, reflect the fact that many patients receive preoperative antiplatelet agents and heparin anticoagulation intraoperatively. Reoperation for the evacuation of a hematoma or control of bleeding following CEA occurs in only 1% of experienced practices (44). Nevertheless, acute airway compromise may occur and opening of the neck at the bedside on rare occasions may obviate the need for the creation of an emergent surgical airway, allowing for an orderly return to the operating room.

Hypertension and Hypotension

Hypertension and hypotension associated with CEA have been attributed to a number of factors. Hypotension and bradycardia are thought to be secondary to increased baroreceptor activity during the dissection of the carotid artery or stimulation of the sinus nerve following the removal of a rigid atherosclerotic plaque. Hypertension may be caused by the interruption of the carotid sinus nerve activity due to its transection or changes in the arterial wall compliance. In an early study (45), severe hypertension complicated 19% of carotid endarterectomies and hypotension affected an additional 28% of cases. Such alterations in blood pressure were associated with a 9% incidence of postoperative neurologic deficits, in contrast to no neurologic complications among normotensive patients. In addition, the evolution of care of the patient who undergoes CEA from an inpatient to an outpatient or during a 23-hour stay visit is primarily dependent on the avoidance of hypo- or hypertension (46). Postoperative hypertension is much more common in chronically hypertensive patients. Patients who have undergone bilateral CEA are particularly prone to develop hypertension, and in addition, appear to lose their normal compensatory respiratory and circulatory responses to hypoxia (47). Because of the potential severity of these complications, hypertension should be controlled and volume deficits corrected in all patients prior to elective CEA (45).

Reports documenting the rates of early complications from large, national, or state databases have gained popularity in recent years. Table 30.3 documents the results of four large studies in which hard end points, such as mortality, stroke, and myocardial infarction rates, are reported (2–5). However, these studies often lack granularity, and do not report on complications such as cranial nerve injury or hematoma rates.

Late complications

Recurrent Carotid Stenosis

Symptomatic recurrence of carotid stenosis occurs in less than 3% of patients, whereas the asymptomatic recurrence rate is between 9% and 12% (48). Two forms of recurrent carotid disease have been identified (49). One type occurs within the first 2 years secondary to neointimal fibroplasia. This lesion is characterized by the proliferation of mesenchymal cells, perhaps of smooth-muscle origin (Fig. 30.2). The second type usually develops after 2 years and represents recurrent atherosclerosis. The mechanisms by which these two forms of recurrent carotid stenosis evolve are unknown, but there is evidence that they represent a continuum and are a consequence of vessel wall injury (50). In this regard, extensive platelet aggregation within the endarterectomized vessel may be associated with the release of various growth factors that act as a stimulus to cell proliferation. Aspirin and other antiplatelet agents may prevent platelet aggregation with adherence to the vessel wall, yet there is little clinical evidence that these drugs prevent carotid stenosis (48). Other factors identified with hypercellular responses after CEA include hypercholesterolemia and female gender (51). The incidence of recurrent carotid stenosis is three times higher in women than it is in men. Recurrent carotid stenosis also occurs more often in patients with diffuse vascular disease and has been most

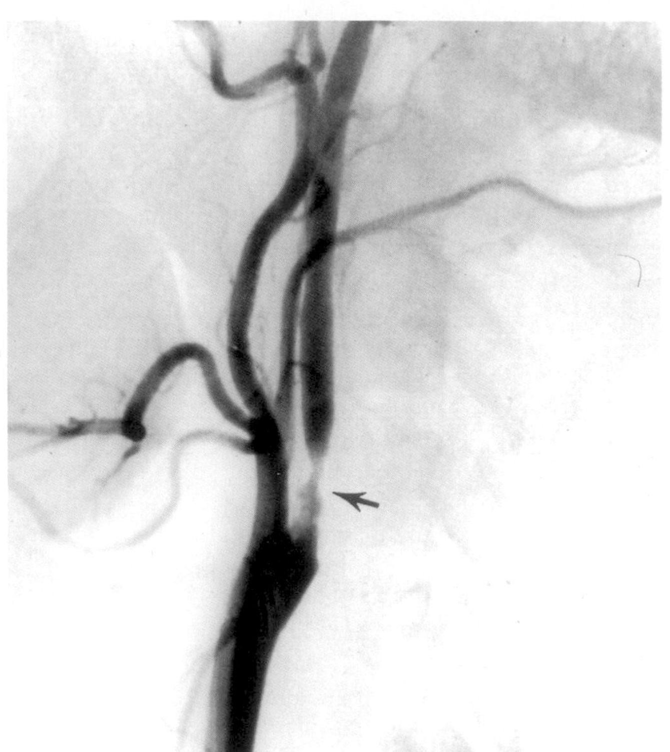

FIGURE 30.2. Recurrent carotid stenosis secondary to intimal fibroplasia following carotid endarterectomy.

Table 30.3 Complication rates from state and national databases following carotid endarterectomy (CEA)

Primary Author	Year of Report	Study Year	CEA (*N*)	Mortality (%)	Stroke (%)	Myocardial Infarction (%)
McPhee	2008	2005	122,986	0.57	1.1	Not stated
Sidawy	2009	2005–2007	3,259	0.73	1.68	0.58
Halm	2009	1998–1999	8,662[a]	1.1	3.1	Not stated
Vogel	2009	2005	73,929	0.26	2.66	2.34

[a]Only white patients are included in this table since cumulative numbers for all races were not included in this report.

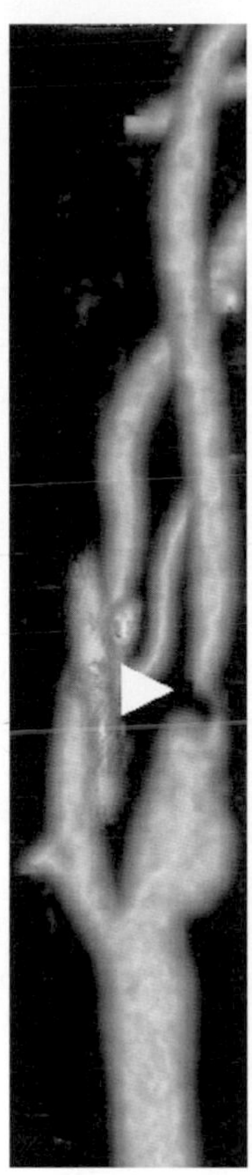

FIGURE 30.3. Computed tomography angiography (CTA) documenting high grade stenosis (*arrow*) distal to a previous carotid endarterectomy (CEA).

striking in those with a history of heavy cigarette smoking (48). Carotid patching has also been documented to decrease the incidence of recurrent carotid stenosis, with autogenous saphenous vein patches outperforming synthetic patches (52).

High-grade stenoses or symptomatic recurrent carotid artery stenoses should be assessed by CT angiography (Fig. 30.3) or conventional cerebral arteriography and treated. Operations for recurrent carotid artery stenosis can be demanding, particularly those that occur within the first 2 years. In these cases, there is usually extensive scarring around the artery, making the dissection challenging. Special attention should be paid to the identification and avoidance of cranial nerve injury. Patch-graft angioplasty is recommended in closing the carotid arteriotomy in reoperations. Replacement of the affected carotid artery with an ePTFE or saphenous vein graft may be necessary (53). Carotid stenting as a means to lessen the risks accompanying reoperation has gained favor in the treatment of recurrent carotid artery stenoses (54).

False Aneurysm

False aneurysm formation following CEA is a particularly rare complication, occurring in less than 0.05% of cases (55). Causes of aneurysm formation include suture line failure, arterial wall degeneration, and infection, particularly of a patch used in the arteriotomy closure (Fig. 30.4). The management of carotid artery false aneurysms usually entails arterial closure with a saphenous vein patch or carotid artery replacement with an interposition vein graft.

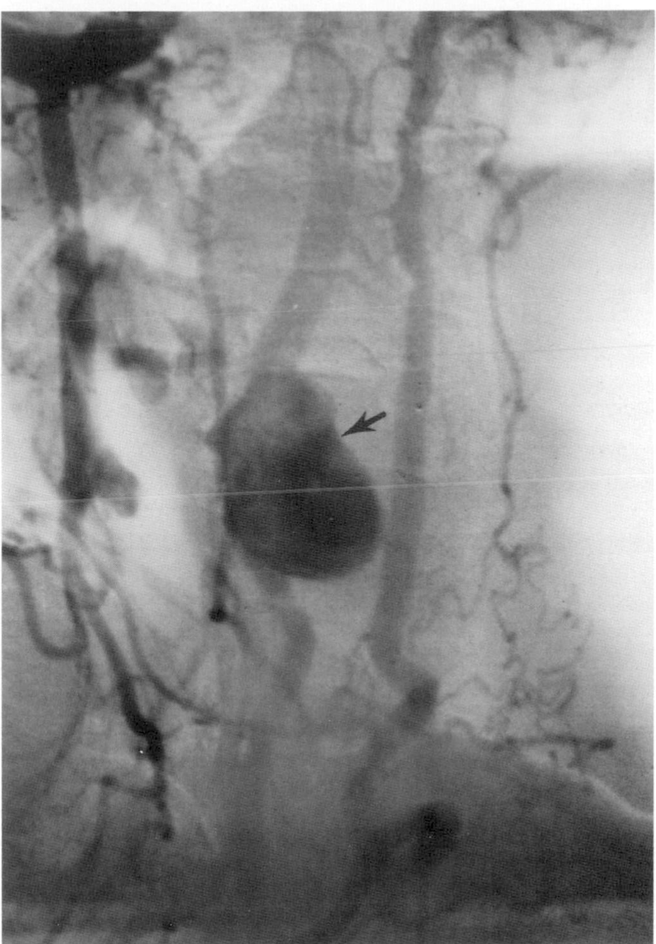

FIGURE 30.4. False aneurysm of right carotid artery following carotid endarterectomy with patch graft closure.

AORTA

Modern open aortic reconstruction is one of the most complex vascular surgery procedures, with significant variation in mortality and morbidity based on both patient and provider variables (56,57). The number of aortic procedures has been impacted by both the aging of society, as well as by the introduction of endovascular aortic repair. The importance of comorbid diseases on mortality associated with elective and emergent abdominal aortic aneurysm (AAA) repair are important and have been well documented in two large population-based studies (58,59). Specific complications (Table 30.4) and complication rates (Table 30.5) are discussed individually (60–63).

Early complications

Myocardial Ischemia and Infarction

Cardiac complications are the most relevant causes of perioperative mortality and late postoperative death following

Table 30.4 Common early and late complications following infrarenal abdominal aortic aneurysm repair

Early
Myocardial infarction
Hemorrhage
Respiratory failure
Renal failure
Embolization
Mesenteric ischemia
Spinal cord ischemia
Ureteral injuries
Chylous ascites
Late
Graft infection (aortoduodenal fistula, anastomotic pseudoaneurysm)
Graft thrombosis
Structural graft failure
Aneurysm proximal/distal to repair
Abdominal wall hernia
Impotence/retrograde ejaculation

aortic surgery (64). Fatal myocardial infarction accounted for 37% of early postoperative deaths among 343 consecutive patients with abdominal aortic aneurysms treated at a major referral center (65). In this regard, severe coronary artery disease was present in 36% of 1,000 patients with AAAs who were subjected to mandatory coronary arteriography before routine aortic surgery. Recent results from the same institution suggests that the rate of this dreaded complication has markedly decreased with only 1% of 1,135 patients sustaining a perioperative myocardial infarction following open AAA repair (62).

Aggressive preoperative cardiac management of patients who are to undergo aortic operations includes selective exercise or chemical stress testing, as well as coronary arteriography (66), and in select cases, it includes preoperative coronary artery angioplasty or bypass. The criteria for pursuing extensive cardiac studies have been well established (67,68). The combined performance of CABG and AAA repair has been reported (69) but can be advocated only in patients with both symptomatic coronary and aneurysm disease. Modern intraoperative and postoperative care (60) includes hemodynamic assessments with Swan-Ganz pulmonary artery catheters and transesophageal echocardiography. Such monitoring has been reported to result in less than a 2% perioperative mortality rate, and more importantly, a 75% 5-year survival rate with only a 5% late cardiac mortality (70). These data contrast with a 25% to 35% cardiac mortality at 5 years following major aortic surgery noted in older series.

Hemorrhage

Hemorrhage may contribute to early morbidity and mortality following elective aortic surgery (71). Certain factors may be associated with excessive operative blood loss during aortic surgery. Venous anomalies, which occur in approximately 5% of cases, such as the duplication of the inferior vena cava, circumferential renal vein, left-sided inferior vena cava, and the retroaortic left renal vein may be easily injured and lead to considerable hemorrhage. The absence of an anterior left renal vein is indicative of a retroaortic left renal vein, which may be torn during the posterior dissection of the proximal infrarenal aorta. Particularly disposed to injury is the posteriorly located small lumbar vein originating from the midportion of the left renal vein. Careful ligation of all vessels transected while exposing the aorta not only reduces operative blood loss but also lessens the incidence of troublesome postoperative hemorrhage. Similarly, careful temperature control and blood component replacement will lessen the incidence of coagulopathies associated with excessive blood loss and the administration of large quantities of banked blood. The benefits of using autotransfusion devices during aortic surgery repair has been supported by some (72), but contested by others (73).

Accurate blood and fluid replacement is important in preventing hypotension associated with aortic unclamping (64). Vasodilators used to decrease peripheral resistance and afterload during aortic cross-clamping should be discontinued prior to declamping so that further decreases in peripheral resistance upon declamping will not result in hypotension. Reperfusion of ischemic extremities releases

Table 30.5 Early complications following intact abdominal aortic aneurysm repair from contemporary series

Primary Author	Year of Report	Study Period	Patients Undergoing Elective Open AAA Repair (*N*)	Mortality (%)	Myocardial Infarction (%)	Acute Renal Failure (%)	Respiratory Failure (%)	Ischemic Colitis (%)
Bertges	2000	1994–1999	314	1.9	2.9	4.5	7.3	1.6
Elkouri	2004	1999–2001	261	1.2	5.4	4.2	7.7	Not stated
Hertzer	2002	1989–1998	1,135	1.2	1	1.7	4	1
Menard	2003	1990–2000	572	1.0	1.2	2.3	5.2[a]	0.2

[a]Number reflects clinically significant pneumonia only, not additional sources of respiratory failure.

vasoactive substances that have an adverse effect on blood pressure, such as lactic acid, potassium, and other vasoactive products, into the systemic circulation (74). An expeditious operation, slow pelvic and lower extremity reperfusion, and good communication with the anesthesiologist should lessen hazardous reperfusion events.

Renal Insufficiency

Renal insufficiency accompanying aortic surgery is more likely to occur with hemorrhagic hypotension and inadequate blood replacement (75). It is associated with more than 30% mortality in the setting of an elective aneurysmectomy (58). Temporary or permanent renal failure affects more than 70% of patients with ruptured AAAs. In this setting, it is associated with a 53% mortality rate for being directly related to total aortic clamp time—the time delay from actual rupture to aneurysm resection—as well as blood loss (76). Renal failure is also a relatively common complication following the resection of thoracoabdominal aneurysms (77). Postoperative dialysis is required in 5% of these patients who have normal preoperative renal function and 17% of those with preoperative serum creatinine levels >2 mg/dL (78). Intraoperative renal artery perfusion with cold balanced salt solutions may have a protective effect in those with impaired preoperative renal function, but it does not appear to protect against disturbances in renal function among patients with normal preoperative function.

Embolization

Lower extremity embolization is a serious complication of aortic surgery, often from the dislodgement of mural debris during operative dissection or from accumulated thrombus in the static column of blood above the aortic clamp (Fig. 30.5). Although larger emboli can often be retrieved with a balloon catheter, smaller atheroembolic particles cannot be removed and will lead to microvascular occlusions, producing cutaneous ischemia including so-called "trash foot" if the digital arteries are affected (79). The frequency of such complications has been generally accepted to range from 2% to 5%.

Technical maneuvers to lessen the complication of embolization during aortic surgery include careful dissection of iliac vessels prior to the clamp application, distal iliac clamp application prior to a proximal aortic clamp application, effective systemic heparin anticoagulation, thorough aspiration of the lumen of the aortic prosthesis prior to implantation to remove any adherent blood or debris, prevention of stagnant blood accumulation in the graft while the anastomoses are being performed, as well as vigorous flushing of the proximal and distal vessels prior to reestablishment of extremity arterial blood flow. Patients with atheroembolism experience extreme pain in the feet and toes associated with an exaggerated inflammatory response to cholesterol emboli. Epidural anesthesia may help to blunt the sympathetic vasoconstrictive response associated with this type of ischemic pain.

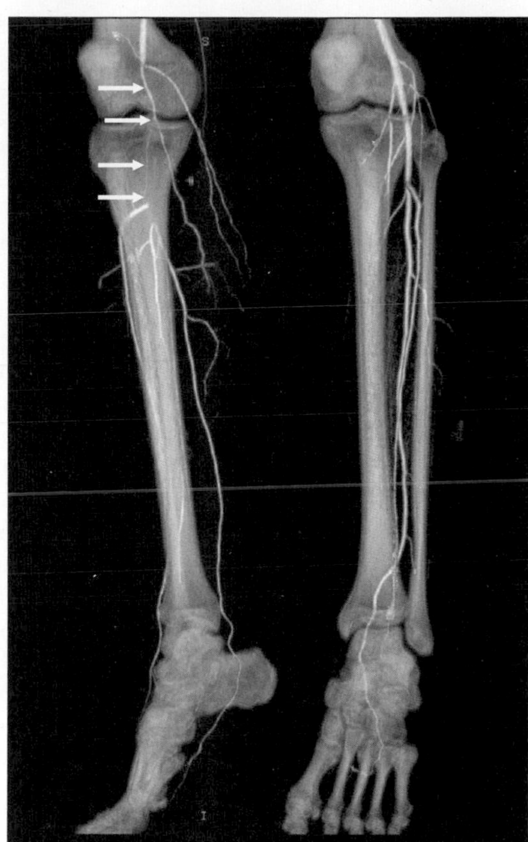

FIGURE 30.5. CTA following aortobifemoral bypass documenting missing popliteal artery, consistent with a decrease in ankle–brachial indices (ABIs), secondary to embolism from debris in the femoral artery.

Colon Ischemia

Colon ischemia has been reported to accompany 0.2% to 10% of AAA repairs (80,81). Intestinal ischemia is less common following aortofemoral bypass or aortoiliac endarterectomy for occlusive disease. A prospective study (82) using a routine colonoscopy documented colon ischemia in 4.3% of elective aortic procedures for occlusive disease, 7.4% for aneurysmal disease, and 60% when treating ruptured AAAs. Overall mortality for colon ischemia in this setting is approximately 50% and approaches 90% with transmural infarction. Colonic ischemia is more likely to accompany aortic resection with improper inferior mesenteric artery ligation, ruptured aneurysms with arterial and venous compression by hematoma within the mesocolon, operative trauma to vessels within the mesocolon, hypotension with diminished perfusion of colon blood vessels, inadequate collaterals to the inferior mesenteric arterial circulation, and damage to collateral vessels when they do exist. The presence of a large meandering mesenteric artery, carrying blood from the left colic branch of the inferior mesenteric to the left branch of the middle colic artery just beyond its origin from the superior mesenteric artery, is indicative of superior mesenteric artery occlusive disease. In such cases, the reconstruction of the superior mesenteric artery or inferior mesenteric artery reimplantation into the vascular graft may be necessary to avoid colon ischemia. Although rarely measured, inferior mesenteric artery back pressure of less than 40 mm Hg in patients undergoing AAA resection also suggests a need to restore antegrade flow in this vessel (83). Routine reimplantation of the inferior mesenteric artery into the aortic graft has been advocated by some, but such does not ensure the prevention of significant mesenteric ischemia (84). Intraoperative Doppler confirmation of blood flow at both the mesenteric and antimesenteric borders of the sigmoid colon is a useful means of confirming the adequacy of collateral blood flow to the colon following aortic reconstruction.

Patients with severe colon ischemia often present 1 to 2 days postoperatively with liquid brown or bloody diarrhea, left-sided abdominal pain, abdominal distension, acidosis, oliguria, and fever. Less severe ischemia may not become apparent until 5 to 7 days after surgery. Any patient who undergoes aortic surgery and develops these signs and symptoms requires urgent colonoscopy. If transmural infarction is suspected, laparotomy and resection of the affected colon should be undertaken with the creation of a proximal colostomy and a Hartmann's pouch or mucous fistula distally. Mucosal ischemia, if not severe, may be managed by hydration, hemodynamic stabilization, and the intravenous administration of antibiotics. Mucosal ischemia may resolve within 7 to 10 days, but close monitoring with repeated colonoscopy is indicated. If deeper structures are affected and perforation does not occur, stricture formation may occur in 6 to 10 weeks. In one study of 472 cases of AAA repair, 33% of the elective mortality was associated with acute gastrointestinal complications, of which ischemic colitis was the most common (80).

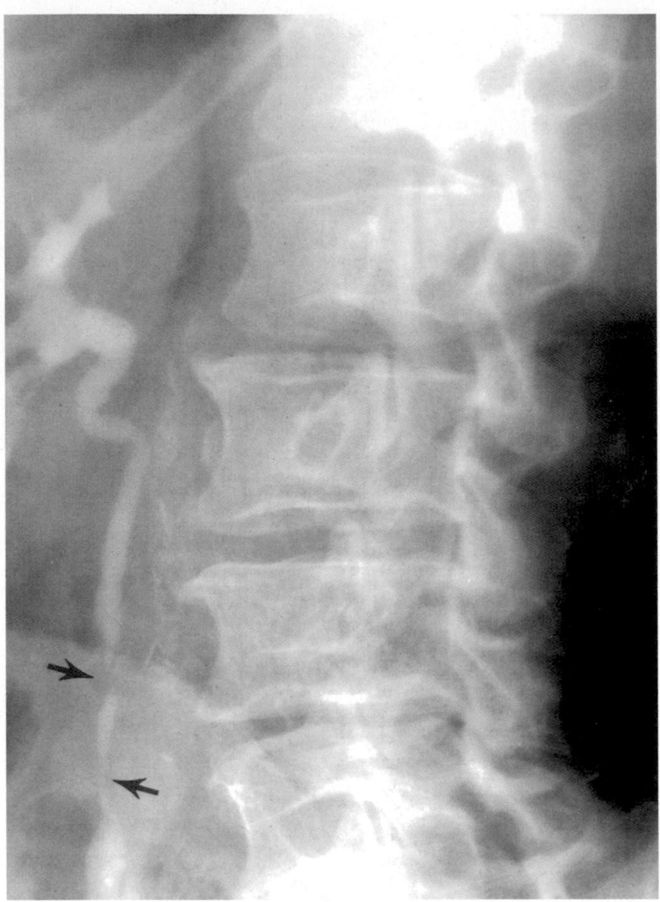

FIGURE 30.6. Ureteral injury (*arrows*) due to excessive dissection and devascularization during aortic reconstruction leading to an ischemic stenosis.

Spinal Cord Ischemia

Spinal cord ischemia, accompanies 0.2% of elective AAA repairs and 2% of emergent repairs of ruptured aneurysms. Spinal cord ischemia is not predictable from preoperative arteriograms (85). Among 51 reported cases of postoperative spinal cord ischemia following abdominal aortic surgery, 45% occurred with ruptured aneurysms, 33% with elective aneurysmectomy, and 20% with treatment for AIOD (86).

Spinal cord ischemia is more common following thoracoabdominal aneurysm repair, occurring in approximately 10% of these procedures, and in more than 40% of patients with aneurysms caused by dissections (78). The primary cause of spinal ischemia has been attributed to the interruption of the cord's blood supply. The clamping of the supraceliac aorta and concomitant hypotension appear to contribute to this complication. The former relates to the aortic origin of the spinal artery of Adamkiewicz, which has been found as high as T8 and as low as L4. Impaired hypogastric artery perfusion, embolization, and postoperative hypotension may also cause lower spinal cord ischemia during abdominal aortic surgery (87).

No universal intervention has been found to protect against spinal cord ischemia. Recent research has centered on the gradient between spinal cord pressure and systemic arterial blood pressure below the aortic cross-clamp. In order to maintain at least a 10 mm Hg gradient, the withdrawal of spinal fluid to decrease intraspinal canal pressure has been advocated (88,89). Spinal cord monitoring, using somatosensory evoked potentials, as well as various drug interventions have also been proposed to lessen the risk of this complication (90,91).

Ureteral Injuries

Ureteral injuries may occur during dissection and repair of large aortic or iliac aneurysms, particularly in the presence of inflammatory aneurysms (92) (Fig. 30.6). Most ureteric injuries are associated with devascularization due to the excessive or injudicious skeletonization of the ureter. The inadvertent inclusion of a portion of the ureteral wall in the suture closure of tissues over the implanted aortic graft is an infrequent cause of ureteral injury. Aortofemoral graft limbs should be tunneled posterior to the ureters so as to prevent compression of the ureters.

Large Administrative Databases

Early complication rates derived from large administrative datasets of patients undergoing open AAA repair may now be compared to complication rates for patients undergoing endovascular AAA repair (EVAR) (Table 30.6) (6–10). It is

Table 30.6 Complication rates from state and national databases following open AAA repair

Primary Author	Year of Report	Study Period	Patients (*N*)	Mortality (%)	Cardiac Complication (%)	Renal Complication (%)	Respiratory Complication (%)	Mesenteric Ischemia (%)
Dillavou	2006	1994–2003	Roughly 28,000/year	Decreased from 5.57 to 3.20	Not stated	Not stated	Not stated	Not stated
Giles	2009	2001–2004	32,056	5.3	Not stated	Not stated	Not stated	Not stated
Schermerhorn	2008	2001–2004	22,830	4.8	9.4	10.9	17.4	2.1
Schwarze	2009	2001–2006	Decreased from 17,784 to 8,451/year	3.19–4.24	7.57–9.68	5.74–11.08	15.2–20.8	Not stated

clear from these reports that, over time, the results of open AAA repair have improved with lower mortality rates. The impact of EVAR on the results of open AAA repair, over time, will be important to continue to follow, as many of the patients who presently undergo open repair are not anatomically appropriate candidates for EVAR. In addition, the training of surgeons to perform open repair will be challenged by the ever increasing use of endovascular technology to manage aortic pathology.

Late complications

Prosthetic Aortic Graft Infection

This complication affects between 1% and 6% of implanted aortic grafts, with an average incidence of 0.7% for aortoiliac grafts and 1.6% for aortofemoral grafts (93). Mortality from infected grafts in the aortoiliac or aortofemoral positions can be as high as 50%. However, in a series of 92 patients with 84 infected aortoiliac or aortofemoral grafts, more than 70% were cured of their infection, with follow-up ranging from 10 months to 12 years (94). In this series, 25% of the patients required amputation, most at a level above the knee. Thus, amputation morbidity remains high, even with successful management of the graft infection.

Factors contributing to graft infection include intraoperative contact of the graft with the skin, contaminated lymphatics, intraoperative breaks in sterile technique, extension from wound sepsis, arterial wall infection, and transient bacteremias. Bacteria are found 43% of the time in aneurysm thrombus and aortic wall specimens cultured during routine AAA repair with the most common organism being *Staphylococcus epidermidis* (95).

A significant increase in graft infection occurs in patients with positive arterial wall cultures undergoing secondary operations. The bacteriology of graft sepsis has changed. In 1977, *Staphylococcus aureus* was the leading pathogen (96), with a shift to *S. epidermidis* as the most likely cause of infection. *S. epidermidis* organisms are sometimes difficult to culture from infected grafts. As such, portions of the grafts should be finely diced up and cultured not only on plates but also in broth following sonication (97). A number of tests may be performed if a diagnosis of graft infection is suspected, including indium-labeled white blood cell imaging, MRI, and CT (Fig. 30.7). Direct operative inspection of the graft suspected to be infected may be required to establish the presence or absence of infection. Failure of graft incorporation, accumulation of perigraft fluid or debris, and a Gram stain providing evidence of bacteria or leukocytes all support the existence of a graft infection.

The traditional means of treating an infected graft is first its removal, followed by secondary revascularization. In most series, this method has been supplanted by revascularization first, either during the same operation as the graft removal or staged 2 to 5 days prior to graft removal (98). Significant differences in mortality or new graft infections do not occur using this latter technique; however, there is a significantly lower rate of extremity amputation. The use of the superficial femoral vein to replace the infected aortic graft has been recently advocated (99). Others have suggested the use of antibiotic-soaked grafts or cryopreserved grafts or extra-anatomic bypasses (100,101).

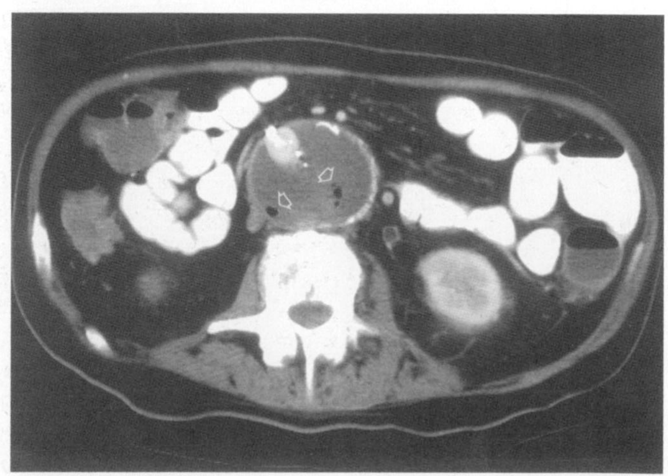

FIGURE 30.7. Infected graft in a redundant aortic aneurysm sac with visible gas bubbles (*white arrow heads*).

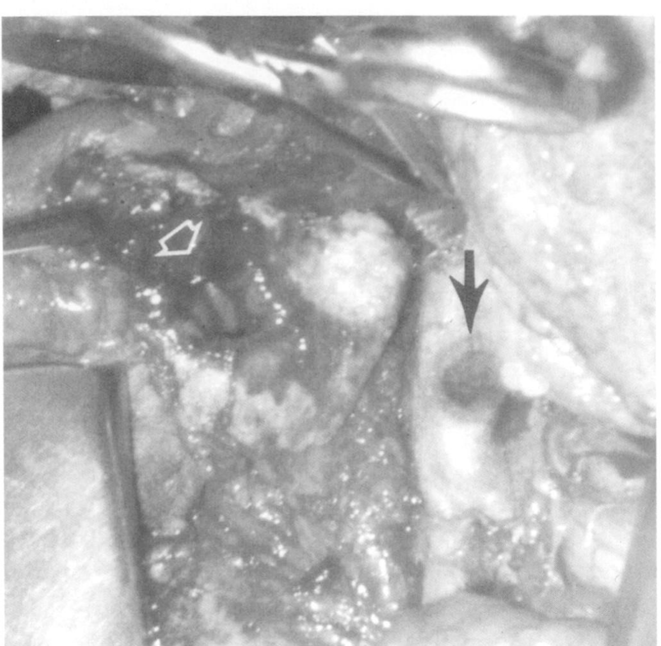

FIGURE 30.8. Bile staining (*solid arrow*) of an infected aortic graft as a consequence of a duodenal erosion (*open arrow*).

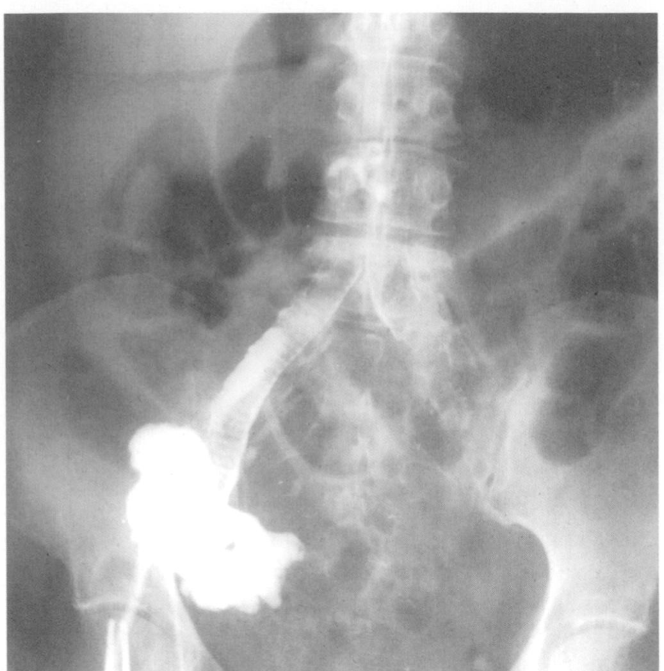

FIGURE 30.10. Infected aortic graft limb with opaque contrast injected through an open sinus tract in the groin. Primary infection was an aortoduodenal erosion.

Aortoenteric graft intestinal erosion is a distinct subcategory of graft infection (Fig. 30.8). This complication often follows a lack of retroperitoneal tissue coverage of the implanted aortic graft during the primary reconstruction (Fig. 30.9). Graft sepsis and intestinal bleeding are usually the first manifestations of this complication. The spread of the graft infection to involve the entire conduit occurs in many cases (Fig. 30.10). In general, the entire prosthetic graft in this setting must be excised.

In the case of an isolated aortobifemoral graft limb infection, after demonstration of good incorporation of the proximal graft limb at the graft bifurcation, the limb alone may be removed leaving the remainder of the graft in place. In this setting, the proximal limb may be divided, soft tissue interposed between the limb and the main body of the graft, and the distal limb removed from the groin after closure of the abdominal incision. If the body of an aortic graft requires removal, the aortic stump must be securely closed with a double layer of monofilament suture and covered with omentum or presacral fascia.

Structural Graft Failure

Serious structural graft failure is rare with modern grafts. Most large prostheses placed in the aortoiliofemoral area function well, exhibiting 85% to 95% long-term patencies. However, fabric prostheses may exhibit friability, inability

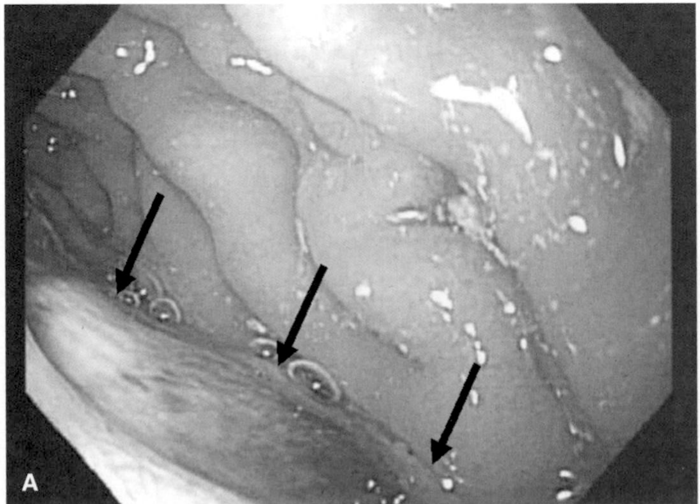

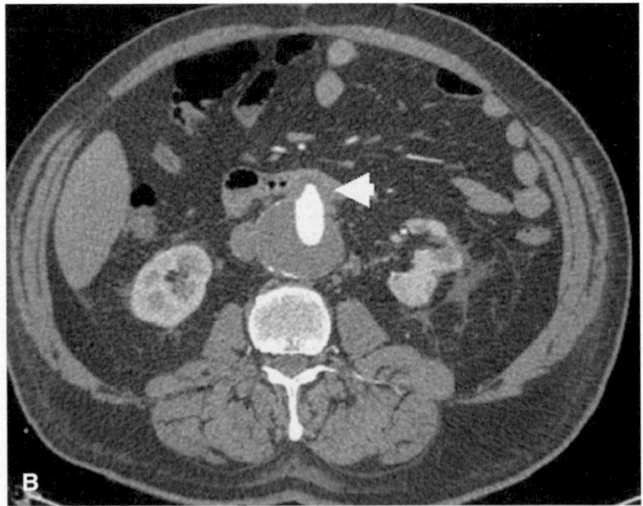

FIGURE 30.9. **A:** Endoscopy (black arrows denote exposed vascular graft). **B:** Confirming CTA, documenting an aortoenteric fistula (*white arrow head*).

to hold sutures, rents in the wall, aneurysm formation, and both early and late dilation (102). Defective grafts have been described for all types of grafts monthly involving Dacron knitted, woven, and velour construction. Structural failures in grafts usually reflect mechanical failures in their construction. Fabricated Dacron grafts, because of their design, have been noted to increase in diameter by approximately 15% to 20% following insertion into the arterial circulation. Anticipated graft dilation such as this must be taken into consideration when choosing a prosthetic graft size for implantation.

Graft Thromboses

Early aortoiliac or aortofemoral graft thromboses are usually technical in nature, including intimal flaps, anastomotic narrowing, graft twisting or kinking, compression of the graft limb by the inguinal ligament, unrecognized inflow disease, inadequate runoff because of unappreciated distal disease, and undiagnosed hypercoagulability (103). Late graft thromboses are usually secondary to progressive downstream atherosclerosis or anastomotic intimal fibrodysplasia (Figs. 30.11 and 30.12).

The most important factor contributing to long-term aortoiliac or aortofemoral graft patency is inadequate outflow. In the case of an aortofemoral bypass for occlusive disease, as opposed to aneurysm disease, this relates to the patency of the deep femoral artery. Progressive atherosclerosis of the superficial femoral or infrapopliteal arteries may contribute to graft thrombosis, particularly in patients who continue to smoke (103). Impaired inflow is a much less common cause of late graft thrombosis (104), and when it does occur, it is most often associated with the low placement of grafts originating from the more terminal aorta. Less frequent causes of late graft thromboses include kinking or excessive angulation of the graft limbs, accumulation of mural thrombus, and pseudoaneurysm formation.

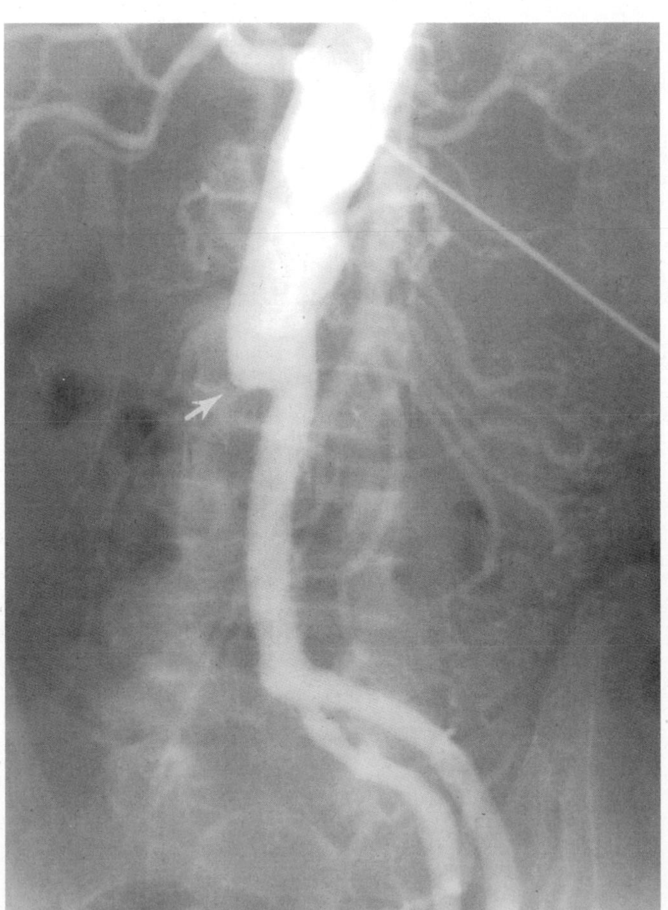

FIGURE 30.11. Late limb occlusion of an aortobifemoral bypass graft.

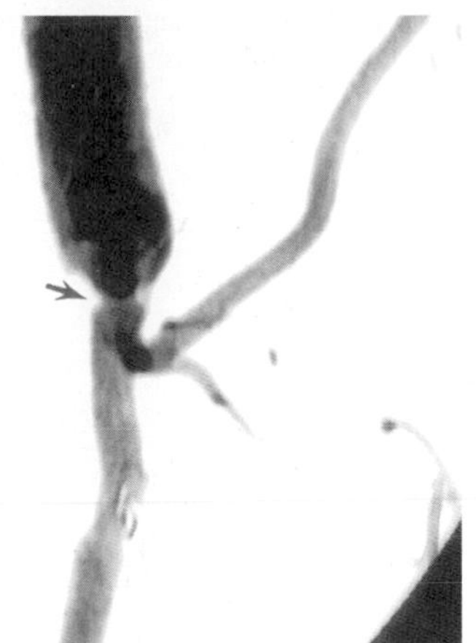

FIGURE 30.12. Intimal hyperplasia resulting in an anastomotic stenosis (*arrow*) of an aortobifemoral bypass graft.

A comprehensive study of 1,748 aortic reconstructions in 1,647 patients with aortoiliac occlusive disease included 1,186 aortofemoral bypasses, 76 aortoiliac bypasses, 176 combined aortoiliac and aortofemoral bypasses, 181 cases of aortoiliac endarterectomy, and 129 remote bypasses (105). Early perioperative or postoperative graft occlusion decreased from 8.3% from 1954 to 1963 to 3.2% from 1974 to 1983. Late anastomotic thromboses affected 13.1% of aortofemoral bypasses, 10.5% of aortoiliac bypasses, 10.8% of bypasses combining aortoiliac and aortofemoral limbs, and 13.8% of aortoiliac endarterectomies. Anastomotic stenoses, defined as a reduction in lumen size to the degree of the threatened thrombosis, occurred in 4.5% of aortofemoral bypasses, 3.9% of aortoiliac bypasses, and 2.2% of aortoiliac endarterectomies. Secondary repair of complications affecting aortofemoral bypass procedures resulted in 77% 5-year patency rates, 77% 10-year patency rates, 73% 15-year patency rates, and 68% 20-year patency rates.

Anastomotic Aneurysms

Anastomotic aneurysms affect up to 6% of all aortoiliac or aortofemoral grafts (Fig. 30.13). In a large experience with 4,214 vascular reconstructions between 1957 and 1974, there was a 1.7% incidence of anastomotic aneurysms, occurring with a 3% incidence in the femoral region, 1.2% in the iliac region, and 0.2% in the aortic region (106). The most common cause of false aneurysm formation was the

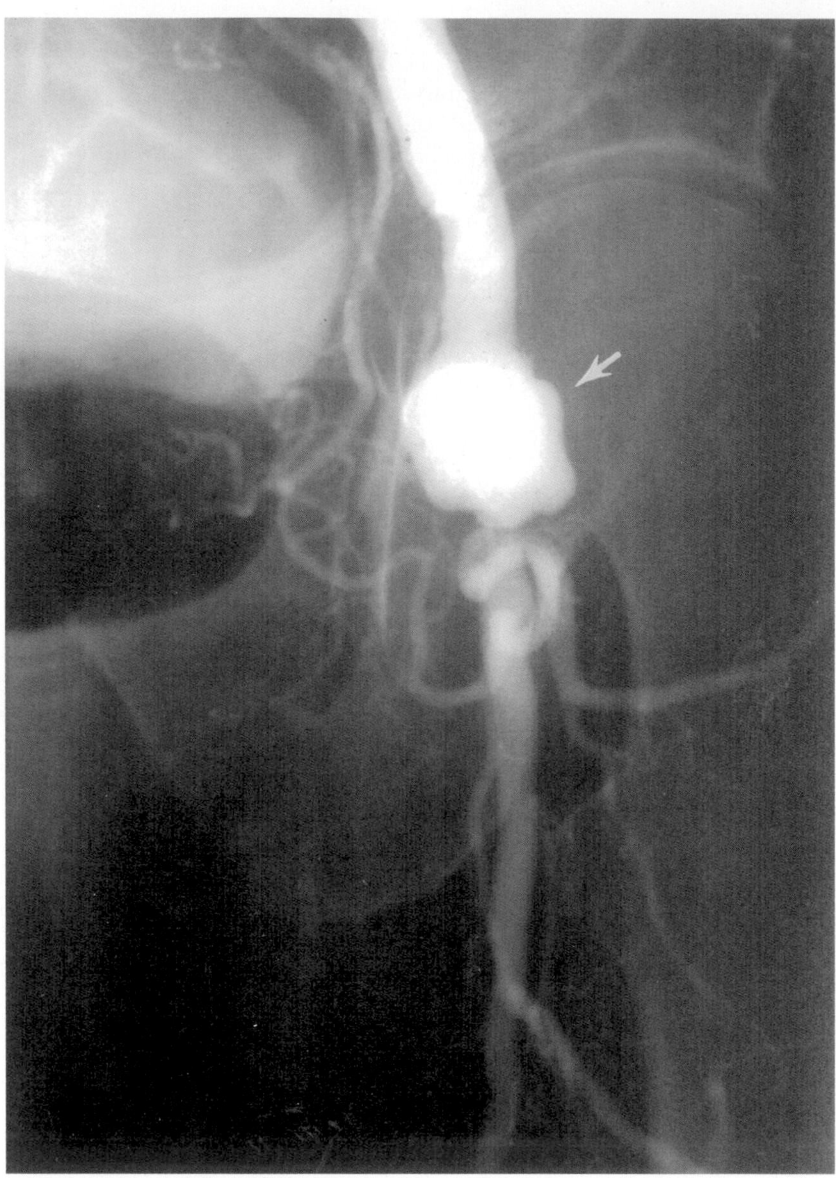

FIGURE 30.13. Femoral artery anastomotic aneurysm (*arrow*) affecting an aortobifemoral bypass graft limb.

structural deficiency of the host vessel, followed by hypertension, mechanical stress, graft or suture defects, and infection. Elective repair of anastomotic aneurysms is successful in >80% of cases, whereas emergency repair is successful in 60% of cases. Late recurrences range from 11% to 14%.

Femoral false aneurysms are usually obvious on a physical examination. If rupture occurs, the vessel can usually be compressed prior to emergency operative intervention. However, aortic false aneurysms may remain silent until they become very large and rupture with life-threatening hemorrhage. Overall mortality for treating anastomotic aneurysms in the femoral region is 3.5%, with an amputation rate of 2.8% (107). Repair of false aortic aneurysms usually involves the insertion of a new segment of graft after debridement or excision of the involved native vessel. Endovascular graft placement in this setting may prove less hazardous (108).

Male Impotence

Iatrogenic sexual dysfunction, including impotence, and retrograde ejaculation has been reported to range from 21% to 88% in men undergoing conventional aortic reconstruction. In a unique experience employing a nerve-sparing approach with minimal aortic dissection and reperfusion of at least one hypogastric vessel, impotence was eliminated and retrograde ejaculation was reduced from 43% to 3% (109). Inasmuch as some 70% to 80% of patients with aortoiliac or aortofemoral arterial occlusive disease may already be impotent, it is important to document the presence or absence of impotence prior to surgery (110).

Vasculogenic impotence involves an inability to sustain an erection (111). Neurogenic impotence refers to the inability to achieve any erection at all. A penile systolic–brachial index below 0.6 is supportive of the presence of vasculogenic impotence. When vasculogenic impotence exists, consideration should be given to restoring internal

Table 30.7 Common early and late complications following lower extremity bypass

Early
Myocardial infarction
Hemorrhage
Bypass graft thrombosis
Lower extremity swelling (lymphocele, venous insufficiency)
Superficial skin infection (SSI)
Late
Graft thrombosis (neointimal hyperplasia 1–24 months, recurrent atherosclerosis (>24 months)
Graft infection
Retained AV fistula

iliac artery blood flow or occasionally performing a more direct revascularization of the penis. In the presence of neurogenic impotence, a penile implant is acceptable treatment. Most patients developing vasculogenic impotence from aortic surgery will not benefit from further revascularization, unless clear evidence of impaired pelvic perfusion exists. However, most will benefit from the newer pharmacologic agents available to treat erectile dysfunction.

LOWER EXTREMITY OCCLUSIVE DISEASE

All patients who undergo lower extremity revascularization should be subjected to rigorous postoperative follow-up (112). Surveillance is considered mandatory to detect impending graft failure, which may occur in 50% of patients. Specific complications (Table 30.7) and complication rates (Table 30.8) accompanying lower extremity bypass deserve note (113–117). Although lower extremity bypass is commonly performed, large administrative databases suggest that the overall mortality for these procedures is not insignificant (Table 30–9) (10,11).

Early complications

Myocardial Ischemia and Infarction

The major cause of early and late death after lower extremity revascularization is myocardial infarction (118). Operative mortality rates between 3% and 5% accompany these procedures and are almost entirely due to perioperative cardiac events. Patients treated for tibial or peroneal occlusive disease have a particularly high incidence of underlying coronary artery disease that underlies these cardiac complications.

Hemorrhage

Hemorrhage occurs after lower extremity revascularization in 1% to 3% of cases (119). Serious hemorrhage is usually secondary to anastomotic bleeding or unligated branches of implanted vein grafts. Less often, bleeding is due to coagulation defects, often related to the excessive administration of heparin and the use of dextran or antiplatelet agents such as aspirin and Plavix.

Bypass Graft Thrombosis

Acute bypass graft thrombosis occurring within 24 hours of surgery affects approximately 5% of lower extremity revascularizations. The most common causes of early graft thromboses are technical, including injury to veins during harvest, intimal flaps from an incomplete endarterectomy or a clamp injury, improper graft tunneling causing twisted or kinked conduits, and grafts placed under excessive tension. Early graft failure is twice as common in bypass grafts placed for limb salvage compared to those used in treating claudication (120). Poor arterial inflow and outflow have also been associated with early graft thromboses, as are infrapopliteal bypasses compared to above-the-knee bypass grafts. Hypovolemia or diminished cardiac output can also contribute to graft thrombosis. A hypercoagulable state may affect approximately 5% of patients undergoing infrainguinal bypass (121), and unexplained acute graft

Table 30.8 Complication rates following lower extremity bypass from contemporary, large, single institutional series

Primary Author	Year of Report	Study Period	Number of Lower Extremity Bypass Procedures (*N*)	Mortality (%)	Myocardial Infarction (%)	Stroke (%)	Perioperative Graft Failure (%)	Postoperative Bleeding (%)
Chew	2001	1983–1999	165[a]	1.8	9[b]	Not stated	11	5.4
Goshima	2004	1990–2002	318	1.3	3.9	1.3	3.5	1.3
Pomposelli	2003	1990–2000	1,032[c]	1.0	3[b]	0.3	4.2	Not stated
Raffetto	2002	Not stated	352	1.1	2.6	0.3	6.8	0.8
Roddy	2003	1968–1999	5,880	3.1	2.9[b]	Not stated	1.8[d]	2.1

[a]Surgical technique using composite vein grafts only.
[b]Percentage also reflects patients with other severe cardiac morbidity, such as congestive heart failure and arrhythmia.
[c]Surgical technique using only the dorsalis pedis artery as the target vessel.
[d]Perioperative graft failure defined as immediate limb loss.

Table **30.9** **Complication rates from large databases following lower extremity bypass**

Primary Author	Year of Report	Study Period	Bypass Procedures (*N*)	Mortality (%)
Aylin	2007	2001–2004	9,661	6.5%
[a]Birkmeyer	2002	1994–1999	Approx. 250,000	4.9–6.1%

thromboses deserve an evaluation for such. The use of statins may lessen lower extremity graft failures (122,123).

Most complications affecting lower extremity revascularizations are correctable if recognized early. In this regard, an objective assessment of the reconstruction in the operating room is critical. Completion angiography has been replaced by intraoperative duplex examination as the most common means of assessing the adequacy of graft placement (124), with standard criteria predictive of early bypass graft failure (117). Immediate postoperative ankle–brachial indices (ABIs) should also be performed to establish a baseline by which to compare future ABI studies.

Lymphoceles and Lymph Drainage

These complications occur most commonly following groin dissection and usually result from lymphatic channel interruption or a transected lymph node. Lymphatic drainage through a surgical incision is usually treated initially with strict bed rest and leg elevation. Frequent applications of sterile dressings or povidone–iodine–soaked gauze to the wound lessens the incidence of wound infection. Patients with small-volume intermittent drainage may be safely managed nonoperatively for short periods by this method, particularly in the absence of an underlying prosthetic graft. The need for operative intervention depends on the magnitude of the leak as well as the type of arterial reconstruction. Large quantities of lymph drainage or the presence of a prosthetic graft that would be at risk for infection necessitate prompt surgical exploration, with identification and ligature of identifiable leaking lymphatics.

Large administrative datasets

Early complication rates documented in large administrative databases are, for the most part, lacking for lower extremity bypasses, perhaps, in part, due to the lack of hard end points that can be easily tracked. Nevertheless, data from these studies document a fairly high mortality rate in these patients, further confirming the systemic nature of atherosclerosis.

Late complications

Late Graft Occlusion

Late (greater than 12 months) occlusion of lower extremity revascularization appears as a result of two distinct pathological entities (125). Those occurring within 12 to 24 months after graft insertion are most often due to neointimal hyperplasia and are usually found at the site of the distal anastomosis (Figs. 30.14 and 30.15). Graft occlusions that occur beyond 24 months are most often due to the progression of atherosclerosis (126). In one study, 87% of graft occlusions secondary to the progression of atherosclerosis occurred beyond the first year of implantation (127).

Graft Infection

Graft infection is a serious complication of lower extremity revascularization. Mortality after lower extremity graft infection averages 9% (128), and more than 50% of patients with this complication require amputation. The incidence of graft infection is three times higher when using synthetic grafts compared to autogenous vein grafts. The overall incidence of infection in expanded polytetrafluoroethylene or Dacron grafts is approximately 3% (128). If only one anastomosis is involved, local treatment with antibiotics, wound debridement, and muscle coverage may be attempted in selected cases. However, total graft excision and revascularization by an alternate route is required in most cases of infected synthetic conduits.

Lower Extremity Edema

Edema is a common and troublesome complication affecting as many as two-thirds of patients after lower extremity revascularization (129,130). Three mechanisms contribute to the development of edema. First, the loss of arteriolar vasoconstriction due to chronic ischemia can lead to uncontrolled hyperemia and increased pressures within the microcirculation, particularly when the leg is dependent. Second, interruption of lymphatic channels often occurs during vascular dissection. Third, the harvesting of the ipsilateral greater saphenous vein as the conduit for a bypass may render some patients with worsening venous insufficiency. Postoperative edema, although often very obvious, is usually self-limited and resolves in 3 to 4 months. Compression therapy in the form of support stockings or elastic wraps may alleviate symptoms in these patients.

Complications of In Situ Saphenous Vein Bypass Reconstructions

These include the persistence of large arteriovenous fistulas (Fig. 30.16), obstruction by residual valve leaflets, vasospasm, and luminal platelet aggregation (131). Although small arteriovenous fistulas are usually of little consequence, large

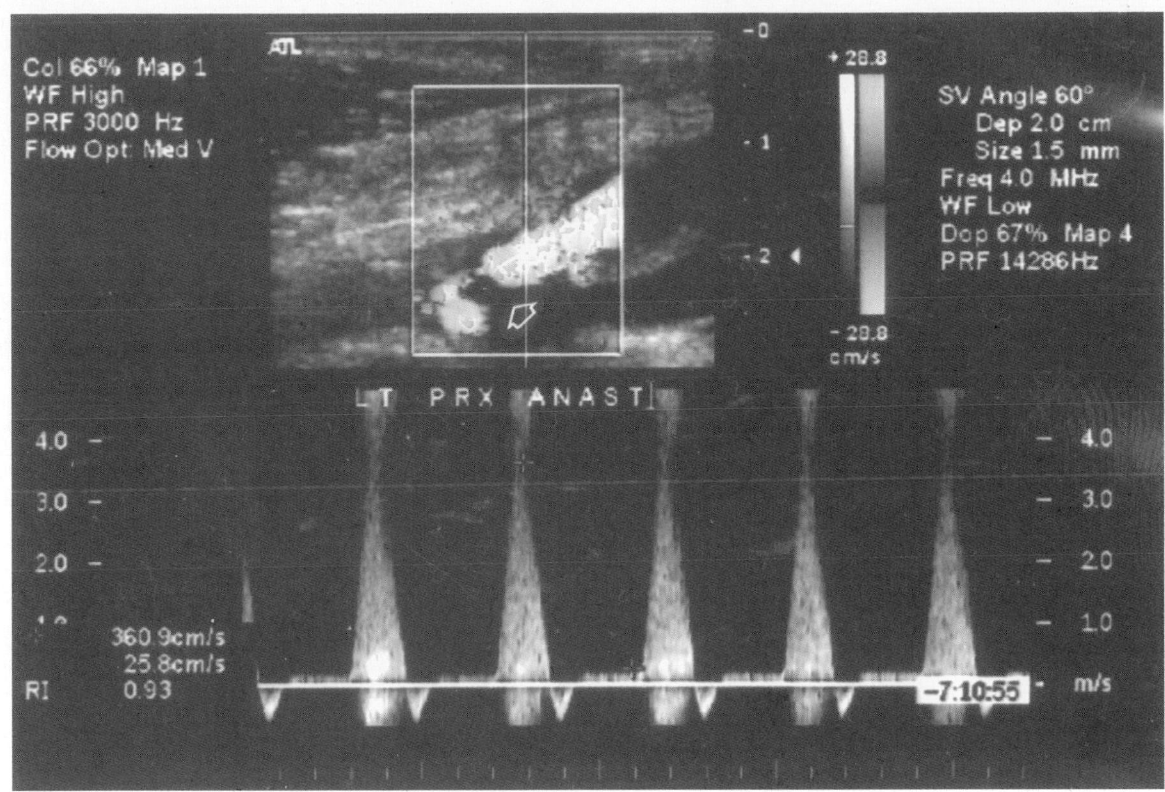

FIGURE 30.14. Femoral popliteal bypass stenosis due to intimal hyperplasia evident by duplex scan on direct image (*arrow*) and elevated blood flow velocities.

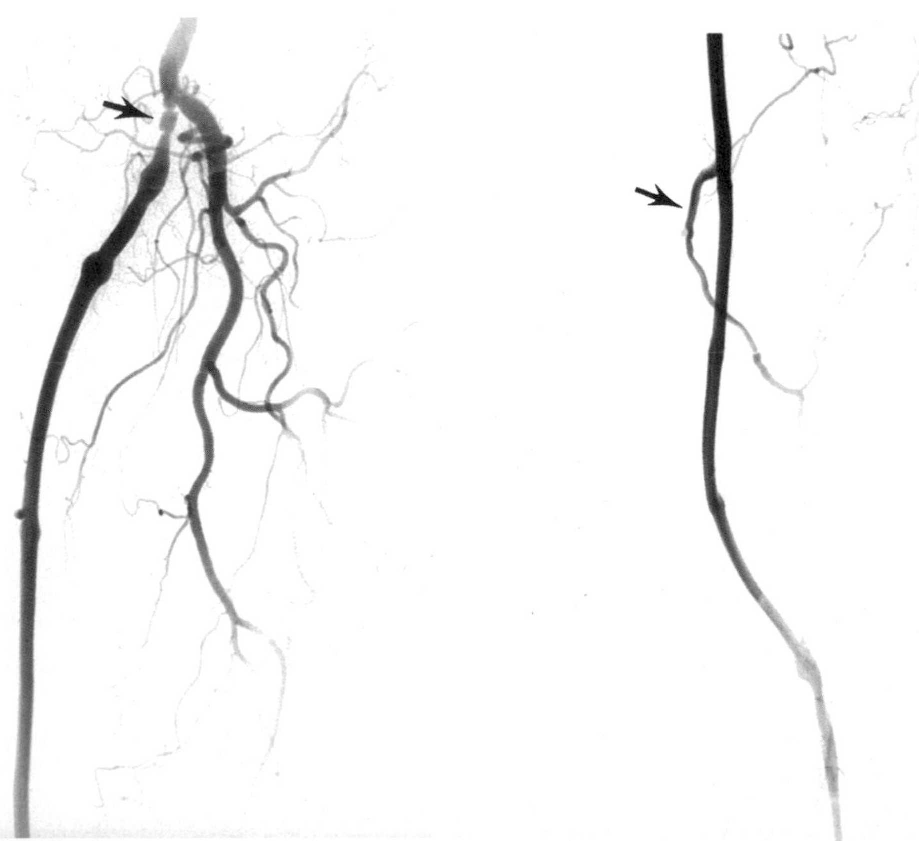

FIGURE 30.15. Femoral artery to popliteal artery venous bypass stenosis (*arrow*) evident on arteriogram.

FIGURE 30.16. Retained vein graft fistula (*arrow*) following *in situ* vein bypass.

fistulas communicating with the deep system require interruption. Fistulas may be identified by intraoperative Doppler examination or intraoperative arteriography. Their late persistence often causes areas of cutaneous erythema and painful induration. Residual competent valve leaflets are a recognized cause of early graft thrombosis when the retrograde passing of a valvulotome or valve cutter compresses the valve leaflet against the vein wall, where it snpaily remains in the open position. Identification of these collapsed leaflets on intraoperative angiography is difficult. Sometimes only direct mechanical manipulation of the vein will cause the leaflet to go into the closed position, allowing identification. Platelet aggregates invariably attach to the damaged endothelium from mechanical or ischemic injury and may, on occasion, require a longitudinal venotomy for removal, followed by vein patch angioplasty to close the defect. Attempts at platelet removal by balloon catheter in this setting may only cause further vein injury and platelet aggregation (131).

REFERENCES

1. Upchurch GR, Dimick JB, Wainess RM, et al. Diffusion of new technology in health care: the case of aorto-iliac occlusive disease. *Surgery* 2004;136(4):812–818.
2. McPhee JT, Schanzer A, Messina LM, et al. Carotid artery stenting has increased rates of postprocedure stroke, death, and resource utilization than does carotid endarterectomy in the United States, 2005. *J Vasc Surg* 2008;48(6):1442–1450, 1450.e1.
3. Sidawy AN, Zwolak RM, White RA, et al. Risk-adjusted 30-day outcomes of carotid stenting and endarterectomy: results from the SVS Vascular Registry. *J Vasc Surg* 2009;49(1):71–79.
4. Halm EA, Tuhrim S, Wang JJ, et al. Racial and ethnic disparities in outcomes and appropriateness of carotid endarterectomy: impact of patient and provider factors. *Stroke* 2009;40(7):2493–2501.
5. Vogel TR, Dombrovskiy VY, Haser PB, et al. Outcomes of carotid artery stenting and endarterectomy in the United States. *J Vasc Surg* 2009;49(2):325–330, discussion 330.
6. Dillavou ED, Muluk SC, Makaroun MS. A decade of change in abdominal aortic aneurysm repair in the United States: Have we improved outcomes equally between men and women? *J Vasc Surg* 2006;43(2):230–238, discussion 238.
7. Giles KA, Schermerhorn ML, O'Malley AJ, et al. Risk prediction for perioperative mortality of endovascular vs open repair of abdominal aortic aneurysms using the Medicare population. *J Vasc Surg* 2009;50(2): 256–262.
8. Schermerhorn ML, O'Malley AJ, Jhaveri A, et al. Endovascular vs. open repair of abdominal aortic aneurysms in the Medicare population. *N Engl J Med* 2008;358(5):464–474.
9. Schwarze ML, Shen Y, Hemmerich J, et al. Age-related trends in utilization and outcome of open and endovascular repair for abdominal aortic aneurysm in the United States, 2001–2006. *J Vasc Surg* 2009; 50(4):722–729.e2.
10. Aylin P, Lees T, Baker S, et al. Descriptive study comparing routine hospital administrative data with the Vascular Society of Great Britain and Ireland's National Vascular Database. *Eur J Vasc Endovasc Surg* 2007;33(4):461–465, discussion 466.
11. Birkmeyer JD, Siewers AE, Finlayson EV, et al. Hospital volume and surgical mortality in the United States. *N Engl J Med* 2002;346(15): 1128–1137.
12. Stanley JC, Messina LM, Wakefield TW. Complications in surgery and trauma. In: Greenfield LJ, eds. *Complications in vascular surgery and trauma*. Philadelphia, PA: JB Lippincott; 1989:359–387.
13. Howard VJ, Voeks JH, Lutsep HL, et al. Does sex matter? Thirty-day stroke and death rates after carotid artery stenting in women versus men: results from the Carotid Revascularization Endarterectomy versus Stenting Trial (CREST) lead-in phase. *Stroke* 2009;40(4): 1140–1147.
14. Gurm HS, Yadav JS, Fayad P, et al. Long-term results of carotid stenting versus endarterectomy in high-risk patients. *N Engl J Med* 2008; 358(15):1572–1579.
15. Stanley JC, Barnes RW, Ernst CB, et al. Vascular surgery in the United States: workforce issues. Report of the Society for Vascular Surgery and the International Society for Cardiovascular Surgery, North American Chapter, Committee on Workforce Issues. *J Vasc Surg* 1996; 23(1):172–181.
16. Moore WS, Barnett HJ, Beebe HG, et al. Guidelines for carotid endarterectomy. A multidisciplinary consensus statement from the Ad Hoc Committee, American Heart Association. *Circulation* 1995; 91(2):566–579.
17. Biller J, Feinberg WM, Castaldo JE, et al. Guidelines for carotid endarterectomy: a statement for healthcare professionals from a Special Writing Group of the Stroke Council, American Heart Association. *Circulation* 1998;97(5):501–509.
18. Cowan JA Jr, Dimick JB, Thompson BG, et al. Surgeon volume as an indicator of outcomes after carotid endarterectomy: an effect independent of specialty practice and hospital volume. *J Am Coll Surg* 2002;195(6):814–821.
19. Ballotta E, Da Giau G, Piccoli A, et al. Durability of carotid endarterectomy for treatment of symptomatic and asymptomatic stenoses. *J Vasc Surg* 2004;40(2):270–278.
20. Conrad MF, Shepard AD, Pandurangi K, et al. Outcome of carotid endarterectomy in African Americans: is race a factor? *J Vasc Surg* 2003;38(1):129–137.
21. Darling RC III, Mehta M, Roddy SP, et al. Eversion carotid endarterectomy: a technical alternative that may obviate patch closure in women. *Cardiovasc Surg* 2003;11(5):347–352.
22. Ecker RD, Pichelmann MA, Meissner I, et al. Durability of carotid endarterectomy. *Stroke* 2003;34(12):2941–2944.
23. Illig KA, Shortell CK, Zhang R, et al. Carotid endarterectomy then and now: outcome and cost-effectiveness of modern practice. *Surgery* 2003;134(4):705–711, discussion 711–712.
24. Debakey ME, Crawford ES, Cooley DA, et al. Cerebral arterial insufficiency: one to 11-year results following arterial reconstructive operation. *Ann Surg* 1965;161:921–945.
25. Hertzer NR, Arison R. Cumulative stroke and survival ten years after carotid endarterectomy. *J Vasc Surg* 1985;2(5):661–668.
26. Perler BA, Burdick JF, Williams GM. The safety of carotid endarterectomy at the time of coronary artery bypass surgery: analysis of results in a high-risk patient population. *J Vasc Surg* 1985;2(4):558–563.
27. Hertzer NR, Loop FD, Beven EG, et al. Surgical staging for simultaneous coronary and carotid disease: a study including prospective randomization. *J Vasc Surg* 1989;9(3):455–463.
28. Ricotta JJ, Peterson, MJ, Char DJ, Current therapy in vascular surgery. In: Ernst CB, Stanley JC. eds. *Management of concomitant carotid and coronary arterial disease*. St. Louis, MO: Mosby; 2001:101–104.
29. Brown KR, Kresowik TF, Chin MH, et al. Multistate population-based outcomes of combined carotid endarterectomy and coronary artery bypass. *J Vasc Surg* 2003;37(1):32–39.
30. Graham AM, Gewertz BL, Zarins CK. Predicting cerebral ischemia during carotid endarterectomy. *Arch Surg* 1986;121(5):595–598.
31. Till JS, Toole JF, Howard VJ, et al. Declining morbidity and mortality of carotid endarterectomy. The Wake Forest University Medical Center experience. *Stroke* 1987;18(5):823–829.
32. Imparato AM, Riles TS, Lamparello PJ, et al. Complications in vascular surgery. In: Bernhard VM, Towne JB, eds. *The management of TIA and acute strokes after carotid endarterectomy*. New York, NY: Grune & Stratton; 1985:725.
33. Moore WS, Hall AD. Carotid artery back pressure: a test of cerebral tolerance to temporary carotid occlusion. *Arch Surg* 1969;99(6):702–710.
34. Hays RJ, Levinson SA, Wylie EJ. Intraoperative measurement of carotid back pressure as a guide to operative management for carotid endarterectomy. *Surgery* 1972;72(6):953–960.
35. Kwaan JH, Peterson GJ, Connolly JE. Stump pressure: an unreliable guide for shunting during carotid endarterectomy. *Arch Surg* 1980; 115(9):1083–1086.
36. Baker JD, Gluecklich B, Watson CW, et al. An evaluation of electroencephalographic monitoring for carotid study. *Surgery* 1975;78(6): 787–794.
37. Pruitt JC. 1009 consecutive carotid endarterectomies using local anesthesia, EEG, and selective shunting with Pruitt-Inahara carotid shunt. *Contemp Surg* 1983;23:49–58.
38. Brooke BS, McGirt MJ, Woodworth GF, et al. Preoperative statin and diuretic use influence the presentation of patients undergoing carotid

endarterectomy: results of a large single-institution case-control study. *J Vasc Surg* 2007;45(2):298–303.
39. Ascher E, Markevich N, Kallakuri S, et al. Intraoperative carotid artery duplex scanning in a modern series of 650 consecutive primary endarterectomy procedures. *J Vasc Surg* 2004;39(2):416–420.
40. Caplan LR, Skillman J, Ojemann R, et al. Intracerebral hemorrhage following carotid endarterectomy: a hypertensive complication? *Stroke* 1978;9(5):457–460.
41. Moulakakis KG, Mylonas SN, Sfyroeras GS, et al. Hyperperfusion syndrome after carotid revascularization. *J Vasc Surg* 2009;49(4): 1060–1068.
42. Hertzer NR. Vascular surgery. In: Rutherford RB, ed. *Postoperative management and complications of extracranial carotid reconstruction*. Philadelphia, PA: W.B. Saunders; 1984:1300.
43. Evans WE, Mendelowitz DS, Liapis C, et al. Motor speech deficit following carotid endarterectomy. *Ann Surg* 1982;196(4):461–464.
44. Thompson JE. Complications of carotid endarterectomy and their prevention. *World J Surg* 1979;3(2):155–165.
45. Bove EL, Fry WJ, Gross WS, et al. Hypotension and hypertension as consequences of baroreceptor dysfunction following carotid endarterectomy. *Surgery* 1979;85(6):633–637.
46. Posner SR, Boxer L, Proctor M, et al. Uncomplicated carotid endarterectomy: factors contributing to blood pressure instability precluding safe early discharge. *Vascular* 2004;12(5):278–284.
47. Wade JG, Larson CP Jr, Hickey RF, et al. Effect of carotid endarterectomy on carotid chemoreceptor and baroreceptor function in man. *N Engl J Med* 1970;282(15):823–829.
48. Clagett GP, Rich NM, McDonald PT, et al. Etiologic factors for recurrent carotid artery stenosis. *Surgery* 1983;93(2):313–318.
49. Stoney RJ, String ST. Recurrent carotid stenosis. *Surgery* 1976;80(6): 705–710.
50. Imparato AM, Bracco A, Kim GE, et al. Intimal and neointimal fibrous proliferation causing failure of arterial reconstructions. *Surgery* 1972; 72(6):1007–1017.
51. Rapp J, Stoney RJ, Complications in vascular surgery. In: Bernhard VM, Towne JB, eds. *Recurrent carotid stenosis*. New York, NY: Grune & Stratton; 1986:767.
52. Archie JP Jr. A fifteen-year experience with carotid endarterectomy after a formal operative protocol requiring highly frequent patch angioplasty. *J Vasc Surg* 2000;31(4):724–735.
53. Roddy SP, Darling RC III, Ozsvath KJ, et al. Choice of material for internal carotid artery bypass grafting: vein or prosthetic? Analysis of 44 procedures. *Cardiovasc Surg* 2002;10(6):540–544.
54. Attigah N, Kulkens S, Deyle C, et al. Redo Surgery or Carotid Stenting for Restenosis after Carotid Endarterectomy: Results of Two Different Treatment Strategies. *Ann Vasc Surg* 2009;24(2):190–195.
55. Reul GJ, Cooley DA. Reoperative arterial surgery. In: Bergan JJ, Yao JST, eds. *False aneurysm of the carotid artery*. New York, NY: Grune & Stratton; 1986:538.
56. Dimick JB, Stanley JC, Axelrod DA, et al. Variation in death rate after abdominal aortic aneurysmectomy in the United States: impact of hospital volume, gender, and age. *Ann Surg* 2002;235(4):579–585.
57. Dimick JB, Upchurch GR Jr. The quality of care for patients with abdominal aortic aneurysms. *Cardiovasc Surg* 2003;11(5):331–336.
58. Katz DJ, Stanley JC, Zelenock GB. Operative mortality rates for intact and ruptured abdominal aortic aneurysms in Michigan: an eleven-year statewide experience. *J Vasc Surg* 1994;19(5):804–815, discussion 816–817.
59. Katz DJ, Stanley JC, Zelenock GB. Gender differences in abdominal aortic aneurysm prevalence, treatment, and outcome. *J Vasc Surg* 1997; 25(3):561–568.
60. Bertges DJ, Rhee RY, Muluk SC, et al. Is routine use of the intensive care unit after elective infrarenal abdominal aortic aneurysm repair necessary? *J Vasc Surg* 2000;32(4):634–642.
61. Elkouri S, Gloviczki P, McKusick MA, et al. Perioperative complications and early outcome after endovascular and open surgical repair of abdominal aortic aneurysms. *J Vasc Surg* 2004;39(3):497–505.
62. Hertzer NR, Mascha EJ, Karafa MT, et al. Open infrarenal abdominal aortic aneurysm repair: the Cleveland Clinic experience from 1989 to 1998. *J Vasc Surg* 2002;35(6):1145–1154.
63. Menard MT, Chew DK, Chan RK, et al. Outcome in patients at high risk after open surgical repair of abdominal aortic aneurysm. *J Vasc Surg* 2003;37(2):285–292.
64. Dauchot PJ, DePalma R, Grum D, et al. Detection and prevention of cardiac dysfunction during aortic surgery. *J Surg Res* 1979;26(5): 574–580.
65. Hertzer NR. Fatal myocardial infarction following abdominal aortic aneurysm resection. Three hundred forty-three patients followed 6–11 years postoperatively. *Ann Surg* 1980;192(5):667–673.
66. Beven EG. Routine coronary angiography in patients undergoing surgery for abdominal aortic aneurysm and lower extremity occlusive disease. *J Vasc Surg* 1986;3(4):682–684.
67. Froehlich JB, Karavite D, Russman PL, et al. American College of Cardiology/American Heart Association preoperative assessment guidelines reduce resource utilization before aortic surgery. *J Vasc Surg* 2002;36(4):758–763.
68. Eagle KA, Brundage BH, Chaitman BR, et al. Guidelines for perioperative cardiovascular evaluation for noncardiac surgery. Report of the American College of Cardiology/American Heart Association Task Force on practice guidelines (committee on perioperative cardiovascular evaluation for noncardiac surgery). *J Am Coll Cardiol* 1996;27(4): 910–948.
69. Ohuchi H, Gojo S, Sato H, et al. Simultaneous abdominal aortic aneurysm repair during the on-pump coronary artery bypass grafting. *Ann Thorac Cardiovasc Surg* 2003;9(6):409–411.
70. Hertzer NR, Young JR, Beven EG, et al. Late results of coronary bypass in patients with infrarenal aortic aneurysms. The Cleveland Clinic Study. *Ann Surg* 1987;205(4):360–367.
71. Diehl JT, Cali RF, Hertzer NR, et al. Complications of abdominal aortic reconstruction. An analysis of perioperative risk factors in 557 patients. *Ann Surg* 1983;197(1):49–56.
72. O'Hara PJ, Hertzer NR, Santilli PH, et al. Intraoperative autotransfusion during abdominal aortic reconstruction. *Am J Surg* 1983;145(2): 215–220.
73. Clagett GP, Valentine RJ, Jackson MR, et al. A randomized trial of intraoperative autotransfusion during aortic surgery. *J Vasc Surg* 1999;29(1):22–30, discussion 30–31.
74. Haimovici H. Vascular emergencies. In: Haimovici H, ed. *Metabolic syndrome secondary to acute arterial occlusions*. East Norwalk, CT: Appleton & Lange; 1982:267.
75. Bush HL Jr. Renal failure following abdominal aortic reconstruction. *Surgery* 1983;93(1 Pt 1):107–109.
76. Wakefield TW, Whitehouse WM Jr, Wu SC, et al. Abdominal aortic aneurysm rupture: statistical analysis of factors affecting outcome of surgical treatment. *Surgery* 1982;91(5):586–596.
77. Hassoun HT, Miller CC III, Huynh TT, et al. Cold visceral perfusion improves early survival in patients with acute renal failure after thoracoabdominal aortic aneurysm repair. *J Vasc Surg* 2004;39(3):506–512.
78. Crawford ES, Crawford JL, Safi HJ, et al. Thoracoabdominal aortic aneurysms: preoperative and intraoperative factors determining immediate and long-term results of operations in 605 patients. *J Vasc Surg* 1986;3(3):389–404.
79. Starr DS, Lawrie GM, Morris GC Jr. Prevention of distal embolism during arterial reconstruction. *Am J Surg* 1979;138(6):764–769.
80. Crowson M, Fielding JW, Black J, et al. Acute gastrointestinal complications of infrarenal aortic aneurysm repair. *Br J Surg* 1984;71(11): 825–828.
81. Zelenock GB, Strodel WE, Knol JA, et al. A prospective study of clinically and endoscopically documented colonic ischemia in 100 patients undergoing aortic reconstructive surgery with aggressive colonic and direct pelvic revascularization, compared with historic controls. *Surgery* 1989;106(4):771–779, discussion 779–780.
82. Hagihara PF, Ernst CB, Griffen WO Jr. Incidence of ischemic colitis following abdominal aortic reconstruction. *Surg Gynecol Obstet* 1979; 149(4):571–573.
83. Ernst CB, Hagihara PF, Daugherty ME, et al. Inferior mesenteric artery stump pressure: a reliable index for safe IMA ligation during abdominal aortic aneurysmectomy. *Ann Surg* 1978;187(6):641–646.
84. Mitchell KM, Valentine RJ. Inferior mesenteric artery reimplantation does not guarantee colon viability in aortic surgery. *J Am Coll Surg* 2002;194(2):151–155.
85. Szilagyi DE, Hageman JH, Smith RF, et al. Spinal cord damage in surgery of the abdominal aorta. *Surgery* 1978;83(1):38–56.
86. Elliott JP, Szilagyi DL, Hageman JH, et al, Complications in vascular surgery. In: Bernhard VM, Towne JB, eds. *Spinal cord ischemia: secondary to surgery of the abdominal aorta*. New York, NY: Grune & Stratton; 1985:291.
87. Picone AL, Green RM, Ricotta JR, et al. Spinal cord ischemia following operations on the abdominal aorta. *J Vasc Surg* 1986;3(1):94–103.
88. McCullough JL, Hollier LH, Nugent M. Paraplegia after thoracic aortic occlusion: influence of cerebrospinal fluid drainage. Experimental and early clinical results. *J Vasc Surg* 1988;7(1):153–160.

89. Acher CW, Wynn MM, Hoch JR, et al. Combined use of cerebral spinal fluid drainage and naloxone reduces the risk of paraplegia in thoracoabdominal aneurysm repair. *J Vasc Surg* 1994;19(2):236–246, discussion 247–248.
90. Laschinger JC, Cunningham JN Jr, Catinella FP, et al. Detection and prevention of intraoperative spinal cord ischemia after cross-clamping of the thoracic aorta: use of somatosensory evoked potentials. *Surgery* 1982;92(6):1109–1117.
91. Joob AW, Dunn C, Miller E, et al. Effect of left atrial to left femoral artery bypass and renin-angiotensin system blockade on renal blood flow and function during and after thoracic aortic occlusion. *J Vasc Surg* 1987;5(2):329–335.
92. Labardini MM, Ratliff RK. The abdominal aortic aneurysm and the ureter. *J Urol* 1967;98(5):590–596.
93. Szilagyi DE, Smith RF, Elliott JP, et al. Infection in arterial reconstruction with synthetic grafts. *Ann Surg* 1972;176(3):321–333.
94. Reilly LM, Altman H, Lusby RJ, et al. Late results following surgical management of vascular graft infection. *J Vasc Surg* 1984;1(1):36–44.
95. Macbeth GA, Rubin JR, McIntyre KE Jr, et al. The relevance of arterial wall microbiology to the treatment of prosthetic graft infections: graft infection vs. arterial infection. *J Vasc Surg* 1984;1(6):750–756.
96. Liekweg WG Jr, Greenfield LJ. Vascular prosthetic infections: collected experience and results of treatment. *Surgery* 1977;81(3): 335–342.
97. Tollefson DF, Bandyk DF, Kaebnick HW, et al. Surface biofilm disruption. Enhanced recovery of microorganisms from vascular prostheses. *Arch Surg* 1987;122(1):38–43.
98. Reilly LM, Stoney RJ, Goldstone J, et al. Improved management of aortic graft infection: the influence of operation sequence and staging. *J Vasc Surg* 1987;5(3):421–431.
99. Clagett GP, Valentine RJ, Hagino RT. Autogenous aortoiliac/femoral reconstruction from superficial femoral-popliteal veins: feasibility and durability. *J Vasc Surg* 1997;25(2):255–266, discussion 267–270.
100. Kieffer E, Gomes D, Chiche L, et al. Allograft replacement for infrarenal aortic graft infection: early and late results in 179 patients. *J Vasc Surg* 2004;39(5):1009–1017.
101. Bandyk DF, Novotney ML, Johnson BL, et al. Use of rifampin-soaked gelatin-sealed polyester grafts for in situ treatment of primary aortic and vascular prosthetic infections. *J Surg Res* 2001;95(1):44–49.
102. Stanley JC, Lindenauer SM, Graham LM, et al. Vascular surgery. A comprehensive review. In: Moore W, eds. *Vascular grafts*. New York, NY: Grune & Stratton; 1986:365–390.
103. Lalka SG, Bernhard VM. Vascular surgery. A comprehensive review. In: Moore W, eds. *Noninfectious complications in vascular surgery*. New York, NY: Grune & Stratton; 1986:959.
104. Brewster DC, Darling RC. Optimal methods of aortoiliac reconstruction. *Surgery* 1978;84(6):739–748.
105. Szilagyi DE, Elliott JP Jr, Smith RF, et al. A thirty-year survey of the reconstructive surgical treatment of aortoiliac occlusive disease. *J Vasc Surg* 1986;3(3):421–436.
106. Szilagyi DE, Smith RF, Elliott JP, et al. Anastomotic aneurysms after vascular reconstruction: problems of incidence, etiology, and treatment. *Surgery* 1975;78(6):800–816.
107. Evans WE, Mendelowitz DS, Liapis C, et al. Complications in vascular surgery. In: Bernhard VM, Towne JB, eds. *Anastomotic femoral false aneurysms*. New York, NY: Grune & Stratton; 1985:205.
108. Berchtold C, Eibl C, Seelig MH, et al. Endovascular treatment and complete regression of an infected abdominal aortic aneurysm. *J Endovasc Ther* 2002;9(4):543–548.
109. Flanigan DP, Schuler JJ, Keifer T, et al. Elimination of iatrogenic impotence and improvement of sexual function after aortoiliac revascularization. *Arch Surg* 1982;117(5):544–550.
110. Nath RL, Menzoian JO, Kaplan KH, et al. The multidisciplinary approach to vasculogenic impotence. *Surgery* 1981;89(1):124–133.
111. DePalma RG, Emsellem HA, Edwards CM, et al. A screening sequence for vasculogenic impotence. *J Vasc Surg* 1987;5(2):228–236.
112. Ferris BL, Mills JL Sr, Hughes JD, et al. Is early postoperative duplex scan surveillance of leg bypass grafts clinically important? *J Vasc Surg* 2003;37(3):495–500.
113. Chew DK, Conte MS, Donaldson MC, et al. Autogenous composite vein bypass graft for infrainguinal arterial reconstruction. *J Vasc Surg* 2001;33(2):259–264, discussion 264–265.
114. Goshima KR, Mills JL Sr, Hughes JD. A new look at outcomes after infrainguinal bypass surgery: traditional reporting standards systematically underestimate the expenditure of effort required to attain limb salvage. *J Vasc Surg* 2004;39(2):330–335.
115. Pomposelli FB, Kansal N, Hamdan AD, et al. A decade of experience with dorsalis pedis artery bypass: analysis of outcome in more than 1000 cases. *J Vasc Surg* 2003;37(2):307–315.
116. Raffetto JD, Chen MN, LaMorte WW, et al. Factors that predict site of outflow target artery anastomosis in infrainguinal revascularization. *J Vasc Surg* 2002;35(6):1093–1099.
117. Roddy SP, Darling RC III, Maharaj D, et al. Gender-related differences in outcome: an analysis of 5880 infrainguinal arterial reconstructions. *J Vasc Surg* 2003;37(2):399–402.
118. Hertzer NR. Fatal myocardial infarction following lower extremity revascularization. Two hundred seventy-three patients followed six to eleven postoperative years. *Ann Surg* 1981;193(4):492–498.
119. Brewster DC. Complications in vascular surgery. In: Bernhard VM, Towne JB, ed. *Early complications of vascular repair below the inguinal ligament*. New York, NY: Grune & Stratton; 1985:37.
120. Brewster DC, LaSalle AJ, Robison JG, et al. Femoropopliteal graft failures. Clinical consequences and success of secondary reconstructions. *Arch Surg* 1983;118(9):1043–1047.
121. Donaldson MC, Mannick JA, Whittemore AD. Causes of primary graft failure after in situ saphenous vein bypass grafting. *J Vasc Surg* 1992;15(1):113–138, discussion 118–120.
122. Henke PK, Blackburn S, Proctor MC, et al. Patients undergoing infrainguinal bypass to treat atherosclerotic vascular disease are underprescribed cardioprotective medications: effect on graft patency, limb salvage, and mortality. *J Vasc Surg* 2004;39(2):357–365.
123. Abbruzzese TA, Havens J, Belkin M, et al. Statin therapy is associated with improved patency of autogenous infrainguinal bypass grafts. *J Vasc Surg* 2004;39(6):1178–1185.
124. Bandyk DF. Reoperative arterial surgery. In: Bergan JJ, Yao JST, ed. *Postoperative surveillance of femorodistal grafts: the application of echo-Doppler (duplex) ultrasonic scanning*. New York, NY: Grune & Stratton; 1986:59.
125. LoGerfo FW, Quist WC, Cantelmo NL, et al. Integrity of vein grafts as a function of initial intimal and medial preservation. *Circulation* 1983; 68(3 Pt 2):II117–II124.
126. Veith FJ, Gupta S, Daly V. Management of early and late thrombosis of expanded polytetrafluoroethylene (PTFE) femoropopliteal bypass grafts: favorable prognosis with appropriate reoperation. *Surgery* 1980;87(5):581–587.
127. Whittemore AD, Clowes AW, Couch NP, et al. Secondary femoropopliteal reconstruction. *Ann Surg* 1981;193(1):35–42.
128. Durham JR, Rubin JR, Malone JM. Reoperative arterial surgery. In: Bergan JJ, Yao JST, eds. *Management of infected infrainguinal bypass grafts*. New York, NY: Grune & Stratton; 1986:359.
129. Schubart PJ, Porter JM. Reoperative arterial surgery. In: Bergan JJ, Yao JST, eds. *Leg edema following femorodistal bypass*. New York, NY: Grune & Stratton; 1986:331.
130. Eickhoff JH, Engell HC. Local regulation of blood flow and the occurrence of edema after arterial reconstruction of the lower limbs. *Ann Surg* 1982;195(4):474–478.
131. Leather RP, Karmody AM, Shah DM, et al. Reoperative arterial surgery. In: Bergan JJ, Yao JST, eds. *The in situ saphenous vein arterial bypass*. New York, NY: Grune & Stratton; 1986:299.

CHAPTER

31

Complications of Venous Disease and Therapy

Thomas W. Wakefield and Peter K. Henke

INCIDENCE, RISK FACTORS, AND CATEGORIES

Deep venous thrombosis (DVT) and pulmonary embolism (PE), together called venous thromboembolism (VTE), are a serious health concern. It has been estimated that there are more than 900,000 cases per year in the US (1). Approximately 300,000 people die of PE yearly and deaths from PE are five times more common than deaths from breast cancer, AIDS, and motor vehicle accidents combined. VTE is the third most common vascular disease after heart disease and stroke. In addition, patients with pain and leg swelling after thrombosis (called *postthrombotic syndrome [PTS]*) suffer poor quality of life due to chronic symptoms. PTS occurs in as many as 30% of patients ovserved over 8 years (2).

Acquired risk factors include age, malignancy, surgery, trauma, immobilization, oral contraceptive use, hormone replacement therapy, pregnancy and the puerperium, obesity, neurological disease, cardiac disease, and antiphospholipid antibodies (3). Genetic risk factors include deficiencies of antithrombin, protein C and protein S, factor V Leiden, prothrombin 20210 A, blood group non-O, hyperhomocysteinemia, dysfibrinogenemia, dysplasminogenemia, reduced heparin cofactor II activity, elevated levels of clotting factors (factors XI, IX, VII, VIII, X, and II), and plasminogen activator inhibitor-1 (4). Hematologic diseases associated with an increased risk of DVT include disseminated intravascular coagulation, heparin-induced thrombocytopenia (HIT), thrombotic thrombocytopenic purpura (TTP), antiphospholipid antibody syndrome, hemolytic uremic syndrome, and myeloproliferative disorders (polycythemia vera and essential thrombocythemia) (5).

When a patient presents with an unprovoked VTE at a young age (age <50 years), unusual site of thrombosis (e.g., mesenteric veins), or if there is a family history of VTE, a work-up for a hypercoagulable state is suggested (Table 31.1) (3,4).

Most cases of DVT affect the lower limb and include the popliteal, femoral, or iliac veins. Presenting symptoms include unilateral limb pain and swelling, but DVT is sometimes silent, with PE as the first manifestation.

Phlegmasia alba dolens/phlegmasia cerulea dolens

Massive iliofemoral DVT may cause phlegmasia alba dolens (the white swollen leg) and phlegmasia cerulea dolens (the blue swollen leg). When capillaries occlude, venous gangrene may result, as arterial inflow becomes obstructed due to extreme venous hypertension. Alternatively, arterial emboli or spasm may occur. The toes on the involved limb turn blue and black, and the skin blisters. Venous gangrene can be differentiated from arterial ischemia by generalized swelling and limb blueness as opposed to the pale, cold limb of acute arterial ischemia. Venous gangrene is often associated with an underlying malignancy, and phlegmasia cerulea dolens virtually always precedes this diagnosis. Amputation rates of 20% to 50% are noted, with PE rates of 12% to 40% and mortality of 20% to 40% (6).

Axillary/subclavian vein thrombosis

Thrombosis of the axillary/subclavian vein is an uncommon event accounting for <5% of all cases of acute DVT. Nevertheless, axillary/subclavian venous thromboses have been associated with PE in up to 10% to 15% of cases and can be the source of significant disability (7). Primary axillary/subclavian vein thrombosis results from intermittent obstruction of the vein in the thoracic outlet (Paget—von Schrötter syndrome) in relatively healthy muscular individuals, with strenuous exercise often precipitating the thrombosis. Thrombosis may also occur in patients with hypercoagulable states. Secondary axillary/subclavian vein thrombosis most commonly results from indwelling catheters or pacemaker wires. Less common secondary causes include congestive heart failure, nephrotic syndrome, mediastinal tumors, and malignancy. Most patients present with pain, edema, and cyanosis of the arm. Superficial venous distension may be apparent in the arm, forearm, shoulder, and anterior chest wall, and this finding can aid in the diagnosis.

Thomas W. Wakefield and Peter K. Henke: Section of Vascular Surgery University of Michigan, Ann Arbor, MI 48109

Table 31.1 Hypercoagulable testing
Standard coagulation tests
Mixing studies (if APTT is elevated)
Antithrombin antigen and activity
Protein C antigen and activity
Protein S antigen
APC resistance test
Factor V genetic analysis
Prothrombin 20210A genetic analysis
Homocysteine level
Antiphospholipid/anticardiolipin antibody screen
Factor VIII levels
Platelet count/platelet aggregation testing
Functional plasminogen
Heparin antibodies

APTT, activated partial thromboplastin time.

Superficial thrombophlebitis

Superficial thrombophlebitis occurs in more than 125,000 patients per year and is associated with varicose veins (VVs), pregnancy, thromboangiitis obliterans (Behçet disease), and indwelling catheters. Complications of superficial thrombophlebitis have been associated with male gender and a history of VTE (8). Clinically, a painful, firm, palpable cord with inflammation and tenderness along the affected vein, and occasionally edema, are noted. There may be a history of venous puncture or intravenous canalization, trauma, physical inactivity, oral contraceptives, malignancy, or infection. The presence of migratory superficial thrombophlebitis suggests the presence of cancer (e.g., carcinoma of the pancreas [Trousseau sign]). The incidence of DVT associated with superficial thrombophlebitis is estimated to be between 0.75% and 40%. The association of a noncontiguous DVT with superficial thrombophlebitis is as high as 25% to 75% in patients who present with involvement of both systems (9). PE, the most lethal and underrecognized complication associated with this entity, occurs from 0% to 17% (10).

Suppurative superficial thrombophlebitis is associated with intravenous catheter use or multiple puncture sites secondary to intravenous drug abuse, most often in the upper extremity. The clinical presentation is similar to that of nonsuppurative superficial thrombophlebitis, although there is often also pyrexia, leukocytosis, and bacteremia. Local intravenous catheter site infections occur in up to 8% of cases, and bacteremia is detected in approximately 1 of every 400 intravenous catheterizations (9). Immunocompromised and burn patients are particularly susceptible to superficial thrombophlebitis.

Hypercoagulability in the setting of superficial thrombophlebitis is not uncommon. The risk of superficial thrombophlebitis in the absence of VVs, malignancy, or autoimmune disorders is approximately 13-fold higher for deficiencies of inhibitors of coagulation (antithrombin, protein C, or protein S), 6-fold higher for factor V Leiden mutation, and 4-fold higher for the prothrombin gene mutation (11). The same indications for hypercoagulable work-up in patients with DVT should be applied to patients with superficial thrombophlebitis (8). This category includes patients *without* an associated history of trauma or inactivity, venipuncture, malignancy, or VVs and *with* severe superficial thrombophlebitis, recurrence, family history, early age at presentation, and resistance to therapy.

VENOUS DISEASE DIAGNOSIS

Deep venous thrombosis

The diagnosis of DVT must be made with confirmatory imaging, as patients will be asymptomatic at presentation in up to 50% of the cases. Patients may complain of a dull ache or pain in the calf or leg. The most common physical finding is edema, although Wells has classified patients into a scoring system that emphasizes the physical presentation. In the Wells criteria, characteristics include the presence of active cancer, paralysis or paresis, recent plaster immobilization of the lower extremity, being recently bedridden for 3 days or more, localized tenderness along the distribution of the deep venous system, the entire leg being swollen, calf swelling that is at least 3 cm larger on the involved side than on the noninvolved side, pitting edema in the symptomatic leg, and a history of DVT (12).

Tests for making the diagnosis of DVT of historical interest include indirect flow examinations. Duplex ultrasound imaging has replaced these tests because of its high sensitivity, specificity, and reproducibility. Duplex ultrasound imaging includes a Doppler flow pattern and a B-mode image. Duplex imaging carries sensitivity and specificity rates >95% (13). According to the Grade criteria for the strength of medical evidence, duplex ultrasound as the test of choice for the diagnosis of DVT is given a 2 C level of evidence (13–15). Magnetic resonance imaging may be helpful to diagnose central pelvic vein and inferior vena cava (IVC) thrombosis, whereas spiral computed tomography (CT) scanning is used when combined with chest imaging during examination for PE (16). Even at the calf level, duplex imaging is an acceptable technique in symptomatic patients. Other advantages of duplex imaging include the fact that the examination is painless, requires no contrast, can be serially repeated, and is safe during pregnancy. The test also identifies other potential causes of a patient's symptoms (14).

A single complete technically adequate negative duplex scan is accurate enough to withhold anticoagulation with minimal long-term adverse thromboembolic complications (17). However, all segments of the leg must have been evaluated successfully. If the duplex scan is indeterminate, treatment may be based on other factors such as biomarkers. Repeat imaging may be performed in 48 to 72 hours or if the patient's symptoms change or worsen. Combining clinical characteristics with a D-dimer assay may decrease the number of negative duplex scans performed (12). Although the use of clinical characteristics and D-dimer levels is useful to rule out thrombosis, the reverse is not true. A positive D-dimer associated with a positive risk assessment is associated with thrombosis in approximately 70% of cases and is not considered good enough to base anticoagulant therapy on (18). Other conditions that may be confused with DVT include lymphedema, muscle strain, and muscle contusion. Iliac vein obstruction can lead to unilateral leg edema and predispose to DVT (May–Thurner syndrome), whereas the presence of a cyst behind the knee may produce unilateral leg pain and edema. Other causes of leg swelling (usually bilateral) include cardiac, renal, or hepatic abnormalities.

Diagnosis of incompetent venous perforators, in planning for venous stasis ulceration treatment, can be accomplished by duplex with a sensitivity >80% (19). Ascending venography may also be of benefit in this regard. The duplex scan can also be used to diagnose femoropopliteal venous reflux reliably, which contributes to primary venous varicosities in 50% (20). Saphenopopliteal reflux should also be documented, as this may contribute to persistent and recurrent venous varicosities.

A definitive diagnosis of chronic venous insufficiency (CVI) is essential for selecting patients who will benefit most from any given intervention. A standard severity classification scoring system that includes a Venous Clinical Severity Score (VCSS) and the more traditional CEAP (Clinical Etiology Anatomic Pathophysiologic) system has been developed (21). The latter is a standard way to categorize venous insufficiency, and it includes etiology and anatomical information. The CEAP classification allows cross-communication between physicians, whereas the VCSS allows for the documentation of therapeutic outcome for any given procedure. It differentiates between reflux and obstructive components that may aid with therapy.

If further interventions are planned, CVI is diagnosed with both duplex ultrasound imaging assessing valvular reflux and air plethysmography (APG). APG is a noninvasive venous assessment that assesses for calf muscle pump function and reflux and obstructive components of venous insufficiency. A recent report suggests this is most sensitive for reflux assessment, both in the deep and superficial systems (22). However, there is no correlation with the parameters of APG and the severity of clinical disease. Similarly, foot venous pressures or ambulatory venous pressure measurements are invasive methods to quantify venous hypertension. A needle is placed in the medial vein of the great toe and pressures are taken both at rest and after calf ejection with compression. Unlike APG, foot venous pressure does correlate with venous clinical severity symptomatology (23). This test may be used for preprocedural and postprocedural quantification of therapy, although it has not gained widespread popularity because of its invasive nature and procedural pain for the patient.

Pulmonary embolism

Almost any pulmonary symptom can mimic a PE. Chest radiograph changes are infrequently present, and hemoptysis represents pulmonary infarction and suggests a far advanced state of abnormality. The diagnostic modalities for PE are in flux. In the most recent past, the tests used included ventilation/perfusion scanning (V/Q) and pulmonary arteriography. Unfortunately, V/Q scanning is diagnostic in only approximately one-third of cases, and pulmonary arteriography may causes morbidity and occasional mortality. Spiral CT scanning has shown significant promise and in many institutions has become the test of choice. Certain biomarkers of cardiac injury, including troponin and brain natriuretic peptide, have now been recognized to be useful in acute PE (24). For example, if the biomarkers are found present, further testing with echocardiography is indicated to determine right ventricular strain and to direct thrombolytic therapy.

VENOUS THROMBOEMBOLISM PROPHYLAXIS

One of the most common yet preventable complications of major surgery and hospital illness is VTE (25). Prevention of VTE has received increased scrutiny from insurers, quality groups and the Joint Commission. Methods for VTE prophylaxis include pharmacologic, mechanical, and combinations thereof (26). The goal is to prevent VTE, while balancing and minimizing bleeding occurrence.

Evidence-based pharmacologic prophylaxis includes low-dose unfractionated heparin (UFH), low-molecular-weight heparin (LMWH), fondaparinux, and warfarin. Enoxaparin and dalteparin are the LMWHs approved by the U.S. Food and Drug Administration (FDA). Prophylactic dosages for enoxaparin are either 30 mg subcutaneously every 12 hours or 40 mg once daily, whereas dalteparin dosage is either 2,500 or 5,000 anti–factor Xa units subcutaneously once daily, and fondaparinux is 2.5 mg SQ qd. Bleeding complications associated with pharmacologic prophylaxis are quite low, generally less than 3% (27). Importantly, aspirin alone is not recommended for prophylaxis.

Mechanical methods of prophylaxis include pneumatic compression devices (PCDs) and graded elastic stockings. Mechanical prophylaxis with PCDs reduces the incidence of DVT (26), although this has not been proven with the same rigor as with pharmacologic agents. The effectiveness of PCDs is based on overcoming venous stasis and increasing lower extremity blood flow and, possibly, by increasing native fibrinolytic activators. Compliance with these devices is a primary issue as they need to be physically on the limb to provide protection, and some clinical conditions prevent this.

Risk stratification

General surgical patients may have an incidence of VTE as high as 25% without prophylaxis, although this is based on historical series (26). Assessment of risk can be done by categorizing broad group risk (26) (Table 31.2) or

Table 31.2 Thromboembolism risk and recommended prophylaxis

Level of Risk	Approximate Risk	Prophylaxis Option
Low		
Minor Surgery	<10%	Non Specific
Mobile inpatients		Early ambulation
Moderate		
Most general, gynecologic, urologic surgeries	10–40%	LMWH, LD-UFH BID or TID, fonda parinux and/or PCD's
Increased age, prior VTE, Malignancy		
High		
Hip and knee arthroplasty	>40%	LMWH, fondaparinux, and PCD's
Major trauma		
Multiple VTE risk factors		

Modified from Geerts, W. et al. Chest 2008.

by a scoring system based on individual patient factors (28) (Table 31.3). The best system for assessing risk is debatable, but recent research suggests utility of the individual scoring system in surgery patient. Regardless of the system used, the important point is to determine each patient's risk and implement appropriate prophylaxis. Computer-generated reminders and standardized order sets seem to improve compliance over time, whereas passive reminders do not (29,30). Further, standardized history and physical examination intakes with "built in" VTE risk assessment may also increase appropriate prophylaxis.

The spectrum of VTE risk ranges from low risk, where no specific VTE prophylaxis outside of early ambulation is indicated, to highest risk where both pharmacological and PCDs are indicated. Specific surgeries have various levels of evidence with different pharmacologic agents and clinical conditions. To summarize the consensus recommendations in general, vascular, urologic, and gynecologic surgeries, prophylactic LDH (5,000 U TID) is as efficacious as LMWH for VTE prophylaxis, although bleeding risk and HIT risk may be higher (Fig. 31.1) (26). In orthopedic patients, fondaparinux is more effective than LDH or LMWH, and is recommended for hip and knee replacement. In a meta-analysis of more than 7,000 patients, there was >50% risk reduction compared with LMWH (begun 12 to 24 hours after surgery) with fondaparinux (begun 6 hours after surgery) (31). Although major bleeding was increased, critical bleeding was not increased. Fondaparinux has also been effective in prophylaxis of general medical patients, of abdominal surgery patients, and for extended prophylaxis after hip fracture (32–34).

In trauma patients without prophylaxis, DVT may occur in up to 50% of high-risk cases, and PE is the third most common cause of death in those surviving beyond the first day. From several series, LMWH is more efficacious than LDH (Fig. 31.2). Specific risk factors in trauma patients include spinal cord injury, lower extremity or pelvic fractures, surgical procedures, advanced age, femoral venous lines or major venous repairs, prolonged immobility, and prolonged duration of hospital stay (35). In trauma patients at high bleeding risk not receiving pharmacologic prophylaxis, duplex ultrasound screening is appropriate when dictated by clinical indications.

Whether presurgical (on call to operating room) versus early postsurgical (≤6 hours after surgery) pharmacologic agent administration is best is not clear, but it is recommended for gynecological surgery but not for orthopedic surgery (26). No clear consensus exists for general surgery patients. The institution of PCDs should be started before surgery begins, although level 1 evidence is lacking supporting this practice.

Placement of a vena caval filter is often done for VTE prophylaxis, but there is no solid evidence for this practice (26). Appropriate indications for vena cava filters include patients with proximal DVT when anticoagulation is contraindicated or when a failure or complication of anticoagulation occurs (36,37). The use of IVC filters strictly for prophylaxis in the highest risk patients requires prospective study, as does the use of retrievable versus permanent filter use.

Prolonged posthospital prophylaxis may decrease overall VTE rates, as some studies suggest that up to one-third of episodes of VTE occur after discharge (29). Specific patient groups that benefit include hip and knee replacement orthopedic patients and those with abdominal or pelvic malignancies (38). For example, evidence suggests that continuation of LMWH is better than placebo for extended 4-week prophylaxis in patients undergoing abdominal and pelvic cancer surgery (39).

Pharmacologic prophylaxis (especially LMWH) in the presence of spinal and epidural catheters may increase the potential of hematoma formation. Factors that may contribute to this problem include coagulopathy, traumatic catheter or needle insertion, repeated insertion attempts, use of continuous epidural catheters, anticoagulant dosage, concurrent administration of medications that increase bleeding, vertebral column abnormalities, older age, and female gender (27). A practical problem also arises in the form of discontinuation of the epidural catheter and starting and stopping pharmacological prophylaxis. Timing of prophylaxis dosing should be kept in mind. Our own practice is to allow approximately 2 hours between prophylaxis agent administration and catheter removal. It is imperative to make sure that the prophylactic agent is not fully discontinued around the time of catheter removal.

STANDARD THERAPY FOR VENOUS THROMBOEMBOLISM

The primary treatment of VTE is systemic anticoagulation, which reduces the risk of PE, extension of thrombosis, and recurrence of thrombosis. Immediate systemic anticoagulation should be achieved, as recurrence rates for VTE are approximately 4- to 6-fold higher if anticoagulation is not therapeutic in the first 24 hours (40). This is less of an issue

Table 31.3 Thrombosis risk factor assessment

Patient's Name:_________________ Age: ___ Sex: ___ Wgt:___lbs

Choose All That Apply

Each Risk Factor Represents 1 Point

- Age 41–60 years
- Minor surgery planned
- History of prior major surgery
- Varicose veins
- History of inflammatory bowel disease
- Swollen legs (current)
- Obesity (BMI >30)
- Acute myocardial infarction (<1 month)
- Congestive heart failure (<1 month)
- Sepsis (<1 month)
- Serious lung disease incl. pneumonia (<1 month)
- Abnormal pulmonary function (COPD)
- Medical patient currently at bed rest
- Leg plaster cast or brace
- Other risk factors____________________

Each Risk Factor Represents 3 Points

- Age over 75 years
- Major surgery lasting 2–3 hours
- BMI >50 (venous stasis syndrome)
- History of SVT, DVT/PE
- Family history of DVT/PE
- Present cancer or chemotherapy
- Positive Factor V Leiden
- Positive Prothrombin 20210A
- Elevated serum homocysteine
- Positive Lupus anticoagulant
- Elevated anticardiolipin antibodies
- Heparin-induced thrombocytopenia (HIT)
- Other thrombophilia
  Type______________________________

Each Risk Factor Represents 2 Points

- Age 60–74 years
- Major surgery (>60 minutes)
- Arthroscopic surgery (>60 minutes)
- Laparoscopic surgery (>60 minutes)
- Previous malignancy
- Central venous access
- Morbid obesity (BMI >40)

Each Risk Factor Represents 5 Points

- Elective major lower extremity arthroplasty
- Hip, pelvis or leg fracture (<1 month)
- Stroke (<1 month)
- Multiple trauma (<1 month)
- Acute spinal cord injury (paralysis) (<1 month)
- Major surgery lasting over 3 hours

For Women Only (Each Represents 1 Point)

- Oral contraceptives or hormone replacement therapy
- Pregnancy or postpartum (<1 month)
- History of unexplained stillborn infant, recurrent spontaneous abortion (≥3), premature birth with toxemia or growth-restricted infant

Total Risk Factor Score ☐

Please see Following Page for Prophylaxis Safety Considerations
Revised May 16, 2006

Prophylaxis Regimen

Total Risk Factor Score	Incidence of DVT	Risk Level	Prophylaxis Regimen
0–1	<10%	Low Risk	No specific measures; early ambulation
2	10–20%	Moderate Risk	ES or IPC or LDUH, or LWMH
3–4	20–40%	High Risk	IPC or LDUH, or LMWH alone *or* in combination with ES or IPC
5 or more	40–80% 1–5% mortality	Highest Risk	Pharmacological: LDUH, LMWH*, Warfarin*, or Fac Xa* alone *or* in combination with ES or IPC

Legend

ES — Elastic Stockings
IPC — Intermittent Pneumatic Compression
LDUH — Low Dose Unfractionated Heparin
LMWH — Low Molecular Weight Heparin
Fac Xa — Factor X Inhibitor

Prophylaxis Safety Considerations: Check box if answer is 'YES'

Anticoagulants: Factors Associated with Increased Bleeding

☐ Is patient experiencing any active bleeding?
☐ Does patient have (or has had history of) heparin-induced thrombocytopenia?
☐ Is patient's platelet count <100,000/mm^3?
☐ Is patient taking oral anticoagulants, platelet inhibitors (e.g., NSAIDS, Clopidigrel, Salicylates)?
☐ Is patient's creatinine clearance abnormal? If yes, please indicate value ___________
If any of the above boxes are checked, the patient may not be a candidate for anticoagulant therapy and you should consider alternative prophylactic measures.

Intermittent Pneumatic Compression (IPC)

☐ Does patient have severe peripheral arterial disease?
☐ Does patient have congestive heart failure?
☐ Does patient have an acute superficial/deep vein thrombosis?
If any of the above boxes are checked, then patient may not be a candidate for intermittent compression therapy and you should consider alternative prophylactic measures.

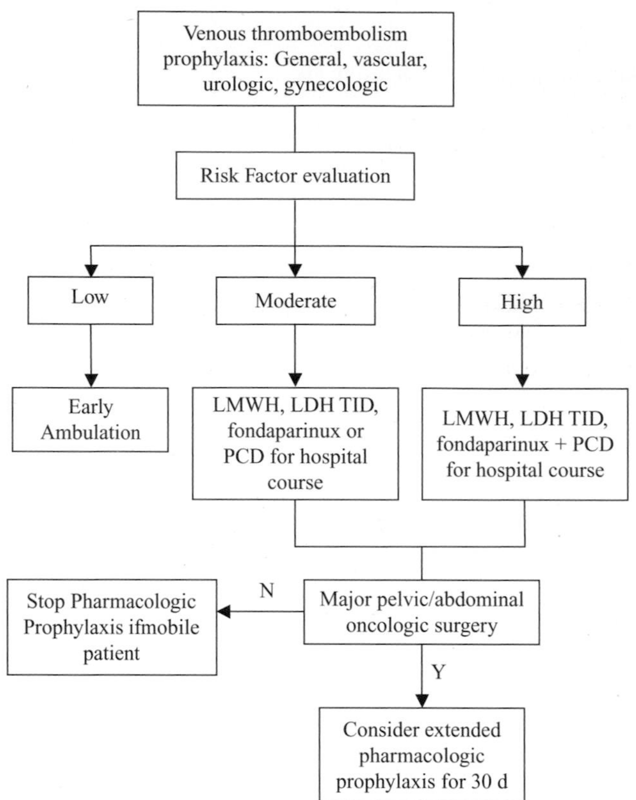

FIGURE 31.1. Algorithm for venous thromboembolism prophylaxis for general, vascular, urologic, and gynecologic patients.

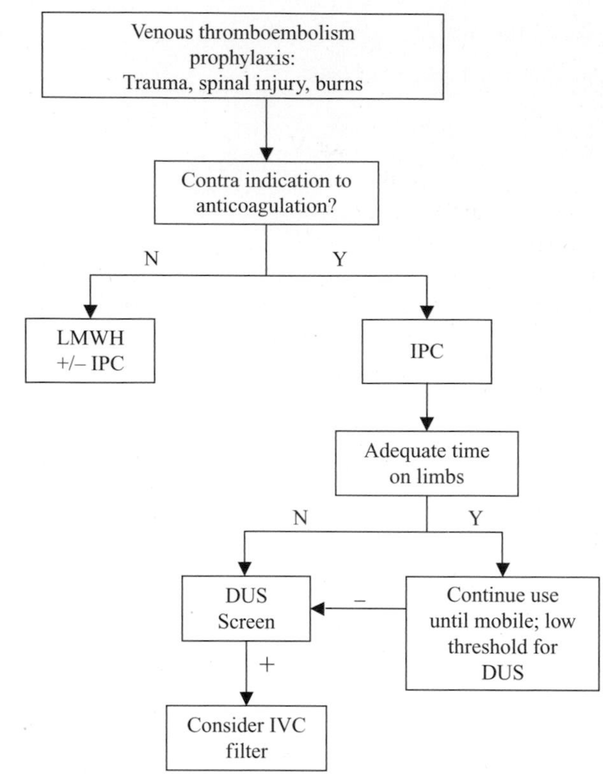

FIGURE 31.2. Algorithm for venous thromboembolism prophylaxis for trauma, spinal injury, and burn patients.

with LMWH as compared with intravenous UFH. In addition, anticoagulation has been shown to prevent the development of fatal PE, both during the initial treatment and after the treatment is complete (41). However, recurrent DVT may still occur in up to one-third of patients over the next 8 years after adequate anticoagulant therapy (42).

Traditionally, systemic intravenous UFH has been undertaken for 5 days during which time oral anticoagulation with vitamin K antagonists (usually warfarin) is instituted. Because the INR is slightly prolonged by heparin preparations and most of the liver coagulant factors have long half-lives, INR's therapeutic for two consecutive days is usually recommended before stopping heparin (43). However, because of the need for intravenous administration, frequent monitoring, and the bleeding risks of UFH, LMWHs have been advanced as primary therapy for VTE. LMWHs, derived from the lower-molecular-weight range of standard heparin, demonstrate less direct thrombin inhibition and more anti–factor Xa inhibition. LMWHs are at least equivalent to UFH, if not slightly superior, regarding thrombus recurrence, with a lower risk for major hemorrhage (44).

LMWHs may be administered subcutaneously, weight-based, and do not require monitoring except in certain circumstances (renal failure, morbid obesity and during pregnancy), and thus they may be given in the outpatient setting (45). The use in the outpatient setting requires a coordinated team approach of many health care providers. There is also early evidence that LMWHs may decrease the incidence of PTS (46). Taking all of the evidence together, LMWHs are preferred over standard UFH for the initial treatment of VTE with a level of evidence 1 A based on the most current American College of Chest Physicians (ACCP) guidelines (47).

Fondaparinux is also efficacious for the treatment of both DVT and PE (26,48,49). Fondaparinux is administered in a weight-based manner—5 mg for weight <50 kg, 7.5 mg for weight 50 to 100 kg, and 10 mg for weight >100 kg. Treatment at least for 5 days with concurrent administration of oral anticoagulation is recommended, until the INR is therapeutic at a level of 2 to 3.

Warfarin should be begun after heparinization is therapeutic, to prevent warfarin-induced skin necrosis, which occurs due to transient hypercoagulability that may occur after warfarin is begun. Warfarin inhibits protein C and protein S before most coagulation factors are inhibited by warfarin. The goal for warfarin is an INR between 2.0 and 3.0. The recommended duration of anticoagulation after a first episode of VTE with an identifiable risk factor(s) is 3 to 6 months (50). Calf level thrombi may be treated with warfarin for 6 to 12 weeks. After a second episode of VTE, the usual recommendation is prolonged warfarin use unless there are other modifying factors. The duration of warfarin usage in other situations is controversial. VTE recurrence is increased in the presence of homozygous factor V Leiden and prothrombin 20210 A mutation, protein C or protein S deficiency, antithrombin deficiency, antiphospholipid antibodies, and unresolved cancer (3). In these conditions, long-term warfarin is recommended, especially with multiple hypercoagulable states. However, heterozygous factor V Leiden and prothrombin 20210 A do not carry the same risk as their homozygous counterparts, and the duration of oral anticoagulation may be shortened. In fact, there may be no increased risk of recurrence with heterozygous factor V Leiden.

Recently, two additional criteria have been used to determine the duration of anticoagulation. One involves the amount of chronic scar tissue in the affected vein. The second and perhaps better-validated criterion involves D-dimer testing obtained 1 month after warfarin administration is stopped (51). If the D-dimer level is elevated above normal, evidence suggests that warfarin should be continued, as this result suggests that the patient is still prothrombotic (52–54). One study demonstrated a statistically significant advantage to resuming warfarin if the D-dimer assay is positive as compared with remaining off warfarin over 1.4-year follow-up (OR 4.26, $p = 0.02$) (55).

Unprovoked VTE requires additional considerations. Most believe that true unprovoked VTE requires >6 months of warfarin administration, but the actual duration is not known. A multicenter trial suggested that for idiopathic DVT, low-dose warfarin (INR, 1.5 to 2.0) was superior to placebo over a 4-year follow-up period with a 64% risk reduction for recurrent DVT (56). However, a second study suggested that full-dose warfarin (INR, 2 to 3) is superior to low-dose warfarin in the same patient group without a difference in bleeding (57). These data together suggest that for inprovoked thrombosis, long-term treatment is desirable at an INR of 2 to 3. In aggregate, criteria for discontinuation of oral anticoagulation are given a level of evidence of 1 A (47,52–54,56,57).

The most common complication of anticoagulation is bleeding, and therapy duration must be balanced against this risk. With UFH, bleeding occurs in approximately 10% of cases over the first 5 days; with warfarin at an INR at 2 to 3, the incidence of major bleeding is approximately 6% per year. When used for patients with VTE, major bleeding has been reported in 0% to 7% of patients and fatal bleeding in 0% to 2% of patients (58). A meta-analysis reported a 9.1% rate of hemorrhagic complications for anticoagulation continued for more than 3 months. To decrease bleeding, oral dose adjustments, the use of anticoagulation clinics, and even home monitoring have been suggested.

Another complication of heparin is HIT. This condition occurs when a heparin-dependent antibody immunoglobulin binds to platelets and activates them, leading to thrombocytopenia and thrombosis (59). HIT occurs in 0.6% to 30% of patients in whom heparin is administered. While morbidity and mortality has been high, early diagnosis and appropriate treatment have decreased these rates (60). HIT usually begins 3 to 14 days after heparin is begun but may occur earlier if the patient has been exposed to heparin in the past. Both bovine and porcine UFH as well as LMWH have been associated with HIT, although the incidence and severity with LMWH is less. Arterial and venous thromboses have been reported, and even small exposures to heparin (heparin coating on indwelling catheters) can cause the syndrome.

The diagnosis of HIT should be suspected when a patient experiences >50% drop in platelet count, when there is a drop in platelet count below 100,000/μL during heparin therapy, or when thrombosis occurs during heparin therapy (61). The most frequently used test to make this diagnosis is an enzyme—linked immunosorbent assay (ELISA) that detects the antiheparin antibody in the patient's plasma. This test is highly sensitive but poorly specific. Another test that can be used is the serotonin release assay, which is more specific but less sensitive than the ELISA test (62). Once the diagnosis is made (or even initially strongly suspected), cessation of heparin is the most important step in treatment. Warfarin should not be started until an adequate alternative anticoagulant has been established, to prevent paradoxical thrombosis. LMWHs cannot be substituted because of high cross–reactivity with standard heparin antibodies. The direct thrombin inhibitors hirudin (lepirudin/Refludan) and argatroban are the treatments now approved by FDA, although other agents such as fondaparinux have been also found to treat this syndrome (63,64). Lepirudin is excreted renally and argatroban is metabolized by the liver. The use of these alternative agents is given 2 C and 1 C levels of evidence (47,61,63,64).

The safety of LMWH compared with that of warfarin has led to a consideration of the long-term use of LMWH as a replacement for oral vitamin K antagonists. Rates of vein recanalization have been reported to be higher in certain venous segments using LMWH versus traditional oral agents. In addition, LMWH in certain cancer patients, when used for 6 months, has been associated with decreased rates of VTE recurrence and even mortality without differences in major bleeding (65).

The use of once-a-day as compared with twice-a-day LMWH dosing has been assessed. In a meta-analysis of more than 1,500 patients with VTE, there were no significant differences in recurrent thromboembolism, thrombosis size, hemorrhagic events, and mortality between once-a-day and twice-a-day dosing (66). However, patients with marked obesity, and those with cancer may still benefit from twice-a-day dosing (67).

ALTERNATIVE/FUTURE MEDICAL TREATMENTS FOR DEEP VENOUS THROMBOSIS/PULMONARY EMBOLISM

Two classes of agents for VTE treatment being developed include direct thrombin inhibitors and specific factor Xa inhibitors. Ximelagatran, a direct thrombin inhibitor, showed great promise a few years ago to replace warfarin. However,

Table 31.4 Comparison of properties of rivaroxaban, aplxaban, and dablgatran etexllate

Property	Rivaroxaban	Aplxaban	Dablgatran Etexllate
Target	Factor Xa	Factor Xa	Thrombin
Route of Administration	Oral	Oral	Oral
Prodrug	No	No	Yes
Bioavailability, %	>80	>50	6
Time to peak drug level, h	3	3	2
Half-life, h	9	9–14	14–17
Frequency of administration	Once-daily	Twice-daily	Once or twice-daily
Drug interactions	Potent CYP3A4 and P-glycoprotein inhibitors	Potent CYP3A4 and P-glycoprotein inhibitors	Proton pump inhibitors
Renal excretion, %	66	25	80
Safe in pregnancy	No	No	No
Antidote	No	No	No

From Gross PL, Weitz JI. New anticoagulants for treatment for venous Thromboembolism. Atheroscler Thromb Vasc Biol 2008;28:384. (Used with permission)

ximelagatran caused an elevation in liver function tests in up to 6% of patients and was not approved. A relative of this drug, dabigatran etexilate, is currently undergoing phase III studies in the prophylaxis and treatment of VTE and has met a noninflammatory target to enoxaparin in prophylaxis for orthopedic procedures. Importantly, there have not been elevations in liver enzyme levels or acute coronary events so far (Table 31.4) (68,69).

Fondaparinux and its relative, idraparinux, are most similar to LMWH, as they target factor Xa without inhibiting thrombin. These subcutaneously administered drugs demonstrate a half-life of 17 hours for fondaparinux and 80 to 130 hours for idraparinux (compared with 4 hours for LMWH) and exhibit no endothelial or protein binding. Neither of these drugs produces thrombocytopenia, and fondaparinux has been suggested as a treatment for HIT.

Idraparinux with the longer half-life in an open-label, noninferiority trial of 2,904 DVT patients and 2,215 PE patients did not meet the noninferiority requirement for PE (70). In addition, in a study of long-term treatment in DVT/PE patients, major bleeding was a significant problem, with three intracranial bleeding episodes noted (70). Idraparinux development has been halted. However, idraparinux is being biotinylated (a drug called *SSR 126517*) so that it can be reversed with avidin, as there is currently no antidote for idraparinux. Phase III trials are under way (71).

New oral anti–factor Xa agents are being developed. Rivaroxaban and apixaban are the two agents furthest along in the development (Table 31.4). Rivaroxaban has 66% renal excretion, whereas apixaban has only 25% renal excretion (68,72). Rivaroxaban is in phase II trials and phase III trails showing good results in the prophylaxis and treatment of DVT, whereas apixaban is in both phase II trials of patients with proximal DVT and phase III trials (68,69,72,73).

Other antithrombotic agents are being evaluated, including oral heparins; other direct thrombin inhibitors such as bivalirudin; defibrinating agents such as ancrod; anti-inflammatory agents such as P-selectin inhibitors; factor VIIa inhibitors; tissue factor pathway inhibitor; and activated protein C (74,75). The use of P-selectin inhibitors is an area of ongoing research in our laboratory. An anti-inflammatory approach uses an antithrombotic agent that does not cause direct anticoagulant activities and presents the possibility of an agent that prevents thrombus amplification without bleeding potential.

VENA CAVA FILTERS

The primary indications for IVC filters include a complication of anticoagulation, a contraindication to anticoagulation, and/or failure of anticoagulation (Table 31.5). Protection from PE has been >95% by using cone-shaped wire-based permanent IVC filters over the past 30 years (76). As the IVC filter has achieved success, its indications have widened. These indications include now a free-floating thrombus tail longer than 5 cm, if anticoagulation risk is excessive (i.e., older patient with DVT or following major trauma), when the risk of PE is very high, and to allow for perioperative epidural anesthesia (77–79). Devices can be either permanent or retrievable.

Filters are placed in an infrarenal location in most cases. However, they may be placed in the suprarenal or the superior vena caval location in certain situations. Suprarenal placement indications include high-lying clot, pregnancy or use in women of childbearing age, or previous filter filled with clot or that has failed. Sepsis is not a contraindication to the use of wire-based filters since the trapped material can be sterilized by antibiotics administration.

Table 31.5 Vena cava filter placement indications and complications

Indications	Complications
Contraindication to anticoagulation Complication of anticoagulation Failure of anticoagulation	Placement • Site bleed/thrombosis • Malposition • Pulmonary embolism • Guidewire entrapment Device • Migration • Occlusion • 1° failure Late • Strut fracture • Penetration • Wire ensnarement (other procedure) • 1° failure

Filters may be placed under x-ray guidance or by using either external ultrasound or intravascular ultrasound. External ultrasound may be ineffective in the face of morbid obesity, overlying bowel gas, or the presence of open abdominal wounds (80). Other than one randomized prospective study on the use of filters as treatment of DVT (which is not how filters are traditionally used), the use of IVC filters is given a 2 C level of evidence based on ACCP guidelines (47,81).

Filter complications are categorized as periprocedural, early device-related, and long-term device-related (Table 31.5) (82,83). Periprocedural complications include bleeding, PE at the time of filter deployment, device-specific misplacement, or inability to insert the device (84). The most common complication is bleeding, but cessation of heparin around the time of insertion can lessen this risk. As the venous system has generally low pressure, the risk of bleeding is not high relative to arterial puncture. The use of gentle firm pressure with sheath removal is important. Periprocedural PE may occur if the filter is deployed through a thrombus (85). Duplex assessment of distal iliac vein thrombus involvement and cavography to assess iliac vein patency can minimize this complication. Conversely, many filters can be placed through jugular or upper arm veins as the delivery systems are now lower profile.

Early device-related complications usually involve filter deployment. As user experience has increased, failure to deploy the filter has become very uncommon. Vena cava filters are generally placed at the level of L2–L3 for IVC placement and T12–L1 for suprarenal filter placement. Misplacement of the filter may occur if cavography or ultrasound imaging is not used. For example, there is a >20-fold increased risk of misplacement if only external bony landmarks are employed (37). If misplacement is evident and the filter's efficacy is thought to be compromised, the decision whether or not to place a more proximal filter needs to be made on an individual basis. No increase in direct thrombotic complications has been observed in patients with two filters (86). For suprarenal filters, no greater complication rate has been found than for the infrarenal location. In a series of 124 consecutive patients with suprarenal Greenfield filters, no renal failure secondary to renal vein thrombosis was documented (87). In patients with malignancy, the risk of thrombotic renal vein occlusion may be higher (88).

Long-term device-related complications, including filter migration, are less common than previously thought, as respiratory variation may account for as much as 20 mm of movement as depicted on plain abdominal radiographs taken at different time points. Current rates of migration of >20 mm rates are 9% to 11% (82). A large IVC (>28 mm diameter) needs to be imaged before the filter is placed, and either bilateral iliac venous filters or a bird's nest IVC filter should be used. Excessive filter tilt is another potential complication. This may occur with strut deployment into a vessel orifice or misplacement of the sheath device at the time of placement. Some reports have suggested that increased filter tilt may decrease the effectiveness of the filter for trapping PE, but little objective data support this contention unless the tilt is >15% off the axial midline (36).

Device failure, defined as recurrent PE despite a technically good placement, may occur in 2% to 5% of patients (37,86,89). One way to decrease this risk is to have the patient concurrently anticoagulated if the patient has a particularly malignant form of hypercoagulability and if there are no contraindications to anticoagulation. For example, if the patient has a limited contraindication to anticoagulation for which the filter is placed but has a persistent risk of VTE, anticoagulation in the setting of a filter is indicated. IVC occlusion after filter placement is a dreaded complication that may occur in the early or late setting and may lead to phlegmasia cerulea dolens in up to 24% of patients who are unable to be anticoagulated (90). Various rates of IVC occlusion have been documented with all filter types and may be highest with the bird's nest filter or the TrapEase-type filter (91–93). The lack of prospective randomized trials with regard to specific filter type, particularly in the long term, limits data about IVC occlusion rates. The best information comes from the Greenfield database, with approximately 3,200 patients older than 27 years, showing an overall IVC occlusion rate of approximately 2% to 4% (86,94). Filter occlusion may be caused by the filter performing its function by trapping a massive PE or as a complication of the filter causing an IVC thrombosis.

When an IVC occludes acutely, the patient may become hypotensive. It is important to differentiate an acute massive PE (filter failure) in a patient with a patent IVC from an occluded IVC and normal pulmonary artery. This distinction can be made by bedside detection of jugular venous distention. If distension is evident, it is likely that the patient has right heart failure and thrombolytics and vasopressor agents may be appropriate (82). However, if the patient has intravascular volume depletion due to an occluded IVC, large volume resuscitation is mandatory. Any patient with an IVC filter who develops sudden lower extremity edema needs an urgent caval duplex examination, and, if technically unsatisfactory, a cavogram.

Several strategies are available to treat IVC occlusion. For an acute thrombus, full anticoagulation with heparin followed by catheter-directed thrombolysis may alleviate the problem. If the thrombus is older, catheter suction embolectomy and dissolution by a mechanical thrombus fragmentation device may be performed (95,96). If occlusion is recent, one may place a protective suprarenal filter and then navigate in the perifilter plane to recanalize the IVC, by using a stent to push the filter against the IVC wall (97).

Chronic occlusions with minimal symptoms should be managed expectantly. If the filter becomes full of thrombus, its effectiveness for trapping PE is markedly reduced and a suprarenal filter needs to be placed, as PE may occur in up to 33% of patients (98).

Prophylactic IVC filters that are placed for patients at high risk for VTE, such as those with major trauma have low to immediate complication rates, and long-term DVT has been documented in up to 44% (99,100). Whether this significant DVT rate would have occurred without filter placement is unknown. Long-term morbidity after prophylactic IVC filter placement is usually due to the development of DVT and subsequent CVI (101). In one series of pediatric patients who had filters placed for prophylaxis from 19 months to 14 years, no PE, IVC thrombosis, or migration was documented (102).

Less common filter complications include ensnared guidewires, either at the time of placement (more common with a jugular approach) or at a remote time, with a wire for another procedure or device (e.g., central venous access) (83,103). The J-wire can become caught by the strut apex fixation. Standard endovascular techniques using snares and catheters to straighten the J-wire allow disengagement. If a wire is placed for venous access and the operator is unaware that a filter is present, significant problems may occur if the wire cannot be pulled out. It is incumbent on the operator to remove the wire carefully, and if retrieval is not easy, fluoroscopy is used to identify where the wire is ensnared. If guidewires are removed forcefully, the filter may fracture and end up in the heart.

Filter strut fracture may be demonstrated at late follow-up by duplex ultrasonography or by a CT scan. Fracture rarely causes a complication, as the struts and the device are well incorporated via attachment sites. Strut fracture is more common in the suprarenal location as greater IVC motion occurs in this area. Penetration of hooks into the aorta or small bowel has been documented but rarely has clinical consequences. Retroperitoneal hemorrhage has been documented (104). Renal penetration with resultant hydronephrosis and small bowel obstruction have been documented only by case reports (105–107). Intracardiac migration of a filter is rare (<0.1%) and usually necessitates either an open surgical procedure or a catheter-based procedure with a snare to remove the filter (108).

THROMBOLYTIC AND SURGICAL PROCEDURES FOR DEEP VENOUS THROMBOSIS AND PULMONARY EMBOLISM

The incidence of CVI after appropriate anticoagulant treatment for DVT has been reported as 23% after 2 years, 28% after 5 years, and 29% after 8 years (42). Thus, the use of thrombolytic agents to rapidly decrease thrombus load may decrease the long-term sequelae. By duplex ultrasound, spontaneous lysis time is 2.3- to 7.3-fold longer in segments that reflux than in segments without reflux (109). Systemic thrombolysis in two small series revealed a decrease in CVI with streptokinase, as opposed to systemic heparin anticoagulation. However, results depend on complete thrombolysis and as the ability to predict complete lysis is poor, combined with its bleeding potential, thrombolysis is used infrequently. However, administration of thrombolytics directly into venous thrombi has increased in popularity and has led to the publication of a national thrombolysis registry (110,111). In 473 patients, 287 of whom underwent follow-up, 312 urokinase infusions in 303 limbs were reported. Venous thrombi were noted in the iliofemoral segment in 71% of cases alone, without IVC involvement in 79%, and including the IVC in 21% of cases. Patients had acute venous thrombosis in approximately two-thirds of cases, 16% had chronic venous thrombosis, and 19% had combined acute and chronic venous thrombosis. Approximately 30% had a prior DVT. Complete thrombolysis was achieved in 31%, whereas partial lysis was achieved in 52% of cases. Acute DVT and no history of DVT predicted success, and complications included major bleeding necessitating blood products in 11% and minor bleeding in 16%. Intracranial hemorrhage rate was 0.2%, subdural hemorrhage rate was 0.2%, and mortality was 0.4%. Patency at 12 months was 79% if lysis was complete, 58% with >50% lysis, and 32% with <50% lysis. Absence of valvular reflux was noted in 72% of cases if there was complete lysis.

Importantly, aggressive therapies have been found to improve the quality of life. A small randomized study demonstrated that thrombolysis is superior to anticoagulation in patients with iliofemoral DVT (112). The use of thrombolytic agents for DVT is now given a 2 B level of evidence (47).

Surgical approaches for PE are indicated for patients with massive PE with hypotension who require large doses of vasopressors. These are often patients in whom thrombolysis has been unsuccessful. The technique of open pulmonary embolectomy is associated with high rates of morbidity and mortality. Today, open pulmonary embolectomy is limited to those who require manual cardiac massage for hypotension or when catheter pulmonary embolectomy fails. In the future, there may be a more expanded role for pulmonary embolectomy (113).

Catheter-directed thrombolysis is well accepted for axillary/subclavian venous thrombosis, particularly effort thrombosis in young patients (114). More rapid thrombolysis decreases long-term risk of swelling and dependence of venous collateralization for outflow (115). Subclavian vein angioplasty and stenting for exertional axillary/subclavian venous thrombosis have been reported (116), but the stents may crimp, migrate, or erode through the vein, given upper shoulder outlet motion. A thoracic outlet decompression procedure is efficacious, as thoracic outlet compression most often causes the underlying venous stenosis. It is important that the patient undergo positional phlebography if the axillary/subclavian axis is patent to confirm extrinsic compression of the axillary and subclavian veins at the thoracic outlet. Generally, thoracic outlet decompression follows thrombolysis. Operative timing, whether immediate or after a delay to allow for the vein wall inflammatory response to subside, is controversial. In cases of secondary axillary/subclavian DVT due to indwelling catheters, anticoagulation along with the removal of the catheter is indicated. The duration of anticoagulation should be individualized, reflecting the patient's thrombotic risk—usually <3 months. Patch venoplasty is also recommended if persistent venous narrowing is present after thoracic outlet decompression. The main complications of thoracic outlet decompression are bleeding, lymphatic leak, infection, recurrent thrombosis, and brachial plexus nerve injury (117).

Thrombolytic therapy for PE remains controversial. Although agents lyse thrombus effectively, recurrence rates and patient mortality have not been improved. However, the original studies were not powered to address this outcome. Results have been optimized when patients are young, the embolus is fresh (<48 hours old), and the embolus is large. Streptokinase, urokinase, and tissue plasminogen activator have all been used (118). These agents rapidly dissolve clot, but by 7 days, the advantages for all three agents decrease. Thus, the benefit of thrombolytic agents for PE appears to be greatest in those 10% of patients who would die as a result of massive PE in the first hour after the PE occurs. However, recent data suggest that thrombolysis may be useful in patients with right ventricular dysfunction without hemodynamic instability and patients with evidence of right heart changes (119–124).

Venous and pulmonary thrombectomy

Iliofemoral venous thrombectomy results in mechanical clearing of the venous circulation and may be combined with the creation of a temporary arteriovenous fistula. Thrombectomy uses a Fogarty balloon catheter passed from the femoral vein during Valsalva maneuvers. The arteriovenous fistula is fashioned such that it can be taken down by nonsurgical endovascular techniques and provides rapid blood flow through the iliac venous system. Complete venography in the operating room is recommended, as back-bleeding is unreliable for the assessment of complete thrombus clearance. Back-bleeding can occur from a disobliterated side-branch only. Recurrence rates less than 20% have been reported. The incidence of PE during the first week after thrombectomy is equivalent to the incidence with only anticoagulation. Thrombectomy has primarily been used for limb-threatening phlegmasia. Clinical success has been reported between 42% and 93% (125). The largest series of 77 legs with a follow-up between 5 and 13 years revealed maintenance of patency but a steady decline in valvular competence (126).

Venous thrombectomy may also be used in situations of significant iliofemoral thrombosis to decrease postthrombotic sequelae when thrombolysis fails or is contraindicated. In the only study comparing iliofemoral venous thrombectomy with anticoagulation (31 patients) with anticoagulation alone (32 patients), iliofemoral vein patency was better (76% vs. 35%), femoropopliteal patency was better (52% vs. 26%), and the clinical outcome was improved at 6 months (40% asymptomatic vs. 7%) (126). At 10 years, the number of patients available for follow-up had decreased to 13 (thrombectomy) and 17 (anticoagulation-alone). Patency remained better in the thrombectomy group (83% vs. 41%), as did the absence of popliteal reflux (78% vs. 43%).

VENOUS VARICOSITIES

VV disease is a common problem. By some estimates, it may account for up to 2% of all health care costs within the United States, a figure that approaches approximately $1 billion annually (127). It is estimated that VVs of the lower extremities are present in 15% to 20% of the population (128).

The exact cause of VVs is not known, although several factors play a role in the etiology. Venous hypertension, valvular incompetence, and reflux from the deep to the superficial system are involved in VV development and propagation. Other factors include genetic and familial predisposition, local hemodynamic forces such as prolonged periods of standing, and circulating levels of estrogen hormones (128). Previous DVT may also predispose to later development of VVs (42).

All patients should receive conservative treatment, including good compression, weight loss, exercise to improve calf muscle pump function, and intermittent leg elevation. Compression includes graded compression stockings, 20 to 30 mm Hg for moderate disease and 30 to 40 mm Hg for more severe disease (129). Randomized controlled trials have demonstrated a 50% reduction in the development of the PTS in patients treated with compression stockings after DVT, and other trials have demonstrated at least symptomatic improvement (130,131). Although it may seem that a compression regimen is difficult to comply with and uncomfortable, studies aimed at evaluating compliance with compression therapy have demonstrated compliance rates of 5 hours a day wearing compression stockings approaching 75%.

When considering operation for venous disease, consideration must be given to both the superficial varicosities and accompanying deep venous reflux. Operation is indicated for superficial venous insufficiency with symptoms of leg heaviness, soreness, swelling, or fatigue. Indications for removal of varicosities include pain over the varicosities, previous thrombophlebitis, and bleeding. Operative management may be useful in the treatment of associated skin changes, including hyperpigmentation and severe venous ulcers, although many ulcers will heal with compression alone. Although the ESCHAR trial demonstrated similar rates of venous ulcer healing in groups treated with conservative management and VV surgery, the group receiving surgical treatment had a significantly reduced rate of recurrence—12% versus 28% (129).

Contraindications to operative treatment for VV disease include the presence of arterial insufficiency as a cause for leg discomfort or primary lymphedema as a source of symptoms. Deep venous obstruction, including active DVT, should prompt postponement of treatment. In addition, active skin infection or pregnancy should delay operative treatment.

Ligation, division, and stripping of the great saphenous vein constitutes the standard, time-tested, tried, and true treatment for VVs. The rationale behind this procedure is that it allows the correction of the reflux present in the limbs of patients suffering from VV disease and decreases recurrence. Formal stripping has a low rate of recurrence and is the most definitive option for correction of saphenous reflux contributing to VV disease. Perhaps the longest follow-up is a series published in 2001, based on clinical assessment and duplex scan of patients who had undergone VV excision 31 to 39 years previously. In this long-term follow-up, the rate of recurrence was 47%. In the Gloucester study, however, the risk of recurrence at up to 12 years was approximately 10% with ligation and stripping compared with nearly 30% for those undergoing ligation only (reactive risk (RR) 2.65, 95% confidence interval [CI] 1.20 to 5.84, $p = 0.012$). Less drastic than total ligation and stripping is ligation and division of the saphenous vein with interruption of specific perforating veins. This procedure allows the preservation of the saphenous vein.

The practice of physically removing the saphenous vein has been almost completely replaced by saphenous vein ablation. Endoluminal ablation of the great saphenous vein, providing functional ablation without requiring formal stripping, was first reported by Boné in 1999, and the first English language report followed, by Navarro, in 2001 (132,133). Endovenous ablation uses a heat source (either a laser emitting diode or a radiofrequency probe) to induce occlusion of the great saphenous vein. In laser ablation, hemoglobin in circulating red blood cells acts as a chromophore. Although some damage is caused to the vein wall directly in the path of the laser, the heat produced by the interaction of the laser with the red blood cells causes the formation of steam bubbles, which lead to thermal injury to the interior of the vein. Endothelium is damaged and denuded, and occlusion of the treated segment ensues (134). In our series of 460 limbs in 364 patients with 443 successful endovenous laser therapy and 135 concomitant procedures we noted 3 limbs (0.7%) with DVT, 32 limbs (7.2%) with saphenofemoral thrombus extension, 11 limbs (2.5%) with superficial thrombophlebitis, and one 1 PE. Bruising was assessed at the first postoperative visit, and data were available for 303 limbs (67.5%). Bruising was minimal in 48 limbs (15.9%), moderate in 77 (25.4%), and no bruising was apparent in 178 (58.7%). There were 9 cases (2.0%) of cellulitis in patients' limbs, 4 (0.9%) of postoperative fluid collections requiring further intervention, 4 (0.9%) of neovascularization and perivenous inflammation, and 2 (0.5%) of paresthesias (135).

In principle, radiofrequency ablation (RFA) is quite similar to laser ablation in that it uses a heat source placed inside the greater saphenous vein to produce vascular and endothelial damage and occlusion of the treated vein. In RFA, direct heating causes contraction of the collagen in the vessel wall and loss of the endothelial lining, to occlude the vein. For both techniques, postoperative application of a compressive dressing is recommended. RFA tends to cause less bruising and pain postprocedure than laser ablation.

As persistence of VVs may be related to the continued presence of incompetent perforating veins, multiple approaches for the correction of incompetent perforating veins have been advocated. One approach that has been used with some success but less commonly used now is subfascial endoscopic perforator ablation. Minimally invasive approaches have gained enthusiasm for the lower leg and calf, as this is a site more prone to the most severe sequelae of venous insufficiency including stasis pigmentation and stasis dermatitis (136). Further operative treatment of perforating veins in the thigh and upper leg is technically simpler and associated with a lower complication rate than similar treatment in the calf. Interruption of perforating veins has been suggested to decrease venous ulcer healing time and increase time to recurrence in legs with severe venous ulceration (136–138).

For the treatment of small (<4 mm) VVs that pose primarily a cosmetic problem, the use of sclerosing agents has been highly effective. This type of treatment, however, is less successful in treating larger varicosities. The underlying concept is that the injected agent damages the vascular endothelium, leading to obliteration of the vein lumen. Many sclerosants have been tried, including sodium morrhuate, sodium tetradecyl sulfate, ethanolamine oleate, and polidocanol. The only sclerosant approved in the United States is sodium tetradecyl sulfate.

In part because traditional sclerotherapy has been unsuccessful in providing adequate closure of larger VVs, the technique of creating a foam for injection has been advocated by some. Currently, there are no foam sclerosants commercially available in the United States; however, a foam may be created by mixing available sclerosants with air. In general, this has been regarded as a relatively safe and effective procedure, and a recent systematic review found a rate of occlusion of 87%, less than that associated with surgery but greater than that typically seen with liquid sclerotherapy. In this analysis, the rate of adverse events was rare, with PE and DVT each occurring in <1% of patients, visual disturbance in 1%, and headache in 4% (139). However, although there have been reports of demonstrated microembolic phenomena during this procedure, serious adverse consequences have been rare (140).

Stab avulsion of superficial varicosities, also referred to as *ambulatory phlebectomy*, remains a staple of treatment for VVs although it is being supplanted in some centers by transilluminated powered phlebectomy. The goal of stab avulsion is the removal of superficial varicosities from the lower extremities. This technique was first described in 1966 and involves making many small incisions over the varicosities and excising them with special hooks.

The complications of open phlebectomy are mostly minor and non–life-threatening. Infection is very rare. An antiseptic leg and groin wash twice the night before surgery is recommended. There is no need for systemic antibiotic prophylaxis. Hematoma and lymphocele occur in <0.5% of cases. Avoiding dissection of the anterior tibial dorsal veins decreases lymphocele formation (141). To decrease the risk of perioperative hematoma, it is important to obtain a careful history of the patient's medications, including herbal supplements, high-dose vitamin E, aspirin, or other anticoagulants, as these may potentiate a hematoma due to venous oozing. Generally, venous hematomas resolve spontaneously and do not require additional surgical therapy or transfusion. Use of a tourniquet may decrease bleeding associated with varicosity excision (142).

As an office procedure, venous varicosity excision has been performed by using tumescent anesthesia where a dilute amount of low-concentration lidocaine (0.5%) with very dilute epinephrine (1:1,000,000) allows for a large area to be anesthetized. Earlier return to usual activities may be an additional benefit (143).

Peripheral nerve injury is the most common complication of open phlebectomy, with approximately 40% to 50% of patients having some hypesthesia in the area of the incisions, usually within the greater saphenous nerve distribution (144,145). Permanent nerve injury occurs approximately 1% of the time. With calf vein excision in the lesser saphenous distribution, the sural nerve is at the greatest risk.

Recurrence of VVs is also a known complication, and some surgeons consider this part of the natural history. Recurrence of VV is thought to occur by recruitment of collaterals or recanalization of the obliterated vein. To avoid this complication, it is important preoperatively to have the patient stand and to mark all the veins to avoid missing any varicosities that disappear once the patient is recumbent. Duplex-directed varicose excision may also decrease incision number and decrease varicosity recurrence by directing excision and ligation of incompetent perforators (146).

Transilluminated powered phlebectomy (TriVex, InaVein, Inc.) is designed as an alternative to stab phlebectomy, with several postulated advantages. This technique involves the use of a handpiece transilluminator and a resector with strong suction (147,148). Tumescent anesthesia is used liberally during this technique, with dermal punches to clear blood and tumescence out of the leg. As this technique occurs under direct vision, more complete excision of the VV clusters will be possible. Second, by using the instruments, which require only the use of fewer incisions, the more minimally invasive procedures will offer a more comfortable and cosmetically pleasing result than the traditional stab phlebectomy. Comparisons of powered phlebectomy and traditional stab avulsion have generally showed similar outcomes, with trends toward more postoperative hematoma formation and discomfort in the immediate postoperative period, but fewer incisions (149,150).

CHRONIC VENOUS INSUFFICIENCY

Preventing complications of CVI is best achieved by appropriate use of compression garments, prevention of recurrent DVT in patients with PTS, and with selective endoluminal or open intervention (Table 31.6) (151). The progression of CVI is slow and progressive. Leg varicosities are the most

Table 31.6 Chronic venous insufficiency preventative measures to reduce complications

Action	Rx	Complications	Level of Evidence
Compression	20–30 mmHg 30–40 mmHg	None major	Ia
Address Superficial venous Incompetence	Saphenous and/or Perforator Ablation	Local skin bruise incisional problems	Ib
Address Venous Iliac Obstruction	Diagnose with MRV/ Venogram Endolumal PTA/stent	Stent Thrombosis Stent malposition	IIb
Prevent Recurrence of DVT	• Adequate duration of anticoagulation • Biomarker evaluation with d-dimer measurement	Bleeding; VTE recurrence	Ib

MRV = magnetic resonance venography; PTA = percutaneous transluminal Angioplasty.

common presentation, followed by edema and leg heaviness, with severe CVI affecting up to 30% of patients and causing most of the associated morbidity (42,152). The pathophysiology of venous ulceration is often related to the failure of DVT resolution and obstruction and less commonly associated with valvular dysfunction without proximal obstruction or incompetent perforators. Risk for PTS is associated with greater initial thrombus burden, the sites of thrombosis (proximal > distal), and inadequate anticoagulation (153).

Standard therapy for venous stasis ulceration includes limb elevation, graded compression, and local wound care. Patient compliance with graded compression is critical for good outcomes (154). The main complications with local venous ulcer therapy are allergic reaction to the agent used and failure of therapy due to intractable venous stasis ulceration.

Compression stockings are cost-effective and are better than routine care for ulcer healing (155), and nonelastic garments may be better than elastic types (156). It is important to decrease local bacterial colonization, promote a granulating wound bed, and provide an environment that allows healing. It is the authors' opinion that the Unna boot is most effective in this regard for a *noninfected* venous stasis ulcer. The wound is protected, and the constant compression of the dressing decreases venous hypertension that impairs healing. Care must be taken to place compression dressings so that the Unna boot is firmly applied but is not so tight as to create skin breakdown. If the patient has evidence of cellulitis, systemic antibiotics are recommended. However, no evidence supports routine antibiotic use for prolonged periods, as this may increase bacterial resistance. Occasionally, ulcers that are long standing (>12 months) should be evaluated for premalignant changes by local punch biopsy.

Multimodality surgical and endoluminal therapy for venous stasis ulceration first needs to address the contribution of the perforating and superficial venous system to this problem (157,158). Evidence suggests surgical treatment of superficial incompetence such as saphenous vein ablation is effective for reducing ulcer recurrence and may be associated with faster healing (129) even if deep insufficiency also exists (135). However, the strongest data are in the prevention of venous ulcer recurrence. Complications related to superficial venous ablation are listed under VV therapy in this chapter.

Subfascial perforator surgery has been advanced to address perforator incompetence (159). This technique involves remote endoscopic access to visualize and ligate the subfascial perforators. While occasionally used, a randomized prospective controlled trial suggested little benefit of this technique over standard compression wound care, except in patients with very large ulcers (160). Thus, this surgical procedure is uncommonly performed. Newer techniques with percutaneous endoluminal perforator ablation may represent a more efficacious approach, but large series are lacking.

The primary therapy for proximal deep vein stenosis or occlusion is endovascular, particularly for obstructive venous pathology. Endovenous angioplasty and stenting is very effective to reduce venous claudication (161), little in stent restenosis or occlusion does occur (162), and this intervention provides excellent durability (163). Endovascular venoplasty and stenting appears to work much better in the iliac vein than in other locations, and it is currently the definitive approach for the patient with iliac vein compression syndrome (May–Thurner syndrome) (164). Major complications include bleeding, wound infection of the incision, and stent thrombosis. The main predictive factors for stent thrombosis include: Male gender (odds ratio [OR] 6.5), recent trauma (OR 5.3), and age <40 years (OR 3.8) (163). Overall, endoluminal therapies can reduce major wound-related morbidity and likely decrease PTS severity by returning prograde venous flow in symptomatic patients.

Results with venous reconstructive surgery for severe manifestations such as pain or persistent ulceration, or both, are better if the etiology is primary valvular dysfunction rather than postphlebitic disease (159,165). Primary valvuloplasty and axillary vein to popliteal vein valve transplants are selectively performed. The efficacy of these techniques is less clear, as evidence outside of case series is unavailable and long-term patient follow-up is scant. Primary complications include bleeding and thrombosis. Adjuncts to decrease these problems include meticulous hemostasis and periprocedural use of PCDs, as well as judicious perioperative anticoagulation. Some investigators advocate the use of intravenous dextran followed by coumadinization (166). Nerve injury and other injuries are quite rare. Long-term arm swelling related to segmental axillary vein removal for popliteal vein valve transplant is minimal as long as the patient has a competent cephalic vein that enters distal to the area where the vein segment with valve is removed. Preoperative arm ascending venography is essential in selecting the axillary venous segment to use and in confirming that a usable valve is present.

Reconstruction of the IVC and iliofemoral veins for venoocclusive disease may also be done in limited settings. By far, the most common procedure is a saphenous vein femorofemoral crossover bypass for chronic iliac venous obstruction. The expectation for venous reconstruction surgery needs to be realistic, as venous physiology makes these repairs much less durable than arterial reconstructions. For nonmalignant IVC occlusion, both venous reconstructive surgery and IVC recanalization by endovascular techniques have been advanced. In one surgical series, 42 patients underwent 44 venous reconstructions (165). Thirty-six patients had limb swelling or venous claudication, 38 had pain, and 14 had venous ulceration. Obstruction was acquired in 40 cases. For therapy, 18 patients had saphenous vein crossover grafts, 17 had ePTFE grafts implanted (8 femorocaval, 5 iliocaval, 3 cross-femoral, and 1 cavoatrial), 6 patients had spiral vein grafts, and 1 patient had a vein patch angioplasty. At 3.5-year mean follow-up, the secondary 3-year patency was 62% (83% Palma and 54% iliocaval and femorocaval grafts). At 2 years, all ePTFE grafts had a 45% patency rate (165). Thrombectomy was required in approximately 7% of patients. Thus, the procedure can be recommended only in properly selected patients (167).

Regarding endovascular interventions, a series of 120 patients over a 10-year period has been reported. In these patients, stenotic segments of the IVC were balloon dilated, and occluded segments were recanalized when feasible and stents placed under intravascular ultrasound (168). Pathology was total occlusion in 14% and stenoses in 86%. Common iliac vein obstruction was concurrent in 93%. Distal reflux was present in 66%. Modifications of the basic stent technique were required in recanalization of total occlusions (four extending up to the atrium), two bilateral stent deployments, and nine IVC filter cases. Stent deployment across the renal and hepatic veins or the contralateral iliac vein had no adverse sequelae. Cumulative stent patency at 2 years was 82%. Complete relief of pain and swelling at 3.5 years was 74% and 51%, respectively. The cumulative rate of complete ulcer healing at 2 years was 63%. Overall clinical outcome was rated as good or excellent in 70% (168).

Surgical reconstruction of the iliofemoral veins and IVC in the setting of malignancy is accepted therapy, although not common. The risks are bleeding and thrombosis. Anticoagulants, perioperative PCDs to maintain brisk venous flow, and arteriovenous fistulae are adjuncts that can be used to improve patency rates although large comparative series are lacking. Referral to a center that has expertise and experience with these cases is probably the most practical measure to ensure fewer complications. In a series of 18 patients, no major morbidity and no mortality occurred, no anticoagulation was used, and overall clinical patency was approximately 80% (169). In another series of 29 procedures for primary (n2) and secondary (n27) IVC tumors in which the IVC was replaced with a large diameter externally supported ePTFE graft in most cases and three patients had arteriovenous fistulae created, only two late graft occlusions occurred at a mean follow-up of 2.8 years. There were 11 late deaths from malignancy. In this series, IVC replacement was at the level of the suprarenal segment of the IVC in 15 patients, at the infrarenal segment of the IVC in 10 patients, at both segments of the IVC in 3 patients, and at the renal vein confluence in 1 patient (170).

REFERENCES

1. Heit JA, Cohen AT, Anderson FJ. Estimated annual number of incident and recurrent, non-fatal venous thromboembolism (VTE) events in the US. *Blood* 2005;106(11):267a.
2. Prandoni P, Lensing AW, Prins MR. Long-term outcomes after deep venous thrombosis of the lower extremities. *Vasc Med* 1998;3(1):57–60.
3. Bauer KA, Rosendaal FR, Heit JA. Hypercoagulability: too many tests, too much conflicting data. *Hematology Am Soc Hematol Educ Program* 2002:353–368.
4. Henke P. Thrombosis due to hypercoagulable states. *Rutherford's textbook of vascular surgery,* 6th ed. Philadelphia, PA: Elsevier 2004;568–78.
5. Andreotti F, Becker RC. Atherothrombotic disorders: new insights from hematology. *Circulation* 2005;111(14):1855–1863.
6. Perkins JM, Magee TR, Galland RB. Phlegmasia caerulea dolens and venous gangrene. *Br J Surg* 1996;83(1):19–23.
7. Prandoni P, Bernardi E. Upper extremity deep vein thrombosis. *Curr Opin Pulm Med* 1999;5(4):222–226.
8. Quenet S, Laporte S, Decousus H, et al. Factors predictive of venous thrombotic complications in patients with isolated superficial vein thrombosis. *J Vasc Surg* 2003;38(5):944–949.
9. Sullivan V, Wakefield TW. Superficial Venous Thrombosis. In: Pearce WH, Yao JST, editors. *Trends in vascular surgery.* Chicago: Precept Press. 2002:463–472.
10. Heit JA, Silverstein MD, Mohr DN, et al. The epidemiology of venous thromboembolism in the community. *Thromb Haemost* 2001;86(1): 452–463.
11. Martinelli I, Cattaneo M, Taioli E, et al. Genetic risk factors for superficial vein thrombosis. *Thromb Haemost* 1999;82(4):1215–1217.
12. Wells PS, Anderson DR, Rodger M, et al. Evaluation of D-dimer in the diagnosis of suspected deep-vein thrombosis. *N Engl J Med* 2003; 349(13):1227–1235.
13. Fowl RJ, Strothman GB, Blebea J, et al. Inappropriate use of venous duplex scans: an analysis of indications and results. *J Vasc Surg* 1996; 23(5):881–885, discussion 885–886.
14. Douglas MG, Sumner DS. Duplex scanning for deep vein thrombosis: has it replaced both phlebography and noninvasive testing? *Semin Vasc Surg* 1996;9(1):3–12.
15. Guyatt G, Schünemann HJ, Cook D, et al. Applying the grades of recommendation for antithrombotic and thrombolytic therapy: the Seventh ACCP Conference on Antithrombotic and Thrombolytic Therapy. *Chest* 2004;126(Suppl):179S–187S.
16. Stein PD, Fowler SE, Goodman LR, et al. Multidetector computed tomography for acute pulmonary embolism. *N Engl J Med* 2006;354 (22):2317–2327.
17. Schellong SM, Schwarz T, Halbritter K, et al. Complete compression ultrasonography of the leg veins as a single test for the diagnosis of deep vein thrombosis. *Thromb Haemost* 2003;89(2):228–234.
18. Cornuz J, Ghali WA, Hayoz D, et al. Clinical prediction of deep venous thrombosis using two risk assessment methods in combination with rapid quantitative D-dimer testing. *Am J Med* 2002;112(3):198–203.
19. Pierik EG, Toonder IM, van Urk H, et al. Validation of duplex ultrasonography in detecting competent and incompetent perforating veins in patients with venous ulceration of the lower leg. *J Vasc Surg* 1997;26(1):49–52.
20. Sakurai T, Matsushita M, Nishikimi N, et al. Hemodynamic assessment of femoropopliteal venous reflux in patients with primary varicose veins. *J Vasc Surg* 1997;26(2):260–264.
21. Rutherford RB, Padberg FT Jr, Comerota AJ, et al. Venous severity scoring: an adjunct to venous outcome assessment. *J Vasc Surg* 2000; 31(6):1307–1312.
22. Criado E, Farber MA, Marston WA, et al. The role of air plethysmography in the diagnosis of chronic venous insufficiency. *J Vasc Surg* 1998;27(4):660–670.
23. Fukuoka M, Okada M, Sugimoto T. Foot venous pressure measurement for evaluation of lower limb venous insufficiency. *J Vasc Surg* 1998;27(4):671–676.
24. Kucher N, Goldhaber SZ. Cardiac biomarkers for risk stratification of patients with acute pulmonary embolism. *Circulation* 2003;108(18): 2191–2194.
25. Cohen AT, Agnelli G, Anderson FA, et al. Venous thromboembolism (VTE) in Europe: the number of VTE events and associated morbidity and mortality. *Thromb Haemost* 2007;98(4):756–764.
26. Geerts W. Antithrombotic and thrombolytic therapy (8th ed: ACCP Guidelines). *Chest.* 2008;133:381s–451s.
27. Schulman S, Beyth RJ, Kearon C, et al. Hemorrhagic complications of anticoagulant and thrombolytic treatment: American College of Chest Physicians Evidence-Based Clinical Practice Guidelines (8th edition). *Chest.* 2008;133(6, Suppl):257S–298S.
28. Caprini JA. Thrombosis risk assessment as a guide to quality patient care. *Dis Mon* 2005;51(2–3):70–78.
29. Kucher N, Koo S, Quiroz R, et al. Electronic alerts to prevent venous thromboembolism among hospitalized patients. *N Engl J Med* 2005; 352(10):969–977.
30. Tooher R, Middleton P, Pham C, et al. A systematic review of strategies to improve prophylaxis for venous thromboembolism in hospitals. *Ann Surg* 2005;241(3):397–415.

31. Turpie AG, Bauer KA, Eriksson BI, et al. Fondaparinux vs enoxaparin for the prevention of venous thromboembolism in major orthopedic surgery: a meta-analysis of 4 randomized double-blind studies. *Arch Intern Med* 2002;162(16):1833–1840.
32. Wolozinsky M, Yavin YY, Cohen AT. Pharmacological prevention of venous thromboembolism in medical patients at risk. *Am J Cardiovasc Drugs* 2005;5(6):409–415.
33. Agnelli G, Bergqvist D, Cohen AT, et al. Randomized clinical trial of postoperative fondaparinux versus perioperative dalteparin for prevention of venous thromboembolism in high-risk abdominal surgery. *Br J Surg* 2005;92(10):1212–1220.
34. Eriksson BI, Lassen MR. Duration of prophylaxis against venous thromboembolism with fondaparinux after hip fracture surgery: a multicenter, randomized, placebo-controlled, double-blind study. *Arch Intern Med* 2003;163(11):1337–1342.
35. Knudson MM, Collins JA, Goodman SB, et al. Thromboembolism following multiple trauma. *J Trauma* 1992;32(1):2–11.
36. Rogers FB, Strindberg G, Shackford SR, et al. Five-year follow-up of prophylactic vena cava filters in high-risk trauma patients. *Arch Surg* 1998;133(4):406–411, discussion 412.
37. Streiff MB. Vena caval filters: a comprehensive review. *Blood* 2000; 95(12):3669–3677.
38. Osborne NH, Wakefield TW, Henke PK. Venous thromboembolism in cancer patients undergoing major surgery. *Ann Surg Oncol* 2008;15(12): 3567–3578.
39. Bergqvist D, Agnelli G, Cohen AT, et al. Duration of prophylaxis against venous thromboembolism with enoxaparin after surgery for cancer. *N Engl J Med* 2002;346(13):975–980.
40. Hull RD, Raskob GE, Brant RF, et al. Relation between the time to achieve the lower limit of the APTT therapeutic range and recurrent venous thromboembolism during heparin treatment for deep vein thrombosis. *Arch Intern Med* 1997;157(22):2562–2568.
41. Douketis JD, Kearon C, Bates S, et al. Risk of fatal pulmonary embolism in patients with treated venous thromboembolism. *JAMA* 1998;279(6):458–462.
42. Prandoni P, Lensing AW, Cogo A, et al. The long-term clinical course of acute deep venous thrombosis. *Ann Intern Med* 1996;125(1):1–7.
43. Bates SM, Ginsberg JS. Clinical practice: treatment of deep-vein thrombosis. *N Engl J Med* 2004;351(3):268–277.
44. van Den Belt AG, Prins MH, Lensing AW, et al. Fixed dose subcutaneous low molecular weight heparins versus adjusted dose unfractionated heparin for venous thromboembolism. *Cochrane Database Syst Rev* 2000(2):CD001100.
45. Ageno W, Turpie AG. Low-molecular-weight heparin in the treatment of pulmonary embolism. *Semin Vasc Surg* 2000;13(3):189–193.
46. Hull RD, Pineo GF, Brant RF, et al. *Am J Med* 2009;122:762–769.
47. Kearon C, Kahn SR, Agnelli G, et al. Antithrombotic therapy for venous thromboembolic disease: American College of Chest Physicians Evidence-Based Clinical Practice Guidelines (8th edition). *Chest* 2008;133(6, Suppl):454S–545S.
48. Buller HR, Davidson BL, Decousus H, et al. Fondaparinux or enoxaparin for the initial treatment of symptomatic deep venous thrombosis: a randomized trial. *Ann Intern Med* 2004;140(11): 867–873.
49. Buller HR, Davidson BL, Decousus H, et al. Subcutaneous fondaparinux versus intravenous unfractionated heparin in the initial treatment of pulmonary embolism. *N Engl J Med* 2003;349(18): 1695–1702.
50. Hyers TM, Agnelli G, Hull RD, et al. Antithrombotic therapy for venous thromboembolic disease. *Chest* 2001;119(1)(Suppl): 176S–193S.
51. Zhu T, Martinez I, Emmerich J. Venous thromboembolism: risk factors for recurrence. *Arterioscler Thromb Vasc Biol* 2009;29(3):298–310.
52. Prandoni P, Lensing AW, Prins MH, et al. Residual venous thrombosis as a predictive factor of recurrent venous thromboembolism. *Ann Intern Med* 2002;137(12):955–960.
53. Hull RD, Marder VJ, Mah AF, et al. Quantitative assessment of thrombus burden predicts the outcome of treatment for venous thrombosis: a systematic review. *Am J Med* 2005;118(5):456–464.
54. Cosmi B, Legnani C, Cini M, et al. D-dimer levels in combination with residual venous obstruction and the risk of recurrence after anticoagulation withdrawal for a first idiopathic deep vein thrombosis. *Thromb Haemost* 2005;94(5):969–974.
55. Palareti G, Cosmi B, Legnani C, et al. D-dimer testing to determine the duration of anticoagulation therapy. *N Engl J Med* 2006;355(17): 1780–1789.
56. Ridker PM, Goldhaber SZ, Danielson E, et al. Long-term, low-intensity warfarin therapy for the prevention of recurrent venous thromboembolism. *N Engl J Med* 2003;348(15):1425–1434.
57. Kearon C, Ginsberg JS, Kovacs MJ, et al. Comparison of low-intensity warfarin therapy with conventional-intensity warfarin therapy for long-term prevention of recurrent venous thromboembolism. *N Engl J Med* 2003;349(7):631–639.
58. Linkins LA, Choi PT, Douketis JD. Clinical impact of bleeding in patients taking oral anticoagulant therapy for venous thromboembolism: a meta-analysis. *Ann Intern Med* 2003;139(11):893–900.
59. Greinacher A, Michels I, Mueller-Eckhardt C. Heparin-associated thrombocytopenia: the antibody is not heparin specific. *Thromb Haemost* 1992;67(5):545–549.
60. Almeida JI, Coats R, Liem TK, et al. Reduced morbidity and mortality rates of the heparin-induced thrombocytopenia syndrome. *J Vasc Surg* 1998;27(2):309–314, discussion 315–316.
61. Alving BM. How I treat heparin-induced thrombocytopenia and thrombosis. *Blood* 2003;101(1):31–37.
62. Baldwin ZK, Spitzer AL, Ng VL, et al. Contemporary standards for the diagnosis and treatment of heparin-induced thrombocytopenia (HIT). *Surgery* 2008;143(3):305–312.
63. Greinacher A, Volpel H, Janssens U, et al. Recombinant hirudin (lepirudin) provides safe and effective anticoagulation in patients with heparin-induced thrombocytopenia: a prospective study. *Circulation* 1999;99(1):73–80.
64. Kovacs MJ. Successful treatment of heparin induced thrombocytopenia (HIT) with fondaparinux. *Thromb Haemost* 2005;93(5):999–1000.
65. Lee AY, Levine MN, Baker RI, et al. Low-molecular-weight heparin versus a coumarin for the prevention of recurrent venous thromboembolism in patients with cancer. *N Engl J Med* 2003;349(2):146–153.
66. van dongen CJ, Mac Gillavry MR, Prins MH. Once versus twice daily LMWH for the initial treatment of venous thromboembolism. *Cochrane Database Syst Rev* 2003;(1):CD003074.
67. Merli G, Spiro TE, Olsson CG, et al. Subcutaneous enoxaparin once or twice daily compared with intravenous unfractionated heparin for treatment of venous thromboembolic disease. *Ann Intern Med* 2001; 134(3):191–202.
68. Gross PL, Weitz JI. New anticoagulants for treatment of venous thromboembolism. *Arterioscler Thromb Vasc Biol* 2008;28(3):380–386.
69. Caprini JA. The future of medical therapy for venous thromboemboli. *Am J Med* 2008;121:S10–S19.
70. Buller HR, Cohen AT, Davidson B, et al. Idraparinux versus standard therapy for venous thromboembolic disease. *N Engl J Med* 2007;357(11): 1094–1104.
71. Spyropoulos AC. Investigational treatments of venous thromboembolism. *Expert Opin Investig Drugs* 2007;16(4):431–440.
72. Agnelli G, Gallus A, Goldhaber SZ, et al. Treatment of proximal deep-vein thrombosis with the oral direct factor Xa inhibitor rivaroxaban (BAY 59-7939): the ODIXa-DVT (Oral Direct Factor Xa Inhibitor BAY 59-7939 in Patients With Acute Symptomatic Deep-Vein Thrombosis) study. *Circulation* 2007;116(2):180–187.
73. Buller HR, Lensing AW, Prins MH, et al. A dose-ranging study evaluating once-daily oral administration of the factor Xa inhibitor rivaroxaban in the treatment of patients with acute symptomatic deep vein thrombosis: the Einstein-DVT Dose-Ranging Study. *Blood* 2008;112(6): 2242–2247.
74. Weitz JI, Hirsh J, Samama MM. New anticoagulant drugs: the Seventh ACCP Conference on Antithrombotic and Thrombolytic Therapy. *Chest* 2004;126(3)(Suppl):265S–286S.
75. Saiah E, Soares C. Small molecule coagulation cascade inhibitors in the clinic. *Curr Top Med Chem* 2005;5(16):1677–1695.
76. Greenfield LJ, Proctor MC. Twenty-year clinical experience with the Greenfield filter. *Cardiovasc Surg* 1995;3(2):199–205.
77. Berry RE, George JE, Shaver WA. Free-floating deep venous thrombosis: a retrospective analysis. *Ann Surg* 1990;211(6):719–722, discussion 722–723.
78. Langan EM III, Miller RS, Casey WJ III, et al. Prophylactic inferior vena cava filters in trauma patients at high risk: follow-up examination and risk/benefit assessment. *J Vasc Surg* 1999;30(3):484–488.
79. Sugerman HJ, Sugerman EL, Wolfe L, et al. Risks and benefits of gastric bypass in morbidly obese patients with severe venous stasis disease. *Ann Surg* 2001;234(1):41–46.
80. Chiou AC. Bedside placement of IVC filters. *Endovasc Today* 2005;4: 60–63.
81. Decousus H, Leizorovicz A, Parent F, et al. A clinical trial of vena caval filters in the prevention of pulmonary embolism in patients with proximal

deep-vein thrombosis: Prevention du Risque d'Embolie Pulmonaire par Interruption Cave Study Group. *N Engl J Med* 1998;338(7):409–415.
82. Greenfield LJ, Proctor MC. Filter complications and their management. *Semin Vasc Surg* 2000;13(3):213–216.
83. Joels CS, Sing RF, Heniford BT. Complications of inferior vena cava filters. *Am Surg* 2003;69(8):654–659.
84. Promisloff RA. Pulmonary embolism after insertion of a Greenfield filter. *J Am Osteopath Assoc* 2002;102(10):558–560.
85. Kinney TB, Rose SC, Lim GW, et al. Fatal paradoxic embolism occurring during IVC filter insertion in a patient with chronic pulmonary thromboembolic disease. *J Vasc Interv Radiol* 2001;12(6):770–772.
86. Greenfield LJ, Proctor MC. Recurrent thromboembolism in patients with vena cava filters. *J Vasc Surg* 2001;33(3):510–514.
87. Henke P, Varma MH, Proctor MC, et al. Suprarenal Greenfield filter placement: the Ann Arbor experience. In: Yao JT, Pearce WH, eds. *Modern trends in vascular surgery*. St. Louis; MO: McGraw-Hill 2000;427–434.
88. Marcy PY, Magne N, Frenay M, et al. Renal failure secondary to thrombotic complications of suprarenal inferior vena cava filter in cancer patients. *Cardiovasc Intervent Radiol* 2001;24(4):257–259.
89. Ferris EJ, McCowan TC, Carver DK, et al. Percutaneous inferior vena caval filters: follow-up of seven designs in 320 patients. *Radiology* 1993;188(3):851–856.
90. Harris EJ Jr, Kinney EV, Harris EJ Sr, et al. Phlegmasia complicating prophylactic percutaneous inferior vena caval interruption: a word of caution. *J Vasc Surg* 1995;22(5):606–611.
91. Thomas JH, Cornell KM, Siegel EL, et al. Vena caval occlusion after bird's nest filter placement. *Am J Surg* 1998;176(6):598–600.
92. MAUDE database. The FDA Web site: www.fda.gov. Updated 2003.
93. Schutzer R, Ascher E, Hingorani A, et al. Preliminary results of the new 6 F TrapEase inferior vena cava filter. *Ann Vasc Surg* 2003;17(1):103–106.
94. Greenfield LJ, Proctor MC. Vena caval filters for the prevention of pulmonary embolism. *N Engl J Med* 1998;339(1):47; author reply 47–48.
95. Reekers JA. Re: current practice of temporary vena cava filter insertion: a multicenter registry. *J Vasc Interv Radiol* 2000;11(10):1363–1364.
96. Poon WL, Luk SH, Yam KY, et al. Mechanical thrombectomy in inferior vena cava thrombosis after caval filter placement: a report of three cases. *Cardiovasc Intervent Radiol* 2002;25(5):440–443.
97. Joshi A, Carr J, Chrisman H, et al. Filter-related, thrombotic occlusion of the inferior vena cava treated with a Gianturco stent. *J Vasc Interv Radiol* 2003;14(3):381–385.
98. Tardy B, Mismetti P, Page Y, et al. Symptomatic inferior vena cava filter thrombosis: clinical study of 30 consecutive cases. *Eur Respir J* 1996;9(10):2012–2016.
99. Wojcik R, Cipolle MD, Fearen I, et al. Long-term follow-up of trauma patients with a vena caval filter. *J Trauma* 2000;49(5):839–843.
100. Greenfield LJ, Proctor MC, Michaels AJ, et al. Prophylactic vena caval filters in trauma: the rest of the story. *J Vasc Surg* 2000;32(3):490–495, discussion 496–497.
101. Patton JH Jr, Fabian TC, Croce MA, et al. Prophylactic Greenfield filters: acute complications and long-term follow-up. *J Trauma* 1996; 41(2):231–236, discussion 236–237.
102. Cahn MD, Rohrer MJ, Martella MB, et al. Long-term follow-up of Greenfield inferior vena cava filter placement in children. *J Vasc Surg* 2001;34(5):820–825.
103. Dardik A, Campbell KA, Yeo CJ, et al. Vena cava filter ensnarement and delayed migration: an unusual series of cases. *J Vasc Surg* 1997; 26(5):869–874.
104. Woodward EB, Farber A, Wagner WH, et al. Delayed retroperitoneal arterial hemorrhage after inferior vena cava (IVC) filter insertion: case report and literature review of caval perforations by IVC filters. *Ann Vasc Surg* 2002;16(2):193–196.
105. Raghavan S, Akhtar A, Bastani B. Migration of inferior vena cava filter into renal hilum. *Nephron* 2002;91(2):333–335.
106. Porcellini M, Stassano P, Musumeci A, et al. Intracardiac migration of nitinol TrapEase vena cava filter and paradoxical embolism. *Eur J Cardiothorac Surg* 2002;22(3):460–461.
107. Jackson Slappy AL, Kennedy RJ, Hakaim AG, et al. Delayed transcaval renal penetration of a Greenfield filter presenting as symptomatic hydronephrosis. *J Urol* 2002;167(4):1778–1779.
108. Loehr SP, Hamilton C, Dyer R. Retrieval of entrapped guide wire in an IVC filter facilitated with use of a myocardial biopsy forceps and snare device. *J Vasc Interv Radiol* 2001;12(9):1116–1119.
109. Meissner MH, Manzo RA, Bergelin RO, et al. Deep venous insufficiency: the relationship between lysis and subsequent reflux. *J Vasc Surg* 1993;18(4):596–605, discussion 606–608.
110. Semba CP, Dake MD. Iliofemoral deep venous thrombosis: aggressive therapy with catheter-directed thrombolysis. *Radiology* 1994;191(2): 487–494.
111. Mewissen MW, Seabrook GR, Meissner MH, et al. Catheter-directed thrombolysis for lower extremity deep venous thrombosis: report of a national multicenter registry. *Radiology* 1999;211(1):39–49.
112. Elsharawy M, Elzayat E. Early results of thrombolysis vs anticoagulation in iliofemoral venous thrombosis: a randomised clinical trial. *Eur J Vasc Endovasc Surg* 2002;24(3):209–214.
113. Meneveau N, Seronde MF, Blonde MC, et al. Management of unsuccessful thrombolysis in acute massive pulmonary embolism. *Chest* 2006;129(4):1043–1050.
114. Meissner MH. Thrombolytic therapy for acute deep vein thrombosis and the venous registry. *Rev Cardiovasc Med* 2002;3(Suppl 2):S53–S60.
115. Sharafuddin MJ, Sun S, Hoballah JJ. Endovascular management of venous thrombotic diseases of the upper torso and extremities. *J Vasc Interv Radiol* 2002;13(10):975–990.
116. Meier GH, Pollak JS, Rosenblatt M, et al. Initial experience with venous stents in exertional axillary-subclavian vein thrombosis. *J Vasc Surg* 1996;24(6):974–981, discussion 981–983.
117. Axelrod DA, Proctor MC, Geisser ME, et al. Outcomes after surgery for thoracic outlet syndrome. *J Vasc Surg* 2001;33(6):1220–1225.
118. Turpie AG. Thrombolytic agents in venous thrombosis. *J Vasc Surg* 1990;12:196.
119. Goldhaber SZ. Pulmonary embolism. *Lancet* 2004;363(9417):1295–1305.
120. Sharma GV, Folland ED, McIntyre KM, et al. Long-term benefit of thrombolytic therapy in patients with pulmonary embolism. *Vasc Med* 2000;5(2):91–95.
121. Goldhaber SZ, Haire WD, Feldstein ML, et al. Alteplase versus heparin in acute pulmonary embolism: randomised trial assessing right-ventricular function and pulmonary perfusion. *Lancet* 1993; 341(8844):507–511.
122. Jerjes-Sanchez C, Ramirez-Rivera A, Arriaga-Nava R, et al. High dose and short-term streptokinase infusion in patients with pulmonary embolism: prospective with seven-year follow-up trial. *J Thromb Thrombolysis* 2001;12(3):237–247.
123. Konstantinides S, Geibel A, Olschewski M, et al. Association between thrombolytic treatment and the prognosis of hemodynamically stable patients with major pulmonary embolism: results of a multicenter registry. *Circulation* 1997;96(3):882–888.
124. Eid-Lidt G, Gaspar J, Sandoval J, et al. Combined clot fragmentation and aspiration in patients with acute pulmonary embolism. *Chest* 2008;134(1):54–60.
125. Eklof B, Kistner RL. Is there a role for thrombectomy in iliofemoral venous thrombosis? *Semin Vasc Surg* 1996;9(1):34–45.
126. Juhan CM, Alimi YS, Barthelemy PJ, et al. Late results of iliofemoral venous thrombectomy. *J Vasc Surg* 1997;25(3):417–422.
127. Patel NP, Labropoulos N, Pappas PJ. Current management of venous ulceration. *Plast Reconstr Surg* 2006;117(7)(Suppl):254S–260S.
128. Beebe-Dimmer JL, Pfeifer JR, Engle JS, et al. The epidemiology of chronic venous insufficiency and varicose veins. *Ann Epidemiol* 2005; 15(3):175–184.
129. Barwell JR, Davies CE, Deacon J, et al. Comparison of surgery and compression with compression alone in chronic venous ulceration (ESCHAR study): randomised controlled trial. *Lancet* 2004;363(9424): 1854–1859.
130. Prandoni P, Lensing AW, Prins MH, et al. Below-knee elastic compression stockings to prevent the post-thrombotic syndrome: a randomized, controlled trial. *Ann Intern Med* 2004;141(4):249–256.
131. Kakkos SK, Daskalopoulou SS, Daskalopoulos ME, et al. Review on the value of graduated elastic compression stockings after deep vein thrombosis. *Thromb Haemost* 2006;96(4):441–445.
132. Bone C. Tratamiento endoluminal de las varices con laser de diodo: estudio preliminary. *Rev Patol Vasc* 1999;5:35–46.
133. Navarro L, Min RJ, Bone C. Endovenous laser: a new minimally invasive method of treatment for varicose veins—preliminary observations using an 810 nm diode laser. *Dermatol Surg* 2001;27(2):117–122.
134. Fan CM, Rox-Anderson R. Endovenous laser ablation: mechanism of action. *Phlebology* 2008;23(5):206–213.
135. Knipp BS, Blackburn SA, Bloom JR, et al. Endovenous laser ablation: venous outcomes and thrombotic complications are independent of the presence of deep venous insufficiency. *J Vasc Surg* 2008;48(6): 1538–1545.
136. Puggioni A, Kalra M, Gloviczki P. Superficial vein surgery and SEPS for chronic venous insufficiency. *Semin Vasc Surg* 2005;18(1): 41–48.

137. Sparks SR, Ballard JL, Bergan JJ, et al. Early benefits of subfascial endoscopic perforator surgery (SEPS) in healing venous ulcers. *Ann Vasc Surg* 1997;11(4):367–373.
138. Kalra M, Gloviczki P. Subfascial endoscopic perforator vein surgery: who benefits? *Semin Vasc Surg* 2002;15(1):39–49.
139. Jia X, Mowatt G, Burr JM, et al. Systematic review of foam sclerotherapy for varicose veins. *Br J Surg* 2007;94(8):925–936.
140. Ceulen RP, Sommer A, Vernooy K. Microembolism during foam sclerotherapy of varicose veins. *N Engl J Med* 2008;358(14):1525–1526.
141. French LE, Braun R, Masouye I, et al. Post-stripping sclerodermiform dermatitis. *Arch Dermatol* 1999;135(11):1387–1391.
142. Rigby K, Palfreyman SJ, Beverley C, et al. Surgery for varicose veins: use of tourniquet. *Cochrane Database Syst Rev* 2009;(4):CD001486.
143. Bergan JJ. Varicose veins: hooks, clamps, and suction: application of new techniques to enhance varicose vein surgery. *Semin Vasc Surg* 2002;15(1):21–26.
144. Goldman M. Complications of sclerotherapy in venous surgery. In: Gloviczki P, Yao JST, eds. *Handbook of venous disorders*, 2nd ed. London, England: Hoddard & Stoughton; 2001.
145. Morrison C, Dalsing MC. Signs and symptoms of saphenous nerve injury after greater saphenous vein stripping: prevalence, severity, and relevance for modern practice. *J Vasc Surg* 2003;38(5):886–890.
146. Criado E, Lujan S, Izquierdo L, et al. Conservative hemodynamic surgery for varicose veins. *Semin Vasc Surg* 2002;15(1):27–33.
147. Scavee V, Theys S, Schoevaerdts JC. Transilluminated powered miniphlebectomy: early clinical experience. *Acta Chir Belg* 2001;101(5): 247–249.
148. Cheshire N, Elias SM, Keagy B, et al. Powered phlebectomy (TriVex) in treatment of varicose veins. *Ann Vasc Surg* 2002;16(4):488–494.
149. Chetter IC, Mylankal KJ, Hughes H, et al. Randomized clinical trial comparing multiple stab incision phlebectomy and transilluminated powered phlebectomy for varicose veins. *Br J Surg* 2006;93(2): 169–174.
150. de Zeeuw R, Wittens C, Loots M, et al. Transilluminated powered phlebectomy accomplished by local tumescent anaesthesia in the treatment of tributary varicose veins: preliminary clinical results. *Phlebology* 2007;22(2):90–94.
151. Bergan JJ, Schmid-Schonbein GW, Smith PD, et al. Chronic venous disease. *N Engl J Med* 2006;355(5):488–498.
152. Kahn SR, Shrier I, Julian JA, et al. Determinants and time course of the postthrombotic syndrome after acute deep venous thrombosis. *Ann Intern Med* 2008;149(10):698–707.
153. Labropoulos N, Waggoner T, Sammis W, et al. The effect of venous thrombus location and extent on the development of post-thrombotic signs and symptoms. *J Vasc Surg* 2008;48(2):407–412.
154. Kunimoto BT. Management and prevention of venous leg ulcers: a literature-guided approach. *Ostomy Wound Manage* 2001;47(6):36–42, 44–39.
155. Korn P, Patel ST, Heller JA, et al. Why insurers should reimburse for compression stockings in patients with chronic venous stasis. *J Vasc Surg* 2002;35(5):950–957.
156. Blecken SR, Villavicencio JL, Kao TC. Comparison of elastic versus nonelastic compression in bilateral venous ulcers: a randomized trial. *J Vasc Surg* 2005;42(6):1150–1155.
157. Padberg FT Jr. Surgical intervention in venous ulceration. *Cardiovasc Surg* 1999;7(1):83–90.
158. Tawes RL, Barron ML, Coello AA, et al. Optimal therapy for advanced chronic venous insufficiency. *J Vasc Surg* 2003;37(3):545–551.
159. Gloviczki P. Subfascial endoscopic perforator vein surgery: indications and results. *Vasc Med* 1999;4(3):173–180.
160. van Gent BW, Hop WC, van Praag MC et al. Conservative versus surgical treatment of venous leg ulcers: a prospective, randomized, multicenter trial. *J Vasc Surg* 2006;44(3):563–571.
161. Delis KT, Bjarnason H, Wennberg PW, et al. Successful iliac vein and inferior vena cava stenting ameliorates venous claudication and improves venous outflow, calf muscle pump function, and clinical status in post-thrombotic syndrome. *Ann Surg* 2007;245(1): 130–139.
162. Neglen P, Hollis KC, Olivier J, et al. Stenting of the venous outflow in chronic venous disease: long-term stent-related outcome, clinical, and hemodynamic result. *J Vasc Surg* 2007;46(5):979–990.
163. Knipp BS, Ferguson E, Williams DM, et al. Factors associated with outcome after interventional treatment of symptomatic iliac vein compression syndrome. *J Vasc Surg* 2007;46(4):743–749.
164. Thorpe P, Osse FS, Dang HP. Endovascular reconstruction for chronic iliac vein and inferior vena cava obstruction. In: Gloviczki P, Yao JST, eds. *Handbook of venous disorders*, 2nd ed. London, England: Hoddard & Stoughton; 2001.
165. Jost CJ, Gloviczki P, Cherry KJ Jr, et al. Surgical reconstruction of iliofemoral veins and the inferior vena cava for nonmalignant occlusive disease. *J Vasc Surg* 2001;33(2):320–327, discussion 327–328.
166. Bergan JJ, Kumins NH, Owens EL, et al. Surgical and endovascular treatment of lower extremity venous insufficiency. *J Vasc Interv Radiol* 2002;13(6):563–568.
167. Alimi YS, DiMauro P, Fabre D, et al. Iliac vein reconstructions to treat acute and chronic venous occlusive disease. *J Vasc Surg* 1997;25(4): 673–681.
168. Raju S, Hollis K, Neglen P. Obstructive lesions of the inferior vena cava: clinical features and endovenous treatment. *J Vasc Surg* 2006; 44(4):820–827.
169. Sarkar R, Eilber FR, Gelabert HA, et al. Prosthetic replacement of the inferior vena cava for malignancy. *J Vasc Surg* 1998;28(1):75–81, discussion 82–83.
170. Bower TC, Nagorney DM, Cherry KJ Jr, et al. Replacement of the inferior vena cava for malignancy: an update. *J Vasc Surg* 2000;31(2):270–281.

CHAPTER

32

Complications of Endovascular Therapy

Matthew J. Eagleton and Sunita D. Srivastava

INTRODUCTION

The number of patients undergoing endovascular interventions is increasing. At some point, most surgeons will manage patients who require an endovascular procedure, or they will be called on to manage one of the complications of an intervention. Outlined in this chapter are the main complications encountered with several of the most common endovascular therapies.

ARTERIAL INTERVENTIONS

Diagnostic angiography

A number of complications can occur during the performance of routine angiography. Most of these complications are not specific to diagnostic angiography but can occur during the performance of any number of vascular interventions. More common complications include those associated with the administration of radiologic contrast agents and injury to the artery used for access.

Contrast nephropathy

Contrast nephropathy is the development of acute renal failure or insufficiency secondary to the parenteral administration of radiologic contrast agents. Contrast nephropathy is the third leading cause of acute renal failure in hospitalized patients (1). The incidence of contrast nephropathy varies widely and depends on the definition of renal insufficiency used by the varying studies (2,3). Contrast nephropathy generally presents as an elevation in serum creatinine 1 to 2 days after dye administration. Creatinine values peak after 3 to 5 days and return to baseline by 7 to 10 days (2,4). The acute renal failure is usually nonoliguric in nature. Urinalysis reveals a range of findings from normal to granular casts, tubular epithelial cells, and protein. The diagnosis of contrast nephropathy is typically easy to make, given the temporal relationship of the onset of renal failure to the contrast load. Other causes of acute renal failure, such as hypovolemia and atheroembolization of the renal arteries, should be excluded.

The pathogenesis of contrast nephropathy is complex and involves a synergistic effect of direct renal tubular epithelial cell toxicity and renal medullary ischemia. Three main factors contribute to its development, including osmotic effects, renal hemodynamic effects, and renal tubular effects (3,5). Contrast media are small molecules that become concentrated in urine up to 100-fold within the first 4 hours after administration. The increase in osmolarity causes an increase in intratubular hydrostatic pressure and decreases filtration pressure in glomeruli, leading to osmotic diuresis and increased sodium and water excretion. The increased sodium load to the macula densa in the distal tubule causes a decrease in the glomerular filtration rate (6). This response is more pronounced with contrast agents that have a high osmolarity compared to those that are iso-osmolar or hypo-osmolar. The osmotic diuresis also places an increased metabolic demand on the distal nephron and may aggravate medullary hypoxia (7).

Contrast agents can cause direct cytotoxicity, leading to contrast nephropathy. Cytotoxicity is suggested by evidence of cell injury on histologic evaluation and by the presence of enzymuria, particularly *N*-acetyl-*β*-glucosaminidase and alkaline phosphatase (8,9).

Contrast agents affect renal blood flow in a biphasic pattern. Initially, there is a brief increase in renal blood flow, followed by a steady decline. Decreased blood flow is due to the induction of renal vasoconstriction caused by rheologic changes, erythrocyte deformability, and the release of a variety of endothelial factors, including endothelin, adenosine, calcium, and oxygen free radicals (6,10–12).

Alterations in renal function are seen in almost every patient who receives a contrast load, but not every patient develops contrast nephropathy (13). There are a variety of risk factors for development of acute renal failure following contrast dye administration (Table 32.1). Alone, chronic renal insufficiency is the most important risk factor; combined with diabetes mellitus, negative effects are synergistic. In one series of 1,800 patients undergoing cardiac catheterization, the rate of contrast nephropathy was 14.5% for all patients. When adjusted for the presence of risk factors, the development of contrast nephropathy increases from 1.2% in patients with no risk factors to 100% in patients with four or more risk factors (14).

Matthew J. Eagleton, Sunita D. Srivastava: Cleveland Clinic Lerner College of Medicine-CWRU, Department of Vascular Surgery, Cleveland, OH 44195

Table 32.1 Risk factors for contrast nephropathy
Chronic renal insufficiency
Diabetes mellitus
Congestive heart failure
High dose contrast agent
Nephrotoxic drugs (i.e., antibiotics)
Agents that decrease renal perfusion (i.e., NSAIDs)

NSAIDs, nonsteroidal anti-inflammatory drugs.

Contrast nephropathy, despite generally resolving over the course of 7 to 10 days, is not a benign complication. Few patients go on to require dialysis, but up to 30% will have residual renal impairment and there is some suggestion that patients affected by contrast nephropathy have increased mortality rates (15,16). Management of these patients is similar to other patients who develop acute renal failure. A thorough investigation should be made to identify contributing factors, such as hypovolemia or nephrotoxic medications, with correction. Monitoring of serum chemistries and assessment of fluid status should be performed.

Although there is no antidote for the nephrotoxic effects of radiologic contrast media, several strategies have been devised with the hope of decreasing morbidity. Nonionic and low-osmolality contrast agents were developed to lower the complications of radiologic dye. These agents are associated with a lower incidence of contrast nephropathy compared to high-osmolarity agents (17). Preprocedural administration of intravenous fluid is a simple, inexpensive measure that treats hypovolemia and should theoretically offer protection to patients who are going to receive radiologic contrast agents. In addition, it appears that isotonic 0.9% normal saline is preferable over hypotonic solutions (18). Dopamine was thought to be protective, given its renal vasodilatory effects, but several studies reveal it to have no effect on the development of contrast nephropathy in patients with underlying risk factors, and in one study, dopamine increased the risk in diabetic patients (19,20). Similarly, selective dopamine A_1 agonists, like fenoldopam mesylate (a potent vasodilator that increases renal plasma flow), have failed to provide significant nephroprotection in larger studies evaluating nephrotoxicity (21). Acetylcysteine is an antioxidant that has been evaluated in several studies for reducing the incidence of contrast nephropathy. A meta-analysis of seven randomized prospective trials comparing orally administered acetylcysteine with hydration alone have shown it to significantly reduce the risk of developing contrast nephropathy in patients with underlying chronic renal insufficiency (22). Most recently, the combination of N-acetyl cysteine (NAC) with volume supplementation by sodium bicarbonate was found to be superior to NAC and saline alone (23). Prostaglandins, specifically prostaglandin E (PGE) and prostaglandin I2 (PGI_2), have attenuated the rise of serum creatinine after contrast administration (24,25). Their major side effects, such as hypotension and nausea, have limited their use. Contrast material can be removed with the use of hemodialysis, which has led some to question whether it could serve to prevent contrast-induced nephropathy. The data supporting this, however, is sparse, and it is not currently recommended routinely.

Puncture site complications

The incidence of puncture site complications ranges from 0.3% to 35% (26–32). Lower rates are associated with diagnostic procedures, while higher rates follow interventional procedures due to the use of larger sheaths (33). Factors that increase the risk of puncture site complications are significant atherosclerotic disease in the artery that is being accessed, obesity, and the use of antithrombotic or fibrinolytic pharmacotherapies (30). The more complex the procedure, the higher the rate of puncture site complications (27). In only 9% of all cases is surgical therapy necessary (26).

Hemorrhage

Hemorrhage is the most common puncture site complication, occurring in 8% of diagnostic procedures and 18% of arterial interventions (26,28–31). Patients present with a painful, pulseless mass at the puncture site. Assessment with duplex ultrasound is necessary to exclude pseudoaneurysm. Hemorrhage may not be obvious on physical exam if the bleeding tracks into the retroperitoneum. In these situations, computed tomography will verify the diagnosis. Management entails application of pressure over the puncture site followed by continued close observation. If hemorrhage persists, surgical intervention is required. Other indications for surgical intervention include significant overlying skin changes and hematoma, causing symptomatic compression of adjacent nervous or venous structures.

Pseudoaneurysm

Diagnostic procedures are associated with the development of pseudoaneurysms at the puncture site in <1% of patients having diagnostic procedures and in up to 5% of those undergoing interventions (26,29,30,32,34). Pseudoaneurysms can be detected by the palpation of a pulsatile mass on physical exam and confirmed by duplex ultrasound. The most common anatomic factor associated with femoral pseudoaneurysm formation is aberrant puncture, entering the vessel in either the external iliac artery or superficial femoral artery (35–38). Both these locations make compression following sheath and catheter removal more difficult and less successful. The use of periprocedural anticoagulation also increases the risk of pseudoaneurysm formation (32). Small pseudoaneurysms (<3 cm) can resolve spontaneously, provided patients are not anticoagulated (32,39).

Persistent pseudoaneurysms and those that cause symptoms require intervention. Untreated lesions may cause pain, neuropathy, arteriovenous fistulas with steal syndrome, or rupture. Treatment was classically performed with surgical repair, and urgent surgical intervention is recommended when there is an expanding pseudoaneurysm, an expanding hematoma, severe pain, femoral nerve compression, or groin infection (39). When surgical repair is required, management can often be accomplished by lateral suture of the arterial communication. With large pseudoaneurysms (<3 cm), proximal control of the distal external iliac artery through a retroperitoneal incision may be required prior to repair.

Recently, nonsurgical treatment of pseudoaneurysms has proven effective. Initial experience was with ultrasound-guided compression of the pseudoaneurysm origin. Compression is applied for ≥30 minutes. Success rates for compression therapy vary and are significantly affected by the presence of ongoing anticoagulation. In anticoagulated patients, failure rates are as high as 41% (34). When anticoagulation is not present, success rates approach 90% (40). An alternative is ultrasound-guided thrombin injection. This therapy has proven effective in >90% of patients, including those with ongoing anticoagulation (34,41). The major risk of this procedure is induction of thrombus in the native vessel and subsequent occlusion or distal embolization. Thrombus occurs in up to 3% of patients undergoing thrombin injection and requires surgical intervention (34). The risk appears to be reduced if high risk lesions are excluded. These include pseudoaneurysms composed of short, wide (>10 mm) necks and those in small-diameter native arteries. The use of covered stents has been described to treat postprocedural pseudoaneurysms, but experience with this modality is not widespread (42,43).

Arteriovenous Fistula

The development of an arteriovenous fistula complicates diagnostic angiography in <1% of cases and interventional procedures in up to 2% of cases (26,30,31). The incidence is higher when the puncture site is more caudal on the femoral artery, due to the juxtaposition of the superficial femoral artery, deep femoral artery, and adjacent veins in this region. On physical examination, a bruit will be heard over the puncture site, and duplex ultrasound easily confirms the diagnosis. Most arteriovenous fistulae spontaneously thrombose (32,39). Patients with this complication can be safely monitored with ultrasound until closure. Indications for intervention include the development of congestive heart failure due to the fistula, limb ischemia, venous insufficiency, or distal embolization. In these instances, surgical intervention is warranted. Employing covered stents to treat the lesion has been described, but their use is not widespread (42,43).

Neuropathy

Nerve injury due to compression from local bleeding is the most common and debilitating complication after transaxillary arteriography. Because of the close proximity of the axillary artery and brachial plexus, even a small hematoma can produce significant nerve compression. Patients can present with sensory and motor deficits that can affect the median, radial, and ulnar nerve distribution. This complication occurs in <1% of transaxillary procedures (31). The incidence of femoral neuropathy after a femoral artery puncture is ~0.2% (44). Femoral neuropathy occurs more frequently with retroperitoneal hemorrhage. Prompt surgical decompression is necessary in patients who have neurologic symptoms to reduce the incidence of prolonged deficits (31,44,45).

Vascular Closure Device Complications

Several devices have been developed over the past decade to assist in arterial puncture site closure. Approaches include collagen plug–mediated devices, suture-mediated devices, and percutaneous placement of metallic "clips" to occlude the arteriotomy site. These devices have shown to significantly decrease the amount of time necessary to obtain hemostasis (46–48), but there remains some controversy as to whether they provide an effective reduction in the complications associated with arterial access. Several reports have shown similar complication rates compared to hemostasis obtained by manual compression (49–52). Some investigators have reported increased complications with closure devices (53,54), while more recently, larger randomized controlled trials suggest that closure devices may be associated with decreased complication rates for both diagnostic and interventional procedures (55). Complications specific to the use of these percutaneous arterial closure devices include embolization of collagen plugs, arterial occlusion, and infection (56–58). These events occur in <2% of device deployments and may be reduced if proper patient selection is employed (58,59).

Catheter and guidewire-related complications

Thrombosis

Arterial thrombosis is rare (<1% of cases) following both diagnostic and interventional procedures (26,29,30). Thrombosis is affected by the size of the catheter in relation to the size of the arterial lumen and the length of the catheter exposed to the blood (60–62). This relationship affects the size of the thrombus that develops on the catheter. Thrombotic complications present with a variety of symptoms. If the region supplied by the occluded artery has a vast collateral blood supply, no significant symptoms may arise and the only finding may be loss of distal palpable pulses. This finding is typical of brachial artery thrombosis following upper extremity arterial access. Most episodes of thrombosis are treated with thrombectomy, but if severe underlying atherosclerotic disease is present, arterial bypass may be required.

Arterial Dissection

Arterial dissection is rare, occurring in <1% of cases (26,29,30). Arterial dissection more frequently occurs after interventional procedures and with antegrade arterial punctures. Occasionally, no intervention is required, especially if a retrograde dissection has occurred. More severe dissections present with complete arterial occlusion and loss of a pulse on physical examination. The surgical procedure required to repair these dissections depends on the defect's extent and location. Short focal lesions can be treated by endarterectomy, but more extensive dissections may require arterial bypass.

Embolization

Embolization complicates diagnostic arteriography and arterial interventions at a rate approaching 6% (26,30). Embolization can result from dislodgment of atheroemboli and the development and embolization of thrombus on the introducer sheath, and it can involve foreign bodies such as sheared-off portions of angiographic catheters. When embolization occurs, the surgeon should consider intervention to prevent sequelae. Options include immediate percutaneous or surgical thrombectomy (or removal of foreign body) and selective thrombolysis (45,63,64). Cholesterol syndrome is due to the dislodgment of cholesterol crystals from atheromatous vessels, particularly the aorta. Cholesterol emboli lodge in small arterioles and most often affect the skin in the form of livedo reticularis, the kidneys resulting in renal failure, and the digits resulting in "blue toe syndrome" (65–67). The incidence and sequelae of embolization during cerebral angiography and carotid artery interventions have been extensively studied and will be discussed in more detail below.

SUPRA-AORTIC INTERVENTIONS

Cerebral angiography

Many of the complications encountered with cerebral angiography are similar to those of routine peripheral or coronary angiography. The consequence of embolization, however, is more profound, as the outcome may be a cerebral vascular accident. Overall complication rates for cerebral angiography parallel peripheral angiography and coronary angiography, ranging from 0.6% to 10% (68–71). Complications include strokes (occurring at an incidence of ~0.5%) and transient ischemic attacks (TIAs) (occurring at an incidence of ~0.4%) (71). The incidence of embolization and subsequent cerebral ischemic event increases if the patients have symptomatic carotid artery stenosis (70,72). Embolization during cerebral angiography, however, is not always symptomatic. Sources of embolization include microscopic air embolization or silent thromboembolism (73,74). Bendszus et al. (75) evaluated diffusion-weighted magnetic resonance imaging before and after angiography to assess embolic events in 100 consecutive patients undergoing diagnostic angiography. In this study, 23% of patients had evidence of embolization without neurologic symptoms. The appearance of lesions was associated with difficult vessel access, higher contrast loads, increased fluoroscopy time, and the use of multiple catheters.

Carotid artery angioplasty and stenting

Technical Proficiency

Carotid procedures represent a more complex level of intervention due to the demanding technical skills required for the procedure. They include the familiarity with smaller profile systems, including monorail delivery systems, variety of cerebral protection devices, and new stent platforms with variable deployment characteristics. The operator must be technically facile at intervening from long distances (femoral artery to internal carotid artery), cannulating a diseased and friable internal carotid artery followed by placement of distal protection device, balloon angioplasty, stent delivery and deployment, and finally capturing the protection device without embolization. Several studies have demonstrated the importance of the clinical operator's proficiency in successful carotid interventions (76,77). Arch anomalies and arch tortuosity are anatomic variables that add to the complexity of the carotid intervention as well as higher incidence of thromboembolic complications due to the more extensive catheter manipulations and disruption of aortic or carotid plaques (78).

Stroke

Stroke is the most feared complication of cerebrovascular interventions. With the growing use of carotid artery stenting, a more thorough evaluation of associated complications is being realized. The incidence of cerebrovascular events following carotid artery stenting varies according to classification schemes. Events are categorized as major strokes, minor strokes, and TIAs.

Technical success in carotid artery stenting approaches 100% (79–83). Thirty-day rates of major stroke range from 1.3% to 3.6%, while rates of minor stroke and TIA range from 0% to 1.3% and from 3.4% to 10.7%, respectively. Patients with severely elevated baseline systolic blood pressure are at higher risk for hemodynamic instability and neurologic events during carotid artery stenting (84).

Unfortunately, it is rare that an operation can correct distal cerebral embolization. Distal thrombolysis should be attempted if arterial occlusion is visualized angiographically, although it is impossible to ascertain whether the occlusion is secondary to atheromatous embolization or thromboembolization. Treatment is continued until lysis is achieved, there is systemic evidence of fibrinolysis, a limiting total dose of thrombolytic has been delivered, or presence of intracranial hemorrhage (85).

Most carotid artery stent-related strokes are due to distal atheroemboli or thromboemboli dislodged at the time of the procedure. In order to decrease the incidence of these complications, several cerebral protection devices have been developed. Several series evaluating the efficacy of cerebral protection devices have shown an 80% reduction in acute neurologic events related to embolism compared to unprotected procedures (86–89). Despite the use of embolic protection devices, however, embolization has been shown to occur postprocedurally for up to 48 hours on diffusion-weighted magnetic resonance imaging (90). Cerebral protection devices are also associated with complications. These complications are infrequent (occurring <1% of the time) and include focal dissection of the internal carotid artery and failure of device deployment. Internal carotid artery vasospasm occurs in up to 15% of patients, half of whom respond to vasodilatory therapy with nitroglycerin (86). In patients in whom occlusive protection devices are used (i.e., balloon occluders and flow reversal systems), transient alterations in mental function are documented in 15% of patients (91). This intolerance to flow arrest is typically resolved with the restoration of intracranial flow (92). The proximal occlusion and flow reversal system has had fewer reports of cerebral hypoperfusion (93). Local vessel interaction with the deployed protection device can also result in complications. Intimal damage due to oversizing of the protection device, spasm, and embolization around the device can result in embolic and thrombotic consequences (94). In addition, excessive debris captured within the device from excessive balloon dilation or bulky disease may result in failure of collapse of the device for retrieval. Manipulations of the device without sheath protection may result in entanglement with the stent struts, detachment of the filter, and potential conversion to open carotid endarterectomy. Early recognition of cerebral protection device problems and troubleshooting are critical to prevent conversions and thromboembolic events. Avoidance of overdilation with balloon angioplasty, aspiration of the full filter basket, maintenance of systemic anticoagulation, and sheath access in the common carotid artery may reduce retrieval problems.

Hemodynamic Instability

Carotid artery angioplasty and stenting involves dilation of the carotid bulb. This maneuver can cause immediate cardiovascular hemodynamic alterations, similar to the blood pressure and heart rate changes associated with carotid endarterectomy. In the review by Ohki et al. (95), nearly one-third of patients had an alteration in heart rate. Ten percent of the patients had transient asystole, while 20% developed transient bradycardia (95). Approximately 30% developed concomitant hypotension, half of whom required infusion of phenylephrine. All underwent monitoring in an intensive care unit. Recently, Hobson et al. (96) published the lead-in phase data for the Carotid Revascularization Endarterectomy versus Stenting Trial (CREST) trial and reported higher rates of complications in carotid stenting with increasing age from stroke and death. Octogenarians were at highest risk with a 12.1% 30-day stroke and death rate from carotid stenting and were reported to have higher incidence of hemodynamic instability during the procedure. Maintenance of adequate intravascular volume, vasopressor use, and avoidance of overdilation with balloon angioplasty and oversized stents may reduce this complication (84,97,98).

Myocardial Infarction and Death

Most patients who undergo carotid artery stenting are considered to be at high operative risk. In one of the first large series, 77% of patients would have been ineligible for the North American Symptomatic Carotid Endarterectomy Trial due to the presence of medical comorbidities (99). Included in this group of comorbidities is significant coronary artery disease, which is present in 80% of patients in some series (81). Despite this level of risk, rates of perioperative myocardial infarction were only 0% to 0.6% (80,82). The 30-day death rates have been reported to be between 0% and 4.5% (60,76,83,100–102). The majority of deaths were related to periprocedural myocardial infarction, fatal stroke, or intracranial hemorrhage.

Restenosis and Late Stroke

The natural history of in-stent restenosis is unknown. A restenosis rate following carotid artery stenting has been reported to be 3% at 1 year (103). Two types of restenosis have been described: narrowing within the stent and stenosis at the end of the stent, often caused by a kink in the artery. Most restenoses are treated with another stent or balloon angioplasty, with one-third developing repeated episodes of recurrent stenosis. Several studies have used life-table analysis to determine long-term restenosis and stroke-free rates. Lal et al. (104) reported an in-stent restenosis rate (restenosis defined as >80% stenosis) of 6.4% at 60 months. Over half of these occurred at ≤15, and none were associated with neurologic deficits. Hobson et al. (83) reported a similar time period of recurrent stenosis. Investigators have reported an 89% freedom from stroke rate at 48 months with a recurrent stenosis rate of 45% (105). At most institutions, asymptomatic patients who develop a restenosis >80% or symptomatic patients who develop a restenosis >50% are considered for reintervention. Reintervention can entail angioplasty, angioplasty with a cutting balloon, repeat carotid artery stenting, and carotid artery resection with interposition graft (81,103, 106).

Brachiocephalic angioplasty and stenting

Embolization and Stroke

The incidence of acute cerebral ischemia following subclavian artery intervention is low. In one series, there was only one incidence of TIA in 76 interventions (107). The risk of vertebral artery embolization is almost negligible due to the "delay" phenomenon described by Ringelstein and Zeumer (108). Following proximal subclavian artery angioplasty, the reversal of flow from retrograde to antegrade does not occur immediately but gradually. Distal embolization involving the brachial artery and left internal mammary artery has been reported in 1.1% of patients (109). Brachial artery embolization can be easily managed with a brachial artery cutdown and embolectomy. Embolization to the left internal mammary artery may have a profound effect in patients who have had coronary artery bypass grafting. Patients may experience acute myocardial infarction and corresponding hemodynamic compromise. Treatment is generally catheter-directed thrombolytic therapy. Although common carotid angioplasty and stenting has been reported with success by several investigators (109,110), higher risks of embolization and stroke have been documented in cases of combined common carotid artery stenting and standard carotid bifurcation endarterectomy (109).

Technical Complications

Technical complications have been described in 11% of patients undergoing treatment of subclavian artery stenosis or occlusion (107,109,111). These complications include stent migration, failure to cross the occlusive lesion, arterial dissection, acute thrombosis, arterial rupture, and inadvertent covering of the vertebral artery. Arterial dissection is treated by placement of a stent. Acute thrombosis is treated with locally delivered thrombolysis and subsequent balloon angioplasty. Arterial rupture is one of the most feared complications of endovascular therapies. Rupture is detected by visualization of contrast extravasation on completion angiogram. Prompt recognition is important in order to avoid exsanguinations or limb loss. An angioplasty balloon can be reinserted and inflated at the site of rupture, providing a tamponade effect (112). Prolonged balloon inflation may be sufficient to provide hemostasis and no further intervention may be necessary. If balloon inflation fails, a treatment option is placement of a covered stent to exclude the artery's ruptured area. This maneuver has proven effective in the treatment of a variety of brachiocephalic injuries and is associated with shorter operative times, less blood loss, and equivalent patency rates compared to open surgery (113).

Not all subclavian artery ruptures following percutaneous transluminal angioplasty (PTA) or stent placement are immediately identified. Disruption may present in a delayed fashion in the form of a pseudoaneurysm. This complication may present with symptoms due to compression on surrounding structures, including the recurrent laryngeal nerve (hoarseness), sympathetic chain (Horner syndrome), and brachial plexus (weakness or paresthesias). Although an endovascular approach may be effective at ameliorating the pseudoaneurysm, symptomatic lesions are best treated with open surgery to accomplish aneurysmal decompression.

Stent Infection

One incidence of subclavian artery stent infection has been described in the literature (114). The patient presented with *Staphylococcus aureus* bacteremia and stigmata of septic emboli to the ipsilateral hand 6 days after stent placement. CT evaluation revealed a phlegmon surrounding the stented portion of the artery; angiography detected a pseudoaneurysm at the site. The patient underwent resection of the affected portion of the artery with autogenous vascular reconstruction. The underlying etiology of the stent infection is unknown, but it was hypothesized that prolonged femoral access and an infected left arm venous access contributed to stent infection.

Mortality

Mortality rates from brachiocephalic interventions are low, reported at 0% to 4.8% (107,109,111,115). Deaths in the immediate postprocedural period (30 days) have rarely been attributable directly to the endovascular procedure. In a few cases, deaths were due to strokes that occurred at the time of angioplasty and stent placement (109). Long-term mortality tends to be unrelated to the brachiocephalic disease but related to coexisting or subsequently developed comorbidities.

Restenosis and Occlusion

Immediate success in the treatment of subclavian artery stenosis is between 95% and 100% (107,111,115,116). Angioplasty alone has a lower success rate (80% to 85%) compared to primary arterial stenting (97% to 100%) (107,111,116,117). Complete occlusion of the vessel and lesions >2 cm correlate with lower success rates. Short-term patency (1 year) is lower in patients who have undergone only angioplasty (76%) compared to patients receiving primary stenting (95%) (116). Longer-term outcomes (4 years) favor primary angioplasty, with a patency rate of 68% compared to a primary patency rate stenting of 59%. This difference was due to the development of in-stent stenosis. The development of restenosis can be due to misplacement of the stent, particularly in ostial lesions. Up to half of patients who develop a restenosis become symptomatic (107). Restenosis can be treated, when necessary, by balloon angioplasty.

AORTOILIAC INTERVENTIONS

Aortoiliac angioplasty and stenting

Technical Complications

Iliac artery PTA and stent placement is technically successful in 95% and 97% of patients, respectively (118). Stenotic segments are more effectively treated than occlusions. Technical complications occur in <6% of interventions and include subintimal dilation, dissection, arterial rupture, inability to cross the lesion, and distal embolization. In one series, 2.8% developed complications requiring surgery and 0.9% required reconstructive bypass (119). Clinically significant distal embolization occurs in 1% of patients undergoing iliac artery PTA and stent placement. Doppler ultrasound has detected silent peripheral embolization in 90% of patients following iliac PTA (120). Symptomatic embolization can be treated by a variety of endovascular methods, including suction thrombectomy and thrombolytic therapy. If these modalities are not successful, surgical thromboembolectomy is necessary.

Iliac artery dissection during PTA is reported in 0.5% to 1% of patients (105,121). Half of these patients developed significant luminal compromise. Dissections can be treated

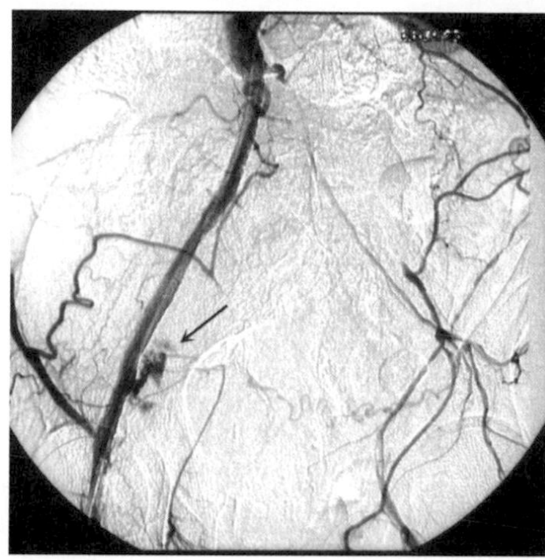

FIGURE 32.1. Angiogram from a patient undergoing iliac artery angioplasty that resulted in a perforation. This is demonstrated by the arrow. The hemorrhage was controlled by brief occlusion of the perforation site with an angioplasty balloon and subsequent placement of an iliac artery stent.

by prolonged balloon inflation to tack down the flap or by placement of an intra-arterial stent. If endovascular therapy is not successful, operative treatments include iliac endarterectomy, iliofemoral bypass, femoral—femoral bypass, and aortobifemoral bypass grafting. Arterial dissection has been reported in 10% of patients undergoing iliac artery stent placement; 70% of the dissections cause hemodynamically significant stenosis requiring an additional stent placement (122).

Vessel injury is related to balloon oversizing and to the degree of arterial calcification. Iliac artery rupture during balloon dilation and stent placement has been reported in 0.9% of cases (123,124). Vessel disruptions can present with uncontained hemorrhage, contained hemorrhage, or pseudoaneurysm formation (Fig. 32.1). The key to initial management is maintenance of endovascular access across the site of disruption with a guidewire. Control of hemorrhage can be obtained with the insertion of an angioplasty balloon to tamponade the site of injury. If prolonged balloon tamponade does not achieve hemostasis, the placement of a covered stent can be used to seal the injury. Uncontrolled hemorrhage warrants emergent surgical intervention, but balloon occlusion proximal to the site of injury can afford some time to prepare for surgery. Risk factors for rupture are similar to those for dissection and include the presence of a high-grade stenosis with heavy calcification. Other risk factors include the use of oversized balloons and manual inflation without manometric control.

Other complications of iliac artery PTA and stent placement include nondeflating angioplasty balloons and stent migration. Modern angioplasty catheters are very reliable, but despite many safeguards, deployment failures can occur. The most common cause of failure of angioplasty balloons is kinking or plugging of the deflation lumen (125). Injection of carbon dioxide or saline can clear the deflation lumen. In addition, a fine wire can be inserted through the inflation lumen. If these techniques are not successful, the balloon can be punctured percutaneously with a 21-gauge needle, depending on the balloon's location and its relationship to surrounding structures.

The exact incidence of iliac stent migration is not known, and this is not a frequently reported complication. Migration is probably not an uncommon complication that occurs when a self-expanding stent abruptly jumps cranially upon deployment (126). Movement may not cause significant morbidity, but it may result in the complete dislodgment of the stent. Unfortunately, once these stents have been deployed, they are difficult to retrieve. Management options for this complication include emergent vascular surgery, observation, stent retrieval using endovascular snares and large introducer sheaths, and aortoiliac bifurcation reconstruction using balloon-expandable stents.

Infection

Stent infection following iliac artery stent placement is rare but has been reported to occur both acutely and in a delayed fashion after several years (127–129). In one case, after thrombolytic therapy and subsequent iliac artery stent placement, the patient developed fever, groin pain, and ipsilateral lower extremity petechiae (128). The patient developed symptoms of systemic inflammatory response with evidence of multisystem organ failure, and *Staphylococcus aureus* grew from blood cultures. Treatment subsequently required excision of the stent and the involved segment of artery, followed by above-the-knee amputation. Another report describes a similar clinical scenario (129). The resected iliac artery revealed severe necrotizing arteritis, and cultures grew *S. aureus* and *S. epidermidis*. Disruption and fracture of the arterial intima and media during angioplasty may predispose this portion of the artery to seeding by bacteria. Bacteria have been shown to colonize a stent surface irreversibly and to prevent tissue incorporation (130). No studies have examined the efficacy of periprocedural antibiotic prophylaxis, but given the seriousness of stent infection, many authors advocate antibiotic use.

Restenosis

Restenosis following iliac artery PTA occurs in 5% to 11% of patients. The incidence of recurrent stenosis and the development of recurrent symptoms depend on the indication for the primary intervention (118,131). Patients treated for limb salvage have higher restenosis and symptom recurrence rates than those treated for claudication. Outcomes are impaired by young age and the presence of poor distal runoff (131,132). Four-year primary patency rates for iliac PTA are 65% for stenosis and 54% for occlusion in patients with claudication and 53% for stenosis and 44% for occlusion in those with limb-threatening ischemia (133). In a meta-analysis evaluating outcomes of iliac artery PTA and stent placement in 1,300 patients, 4-year primary patency rates were 77% for stenotic lesions treated with iliac stenting and 61% for occlusive lesions in patients with claudication and were 67% for stenotic lesions treated with iliac stenting and 53% for occlusive lesions in patients with limb-threatening ischemia (133). The risk of long-term failure was reduced by 39% after stent placement compared to PTA alone. Despite this, limb salvage rates are reported as high as 97% in follow-up (134). Iliac artery stent patency rates are significantly lower in women and in patients with renal insufficiency, diabetes, and/or critical ischemia (134,135) but do not appear to be affected by TransAtlantic InterSociety Consensus (TASC) classification (134).

Late iliac artery thrombosis can develop in 10% of patients (122). Most of these lesions can be treated with thrombolytic therapy followed by repeat angioplasty of in-stent restenosis or endovascular or surgical therapy for more distally occlusive lesions. Patency is reported to be 87% at 1 year (136). Prospective studies reveal that elevated plasma fibrinogen levels are a major risk factor for arterial thrombosis and iliac artery stent restenosis (137).

Mortality

Mortality rates following PTA and stenting of the iliac artery are low and range from 0% to 1.2% (119,123,138). Some mortalities have been directly attributable to the intervention. These include deaths from overwhelming cholesterol embolization, the development of septicemia following reperfusion of ischemic limbs, and contrast reaction.

Aortic endografts for aneurysmal disease

Iliac Artery Rupture

The primary mode of placement of aortic endografts is via a femoral artery cutdown and deployment of grafts through the iliac artery system and into the aorta. Disease, such as atherosclerosis, or tortuosity can lead to complications involving the iliac artery during placement. If the delivery system used to place the endograft is significantly larger than the iliac artery, the vessel can rupture during placement. Iliac artery rupture has been reported in 1% to 2% of cases (139,140). Several maneuvers can be used to traverse complex iliac arteries. Iliac artery stenosis can be predilated with balloon angioplasty to allow safe passage of the delivery system. Preprocedural stenting of the iliac arteries is generally dissuaded as it makes placement prohibitive. If tortuous iliac arteries are present, the use of a stiff guidewire may help reduce the tortuosity and allow easier access (Fig. 32.2). In some instances, the use of two stiff guidewires (also known as a "buddy wire") may straighten the

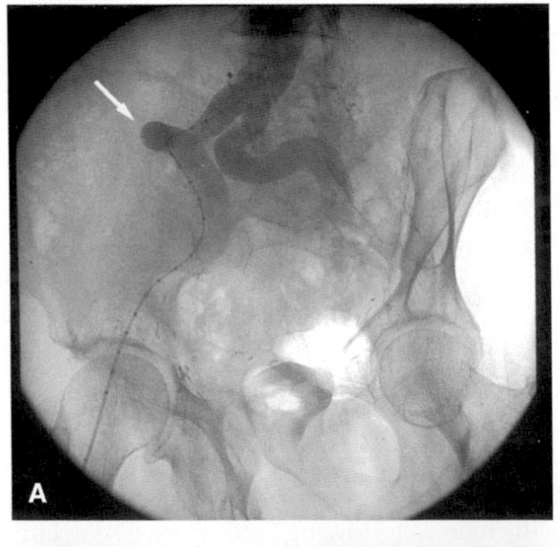

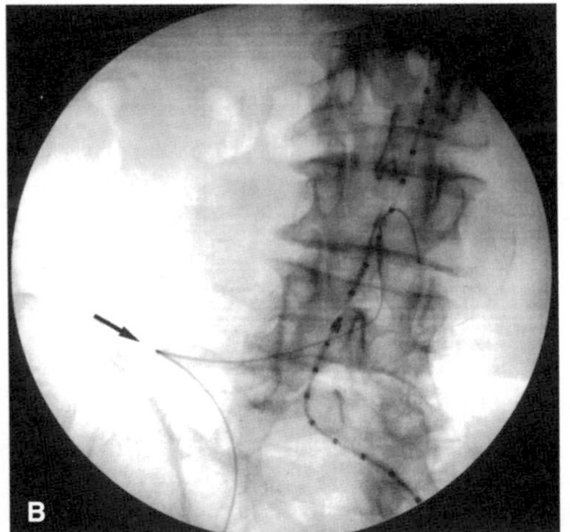

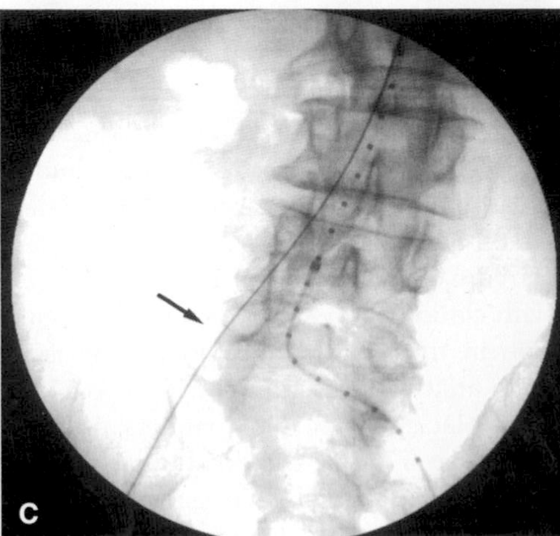

FIGURE 32.2. Angiogram from a patient undergoing endograft repair of an abdominal aortic aneurysm. **A:** The preoperative study revealed tortuous iliac arteries (*arrow*). **B:** Placement of a "floppy" guidewire allows the iliac artery to retain a tortuous course (*arrow*). **C:** Placement of a stiff wire causes the iliac artery system to straighten.

tortuosity. If these techniques do not allow adequate placement of the endograft, an iliac artery conduit can be used. This technique involves the suturing of a prosthetic graft to the midcommon iliac artery. The endograft is placed through the prosthetic graft and common iliac artery, and the iliac limb of the graft is seated in the prosthetic graft. The distal limb of the prosthetic graft is then anastomosed to the common femoral artery. The distal end of the common iliac artery is oversewn to allow retrograde flow through the external iliac artery and into the hypogastric artery.

Pelvic Ischemia

Iliac artery aneurysms coexist with abdominal aortic aneurysms (AAAs) in up to 30% of patients undergoing endograft repair (141–145). This circumstance can present a problem with aortic endograft placement, as the iliac arteries may be too large for the iliac limbs to form a seal. In these situations, the iliac limb of the aortic endograft may be parked in the external iliac artery, covering the hypogastric artery. If this is a planned event, the hypogastric artery is often embolized preoperatively to cause its occlusion and prevent an endoleak. The presence of an internal iliac artery aneurysm would necessitate the same treatment. Rarely, bilateral hypogastric artery embolization is required, usually performed in a staged fashion.

Complications from hypogastric artery embolization can occur in up to 50% of patients (142). Buttock claudication is the predominant complaint after hypogastric artery occlusion. Buttock claudication occurs in 12% to 50% of patients, but few have symptoms that persist beyond several months (141–145). Up to 25% of men complain of new onset erectile dysfunction (144,145). Significant pelvic devascularization leading to colonic ischemia requiring bowel resection is of theoretical concern, but this entity has not been described in any of the larger series. Patients requiring embolization of the more distal branches of the hypogastric artery are at a higher risk of developing pelvic symptoms (146). Bilateral hypogastric artery embolization has not been associated with increased symptoms when compared to unilateral embolization (142,143,145). Coil embolization of the hypogastric artery can be avoided altogether if it is not aneurysmal. If as little as 5 mm of normal diameter common iliac artery is present prior to its bifurcation and there is 15 mm of acceptable artery distal to the bifurcation, coil embolization of the internal iliac artery is not necessary in order to obtain a distal iliac artery seal (147).

Endoleaks

An endoleak is the persistence of blood flow outside of the endograft within the aneurysm sac (AS) (148). Endoleaks are classified according to their etiology. Five types of endoleaks have been described (Table 32.2) (149,150). A type I endoleak (Fig. 32.3) arises from inadequate sealing at either the proximal aortic (allowing antegrade flow) or distal iliac (allowing retrograde flow) attachment sites. Type II endoleaks (Fig. 32.4) arise from patent aortic branch vessels. Such vessels include patent lumbar arteries or the inferior mesenteric artery. These allow retrograde flow into the AS, continued pressurization, and potential risk for rupture. Type III endoleaks develop from defects in the fabric of the graft or at the junction zone between modular components (Fig. 32.5).

Table 32.2 Types of endoleaks

Type I	Inadequate sealing at either the proximal aortic or distal iliac landing zones. Allows antegrade or retrograde flow into the aneurysm sac.
Type II	Patent aortic branch vessel (i.e., lumbar artery) providing retrograde flow into the aneurysm sac.
Type III	Defects in the fabric of the graft or at the junction zone between modular components providing flow into the aneurysm sac.
Type IV	Diffuse leaking of blood between the interstices of the fabric or where the graft is sutured to the stents.
Type V (controversial)	Aneurysm sac pressurized and enlarges despite no identifiable blood flow into the sac.

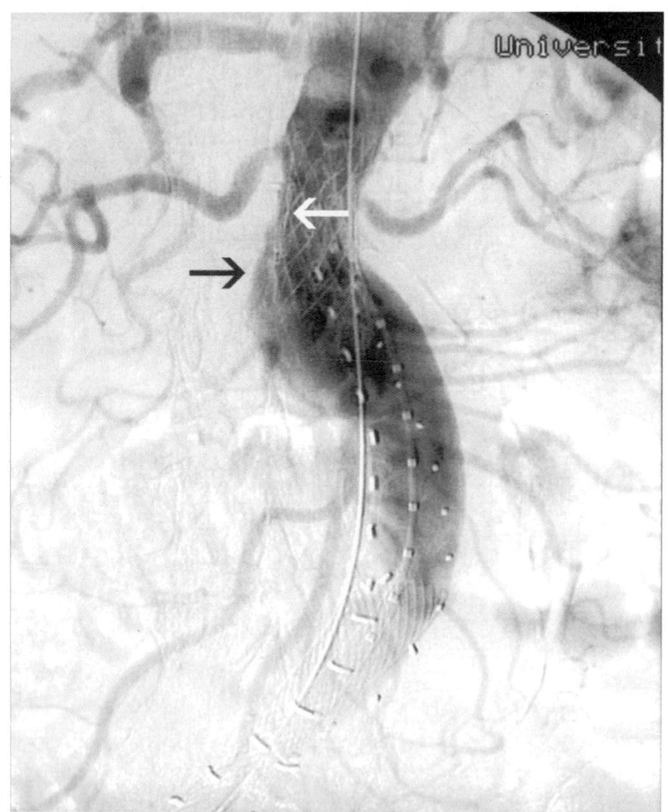

FIGURE 32.3. Aortogram demonstrating a type I endoleak. The white arrow demonstrates the lateral aspect of the stent graft. The black arrow points to contrast leaking around the proximal seal of the endograft, filling the aneurysm sac.

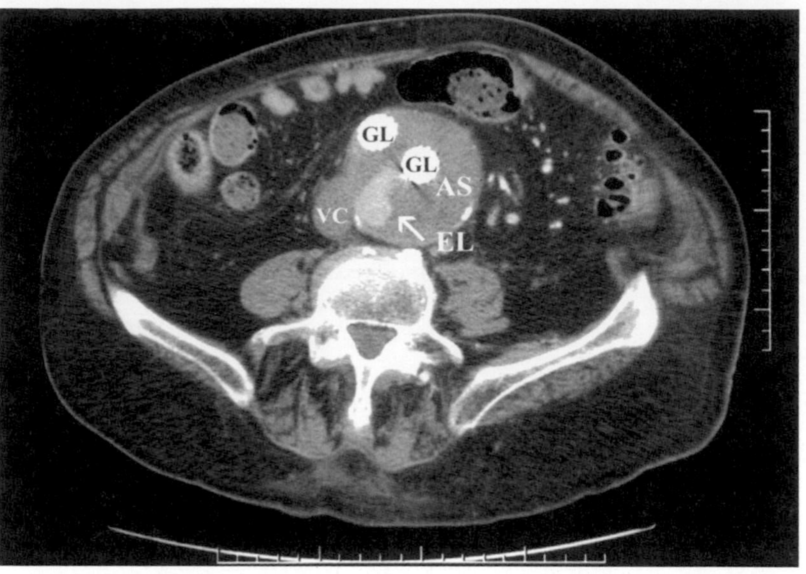

FIGURE 32.4. CT scan demonstrating a type II endoleak. GL represents the graft limbs, and AS is the aortic sac. There is contrast outside the graft limbs within the aneurysm sac that is characteristic of a type II endoleak (EL). This patient had an expanding aneurysm, and selective angiography revealed a patent inferior mesenteric artery. This artery was embolized and there was subsequent regression of the aneurysm size.

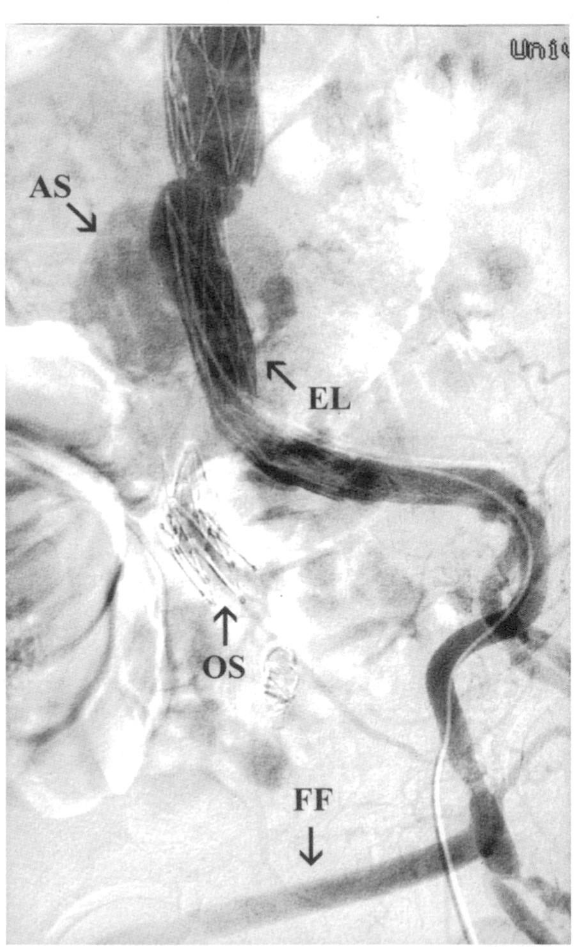

FIGURE 32.5. Aortogram demonstrating a type III endoleak (EL). This patient had a homemade graft inserted that was of aorto-uni-iliac design. There is an occluding stent in the contralateral iliac artery (OS) with a femoral–femoral bypass graft (FF). The patient presented 5 years after the initial graft insertion with back pain and acute expansion of the aneurysm sac (AS). Aortogram reveals a leak from the body of the graft (EL) filling the AS. The endograft was relined with a new graft that sealed the endoleak.

Type IV endoleaks develop secondary to diffuse leaking of blood between the interstices of the fabric or where the graft is sutured to a stent. Type V endoleaks occur when the AS remains pressurized and the aneurysm enlarges, but no flow can be demonstrated within the AS using currently available imaging modalities. A type V endoleak is one in which the defect is large enough to allow blood flow into the sac and to transmit pressure to the sac, but the exit site is not present or too small to be detected by conventional imaging techniques (151).

Type I and type III endoleaks are associated with a significant risk of aneurysm enlargement and possible rupture. These endoleaks should be treated if they are detected (152,153). Treatment may be accomplished by the placement of additional endograft components, including a proximal aortic extension cuff or an additional iliac limb. If the leak is a proximal type I endoleak and the graft is juxtaposed to the inferior border of the renal arteries, a large balloon-expandable stent can be placed in the proximal aspect of the endograft to increase radial force, causing better juxtaposition of the graft to the aortic wall. If less-invasive interventions are unsuccessful at treating these types of endoleaks, removal of the endograft with conventional surgical repair is indicated. Fabric tears are easily managed if the site of the leak is localized. This complication can be managed by placement of an aortic cuff or an iliac extension to cover the hole. If the leak is more diffuse, the entire endograft can be relined or the device can be explanted.

Type II endoleaks are rarely associated with aneurysm rupture (154). At least 10% to 15% of patients will be identified with a type II endoleak during the endograft's lifespan (155–158). Chronic anticoagulation therapy is not associated with an increased risk of type II endoleak formation, but type II leaks are less likely to spontaneously resolve if the patient requires warfarin (159). No intervention is generally undertaken when a type II endoleak is diagnosed unless it is associated with an increase in aneurysm size or associated with aortic pulsatility on physical examination. In these situations, arteriography is required to identify the source of the endoleak. An aortogram is performed, followed by selective injections into each iliac limb, the superior mesenteric artery, and hypogastric arteries. Superselective arterial access is then obtained, which allows embolization of the feeding vessels. Alternatively, direct sac puncture can be performed with embolization of the feeding vessels (160). The sac is then filled with glue, coils, or other embolization material.

Endograft Structural Failure

One of the most worrisome long-term complications associated with aortic endografting is material failure. Structural failure is difficult to identify as patients are often asymptomatic and may not present with acute changes. Three modes of structural failure have been described in aortic endografting, involving fabric erosion, suture disruption, and metal fracture (161). The development of endoleaks secondary to graft erosion has been documented in first-generation grafts (Fig. 32.5) (162,163). Areas of graft erosion are hypothesized to be secondary to the interaction of the stent material with the fabric. Repeated aortic pulsations cause friction between the stent and the fabric, causing eventual graft deterioration and the development of a type III endoleak. In many aortic endografts, the graft material is attached to a metal skeleton with sutures. In several series in which patients developed new endoleaks, a graft explantation suture disruption was discovered within the graft (164,165). The mechanism leading to suture disruption is similar to graft erosion. It is not known, however, if suture disruption directly leads to endograft failure or if the resultant destabilization of the graft results in further deterioration.

The most common structural problem identified with aortic endograft systems has been metallic stent fracture (166). Jacobs et al. (166) reported the outcome of 686 patients who underwent endovascular aneurysm repair. Sixty patients had material failure. Three-fourths of these failures were due to metallic stent fracture. Metal failure was caused by two processes: stress fatigue and metal corrosion. Stress fatigue resulted from repeated aortic pulsations. Metal corrosion occurs predominantly in nitinol stents (167). More recent stent-graft designs have improved nitinol processing and do not exhibit the same extent of corrosion (168–170).

Limb Thrombosis

Endograft limb thrombosis after endovascular aortic endografting occurs in 11% of patients (171–176). A variety of factors have been hypothesized to place patients at increased risk for limb thrombosis. The lack of metallic support within the limbs of endografts has been suggested to increase risk for thrombosis. In one series, 5% of supported limbs required a subsequent intervention to maintain patency while 44% of unsupported limbs required this degree of intervention (173). Oversizing of the graft limb also increases the risk of thrombosis. The infolding of the graft material due to the oversizing decreases the inner diameter, which increases the incidence of thrombosis (174). Extension of the iliac limb into the external iliac artery may place the limb at increased risk of thrombosis due to size mismatch between the graft and the smaller external iliac artery. Damage to the external iliac artery or femoral artery at the time of graft placement (i.e., dissection) can subsequently cause an outflow obstruction and graft limb thrombosis (171).

Management of patients with limb thrombosis depends on the severity of the induced ischemia. Nearly one-third of patients present with mild symptoms and require no intervention (172). Most patients, however, present with more severe ischemia and require a femoral—femoral bypass in order to reperfuse the affected limb. Few patients are successfully treated with thrombolysis or graft thrombectomy followed by endovascular repair. Most episodes of graft limb thrombosis present within the first 6 months; no limb occlusions have been described after 30 months (171–173,177).

Graft Migration

Distal stent-graft migration complicates abdominal aortic endografting in 9% to 45% of patients. Migration is a risk for developing a type I endoleak and delayed rupture or late conversion to open repair (178). The pathophysiology of endograft migration is complex, but blood flow is the main displacing force (179). As the tube of the endograft curves, the change in velocity of the blood causes an increase in the displacement force. Resistance to migration is afforded by friction between the graft and the aortic wall and by the graft's columnar strength. Barbs or hooks encompassed in graft design may provide some additional protection (180).

Angulation of the aortic neck may decrease the frictional force and increase the risk of graft migration (178,181). Other hypotheses about the cause of device migration have focused on the morphologic changes in the aneurysm and aortic neck after endovascular AAA repair. Aortic neck dilation, longitudinal sac shrinkage, and graft shortening have been described (182–185). The aortic neck has been documented to significantly dilate during the first 2 years after endograft repair (186). In a review in which the incidence of graft migration was 15%, the two independent risk factors for endograft migration were neck dilation following repair and a baseline AAA size of >55 mm. Others have argued that neck dilation is not a significant event if adequate graft oversizing was performed at initial endograft placement (187).

Technical Complications and Conversion to Open Surgery

Technical complications have been described in up to one-fourth of endograft placements (188). The occurrence of critical events is independent of operator experience, perhaps reflecting the fact that more anatomically difficult cases are attempted with increasing experience (189). Deployment difficulties include graft foreshortening necessitating the placement of additional distal covered extensions, suprarenal graft displacement, infrarenal graft displacement, and device-related issues such as iliac limb kinking or twisting. Conversion to open surgery has been reported in only 1% to 3% of patients during endograft repair (153,158,190,191). According to the Eurostar registry, however, 18% of patients with endograft placement required a secondary intervention (192). Most of these interventions (76%) were through a transfemoral approach, while the rest required a transabdominal (12%) or extra-anatomic (11%) approach. The rates of freedom from intervention at 1, 3, and 4 years were 89%, 67%, and 62%, respectively. Other large series have mirrored these results (175,177).

Aneurysm Rupture

The risk of rupture following aneurysm repair is low. One series reports a freedom from risk of rupture of 98.7% at 2 years (193). In another series the risk of rupture approached 1% per year (158). The presence of an endoleak and the development of graft migration increase the risk of subsequent AAA rupture.

Mortality

Aortic endograft repair of AAA is associated with a low mortality rate in the range of 1% to 3% (153,158,177,191). Most deaths are related to cardiovascular morbidity. Two large randomized, prospective trials have compared outcomes of endovascular aneurysm repair (EVAR) with those of conventional open surgery for AAA. These studies have demonstrated that EVAR is associated with lower perioperative mortality rates compared to open surgery (1.7% and 1.2% vs. 4.7% and 4.6%) (194,195). The survival advantage, however, is lost at long-term follow-up with 2-year and 4-year mortality rates being similar between the two groups (2-year: 11% vs. 11% and 4-year: 26% vs. 29%). More patients undergoing EVAR (41%), however, required an additional intervention during the follow-up period, compared to only 9% of the surgical arm (194). The need for further interventions, even if performed percutaneously, has been associated with an increased mortality. In one series, up to 8% of patients undergoing a secondary intervention died, and this mortality rose to 18% if a transabdominal approach was necessary (177).

Thoracic Aortic Stent Graft

The use of thoracic aortic stent grafts (thoracic endovascular aortic repair [TEVAR]) to treat thoracic aortic aneurysm, while early in its commercialization, has become mainstream. Many of the acute complications associated with placement of the thoracic aortic stent grafts are the same as those encountered with placement of abdominal grafts. Neurologic complications are one of the most concerning complications associated with TEVAR. During placement of the thoracic stent graft, there is wire, catheter, and device manipulation within the aortic arch, which can lead to cerebral embolization and stroke. Stroke rates occur in 3% to 5% of patients undergoing TEVAR, and it occurs more readily in those patients in whom the stent graft is placed proximal to the left subclavian artery (196). Another catastrophic neurologic complication associated with thoracic aortic surgery is the development of paraplegia, and TEVAR is not immune to this complication. TEVAR, however, is associated with lower rates of paraplegia when compared to conventional surgery (6.2% vs. 13%, $p < 0.007$) (197). The primary factor associated with the development of spinal cord ischemia is the extent of the aorta covered with the stent graft (198). Protective measures, such as maintaining adequate blood pressure and spinal fluid drainage, may help to protect against this devastating complication.

Stent collapse is another complication that appears to be more significant in thoracic aortic stent grafting compared with EVAR. This occurs when thoracic aortic stent grafts are placed in young patients who have acute angulation of the aortic arch and have aortic diameters that are significantly smaller than available stent grafts. This scenario typically occurs in the setting of traumatic aortic transection. When the stent grafts are oversized and placed in an acute angulation, like the aortic arch, they are prone to kink or compress, resulting in acute aortic occlusion, or a functional aortic coarctation (Fig. 32.6). This complication is usually treated with extra-anatomic bypass to the great arch vessels and extension of the endograft landing zone more proximally into a straighter portion of the aorta. Alternatively, arch replacement may be necessary. The development of more

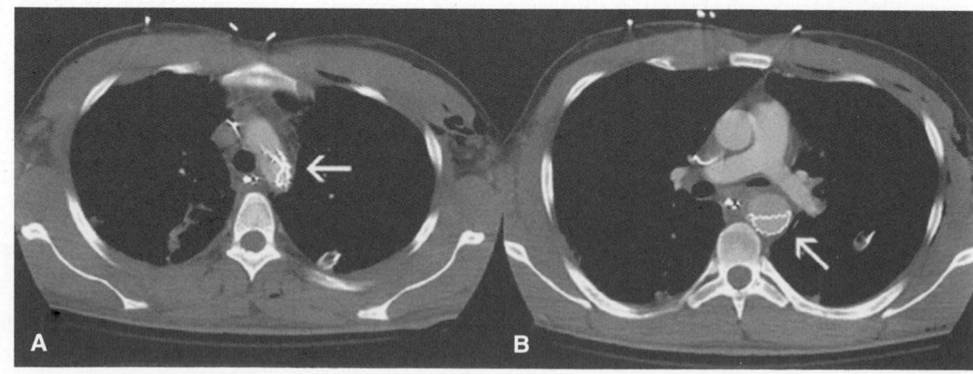

FIGURE 32.6. CT scan from a patient that was treated with a thoracic aortic stent graft for a traumatic aortic dissection. The available graft was significantly larger than the aortic diameter, and it did not accommodate the acute aortic arch angulation. This resulted in a kinked thoracic aortic endograft (**A**, *arrow*). Distal to the kink, the graft was not able to fully expand (**B**, *arrow*) and the patient had a function aortic coarctation. The lesion was treated with an extra-anatomic bypass to the great arch vessels and subsequent extension of the endograft into a more suitable landing zone.

advanced endografting systems, and appropriate device sizing, will help to avoid this complication.

Endoleaks also complicate TEVAR and are classified in a similar fashion (Table 32.2). Endoleak rate after TEVAR has been reported from 4% to 26% (197,199,200), and by life-table analysis, >90% of patients will be free from primary endoleak during 30 months of follow-up (201). Endoleaks tend to be more type I and type III leaks, with fewer type II leaks (202). AS enlargement is more common in stent graft treatment of thoracic aneurysms and has been reported in 7% to 14% of patients at 1 year (202). Long-term data for this complication, however, is lacking given the relative immaturity of the procedure.

As the use thoracic aortic endograft increases and larger volumes of long-term data become available, a more thorough understanding of the long-term complications will be assessed.

Mesenteric artery angioplasty and stenting

Technical Complications

Primary technical success for mesenteric interventions has been reported at 63% to 81% for PTA and 96% to 100% for primary stenting, with overall clinical success (as measured by resolution or significant reduction in symptoms) in up to 88% of patients (203–205). Unsuccessful PTA is managed with subsequent stent placement. In one series, 50% of the immediate clinical failures were due to misdiagnosis of chronic mesenteric ischemia, and in the follow-up period, underlying gastrointestinal cancer was identified (203). Clinical success was not attributable to the number of mesenteric vessels that were treated. Complications described at the site of PTA include arterial dissection, which is managed with placement of a stent in some cases and observation alone in others (204). Episodes of postprocedural bowel ischemia have been described, affecting 7% to 8% of patients undergoing mesenteric artery endovascular therapy (206,207). The etiology of this complication, presumed to be embolization, dissection, or the underlying reason for mesenteric intervention, has not been explained.

Restenosis

Approximately 15% to 20% of patients who have had a successful endovascular mesenteric intervention have recurrent symptoms, generally occurring within the first year (203–206). In most cases, recurrent symptoms are due to the development of restenosis, which can be treated with repeat PTA and, if necessary, secondary stent placement. Primary and assisted primary patency rates for mesenteric stent placement have been reported to be 70% and 90%, respectively, at 18 months (205). If endovascular therapy continues to fail, surgical revascularization should be performed—provided the patient is an acceptable operative candidate.

Mortality

Mortality rates associated with mesenteric PTA and stent placement have been reported to be between 0% and 11% (203,205,206). In all cases of early mortality, death was attributable to bowel ischemia. Five-year survival rates approach 70% and do not depend on whether the patients underwent primary PTA or stenting, the number of mesenteric vessels treated, or whether the superior mesenteric artery, specifically, had an intervention performed upon it (203).

Renal artery angioplasty and stenting

Technical Complications

Renal artery stenting is associated with technical success rates between 91% and 98% (208,209). Complications associated with renal artery PTA and stenting include renal artery rupture (1.7%), aortic dissection at the level of the renal artery (2.2%), flow-limiting renal artery dissection (1.1%), and renal artery thromboembolism (1.1%) (208). Renal artery rupture, if diagnosed at the time of occurrence, can be managed with reversal of anticoagulation and tamponade of the rupture site with inflation of an angioplasty balloon. Rupture is not always identified at the time of the procedure and may present in a delayed fashion with hypotension, drop in hematocrit, and the development of a perinephric hematoma on imaging studies. Depending on the patient's hemodynamic stability, the delayed diagnosis of renal artery rupture may require no further intervention. In cases of uncontrolled hemorrhage or failure of less-invasive therapies, operative repair of the ruptured renal artery is required. Treatment may require a simple arterial repair, arterial reconstruction, or nephrectomy.

Renal artery dissection can be managed by placement of additional stents if dissection involves the main renal artery. When the dissection involves a branch vessel, the problem becomes more difficult to manage and may result in infarction of the portion of the kidney supplied by that branch. Renal artery thrombosis and embolism may be treated with suction thrombectomy or the administration of a thrombolytic agent. Some instances of acute renal artery thrombosis during the procedure require acute surgical revascularization (209). Stent dislodgment has been reported in 2% of patients undergoing renal stent placement (210). Two-thirds of these patients required abortion of the endovascular procedure and conversion to surgical repair. The others had the stents retrieved with the use of an endovascular snare. Failure to use a guiding sheath has been identified as a risk for stent dislodgment during placement.

Renal Function Complications

Approximately 6% to 25% of patients undergoing renal artery PTA and stent placement have an elevation in serum creatinine lasting >30 days (208,209). Over half of these patients required hemodialysis, but not all required long-term dialysis. The etiology of acute renal failure is variable and in some instances is due to distal renal artery embolization or branch vessel thrombosis resulting in renal infarction. Renal infarction has been documented in ~3% of patients.

Infection

Stent infections are not common complications. Several incidences of renal artery stent infection have been described (211–213). The common bacteria in all these cases was *S. aureus*, but in two of the case reports, at least one additional bacterium was isolated from blood cultures, including *Proteus mirabilis* and *Klebsiella pneumoniae*. Risk factors for the development of renal artery stent infection do not differ from risk factors for all stent infections. These include breaks in sterile technique, repeated puncture of the same vessel for arterial access, reuse of an indwelling catheter, increased procedure time, and puncture site hematoma formation (186). Patients present with fever, local pain, and leukocytosis. If bacteremia is associated with a particularly virulent pathogen, patients may present with a profound systemic inflammatory response manifested by hypotension, tachycardia, and multisystem organ failure. An intrarenal abscess may form due to embolization from the infected stent. CT scans are sensitive for the diagnosis of stent infection and show an intense inflammatory response around the affected stent and renal artery. Renal artery pseudoaneurysm formation is associated with the renal artery stent infection (212,213). Death secondary to overwhelming infection has been described as a result of renal artery stent infection (213). Treatment involves intravenous antibiotic administration and resuscitation guided by the clinical scenario. Resection of the infected stent is mandatory, including removal of surrounding infected and devitalized tissue. Excision is followed by autogenous renal artery reconstruction. Some interventionalists recommend the routine use of prophylactic antibiotics prior to renal PTA and stenting (212).

Restenosis

Follow-up angiography is not routine after renal artery PTA or stenting. Patients are reevaluated if they develop worsening renal function or hypertension. In one series, 20.5% of patients developed worsening renal function or hypertension after initially having a positive clinical response to endovascular therapy (209). When these cases underwent angiography, 14 of the 15 patients had evidence of significant in-stent restenosis. Half of these lesions were successfully treated with either angioplasty alone, repeat stent placement, or open surgery. The other half had no intervention, as the degree of restenosis was <50%. Other series have reported restenosis rates ranging between 11% and 44% at 2 years (214,215). Restenosis is secondary to either intimal hyperplasia or progression of atherosclerosis.

Mortality

Thirty-day mortality rates following renal artery PTA and stent are low, between 0% and 1.4% (208–210,216). Mortality has not been directly associated with the renal artery intervention, but to complications from comorbidities.

LOWER EXTREMITY INTERVENTIONS

Femoropopliteal angioplasty and stenting

Technical Complications

Initial technical success of femoropopliteal PTA is between 76% and 95% (217–221). Failure is mainly attributable to the inability to cross occlusions and tight stenoses, inability to inflate the angioplasty balloon, or inability to enter the patent distal lumen. Early failures <24 hours occur in 23% of patients (218).

Complications occurring during PTA include arterial disruption, thrombosis, distal embolization, and arterial dissection. Complications occur more frequently in femoropopliteal interventions compared to iliac artery interventions (13% of cases), and half of these complications are significant enough to require operation, transfusion, or an extended hospital stay. Arterial disruption can present with the development of hematoma, pseudoaneurysm, or arteriovenous fistula. Management includes reversal of anticoagulation and the use of a balloon catheter to occlude the arterial injury. The use of covered stents has been described to effectively treat this complication (222). Operative intervention may be required if bleeding is not controlled.

Embolization can occur from thrombus or atheromatous debris from disrupted plaque. Treatment involves the administration of catheter-directed thrombolytic therapy or surgical thromboembolectomy (Fig. 32.7). Acute thrombosis at the angioplasty site has been described in 2.5% of patients and generally occurs at sites of plaque ulceration (219). As with embolization, thromboses are generally treated with thrombolytic therapy and, if not successful, open thrombectomy. Arterial dissection can also occur following PTA. This complication is often treated with the placement of an intra-arterial stent (Fig. 32.8). Most of the complications related to PTA are best managed by arterial bypass. Complication rates depend on the indication for intervention and the patient's age. Older patients and those who were treated for limb-threatening ischemia have worse outcomes.

Technical success following femoropopliteal artery stenting is reported to be 92% (223). In one series, 27% of cases of femoropopliteal recanalization were complicated by immediate thrombosis requiring thrombolytic therapy (224). One-fifth of these patients could not have patency reestablished. Distal embolization has been reported in 10% of the patients and is treated as outlined earlier (225).

Patency and Amputation

Primary patency rates for femoropopliteal interventions have been reported as 43% to 58% at 1 year, 41% to 46% at 2 years, 38% to 41% at 3 years, and 26% to 38% at 5 years (218–220,226–228). Several factors have been shown to affect outcome of femoropopliteal angioplasty. The length of the lesion has a negative effect on long-term patency. Lofberg et al. (228) evaluated outcomes of 92 patients who

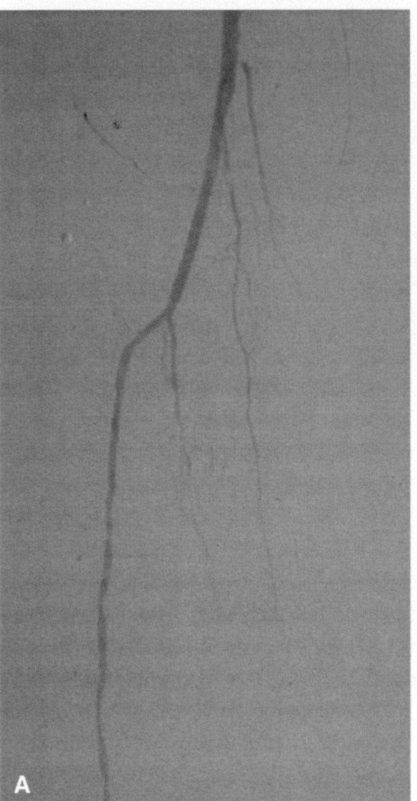

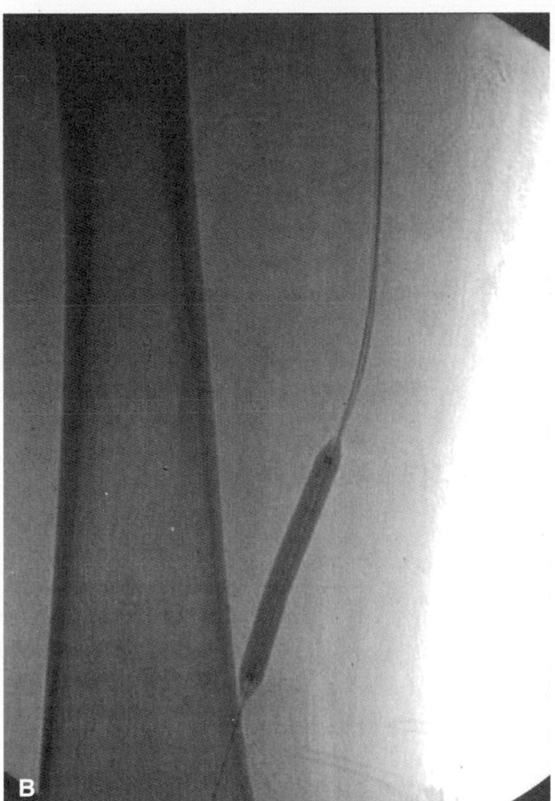

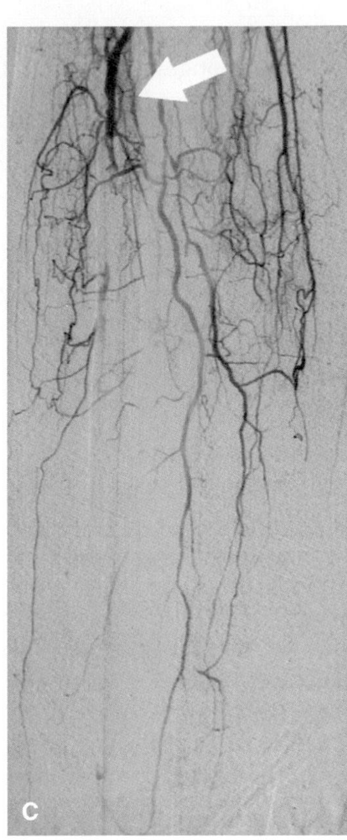

FIGURE 32.7. **A:** Lower extremity angiogram revealing the outflow tract of a patient with a more proximal popliteal artery stenosis. **B:** This lesion underwent primary balloon angioplasty. Postprocedure ankle-brachial index measurements were significantly lower than those taken before the procedure. **C:** Repeat angiography revealed a thromboembolus occluding the outflow tract. Attempts at thrombolysis were unsuccessful and the patient underwent popliteal thromboembolectomy.

underwent 121 PTA procedures. They reported a primary patency at 5 years of only 12% in those with occlusions >5 cm and 32% in those with occlusions <5 cm. Similar results were found by Matsi et al. (227), but they had some success with PTA of lesions up to 10 cm in length. Others have shown that treatment of patients with stenoses faired better than those with occlusions, and those with claudication faired better than those with limb-threatening ischemia (226). The quality of outflow also affects outcome (220). The occurrence of a complication at the time of initial PTA also adversely affects long-term results. Limb salvage is 86% to 91% at 5 years.

In-stent restenosis, as evaluated by intravascular ultrasound, is caused by neointimal hyperplasia and stent

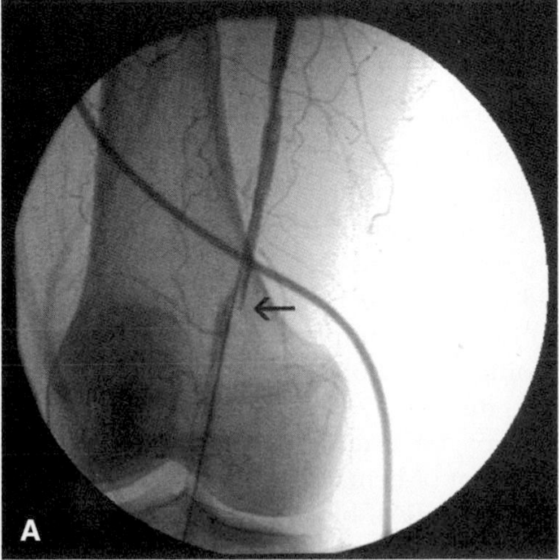

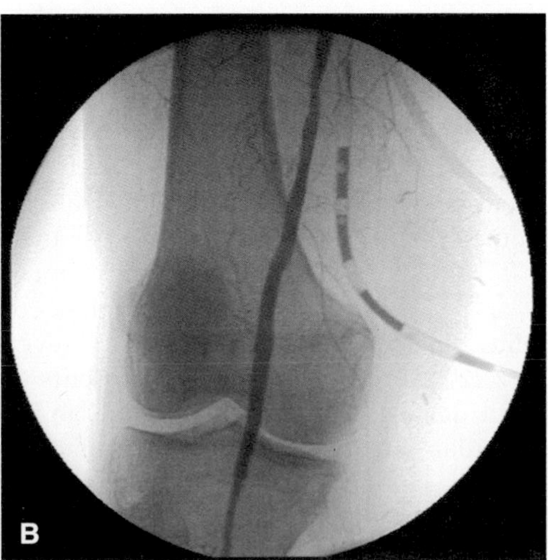

FIGURE 32.8. **A:** Angiogram of a patient who underwent balloon angioplasty of a popliteal artery stenosis. This resulted in an arterial dissection that occluded flow in the vessel. **B:** Placement of an intra-arterial stent successfully treated the dissection.

remodeling, leading to lumen area reduction (229). The extent of changes is most significant at stent edges. Patency may be improved by the use of expanded polytetrafluoroethylene (ePTFE) stent-graft relative to bare stents (230). Saxon et al. (230) reported the largest experience as part of a US multicenter, prospective, randomized trial of PTA versus PTA and ePTFE-covered stents. The total number of patients treated was only 28, with 13 patients receiving PTA alone and 15 patients randomized to PTA and covered stent placement. At 2-year follow-up, primary patency in the covered stent group was 87%, whereas in the PTA alone group, it was only 25% ($p = 0.002$). Further investigation is certainly warranted into the application of this technology. In addition, drug-eluting stents are being investigated for the treatment of femoropopliteal disease. One such study evaluated the use of sirolimus-eluting stents (231). Sirolimus acts as an anti-inflammatory and cytostatic antiproliferative agent that diminishes smooth muscle cell proliferation, which may prevent the development of neointimal hyperplasia. Duda et al. (231) reported on the outcome of 36 patients recruited for the participation in a randomized, double-blind, prospective trial evaluating drug-eluting stents versus uncoated stents in the treatment of femoropopliteal occlusive disease. The in-stent mean lumen diameter was significantly larger in the sirolimus-eluting stent group compared with the uncoated stent at 6 months. Long-term patency rates are not yet known, and further investigation with this stent, as well as others, is underway.

Alternatives to PTA and stenting have been developed for percutaneous intervention of the lower extremity arterial tree, specifically utilizing debulking technologies. Mechanical atherectomy uses either a rotational blade or a "plane"-like device that shaves the atherosclerotic debris from the arterial wall. Most of the results for these devices is presented in small retrospective series or registry data, with the primary end point evaluated often being freedom from target vessel revascularization. Zeller et al. (232) reported a 76% technical success rate with these devices (defined as obtaining <30% residual stenosis). Over half of these lesions, however, required adjunctive balloon angioplasty or stent placement. The majority of data, however, come from the self-reported multicenter Treating Peripherls with SilverHawk: Outcomes Collection (TALON) registry (233). Similar to other series, there was 74% technical success rate, but only one-quarter required an adjunctive procedure. Freedom from target vessel revascularization was 80% at 12 months. Multiple lesions and increasing Rutherford stage were predictors of less-favorable outcomes.

Mortality

Mortality rates after femoropopliteal intervention are low, ranging between 0% and 4.3% (217,220,223,227). Deaths are often related to comorbidities, but death from complications directly related to endovascular therapy has been described, including retroperitoneal hemorrhage (234). Survival rates at 5 years are 51% to 73%, with at least a 6% per year mortality.

Tibial angioplasty and stenting

Few studies provide enough data to adequately evaluate complications following endovascular intervention in the tibial arteries. Technical success has been described in 87% to 92% of patients (235,236). Complications related to tibial PTA include the need for emergency vascular surgery (0.7% of patients), procedurally related deaths (0.4%), amputation (0.4%), and the development of compartment syndrome after tibial recanalization (0.4% of cases) (235). Limb salvage was reported in 91% of these limbs, but 5-year survival was only 31%. The two largest series reported on the outcomes of tibial PTA were reported by Faglia et al. (236) in 2002 and by Dorros et al. (235) in 2001. Faglia et al. reported on the outcomes of 191 tibial PTA procedures performed in patients with critical limb ischemia (rest pain or tissue loss). Clinical recurrence occurred in 7.3% of patients at a mean time to recurrence of 4.6 months. The majority of these recurrences were successfully treated with repeat angioplasty. Major amputation was required in only 5.2% of patients. Dorros et al. reported on the outcome of 270 PTA procedures in patients with critical limb ischemia. Over a 5-year follow-up, only 8% required a subsequent surgical revascularization and only 9% required a major amputation. Survival, however, was only 56% at 5 years. In some centers, tibial PTA for isolated tibial lesions is being considered as the primary intervention prior to tibial artery bypass, particularly in patients with multiple comorbidities.

More recently, Giles et al. (237) reported the results infrapopliteal angioplasty in 176 limbs from 163 patients. In this series, technical success was achieved in 93% of the cases. At 1 and 2 years, primary patency was 53% and 51%, respectively, while freedom from secondary restenosis and reintervention were 63% and 61%, respectively. Patients with less severe and less extensive disease faired better than those with more extensive disease. As more experience is gained with this procedure, a better understanding of its outcomes and its potential applications will be attained.

Thrombolysis

Thrombolytic therapy is used to treat acute arterial or venous occlusions. The main risk associated with thrombolytic therapy is bleeding. A variety of agents is used for thrombolytic therapy, including streptokinase derivatives, urokinase compounds (UK), tissue plasminogen activator, and its recombinant forms (rt-PA). An analysis of data collected in a prospective single-institution registry revealed an overall complication rate of 55.9% in patients undergoing thrombolytic therapy for both arterial and venous disease (238). In patients receiving thrombolytic therapy for arterial disease, complications included development of hematoma or pseudoaneurysm (30.6% UK vs. 57.7% rt-PA), bleeding requiring transfusion (11.9% UK vs. 18.7% rt-PA), and intracranial bleeding

(0.8% UK vs. 3.3% rt-PA). Mortality rates were 2.9% for UK and 1.6% for rt-PA.

In patients being treated for venous disease, the complications reported were hematoma formation (18.4% UK vs. 28.6% rt-PA) and bleeding requiring transfusion (14.3% UK vs. 42.9% rt-PA). There were no episodes of intracranial bleeding in venous patients, but mortality rates were 2% for UK compared to 19% for rt-PA. The causes of mortality were not reported in the venous group, but in the arterial group, some were related to the development of intracranial hemorrhage. There are fewer complications with the use of thrombolytic therapy to treat venous disease, and there appears to be fewer complications with the use of UK compared to rt-PA.

Two major randomized prospective trials have evaluated the use of thrombolytic therapy for lower extremity ischemia: Surgery versus Thrombolysis for Ischemia of the Lower Extremity (STILE) (239) and Thrombolysis or Peripheral Artery Surgery (TOPAS) (240). In these trials, complications occurred with an incidence of 22% to 41% and included hemorrhage, distal embolization, and catheter-related problems. Life-threatening hemorrhage occurred in 6.2% of patients undergoing thrombolytic therapy in the STILE trial and in 12.5% of patients treated with thrombolytics in the TOPAS trial. The TOPAS trial did show that when aspirin and therapeutic heparin were withheld during thrombolytic therapy, the rate of intracranial hemorrhage decreased from 5% to 0.5% (208). Aggressive control of hypertension is also beneficial in decreasing the risk of intracranial hemorrhage (241). Distal embolization occurred in 14% of cases. Embolization is generally self-limiting; as the thrombolysis progresses, the embolization is cleared. Embolization requiring surgery occurs in ~2% of cases.

In order to minimize the risks of thrombolytic therapy, several criteria have been accepted as contraindications (Table 32.3). The use of micropuncture needles and small catheters may decrease the risk of bleeding complications. Monitoring of laboratory values, such as fibrinogen level, have been of no value in predicting which patients are at increased risk of bleeding (241). In the presence of hemorrhage, heparin and thrombolytic agent should be discontinued. If necessary, thrombolytic agents can be reversed with cryoprecipitate, fresh frozen plasma, tranexamic acid, aminocaproic acid, or aprotinin. These interventions are rarely necessary, as most thrombolytic agents have short half-lives in the range of minutes.

Table 32.3 Contraindications to thrombolytic therapy

Absolute Contraindications
Stroke or transient ischemic attack within the past 2 months
Gastrointestinal bleeding within the past 10 days
Neurosurgery or intracranial trauma within the past 3 months
Relatively Major Contraindications
Cardiopulmonary resuscitation within the past 10 days
Major nonvascular surgery or trauma within the past 10 days
Uncontrolled hypertension
Intracranial tumor
Recent eye surgery

VENOUS INTERVENTIONS

Vena cava filters

Technical Complications

Complications during placement of an inferior vena cava (IVC) filter are rare. Problems can include bleeding, embolism, inability to insert the device, misplacement, migration, and guidewire entrapment. Embolism is a rare occurrence, but it can occur if the device is inserted through deep venous thrombosis. If it is suspected that thrombus is lining the IVC or involves both of the iliac veins, an alternative approach places the filter through the internal jugular vein. Occasionally, IVC filter placement is hindered by difficulty in passing the filter through the iliac venous system. This problem is particularly difficult for the left iliac venous system. With newer delivery systems that provide a lower profile and increased flexibility, this complication is rare.

Acute migration of IVC filters occurs when there is lack of apposition to the caval wall with cranial displacement. Possible mechanisms for this complication include the deployment of the filter into thrombus, preventing the limb from attaching to the caval wall or placement in an IVC that is larger than the filter (242). Few IVC filters are approved for placement in vena cavas >28 mm, making this an important anatomic characteristic to identify. Filter migration (movement of >10 mm) has been described in 30% to 76% of filter placements (243). Improved stent designs have lowered this risk to between 3% and 10%. In some instances, the device fails to open at the time of release. This phenomenon has been described in 2% to 42% of cases, depending on the brand of filter used (242,244). Migrated filters can occasionally be left in place, or they may be snared and removed through a large sheath, often requiring a vein cutdown for complete removal.

Postdeployment Complications

Excessive tilt of a filter is another potential complication. Failure to adequately locate the renal veins prior to placement increases the risk of this complication as filter struts lodged in the orifice of a branching vein will offset the filter's alignment. Excessive filter tilting increases the risk of subsequent pulmonary embolism (245). If a filter is tilted by >14 degrees, a second filter should be placed above the level of the initial filter.

Recurrent pulmonary embolism is one of the most serious complications of filter placement, reported in 2% to 5% of Greenfield filters (242). This complication is most often seen in patients who have a malignancy and remain with a hypercoagulable state. In 1% to 2% of patients, the filter traps a massive thrombus, filling the volume of the filter with clot and leading to IVC occlusion. These patients can present with evidence of acute caval occlusion and subsequent decreased cardiac preload. Affected patients will have hypotension and lower extremity swelling. These cases can be distinguished from recurrent acute PE, as that may present with hypotension but will have increased jugular distension. Cavography can confirm the diagnosis, and thrombolytic therapy may be used to restore patency. If the patient is asymptomatic, no intervention is required, as most clots will lyse spontaneously (242).

Full-thickness erosion of filter struts is seen infrequently. This problem may be caused by an inflammatory response of the caval wall to the struts. Rates of strut perforation are surprisingly high and have been reported in 30% to 95% of filters (243). Most cases of perforation remain asymptomatic, but erosion into surrounding structures has been described (246). These structures have included the duodenum and aorta and have resulted in ulceration, hemorrhage, arteriovenous fistula, and heart failure. These serious complications require surgical intervention.

Venous angioplasty and stenting

Technical complications during venous PTA and stent placement are rare. In a large series of patients treated for chronic venous insufficiency, no technical complications occurred and all lesions were technically successfully treated (247). Forty-four of 304 limbs treated, however, required reintervention in the follow-up period due to symptomatic restenosis. Primary patency of these stents at 24 months was 71%, with an assisted patency rate of 97%. No deaths were associated with this procedure, nor were any deaths evident in the follow-up period. Patency rates are lower in those venous segments that required recanalization due to complete occlusion (248). Patients treated for the May—Thurner syndrome have similarly negligible complication rates and comparable patency rates (249). Complications associated with stenting of the superior vena cava in the superior vena cava syndrome have been described in case reports and in one instance was associated with cardiac tamponade.

Endovascular therapy for pulmonary embolism

Technical Failure

The most common complication in endovascular treatment of pulmonary embolism is failure to resolve the thromboembolus. Technical failures occur in 5% to 39% of cases. Most reports indicate that the success of endovascular therapy is directly related to the age of the pulmonary embolism. Greenfield et al. noted that embolectomy success was highest for major pulmonary embolism and massive acute pulmonary embolism (100% and 82% success, respectively) and worst for chronic pulmonary embolism (56% success) (250). In most series, failed procedures occurred in patients who had a history of previous pulmonary embolism, who had elevated pulmonary artery pressure suggestive of chronic pulmonary embolism, or who had chronic thrombus found at the time of pulmonary embolectomy (251). Endovascular therapy for pulmonary embolism is less effective in patients who are >72 hours beyond the initial event and should be performed only in patients with a recent pulmonary embolism and a pulmonary artery pressure <50 mm Hg. Most initial treatment failures require operative thromboembolectomy, or the patients succumb to the hemodynamic compromise induced by the pulmonary embolism. Perforation of the pulmonary artery is a rare occurrence and has only been described twice in the Greenfield series (250). In one instance, the complication was believed to be secondary to the suction pulmonary embolectomy device, and with subsequent modifications, no perforations have been described.

Mortality

Mortality rates mirror treatment failure rates and range from 5% to 28%. Initial problems with cardiac arrest were attributed to large volume contrast bolus injections into the main pulmonary artery (250). Most short-term deaths are secondary to cardiovascular collapse secondary to irreversible right heart failure (250–252). Other causes of death include intracerebral hemorrhage, sepsis, and multisystem organ failure. Survival is directly attributable to the procedure's success. Short-term mortality rates are as high as 73% in patients with failure of thrombus resolution but decrease to 17% with successful treatment (250).

Recurrent Thromboembolism

The incidence of recurrent deep venous thrombosis (4%) and recurrent pulmonary embolism (4%) has been described in only one study (250). These episodes occurred prior to the development of percutaneous placed vena cava filters. The episodes of recurrent pulmonary embolism presented in the interval between pulmonary embolectomy and subsequent vena cava clip placement—which was performed in the operating room as a separate procedure. The placement of a vena cava filter at the time of pulmonary embolectomy, as well as the use of heparin anticoagulation, is beneficial in preventing the risk of recurrent pulmonary embolism.

CONCLUSIONS

Endovascular therapies are becoming more prevalent. Many of the complications that occur are similar among the different interventions. An understanding of the potential adverse events is helpful to the surgeon who is either requesting the intervention or performing it. Most of the complications can be managed in a noninvasive fashion, but when they cannot be, conventional surgery is required.

REFERENCES

1. Hou S, Bushinksy D, Wish J, et al. Hospital-acquired renal insufficiency: a prospective study. *Am J Med* 1983;74:243–248.
2. Murphy S, Barrett B, Parfrey P. Contrast nephropathy. *J Am Soc Nephrol* 2000;11:177–182.
3. Berg K. Nephrotoxicity related to contrast media. *Scand J Urol Nephrol* 2000;34:317–322.
4. Solomon R. Nephrology forum: contrast-medium-induced acute renal failure. *Kidney Int* 1998;53:230–242.
5. Barrett B. Contrast nephropathy. *J Am Soc Nephrol* 1994;5:125–137.
6. Katzberg R. Urography in the 21st century: new contrast media, renal handling, imaging characteristics, and nephrotoxicity. *Radiology* 1997; 204:297–312.
7. Liss P, Nygren A, Olsson U, et al. Effect of contrast media and mannitol on renal medullary blood flow and red cell aggregation in the rat kidney. *Kidney Int* 1996;49:1268–1275.
8. Berg K, Jakobsen J. Nephrotoxicity related to x-ray contrast media. *Adv X-ray Contrast* 1993;1:10–18.
9. Rudnick M, Berns J, Cohen R, et al. Contrast media-associated nephrotoxicity. *Semin Nephrol* 1997;17:15–26.
10. Cantley L, Spokes K, Clark B, et al. Role of endothelin and prostaglandins in radiocontrast-induced renal artery constriction. *Kidney Int* 1993;44: 1217–1223.
11. Bakris G, Burnett J. A role for calcium in radiocontrast-induced reduction in renal hemodynamics. *Kidney Int* 1985;27:465–468.
12. Bakris G, Lass N, Osama Gaber A, et al. Radiocontrast medium-induced decline in renal function: a role for oxygen free radicals. *Am J Physiol* 1990;258:F115–F120.
13. Katholi R, Taylor G, McCann W, et al. Nephrotoxicity from contrast media: attenuation with theophylline. *Radiology* 1995;195:17–22.
14. Rich M, Crecelius C. Incidence, risk factors, and clinical course of acute renal insufficiency after cardiac catheterization in patients 70 years of age or older. *Arch Intern Med* 1995;150:1237–1242.
15. Porter G. Contrast-associated nephropathy. *Am J Cardiol* 1989;64: 22E–26E.
16. Levy E, Viscoli C, Horwitz R. The effect of acute renal failure on mortality: a cohort analysis. *J Am Med Assoc* 1996;275:1489–1494.
17. Rudnick M, Goldfarb S, Wexler L, et al. Nephrotoxicity of ionic and nonionic contrast media in 1196 patients: a randomized trial. *Kidney Int* 1995;47:254–261.
18. Mueller C, Buerkle G, Buettner H. Prevention of contrast media-associated nephropathy: randomized comparison of 2 hydration regimens in 1620 patients undergoing coronary angiography. *Arch Intern Med* 2002;162:329–336.
19. Weisberg L, Kurnik P, Kurnik B. Dopamine and renal blood flow in radiocontrast-induced nephropathy in humans. *Ren Fail* 1993;15:61–68.
20. Abizaid A, Clark C, Mintz G, et al. Effects of dopamine and aminophylline on contrast-induced acute renal failure after coronary angioplasty in patients with preexisting renal insufficiency. *Am J Cardiol* 1999;83:260–263.
21. Tumlin J, Finkel K, Murray P, et al. Fenoldopam mesylate in early acute tubular necrosis: a randomized, double-blind, placebo-controlled clinical trial. *Am J Kidney Dis* 2005;46:26–34.
22. Birck R, Krzossok S, Markowetz F, et al. Acetylcysteine for prevention of contrast nephropathy: meta-analysis. *Lancet* 2003;362:598–603.
23. Briguori C, Airoldi F, D'Andrea D, et al. Renal insufficiency following contrast media administration trial (REMEDIAL). *Circulation* 2007;115: 1211–1217.
24. Koch J, Plum J, Grabensee B, et al. Prostaglandin E1: a new agent for the prevention of renal dysfunction in high risk patients caused by radiocontrast media? *Nephrol Diol Transplant* 2000;15:43–49.
25. Spargias K, Adreanides E, Glamouzis G, et al. Iloprost for prevention of contrast-mediated nephropathy in high-risk patients undergoing a coronary procedure. Results of a randomized pilot study. *Eur J Clin Pharmacol* 2006;62:589–595.
26. Messina L, Brothers T, Wakefield T, et al. Clinical characteristics and surgical management of vascular complications in patients undergoing cardiac catheterization: interventional versus diagnostic procedures. *J Vasc Surg* 1991;13:593–600.
27. Muller D, Podd J, Shamir K, et al. Vascular access site complications in the era of complex percutaneous coronary interventions. *Circulation* 1990;82:510.
28. Young N, Chi K-K, Ajaka J, et al. Complications with outpatient angiography and interventional procedures. *Cardiovasc Intervent Radiol* 2002;25:123–126.
29. Franco C, Goldsmith J, Veith F, et al. Management of arterial injuries produced by percutaneous femoral procedures. *Surgery* 1993;113:419–425.
30. Cragg A, Nakagawa N, Smith T, et al. Hematoma formation after diagnostic angiography: effect of catheter size. *J Vasc Interv Radiol* 1991; 2:231–233.
31. Chitwood R, Shepard A, Shetty P, et al. Surgical complications of transaxillary arteriography: a case-control study. *J Vasc Surg* 1996;23: 844–850.
32. Kresowick T, Khoury M, Miller B, et al. A prospective study of the incidence and natural history of femoral vascular complications after percutaneous transluminal coronary angioplasty. *J Vasc Surg* 1991;13: 328–336.
33. Dowling K, Todd D, Siskin G, et al. Early ambulation after diagnostic angiography using 4-F catheters and sheaths: a feasibility study. *J Endovasc Ther* 2002;9:618–621.
34. Lönn L, Olmarker A, Gertrud K, et al. Treatment of femoral pseudoaneurysm. Percutaneous US-guided thrombin injection versus US-guided compression. *Acta Radiol* 2002;43:396–400.
35. Spies J, Berlin L. Complications of femoral artery puncture. *AJR Am J Roentgenol* 1998;170:9–11.
36. Lilly M, Reichman W, Srazen A, et al. Anatomic and clinical factors associated with complications of transfemoral arteriography. *Ann Vasc Surg* 1990;4:264–269.
37. Altin R, Flicker S, Naidech H. Pseudoaneurysm and arteriovenous fistula after femoral catheterization: association with low femoral punctures. *Am J Radiol* 1989;152:629–631.
38. Rapoport S, Sniderman K, Morse S, et al. Pseudoaneurysm: a complication of faulty technique in femoral arterial puncture. *Radiology* 1985; 154:529–530.
39. Toursarkissian B, Allen B, Petrinec D, et al. Spontaneous closure of selected iatrogenic pseudoaneurysms and arteriovenous fistulae. *J Vasc Surg* 1997;25:803–809.
40. Cox G, Young J, Gray B, et al. Ultrasound-guided compression of postcatheterization pseudoaneurysms: results of treatment in one hundred cases. *J Vasc Surg* 1994;19:683–686.
41. Elford J, Burrell C, Freeman S, et al. Human thrombin injection for the percutaneous treatment of iatrogenic pseudoaneurysms. *Cardiovasc Intervent Radiol* 2002;25:115–118.
42. Waigand J, Uhlich F, Gross M, et al. Percutaneous treatment of pseudoaneurysm and arteriovenous fistulas after invasive vascular procedures. *Catheter Cardiovasc Interv* 1999;47:157–164.
43. Thalhammer C, Kirchherr A, Uhlich F, et al. Postcatheterization pseudoaneurysm and arteriovenous fistulas: repair with percutaneous implantation of endovascular covered stents. *Radiology* 2000;214: 127–131.
44. Kent K, Mosucci M, Gallagher S, et al. Neuropathy after cardiac catheterization: incidence, clinical patterns, and long-term outcome. *J Vasc Surg* 1994;19:1008–1014.
45. Mills J, Wiedeman J, Robison J, et al. Minimizing mortality and morbidity from iatrogenic arterial injuries: the need for early recognition and prompt repair. *J Vasc Surg* 1986;4:22–27.
46. Tron C, Koning R, Eltchaninoff H, et al. A randomized comparison of a percutaneous suture device versus manual compression for femoral artery hemostasis after PTCA. *J Intervent Cardiol* 2003;16:217–221.
47. Sanborn T, Gibbs H, Brinker J, et al. A multicenter randomized trial comparing a percutaneous collagen hemostasis device with conventional manual compression after diagnostic angiography and angioplasty. *J Am Coll Cardiol* 1993;22:1273–1279.
48. Wetter D, Rickli H, von Smekal A, et al. Early sheath removal after coronary artery interventions with use of a suture-mediated closure device: clinical outcome and results of Doppler US evaluation. *J Vasc Interv Radiol* 2000;11:1033–1037.
49. Michalis L, Rees M, Patsouras D, et al. A prospective randomized trial comparing the safety and efficacy of three commercially available closure devices (Angioseal, Vasoseal and Duett). *Cardiovasc Intervent Radiol* 2002;25:423–429.
50. Kornowski R, Brandes S, Teplitsky I, et al. Safety and efficacy of a 6 French perclose arterial suturing device following percutaneous coronary interventions: a pilot evaluation. *J Invasive Cardiol* 2002;14: 741–745.
51. Sesana M, Vaghetti M, Albiero R, et al. Effectiveness and complications of vascular access closure devices after interventional procedures. *J Invasive Cardiol* 2000;12:395–399.
52. Meyerson S, Feldman T, Desai T, et al. Angiographic access site complications in the era of arterial closure devices. *Vasc Endovasc Ther* 2002;36:137–144.

53. Starnes B, O'Donnell S, Gillespie D, et al. Percutaneous arterial closure in peripheral vascular disease: a prospective randomized evaluation of the Perclose device. *J Vasc Surg* 2003;38:263–271.
54. Dangas G, Mehran R, Kokolis S, et al. Vascular complications after percutaneous coronary interventions following hemostasis with manual compression versus arteriotomy closure devices. *J Am Coll Cardiol* 2001;38:638–641.
55. Arora N, Matheny M, Sepke C, et al. A propensity analysis of the risk of vascular complications after cardiac catheterization procedures with the use of vascular closure devices. *Am Heart J* 2007;153:606–611.
56. Goyen M, Manz S, Kroger K, et al. Interventional therapy of vascular complications caused by the hemostatic puncture closure device angio-seal. *Catheter Cardiovasc Interv* 2000;49:142–147.
57. Carere R, Webb J, Miyagishima R, et al. Groin complications associated with collagen plug closure of femoral arterial puncture sites in anticoagulated patients. *Catheter Cardiovasc Diag* 1998;43:124–129.
58. Hoffer E, Bloch R. Percutaneous arterial closure device. *J Vasc Interv Radiol* 2003;14:865–885.
59. Goodney P, Chang R, Cronenwett J. A percutaneous arterial closure protocol can decrease complications after endovascular interventions in vascular surgery patients. *J Vasc Surg* 2008;48:1481–1488.
60. Egglin T, O'Moore P, Feinstein A, et al. Complications of peripheral angiography: a new system to identify patients at increased risk. *J Vasc Surg* 1995;22:787–794.
61. Dawson P, Strickland N. Thromboembolic phenomena in clinical angiography: a role of materials and techniques. *J Vasc Interv Radiol* 1991;2:125.
62. Formanek G, Frech R, Amplatz K. Arterial thrombus formation during clinical percutaneous catheterization. *Circulation* 1970;41:833–839.
63. van Andel G. Arterial occlusion following angiography. *Br J Radiol* 1980;53:747–753.
64. Bolasny B, Killen D. Surgical management of arterial injuries secondary to angiography. *Ann Surg* 1971;174:962–964.
65. Fine M, Kapoor W, Falanga V. Cholesterol crystal embolization: a review of 221 cases in the English literature. Angiology 1987;38:769–784.
66. Deschamps P, Leroy D, Mandard J, et al. Cholesterol embolism in the lower limbs. *Br J Dermatol* 1977;97:93–97.
67. Hendricks I, Monti M, Manasse E, et al. Severe cutaneous cholesterol emboli syndrome after coronary angiography. *Eur J Cardiothorac Surg* 1999;15:215–217.
68. Dion J, Gates P, Fox A, et al. Clinical events following neuroangiography: a prospective study. *Stroke* 1987;18:997–1004.
69. Hankey G, Warlow C, Sellar R. Cerebral angiographic risk in mild cerebrovascular disease. *Stroke* 1990;21(2):209–222.
70. Davies K, Humphrey P. Complications of cerebral angiography in patients with symptomatic carotid territory ischemia screened by carotid ultrasound. *J Neurol Neurosurg Psychiatry* 1993;56:967–972.
71. Johnston D, Chapman K, Goldstein L. Low rate of complications of cerebral angiography in routine clinical practice. *Neurology* 2001;57:2012–2014.
72. Theodotou B, Whaley R, Mahaley M. Complications following transfemoral cerebral angiography for cerebral ischemia: report of 159 angiograms and correlation with surgical risk. *Surg Neurol* 1987;28:90–92.
73. Markus H, Loh A, Israel D, et al. Microscopic air embolism during cerebral angiography and strategies for its avoidance. *Lancet* 1993;341:784–787.
74. Woolfenden A, O'Brien M, Schwartzberg R, et al. Diffusion-weighted MRI in transient global amnesia precipitated by cerebral angiography. *Stroke* 1997;28:2311–2314.
75. Bendszus M, Koltzenburg M, Burger R, et al. Silent embolization in diagnostic cerebral angiography and neurointerventional procedures: a prospective study. *Lancet* 1999;354:1594–1597.
76. Wholey MH, Wholey M, Bergeron P, et al. Current global status of carotid stent placement. *Catheter Cardiovasc Diag* 1998;44:1–6.
77. Mas JL, Chatellier GB, Beyssen B, et al. Endarterectomy versus stenting in patients with symptomatic severe carotid stenosis. *N Engl J Med* 2006;355:1660–1671.
78. Faggioli G, Ferri M, Freyrie A, et al. Aortic arch anomalies are associated with increased risk of neurological events in carotid stent procedures. *Eur J Vasc Endovasc Surg* 2007;33:436–441.
79. Roubin G, Yadav S, Vitek J. Carotid stent-supported angioplasty: a neurovascular intervention to prevent stroke. *Am J Cardiol* 1998;78:8–12.
80. Malek A, Higashida R, Phatouros C, et al. Stent angioplasty for cervical carotid artery stenosis in high-risk symptomatic NASCET-ineligible patients. *Stroke* 2000;31:3029–3033.
81. Ross C, Naslund T, Ranval T. Carotid stent-assisted angioplasty: the newest addition to the surgeons' armamentarium in the management of carotid occlusive disease. *Am Surg* 2002;68:967–975.
82. New G, Iyer S, Dietrich E, et al. Safety, efficacy, and durability of carotid artery stenting for restenosis following carotid endarterectomy: a multicenter study. *J Endovasc Ther* 2000;7:345–352.
83. Hobson RI, Lal B, Chaktoura E, et al. Carotid artery stenting: analysis of data for 105 patients at high risk. *J Vasc Surg* 2003;37:1234–1239.
84. Howell M, Krajcer Z, Dougherty K, et al. Correlation of periprocedural systolic blood pressure changes with neurologic events in high-risk carotid stent patients. *J Endovasc Ther* 2002;9:810–816.
85. Schwarten D. Extracranial brachiocephalic angioplasty. In: Baum S, Pentecost M, eds. *Abram's angiography: interventional radiology*. Boston, MA: Brown and Company; 1997:339–355.
86. Castriota F, Cremonesi A, Manetti R, et al. Impact of cerebral protection devices on early outcome of carotid stenting. *J Endovasc Ther* 2002;9:786–792.
87. Wilentz J, Chati Z, Krafft V, et al. Retinal embolization during carotid angioplasty and stenting: mechanisms and role of cerebral protection systems. *Catheter Cardiovasc Diagn* 2002;56:320–327.
88. Macdonald S, McKevitt F, Venables G, et al. Neurologic outcomes after carotid stenting protected with NeuroShield filter compared to unprotected stenting. *J Endovasc Ther* 2002;9:777–785.
89. Martin J-B, Pache J-C, Treggiari-Venzi M, et al. Role of the distal balloon protection technique in the prevention of cerebral embolic event during carotid stent placement. *Stroke* 2001;32:479–484.
90. Rapp J, Wakil L, Sawhney R, et al. Subclinical embolization after carotid artery stenting: new lesions on diffusion-weighted magnetic resonance imaging occur postprocedure. *J Vasc Surg* 2007;45:867–872.
91. Cremonesi A, Manetti R, Setacci F, et al. Protected carotid stenting: clinical advantages and complications of embolic protection devices in 442 consecutive patients. *Stroke* 2003;34:1936–1943.
92. Chaer R, Trocciola S, DeRubertis B, et al. Cerebral ischemia associated with PercuSurge balloon occlusion balloon during carotid stenting: incidence and possible mechanisms. *J Vasc Surg* 2006;43:946–952.
93. Parodi J, Ferreira LM, Sicard G, et al. Cerebral protection during carotid stenting using flow reversal. *J Vasc Surg* 2005;41:416–422.
94. Eskandari M. Preventable complications of carotid stenting. *Perspect Vasc Surg Endovasc Ther* 2008;20(1):17–25.
95. Ohki T, Veith F, Grenell S, et al. Initial experience with cerebral protection devices to prevent embolization during carotid stenting. *J Vasc Surg* 2002;36:1175–1185.
96. Hobson RI, Howard V, Roubin G, et al. Carotid artery stenting is associated with increased complications in octogenarians: 30 day stroke and death rates in the CREST lead in phase. *J Vasc Surg* 2004;40:1106–1111.
97. Dangas G, Laird JR, Satler LF, et al. Postprocedural hypotension after carotid artery stent placement: predictors and short- and long-term clinical outcomes. *Radiology* 2000;190:691–695.
98. Qureshi AI, Luft AR, Sharma M. Frequency and determinants of postprocedural hemodynamic instability after carotid angioplasty and stenting. *Stroke* 1999;30:2086–2093.
99. Yadav J, Roubin G, Iyer S, et al. Elective stenting of the extracranial carotid arteries. *Circulation* 1997;95:376–381.
100. Bergeron P, Becquemin J-P, Jausseran J-M, et al. Percutaneous stenting of the internal carotid artery: the European CAST-1 study. *J Endovasc Surg* 1999;6:155–159.
101. Henry M, Amor M, Masson I, et al. Angioplasty and stenting of the extracranial carotid arteries. *J Endovasc Surg* 1998;5:293–304.
102. Al-Mubarak N, Roubin G, Gomez C, et al. Carotid artery stenting in patients with high neurologic risks. *Am J Cardiol* 1999;83:1411–1413.
103. Willfort-Ehringer A, Ahmadi R, Gschwadtner M, et al. Single-center experience with carotid stent restenosis. *J Endovasc Ther* 2002;9:299–307.
104. Lal B, Hobson RI, Goldstein J, et al. In-stent recurrent stenosis after carotid artery stenting: life table analysis and clinical relevance. *J Vasc Surg* 2003;38:1162–1169.
105. Becker G, Palmaz J, Rees C, et al. Angioplasty-induced dissections in human iliac arteries: management with Palmaz balloon-expandable intraluminal stents. *Radiology* 1990;176:31–38.
106. Bendok B, Roubin G, Katzen B, et al. Cutting balloon to treat carotid in-stent stenosis: technical note. *J Invasive Cardiol* 2003;15:227–232.

107. Rodriguez-Lopez J, Werner A, Martinez R, et al. Stenting for atherosclerotic occlusive disease of the subclavian artery. *Ann Vasc Surg* 1999;13:254–260.
108. Ringelstein E, Zeumer H. Delayed reversal of vertebral artery blood flow following percutaneous transluminal angioplasty for subclavian steal syndrome. *Neuroradiology* 1984;26:189–198.
109. Sullivan T, Gray B, Bacharach J, et al. Angioplasty and primary stenting of the subclavian, innominate, and common carotid arteries in 83 patients. *J Vasc Surg* 1998;28:1059–1065.
110. Queral L, Criado F. The treatment of focal aortic arch branch lesions with Palmaz stents. *J Vasc Surg* 1996;23:368–375.
111. Al-Mubarak N, Liu M, Dean L, et al. Immediate and late outcomes of subclavian artery stenting. *Catheter Cardiovasc Interv* 1999;46:169–172.
112. Lin P, Bush R, Weiss V, et al. Subclavian artery disruption resulting from endovascular intervention: treatment options. *J Vasc Surg* 2000; 32:607–611.
113. Xenos E, Freeman M, Stevens S, et al. Covered stents for injuries of subclavian and axillary arteries. *J Vasc Surg* 2003;38:451–454.
114. Malek A, Higashida R, Reilly L, et al. Subclavian arteritis and pseudoaneurysm formation secondary to stent infection. *Cardiovasc Intervent Radiol* 2000;23:57–60.
115. Hadjipetrou P, Cox S, Piemonte T, et al. Percutaneous revascularization of atherosclerotic obstruction of aortic arch vessels. *J Am Coll Cardiol* 1999;33:1238–1245.
116. Schillinger M, Haumer M, Schillenger S, et al. Risk stratification for subclavian artery angioplasty: is there an increased rate of restenosis after stent implantation? *J Endovasc Ther* 2001;8:550–557.
117. Korner M, Baumgartner I, Do D, et al. PTA of the subclavian and innominate arteries: long-term results. *Vasa* 1999;28:117–122.
118. Tegtmeyer C, Hartwell G, Selby J, et al. Results and complications of angioplasty in aortoiliac disease. *Circulation* 1991;83:I53–I60.
119. Belli A, Cumberland D, Knox A, et al. Results and complications of angioplasty in aortoiliac disease. *Clin Radiol* 1990;41:380–383.
120. Al-Hamali S, Baskerville P, Fraser S, et al. Detection of distal emboli in patients with peripheral arterial stenosis before and after iliac angioplasty: a prospective study. *J Vasc Surg* 1999;29:345–351.
121. Gardiner GA Jr, Meyerovitz M, Stokes K, et al. Complications of transluminal angioplasty. *Radiology* 1986;159:201–208.
122. Ballard J, Sparks S, Taylor F, et al. Complications of iliac artery stent deployment. *J Vasc Surg* 1996;24:545–555.
123. Palmaz J, Laborde J, Rivera F, et al. Stenting of the iliac arteries with the Palmaz stent: experience from a multicenter trial. *Cardiovasc Intervent Radiol* 1992;15:291–297.
124. Allaire E, Melliere D, Poussier B, et al. Iliac artery rupture during balloon dilatation: what treatment? *Ann Vasc Surg* 2003;17:306–314.
125. Trost D, Jagust M, Weiss M, et al. Percutaneous puncture of nondeflating angioplasty balloons. *J Vasc Interv Radiol* 1999;10:924–926.
126. Parham W, Puri S, Bitar S, et al. Management of iliac stent movement complicating peripheral vascular intervention: a rescue technique when stent deployment malfunctions. *J Invasive Cardiol* 2003;15:277–279.
127. Bunt T, Gill H, Smith D, et al. Infection of a chronically implanted iliac artery stent. *Ann Vasc Surg* 1997;11:529–532.
128. Deiparine M, Ballard J, Taylor F, et al. Endovascular stent infection. *J Vasc Surg* 1996;23:529–533.
129. Therasse E, Soulez G, Cartier P, et al. Infection with fatal outcome after endovascular metallic stent. *Radiology* 1994;192:363–365.
130. Palmaz J. Intravascular stents: tissue—stent interaction and design consideration. *Am J Roentgenol* 1993;160:613–618.
131. Johnston K, Rae M, Hogg-Johnston S, et al. 5-Year results of a prospective study of percutaneous transluminal angioplasty. *Ann Surg* 1987;206: 403–413.
132. Yasuhara H, Shigematsu H, Muto T. Risk factors for restenosis after balloon angioplasty in focal iliac stenosis. *Surgery* 1998;123:658–665.
133. Bosch J, Hunink M. Meta-analysis of the results of percutaneous transluminal angioplasty and stent placement for aortoiliac occlusive disease. *Radiology* 1997;204:87–96.
134. Leville C, Kashyap V, Clair D, et al. Endovascular management of iliac artery occlusions: extending treatment to TransAtlantic Inter-Society Consensus class C and D patients. *J Vasc Surg* 2006;43:32–39.
135. Timaran C, Stevens S, Freeman M, et al. Predictors for adverse outcome after iliac angioplasty and stenting for limb-threatening ischemia. *J Vasc Surg* 2002;36:507–513.
136. Vorwerk D, Guenther R, Schurmann K, et al. Late reobstruction in iliac arterial stents: percutaneous treatment. *Radiology* 1995;197: 479–483.
137. Schillinger M, Exner M, Mlekusch W, et al. Fibrinogen predicts restenosis after endovascular treatment of the iliac arteries. *Thromb Haemost* 2002;87:959–965.
138. Murphy K, Encarnacion C, Le V, et al. Iliac artery stent placement with the Palmaz stent: follow-up study. *J Vasc Interv Radiol* 1995;6: 321–329.
139. Zarins C, White R, Schwarten D, et al. AneuRx stent graft versus open surgical repair of abdominal aortic aneurysms: multicenter prospective clinical trial. *J Vasc Surg* 1999;29:292–305.
140. May J, White G, Waugh R, et al. Improved survival after endoluminal repair with second-generation prostheses compared with open repair in the treatment of abdominal aortic aneurysms: a 5-year concurrent comparison using life table method. *J Vasc Surg* 2001;33:S21–S26.
141. Lee W, O'Dorisio J, Wolf Y, et al. Outcome after unilateral hypogastric artery occlusion during endovascular aneurysm repair. *J Vasc Surg* 2001;33:921–926.
142. Wolpert L, Dittrich K, Hallisey M, et al. Hypogastric artery embolization in endovascular abdominal aortic aneurysm repair. *J Vasc Surg* 2001;33:1193–1198.
143. Criado F, Wilson E, Velazquez O, et al. Safety of coil embolization of the internal iliac artery in endovascular grafting of abdominal aortic aneurysms. *J Vasc Surg* 2000;32:684–688.
144. Schoder M, Zaunbauer L, Holzenbein T, et al. Internal iliac artery embolization before endovascular repair of abdominal aortic aneurysms: frequency, efficacy, and clinical results. *Am J Radiol* 2001;177: 599–605.
145. Mehta M, Veith F, Ohki T, et al. Unilateral and bilateral hypogastric artery interruption during aortoiliac aneurysm repair in 154 patients: a relatively innocuous procedure. *J Vasc Surg* 2001;33:S27–S32.
146. Kritpracha B, Pigott J, Price C, et al. Distal internal iliac artery embolization: a procedure to avoid. *J Vasc Surg* 2003;37:943–948.
147. Wyers M, Shermerhorn M, Fillinger M, et al. Internal iliac occlusion without coil embolization during endovascular abdominal aortic aneurysm repair. *J Vasc Surg* 2002;36:1138–1145.
148. White G, Yu W, May J. Endoleak: a proposed new terminology to describe incomplete aneurysm exclusion by an endoluminal graft. *J Endovasc Surg* 1996;3:124–125.
149. White G, May J, Waugh R, et al. Type I and type II endoleaks: a more useful classification for reporting results of endoluminal AAA repair. *J Endovasc Surg* 1998;5:189–191.
150. White G, May J, Waugh R, et al. Type III and type IV endoleaks: toward a complete definition of blood flow in the sac after endoluminal AAA repair. *J Endovasc Surg* 1998;5:305–309.
151. Ouriel K, Greenberg R, Clair D. Endovascular treatment of aortic aneurysm. *Curr Probl Surg* 2002;39:233.
152. Zarins C, White R, Hodgson K, et al. Endoleak as a predictor of outcome after endovascular aneurysm repair: AneuRx multicenter clinical trial. J Vasc Surg 2000;32:90–107.
153. Holzenbein T, Kretschmer G, Thurnher S, et al. Midterm durability of abdominal aortic aneurysm endograft repair: a word of caution. *J Vasc Surg* 2001;33:S46–S54.
154. Buth J, Harris P, van Marrewijk C, et al. The significance and management of different types of endoleaks. *Semin Vasc Surg* 2003;16:95–102.
155. Chuter T, Faruqi R, Sawhney R, et al. Endoleak after endovascular repair of abdominal aortic aneurysm. *J Vasc Surg* 2001;34:98–105.
156. Buth J, Laheji R. Early complications and endoleaks after endovascular abdominal aortic aneurysm repair: report of a multicenter study. *J Vasc Surg* 2000;31:134–146.
157. Dattilo J, Brewster D, Fan C-M, et al. Clinical failures of endovascular abdominal aortic aneurysm repair: incidence, causes, and management. *J Vasc Surg* 2002;35:1137–1144.
158. Zarins C. The US AneuRx clinical trial: 6-year clinical update. *J Vasc Surg* 2002;37:904–908.
159. Fairman R, Carpenter J, Baum R, et al. Potential impact of therapeutic warfarin treatment on type II endoleaks and sac shrinkage rates on midterm follow-up examination. *J Vasc Surg* 2002;35:679–685.
160. Baum R, Carpenter J, Cope C, et al. Aneurysm sac pressure measurements after endovascular repair of abdominal aortic aneurysms. *J Vasc Surg* 2001;33:32–41.
161. Jacobs T, Teodorescu V, Morrissey N, et al. The endovascular repair of abdominal aortic aneurysm: an update analysis of structural failure modes of endovascular grafts. *Semin Vasc Surg* 2003;16:103–112.
162. Stelter W, Umscheid T, Ziegler P. Three-year experience with modular stent-graft devices for endovascular AAA treatment. *J Endovasc Surg* 1997;4:362–369.

163. Beebe H, Cronenwett J, Katzen B, et al. Results of an aortic endograft trial: impact of device failure beyond 12 months. *J Vasc Surg* 2001;33: S55–S63.
164. Alimi Y, Chakfe N, Rivoal E, et al. Rupture of an abdominal aortic aneurysm after endovascular graft placement and aneurysm size reduction. *J Vasc Surg* 1998;28:178–183.
165. Riepe G, Heilberger P, Umschield T, et al. Frame dislocation of body middle rings in endovascular stent tube grafts. *J Endovasc Surg* 1999; 17:28–34.
166. Jacobs T, Won J, Graveraux E, et al. Mechanical failure of prosthetic human implants: a 10-year experience with aortic stent graft devices. *J Vasc Surg* 2003;37:16–26.
167. Heintz C, Riepe G, Birken L. Corroded nitinol wires in explanted aortic endografts: an important mechanism of failure? *J Endovasc Ther* 2001;8:248–253.
168. Trepanier C, Tabrizian M, Yahia L, et al. Effect of modification of oxide layer on NiTi stent corrosion resistance. *J Biomed Mater Res B Appl Biomater* 1998;43:433–440.
169. Duerig T, Pelton A, Stöckel D. An overview of nitinol medical applications. *Mater Sci Eng A Struct Mater* 1999;273–275:149–160.
170. Starosvetsky E, Gotman I. Corrosion behavior of titanium nitride coated Ni—Ti shape memory surgical alloy. *Biomaterials* 2001;22: 1853–1859.
171. Fairman R, Baum R, Carpenter J, et al. Limb interventions in patients undergoing treatment with an unsupported bifurcated aortic endograft system: a review of the phase II EVT trial. *J Vasc Surg* 2002;36: 118–126.
172. Carroccio A, Faries P, Morrissey N, et al. Predicting iliac limb occlusion after bifurcated aortic stent grafting: anatomic and device-related causes. *J Vasc Surg* 2002;36:679–684.
173. Baum R, Shetty S, Carpenter J, et al. Limb kinking in supported and unsupported abdominal aortic stent-grafts. *J Vasc Interv Radiol* 2000; 11:1165–1171.
174. Amesur N, Zajko A, Orons P, et al. Endovascular treatment of iliac limb stenoses or occlusion in 31 patients treated with the Ancure endograft. *J Vasc Interv Radiol* 2000;11:421–428.
175. Ohki T, Veith F, Shaw P, et al. Increasing incidence of midterm and long-term complications after endovascular graft repair of abdominal aortic aneurysms: a note of caution based on a 9-year experience. *Ann Surg* 2001;234:323–335.
176. Carpenter J, Neschis D, Fairman R, et al. Failure of endovascular abdominal aortic aneurysm graft limbs. *J Vasc Surg* 2001;33:296–303.
177. Sampram E, Karafa M, Mascha E, et al. Nature, frequency, and predictors of secondary procedures after endovascular repair of abdominal aortic aneurysm. *J Vasc Surg* 2003;37:930–937.
178. Cao P, Verzini F, Zannetti S, et al. Device migration after endoluminal abdominal aortic aneurysm repair: analysis of 113 cases with a minimum follow-up period of 2 years. *J Vasc Surg* 2002;35:229–235.
179. Lawrence-Brown M, Semmens J, Hartley D, et al. How is durability related to patient selection and graft design with endoluminal grafting for abdominal aortic aneurysm? In: Greenlaugh R, ed. *The durability of vascular and endovascular surgery*. London: WB Saunders; 1999: 375–385.
180. Resch T, Malina M, Lindblad B, et al. The impact of stent design on proximal stent-graft fixation in the abdominal aorta: an experimental study. *Eur J Vasc Endovasc Surg* 2000;20:190–195.
181. Albertini J-N, Kalliafas S, Travis S, et al. Anatomical risk factors for proximal perigraft endoleak and graft migration following endovascular repair of abdominal aortic aneurysms. *Eur J Vasc Endovasc Surg* 2000;19:308–312.
182. Resch T, Ivancev K, Brunkwall J, et al. Distal migration of stent-grafts after endovascular repair of abdominal aortic aneurysms. *J Vasc Interv Radiol* 1997;10:257–264.
183. Harris P, Brennan J, Martin J, et al. Longitudinal aneurysm shrinkage following endovascular aortic aneurysm repair: a source of intermediate and late complications. *J Endovasc Surg* 1999;6:11–16.
184. White G, May J, Waugh R, et al. Shortening of endografts during deployment in endovascular AAA repair. *J Endovasc Ther* 1999;6:4–10.
185. Prinssen M, Wever J, Mali W, et al. Concerns for the durability of the proximal abdominal aortic aneurysm endograft fixation from a 2-year and 3-year longitudinal computed tomography angiography study. *J Vasc Surg* 2001;33:S64–S69.
186. Badran M, Gould D, Raza I, et al. Aneurysm neck diameter after endovascular repair of abdominal aortic aneurysms. *J Vasc Interv Radiol* 2002;13:887–892.
187. Lee J, Lee J, Aziz I, et al. Stent-graft migration following endovascular repair of aneurysms with large proximal necks: anatomical risk factors and long-term sequelae. *J Endovasc Ther* 2002;9:652–664.
188. Naslund T, Edwards W, Neuzil D, et al. Technical complications of endovascular abdominal aortic aneurysm repair. *J Vasc Surg* 1997;26: 502–510.
189. Fairman R, Velazquez O, Baum R, et al. Endovascular repair of aortic aneurysms: critical events and adjunctive procedures. *J Vasc Surg* 2001;33:1226–1232.
190. Moore W, Matsumura J, Makaroun M, et al. Five-year interim comparison of the Guidant bifurcated endograft with open repair of abdominal aortic aneurysm. *J Vasc Surg* 2003;38:46–55.
191. Becker G, Kovacs M, Mathison M, et al. Risk stratification and outcomes of transluminal endografting for abdominal aortic aneurysm: 7-year experience and long-term follow-up. *J Vasc Interv Radiol* 2003;12:1033–1046.
192. Laheji R, Buth J, Harris P, et al. Need for secondary interventions after endovascular repair of abdominal aortic aneurysms. Intermediate-term follow-up results of a European collaborative registry (EUROSTAR). *Br J Surg* 2000;87:1666–1673.
193. Ouriel K, Clair D, Greenberg R, et al. Endovascular repair of abdominal aortic aneurysms: device-specific outcome. *J Vasc Surg* 2003;37: 991–998.
194. EVAR Trial Participants. Endovascular aneurysm repair versus open repair in patients with abdominal aortic aneurysm (EVAR trial 1): randomised controlled trial. *Lancet* 2005;365:2179–2186.
195. Blankensteijn J, de Jong S, Prinssen M, et al. Two-year outcomes after conventional or endovascular repair of abdominal aortic aneurysms. *N Engl J Med* 2005;352:2398–2405.
196. Criado F, Abul-Khoudoud O, Domer G, et al. Endovascular repair of the thoracic aorta: lessons learned. *Ann Thorac Surg* 2005;80:857–863.
197. Makaroun M, Dillavou E, Wheatley G, et al. Gore TAG Investigators: Five-year results of endovascular treatment with the Gore TAG device compared with open repair of thoracic aortic aneurysms. *J Vasc Surg* 2008;47:912–918.
198. Greenberg R, Lu Q, Roselli E, et al. Contemporary analysis of descending thoracic and thoracoabdominal aneurysm repair. A comparison of endovascular and open techniques. *Circulation* 2008;118: 808–817.
199. Matsumura J, Cambria R, Dake M, et al. International controlled clinical trial of thoracic endovascular aneurysm repair with the Zenith TX2 endovascular graft: 1-year results. *J Vasc Surg* 2008;47:247–257.
200. Fairman R, Farber M, Kwolek C, et al. Pivotal results of the Medtronic Vascular Talent Thoracic Stent Graft System for patients with thoracic aortic disease: the VALOR trial. *J Vasc Surg* 2008;48:546–554.
201. Morales J, Greenberg R, Morales C, et al. Thoracic aortic lesions treated with Zenith TX1 and TX2 thoracic devices: intermediate and long-term outcomes. *J Vasc Surg* 2008;48:54–63.
202. Chaer R, Makaroun M. Late failure after endovascular repair of descending thoracic aneurysms. *Sem Vasc Surg* 2009;22:81–86.
203. Matsumoto A, Angle J, Spinosa D, et al. Percutaneous transluminal angioplasty and stenting in the treatment of chronic mesenteric ischemia: results and longterm followup. *J Am Coll Surg* 2002;194(1, Suppl):S22–S31.
204. Steinmetz E, Tatou E, Favier-Blavoux C, et al. Endovascular treatment as first choice in chronic intestinal ischemia. *Ann Vasc Surg* 2002;16:693–699.
205. Sharafuddin M, Olson C, Sun S, et al. Endovascular treatment of celiac and mesenteric arteries stenoses: application and results. *J Vasc Surg* 2003;38:692–698.
206. Kasirajan K, Dolmatch B, Ouriel K, et al. Delayed onset of ascending paralysis after thoracic aortic stent graft deployment. *J Vasc Surg* 2000; 38:692–698.
207. Sheeran S, Murphy T, Khwaja A, et al. Stent placement for treatment of mesenteric artery stenoses or occlusions. *J Vasc Interv Radiol* 1999; 10:861–867.
208. Ivanovic V, McKusick M, Johnson CI, et al. Renal artery stent placement: complications at a single tertiary care center. *J Vasc Interv Radiol* 2003;14:217–225.
209. Bush R, Najibi S, MacDonald J, et al. Endovascular revascularization of renal artery stenosis: technical and clinical results. *J Vasc Surg* 2001; 33:1041–1049.
210. Bakker J, Goffette P, Henry M, et al. The Erasme study: a multicenter study on the safety and technical results of the Palmaz stent used for the treatment of atherosclerotic ostial renal artery stenosis. *Cardiovasc Intervent Radiol* 1999;22:468–474.

211. DeMaioribus C, Anderson C, Popham S, et al. Mycotic renal artery degeneration and systemic sepsis caused by infected renal artery stent. *J Vasc Surg* 1998;28:547–550.
212. Deitch J, Hansen K, Regan J, et al. Infected renal artery pseudoaneurysm and mycotic aortic aneurysm after percutaneous transluminal renal artery angioplasty and stent placement in a patient with a solitary kidney. *J Vasc Surg* 1998;28:340–344.
213. Bukhari R, Muck P, Schlueter F, et al. Bilateral renal artery stent infection and pseudoaneurysm formation. *J Vasc Interv Radiol* 2000;11:337–341.
214. Henry M, Amor M, Henry I, et al. Stents in the treatment of renal artery stenosis: long-term follow-up. *J Endovasc Surg* 1999;6:42–51.
215. Tullis M, Zierler R, Glickerman D, et al. Results of percutaneous transluminal angioplasty for atherosclerotic renal artery stenosis: a follow-up study with duplex ultrasonography. *J Vasc Surg* 1997;25:46–54.
216. Kashyap V, Sepulveda R, Bena J, et al. The management of renal artery atherosclerosis for renal salvage: does stenting help? *J Vasc Surg* 2007;45:101–109.
217. Hunink M, Donaldson M, Meyerovitz M, et al. Risks and benefits of femoropopliteal percutaneous balloon angioplasty. *J Vasc Surg* 1993;17: 183–194.
218. Stanley B, Teague B, Raptis S, et al. Efficacy of balloon angioplasty of the superficial femoral artery and popliteal artery in the relief of leg ischemia. *J Vasc Surg* 1996;23:679–685.
219. Golledge J, Ferguson K, Ellis M, et al. Outcomes of femoropopliteal angioplasty. *Ann Surg* 1999;229:146–153.
220. Johnston K. Femoral and popliteal arteries: reanalysis of results of balloon angioplasty. *Radiology* 1992;183:767–771.
221. Bolia A, Miles K, Brennan J, et al. Percutaneous transluminal angioplasty of occlusions of the femoral and popliteal arteries by subintimal dissection. *Cardiovasc Intervent Radiol* 1990;13:357–364.
222. Werner G, Ferrari M, Figulla H. Superficial femoral artery rupture after balloon angioplasty: treatment with implantation of a balloon-expandable graft. *J Vasc Interv Radiol* 1999;10:1115–1117.
223. Cheng S, Ting A, Wong J. Endovascular stenting of superficial femoral artery stenosis and occlusions: results and risk factor analysis. *Cardiovasc Surg* 2001;9:133–140.
224. Gordon I, Conroy R, Arefi M, et al. Three-year outcome of endovascular treatment of superficial femoral artery occlusion. *Arch Surg* 2001;136: 221–228.
225. Strecker E, Boos I, Gottman D. Femoropopliteal artery stent placement: evaluation of long-term success. *Radiology* 1997;205:375–383.
226. Matsi P, Manninen H, Vanninen R, et al. Femoropopliteal angioplasty in patients with claudication: primary and secondary patency in 140 limbs with 1–3-year follow up. *Radiology* 1994;191:727–733.
227. Matsi P, Manninen H, Soder H, et al. Percutaneous transluminal angioplasty in femoral artery occlusions: primary and long-term results in 107 claudicant patients using femoral and popliteal catheterization techniques. *Clin Radiol* 1995;50:237–244.
228. Lofberg A, Karacagil S, Ljungman C, et al. Percutaneous transluminal angioplasty of the femoropopliteal arteries in limbs with chronic lower limb ischemia. *J Vasc Surg* 2001;34:114–121.
229. van Lankeren W, Gussenhoven E, van Kints M, et al. Stent remodeling contributes to femoropopliteal artery restenosis: an intravascular ultrasound study. *J Vasc Surg* 1997;25:753–756.
230. Saxon R, Coffman J, Gooding J, et al. Long-term results of ePTFE stent-graft versus angioplasty in the femoropopliteal artery: single center experience from a prospective, randomized trial. *J Vasc Interv Radiol* 2003;14:303–311.
231. Duda S, Bosiers M, Pusich B, et al. Endovascular treatment of peripheral artery disease with expanded PTFE-covered nitinol stents: interim analysis from a prospective controlled study. *Cardiovasc Intervent Radiol* 2002;25:413–418.
232. Zeller T, Rastan A, Schwarzwalder U, et al. Percutaneous peripheral atherectomy of femoropoliteal stenoses using a new-generation device: six-month results from a single-center experience. *J Endovasc Ther* 2004;11:676–668.
233. Ramaiah V, Gammon R, Kiesz S, et al. Midterm outcomes from the TALON registry: treating peripherals with SilverHawk: outcomes collection. *J Endovasc Ther* 2006;13:592–602.
234. Conroy R, Gordon I, Tobis J, et al. Angioplasty and stent placement in chronic occlusion of the superficial femoral artery: technique and results. *J Vasc Interv Radiol* 2000;11:1009–1020.
235. Dorros G, Jaff M, Dorros A, et al. Tibioperoneal (outflow lesion) angioplasty can be used as primary treatment in 235 patients with critical limb ischemia: five-year follow up. *Circulation* 2001;104: 2057–2062.
236. Faglia E, Mantero M, Caminiti M, et al. Extensive use of peripheral angioplasty, particularly infrapopliteal, in the treatment of ischaemic diabetic foot ulcers: clinical results of a multicentric study of 221 consecutive diabetic subjects. *J Intern Med* 2002;252:225–232.
237. Giles K, Pomposelli F, Hamdan A, et al. Infrapopliteal angioplasty for critical limb ischemia: relation of TransAtlantic InterSociety Consensus class to outcome in 176 limbs. *J Vasc Surg* 2008;48:128–136.
238. Ouriel K, Gray B, Clair D, et al. Complications associated with the use of urokinase and recombinant tissue plasminogen activator for catheter-directed peripheral arterial and venous thrombolysis. *J Vasc Interv Radiol* 2000;11:295–298.
239. The STILE Investigators. Results of a prospective randomized trial evaluating surgery versus thrombolysis for ischemia of the lower extremity. *Ann Surg* 1994;220:251–268.
240. Ouriel K, Veith F, Sasahara A. A comparison of recombinant urokinase with vascular surgery as initial treatment for acute arterial occlusion of the legs. *N Engl J Med* 1998;338:1105–1111.
241. McNamara T, Goodwin S, Kandarpa K. Complications of thrombolysis. *Semin Interv Radiol* 2000;11:134–144.
242. Greenfield L, Proctor M. Filter complications and their management. *Semin Vasc Surg* 2000;13:213–216.
243. Joels C, Sing R, Haniford B. Complications of inferior vena cava filters. *Am Surg* 2003;69:654–659.
244. Reed R, Teitelbaum G, Taylor F, et al. Incomplete opening of LGM (VenaTech) filters inserted via transjugular approach. *J Vasc Interv Radiol* 1991;2:441–445.
245. Rogers F, Strindberg G, Shackford S, et al. Five-year follow-up of prophylactic vena cava filters in high-risk trauma patients. *Arch Surg* 1998;133:406–412.
246. Campbell J, Calcagno D. Aortic pseudoaneurysm from aortic perforation with a bird's nest vena cava filter. *J Vasc Surg* 2003;38:596–599.
247. Raju S, Owen S, Neglen P. The clinical impact of iliac venous stents in the management of chronic venous insufficiency. *J Vasc Surg* 2002;35: 8–15.
248. Raju S, McAllister S, Neglen P. Recanalization of totally occluded iliac and adjacent venous segments. *J Vasc Surg* 2002;36:903–911.
249. Lamont J, Pearl G, Patetsios P, et al. Prospective evaluation of endoluminal venous stents in the treatment of the May—Thurner syndrome. *Ann Vasc Surg* 2002;16:61–64.
250. Greenfield L, Proctor M, Williams D, et al. Long-term experience with transvenous catheter pulmonary embolectomy. *J Vasc Surg* 1993;18: 450–458.
251. Timsit F, Reynaud P, Meyer G, et al. Pulmonary embolectomy by catheter device in massive pulmonary embolism. *Chest* 1991;100: 655–658.
252. De Gregario M, Gimeno M, Mainar A, et al. Mechanical and enzymatic thrombolysis for massive pulmonary embolism. *J Vasc Interv Radiol* 2002;13:163–169.

PART

V

Complications of Gastrointestinal Surgery

CHAPTER

33

Complications of Gastric Surgery

Michael W. Mulholland

Gastric operations constitute an increasingly large proportion of the general surgical workload. Although the incidences of complicated peptic ulceration and gastric cancer have declined significantly over the past several decades, gastric operations for treatment of morbid obesity have undergone explosive growth. Complications from gastric operations are common and frequently severe.

Nationwide trends for complications of gastric surgery are clearest in how they relate to the treatment of gastric cancer. Epidemiologic studies in the United States demonstrate that gastric cancer has decreased in incidence over the last two decades (1). Despite this reduction in incidence, gastric cancer remains one of the most common causes of cancer-related deaths in the United States, and surgical resection offers the only chance of cure (1–4).

In one recent study, the overall incidence of gastric cancer and subsequent gastric resection was reported to have declined from 1988 to 2000 (5). Use of a nationwide database has shown that the number of patients with a discharge diagnosis of gastric cancer decreased from 25 cases per 100,000 U.S. adults in 1988 to 20 cases per 100,000 in 2000 (Fig. 33.1). These results were mirrored by declining rates of gastric resection, with a 29% decrease from 5.6 cases per 100,000 adults in 1988 to 4.0 cases per 100,000 in 2000 (Fig. 33.1). The overall proportion of hospitalized gastric cancer patients undergoing gastric resection remained constant at approximately 22%.

Gastric resection for cancer has a relatively high rate of postoperative complication and operative mortality. Inpatient mortality did not significantly change over the 1988–2000 timeframe, with an overall mortality rate of 7.4% for the nationwide group. Rates of adverse outcomes were not uniform but varied in relation to hospital experience with the operation. Low volume centers had an 8.3% mortality rate, medium volume hospitals had a 7.1% mortality rate, and high volume centers had a 6.5% mortality rate (Fig. 33.2). The safety of gastric resection improved from 1988 to 2000 at high volume medical centers, with the mortality rate decreasing from 7.1% between 1988 and 1992, to 6.5% between 1993 and 1996, to 5.8% between 1997 and 2000. A decline in mortality was not observed at low or medium volume hospitals.

Michael W. Mulholland: Professor and Chairman, Department of Surgery, University of Michigan Medical School, Ann Arbor, MI

Despite stagnant overall mortality rates, patients are spending less time in the hospital after gastric resection. The decrease in length of stay suggests improved efficiency and better use of resources over time. Shorter hospital stays may also result from the cost-saving efforts of healthcare payers during the same interval (Fig. 33.3).

Laparoscopic approaches to gastric surgery are increasingly common. Laparoscopic gastric bypass has become standard for the surgical treatment of morbid obesity. In adults, laparoscopic gastrectomy for treatment of gastric cancer is practiced in a few specialized centers. Laparoscopic pyloromyotomy for pyloric stenosis has become widespread in pediatric surgical practice. Several studies comparing open and laparoscopic pyloromyotomy have reported comparable complication rates (6–8). A recent meta-analysis comparing these two approaches concluded that perforation and incomplete division of the hypertrophied muscle were more frequent with laparoscopic pyloromyotomy (9). Operative times were similar but time to oral feeding and hospital stay were shorter with the laparoscopic method. Experience is important. In a recent report, a 5.4-fold increased risk of mucosal perforation or incomplete pyloromyotomy was noted when the operation was performed by a general surgery resident as compared to when performed by a more senior pediatric surgery trainee (10).

PEPTIC ULCERATION

Hemorrhage

Although peptic ulcer disease remains a major worldwide health problem, the United States has experienced a decline in both the incidence of uncomplicated ulceration and the rate of hospitalization for complicated disease (11). Bleeding, perforation, and obstruction are the three major complications of peptic ulcer, with bleeding the most common. Despite appreciation of the role of *Helicobacter pylori* infection in peptic ulcer pathogenesis and improvements in therapeutic endoscopy, mortality from bleeding ulcers has remained stable (8% to 10%) over the past 30 years (11–13). Contemporary patients are increasingly elderly and frequently have coexisting illnesses. Advanced age and the existence of concurrent illness are the most important prognostic factors in patients with bleeding peptic ulcers. Patients older than 60 years have a significantly higher mortality than

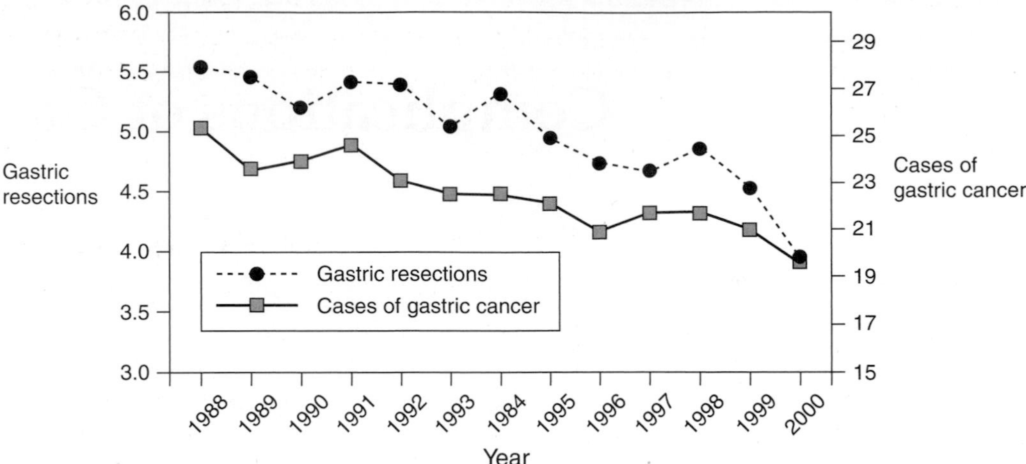

FIGURE 33.1. Incidence of gastric cancer and gastric cancer resection in the United States, per 100,000 adults, from 1988 through 2000.

those younger than 60 years. The presence and number of comorbidities are closely related to mortality (14–18).

Pathogenesis

Infection with the gram-negative bacterium, *H. pylori,* is very strongly linked to the development of peptic ulceration. This infectious association has fundamentally changed the treatment of patients with peptic disease. Although *H. pylori* infection rates have wide geographic variability, the organism is present in as much as 30% to 50% of the population. Most infected individuals remain without symptoms; only 6% to 20% of colonized individuals develop peptic ulcer disease (19). Conversely, *H. pylori* is present in >90% of patients with ulcer disease. Surprisingly, the prevalence of *H. pylori* is 15% to 20% lower in patients with ulcer hemorrhage relative to patients with nonbleeding ulcers (4,20). The significance of this negative correlation is unknown.

Several distinct observations suggest that *H. pylori* is a factor in the pathogenesis of duodenal ulceration. *H. pylori* is the most common cause of chronic active gastritis, characterized by nonerosive inflammation of the gastric mucosa. Antral gastritis is nearly always present in patients with duodenal ulcer; *H. pylori* can be isolated from gastric mucosa in most cases. Gastric metaplasia is very common in the duodenal epithelium surrounding areas of ulceration. Because *H. pylori* binds only to gastric-type epithelium, metaplastic gastric epithelium can be colonized by *H. pylori* from gastric sources. Gastric metaplasia of the duodenal bulb is the means by which antral gastritis with *H. pylori* is converted to active chronic duodenitis. Eradication of *H. pylori* with antimicrobials leads to ulcer healing rates superior to those seen with acid suppressing agents. Relapse of duodenal ulcer after antimicrobial therapy is preceded by reinfection of the gastric mucosa by *H. pylori.*

Helicobacter pylori is the most common bacterial infection worldwide. *H. pylori* infection is usually acquired in childhood and lasts lifelong in the absence of specific therapy. Epidemiologic studies suggest the *H. pylori* infection occurs via person-to-person contact, usually among family

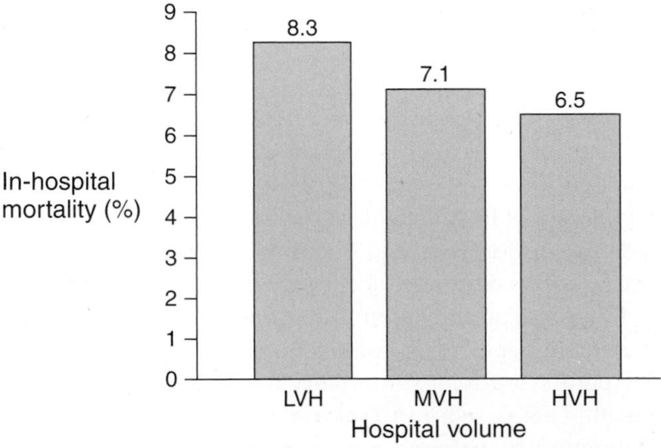

FIGURE 33.2. In-hospital mortality as a function of varying hospital volume. Low hospital volumes are defined as performing four or fewer resections per year. Medium volume hospitals are defined as performing five to eight resections per year. High volume hospitals are defined as performing nine or more resections per year.

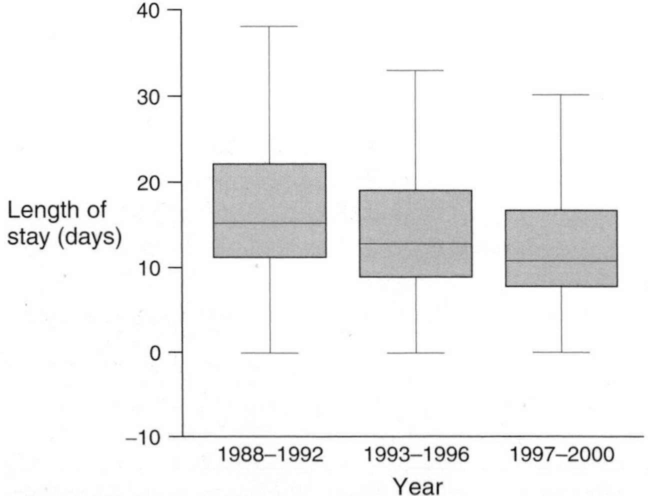

FIGURE 33.3. Length of stay after gastric resection by time period from 1988 through 2000.

members. Transmission is believed to occur during a bout of gastroenteritis; the highest risk is associated with vomiting.

Helicobacter pylori is the only human bacterium known to infect the stomach (21). To avoid the bactericidal activity of the acidic stomach, the organism has evolved mechanisms to move within the gastric environment, to adhere to gastric mucosa, and to abrogate the harmful effects of acid. More than 300 genes of *H. pylori* are regulated by acid.

All strains of *H. pylori* cause persistent infection and all strains induce gastric inflammation.

Bacterial virulence factors including vacuolating cytotoxin A (VacA) and cytotoxin-associated gene A (CagA) are closely associated with the ability of *H. pylori* to cause mucosal damage (22). VacA is a pore-forming cytotoxin of 88 kilodaltons. Upon release from the bacterium, the protein moves to the host cell membrane where it forms a ring structure (22). The ring complex inserts into the membrane of the host cell creating a pore. VacA pores are permeable to anions and small neutral molecules, including urea.

VacA also inserts into endosomal membranes leading to osmotic swelling. Pore formation in mitochondrial membranes induces gastric cell death through apoptosis.

The second major virulence factor in *H. pylori* is CagA. The CagA gene is part of a region of DNA that is termed a pathogenicity island. The genes adjacent to the CagA gene encode proteins that function as microscopic needles for the transfer of bacterial products into host gastric cells.

After CagA protein is transferred to host cells, it becomes phosphorylated on tyrosine residues by host cell kinases. Phosphorylated CagA activates a number of cellular signaling pathways involved in cellular polarity, cytoskeletal protein function, and cellular proliferation and differentiation. Infected gastric cells become more elongated, apical junctions between cells are disrupted, gaps develop between epithelial cells, and epithelial barrier function is lost. Disturbance of cellular function promotes apoptosis, affects epithelia restitution, and may inhibit ulcer healing.

With mucosal colonization, a variety of bacterial and host responses are elicited. *H. pylori* produces the enzyme urease. Urease hydrolyzes urea to produce ammonia, which, in turn, increases luminal pH, thus providing a favorable microenvironment for *H. pylori* survival. Urease production appears to be crucial to the pathogenicity of *H. pylori*; mutants of *H. pylori* that do not produce urease are unable to establish colonization. The bacterium attaches to the gastric epithelium beneath the mucous layer. Following attachment, *H. pylori* causes direct cellular injury and changes gastric secretory physiology.

H. pylori infection produces abnormalities in gastric acid secretion (Table 33.1). Levels of serum gastrin are elevated in patients infected with *H. pylori*. Hypergastrinemia secondary to *H. pylori* infection occurs in response to the cytokines tumor necrosis factor-α and interleukin-8, which are produced in response to mucosal infection. Local secretion of the inhibitory hormone somatostatin is also diminished. The imbalances in gastrin and somatostatin production are manifested clinically as elevated basal and maximal acid outputs. Abnormalities in gastric secretion disappear after *H. pylori* eradication, supporting the idea that infection is the cause of increased acid production (23).

Table 33.1 Gastric secretory responses to *Helicobacter pylori* infection

Acid secretion
Increased basal acid output
Increased maximal acid output
Increased responsiveness to gastrin-releasing peptide
Hormonal
Increased basal gastrin levels
Increased meal induced gastrin release
Decreased acid inhibition by cholecystokinin
Decreased antral distension inhibition of gastrin release
Duodenal bicarbonate secretion
Decreased mucosal bicarbonate secretion

Nonsteroidal anti-inflammatory drugs (NSAIDs) are ubiquitous and have been associated with both gastric and duodenal ulcer diseases. The inhibitory effect of NSAIDs upon prostaglandin production in the gastric mucosa is the cause of NSAID ulcerogenic actions. NSAID use is an important risk factor for ulcer hemorrhage, and NSAIDs significantly increase the risk of bleeding in *H. pylori*–infected individuals (24). Ingestion of NSAIDs is associated with a twofold increase in risk of bleeding in patients who are infected with *H. pylori* relative to patients who are *H. pylori*-negative (17). Only 10% of patients with bleeding ulcers are both *H. pylori*-negative and without a history of NSAID exposure (20).

Endoscopic Treatment

Peptic ulcer disease constitutes a significant proportion of upper gastrointestinal (GI) hemorrhage. A widely variable proportion of patients (20% to 68%) present with melena, while 14% to 30% develop hematemesis and 18% to 50% present with both hematemesis and melena (11,13,25). Initial management is focused on stabilization and then upon diagnosis. Patients should be aggressively resuscitated with intravenous fluids and blood components. Patients presenting with shock, elderly patients (>60 years), and those with recurrent bleeding are at increased risk of death and should be treated in an intensive care unit (14–18). A nasogastric tube should be inserted and the stomach lavaged with warm saline. Lavage is not effective in stopping bleeding; it is performed to allow subsequent endoscopic visualization of the bleeding site. The use of intravenous histamine$_2$-blockers for acute ulcer bleeding has not been shown to be beneficial (11,26,27). Proton pump inhibitors may improve outcomes in patients with bleeding ulcers (28–30). However, these drugs should not be considered the crucial aspect of therapy during the acute episode.

Table 33.2 Endoscopic ulcer appearance and risk of recurrent hemorrhage

Risk	Appearance	Recurrent Bleeding
Low	Clean base Flat spot	0%–15%
High	Adherent clot Nonbleeding visible vessel Active hemorrhage	40%–90%

Upper GI endoscopy, not contrast radiography, is the preferred diagnostic modality for upper GI hemorrhage. Endoscopy can define the nature and site of the bleeding lesion. Endoscopic findings also provide information that predicts the risk of recurrent bleeding (Table 33.2). Endoscopic therapy, performed immediately, defines the nature of the bleeding lesion and is effective in most patients (>80%). When necessary, tissue biopsy can be obtained for histology and for the diagnosis of *H. pylori* infection.

Endoscopy should not be performed until patients have been hemodynamically stabilized. Following resuscitation, endoscopy should be performed emergently in high-risk patients such as the elderly, those with significant blood loss, and patients experiencing rebleeding episodes. Performance of initial endoscopy within 24 hours of the bleeding episode has been associated with improved outcome (31).

The endoscopic appearance of the ulcer bed and ulcer size provide information that predicts the likelihood of rebleeding. Ulcers are categorized on the basis of endoscopic appearances: clean base, flat spot, adherent clot, nonbleeding visible vessel, or active bleeding. Each of these appearances is associated with a defined risk of rebleeding (Table 33.2). Although patients with clean base ulcers have a very low recurrent bleeding rate, those with visible vessels or active bleeding have recurrent bleeding rates of 43% and 55%, respectively (4,32–34). Because of the risk of recurrent hemorrhage associated with these endoscopic findings, patients who have a nonbleeding visible vessel or active bleeding at the time of endoscopy should undergo immediate endoscopic therapy (34). For patients with low risk visual findings, endoscopic therapy is not recommended, as intervention has not been shown to reduce the already low risk of rebleeding (34).

Endoscopic therapy options include thermal coagulation and injection of vessel sclerosants or vasoconstrictor agents. Thermal coagulation involves direct application of heat or electrocoagulation to the bleeding site. The electrocoagulation device or heat probe is passed through the endoscope and positioned so that it overlies the visible bleeding vessel. Initial hemostasis is accomplished by direct vessel compression with coaptation of vessel walls. Energy is applied to produce tissue coagulation.

Endoscopic injection therapy involves injection of solutions into the base of the ulcer, resulting in tamponade, vasoconstriction, and eventual sclerosis of the ulcer bed and surrounding blood vessels. A dilute solution (1:10,000) of epinephrine is most commonly used for this purpose. Other injection agents include polidocanol, ethanol, and thrombin. With either heater probe or injection, the initial success rate is estimated at 75% to 90% (26,34,35). Complications, either immediate bleeding or perforation, have been reported in <1% of cases (11,34).

The major complication of endoscopic therapy is delayed rebleeding, occurring after approximately 10% to 30% of initial endoscopic hemostasis cases (11,25,26,36). Almost all patients who rebleed after endoscopic therapy do so within 96 hours of the initial endoscopic procedure (25). In one report, all fatal rebleeding events occurred within the first 24 hours of the initial bleeding episode (37). High-risk patients include those with hemodynamic instability, comorbid disease, or visible ulcer vessels, and they should be monitored in an intensive care unit. Patients with limited bleeding and low risk findings, such as a clean ulcer base on endoscopy, may be discharged within 24 hours.

Surgery has been the usual treatment in case of failure of endoscopic therapy. Recent data suggest that endoscopic retreatment is also a safe alternative (36). Endoscopic retreatment has a success rate of 50% to 70% in patients who rebleed after initial endoscopic therapy. Endoscopic retreatment must be employed with caution. The perforation rate during endoscopic retreatment is increased, and a significant delay in definitive therapy must not occur for those patients who fail the second attempt at endoscopic hemostasis.

Surgical treatment of rebleeding should be considered for patients who are at highest risk for continued bleeding, including patients with large ulcers and large bleeding vessels, the elderly (>60), patients with active hemorrhage, and patients who develop hypotension. These factors have been associated with failure of endoscopic therapy (14,37,38).

Operative Treatment

Operative therapy is indicated when endoscopic therapy is either not possible or unsuccessful or when bleeding is so rapid that endoscopy is not feasible. Because the indications for surgical therapy are identical to those for endoscopic therapy, a surgeon should be consulted for the care of every patient with upper GI hemorrhage from the outset (Table 33.3). Patient characteristics such as advanced age (>60 years) and the presence of significant comorbid

Table 33.3 Indications for operation in bleeding peptic ulceration

Continuous or recurrent hemorrhage
Ongoing transfusion requirement
Hypotension
Age >60 years with ongoing hemorrhage
Failed endoscopic hemostasis
Ulcer inaccessible to endoscopic therapy

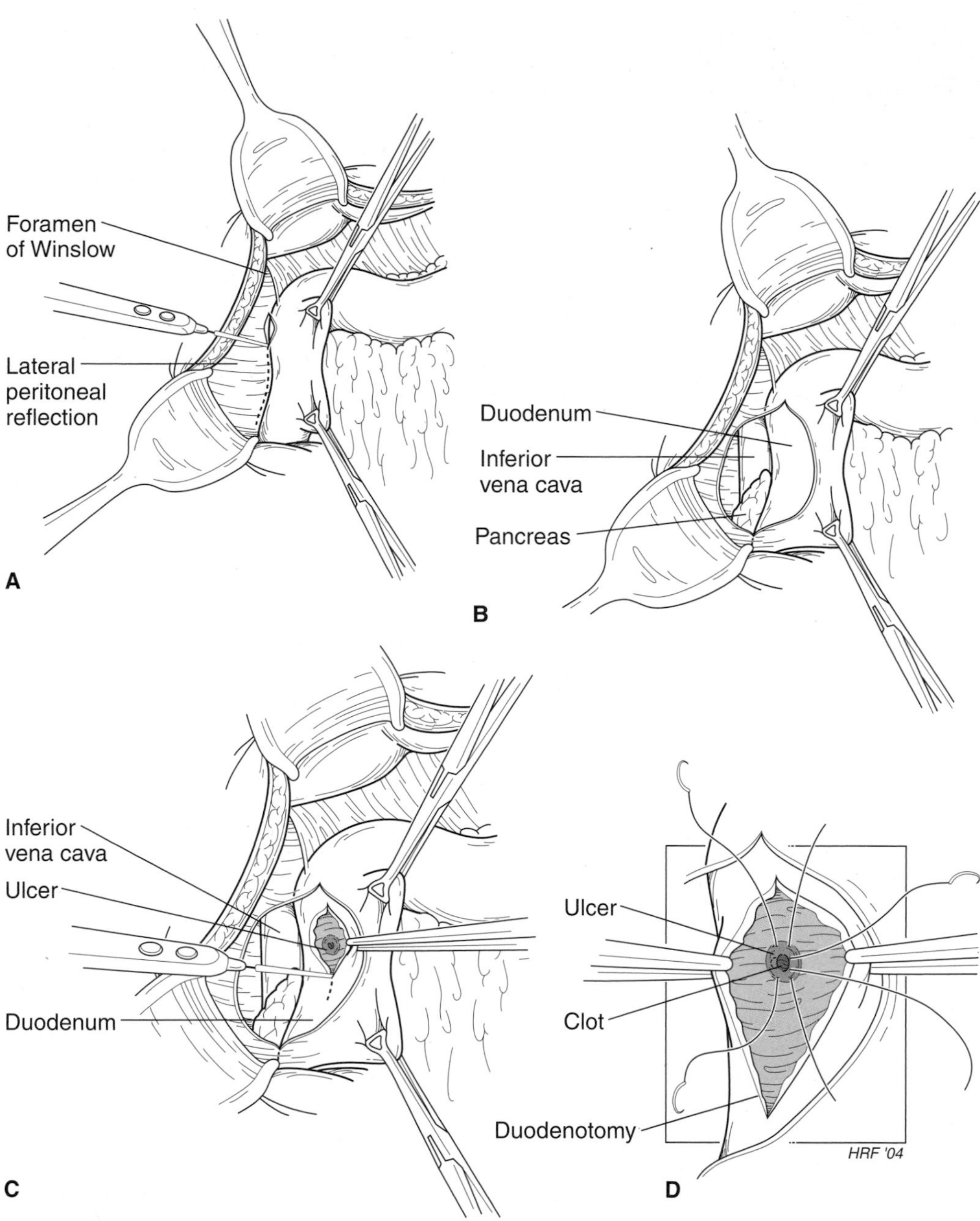

FIGURE 33.4. Operative maneuvers in management of bleeding duodenal ulcer. **A:** The duodenum is mobilized from the retroperitoneum by a Kocher maneuver. **B:** As the duodenum is reflected anteriorly, the retroperitoneal duodenum, the posterior aspect of the pancreatic head, and the inferior vena cava are visualized. **C:** Direct visualization of the ulcer is obtained by a longitudinal duodenotomy. **D:** Circumferential sutures are used to control vessels entering the ulcer base peripherally. Vessels entering perpendicularly are controlled using a U-stitch.

disease predict a superior outcome with early surgery (18,26). Elderly patients or those with cardiovascular compromise cannot sustain repetitive hypotension or the episodic anemia related to delayed surgical therapy.

When surgery is performed for hemorrhage, there are two therapeutic goals. First, the bleeding must be controlled. Second, therapy that minimizes ulcer recurrence should be provided. Direct suture ligature of the ulcer or bleeding site is used to control hemorrhage. When the site of ulcer bleeding is a gastric ulcer, the ulcer should be resected. In addition to hemostasis, ulcer resection provides gastric tissue for histology to evaluate for the presence of gastric cancer. For ulcers located on the lesser curve of the stomach near the gastroesophageal junction, resection may be hazardous and direct suture ligature of the ulcer base is more appropriate, with biopsy to exclude cancer.

For bleeding duodenal ulcers, a Kocher maneuver is first performed to mobilize the duodenum from the retroperitoneum (Fig. 33.4). Through a duodenotomy, the bleeding vessel at the base of the ulcer is visualized and ligated. In placing sutures, care should be taken to avoid the common bile duct as it passes deep to the first and second portions of the duodenum.

After hemostasis is achieved, a decision must be made about the performance of a definitive antiulcer procedure. The surgical literature on this issue predates the current understanding of the pathogenetic role of *H. pylori* in ulcer disease. Currently available but dated literature suggests that the performance of an antiulcer procedure in addition to oversewing the ulcer produces a lower rate of rebleeding compared to oversewing of the ulcer alone. Postoperative morbidity and mortality are reported to be similar (39,40).

Table **33.4** Results of elective operation for peptic ulcer

Procedure	Mortality	Recurrent Ulcer	Dumping
Truncal vagotomy	1%	10%–12%	1%–10%
Proximal gastric vagotomy	0.5%	8%–20%	2%–3%
Truncal vagotomy and antrectomy	1%	1%	10%–20%

However, these studies are flawed in that they do not address the effect of *H. pylori* eradication on bleeding recurrence after surgery.

In the past, vagotomy and pyloroplasty had been recommended in hemodynamically unstable patients when the operative goals need to be achieved expeditiously. When performed electively, operative mortality approximates 1% and ulcer recurrence rates average 10% to 12% (Table 33.4). The incidence of dumping, a syndrome of postprandial flushing and vasomotor effects, ranges from 1% to 10% (41,42). Elective highly selective vagotomy is also associated with low mortality but with somewhat higher recurrence rates of 10% to 15%. In most series, highly selective vagotomy has fewer postoperative symptoms, with an incidence of dumping of <5%. Elective vagotomy and antrectomy is associated with an ulcer recurrence rate of 1% (41,42).

Not surprisingly, surgical results are less salutary when hemorrhage prompts urgent operation. When performed emergently, vagotomy and pyloroplasty has a recurrent bleeding rate of 17%, with a duodenal leak rate of 3%. Vagotomy and gastrectomy has a lower rebleeding rate of 3%, but a significantly higher frequency of duodenal leak at 13%. Rates of reoperations for bleeding and overall mortality are similar for these two procedures (43).

Prevention of recurrent bleeding requires treatment of underlying *H. pylori* infection and discontinuation of NSAIDs. With anti-*H. pylori* therapy and avoidance of NSAIDs, a 95% ulcer cure rate for uncomplicated peptic ulcers has been reported. The combination of omeprazole, amoxicillin, and clarithromycin has been most widely used and is associated with elimination of *H. pylori* in 90% of patients. An alternative regimen combines omeprazole, metronidazole, and either amoxicillin or clarithromycin. When NSAIDs cannot be discontinued, use of the synthetic prostaglandin analog Misoprostol decreases the incidence of recurrent bleeding, especially in the elderly (44,45).

Data from a number of controlled trials are now available, demonstrating that for patients with bleeding as a complication of *H. pylori*-positive ulcers, eradication of infection prevents recurrent ulceration and bleeding. Two randomized trials have reported the results of treatment of *H. pylori* in patients following duodenal ulcer hemorrhage (46,47). Patients treated with antibiotics had a 0% incidence of recurrent bleeding during the year following treatment, while 33% and 27% rates of repeat bleeding were noted in control groups. Two additional trials have compared recurrent bleeding during maintenance ranitidine therapy (11% to 13%) to bleeding subsequent to *H. pylori* eradication (2% to 5%) (48,49). Although it seems likely that effective antibiotic therapy would eliminate duodenal ulcer disease in postoperative patients and thus permit more limited surgical therapy for control of hemorrhage, this approach has not yet been subjected to clinical trial.

Perforation

Hospitalization rates for duodenal ulcer perforation have not decreased with the introduction of powerful antisecretory drugs or with antibiotic treatment of peptic ulcer. In the majority of affected patients, perforation is the first manifestation of duodenal ulcer disease.

The patient usually experiences sudden, severe epigastric pain, followed shortly by diffuse abdominal pain. Chemical irritation of the parietal peritoneum by acidic gastric contents causes severe pain. If there is contact between the gastric contents and the diaphragm, the patient will also experience referred pain in the area of the right scapula. Respiration worsens symptoms. Physical examination typically reveals a silent abdomen with muscular rigidity and epigastric tenderness. Moderate fever and tachycardia are often present; hypotension is initially unusual. Laboratory examination reveals leukocytosis. Hyperamylasemia, attributed to absorption of duodenal contents from the peritoneal cavity, is common. Upright abdominal films demonstrate pneumoperitoneum in 80% of cases. If pneumoperitoneum is absent, computed tomography (CT) with oral contrast may be used to demonstrate perforation.

The fasting human stomach contains 10^2 to 10^3 organisms; oral bacteria, including lactobacilli and aerobic streptococci, predominate. Infectious complications associated with duodenal perforation are closely related to the length of time that elapses before definitive treatment. Peritoneal cultures obtained between 6 to 12 hours of perforation are positive in <50% of cases, but culture positivity increases rapidly thereafter. Beyond 24 hours coliforms and fungal species are increasingly frequent.

Nonoperative management of perforated duodenal ulcer is rarely justified in modern medical practice. Reports of nonoperative management are highly biased by exclusion of patients with gastric ulcer, perforations of >24 hours duration, clinical deterioration, associated shock, diagnostic uncertainty, or comorbid medical illnesses (50). In one report, initial treatment with intravenous fluids, nasogastric suction, and antibiotics was coupled with contrast radiography to evaluate for intraperitoneal leakage of gastric contents. Lack of clinical improvement was an indication for emergent operation. In this series, 28% of patients initially managed nonoperatively had clinical deterioration within 24 hours, and perforated neoplasms were discovered in 27% of patients initially treated for perforated ulcers. Older patients were less likely to improve with nonoperative treatment. Hospitalization was 35% longer in the group treated nonoperatively.

Risk factors that predict operative mortality include concurrent medical comorbidity, preoperative shock, and longstanding perforation (>48 hours) (51). If these factors are absent, ulcer operation may be performed with predictably low mortality and acceptable morbidity. If one or more risk factors are present, the risk of death increases progressively. Patients with zero, one, two, or three risk factors have been reported to have mortality rates of 0%, 10%, 46%, and 100%, respectively (51). In a recent multivariate analysis, age >65 years, American Society of Anesthesiologists (ASA) stage III or IV, and a delay of surgery beyond 24 hours after onset of symptoms predicted mortality (52). When all three risk factors were present, mortality was 61%.

Operative treatment of perforated duodenal ulcer has four goals: patient safety, peritoneal debridement, closure of the perforation, and alteration of the ulcer diathesis so that the risk of recurrent ulceration is minimized. For most patients peritoneal cleansing can be achieved by either laparoscopy or laparotomy. Laparoscopic closure of duodenal perforation is usually confined to those with a solitary prepyloric ulcer located anteriorly (52). Most reports of laparoscopic repair have employed either omental patching or fibrin glue repair. Perforated ulcers with larger defects or those with destruction of the proximal duodenum or penetration into adjacent organs require laparotomy and resectional therapy.

Laparoscopic repair of duodenal perforation and open repair have been compared in two prospective trials (53,54). Laparoscopic repair requires significantly longer operative time (Table 33.5). Postoperative analgesic requirements are fewer with laparoscopy. No significant differences were noted between these techniques in duration of nasogastric suction, intravenous infusion, and hospital stay; time to resumption of oral diet; reoperation rate; morbidity; or mortality.

Two meta-analyses of surgical treatment of perforated peptic ulcer have compared open surgical therapy with laparoscopic approaches (22,55). In terms of operative time, there is no clear superiority of one approach over the other, but all trials reported after 2001 have favored laparoscopic repair. While analgesic use in hospitals is less for laparoscopically treated patients, the more important variable of hospital length of stay was not significantly shorter for these patients. Overall rates of postoperative complications were not statistically different for the two approaches. A lower rate of wound infection in the laparoscopic group approached significance. Return to normal daily activities and work favored the laparoscopic group. The pooled estimate of mortality favored laparoscopic repair.

Table 33.5 Comparison of laparoscopic and open repair of perforated duodenal ulcer

Mortality	Similar
Morbidity	Similar
Analgesics requirements	Less for laparoscopy
Operative time	Shorter for laparotomy
Duration of NG suction	Similar
Duration of IV infusion	Similar
Time to oral intake	Similar
Hospital stay	Similar
Reoperation rate	Similar

NG, nasogastric; IV, intravenous.

Omental patch closure of perforated duodenal ulcer alone is not adequate treatment. Because the underlying ulcer diathesis is not altered, simple patch closure is followed by an ulcer recurrence rate of 61% at a mean of 20 months (47). *H. pylori* eradication following omental patching reduces ulcer recurrence to <5%.

Complications are more frequent and more severe when large duodenal defects or penetration into other organs require resectional therapy. Postoperative morbidity has been reported in 9% of patients with small anterior perforations and in 22% to 34% of those with complicated defects (56).

Postoperative Hemorrhage

Unrecognized injury to the spleen is the most common cause of postoperative hemorrhage after operations on the stomach or duodenum. Splenic hemorrhage occurs as a result of capsular injury from traction on splenic attachments or from inappropriately placed retractors. Failure to properly ligate short gastric vessels during dissection of the greater curvature of the stomach can also lead to splenic hemorrhage. In several series of splenectomy, inadvertent injury during upper abdominal surgery is among the most common indications for splenectomy. In addition to the dangers of hypovolemia, splenectomy increases the incidence of pancreatic fistula, pancreatitis, and septic complications, including subphrenic abscess. Following vagotomy, vessels in proximity to the esophagus may be the source of bleeding.

Intraluminal hemorrhage most commonly represents suture line bleeding from submucosal arterioles and veins. Gastric lavage with warmed saline via the nasogastric tube is used to clear the stomach of clots as a prelude to endoscopy. Endoscopic hemostasis, similar in technique to that described for bleeding ulcers, is usually successful. Uncontrolled hemorrhage is an indication for reoperation.

Gastric Outlet Obstruction

Gastric outlet obstruction and small bowel obstruction are relatively frequent following gastric resection, occurring in 3% to 5% of cases. The major cause of anastomotic obstruction in the early postoperative period is inflammation adjacent to the anastomosis, secondary to subclinical suture line leakage or ischemia. Chronic gastric outlet obstruction is often the consequence of perianastomotic ulceration with resultant cicatrization. Pain is not usually prominent in gastric outlet obstruction. Recurrent vomiting or persistently elevated nasogastric tube output suggests the diagnosis. Fiberoptic endoscopy should be used when gastric outlet obstruction is considered to evaluate anastomotic patency.

If the patient has a Billroth II anastomosis, the patency of each limb must be evaluated. An open anastomosis favors delay in reoperation and support of nutritional needs with parenteral alimentation.

Mechanical small bowel obstruction may occur following Billroth II gastrojejunostomy, performed either retrocolic or antecolic. When gastrojejunostomy is performed in a retrocolic position, obstruction may be due to occlusion of the anastomosis by the transverse mesocolon (Fig. 33.5). The stomach may retract upward, resulting in pinching of one or both jejunal limbs by a relatively unyielding mesentery. This complication may be avoided by suturing the transverse mesentery to the stomach at least 2 cm superior to the anastomosis. The exposure for this maneuver is best achieved inferior to the transverse colon. Volvulus of the proximal or distal limbs of the gastrojejunostomy is possible following Billroth II reconstruction, more commonly when the anastomosis is antecolic.

The afferent loop syndrome is a condition caused by partial obstruction of the proximal limb of a gastrojejunostomy. Obstruction may be caused by kinking or torsion of the anastomosis, obstruction by the transverse mesentery, internal hernia, or recurrent ulceration (Fig. 33.6). Partial obstruction results in intermittent dilatation of the duodenum and

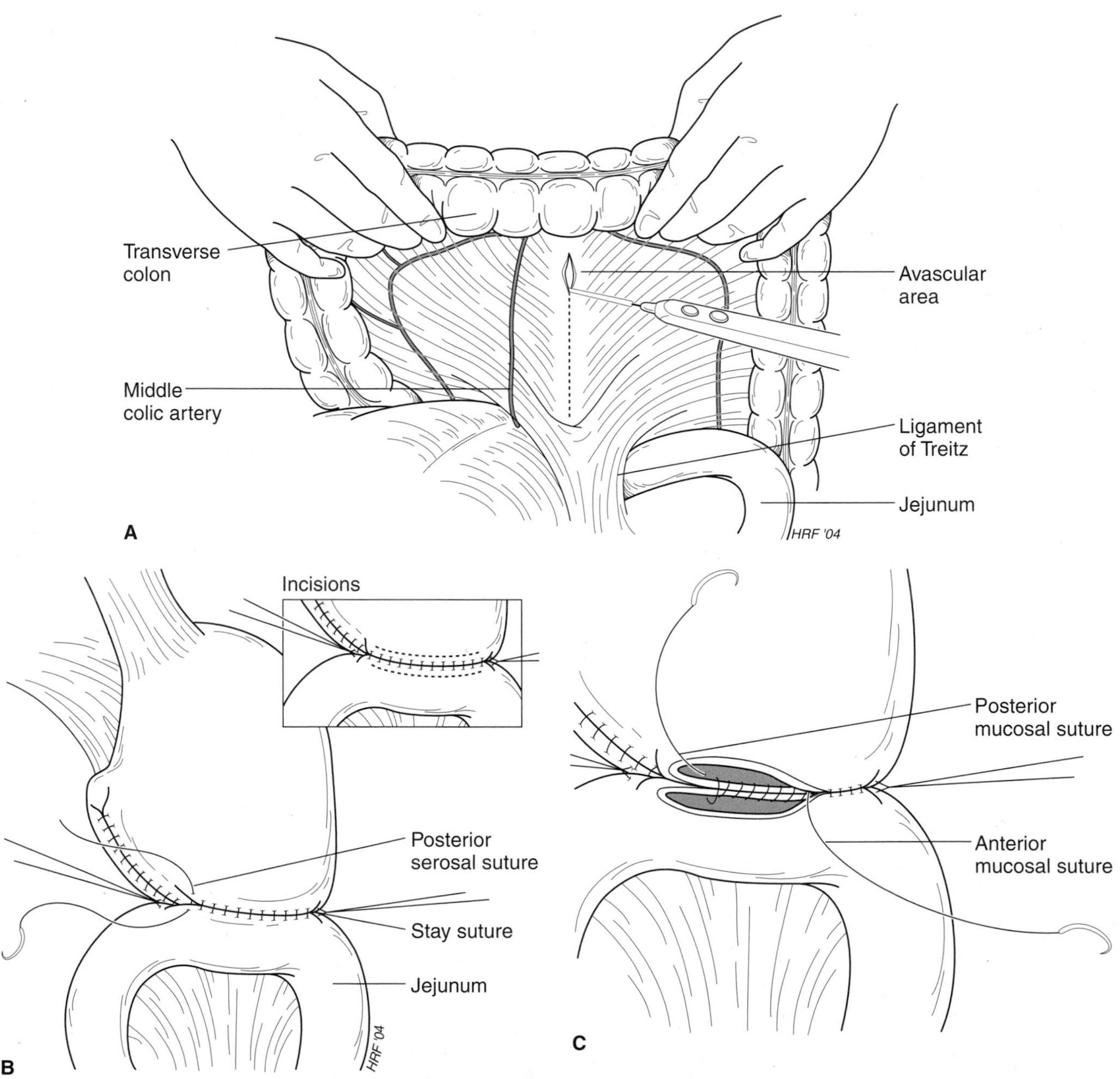

FIGURE 33.5. Construction of gastrojejunostomy. **A:** The transverse colon is retracted upward, and the vascular arcades within the transverse mesocolon are identified. An avascular area to the left of the middle colic vessels is chosen as the site for incision. An incision large enough to deliver the jejunum to the stomach is created. **B:** Interrupted 3-0 seromuscular sutures are placed and tied. Electrocautery is used to create equal length incisions in the stomach and jejunum. **C:** A continuous mucosal suture of absorbable material is begun posteriorly and is continued along the anterior portion of the anastomosis.

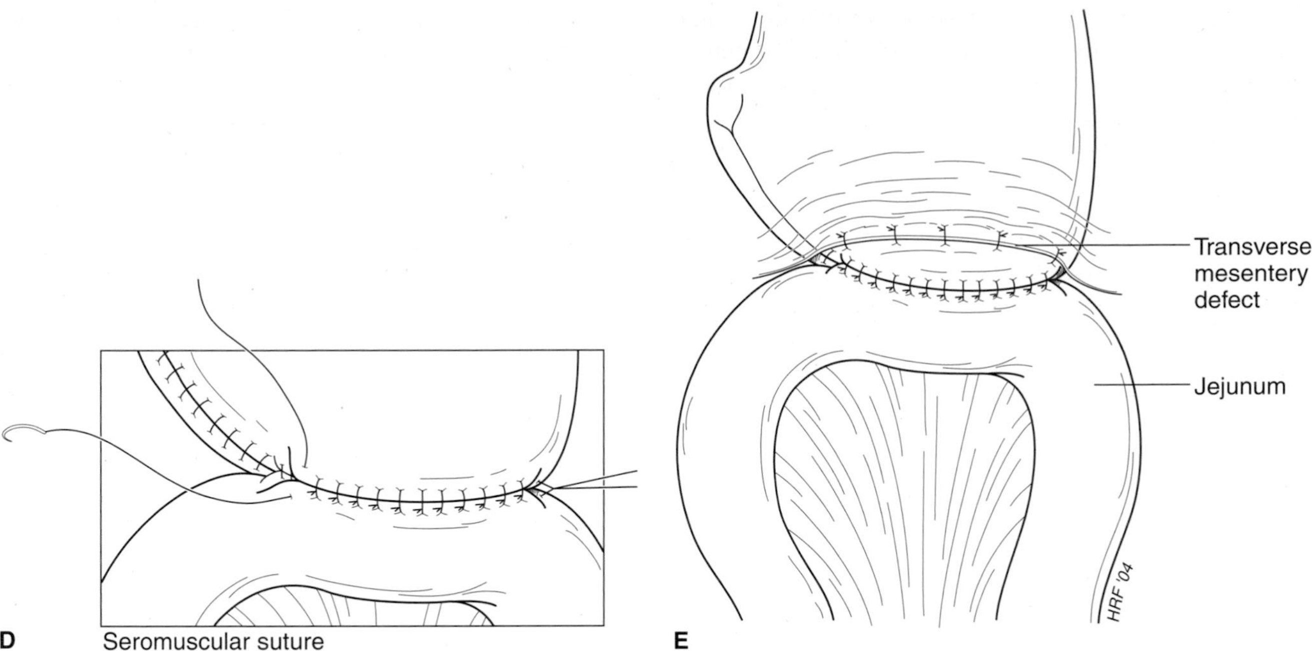

FIGURE 33.5. (*Continued*) **D:** Interrupted seromuscular sutures are used to complete the anterior portion of the double layer of anastomosis. **E:** The completed gastrojejunal anastomosis should be positioned beneath the transverse mesocolon to prevent angulation or obstruction of the efferent or afferent jejunal limbs. The mesenteric defect is secured through the gastric wall with interrupted sutures.

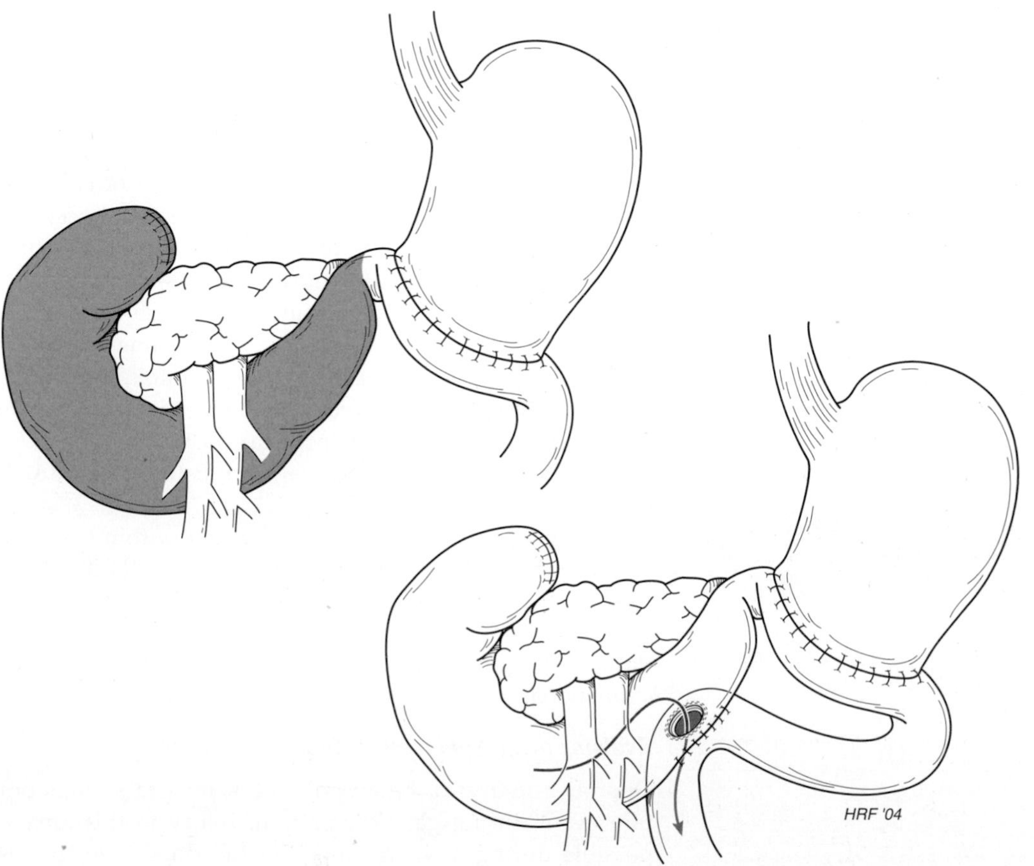

FIGURE 33.6. Afferent loop obstruction can be caused by kinking at the gastrojejunal anastomosis.

proximal jejunum, with periodic release of pancreatic and biliary secretion into the stomach. Afferent loop obstruction occurring in the immediate postoperative period causes severe and unrelenting epigastric pain. Acute afferent loop obstruction is a surgical emergency because, if unrelieved, obstruction can cause duodenal stump leakage. The dilated loop can be visualized on abdominal CT scan; the obstructed limb will not contain orally ingested contrast. Mechanical stasis in the duodenum may cause elevation in serum amylase values and may be confused with postoperative pancreatitis. Acute afferent loop obstruction requires urgent reoperation because of the possibility of perforation.

Jejunogastric intussusception is an unusual cause of gastric outlet obstruction, occurring in <1% of cases (57). In more than three-fourths of patients, the efferent limb is the source of the intussusception. Urgent endoscopy reveals a friable, bluish mass originating from the orifice of the efferent limb. Abdominal CT scan demonstrates a mass within the stomach with a layered, onion-skin-like appearance. Urgent operative reduction of the intussusception is indicated due to the potential for ischemic necrosis of the intussusceptum.

Postsurgical Gastroparesis

Postsurgical gastroparesis is a chronic complication of gastric surgery characterized by disruption of the normal mechanisms of gastric motility (58). Affected patients have postprandial pain, nausea, and vomiting; most have difficulty maintaining adequate oral nutrition. The incidence of motility disturbances following gastric surgery is poorly defined; abnormalities in gastric emptying have been recorded in 30% of patients following truncal vagotomy and Roux-en-Y gastrectomy (58–60).

The pathogenesis of postsurgical gastroparesis is unknown. Lack of vagal tone, abnormalities of neuromuscular coordination, disordered smooth muscle function, and motor abnormalities of the Roux-en-Y limb have been postulated but remain unproven. Histologic examination of the dysfunctional stomach usually reveals no abnormality (58).

The diagnosis of postsurgical gastroparesis requires the absence of anatomic obstruction, including anastomotic stricture and efferent limb obstruction (Table 33.6). Fiberoptic endoscopy of the gastric remnant is a strict requirement. Contrast studies of the small intestine are useful to exclude distal obstruction or generalized intestinal hypomotility. Radionuclide solid phase gastric emptying studies are used to evaluate gastric function and to provide a quantitative measure of the effectiveness of medical therapy.

Table 33.6 Requirements for diagnosis of postsurgical gastroparesis

1. Prior history of gastric resection, usually with vagotomy
2. Upper endoscopy to exclude anastomotic obstruction, efferent limb obstruction, jejunogastric intussusception
3. Exclusion of hypothyroidism, diabetes mellitus
4. Exclusion of medical disorders such as scleroderma, amyloidosis, muscular dystrophy
5. Contrast study of small intestine
6. Solid phase gastric emptying study

Endocrine disturbances can cause disordered gastric emptying. Hypothyroidism and diabetes mellitus are prominent examples. A variety of diseases, including amyloidosis, scleroderma, muscular dystrophy, myasthenia gravis, and psoriasis, can alter gastric emptying. Medications that affect gastric emptying should be discontinued, including narcotics, anticholinergics, and L-dopa. Patients should receive a prolonged trial of prokinetic drug therapy.

Patients who meet these criteria and fail to respond to aggressive medical management are candidates for operative treatment. Total or near-total gastrectomy with Roux-en-Y gastrojejunostomy has been reported as a treatment for postsurgical gastroparesis (58). At a mean follow-up of 56 months, 78% of patients reported symptomatic improvement. For 7% of patients there had been no change in their condition, and for 15% symptoms had worsened. No postoperative deaths were reported for 52 patients. Postoperative complications were noted in 29%, with wound infection, prolonged ileus, and pneumonia the most frequent.

Duodenal Fistula

Duodenal fistula may be a complication of gastric resection, particularly when the duodenum is closed and gastrojejunal reconstruction performed. The duodenal stump may dehisce at the site of closure, an end fistula, or the duodenum may perforate laterally, causing a lateral fistula. Duodenal fistulas are particularly morbid because of the high fluid volume lost and because of the escape of pancreatic and biliary secretions into the peritoneal cavity. Once fistulization has occurred, attempts at immediate operative closure are futile. Initial management is concerned with treatment of sepsis, control of intraperitoneal leakage, and skin protection at any site of external drainage. Percutaneous transhepatic duodenal drainage has been reported as a method to externally drain pancreatic-biliary secretions in the presence of duodenal fistulization (61). Parenteral alimentation is necessary to maintain a positive nitrogen balance in the weeks required for spontaneous closure or reoperation. When distal obstruction exists in the afferent jejunal limb, spontaneous fistula closure will not occur.

If spontaneous closure does not occur within 6 weeks, operative repair is justified. If a portion of the duodenum is missing or nonviable, duodenal reconstruction is required. The most widely accepted method is construction of a Roux-en-Y jejunal segment to close the duodenal defect via a functional side-to-end duodenojejunostomy.

Avulsion of the Sphincter of Oddi

Operative injury to the ampulla of Vater is a serious but rare event during gastric resection. Injury to this area is possible during any operation on the duodenum but is

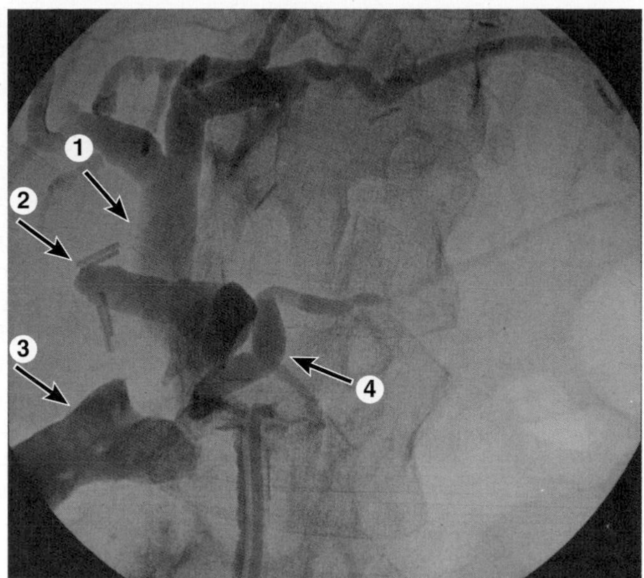

FIGURE 33.7. Avulsion of the ampulla of Vater demonstrated by percutaneous transhepatic cholangiography (PTC). Injection of the PTC catheter demonstrates free flow of contrast into the subhepatic space. The common biliary-pancreatic channel also provides a pancreatogram. Severe inflammatory changes in the subhepatic space were treated by external drainage and parenteral hyperalimentation. The patient ultimately required pancreaticoduodenectomy for correction of the defect. 1, common bile duct; 2, cystic duct stump; 3, subhepatic collection; 4, pancreatic duct.

most frequent in the presence of scarring or inflammation that causes secondary shortening of the duodenal bulb (62). The injury occurs during dissection between the duodenum and pancreas prior to duodenal transection. Most injuries can be recognized by the sudden appearance of bile in the operative field. Postoperatively, the injury causes collection of bile and pancreatic secretions in the subhepatic space (Fig. 33.7). If disconnection of the ampulla is recognized intraoperatively, the duodenal stump may be mobilized further and brought over the ampulla. The ampulla or the individual bile and pancreatic ducts may then be reimplanted. A Roux-en-Y limb of jejunum may also be created for this purpose. When discovered postoperatively, inflammatory changes make ductal reimplantation impractical and pancreaticoduodenectomy becomes necessary.

Dumping

The term *dumping* defines a postoperative syndrome with both GI and vasomotor components. The cause of dumping relates to the unregulated entry of ingested food into the proximal small bowel after vagotomy and either resection or division of the pyloric sphincter (Table 33.7). Early dumping symptoms occur within 1 hour of a meal and include nausea, epigastric discomfort, and palpitations. Severely symptomatic patients may also have dizziness or syncope. Late dumping symptoms follow a meal by 1 to 3 hours and may include reactive hypoglycemia.

Although 5% to 10% of patients experience mild dumping symptoms in the early postoperative period, minor dietary alterations and the passage of time bring improvement in approximately 60% (63). The somatostatin analogue octreotide has been reported to improve dumping symptoms when 50 to 100 μg is administered subcutaneously prior to a meal. The beneficial effects of octreotide on vasomotor symptoms of dumping are due to pressor effects of the compound on splanchnic vessels and inhibition of the release of vasoactive peptides from the gut. Octreotide also decreases peak plasma insulin levels and slows intestinal transit. The systemic effects of octreotide include blunting changes in pulse, systolic blood pressure, and packed red cell volume during early dumping and preventing decreases in serum glucose concentration during late dumping.

Table **33.7** **Features of early dumping syndrome**

Cardiovascular	Gastrointestinal
Tachycardia	Nausea
Palpitations	Colic and cramping
Dizziness	Abdominal pain
Syncope	Diarrhea
Sweating	
Flushing	

Cancer in the Gastric Remnant

A growing number of reports suggest that gastric cancer is more likely to develop in individuals who have undergone previous partial gastrectomy. The clearest risk factor for the development of gastric cancer after gastrectomy is the time interval following surgery. A decreased risk of gastric cancer has been observed during the first 15 years after gastrectomy. Cancer reduction is likely due to the removal of at-risk mucosa from the distal stomach. In contrast, patients from 15 to 20 years after gastric resection for ulcer disease have a relative risk for gastric cancer that is three to five times that of the age-matched and sex-matched general population (64,65).

The molecular mechanisms that underlie development of neoplasia in the remnant stomach are unknown. Decreased luminal pH, permitting bacterial overgrowth with increased production of *N*-nitroso carcinogens, and reflux of bile acids into the stomach have been postulated to promote cancer development. The effects of each are unproven. Vagotomy does not appear to promote cancer development. A Swedish population-based study of 7,198 vagotomized patients followed for 9 to 18 years did not reveal increased risk (66). Prognosis is usually guarded because many gastric remnant cancers are diagnosed at an advanced stage (67,68). Reported 5-year survival ranges from 7% to 33%.

GASTRIC CANCER

In the United States, gastric cancer remains among the top ten causes of cancer-related deaths for both men and women. Although the incidence of gastric cancer has declined in the United States, approximately 22,000 new cases of gastric cancer were reported in 2000 (69).

Pathogenesis

Gastric cancer risk is increased in stomachs that contain polyps. Risk is related to polyp histology, size, and number. Hyperplastic gastric polyps are considered to have no neoplastic potential. In contrast, adenomatous polyps have a definite risk for development of malignancy (70). The risk is greatest for polyps >2 cm in diameter. Multiple adenomatous polyps further increase the risk of cancer. Although nitrites in the diet have been demonstrated to have a role in gastric carcinogenesis in animals, specific human dietary constituents that promote tumor formation have not been identified.

Long-term infestation with the organism *H. pylori* appears to predispose to subsequent development of gastric carcinoma. *H. pylori* is unequivocally associated with the development of chronic gastritis, and regions of the world with high rates of gastric adenocarcinoma also have a high prevalence of *H. pylori* infection. Childhood acquisition of *H. pylori* infection appears to be linked to the subsequent development of premalignant lesions and invasive cancer. In the United States, seropositivity for *H. pylori* increases the risk for cancer development approximately threefold, and in Japanese American males in Hawaii, *H. pylori*-positive subjects demonstrate a sixfold increase in incidence (71,72). *H. pylori* infection is associated with development of adenocarcinoma of both major histologic types and with tumors arising in the body or antrum of the stomach. *H. pylori* infection is not a significant risk factor for cancers of the gastroesophageal junction; these tumors are frequently associated with mucosal abnormalities of Barrett esophagus. However, infection with *H. pylori* alone cannot explain the development of gastric cancer. In North America, approximately 50% of adults older than 50 are seropositive for *H. pylori*, yet only a small fraction develop gastric cancer.

Diagnosis

The most common symptoms of gastric cancer are not specific and include pain, anorexia, and weight loss. These symptoms resemble those of a number of nonneoplastic gastroduodenal diseases, especially benign peptic ulcer. Fiberoptic endoscopy is the definitive diagnostic method when gastric cancer is suspected, and only gastric biopsy can definitively differentiate benign from malignant gastric ulcers. Accuracy of diagnosis can exceed 95% if multiple biopsy specimens are obtained.

Cross-sectional imaging, most commonly CT, has been used to assess extragastric spread. When performed with ingestion of oral contrast, CT reliably demonstrates infiltration of the gastric wall by tumor, gastric ulceration, and hepatic metastasis. The technique is less specific with regard to invasion of adjacent organs and in assessing for presence of lymphatic metastases.

Endoscopic ultrasound is useful to characterize subepithelial lesions that may be confused with gastric cancer. Ultrasound-directed biopsy of submucosal tumors is possible. Endoscopic ultrasound can assess the depth of gastric wall penetration by gastric cancer and demonstrates good correlation with intraoperative assessment and histologic findings. Perigastric lymph nodes involved with tumor are reliably identified and may be biopsied with ultrasound guidance. Because endoscopic ultrasound has a limited depth of tissue penetration, hepatic metastases are not detectable; this limitation hinders complete preoperative staging of gastric cancer patients.

Surgical Therapy

Surgical resection is the only curative treatment for gastric cancer, but in the United States advanced disease at the time of diagnosis prevents curative resection for most patients. The surgical objectives in gastric cancer are to attempt cure in patients with localized tumor and to provide palliation that is both effective and safe for patients with advanced malignancy. Operative treatment of gastric adenocarcinoma has focused on the detection of metastatic disease, the limits of gastric resection for potentially curable lesions, the extent of perigastric lymphadenectomy, the role of splenectomy, and the management of directly involved adjacent organs.

Laparoscopy

The ability of cross-sectional imaging to detect metastatic disease is less sensitive when tumor involves the surface of the liver, the omentum, and the peritoneal surfaces. These are common sites for gastric cancer metastasis that are amenable to laparoscopic examination. Diagnostic laparoscopy can be combined with laparoscopic ultrasound. Preoperative endoscopic ultrasound and laparoscopic ultrasound are complimentary techniques. When combined, a 100% sensitivity in detecting inoperable tumors has been reported (73).

Detection of incurable lesions is important because the mean life expectancy of affected patients is 3 to 9 months. Most patients with metastasis can be treated without the need for palliative surgical resection. In one recent study, no patients deemed incurable by laparoscopy required subsequent operation (74).

Resection

Over the past decade the surgical treatment of gastric cancer has diverged, with minimally invasive approaches for early cancers and increasingly radical operations for advanced tumors. The greatest experience with early gastric cancer has been reported by Japanese surgeons. The Japanese Gastric Cancer Association defines early gastric cancer as a tumor in which invasion is restricted to the mucosa or submucosa regardless of the presence or absence of lymph node metastasis (75). For tumors confined to the mucosa, lymphatic metastasis is present in 1% to 3% of cases; with submucosal involvement the rate of nodal positivity increases to between 14% and 20% (76,77).

Endoscopic mucosal resection has been reported for well-differentiated mucosal tumors of <3 cm without ulceration. Most series have been restricted to well-differentiated adenocarcinomas or adenomas of less than 30 mm size, endoscopic ultrasound findings consistent with an intramucosal lesion, and absence of ulceration (78). Thrombocytopenia, the need for anticoagulation, and significant comorbidities have been contraindications. The endoscopic technique is enhanced by the submucosal injection of viscous compounds such as hyaluronic acid, glycerol, hydroxypropyl methylcellulose, or fibrinogen to elevate the mucosa. Electrosurgical knives of various configurations have been developed to enable en bloc resection.

Because local recurrence is more common with piecemeal resection, removal of the tumor as a single specimen is crucial. Procedure times are longer and complications such as perforation are more common if the lesion is located in the upper third of the stomach, is larger than 20 mm, or exhibits ulceration (79). Bleeding during resection is common, but almost always easily controlled endoscopically. Proton pump inhibitor administration increases safety (80). Experience is important. Procedure times improve after endoscopists have performed 30 interventions (79).

In a series of 445 patients, 5% experienced postoperative bleeding or perforation (81). In 17%, histologic examination revealed submucosal invasion necessitating further operative treatment. Additional analysis, which suggests underdiagnosis of tumor invasion in 45% and missed lymphatic metastasis in 9%, urges continued study before acceptance of this technique (82).

Laparoscopic gastrectomy has also been reported for treatment of gastric malignancy, with purported advantages of reduced pain, shorter hospitalization, and improved quality of life (83). Long-term cancer control rates for laparoscopic gastrectomy have not yet been reported by controlled clinical trial. In one series of 43 cases of laparoscopic gastrectomy, a relatively high incidence of positive surgical margins, local recurrence, and gastric remnant cancer were reported (84). In contrast, laparoscopic gastrectomy for treatment of GI stromal tumors achieved adequate oncologic control in 98% of patients (85).

The extent of gastric resection is determined by the need to obtain a resection margin free of microscopic disease. Gastric cancer frequently demonstrates intramural spread due to the extensive intramural capillary and lymphatic network within the stomach. Microscopic involvement of the resection margin by tumor cells is associated with decreased survival (86). Patients with histologically positive margins of resection are at highest risk to develop recurrent disease, with positive margins strongly correlated with development of anastomotic recurrence. Retrospective studies suggest that a 6-cm distance from the tumor mass to the point of resection is associated with the lowest rate of anastomotic recurrence. Larger margins have not improved survival.

Advancements in operative technique and in postoperative physiologic support have improved results of major gastric resection during the past three decades. Increasingly radical gastric operations can be performed with acceptable morbidity and low mortality. The risk of postoperative mortality is very clearly related to age, with several reports indicating a twofold to fivefold increase in mortality for patients older than 70 (87). Although mortality risk is not significantly different for subtotal gastrectomy and total gastrectomy in patients younger than 70, for older patients, total gastrectomy doubles mortality. Mortality rates for total gastrectomy now range from 2% to 7% (88,89).

Because gastric cancer metastasizes so frequently to lymph nodes, radical extirpation of perigastric lymph nodes has been advocated as a therapeutic maneuver (90). The therapeutic benefit of extended lymphadenectomy in the treatment of gastric adenocarcinoma was derived initially from retrospective experiences and remains controversial. The first favorable experience was reported by the Japanese Research Society for Gastric Cancer (91,92). In the original Japanese system, resections were characterized as follows:

R1—resection of stomach, omentum, and perigastric lymph nodes;

R2—resection of stomach, omentum, and en bloc removal of the superior leaf of the transverse mesocolon, the pancreatic capsule, and lymph nodes along the branches of the celiac artery and in the infraduodenal and supraduodenal areas;

R3—resection of the above structures, plus lymph nodes along the aorta and esophagus, along with the spleen, the tail of the pancreas, and skeletonization of vessels in the portahepatis.

The current Japanese classification system is based on anatomical location of lymph nodes. Upper abdominal nodes are grouped into four levels (N1–N4) relative to the location of the primary tumor. The extent of lymphadenectomy corresponds to the level of nodal dissection, with higher levels of dissection involving nodes at greater remove from the primary tumor.

Only retrospective studies of extended perigastric lymphadenectomy have been reported from Japan. Stage for stage, initial reports suggested an improvement of 10% for patients treated with R2 or R3 operations (91–94). The benefits of extended lymphadenectomy have not been confirmed in observational studies from centers outside Japan.

Randomized trials have also failed to demonstrate a survival advantage for extended lymphadenectomy when entire patient populations were analyzed (95–99).

An effect of extended lymphadenectomy that may mitigate survival advantage is the "upstaging" of tumors. As additional lymph nodes are removed, additional micrometastatic disease is discovered. Patients are consequently placed in higher stage categories with more accurate, although worse, prognosis (100). Patients who do not undergo extended lymphadenectomy have micrometastases, which are undetected and, because of progressive tumor growth and recurrence, will decrease the survivorship of the staging group to which they are assigned.

The safety of extended lymphadenectomy is controversial. Reports from a national Japanese registry indicate a contemporary mortality of <1% (101). Similarly, low mortality risks have been reported from multi-institutional trials in Italy and Germany (100,102). In contrast, reports from the United States, Britain, and the Netherlands have indicated increased short-term morbidity and in-hospital mortality (96–100).

Histologically positive lymph nodes may be present in the splenic hilum and along the splenic artery, and splenectomy has been routinely practiced in some centers, especially in Japan. Splenectomy has not been demonstrated to improve survival for similarly staged patients (103,104). Splenectomy has a clearly adverse effect on postoperative morbidity and mortality. Septic complications due to pancreatic fistula and abscess formation are the major causes of morbidity (105). Splenectomy is not indicated unless the tumor directly invades the spleen or involves splenic hilar lymph nodes.

Resection of the tail of the pancreas does not improve survival. In a large British trial, both morbidity and mortality were doubled when distal pancreatectomy was part of the operation (98). Similar results have been reported in smaller observational series. Pancreatectomy is indicated only if there is direct invasion of the distal pancreas by the primary tumor. Resection of adjacent organs, most commonly the distal pancreas or transverse colon, may be required for local control if direct invasion is present. In these patients, operative morbidity is increased and long-term survival approximates 25% (106).

Total gastrectomy is performed almost exclusively in the context of gastric cancer. This procedure is indicated for gastric tumors at the esophagogastric junction, in the proximal stomach, and along the proximal lesser curvature. For patients with carcinoma of the gastric cardia, esophagectomy has no survival advantage when added to total gastrectomy if tumor resection can be achieved (107). Moreover, addition of esophagectomy is associated with significantly higher morbidity.

The most important complication of total gastrectomy is anastomotic leak at the esophagojejunal anastomosis (Fig. 33.8). In two randomized trials, anastomotic failure was observed in 7% and 11% of patients who underwent total gastrectomy (108,109). Anastomotic leak may be heralded by unexplained tachycardia without fever or leukocytosis.

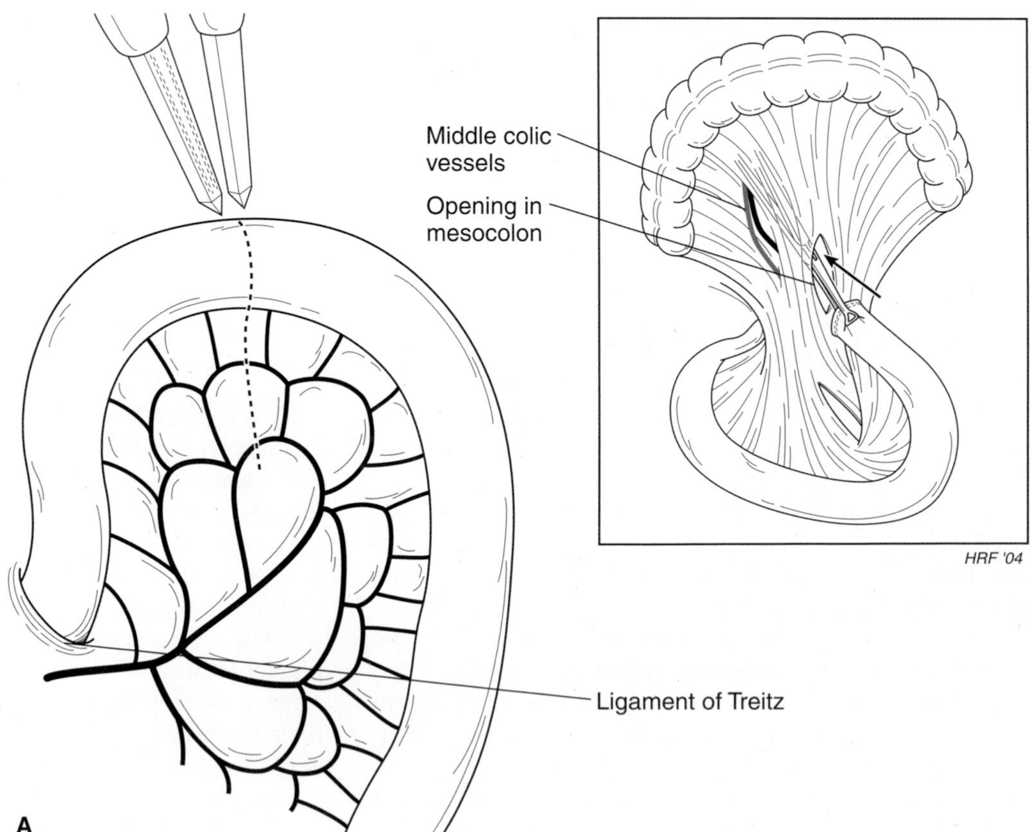

FIGURE 33.8. Creation of a stapled esophagojejunostomy. **A:** The proximal jejunum is divided creating a Roux limb. An opening is made in the transverse mesocolon to the left of the middle colic vessels. The distal end of the transected jejunum is passed retrocolically to the area of the distal esophagus.

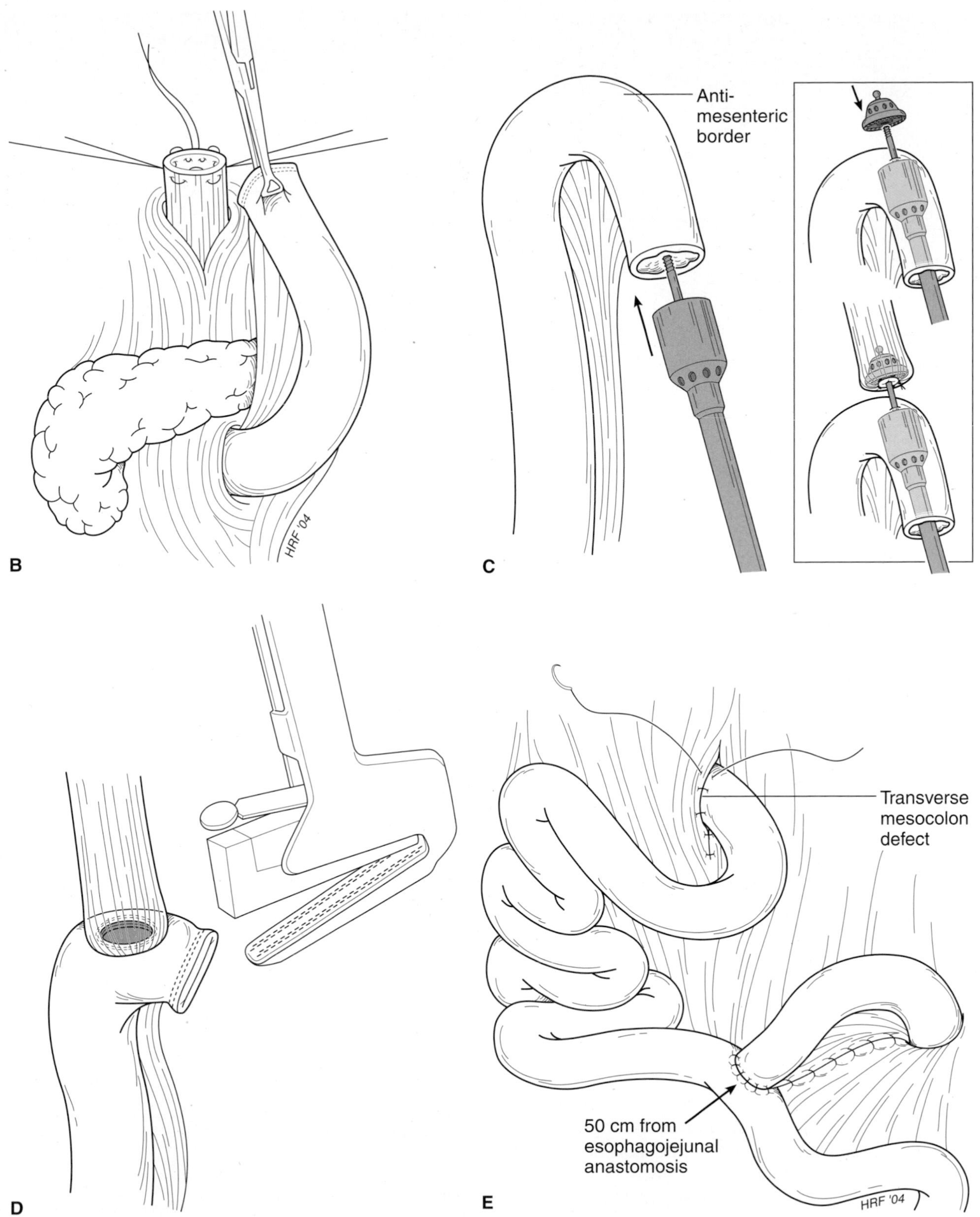

FIGURE 33.8. (*Continued*) **B:** The jejunal limb is approximated to the esophagus without angulation or tension. The stapled jejunal closure is excised to allow introduction of an EEA-type stapling device. **C:** An EEA stapling device is introduced into the opened end of the Roux-en-Y limb and positioned along the antimesenteric border of the jejunum. The anvil is reattached. The anvil is inserted into the distal esophagus, and a previously placed purse string suture is tied. When the EEA device is fired, an end-to-side esophagojejunal anastomosis is created. **D:** After withdrawal of the EEA stapler, the open end of the jejunal limb is closed with an application of a TA stapler. With the surgeon's guidance, a nasogastric tube is placed across the anastomosis. Anastomotic integrity is insured by observing for bubbles in a saline-filled operative field as the anesthesiologist insufflates air through the nasogastric tube. The jejunum is occluded to permit anastomotic distention. **E:** Intestinal continuity is restored through an end-to-side enteroenterostomy 50 cm distal to the esophagojejunal anastomosis. The mesenteric defect in the transverse mesocolon is approximated to the jejunal limb with interrupted sutures.

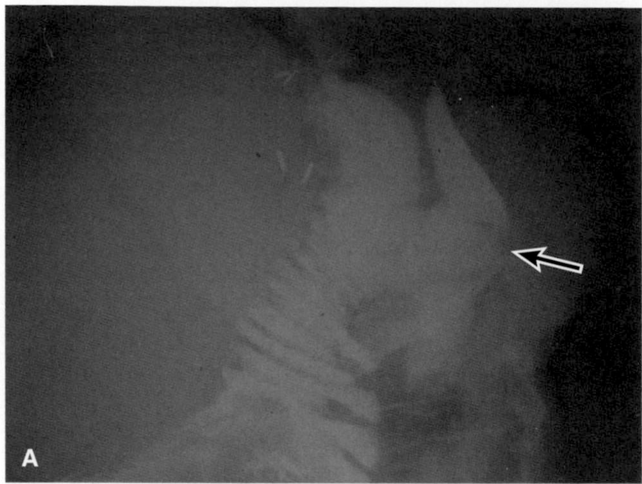
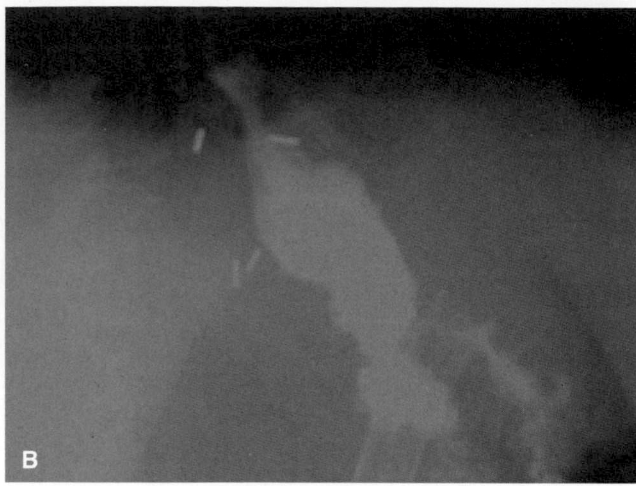

FIGURE 33.9. (A) Water-soluble contrast study demonstrating a contained leak at an esophagojejunal anastomosis (*arrow*). (B) Anastomosis after healing of leak.

Water-soluble contrast radiography should be used to confirm leakage (110) (Fig. 33.9). Intraluminal suction decompression and perianastomotic drainage may be used to create a controlled fistula with expectant fistula closure. Severe surrounding inflammation usually prohibits direct operative repair. Anastomotic dehiscence contributes substantially to the reported operative mortality of total gastrectomy (108,109).

The performance of total gastrectomy creates a substantial postoperative nutritional challenge. Reconstruction with a variety of small intestinal pouch configurations has been reported in observational series (111,112). No controlled data currently exist to prefer pouch reconstruction to simple Roux-en-Y esophagojejunostomy.

MORBID OBESITY

Obesity is epidemic in the United States. An estimated 20% of Americans are obese, a proportion that has risen annually for each of the past 10 years. Obesity is a major public health problem in Canada, Western Europe, and New Zealand, and many nonwestern countries are also reporting an increasing prevalence of obesity.

Degrees of obesity are quantified on the basis of body mass index (BMI), expressed as weight in kilograms per (height in meters)^2. An optimal BMI of 20 to 25 kg/m^2 has been determined actuarially with an initial sample size of approximately 20,000 individuals and life table analysis of 4.2 million individuals followed for 17 years (113). A BMI >40 kg/m^2 defines morbid obesity. A BMI of 35 kg/m^2 may be accepted as morbid obesity in the presence of obesity-related complications such as diabetes mellitus. Approximately 4 million Americans have a BMI between 35 and 40 kg/m^2; another 1.5 million have a BMI of >40 kg/m^2.

Severe obesity is classified as "morbid" because of the strong association with secondary obesity-related diseases. Morbid obesity is associated with increased risk of hypertension, noninsulin-dependent diabetes mellitus, hypertrophic cardiomyopathy, dyslipidemia, pulmonary insufficiency, sleep apnea, and several types of cancer (Table 33.8). Socioeconomic impairment and psychosocial disorders are also increased in morbidly obese individuals. Morbid obesity has an increased risk of premature mortality.

Weight loss reduces the risks of obesity-related comorbidities. For obese patients, weight reduction by as little as 5% to 10% of initial weight produces measurable improvements in glucose intolerance, hypertension, and lipid abnormalities.

Behavioral interventions and dietary modification are sometimes effective in moderate obesity. These measures

Table **33.8** Obesity-related health sequelae
Hypertension
Accelerated atherosclerosis
Hypertrophic cardiomyopathy
Dyslipidemia
Diabetes mellitus
Alveolar hypoventilation
Sleep apnea
Hepatic steatosis
Deep vein thrombosis
Venous stasis ulcers
Pulmonary embolism
Gastroesophageal reflux
Hernias
Degenerative joint disease
Female urinary incontinence
Female hirsutism
Amenorrhea
Intertriginous dermatitis
Carcinoma of uterus, breast, prostate, and colon

are ineffective in morbid obesity, with recidivism rates of 95% within 1 year. To date no pharmacologic agents have been developed that are both effective and safe for the treatment of obesity. In 1991, a National Institutes of Health Consensus Development Panel recommended operative intervention for morbidly obese individuals (BMI of >40 kg/m^2) on the basis that weight reduction by nonsurgical techniques was seldom achieved. The panel also recommended consideration of surgery for less severely obese individuals (BMI of 35 to 40 kg/m^2) with comorbid conditions such as diabetes mellitus or sleep apnea.

Postoperative success requires careful patient selection. In addition to the presence of severe obesity as defined above, the patient must provide evidence of failure to lose weight under medical supervision and the motivation and emotional reserve necessary to undergo the surgical procedure and subsequent lifestyle changes. Comorbid conditions should be sought and treated. Psychiatric evaluation is often useful.

Contemporary bariatric procedures all involve a degree of gastric restriction (Fig. 33.10). Roux-en-Y gastric bypass, the most common procedure in North America, involves creating a small pouch of the proximal stomach, drained via a segment of the proximal jejunum. In this procedure, the distal stomach and duodenum are bypassed. Gastric restriction is augmented by malabsorption in the biliopancreatic diversion procedure. The latter procedure has been further modified with duodenal switch.

The small volume of the gastric reservoir limits oral intake, and the major factor causing weight loss after bariatric procedures is reduced caloric ingestion. In gastric bypass, the small outlet from the gastric pouch may also retard gastric emptying. In each of the illustrated procedures, the dumping syndrome may occur, inhibiting ingestion of calorie-dense foods. Biliopancreatic diversion is designed to induce malabsorption to further augment the effects of gastric restriction. Bile and pancreatic secretions do not mix with food until the terminal ileum, limiting the time and mucosal surface area for digestion and absorption.

A broad experience has accumulated with the surgical treatment of morbid obesity. Three randomized studies and numerous nonrandomized studies have been published since 1986 that examine the efficacy of gastric bypass. The reports prior to 2000 relate to procedures performed via laparotomy. At 24 months after operation, a mean of 60% of excess weight is lost. For most patients, weight loss is maximal between 1 and 2 years postoperatively, with a mean 13-pound regain between 2 and 5 years and stability thereafter (114). A recent report of biliopancreatic diversion demonstrated average excess weight loss of 75% (115). Follow-up ranged from 1 to 21 years.

Surgically induced weight loss is effective in reducing cardiovascular risk. At 2 years, surgically treated patients demonstrated significant improvements in hypertension, diabetes mellitus, hyperinsulinemia, hypertriglyceridemia, and levels of high-density lipoprotein cholesterol. A 32-fold reduction in diabetic risk factors was observed at 2 years (116). This effect was persistent. At an 8-year follow-up, the incidence of diabetes was five times lower in the surgical group relative to unoperated controls.

Relative to nonobese subjects, systolic and diastolic blood pressure are increased in obesity. Left ventricular mass and wall thickness are increased; ejection fraction and diastolic function are decreased in obese subjects. One year after surgery, each of these parameters is improved. The greater the weight loss, the greater the reduction in left ventricular mass and the greater the improvement in diastolic function.

Pulmonary function is improved with surgical weight reduction. The percentage of patients reporting physical inactivity is decreased by two-thirds. Sleep apnea, present in 23% of surgically treated patients preoperatively, was observed in 8% after 2 years (117). No change in frequency of sleep apnea was observed in the control group.

Questionnaire data suggest that weight reduction has beneficial economic consequences. Workdays lost to illness or disability are reduced in years 2 to 5 following surgery. Quality of life instruments record improvement in psychosocial scales. The greater the weight loss, the greater the improvement.

Intraoperative Management

Specially designed operating tables are required for bariatric surgery. Standard operating room tables have a maximum weight limit of 200 kg, while those developed specifically for bariatric procedures are capable of holding 450 kg. Because most bariatric procedures require tilting of the table, efforts must be made to assure that the patient does not slip on its surface. A so-called bean bag, a soft pad filled with thousands of small plastic pellets, is useful for this purpose. The bean bag is molded to the patient's body and, with application of suction, firmly conforms to the patient's contours.

Pressure sores and neural injuries are more common in obese surgical patients, especially diabetics and the super obese. Injuries to the ulnar nerve and the lateral femoral cutaneous nerve are most common. In most instances, injury caused by malpositioning or stretch is neurapraxic and reversible. Padded protection of pressure areas is crucial.

Intraoperative blood pressure measurements will be falsely increased if an inappropriately small blood pressure cuff is used. The cuff bladder should ideally encircle the entire arm, but it must be at least of 75% of arm circumference. Accurate noninvasive blood pressure measurements may be obtained from the ankle or wrist. Invasive arterial monitoring should be used in the super obese.

Pneumoperitoneum used during laparoscopy may adversely affect systemic circulation in obese patients, and use of the Trendelenburg position may exacerbate circulatory changes. Elevated intra-abdominal pressure increases systemic vascular resistance. For intra-abdominal pressures <10 mm Hg, venous return to the right heart increases due to decreased splanchnic blood pooling. As intra-abdominal

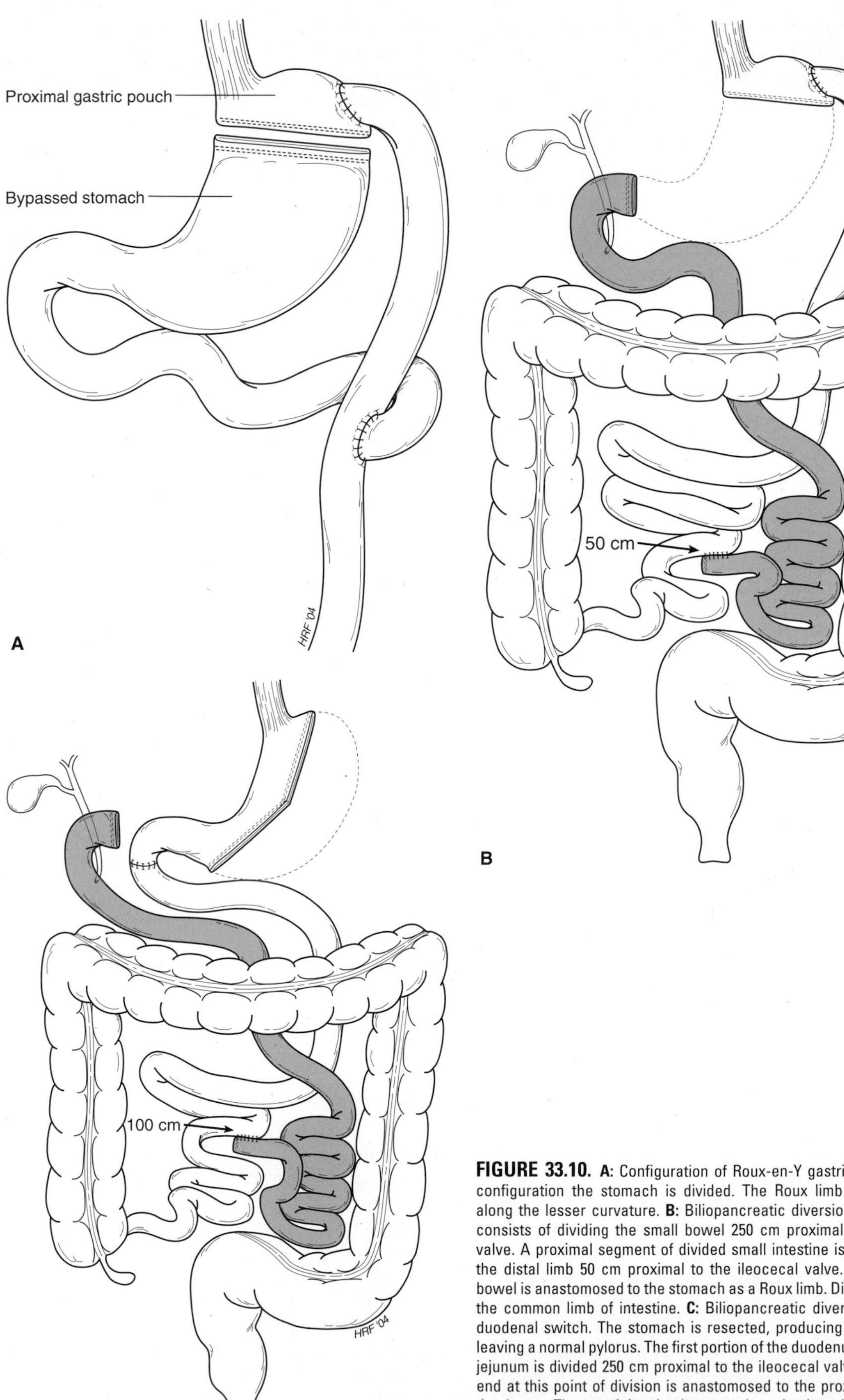

FIGURE 33.10. **A:** Configuration of Roux-en-Y gastric bypass. In this configuration the stomach is divided. The Roux limb is anastomosed along the lesser curvature. **B:** Biliopancreatic diversion. This operation consists of dividing the small bowel 250 cm proximal to the ileocecal valve. A proximal segment of divided small intestine is anastomosed to the distal limb 50 cm proximal to the ileocecal valve. The distal small bowel is anastomosed to the stomach as a Roux limb. Digestion occurs in the common limb of intestine. **C:** Biliopancreatic diversion modified by duodenal switch. The stomach is resected, producing early satiety but leaving a normal pylorus. The first portion of the duodenum is divided. The jejunum is divided 250 cm proximal to the ileocecal valve, and the distal end at this point of division is anastomosed to the proximal segment of duodenum. The remaining duodenum and proximal small bowel are anastomosed to the ileum 100 cm proximal to the ileocecal valve.

pressure increases to >20 mm Hg, inferior vena caval compression decreases venous return and consequently diminishes cardiac output. Renal blood flow decreases when intra-abdominal pressure exceeds 20 mm Hg, and glomerular filtration rate drops. Hypovolemia accentuates these changes at higher intra-abdominal pressures. Both obesity and pneumoperitoneum adversely affect respiratory mechanics.

Postoperative Complications

The largest number of reported experiences with bariatric surgery relate to operations performed by laparotomy. Collectively, these reports illustrate that for Roux-en-Y gastric bypass, 30-day mortality ranges from 0.3% to 2% (118). Overall complication rates range from 20% to 40%. The most frequent acute postoperative complications include deep vein thrombosis (DVT), pulmonary embolism, anastomotic leakage, and wound infection. Late complications include stomal stenosis, staple line dehiscence, and marginal ulceration. Micronutrient deficiencies have also been reported long-term.

Laparoscopic gastric bypass is associated with a postoperative mortality rate of 0% to 1.7%, similar to the rate observed when the operation is performed via laparotomy (117). Contemporary reports of laparoscopic Roux-en-Y gastric bypass demonstrate very low mortality rates and progressive declines in postoperative complications (118). Laparoscopic bariatric surgery requires advanced laparoscopic skills, and many observers have commented upon an extended "learning curve" not accounted for by current mortality statistics. The range of postoperative complications recorded with open gastric bypass has also been noted for procedures performed laparoscopically.

Deep Venous Thrombosis

Overall, the most common cause of death postoperatively is pulmonary embolism. DVT occurs in approximately 2% of patients treated via open operation or laparoscopically (119). Immobility, venous stasis, and the effects of pneumoperitoneum may contribute to thrombus formation. Physical examination is not diagnostically reliable. Doppler examination is the preferred initial diagnostic test. Controlled trials are not available establishing a standard of care for DVT prophylaxis in bariatric surgery. Sequential compression stockings and injection of either subcutaneous heparin or low-molecular weight heparin are recommended. The consequences of pulmonary embolism are more severe in bariatric patients relative to the general population. The hypoventilation syndrome and *cor pulmonale* are increased in obese patients. Both diminish functional cardiac reserve.

Anastomotic Dehiscence

Anastomotic dehiscence or suture line leak has been reported in 1.2% of patients undergoing open gastric bypass (120). This complication occurs in 3% to 6% of cases performed laparoscopically but diminishes with surgeon experience (121,122). The diagnosis of postoperative peritonitis is more difficult in morbidly obese patients. Tachycardia, worsening abdominal or back pain, and hiccups may be the only signs. Concern mandates radiologic investigation with a water-soluble contrast agent. If a leak is confirmed that communicates freely with the peritoneal cavity, the defect should be closed if feasible and the upper abdomen should be externally drained. A gastrostomy tube should be placed in the distal, excluded stomach. In selected cases of leak in which the extravasation is contained, conservative, nonoperative management can be successful (123).

Acute gastric distension of the bypassed distal stomach may occur after either open or laparoscopic gastric bypass. Acute distention may be a result of postoperative peritonitis or as a mechanical consequence of an obstructed enteroenterostomy. Continuous abdominal pain, distension, and hiccups are frequently associated signs. Plain abdominal x-rays or CT demonstrate massive gastric dilatation, often with an air-fluid level. Acute gastric distention must be treated emergently because of the potential for ischemic necrosis of the stomach. Percutaneous or operative gastrostomy decompression is therapeutic.

Incisional Hernia

Postoperative incisional hernias are a major problem in open bariatric surgery, occurring in approximately 20% of cases. A prior incisional hernia doubles this risk. Port site incisional hernias have been reported in 0% to 0.5% of patients after laparoscopic gastric bypass, representing the clearest advantage of the laparoscopic approach (117).

Cholelithiasis

Rapid weight loss, by either dietary means or following surgery, is associated with an increased risk of cholelithiasis. Half of patients following bariatric surgery will demonstrate gall bladder sludge; one-third will develop symptomatic gallstones. The use of prophylactic ursodiol for 6 months following gastric bypass reduced the incidence of symptomatic gallstones to 2% (124). Many surgeons have used the high incidence of postoperative cholelithiasis to justify prophylactic cholecystectomy at the time of gastric bypass. No controlled trial exists to support or refute this practice.

Stomal Complications

The gastrojejunal anastomosis that drains the proximal gastric pouch in gastric bypass is intentionally small at 1 cm. Larger stomas do not create enough restriction of food passage and are not associated with adequate weight loss. As a consequence, stomal stenosis is relatively common, occurring in 12% of cases (125). Affected patients develop early satiety, recurrent vomiting, and upper abdominal pain. Thiamine deficiency has been linked to persistent vomiting, with disturbances in vision and gait (126,127). Stomal stenosis may also cause symptoms of gastroesophageal reflux.

Upper endoscopy is the preferred means of investigation; contrast radiographs are not demonstrative of the degree of stenosis. Most patients with gastrojejunal stenosis after gastric bypass will respond to endoscopic dilatation.

Stomal ulceration may also cause stomal stenosis. The rate of gastrojejunal stomal ulcer approximates 10%. The etiology of stomal ulceration is often multifactorial, including acid secretion by parietal cells in the proximal pouch, ischemia of the jejunal limb, and NSAID use. Failure to heal with proton pump inhibitors and elimination of NSAIDs suggests jejunal ischemia; mucosal biopsies are confirmatory. Prolonged ulceration causes mechanical obstruction because of chronic cicatrization.

Staple line disruption is a complication of gastric bypass techniques in which the stomach is not divided. This complication is suggested by recurrent weight gain after weight loss stabilization. Correction requires reoperation to restaple and divide the stomach. Staple line disruption occurs in 1% of patients.

Nutrient deficiencies are anticipated after Roux-en-Y gastric bypass because the distal stomach and duodenum are bypassed. Defective absorption of vitamin B_{12}, folate, iron, and calcium are sufficiently common to warrant routine postoperative supplementation. Biliopancreatic diversion worsens micronutrient deficiencies because of the more severe anatomic rearrangement. Steatorrhea is universal and high dose calcium supplementation and monthly intramuscular vitamin D are required to prevent metabolic bone disease. Protein malnutrition is the most severe complication of biliopancreatic diversion.

REFERENCES

1. American Cancer Society. Cancer facts and figures. Available at: www.cancer.org.
2. Terry MB, Gaudet MM, Gammon MD. The epidemiology of gastric cancer. *Semin Radiat Oncol* 2002;12:111–127.
3. Martin RC II, Jaques DP, Brennan MF, et al. Extended local resection for advanced gastric cancer: increased survival versus increased morbidity. *Ann Surg* 2002;236:159–165.
4. Schwarz RE, Zagala-Nevarez K. Gastrectomy circumstances that influence early postoperative outcome. *Hepatogastroenterology* 2002;49: 1742–1746.
5. Wainess RM, Dimick JB, Upchurch GR, et al. Epidemiology of surgically treated gastric cancer in the United States, 1988–2000. *J Gastrointest Surg* 2003;7:879–883.
6. St Peter SD, Holcomb GW III, Calkins CM, et al. Open versus laparoscopic pyloromyotomy for pyloric stenosis: a prospective, randomized trial. *Ann Surg* 2006;244:363–370.
7. Yagmurlu A, Barnhart DC, Vernon A, et al. Comparison of the incidence of complications in open and laparoscopic pyloromyotomy: a concurrent single institution series. *J Pediatr Surg* 2004;39: 292–296.
8. Alain JL, Grousseau D, Terrier G. Extramucosal pyloromyotomy by laparoscopy. *Surg Endosc* 1991;5:174–175.
9. Hall NJ, Van Der Zee J, Tan HL, et al. Meta-analysis of laparoscopic versus open pyloromyotomy. *Ann Surg* 2004;240:774–778.
10. Haricharan RN, Aprahamian CJ, Celik A, et al. Laparoscopic pyloromyotomy: effect of resident training on complications. *J Pediatr Surg* 2008;43:97–101.
11. Laine L, Peterson WL. Bleeding peptic ulcer. *N Engl J Med* 1994;331: 717–727.
12. Silverstein FE, Gilbert DA, Tedesco FJ, et al. The national ASGE survey on upper gastrointestinal bleeding. *Gastrointest Endosc* 1981;27: 73–79.
13. Gilbert DA. Epidemiology of upper gastrointestinal bleeding. *Gastrointest Endosc* 1990;36(Suppl 5):8–13.
14. Branicki FJ, Boey J, Fok PJ, et al. Bleeding duodenal ulcer—a prospective evaluation of risk factors for rebleeding and death. *Ann Surg* 1990;211:411–418.
15. Mueller X, Rothenbuehler J, Amery A, et al. Factors predisposing to further hemorrhage and mortality after peptic ulcer bleeding. *J Am Coll Surg* 1994;179:457–461.
16. Branicki FJ, Coleman SY, Folk PJ, et al. Bleeding peptic ulcer: a prospective evaluation of risk factors for rebleeding and mortality. *World J Surg* 1990;14:262–270.
17. Larson G, Schmidt T, Gott J, et al. Upper gastrointestinal bleeding: predictors of outcome. *Surgery* 1986;100:765–772.
18. Imhof M, Schroders C, Ohmann C, et al. Impact of early operation on the mortality from bleeding peptic ulcer—ten years' experience. *Dig Surg* 1998;15:308–314.
19. Feldman RA, Eccersley AJ, Hardie JM. Epidemiology of *Helicobacter pylori*: acquisition, transmission, population prevalence and disease-to-infection ratio. *Br Med Bull* 1998;54:39–53.
20. Vaira D, Menegatti M, Miglioli M. What is the role of *Helicobacter pylori* in complicated peptic ulcer disease? *Gastroenterology* 1997;113: S78–S84.
21. Boey J, Choi SKY, Alagaratnam TT, et al. Risk stratification for perforated duodenal ulcers: a prospective validation of predictive factors. *Ann Surg* 1987;205:22–28.
22. Sanabria AE, Morales CH, Villegas MI. Laparoscopic repair of perforated peptic ulcer disease. *Cochrane Database Syst Rev* 2005;(4): CD004778.
23. El-Omar EM, Penman ID, Ardill JE, et al. *Helicobacter pylori* infection and abnormalities of acid secretion in patients with duodenal ulcer disease. *Gastroenterology* 1995;109:681–691.
24. Aalykke C, Lauritsen JM, Hallas J, et al. *Helicobacter pylori* and risk of ulcer bleeding among users of nonsteroidal anti-inflammatory drugs: a case-control study. *Gastroenterology* 1999;116:1305–1309.
25. Hay JA, Lyubashevsky E, Elashoff J, et al. Upper gastrointestinal hemorrhage clinical guideline—determining the optimal hospital length of stay. *Am J Med* 1996;100:313–322.
26. Jiranek GC, Kozarek RA. A cost-effective approach to the patient with peptic ulcer bleeding. *Surg Clin North Am* 1996;76:83–103.
27. Collins R, Langman M. Treatment with histamine H_2 antagonists in acute upper gastrointestinal hemorrhage: implications of randomized trials. *N Engl J Med* 1985;313:660–666.
28. Khuroo MS, Yattoo GN, Javid G, et al. A comparison of omeprazole and placebo for bleeding peptic ulcer. *N Engl J Med* 1997;336: 1054–1058.
29. Peterson WL, Cook DJ. Antisecretory therapy for bleeding peptic ulcer. *JAMA* 1998;280:877–878.
30. Lau JYW, Sung JJY, Lee KKC, et al. Effect of intravenous omeprazole on recurrent bleeding after endoscopic treatment of bleeding peptic ulcers. *N Engl J Med* 2000;343:310–316.
31. Cooper GS, Chak A, Way LE, et al. Early endoscopy in upper gastrointestinal hemorrhage: associations with recurrent bleeding, surgery, and length of hospital stay. *Gastrointest Endosc* 1999;49: 145–152.
32. Laine L, Cohen H, Brodhead J, et al. Prospective evaluation of immediate versus delayed refeeding and prognostic value of endoscopy in patients with upper gastrointestinal hemorrhage. *Gastroenterology* 1992;102:314–316.
33. Lin HJ, Wang K, Perng CL, et al. Natural history of bleeding peptic ulcers with a tightly adherent clot: a prospective observation. *Gastrointest Endosc* 1996;43:470–473.
34. Cook DJ, Guyatt GH, Salena BJ, et al. Endoscopic therapy for acute nonvariceal upper gastrointestinal hemorrhage: a meta-analysis. *Gastroenterology* 1992;102:139–148.
35. Kubba AK, Palmer KR. Role of endoscopic injection therapy in the treatment of bleeding peptic ulcer. *Br J Surg* 1996;83:461–468.
36. Lau JY, Sung JJ, Lam Y, et al. Endoscopic retreatment compared with surgery in patients with recurrent bleeding after initial endoscopic control of bleeding ulcers. *N Engl J Med* 1999;340:751–756.
37. Hsu P, Lai K, Lin X, et al. When to discharge patients with bleeding peptic ulcers: a prospective study of residual risk of rebleeding. *Gastrointest Endosc* 1996;44:382–387.
38. Brullet E, Campo R, Calvet X, et al. Factors related to the failure of endoscopic injection therapy for bleeding gastric ulcer. *Gut* 1996;39: 155–158.
39. Poxon VA, Keighley MRB, Dykes PW, et al. Comparison of minimal and conventional surgery in patients with bleeding peptic ulcer: a multicentre trial. *Br J Surg* 1991;78:1344–1345.

40. Millat B, Hay JM, Valleur P, et al. Emergency surgical treatment for bleeding duodenal ulcer: oversewing plus vagotomy versus gastric resection, a controlled randomized trial. *World J Surg* 1993;17: 568–574.
41. Mulholland MW, Debas HT. Chronic duodenal and gastric ulcer. *Surg Clin North Am* 1987;67:489–507.
42. Johnston D, Blackett RL. Recurrent peptic ulcers. *World J Surg* 1987;11: 274–282.
43. Millat B, Fingerhut A, Borie F. Surgical treatment of complicated duodenal ulcers: controlled trials. *World J Surg* 2000;24:299–306.
44. Graham DY, White RH, Moreland LW, et al. Duodenal and gastric ulcer prevention with misoprostol in arthritis patients taking NSAIDs. *Ann Intern Med* 1993;119:257–262.
45. Silverstein FE, Graham DY, Senior JR, et al. Misoprostol reduces serious gastrointestinal complications in patients with rheumatoid arthritis receiving nonsteroidal anti-inflammatory drugs: a randomized, double-blind, placebo-controlled trial. *Ann Intern Med* 1995;123: 241–249.
46. Rokkas T, Karameris A, Mavrogeorgis A, et al. Eradication of *Helicobacter pylori* reduces the possibility of rebleeding in peptic ulcer disease. *Gastrointest Endosc* 1995;41:1–4.
47. Jaspersen D, Koerner T, Schorr W, et al. *Helicobacter pylori* eradication reduces the rate of rebleeding in ulcer hemorrhage. *Gastrointest Endosc* 1995;41:5–7.
48. Santander C, Gravalos RG, Cedenilla AG, et al. Maintenance treatment vs *Helicobacter pylori* eradication in preventing re-bleeding of the peptic ulcer disease: a clinical trial and follow up for two years. *Gastroenterology* 1995;108:A208.
49. Maier M, Sohilling D, Dorlars D, et al. Eradication of Helicobacter pylori or H_2 blocker maintenance therapy after peptic ulcer bleeding: a prospective randomized trial. *Gastroenterology* 1995;108:A156.
50. Crofts TJ, Park KGM, Steele RJC, et al. A randomized trial of nonoperative treatment for perforated peptic ulcer. *N Engl J Med* 1989;320:970.
51. Boey J, Wong J, Ong GB. A prospective study of operative risk factors in perforated duodenal ulcers. *Ann Surg* 1982;195:265.
52. Kujath P, Schwandner O, Bruch H-P. Morbidity and mortality of perforated peptic gastroduodenal ulcer following emergency surgery. *Langenbecks Arch Surg* 2002;387:298–302.
53. Lau WY, Leung KL, Kwong KH, et al. A randomized study comparing laparoscopic versus open repair of perforated peptic ulcer using suture or sutureless technique. *Ann Surg* 1996;224:131.
54. Lau WY, Leung KL, Zhu XL, et al. Laparoscopic repair of perforated peptic ulcer. *Br J Surg* 1995;82:814.
55. Lunevicius R, Morkevicius M. Systematic review comparing laparoscopic and open repair for perforated peptic ulcer. *Br J Surg* 2005;92: 1195–1207.
56. Boey J, Lee NW, Koo J, et al. Immediate definitive surgery for perforated duodenal ulcers: a prospective controlled trial. *Ann Surg* 1982; 196:338.
57. Ren P, Huang J, Shin J, et al. Jejunojejunogastric intussusception: a rare intussusception in an adult patient after gastric surgery. *Gastrointest Endosc* 2002;56(2):296–298.
58. Eckhauser FE, Conrad M, Knol J, et al. Safety and long-term durability of completion gastrectomy in 81 patients with postsurgical gastroparesis syndrome. *Am Surgeon* 1998;64:1–7.
59. McCallum RW, Polpalle SC, Schirmer B. Completion gastrectomy for refractory gastroparesis following surgery for peptic ulcer disease, long-term follow-up with subjective and objective parameters. *Dig Dis Sci* 1991;36(11):1556–1561.
60. Cohen AM, Ottinger LW. Delayed gastric emptying following gastrectomy. *Ann Surg* 1976;184(6):689–696.
61. Zarzour JG, Christein JD, Drelichman ER, et al. Percutaneous transhepatic duodenal diversion for the management of duodenal fistulas. *J Gastrointest Surg* 2008;12:1103–1109.
62. Rodkey GV. Safe management of the impossible duodenum, risk avoidance in surgery of peptic ulcer. *Arch Surg* 1988;123:558–562.
63. Eldh J, Kewenter J, Kock NG, et al. Long-term results of surgical treatment for dumping after partial gastrectomy. *Br J Surg* 1974;61: 90–93.
64. Hansson L. Risk of stomach cancer in patients with peptic ulcer disease. *World J Surg* 2000;24:315–320.
65. Tersmette AC, Giardiello FM, Tytgat GNJ, et al. Carcinogenesis after remote peptic ulcer surgery: the long-term prognosis of partial gastrectomy. *Gastroenterology* 1991;101:148–153.
66. Lundegårdh G, Ekbom A, McLaughlin JK, et al. Gastric cancer risk after vagotomy. *Gut* 1994;35:946.
67. Holstein C. Long-term prognosis after partial gastrectomy for gastroduodenal ulcer. *World J Surg* 2000;24:307–314.
68. Safatle-Riberio AV, Riberio U, Reynolds JC. Gastric stump cancer: what is the risk? *Dig Dis* 1998;16:159–168.
69. Boring CC, Squires TS, Tong T. Cancer Statistics 1993. *CA Cancer J Clin* 1993;43:19.
70. Harju E. Gastric polyposis and malignancy. *Br J Surg* 1986;73:532–533.
71. Parsonnet J, Friedman GD, Vandersteen DP, et al. *Helicobacter pylori* infection and the risk of gastric carcinoma. *N Engl J Med* 1991;325: 1127–1131.
72. Nomura A, Stemmermann GN, Chyou P-H, et al. *Helicobacter pylori* infection and gastric carcinoma among Japanese Americans in Hawaii. *N Engl J Med* 1991;325:1132–1136.
73. Mortensen MB, Scheel-Hincke JD, Madsen MR, et al. Combined endoscopy ultrasonography and laparoscopic ultrasonography in the pretherapeutic assessment of resectability in patients with upper gastrointestinal malignancies. *Scand J Gastroenteral* 1996;31:1115–1119.
74. Burke EC, Karpeh MS Jr, Conlou KC. Laparoscopy in the management of gastric adenocarcinoma. *Ann Surg* 1997;225:262–267.
75. Adachi Y, Shiraishi N, Kitano S. Modern treatment of early gastric cancer: review of the Japanese experience. *Dig Surg* 2002;19:333–339.
76. Nakamura K, Morisaki T, Sugitani A, et al. An early gastric carcinoma treatment strategy based on analysis of lymph node metastasis. *Cancer* 1999;85:1500–1505.
77. Kunisaki C, Shimada H, Takahaski M, et al. Prognostic factors in early gastric cancer. *Hepatogastroenterology* 2001;48:294–298.
78. Lee S-H, Park J-H, Park DH, et al. Clinical efficacy of EMR with submucosal injection of a fibrinogen mixture: a prospective randomized trial. *Gastointest Endosc* 2006;64:691–696.
79. Imagawa A, Okada H, Kawahara Y, et al. Endoscopic submucosal dissection for early gastric cancer: results and degrees of technical difficulty as well as success. *Endoscopy* 2006;38:987–990.
80. Watanabe Y, Kato N, Maehata t, et al. Safer endoscopic gastric mucosal resection: prospective proton pump inhibitor administration. *J Gastroent Hepatol* 2006;21:1675–1680.
81. Ono H, Kondo H, Gotoda T, et al. Endoscopic mucosal resection of treatment of early gastric cancer. *Gut* 2001;48:225–229.
82. Korenaga D, Orita H, Mackawa S, et al. Pathological appearance of the stomach after endoscopic mucosal resection for early gastric cancer. *Br J Surg* 1997;84:1563–1566.
83. Cuschieri A. Laparoscopic gastric resection. *Surg Clin North Am* 2000; 80(4):1269–1284.
84. Nokaki I, Kubo Y, Kurita A, et al. Long-term outcome after laparoscopic wedge resection for early gastric cancer. *Surg Endosc* 2008;22: 2665–2669.
85. Sexton JA, Pierce RA, Halpin VJ, et al. Laparoscopic gastric resection for gastrointestinal stromal tumors. *Surg Endosc* 2008;22:2583–2587.
86. Wanebo HJ, Kennedy BJ, Chmiel J, et al. Cancer of the stomach: a patient care study by the American College of Surgeons. *Ann Surg* 1993;218:583–592.
87. Kranenbarg EK, van de Velde CJH. Gastric cancer in the elderly. *Eur J Surg Oncol* 1998;24:384–390.
88. Bittner R, Butters M, Ulrich M, et al. Total gastrectomy: updated operative mortality and long-term survival with particular reference to patients older than 70 years of age. *Ann Surg* 1996;224:37–42.
89. Schwarz R, Karpeh MS, Brennan MF. Factors predicting hospitalization after operative treatment for gastric carcinoma in patients older than 70 years. *J Am Coll Surg* 1997;184:9–15.
90. Shiu MH, Moore E, Sanders M, et al. Influence of the extent of resection on survival after curative treatment of gastric cancer: a retrospective multivariate analysis. *Arch Surg* 1987;122:1347–1351.
91. Maruyama K, Okabayashi K, Kinoshita T. Progress in gastric cancer in Japan and its limit of radicality. *World J Surg* 1987;11:418–425.
92. Noguchi Y, Imada T, Matsumoto A, et al. Radical surgery for gastric cancer: a review of the Japanese experience. *Cancer* 1989;64: 2053–2062.
93. Adachi Y, Kamakura T, Mori M, et al. Role of lymph node dissection and splenectomy in node-positive gastric carcinoma. *Surgery* 1994;116: 837–841.
94. Baba H, Maehara Y, Takeuchi H, et al. Effect of lymph node dissection on the prognosis in patients with node-negative early gastric cancer. *Surgery* 1994;117:165–169.
95. Maeta M, Yamashiro H, Saito S, et al. A prospective plot study of extended (D3) and superextended para-aortic lymphadenectomy (D4) in patients with T3 or T4 gastric cancer managed by total gastrectomy. *Surgery* 1999;125:325–331.

96. Robertson CS, Chung SCS, Woods SDS, et al. A prospective randomized trial comparing R1 subtotal gastrectomy with R3 total gastrectomy for antral cancer. *Ann Surg* 1994;220:176–182.
97. Bonekamp JJ, Hermans J, van de Velde CJH. Extended lymph-node dissection for gastric cancer. *N Engl J Med* 1999;340:908–914.
98. Cushieri A, Fayers P, Fielding J, et al. Postoperative morbidity and mortality after D1 and D2 resections for gastric cancer. *Lancet* 1996; 347:995–999.
99. Siewert JR, Bottcher K, Stein HJ, et al. Relevant prognostic factors in gastric cancer: ten-year results of the German gastric cancer study. *Ann Surg* 1998;228:449–461.
100. Kodera Y, Yamamura Y, Shimizu Y, et al. The number of metastatic lymph nodes: a promising prognostic determinant for gastric carcinoma in the latest edition of the TNM classification. *J Am Coll Surg* 1998;187:579–603.
101. Lee JS, Douglass HO. D2 dissection for gastric cancer. *Surg Oncol* 1997;6(4):215–225.
102. Pacelli F, Doglietto GB, Bellantone R, et al. Extensive versus limited lymph node dissection for gastric cancer: a comparative study of 320 patients. *Br J Surg* 1993;80:1153–1156.
103. Stipa S, DiGiorgio A, Ferri M, et al. Results of curative gastrectomy for carcinoma. *J Am Coll Surg* 1994;179:567–572.
104. Otsuji E, Yamaguchi T, Sawai K, et al. End results of simultaneous splenectomy in patients undergoing total gastrectomy for gastric cancer. *Surgery* 1996;120:40–44.
105. Weitz J, Jaques DP, Brennan M, et al. Association of splenectomy with postoperative complications in patients with proximal gastric and gastroesophageal junction cancer. *Ann Surg Oncol* 2004;11:682–689.
106. Shchepotin IB, Chorny VA, Nauta RJ, et al. Extended surgical resection in T4 gastric cancer. *Am J Surg* 1998;175:123–126.
107. Stein HJ, Feith M, Siewert JR. Cancer of the esophagogastric junction. *Surg Oncol* 2000;9:35–41.
108. Bonenkamp JJ, Songun I, Hermans J, et al. Randomized comparison of morbidity after D1 and D2 dissection for gastric cancer in 996 Dutch patients. *Lancet* 1995;345:745–748.
109. Roder JD, Böttchen K, Siewert JR, et al. Prognostic factors in gastric carcinoma: results of the German gastric carcinoma study 1992. *Cancer* 1993;72:2089–2097.
110. Hogan BA, Winter D, Broe D, et al. Prospective trial comparing contrast swallow, computed tomography and endoscopy t identify anastomotic leak following oesophageal surgery. *Surg Endosc* 2008;22:767–771.
111. Nakane Y, Okumura S, Akehira K, et al. Jejunal pouch reconstruction after total gastrectomy for cancer: a randomized controlled trial. *Ann Surg* 1995;222(1):27–35.
112. Espat NJ, Karpeh M. Reconstruction following total gastrectomy: a review and summary of the randomized prospective clinical trials. *Surg Oncol* 1999;7:65–69.
113. Deitel M. Surgery for morbid obesity: a review. *Eur J Gastroenterol Hepatol* 1999;11(2):57–61.
114. Pories WJ, Swanson MS, MacDonald KG, et al. Who would have thought it? An operation proves to be the most effective therapy for adult-onset diabetes mellitus. *Ann Surg* 1995;222:339–352.
115. Scopinaro N, Adami GF, Marinari GM, et al. Biliopancreatic diversion. *World J Surg* 1998;22:936–946.
116. Sjöström L. Surgical intervention as a strategy for treatment of obesity. *Endocrinology* 2000;13(2):213–320.
117. Schauer PR, Ikramuddin S. Laparoscopic surgery for morbid obesity. *Obes Surg* 2001;81(5):1145–1179.
118. Maher JW, Hawver LM, Pucci A, et al. Four hundred fifty consecutive laparoscopic Roux-en-y gastric bypasses with no mortality and declining leak rates and lengths of stay in a bariatric training program. *J Am Coll Surg* 2008;206:940–944.
119. Byrne TK. Complications of surgery for obesity. *Obes Surg* 2001;81(5): 1181–1193.
120. Surgerman HJ. Gastric surgery for morbid obesity. In: Zinner MJ, ed. *Maingot abdominal operations*, 10th ed. Stamford CT: Appleton & Lange; 1997.
121. Wittgrove AC, Clark GW. Laparoscopic gastric bypass, Roux-en-Y-500 patients: technique and results with 3–6 month follow up. *Obes Surg* 2000;10:233–239.
122. Lee S, Carmody B, Wolfe L, et al. Effect of location and speed of diagnosis on anastomotic leak outcome in 3828 gastric bypass cases. *J Gastrointest Surg* 2007;11:708–713.
123. Csendes A, Burdiles P, Burgos AM, et al. Conservative management of anastomotic leaks after 557 open gastric bypasses. *Obes Surg* 2005;15: 1252–1256.
124. Sugerman HJ, Brewer WH, Shiffman ML, et al. A multicenter, placebo-controlled, randomized, double-blinded, prospective trial of prophylactic ursodiol for the prevention of gallstone formation following gastric-bypass induced rapid weight loss. *Am J Surg* 1995;169:91–97.
125. Sanayal AJ, Sugerman HJ, Kellum JM, et al. Stomal complications of gastric bypass: incidence and outcome of therapy. *Am J Gastroenterol* 1992;87:1165–1169.
126. Kramer LD, Locke GE. Wernicke's encephalopathy: complication of gastric plication. *J Clin Gastroenterol* 1987;9:549–552.
127. Mason ME, Jalagani H, Vinik AI, Metabolic complications of bariatric surgery: diagnosis and management issues. *Gastroenterol Clin N Am* 2005;34:25–33.

CHAPTER

34

Complications of Hepatic Surgery

Theodore H. Welling and James A. Knol

Over the past 30 years, advances in preoperative evaluation, anesthetic management, surgical technique, and postoperative care have allowed for expanding indications for performance of major and minor liver resections for a variety of surgical diseases affecting the liver (Table 34.1). Surgical therapy may be an adjunct or the primary therapy, depending on the disease. The mortality associated with hepatic surgery or resection has declined from about 30% in past years to less than 1% to 4% at high volume institutions, depending on the complexity of the procedure and concomitant liver disease (1). However, knowledge regarding the potential complications is important, because hepatic surgery and resection continue to be associated with about a 40% morbidity rate (2). Hepatic surgical complications encompass a wide spectrum (Table 34.2). Complications specific to the liver relate to the liver's high blood flow, glucose homeostasis and protein anabolism, synthesis of clotting factors, clearance and deactivation of toxins, synthesis and drainage of bile, and role in protection from infectious agents entering the portal circulation through the gastrointestinal (GI) tract.

PATIENT SELECTION

Knowledge of hepatic surgical complications demands that there be appropriate preoperative evaluation to balance the risks of these complications and mortality against potential benefits. In Western countries most liver resections are performed for metastatic colorectal cancer, with about 20% performed for primary hepatobiliary cancer and 10% for benign disease (1). The indications for operations for these various diseases will not be covered here, but they do play a role in a discussion of surgical complications. If surgical therapy does not appear justified, other therapies such as ablative strategies, chemoembolization, radiation, or chemotherapy may offer significant therapeutic advantage or the possibility of downstaging disease such that a safer operation is possible. The indications for operation must be appropriate to justify any operation with associated complications and possible mortality.

Theodore H. Welling*, James A. Knol:** Sections of Transplantation* and General Surgery**, Department of Surgery, University of Michigan Health System

Selection of patients for hepatic resection requires appropriate radiologic workup or staging to eliminate patients for whom cure or significant palliation is not possible. Multiphase (arterial, portal venous, and hepatic venous) computed tomography (CT), or magnetic resonance imaging (MRI), is requisite in determining the extent of tumor in the liver, relationships to the vasculature of the liver, and whether a resection to remove the tumor will spare adequate parenchyma (residual liver remnant) to allow postoperative survival. This type of imaging also allows for optimal detection of disease and assistance in the differential diagnosis of liver masses. In general, if a liver tumor appears resectable, biopsy should be avoided, unless the biopsy will change the decision about whether to operate. Biopsy risks dissemination of tumor within the needle tract or to the peritoneal surfaces.

The patient's overall health and the extent of comorbid disease are significant factors predicting overall complications following hepatic surgery. In a recent large series the rate of pulmonary complications was 21% and the rate of cardiovascular complications was 10% (1). Morbidity and mortality for right hepatic lobectomy have been shown to correlate strongly with preoperative APACHE II scores (3), as has the American Society of Anesthesiologists (ASA) Classification score (4), emphasizing the need for appropriate optimization of patient health and selection.

The liver's health is the final major determinant in selection of patients for liver surgery. Cirrhosis increases the mortality associated with any operation and anesthesia, and an operation that decreases the amount of residual functioning liver further increases that risk (5). The presence of cirrhosis can raise the mortality rate following hepatic resection to as high as 4.7%, whereas the mortality rate following hepatic lobectomy in the absence of liver disease is 2.6% or less (6). Signs of severe cirrhosis include jaundice, ascites, and malnutrition, with laboratory correlates including bilirubin above 2 mg/dL, serum albumin less than 3 g/dL, and a platelet count less than 100,000 per μL. CT or MRI may show a relatively small liver with notching of the surface and, often, relative atrophy of the right lobe and hypertrophy of the left lateral segment and caudate lobe. A preliminary discriminator is the Child– Pugh score; all patients with grade C and most with grade B are not considered satisfactory candidates for operation. The

Table 34.1 Surgical diseases of the liver

Neoplasm—benign	Hepatic adenoma Focal nodular hyperplasia, symptomatic Hemangioma, symptomatic Biliary cystadenoma Hemangioendothelioma
Neoplasm—malignant	Hepatocellular carcinoma Intrahepatic cholangiocarcinoma Hilar cholangiocarcinoma Gallbladder cancer Hepatoblastoma Hemangioendothelioma Direct invasion by adjacent cancers—stomach, colon, renal, adrenal, vena caval Metastases—colorectal and highly selected: neuroendocrine, melanoma, gastrointestinal stromal tumor, endometrial, breast, stomach
Biliary disease	Intrahepatic or high extrahepatic bile duct stricture Intrahepatic bile duct stones Intrahepatic bile duct cysts (Caroli disease) Biliary fistula
Infection	Pyogenic abscess Echinococcal abscess Amebic abscess
Vascular disease	Hepatic artery aneurysm or pseudoaneurysm Biliary-arterial or biliary-venous fistula Arterial-portal fistula or arterial-hepatic venous fistula

Model for End-stage Liver Disease (MELD) score has been shown to be more predictive of worse outcomes, with patients with scores of greater than or equal to 9 experiencing as high as 29% perioperative mortality, depending on extent of resection (4). The presence of portal hypertension, as diagnosed by elevated hepatic vein pressure gradient or depressed platelet count, predicts persistent hepatic decompensation in over 75% of patients postresection (7). A variety of other methods have been proposed to predict which patients with liver disease are candidates for resection and how much of the diseased liver may safely be removed or ablated (8–10). Severe fibrosis, jaundice due to causes other than cirrhosis, steatosis greater than 30%, and a history of chemotherapy, particularly hepatic artery infusion therapy, are other indicators of a damaged liver and increase the risk of resection or ablation (11,12).

Table 34.2 Complications of liver surgery

Liver Surgery	
Intraoperative hemorrhage	Postoperative hemorrhage
Intrahepatic hematoma	Postoperative coagulopathy
Liver failure	Perihepatic abscess
Biliary fistula	Biliary stricture
Biloma	Bile peritonitis
Cholangitis	Hepatic abscess
Wound infection	Pneumonia
Hemobilia	Hepatic necrosis
Hepatic artery thrombosis	Portal vein thrombosis/insufficiency
Intraoperative air embolus	Hepatic vein thrombosis/insufficiency
Ascites	Peritonitis
Gastrointestinal bleeding	Pleural effusion
Special to Ablation Procedures	
Myoglobinuria	Thermal injury to surrounding structures

Table 34.3 Intrahepatic liver volume ratios based on CT scan for normal livers

Segments	Percent of Total Liver Volume
Right liver	65 ± 7 (49–82)
Left liver	33 ± 7 (17–49)
Segment IV	17 ± 4 (10–29)
Bisegment II + III	16 ± 4 (5–27)
Segment I	2 ± 0 (1–3)

Adapted from Abdalla EK, Denys A, Chevalier P, et al. Total and segmental liver volume variations: implications for liver surgery. *Surgery* 2004;135:414–420.

Preservation of remaining liver health following liver resection is of paramount importance. Resection planning requires estimation of the postresection functioning liver remnant. Postoperative liver dysfunction is significantly increased in patients with normal liver function when the liver remnant is less than 25% of the initial liver volume (13). In the normal liver there is variation in the proportions of the hepatic segments that comprise the usual anatomic liver resections (Table 34.3) (14). The experienced liver surgeon can make some estimates on the basis of the imaging studies. However, volumetric analysis should be done in patients with a normal liver in whom an extended lobectomy is planned or in patients with damaged livers in whom any resection or ablation equivalent or greater than a single liver segment is anticipated (15). In addition, in patients for whom there is a possibility of preexisting liver damage, biopsy from the area of the potential remnant liver should be considered in order to confirm the presence or absence of liver disease.

For patients in whom resection or ablation cannot be executed because of the threat of small functioning liver remnant, inducing hypertrophy in the liver that is to be preserved may be attempted. Hypertrophy is most often induced by percutaneous portal vein embolization to the liver that is to be resected, with operation following at 4 to 6 weeks following embolization (16,17). Patients in whom preoperative portal vein embolization should be considered are listed in Table 34.4. High dose focal liver irradiation also induces hypertrophy in the unirradiated liver. Operative portal vein ligation will also cause hypertrophy in the opposite liver lobe but with more complications relative to percutaneous embolization. Finally,

Table 34.4 Indications for preoperative portal vein embolization

Patients with underlying normal liver
Future liver remnant volume less than 30%
Major hepatectomy associated with gastrointestinal procedure
Resection of bilobar tumors, including a major hepatectomy
Patients with diseased liver
Cirrhosis
Severe fibrosis
Jaundice
Steatosis greater than 30%
Chemotherapy

From Clavien PA, Emond J, Vauthey JN, et al. Protection of the liver during hepatic surgery. *J Gastrointest Surg* 2004;8:313–327.

planned two-stage hepatectomy for tumor has been reported as a means of resecting all tumors, and avoids a small functioning remnant liver (18).

COMPLICATIONS OF HEPATIC SURGERY

The complications of hepatic surgery can be variously categorized. For the surgeon they are most usefully divided into intraoperative and postoperative complications.

Intraoperative complications

Intraoperative complications can be lethal during hepatic surgery or in the early, intermediate, or late postoperative periods. Decisions made before and during the operation and the conduct of the operation are significant factors in the incidence and severity of intraoperative and postoperative complications. The major complications occurring during operation are bleeding, vascular injury, air embolus, and biliary injury.

Preexisting Bleeding

Preexisting bleeding associated with hepatic surgery is generally from blunt or penetrating injury or from rupture of a tumor. Rupture of a benign tumor resulting in bleeding is almost exclusively due to hepatic adenoma, with only extremely rare case reports of rupture of hepatic hemangiomas, spontaneously or associated with blunt trauma, or from focal nodular hyperplasia. Rupture of malignant tumor with bleeding is almost always due to hepatocellular carcinoma. Bleeding from liver metastases is vanishingly rare.

The principles and methods for dealing with hepatic bleeding from trauma are not this chapter's topic. The approach is based on classification of the injury and is aimed at control of bleeding. Initial maneuvers are four: (a) packing of the liver with pressure, (b) achieving cardiovascular resuscitation with fluid and blood products, (c) maintaining body temperature, and (d) normalizing coagulation as much as possible. Control of bleeding proceeds from less to more invasive, performing the minimum to achieve bleeding control. Removal of devitalized liver tissue and provision of adequate drainage for bile duct disruption are the other major imperatives in the management of traumatic liver injuries.

Operation for bleeding after a percutaneous biopsy should be individualized, based on the indications for the biopsy. Bleeding from liver tissue at the site of needle entry can almost always be stopped with pressure, combined with fulguration, or with horizontal mattress suture of the needle entrance site at the liver capsule. If the bleeding is coming from a hemangioma at the liver's surface, where the needle punctured the tumor, bleeding may be stopped with pressure or with a gently placed horizontal mattress suture around the needle entrance site, but it may occasionally require resection of the tumor by enucleation. Bleeding from other tumors can usually be stopped with pressure, cautery (at high settings), argon plasma coagulation, or suture, and rarely requires resection. However, depending on the surgeon's experience, resection may be the preferred route. In some cases arterial bleeding from within the liver may not readily stop with pressure and can result in intrahepatic hematoma. Packing, closing the abdomen, and emergent angiography with embolization are the preferred steps in such a case.

Frequently, a tumor that ruptures into the peritoneal cavity or produces intracapsular hematoma will stop bleeding spontaneously, and operation can be done on an urgent rather than emergent basis. A history of prolonged oral contraceptive use in a woman is a strong predictor of hepatic adenoma, whereas a history of hepatitis B or C or cirrhosis indicates that hepatocellular cancer is likely to be the cause of bleeding. Abnormal laboratory studies, including hepatitis serologies, liver function studies, and alpha-fetoprotein suggest cirrhosis and hepatocellular cancer. If the situation allows, liver imaging should be done to delineate the tumor causing the bleeding. CT or MRI should be done with contrast, including arterial phase imaging. Tumors that rupture are usually hypervascular and are best demonstrated by arterial phase imaging. Noncontrast scans and contrast scans in the portal venous phase are likely to be confusing if there is intrahepatic or subcapsular hemorrhage, with difficulty distinguishing between tumor and intrahepatic hematoma. Because the tumor's pathology is not likely to be fully certain at operation, the operative approach should be that for a malignant tumor, with preference to formal resection as opposed to enucleation.

Intraoperative Bleeding

Intraoperative bleeding with liver operations, as with all operations, should be kept to a minimum, and a number of measures can be employed to facilitate minimizing blood loss. The extent of blood transfusion has been correlated with postoperative morbidity and mortality in liver surgery (19). Increasing level of blood transfusion has also been inversely correlated with tumor-free survival after liver resection for malignancy (19–21), with a recent study on hepatocellular carcinoma patients demonstrating

Table 34.5 Sources of extrahepatic blood loss

Sources of extrahepatic blood loss
Liver capsule transgression
Diaphragm injury
Hepatic vein injury
Vena caval injury
Phrenic vein injury
Variceal injury
Right adrenal vein injury
Right adrenal gland injury
Portal vein injury
Hepatic artery injury

increased intraoperative blood loss as an independent risk factor for tumor recurrence and disease specific survival (22). Blood loss that occurs before transecting the liver can be insidiously large—sometimes the major source of blood loss for the operation. Some of this blood loss is under the surgeon's control, but some perihepatic blood loss can be due to disease factors.

Technical Factors

Technical factors leading to perihepatic blood loss in liver surgery are listed in Table 34.5. Experience, knowledge of the anatomy, and a commitment to limited blood loss are important to minimize loss from these sources. Achieving as much exposure or visualization as possible, with an appropriately large incision, appropriate retraction, and visualization if done laparoscopically, is also important for minimizing blood loss in this stage of the liver operation. Exposure may be particularly difficult in the deep-chested patient, in patients whose liver lies superior to the costal margin, in patients with large tumors, and in patients with large livers.

The usual sources of massive intraoperative bleeding and, occasionally, postoperative bleeding are the hepatic veins and the vena cava. Injuries occur at margins of the liver at the mobilization stage or at the margins of or within the liver during transection of the liver. Bleeding from these vessels during the mobilization stage is almost always technical and avoidable, except in the reoperative setting, where there may be dense scarring adjacent to the major vessels, making the dissection and control extremely difficult. Although these veins are relatively tough, avoidance of excessive traction or torsion on the venous structures is necessary to avoid tearing. Suture ligature, suture closure, or vascular staple closure of medium and large tributaries of the cava are more secure than clips and standard ligatures, which have a tendency to brush or roll off during manipulations of the liver and with traction on the vena cava. If a tear develops in the vena cava, or a clamp slips off a large tributary after its division, finger occlusion and then serial placement of Babcock or Alice clamps on the vessel across the opening can usually bring a large opening under quick control. The clamps are removed sequentially as the opening is closed with suture.

Portal Hypertension

Some liver operations must be performed in the presence of portal hypertension. The critical areas to be addressed to minimize blood loss are the abdominal wall, intra-abdominal adhesions of the omentum, the liver hilum, the gastrohepatic ligament, and the retroperitoneum inferior to the liver hilum. Adhesions of omentum to the abdominal wall and to the area of the liver hilum are common routes of portosystemic decompression and are likely to contain large, relatively delicate vessels with blood at pressure above the normal splanchnic venous pressure. These adhesions should be taken down carefully. Large variceal vessels are often present in the gastrohepatic ligament, which should also be taken down between clamps or heat coagulation sealing, remembering to evaluate for the presence of a replaced left hepatic artery crossing the ligament. Large collaterals may be found in the retroperitoneum adjacent or anterior to the infrahepatic vena cava, with the feeding vessels occasionally coming from the liver hilum. Particularly when portal hypertension is associated with portal vein thrombosis, there will be large fragile collateral vessels in the hepatoduodenal ligament. Attachments between the diaphragm and the liver are much less likely to have collaterals as a manifestation of portosystemic shunting.

Reoperative Surgery

Reoperative liver surgery is usually associated with increased perihepatic blood loss because of the density of liver adhesions to the diaphragm, retroperitoneum, and right adrenal gland. There is difficulty staying out of the liver and out of the diaphragm and adrenal gland when attempting to dissect those structures from each other. Judicious use of the cautery and good exposure can minimize blood loss. Special care should be exercised when approaching the liver hilum and the regions of the vena cava and the termini of the hepatic veins.

Hepatic Bleeding

Transection of liver tissue can be associated with significant blood loss. Mortality from intraoperative bleeding continues to be reported, but rarely, although blood loss with major resections often requires one to three transfusions either intraoperatively or postoperatively. In recent series transfusion outliers continue to be ten units of blood loss or more (5,19).

Control of minor bleeding points on the raw liver surface is best addressed with pressure or cautery during liver transection. Major bleeding points are best controlled with suture technique. Where there is a side opening in a vessel, such as where a branch has been avulsed, it is preferable to directly close the opening in the vessel with fine suture rather than to include the entire vessel in a mass suture ligature. An end-bleeding vessel that has retracted into the liver parenchyma can be controlled with a figure-8 or horizontal mattress

Table 34.6 Factors in blood loss during liver transection
Unsatisfactory exposure
High central venous pressure
Large tumor
Large liver
Close proximity of tumor to large intrahepatic vessels
Coagulopathy
Inexperienced surgeon
Inexperienced surgical assistants
Improper equipment
Inappropriate operative approach

suture into the surrounding parenchyma, tied only tight enough to occlude the vessel. Control of the cut liver edge with large mattress sutures is also a helpful way to control bleeding in situations where those sutures will not occlude important blood inflow, bile drainage, or hepatic venous drainage of the liver remnant and where the sutures are placed relatively close to the liver edge. A similar effect can be achieved using a stapler to divide the liver parenchyma where the liver thickness will accommodate its use (3 cm in normal liver). Because liver bleeding is frequently from low-pressure vessels, control of bleeding with packing is commonly used for brief periods during an operation, but packing can be prolonged for up to 72 hours and can be very useful in the case of an unstable patient or a patient with coagulopathy. Hemostatic agents, such as crystallized collagen or coagulating liquids or sprays, cautery at high settings, and the argon plasma coagulator are all useful methods for dealing with diffuse bleeding from the raw liver surface. Sewing omentum or peritoneum over the raw surface has not proven effective in stopping bleeding (23).

Factors that are associated with large operative blood loss are listed in Table 34.6. As many of these factors as possible should be controlled to minimize bleeding. Control of blood loss while transecting the liver can usually be achieved to a remarkable extent. This control involves both liver blood flow control and the use of transection methods that improve exposure of vessels.

Liver Blood Flow Control to Minimize Blood Loss

Inflow occlusion is the primary method by which blood flow control is achieved. There are a variety of methods of performing inflow occlusion. General inflow occlusion is exemplified by the Pringle maneuver, which clamps the hepatoduodenal ligament at the foramen of Winslow. More selective means include occlusion of portal flow to a particular portal segment using ultrasound-guided placement of a balloon catheter or dissecting and occluding by ligature or stapling the portal triad to only the particular portion of the liver to be resected. The potential for accessory arterial inflow must be recognized, particularly in a replaced or accessory left hepatic artery crossing the gastrohepatic ligament. Because blood loss from the hepatic veins and their tributaries will still occur with inflow occlusion, maintaining a relatively low central venous pressure will help in limiting blood loss during transection (24,25).

Partial vascular exclusion can be performed on a part of the liver and can very effectively limit blood loss, as long as dissection remains within the excluded portion. This method is particularly applicable in the liver with cirrhosis or in other conditions in which the functioning residual liver is small or compromised and when the added insult of warm ischemia could be hazardous. For selective inflow occlusion, facility with intraoperative ultrasound is essential for identifying the appropriate pedicle to be occluded and the position of that pedicle.

Blood loss during liver transection can be nearly completely eliminated by total vascular exclusion, comprising complete inflow and outflow vascular occlusion of the liver. The blood that is lost is only that within vessels in the liver. Total vascular exclusion is accomplished by (a) establishing inflow occlusion, remembering that accessory hepatic arteries may be present, (b) occluding the infrahepatic vena cava, and (c) occluding the suprahepatic vena cava. A method that excludes the right adrenal vein and lumbar veins requires mobilizing the right lobe of the liver, establishing a window posterior to the suprahepatic vena cava, dividing peritoneal attachments between the caudate lobe and the left aspect of the vena cava to mobilize the caudate lobe anteriorly, and then placing an infrahepatic clamp with its tip in the window behind the suprahepatic vena cava. A major consideration with total hepatic vascular exclusion is that cardiac venous return may be compromised, resulting in hypotension when total vascular exclusion is implemented. Hypotension can usually be avoided if the central venous pressure is raised to about 12 mm Hg prior to placing the vena cava clamps. An advantage of this method is that resection or dissection in the liver around the junction of the major hepatic veins can be more safely performed; injuries to those veins can be repaired in a relatively bloodless field. Disadvantages include the need to push up the central venous pressure, the more extensive dissection that must be done to place the clamps, and the possibility that a greater warm ischemic injury may occur to the residual liver segment than would occur with inflow occlusion alone (26).

Liver Transection Methods to Minimize Blood Loss

Early liver surgery made use of the finger-fracture technique, in which the liver parenchyma was crushed between the fingers, leaving behind the more fibrous vessels and bile ducts for control by ligature, clips, staples, or heat coagulation-sealing. Finger-fracture, although still occasionally useful, and the most rapid way of transecting liver short of sharp transection, tends to tear the hepatic venous structures because they contain less connective tissue in the wall. The technique may tear the smaller vascular and biliary structures before they can be controlled and is less effective in livers that have developed fibrosis.

Several methods are commonly in use to transect liver in a way that permits encountered nonparenchymal structures to be controlled. The clamp-crush technique uses an instrument, usually with multiple small teeth—such as a vascular clamp—to crush the parenchyma in small bites. The crushed parenchyma is subsequently aspirated away, and the exposed vascular and biliary structures are ligated. The Cavitron ultrasonic aspirator (CUSA) technique uses high-energy ultrasound transmitted to a suction tip through a special handpiece. Hydrodissection uses a fine high-pressure water jet to disrupt the parenchyma. With the CUSA and hydrodissection, the disrupted parenchyma is immediately aspirated through the handpiece, exposing the more fibrous vessels and bile ducts. These latter two techniques are less efficient in fibrotic and cirrhotic livers. Recently, with the development of techniques for laparoscopic liver resection, high frequency sonic scalpel, bipolar technology, and linear cutting staplers have shown applicability in selected circumstances (27). In addition, precoagulation devices have proven to be effective by application to the line of liver division before formal hepatic transection (28,29). These modern techniques are much more effective in maintaining a bloodless field during liver transection compared to finger-fracture with no apparent increase in biliary complications. With a bloodless field and exposure of structures, these methods permit recognition of the internal liver anatomy during transection, leading to less chance of misdirection during liver transection.

Mapping of the position of the major vessels within the liver by intraoperative ultrasound can significantly affect blood loss associated with liver transection. Major resections approach the central or right hepatic veins, which, because they are not generally occluded during liver transection, can be a major source of blood loss if injured. Maintaining a centimeter or two distance from these vessels, when possible, avoids avulsion of small and medium-sized tributaries, which tends to occur when the dissection is carried immediately adjacent to these large veins.

Cryoablation

Two sources of intraoperative bleeding that are not common to other liver operations occur with cryoablation. The major source of blood loss as a complication of liver cryoablation is cracking of the liver parenchyma at the margins of the ice-ball as it thaws. Intraparenchymal bleeding adjacent to the thawed ice-ball is not a common problem. If the ice-ball is at the surface of the liver, during the freezing phase, because water expands as it freezes, the capsule or surface will often fracture. When the ice-ball thaws, there is a risk of bleeding at these fractures. The liver can also be avulsed from the ice-ball if care is not taken, resulting in vessel tears. Care in handling the frozen and postfrozen portion of the liver, observation until the surface has thawed before closing the abdomen, and the use of surface- coating hemostatic agents are preventative measures. Treatment for the bleeding includes packing, correction of coagulopathy, procoagulation agents, and judicious suture placement.

The other source of intraoperative bleeding after cryoablation is through the cryoprobe tract after the probe is withdrawn. Two measures prevent bleeding through this tract. The first, and most important, is to avoid placing the initial needle and guidewire for the dilator and sheath through, or in close proximity to, large vessels. The second is to slide the sheath back into the tract over the probe before withdrawing the probe, then to withdraw the probe, and then to pack the tract with small particles of Gelfoam while gradually withdrawing the sheath. However, radiofrequency ablation (RFA) is currently the more accepted ablative strategy for appropriately selected tumors and avoids the occasional bleeding associated with the cryotherapy ablative technique.

Vascular Injuries

A normal liver can survive permanent interruption of arterial inflow if there is normal flow through the portal vein and there is no additional hepatocellular injury due to associated prolonged warm ischemia or decreased splanchnic blood flow secondary to hypotension or due to the use of vasopressors. If the attachments of the liver to the diaphragm and the retroperitoneum remain intact, collateral arterial flow has been demonstrated within 24 hours of ligation of the main arterial inflow. In over 85% of instances, either the right or the left hepatic artery can be ligated and there will be establishment of intrahepatic arterial collaterals to the dearterialized side immediately or within days (30).

A normal liver can also usually withstand portal vein interruption if arterial flow remains intact and there is no hypotension, decreased splanchnic arterial blood flow, or hepatocellular injury from warm ischemia. However, occlusion of both arterial and venous blood supplies leads to rapid hepatic necrosis and acute liver failure. A diseased liver may not tolerate decreased blood flow from interruption of either portal or hepatic arterial sources.

Intraoperative complete liver devascularization is a technical issue. Care in dissection in the subhepatic area, continual evaluation of orientation when dissecting in the area of the liver hilum, and identification of the principal arteries by palpation for pulses in the hepatoduodenal ligament will help prevent hilar vascular injuries. The principles of dissecting the arteries from "large and known to the smaller and nonpalpable" and from anterior inferior left to superior and right will also help to prevent injury to arterial structures. Use of intraoperative ultrasound in the hilum can help define the location of the portal vein in the difficult hilum. The portal vein, in addition, has a very consistent posterior position in the hepatoduodenal ligament, unlike the arteries, which are variable in position and course.

If division of the portal vein or arterial supply, or both, in the hepatoduodenal ligament is discovered intraoperatively, salvage requires immediate revascularization. For the surgeon inexperienced in vascular reconstruction, assistance of a liver transplant surgeon or vascular surgeon should be immediately enlisted. The portal vein should be repaired first, because the portal vein is the greater source of blood flow to the hepatocytes (60% to 70%) than the artery. End-to-end repair can often be done, particularly if the duodenum is kocherized, but vein graft may be required. Internal jugular vein, external iliac vein, left renal vein, saphenous vein, or pericardial patch can be used as either conduit or patch material depending on the situation. Externally supported polytetrafluoroethylene (PTFE) graft has been used but is not the first choice. Repair or anastomosis is usually performed with a running fine polypropylene monofilament suture. Arterial repair should be performed with a spatulated repair using fine polypropylene suture. Reversed saphenous vein can be used for graft if necessary. Additional mobility of the proximal artery can be obtained in some cases by dividing the gastroduodenal artery. Ideally, the patient should be heparinized for the repair and started on aspirin postoperatively.

Injury of the Glisson sheath-encased portal trinity within the liver can occur. Injury at this level is difficult to treat because there is often combined injury to the portal vein, the accompanying artery, and the accompanying bile duct. The best course is usually to suture repair or ligate the injured vessels and observe briefly to determine how much liver is affected, leaving the bile duct initially unrepaired. If a large amount of liver appears devascularized, further attempts should be made to repair the vessels, especially the portal vein. Resection may be advisable based on subsequent residual functioning liver volume. Once a decision has been made with regard to salvage versus resection, bile duct primary repair, biliary enteric anastomosis, or liver resection should be performed.

When there is irretrievable liver devascularization, the only option may be emergency liver transplant. Bleeding should be controlled as much as possible, and contact with a transplant center and with a liver transplant surgeon at that center should be carried out immediately. Survival for anhepatic patients is usually less than 72 hours.

Maintenance of venous drainage from the residual liver remnant also demands planning and continued intraoperative attention. Liver tissue without venous drainage will not remain viable. Protection of venous drainage includes evaluation for the course of the major hepatic veins, crossing them with resection only in a planned fashion, and evaluation for accessory hepatic veins, which may allow partial lobe resections and/or dividing a major hepatic vein. In extreme cases vein grafts can be used to replace resected segments of major veins (31). Care for venous drainage must avoid occluding residual hepatic veins with ill-placed sutures into the hepatic parenchyma in an attempt to control bleeding.

Bile Duct Injuries

Injury to the extrahepatic bile ducts associated with liver surgery can be irreparable and the etiology of mortality due to acute hepatic failure. The bile ducts, particularly at the hilar plate, are more easily disrupted than the vessels and are usually more difficult to dissect individually at that level. There is some variation in the branching pattern, such that in a small percentage of cases there is a tributary from the right liver draining into the left main duct. Less frequently there may be a tributary from the left liver draining into the right duct (32). Ligation or injury to the remaining bile ducts after a major resection may not always be apparent, so that great care should be exercised in identifying and dissecting the bile ducts at the hilum. With lobectomy or trisegmentectomy, if there is distance between tumor and the hilum it is safer to dissect the bile ducts in a Glissonian fashion—that is, to dissect into the liver substance slightly away from the liver hilum outside the Glisson capsule and to divide the particular duct somewhat away from the actual main bile duct bifurcation (33). Even if the vessels are divided at the hilum, division of the bile duct can be delayed until the liver parenchyma is divided at the hilum, when the branching pattern can be demonstrated as the parenchyma is dissected away. This approach is also useful in dissection for hilar cholangiocarcinoma, where later division of the bile duct may allow for more margin on the tumor.

Operative injury to intrahepatic bile ducts occurs almost exclusively when operation is carried out with disregard for the liver's internal anatomy. However, resections involving the hilus (central liver resections and caudate resections) are noted to be at higher risk of biliary complications such as leaks, raising the incidence from less than 4% to as high as 10% to 15% (34). The biliary drainage to a segment or segments of liver may be occluded or divided within the liver. With incision into or through the liver, intrahepatic biliary injury will occur if a line of division of the liver crosses the plane of biliary drainage without removing the portion of liver that is served by that biliary drainage. Intrahepatic biliary injury can also occur with placement of probes for cryoablation or radiofrequency ablation, with placement of catheters into the liver for biliary drainage or abscess drainage, or with needle liver biopsy.

If the bile ducts in the isolated segment are completely occluded, and provided that the bile within the isolated segment remains sterile, the result is that the isolated segment of liver will atrophy. However, if the segment of liver associated with an obstructed bile duct is an important component of the functioning liver remnant, the patient may experience postoperative liver failure. If the bile within an isolated bile duct is not sterile, a liver abscess is likely to result. If a bile duct in an isolated segment is not adequately occluded, more so with incision through the liver than with needle or probe bile duct injury, a persistent bile leak from the surface of the liver is likely.

Avoidance of bile duct injury is the best practice and is based on knowledge of liver internal anatomy, demonstrated by intraoperative ultrasound. Successful primary repair of intrahepatic or extrahepatic bile ducts may be possible when the ducts are of relatively large caliber (≥3 mm diameter) and the injury does not involve greater than 50% of the circumference of the bile duct. In larger hepatic ducts with >50% circumference injury, bile drainage should be established into a Roux-en-Y limb of intestine. Stenting of injured intrahepatic bile ducts may be used to achieve temporary but not permanent drainage.

Air Embolism

Air embolism is a risk during procedures involving division of the hepatic parenchyma. Because of relatively low pressure in the hepatic veins there is the risk of air being drawn into the vein and blood flow carrying that air through the right heart and into the pulmonary arteries. The air, if voluminous enough, can cause blockage of pulmonary artery blood flow. More feared is air that crosses an atrial septal defect and passes into the arterial circulation to the coronary arteries or the cerebral circulation, with potentially devastating effects. In practice, the risk of air embolism is not very great during open operations on the liver because patients are maintained on positive pressure ventilation during general anesthesia. The central venous pressure is therefore always greater than zero, and blood exits the openings in the veins rather than air being drawn in. The veins are very thin-walled and collapse to a great degree when central venous pressure drops. Operating in the reverse-Trendelenburg position does decrease central venous pressure, but usually not so far as to result in air embolism. If there is significant blood loss and decreasing central venous pressure, considering moving into a flat position is prudent.

The risk of CO_2 embolus is much more significant with laparoscopic liver surgery because the pressure of the CO_2 within the peritoneal cavity is usually higher than the central venous pressure. Although reports of air embolus occurring with laparoscopic procedures on other organs exist, none exist for laparoscopic liver resection. A single study addressing this issue did not cause any significant or planned openings into a major hepatic vein or the suprahepatic vena cava; so while the complication is possible, its incidence is unknown (35).

Treatment for air embolus intraoperatively includes placement of the patient in Trendelenburg position, aspiration of air through a central line, use of 100% inspired oxygen, restoration of central venous pressure, and closure or occlusion of the opening through which the air entered the circulation. Although recommended with air embolus, turning the patient on the left side is less feasible intraoperatively.

Diaphragmatic Injury

Occasionally a portion of the diaphragm must be resected while removing a hepatic tumor. With care, injury to the lung can be avoided, although infrequently the lung is adherent to the process at the diaphragm. If no injury to the lung occurs, there usually is no compromise in respiratory function during the operation. Lung volume can be compromised if large amounts of fluid fill the pleural space, leaving decreased chest volume for lung expansion, or if the opening in the diaphragm is so small that air entering the pleural space is entrapped, causing a tension pneumothorax.

There is usually no problem with leaving the diaphragm open until after the liver resection is completed. The diaphragmatic repair rarely requires prosthetic placement. The opening should be repaired using permanent suture usually with a running technique. Clot and fluid should be evacuated from the pleural space before and during the repair. Usually a chest tube is not required, if residual air is aspirated from the chest cavity with a catheter through the defect while the anesthetist supplies forced inspiration. The catheter is withdrawn on suction as the last suture is tied.

Postoperative complications

Fulminant Hepatic Failure

Fulminant hepatic failure is defined as the development of hepatic encephalopathy within 8 weeks of the patient being healthy. The most common cause of fulminant hepatic failure following liver resection is a small functioning liver remnant. Other etiologies include liver devascularization, interruption of venous drainage from the liver, excessive liver warm ischemia, major bile duct obstruction, halogenated anesthetic agents, viral infections with hepatitis B, and reactions to certain drugs. The hallmark of postoperative liver failure is a persistently rising bilirubin, coagulopathy, and encephalopathy. This can be accompanied by acidosis, renal failure, and hypoglycemia. It is important during this situation to evaluate for unrecognized vascular injuries that could be contributing to the liver failure with the use of duplex ultrasound, CT angiography, or MRI. Acute high grade obstruction of the biliary tree should also be investigated by use of magnetic resonance cholangiopancreatography (MRCP), endoscopic retrograde cholangiopancreatography (ERCP), or percutaneous transhepatic cholangiography (PTC) depending on anatomical factors and overall index of suspicion. Currently there is no treatment for postoperative fulminant liver failure other than supportive care allowing for hopeful return of liver function and recovery. Otherwise transplantation needs to be considered depending on ongoing oncologic or infectious issues. In these circumstances, bioartificial liver methods have been used in trials as bridges to transplant; however, their efficacy is still unclear (36).

Hepatic Insufficiency

Liver regeneration can replace the removed liver to a varying extent, depending on the liver's health, but it does not do so instantaneously. In a normal liver full regenerative replacement after a major liver resection occurs in about 6 months with over 80% of this occurring over a 6 to 8 week period. A damaged liver regenerates less rapidly and less fully. A guideline has been that in the normal liver, a liver remnant of 25% to 30% of the initial liver volume is compatible with survival; with Child A cirrhosis a liver remnant of 40% to 50% of the initial liver volume is compatible with survival; and with intermediate levels of liver injury, such as with fatty liver, a liver remnant of 40% of the initial liver volume is compatible with survival (16,37). The amount of residual functioning liver volume is also influenced by technical factors resulting from the operation: injury to the liver by warm ischemia, adequacy of vascular supply to the remaining liver volume, venous drainage from the remaining liver volume, and biliary drainage. These factors can all influence the degree of hepatic insufficiency postresection. Additionally, a recent study has suggested that laparoscopic liver resection may result in a decreased incidence of hepatic decompensation in cirrhotic patients with similar oncologic outcomes (38).

Subacute hepatic failure is defined as the onset of hepatic coma at greater than 8 weeks from a healthy state. Etiologies associated with liver operations include small functioning liver remnant, hepatitis B from transfusion or reactivation associated with the operation (39), and partial bile duct obstruction, caused by unrelieved choledocholithiasis, hepatolithiasis, or progressive stricture due to ischemia or thermal injury. Chronic liver failure can continue to progress, usually in cases involving those with chronic liver disease or cirrhosis.

Should hepatic insufficiency develop, measures must be undertaken to limit the consequences of this state, such as management of ascites with the use of sodium restriction and diuretics and management of encephalopathy by the use of agents to minimize intestinal flora. Factors in the formation of ascites include a decrease in serum colloid osmotic pressure and an increase in portal venous pressure. Serum albumin, the major determinant of serum colloid osmotic pressure, is usually severely depressed after major liver resection—to as low as 1.6 g/dL, with recovery over several weeks to months. With liver resection of greater than 30%, there is an increase in portal venous pressure (40,41). Complications of ascites include ascitic leak from incisions. Pressure phenomena may occur, including abdominal pain due to the distention, early satiety and vomiting due to compression of the stomach and intestines, and abdominal compartment syndrome. Infected ascites, secondary to contamination through drain tracts, incisions, or from paracenteses, may also occur.

In patients with cirrhosis and in those with major liver resection, immediate postoperative treatment with spironolactone and avoidance of high postoperative central venous pressure (which is a partial determinant of portal venous pressure) may help to decrease the rate of formation of ascites. Paracentesis may be required in cases of suspected infected ascites (diagnostic) or in cases of compressive symptoms (therapeutic) and should be performed under ultrasound guidance. Drains in patients with ascites should be avoided and, if placed, should be removed early and the tract closed to prevent ascitic leak. Indeed, a randomized prospective trial showed that use of drains in cirrhotic patients with ascites resulted in higher infectious complication rates (42).

Warm Ischemia

Warm ischemia is associated with injury to liver cells. Warm ischemia causes a postoperative rise in transaminases, which usually peak at about 24 to 48 hours; this increase is proportional to the length of the warm ischemia and the overall health of the liver remnant. Most liver surgeons use inflow occlusion to decrease blood loss during resection, and they often use it when doing intraoperative liver ablations. Limiting the duration of each individual event of liver inflow occlusion seems to decrease the postoperative transaminase rise, but this practice demands multiple periods of reperfusion and prolongs the time of transection, and it sometimes increases blood loss. Recently there has been a trend toward "ischemic preconditioning," using an initial 10-minute period of warm ischemia followed by a 10-minute period of reperfusion, after which a continuous longer stretch of warm ischemia seems to cause less liver cell injury than the same duration of warm ischemia without the "ischemic preconditioning" (43). The benefits are greatest in younger patients, for longer duration hepatic inflow occlusions, for resections in which over 50% of the liver is resected, and when there is liver steatosis. It has also been reported that warm ischemia is better tolerated with only inflow occlusion as compared to total hepatic vascular exclusion. It is postulated that there is some liver cell perfusion retrograde via the hepatic veins when there is inflow occlusion without outflow occlusion (26).

The tolerated length of warm ischemia is related to the residual functioning liver volume, but few data directly correlate those two parameters. For a right hepatic lobectomy in a normal liver (averaging about 65% resection), warm ischemia is tolerated for 60 minutes without intermittent reperfusion (44). With cirrhosis, warm ischemia can be tolerated up to 30 minutes. However, most liver surgeons who operate frequently on cirrhotic livers maintain inflow occlusion for only 15 to 20 minutes, interspersed with periods of 5 to 10 minutes of reperfusion.

Liver Devascularization

Fulminant hepatic failure will occur rapidly with total devascularization of a normal liver and occurs with less than total devascularization of a cirrhotic or otherwise damaged liver. Intraoperatively recognized devascularization is discussed above. Unrecognized devascularization can occur intraoperatively, and postoperative portal venous or hepatic artery thrombosis can occur due to operative injury or due to a hypercoagulable state. Avoidance of devascularization postoperatively includes respectful handling of the hilar blood vessels during operation and investigation of any suspected hypercoagulable states preoperatively so that appropriate postoperative prophylaxis may be implemented. Thrombosis of major hepatic arteries or the portal vein postoperatively may be detected by power Doppler ultrasound, arterial and portal venous phase CT, or MRI. With early detection of hepatic artery or portal vein thrombosis and evidence of compromised liver function, treatment with catheter-directed thrombolysis, operative thrombectomy, and/or vascular repair may be lifesaving (45).

Biloma

An intra-abdominal collection of bile, or biloma, occurs in about 3% of patients after major liver resection, and to a lesser extent after minor liver resection or with drainage of liver abscess (1). Partial excision or enucleation of a biliary cystadenoma also has a moderate risk of biloma. Biloma can be lessened by meticulous detection and closure of all sites of bile drainage on the raw surface of the liver. Placing drains at the time of operation does not lessen bile leak-associated complications, but drainage with a closed system is more likely to convert a biloma to a biliary fistula as well as to avoid an infected biloma or bile peritonitis.

Symptoms and signs of uninfected biloma may be minimal. There may be right upper quadrant or epigastric discomfort and tenderness, rarely a palpable mass, and often a minor rise in serum bilirubin. Diagnosis is by ultrasonography or CT, combined with diagnostic aspiration of bilious fluid. Treatment is tube drainage, which is usually possible percutaneously. Persistent bile drainage indicates a biliary fistula. Fever, tachycardia, and abdominal pain may develop in cases of an infected biloma. The treatment is antibiotics and percutaneous tube drainage.

Bile Peritonitis

Bile peritonitis results from bile accessing the general peritoneal cavity rather than being walled off into a discrete collection. Bile peritonitis is usually associated with insidious onset of symptoms, including ileus, malaise, abdominal distention, and, eventually, peritoneal signs. The initial peritonitis is chemical, but often bacteria are present and infectious peritonitis subsequently develops. Making the diagnosis of bile peritonitis requires an awareness of the subtlety of initial symptoms and signs and an abdominal ultrasound or CT demonstrating intra-abdominal fluid, confirmed by aspiration of bile. Appropriate placement of closed suction drains following liver operations can usually prevent bile peritonitis. The drains should be left in place for 3 to 4 days to allow any bile leakage to become manifest. Drain fluid should be checked for bile before removing the drain.

Treatment of bile peritonitis requires drainage of the leaking bile. Treatment often also requires decompression of the biliary tree by endobiliary stent or percutaneous transhepatic biliary drain. In cases where the leaking biliary system is not in continuity with the main biliary tree, draining the main bile ducts will not be effective in decreasing the bile leak (see the following section, "Biliary Fistula"). Although drainage of biliary ascites may be possible percutaneously, effective drainage may require laparotomy, evacuation of bile, irrigation of the abdomen, and directed placement of drains.

Biliary Fistula

Postoperative biliary fistula is most frequently a biliary-cutaneous fistula, as represented by bile drainage through an operatively placed drain. A biliary-cutaneous fistula can also occur through a drain site after removal of the drain or through the operative wound or laparoscopic port sites. Occasionally, undrained bile, usually infected, will erode through the diaphragm into a bronchus or into a gastrointestinal viscus. Persistent biliary fistula is almost always associated with a bile duct that has no free-flowing drainage to the intestine. Such situations include bile drainage from an excluded biliary system (Fig. 34.1) or from a source proximal to an obstructed bile duct. Etiologies of bile duct obstruction include iatrogenic occlusion (clip, ligature, thermal injury),

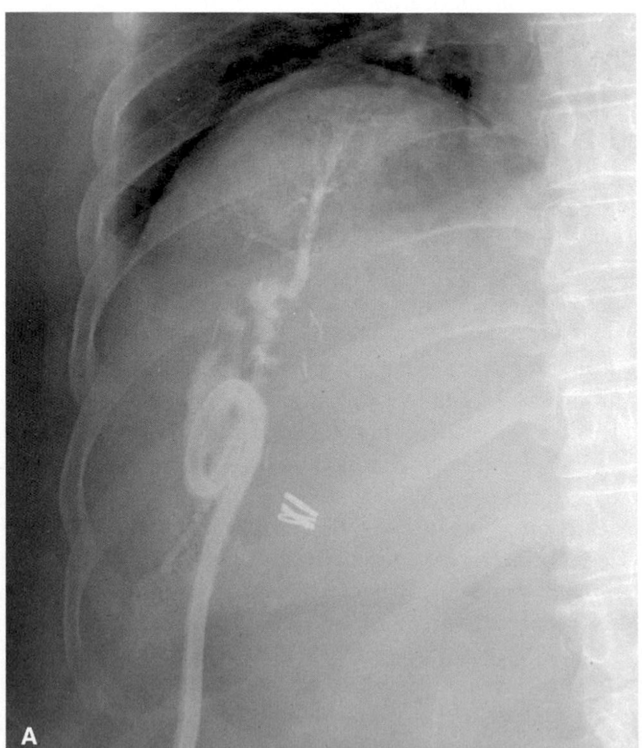

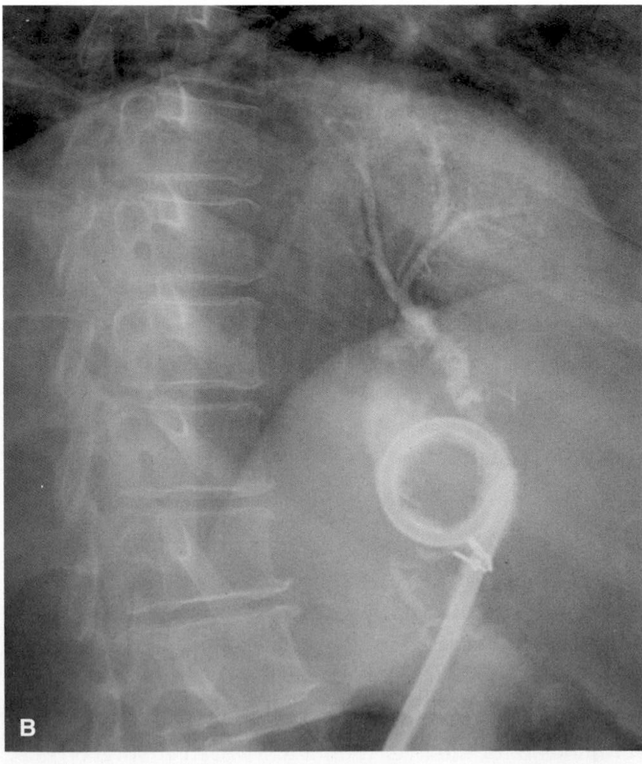

FIGURE 34.1. Isolated bile duct after nonanatomic liver resection. **A:** anteroposterior view; **B:** lateral view.

bile duct stone, bile duct hematoma, tumor involving the bile duct or compressing the bile duct, bile duct parasite, inflammatory-associated stenosis, or ischemic or radiation-associated stricture.

Postoperative bile fistula, if confined to a drain, should not be treated by early drain withdrawal (46). The drain should be left in place long enough to allow formation of a fibrous tract around the drain—4 to 6 weeks, or longer if the patient is malnourished or on steroids. In the majority of cases the fistula will heal by 4 weeks without any additional interventions. If bile leakage continues, the etiology of the drainage is one of the conditions listed above, or the drain may be lying immediately on the leak point, preventing healing. The safest course with persistent bile drainage is to perform a radiocontrast drain injection study, with gravity or very gently injected instillation of contrast to determine: (a) if the drain is immediately against the opening in the biliary tree, (b) if there is an isolated biliary segment, and (c) if there is distal obstruction of the visualized biliary tree. With the first circumstance, withdrawal of the drain beyond the point of contact with the biliary tree will permit scar to close the opening in the biliary tree, and usually the bile leak will resolve, after which the drain can be gradually withdrawn. Alternatively, ERCP with stent and sphincterotomy may be performed to allow the bile to preferentially flow into the duodenum rather than into the drain allowing subsequent drain removal and healing of the biliary leak.

When an isolated segment of bile duct is found, the problem is more difficult. By this point the bile may have become contaminated with bacteria. Although withdrawal of the drain after a drain tract has formed may result in closure of the fistula, there is also a chance that fistula will recur or that cholangitis or liver abscess, or both, will result. Measures that have been successful for treatment of the isolated biliary segment include injection with tetracycline or with fibrin glue. In cases in which treatment by these measures fails, reoperation with resection of the isolated biliary segment may be required. If the bile duct draining the isolated segment is large and a 1-cm or larger mucosa-to-mucosa anastomosis can be created, Roux-en-Y biliary-enteric reconstruction is an option.

When distal obstruction of the biliary tree is responsible for persistent biliary fistula, the focus of treatment should be directed to the distal stricture (discussed below), the successful treatment of which usually allows resolution of the fistula (47).

If the bile drainage is not through a drain, investigation should begin with CT, looking for parahepatic fluid collection, intrahepatic fluid collection, and biliary tract dilation denoting biliary obstruction. Extrahepatic fluid should be sampled by image-guided needle aspiration and drained if purulent or bilious. The treatment of the drain is then as outlined above. If there is evidence of distal biliary obstruction, further evaluation with MRCP, PTC, or ERCP is indicated. Percutaneous or endobiliary stent placement might be indicated for temporary relief of the obstruction to promote resolution of the fistula.

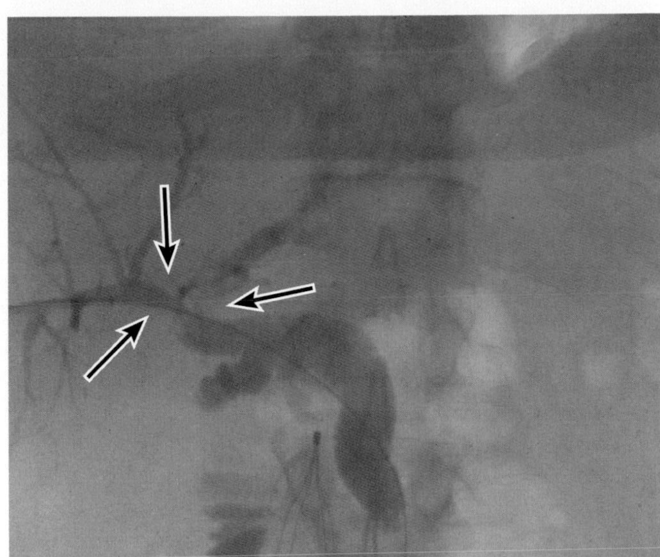

FIGURE 34.2. Ischemic bile duct injury after ligation of hepatic arterial blood supply. The arrows outline the area of ischemic stricture.

Biliary Stricture or Obstruction

Biliary stricture following operation or surgical intervention may result from mechanical injury by a scalpel, biopsy needle, ablation probe, or drainage catheter; from thermal injury with cautery, laser, radiofrequency ablation, cryoablation, or laser probe ablation; from ischemia due to devascularization of the bile duct (Fig. 34.2); or from chemical injury with hypertonic saline or formalin or other chemical scolicidal solution in the treatment of echinococcal cyst. Avoidance of bile duct stricture should always be the goal, because treatment may be very complicated and the potential complications associated with bile duct stricture can be devastating. The first and major step in avoidance of bile duct strictures is recognition of the variety of mechanisms that can cause these problems and care in the use of such modalities.

The results of bile duct stricture are varied and depend on whether there is complete or partial obstruction and on the proportion of liver that is involved. High-grade stricture obstructing bile egress from the entire liver is associated with jaundice and, if unalleviated, liver failure. In situations in which the bile is sterile and the liver parenchyma is relatively normal, high-grade stricture of bile ducts proximal to the main bile duct may prove innocuous. The liver subserved by the obstructed bile duct will atrophy, and the liver with normal bile duct drainage will hypertrophy. If the portion of liver subserved by the obstructed bile duct is small, the damage in the sterile situation is likely to be insignificant. Even with up to 50% of the liver substance obstructed, in the absence of infection, early symptoms or signs are unlikely. Intrahepatic stone formation is unlikely, because at a pressure of 40 mm Hg, bile formation in the associated hepatocytes stops and the components necessary to form stones are absent. Although serum alkaline phosphatase will be elevated in such a situation, the bilirubin will often rise only mildly. The two potential complications are (a) infection of the bile in the obstructed biliary tree, with resulting cholangitis, liver abscess, or both, and (b) increased risk of cholangiocarcinoma associated with chronically obstructed bile ducts.

Obstructions that are not high-grade are more likely to be associated with intrahepatic duct stone formation. Whether there is an increased risk of cholangitis with intrahepatic duct stone formation is unknown. Intrahepatic bile duct stone formation is likely to worsen the effects of a low-grade stricture, potentially converting it to the equivalent of a high-grade stricture.

Low-grade stricture of the main bile duct or of the drainage to many portions of the liver is likely to result in secondary biliary cirrhosis. The progress to secondary biliary cirrhosis may be occult, the risk of the occurrence denoted only by an elevated alkaline phosphatase. Liver biopsy may be the only method to determine whether cirrhosis has developed. Because the occurrence of secondary biliary cirrhosis is variable, persistently elevated alkaline phosphatase should prompt investigation by imaging studies looking for intrahepatic bile duct dilation.

Early treatment of bile duct stricture is important before atrophy or secondary biliary cirrhosis occurs and consists of reestablishment of free, low-pressure drainage from the affected bile ducts. Treatments for stricture include balloon cholangioplasty via ERCP or PTC combined with plastic external, internal, or internal/external drains/stents, or biliary-enteric anastomosis. Stents have a limited lifetime (usually less than 16 weeks) because of buildup of bile salts and proteinaceous material on the plastic, with occlusion and reobstruction and/or cholangitis. Internal expandable metal stents have a longer lifetime, but have a maximal useful effectiveness with benign strictures of about 5 years (48) and cannot be changed. For strictures that cannot be adequately treated with balloon cholangioplasty, biliary-enteric anastomosis should be performed, if possible. For strictures that cannot be adequately treated with serial dilations or biliary-enteric anastomosis, consideration should be given to resection of the affected portion of the liver, if an adequate liver remnant can be left. Such a resection avoids the risk of recurrent cholangitis and liver abscess and the more distant risk of cholangiocarcinoma.

Hemobilia

Hemobilia, bleeding into the bile ducts, can occur after liver resection from direct trauma, such as with core needle biopsy during a procedure on the liver, abscess eroding into both bile duct and adjacent vessel, communication of bile duct and vessel within a postoperative hematoma, arterial pseudoaneurysm rupturing into a bile duct, or injury to both bile duct and a vessel due to radiofrequency ablation, cryoablation, or laser ablation of a liver lesion. Etiologies also include bleeding from tumor within bile ducts, such as hepatocellular carcinoma or bile duct malignancies.

Manifestations are most commonly right upper quadrant pain, jaundice, and hematemesis, but also include occult unexplained blood loss, melena or hematochezia, hyperbilirubinemia, and acute pancreatitis. With significant hemobilia, the feeding vessel is more often an artery than a portal vein branch or a hepatic vein branch. Arterial pressure is more likely to cause continued bleeding despite increased biliary pressures associated with the formation of clot in the bile ducts.

Diagnosis is made by a combination of studies in correlation with symptoms: finding blood in the stool or hematemesis, without a lesion to explain the bleeding in the gastrointestinal tract on endoscopy; by observing blood coming from the papilla of Vater on upper endoscopy; by biliary dilation on ultrasound or CT with high-density material within the bile ducts; by demonstration of irregular filling defects in the bile ducts on cholangiography; with demonstration of entry of contrast into a vessel on cholangiography; and by demonstration of hepatic artery pseudo-aneurysm or contrast entering the biliary tree on visceral angiography. Resolution can be spontaneous; however, treatment of persistent or massive hemobilia by hepatic artery embolization is usually effective. Quite infrequently, hepatic artery ligation or hepatic resection of the affected area of liver is required.

Cholangitis

If there is no free bile drainage postoperatively after liver surgery and if the biliary tree has been seeded with organisms, cholangitis can occur. Most critical in treating and avoiding cholangitis is the intraoperative establishment and postoperative maintenance of adequate biliary drainage. At operation, that goal includes assessment of biliary drainage, removal of obstructing debris such as stones, and constructing a generous anastomosis whenever possible. Treatment of early postoperative cholangitis is with antibiotics and institution of free biliary drainage.

Cholangitis may occur at months to years after liver surgery, usually resulting from restricted drainage of contaminated bile with the most common etiologies being listed in Table 34.7. Investigation should include determination of serum alkaline phosphatase levels and bilirubin. Evaluation

Table **34.7** Etiologies of cholangitis after liver surgery
Common bile duct stones
Benign biliary stricture
Malignant biliary stricture
Biliary-enteric anastomotic stricture
Biliary-enteric stent
Percutaneous transhepatic biliary drain
Percutaneous transhepatic cholangiography
Endoscopic retrograde cholangiography
Biliary-enteric fistula
Common bile duct parasites
Recurrent pyogenic cholangitis

also requires imaging—first, of the biliary tree to assess for site(s) of stricture and for the presence of biliary stones; second, of the surrounding structures to detect extrinsic tissue causing biliary obstruction, such as intrahepatic or extrahepatic tumor, lymphadenopathy, pseudocyst, or abscess; and, third, of the liver to survey for hepatic abscess and for partial liver atrophy. Ultrasonography should serve as an initial screen. If cholangitis is suspected, CT or MRI/MRCP should be performed.

The long-term solution to cholangitis is to obtain adequate and permanent biliary drainage. Because of the variety of etiologies, there is no single solution. Occasionally, symptoms and signs of cholangitis will occur in some individuals without evidence of inadequate biliary drainage. In these individuals supportive treatment is all that can be offered, but reevaluation should be carried out at intervals if symptoms and signs continue.

Intrahepatic Abscess

Intrahepatic abscess may result as a complication of liver surgery when there is cholangitis, when there is focal bile duct obstruction with the obstructed bile duct becoming secondarily infected, or when an intrahepatic hematoma becomes secondarily infected. If limited in number and less than 2 to 3 cm in size, hepatic abscesses may be drained percutaneously and treated with antibiotics. Smaller abscesses will often resolve with antibiotic treatment alone. Investigation for obstructed bile ducts should be undertaken whenever hepatic abscess occurs, but treatment should not await this evaluation. When there is no resolution of the abscess or there is occurrence of additional abscesses, reevaluation should be considered. Occasionally, operative drainage is required for multiple abscesses or failure of percutaneous therapy.

Parahepatic Abscess

Parahepatic abscess occurs rarely and is usually associated with factors such as an infected biloma or infected hematoma. Meticulous hemostasis, closure of any sites of bile leakage, and avoidance of postoperative coagulopathy are the primary means of preventing parahepatic abscess. Placement of closed suction drains, maintained for only a limited time postoperatively, may decrease the incidence of infected biloma as the source of parahepatic abscess. Treatment of parahepatic abscess is percutaneous drainage and antibiotics, similar to the treatment of other postoperative intra-abdominal abscesses.

Renal Failure

Renal failure as a complication of liver surgery may have a number of etiologies, including hypotension due to blood loss or sepsis, toxic injury from nephrotoxic drugs, inadequate fluid administration or excessive fluid loss with diuretic use, or, uncommonly, hepatorenal syndrome in patients with cirrhosis or liver failure. Characteristic of the hepatorenal syndrome are a urine sodium concentration of less than 10 mEq/L, high urine osmolality, and high urine-to-plasma ratios of creatinine. The diagnosis and treatment of the common causes of renal failure are those employed in the postoperative setting and are not unique to liver surgery. Hepatorenal syndrome has no well-established mechanism, although elevation of various cytokines, including endothelin-1, and decreases in certain prostaglandins have been implicated. Hepatorenal syndrome is invariably lethal after liver surgery unless treated by liver transplantation.

Gastrointestinal Bleeding

GI bleeding after liver surgery in the noncirrhotic patient occurs in less than 1% of patients (1) and is predominantly due to gastric erosions or ulceration associated with postoperative sepsis. Stress ulceration can largely be avoided with agents that maintain the postoperative gastric pH greater than 5, such as H_2-blockers or proton pump inhibitors. Other etiologies include postoperative coagulopathy and hemobilia. In patients with cirrhosis with portal hypertension, bleeding may also occur from esophagogastric varices or from portal gastropathy.

SUMMARY

Liver surgery and procedures can be done safely at institutions where high volumes of such surgery are performed. Safety involves experience with the patient evaluation, selection for procedures, performance of the operations, and postoperative care. Safety also involves recognition of possible complications associated with procedures, avoidance whenever possible, and expeditious treatment of complications when they occur.

REFERENCES

1. Jarnagin WR, Gonen M, Fong Y, et al. Improvement in perioperative outcome after hepatic resection: analysis of 1,803 consecutive cases over the past decade. *Ann Surg* 2002;236:397–406; discussion 406–397.
2. McKay A, You I, Bigam D, et al. Impact of surgeon training on outcomes after resective hepatic surgery. *Ann Surg Oncol* 2008;15:1348–1355.
3. Gagner M, Franco D, Vons C, et al. Analysis of morbidity and mortality rates in right hepatectomy with the preoperative APACHE II score. *Surgery* 1991;110:487–492.
4. Teh SH, Christein J, Donohue J, et al. Hepatic resection of hepatocellular carcinoma in patients with cirrhosis: Model of End-Stage Liver Disease (MELD) score predicts perioperative mortality. *J Gastrointest Surg* 2005;9:1207–1215; discussion 1215.
5. Belghiti J, Hiramatsu K, Benoist S, et al. Seven hundred forty-seven hepatectomies in the 1990s: an update to evaluate the actual risk of liver resection. *J Am Coll Surg* 2000;191(1):38–46.
6. Asiyanbola B, Chang D, Gleisner AL, et al. Operative mortality after hepatic resection: are literature-based rates broadly applicable? *J Gastrointest Surg* 2008;12:842–851.
7. Bruix J, Castells A, Bosch J, et al. Surgical resection of hepatocellular carcinoma in cirrhotic patients: prognostic value of preoperative portal pressure. *Gastroenterology* 1996;111:1018–1022.
8. Hashimoto M, Watanabe G. Hepatic parenchymal cell volume and the indocyanine green tolerance test. *J Surg Res* 2000;92:222–227.
9. Wakabayashi H, Ishimura K, Izuishi K, et al. Evaluation of liver function for hepatic resection for hepatocellular carcinoma in the liver with damaged parenchyma. *J Surg Res* 2004;116:248–252.
10. Hemming AW, Gallinger S, Greig PD, et al. The hippurate ratio as an indicator of functional hepatic reserve for resection of hepatocellular carcinoma in cirrhotic patients. *J Gastrointest Surg* 2001;5:316–321.

consequence, but all concerning symptoms following cholecystectomy should be thoroughly investigated to determine that the patient does not have a biliary injury. Taking the approach that any postcholecystectomy problem could represent, a biliary injury will serve surgeons well, as these complications are much easier to manage the more efficiently they are diagnosed sparing the patient the risk of sepsis and liver dysfunction .

BILE DUCT INJURY FROM CHOLECYSTECTOMY

Mechanism and prevention of bile duct injury

Thanks to the research of expert surgeons such as Way, Strasberg, and others, the mechanism responsible for bile duct injury during laparoscopic cholecystectomy has been well studied and described (10,15–17). Bile duct injury is created by a misidentification of the anatomy, often facilitated by a "perceptual illusion" that leads to erroneous assumptions about the anatomy of the structures contained within the triangle of Calot (17). The common feature of this error in perception is misidentification of the common bile duct as the cystic duct, a mistake also described as the "hidden cystic duct" syndrome that appears to be facilitated by use of the infundibular technique of laparoscopic cholecystectomy (18). This error in correctly identifying the anatomy of the triangle of Calot can lead to what is referred to as the "classic" bile duct injury (19) clipping and division of the common bile duct, followed by further traction on the gallbladder, which leads to a second, higher injury with division of the common hepatic duct, often near the bifurcation. This second division of the duct, if noticed by the operating surgeon, is often described in the operative note as a second cystic duct or an accessory duct. In some cases, the right hepatic artery is also injured during this process.

Other described mechanisms of injury are listed in Table 35.1 and include "tenting," in which the common bile duct is pulled laterally while the cystic duct is being clipped and is inadvertently caught in the clip, narrowing the common bile duct; thermal injuries due to inappropriate use of cautery; excessive application of clips to control bleeding in the triangle of Calot; and injury to an aberrant or low-inserting right hepatic duct (17,20). All these injuries seem to result from a similar anatomic misperception, specifically the error of unknowingly dissecting too closely to either the common hepatic or right hepatic duct when the surgeon believes he or she has ample room for dissection (17).

Clearly, the most effective means of addressing bile duct injury is prevention, particularly now that the mechanism of injury has been well described. To that end, it is worth considering the methods commonly described for accurate cystic duct identification. The first, or "infundibular," method involves dissection of the cystic duct along its anterior and posterior aspects in the triangle of Calot. Confirmation of the anatomy is noted by seeing a "flair" as the cystic duct widens to become the infundibulum of the gallbladder neck. This technique is widely used and is endorsed by many major surgical texts (21,22). It is favored, particularly by surgeons with limited laparoscopic experience, as it often requires minimal dissection and mobilization of the gallbladder prior to controlling the cystic duct. Unfortunately, in the study that described the "hidden cystic duct syndrome," 17 of 21 common bile duct injuries were sustained when using the infundibular technique (18). In acute cholecystitis, the cystic duct is often hidden behind an inflamed gallbladder neck. Other factors that may contribute to a hidden cystic duct include large impacted stones, a short or absent cystic duct, and adhesions between the gallbladder neck and the common duct, such that the cystic duct is obscured.

Given these limitations to the infundibular technique, many surgeons believe that the "critical view" technique is the preferred method of laparoscopic cholecystectomy (10,18,23,24). In this method, the triangle of Calot is completely cleared of fibrous and fatty tissues so that only the cystic duct and artery are visible, as displayed in Figure 35.1.

Table 35.1 Mechanisms of biliary injury during laparoscopic cholecystectomy

Misidentification of anatomic structures • Failure to achieve the critical view of safety • Common bile duct misidentified as the cystic duct • Aberrant right hepatic duct mistaken for the cystic duct • Ligation of right hepatic artery intending to ligate cystic artery
Technical mechanisms • Inadequately occluded cystic duct • Use of cautery too close to portal structures • Tenting of cystic duct during dissection and/or application of clips • Overuse of clips to control bleeding • Improper portal dissection

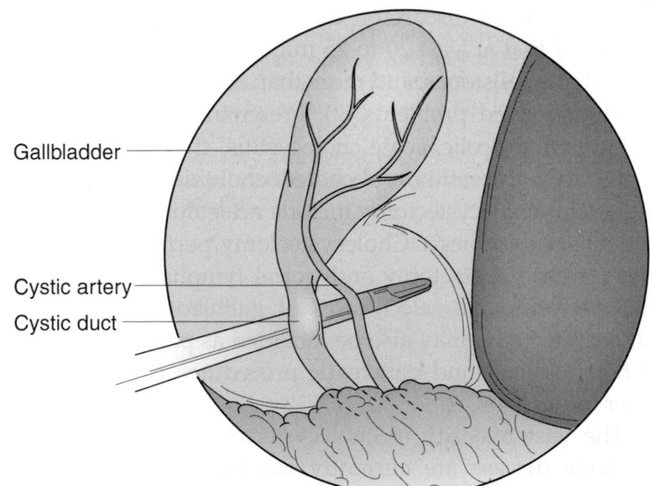

FIGURE 35.1. The critical view of safety, created by full dissection of the structures in the triangle of Calot and mobilization of the infundibulum completely off the cystic plate. Note there are only two structures clearly entering the gallbladder, the cystic duct, and the cystic artery, and the liver is seen clearly through the triangle of Calot. (Reproduced with permission from Greenfield LJ, Mulholland MW. *Greenfield's surgery: scientific principles and practice*, 5th ed. Philadelphia, PA: Lippincott Williams & Wilkins; 2006: Chapter 60.)

To facilitate this dissection and enhance visualization, the peritoneum between the liver and the infundibulum is opened completely. This separates the gallbladder completely from the cystic plate – the adventitial tissue that is opposed to the nonperitonealized portion of the gallbladder. This allows the infundibulum to be moved anteriorly and posteriorly easily and broadens Calot's triangle. After this dissection, the cystic plate and surrounding liver should be visible easily through Calot's triangle. With this view achieved, the two structures inserting on the gallbladder can only be the cystic duct and cystic artery. If this view is not achieved, the dissection is stopped and a cholangiogram is obtained to define the anatomy or the procedure is converted to open. Reasons that the critical view may not be achieved include aberrant biliary anatomy, such as an absent or extremely short cystic duct, or inflammation that obliterates the space between the cystic duct and hepatic duct. Both these factors are associated with an increased risk of bile duct injury and should cause the surgeon to pause and reconsider the surgical approach.

While no data from randomized clinical trials are available to support the superiority of the critical view technique for prevention of bile duct injury, large series do support its safety and efficacy. In a study of more than 3,000 patients from the Netherlands who underwent laparoscopic cholecystectomy using the critical view technique, a single bile duct injury was noted (for an injury rate of 0.003%) (25). Single-institution studies where documentation of the technique was even more stringent have confirmed similar low rates of bile duct injury (26,27). The importance and simplicity of the critical view once achieved have been increasingly recognized in the surgical literature, and photo or video documentation of the critical view as an essential portion of the operative record has been advocated (24,28,29).

Use of intraoperative cholangiography

The role for intraoperative cholangiography (IOC), and its ability to prevent bile duct injury, has been debated since the introduction of the technique. Flum et al. (30) demonstrated that not using IOC was associated with a higher rate of bile duct injury. After adjusting for patient and surgeon covariates, Medicare beneficiaries appeared 71% more likely to sustain a bile duct injury during cholecystectomy if IOC was not performed. Based on these compelling data and other single-institution series, IOC has been proposed as a method to avoid bile duct injury. Others have suggested that IOC allows for the earlier recognition of bile duct injury with limitation of associated morbidity (14,31,32). In addition, use of IOC as a method to prevent bile duct injury has been suggested to be cost-effective, as prevention of even a single bile duct injury saves extensive personal and financial costs for the individual patient (33).

In contrast, other data suggest that IOC may not prevent bile duct injury and is not a substitute for careful surgical technique, such as obtaining the critical view of safety. Unfortunately, IOC may be performed even in cases where a bile duct injury is sustained, and the cholangiogram interpreted incorrectly, which emphasizes that its use is not equivalent with absolute prevention of bile duct injury (17). One study even suggested that IOC may be associated with creation of a bile duct injury in rare cases, occurring at about the same frequency as bile duct injury in large series (0.4%) (34). A prospective trial of routine IOC demonstrated no impact of the test on the rate of major bile duct injury, but clearly showed the increased cost and operative time associated with IOC (35–38). A recent analysis of national patterns of the use of IOC suggests that it is not utilized at all in some hospitals performing cholecystectomy and is associated with more than $700 in additional charges per case, making it not cost-effective to prevent bile duct injury (39). More recent studies have questioned the role of routine IOC when the critical view technique is employed and have argued for the use of selective IOC in cases when the critical view cannot be achieved (23,40,41). Selective use of IOC is arguably the preferred application of this technique for experienced surgeons, though a compelling argument can be made for surgeons to routinely perform IOC while early in their learning curve with laparoscopic cholecystectomy and for IOC to be routinely taught to surgical trainees. Clearly, it is a technique that all surgeons performing biliary tract procedures should be able to complete efficiently and interpret accurately. Ironically, evidence suggests that inexperienced surgeons and those in academic positions teaching residents are exactly those surgeons least likely to use IOC (42).

While the role of IOC in prevention of bile duct injury is debatable, selective IOC has more clear indications in the detection and management of choledocholithiasis. Accepted indications for IOC include abnormal liver profile at the time of cholecystectomy [elevated aspartate aminotransferase (AST), alanine aminotransferase (ALT), alkaline phosphatase, and/or bilirubin], unsuccessful preoperative endoscopic retrograde cholangiopancreatography (ERCP) for choledocholithiasis, and the intraoperative recognition of aberrant anatomy or suspected injury, as discussed earlier. Other indications where selective IOC should be strongly considered include a history of biliary pancreatitis without previous ERCP, dilated common bile duct on preoperative imaging that has not been evaluated via ERCP, and a previous history of jaundice without ERCP. Some surgeons have advocated for the use of preoperative magnetic resonance cholangiopancreatography (MRCP), with IOC reserved for patients with abnormal or equivocal MRCP (41,43). MRCP appears to have a high correlation with the findings upon performance of IOC and may prevent the added cost, operative time, and low risk of biliary injury associated with IOC (44).

A potential alternative to IOC is intraoperative ultrasonography (IOUS). This technique offers the advantages of cholangiography but is noninvasive, repeatable, fast, and inexpensive. Its limitations are that it is clearly dependent on an experienced user, high-resolution equipment, and a standard and reproducible technique. Surgical trainees are not routinely taught IOUS, and many of their superiors may not have incorporated it in their practice, therefore limiting the propagation of the technique. Nevertheless, comparative series suggest that in experienced hands, IOUS offers equivalent or superior sensitivity and specificity in the detection of common bile duct stones to IOC, with no increased risk of bile duct injury (45–49). IOUS may eventually replace the use of IOC for many indications (50), akin to the transition that has occurred away from ERCP toward initial endoscopic ultrasound (EUS) for evaluation for distal biliary obstruction.

Diagnosis of bile duct injury following cholecystectomy

Intraoperative Diagnosis of Bile Duct Injury

Recognition of a biliary injury during cholecystectomy can be a distressing scenario for any surgeon. As described earlier, most biliary injuries are the result of a misperception of anatomy that persists until the injury is recognized, so surgeons who find themselves in this situation are often surprised, as well as fearful of the morbidity that their patients may suffer. Even experienced surgeons should call a colleague into the operating room for assistance and counsel. Even if a hepatobiliary surgeon is not available, a second surgeon with a new perspective and more objectivity about the individual case can assist greatly in intraoperative decision-making and surgical management. As soon as a bile duct injury is suspected, an IOC should be performed. Depending on the point in the cholecystectomy when the injury was recognized, cannulation of a ductal structure may be difficult and itself requires conversion to a laparotomy. Inability to perform a cholangiogram and confusion about the anatomy should always prompt conversion to a laparotomy. In the rare case where a bile duct injury is recognized and confirmed by IOC while still laparoscopic and the primary surgeon is not comfortable performing the repair, laparoscopic placement of subhepatic drains with immediate transfer to a hepatobiliary surgeon and center is appropriate.

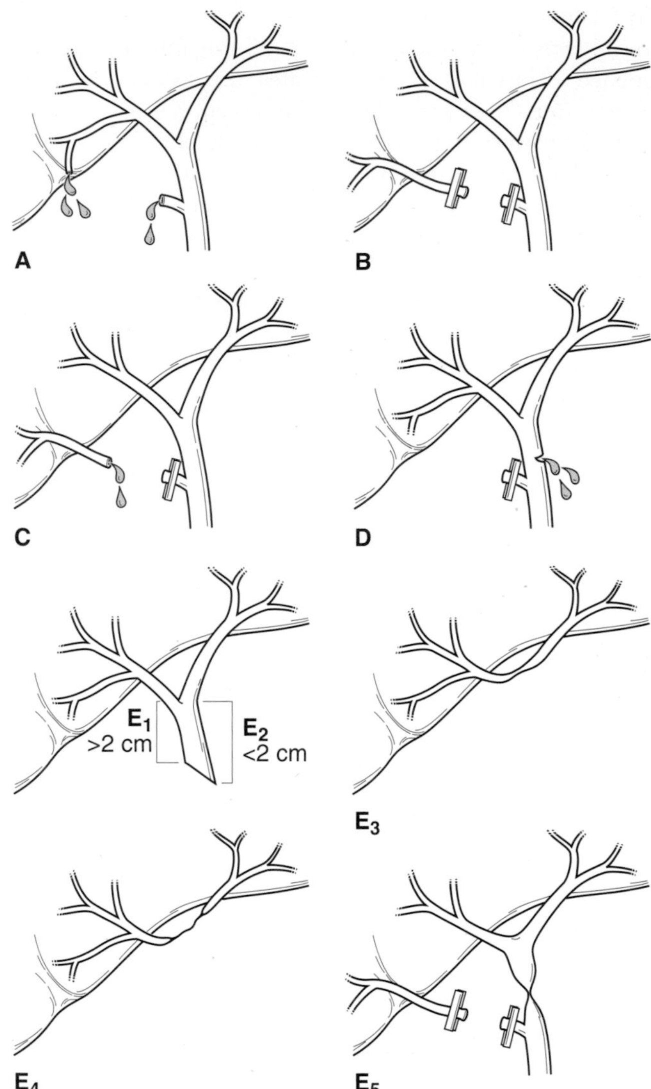

FIGURE 35.2. The Bismuth–Strasberg classification of biliary injuries following laparoscopic cholecystectomy. (Reproduced with permission from Winslow ER, Fialkowski EA, Linehan DC, et al. "Sideways": results of repair of biliary injuries using a policy of side-to-side hepatico-jejunostomy. *Ann Surg* 2009;249(3):426–434.)

Once IOC confirms a bile duct injury, attention needs to be paid to the condition of the patient and the extent of the injury. Bile duct injuries can occur in the setting of a lengthy or difficult dissection, so consideration of the patient's anesthetic course, control of bleeding, and degree of resuscitation should be discussed. If the decision is made to repair the injury at the time of the index operation, the anesthetic and operative staff should be alerted of the need for additional operative time and any additional equipment that may be needed (retractors, biliary catheters, fine sutures, instruments, etc.). Once the patient's stability is assured, the surgeon should turn to carefully and methodically defining the classification of the biliary injury (see Fig. 35.2) and assessing for any associated vascular injury. Additional dissection may be needed to define the portal structures, but this should be done cautiously, especially if repair is not going to occur at the index operation. IOUS with liver duplex examination can be quite helpful in documenting hepatic arterial and portal venous inflow to both lobes of the liver, which can offer delineation of the degree and significance of any associated vascular injury.

The decision to proceed with repair of a biliary injury at the primary operation should be made carefully. Studies have documented that one of the risk factors for poor outcomes following repair of a bile duct injury following cholecystectomy is repair by the primary surgeon (11,51,52), which reflects not only the lack of advanced hepatobiliary experience among most surgeons performing laparoscopic cholecystectomy but also the judgment and insight that may be compromised by the emotions of a recognized injury. Surgeon experience is not the only consideration, as thought should be given to the availability of resources that may be necessary in the postoperative period to assist in management of these complicated patients, including but not limited to intensive care resources, advanced endoscopists, and interventional radiology. Technical factors related to the injury should also be considered. Injuries that involve the hepatic duct bifurcation or higher, injuries with associated vascular compromise, and biliary injuries made with thermal energy (as opposed to sharp dissection) should all be considered relative contraindications to repair at the primary operation either due to their complexity (high or segmental ductal injuries) or due to the possibility of the injury evolving further (in the case of thermal injuries and those with associated hepatic arterial ligation). One final consideration is that most hepatobiliary surgeons prefer to encounter these injuries in as undisturbed a field as possible, where they can guide the additional dissection, and the results of repair are clearly better than when having to redo a previous repair. It is better to decide early to refer the patient to a hepatobiliary surgeon than to make that decision after having attempted a suboptimal repair.

If the decision is made not to repair the injury at the primary operation, drains should be placed and arrangements made for immediate transfer to a hepatobiliary center. In the case of a complete transaction with ligation, it is not necessary to "undo" the ligation. Removing sutures and clips can be difficult and associated with bleeding, which then requires additional maneuvers to control. Leaving the biliary system obstructed in the short term does not typically cause immediate morbidity and may even facilitate the placement of transhepatic catheters if the biliary system dilates proximally. If the hepatic duct is open and draining, a red rubber catheter or silastic feeding tube may be placed into the proximal duct in an effort to control the biliary outflow. Again, excessive maneuvers to suture in a tube, place a balloon catheter, or other involved means to control biliary drainage are well intended but may be associated with further injury to the remnant duct, which potentially shortens the amount of hepatic duct available to the repairing surgeon (53). Leaving large (10 French or greater) subhepatic biliary drains is often perfectly adequate to control biliary effluent for the time of transfer until definitive repair or drainage can be achieved.

Postoperative Diagnosis of Biliary Injury

Bile duct injuries following cholecystectomy can present in an early or late manner, and the severity of their presentation is often dependent on the degree of injury. Early symptoms that should prompt further evaluation include fever, nausea, emesis, abdominal pain, and malaise. Bilious drainage from a surgical drain or from an incision is always abnormal and diagnostic of a biliary leak. Even in the case of injuries associated with complete ligation of the extrahepatic biliary drainage, jaundice may not occur as abdominal pain and other symptoms will often lead patients to seek care before their bilirubin has had time to rise significantly. Laboratory evaluation may be underwhelming, though a leukocytosis may be present. The abnormalities of the liver profile may be subtle—total bilirubin may be normal or only slightly elevated (2 to 4 mg/dL) in the case of a complete biliary transaction with free leak. Reabsorption of bile from the peritoneum may elevate the bilirubin slightly. Marked elevation of the AST and ALT is usually not present and should raise concern of an associated vascular injury when present. Biliary injuries are typically not associated with significant abnormalities of the amylase and lipase. When these values are elevated following cholecystectomy, especially in concert with an abnormal liver profile, a retained common bile duct stone rather than a bile duct injury may be the problem.

A heightened awareness of bile duct injury should be maintained in all patients with early problems following cholecystectomy, with efforts made to confirm or refute that diagnosis made efficiently. Postcholecystectomy pain that appears out of proportion to the usual pain following a laparoscopic procedure, or presents in a delayed fashion after the initial postoperative discomfort has resolved, deserves a thorough investigation. A careful interval history and physical exam, and laboratory studies as indicated, are important. Mistakes may be made when managing such patients over the phone, or through midlevel providers, when a clinic visit often is all that is needed to distinguish incisional pain or abdominal wall bruising from a more serious problem. Initial focus should be on the appropriate resuscitation and stabilization of the patient, as both cholangitis and infected extravasated bile can lead to profound sepsis (54,55). Broad spectrum antibiotics should be administered efficiently if either of these diagnoses are suspected or confirmed.

Initial diagnostic imaging may include ultrasound, to assess for perihepatic fluid collections and biliary ductal dilatation, or computed tomography (CT) in select patients. If identified, significant perihepatic collections may be percutaneously drained. If bilious, a biliary leak is diagnosed and the evaluation should proceed with direct cholangiography either by ERCP or by percutaneous transhepatic cholangiography (PTC). If the fluid visualized on ultrasound or CT is not easily drained, or if the question of a biliary injury is still open, a hepatobiliary imino-diacetic acid (HIDA) scan may be performed. HIDA scans can detect extravasation of biliary drainage and may also demonstrate failure of bile excreted from the liver to enter the duodenum. Further anatomic detail is not available from HIDA scans, but it may be sufficient to confirm a suspicion of biliary injury before proceeding to more invasive means of cholangiography. CT angiography, with dual arterial and portal venous phases, can be used to define associated vascular injury.

ERCP by a skilled endoscopist is often the best initial invasive study in a patient with a suspected biliary injury. In injuries where the connection of the extrahepatic biliary tree to the duodenum is still intact, ERCP may be diagnostic and therapeutic. Endoscopic sphincterotomy and placement of an endobiliary stent are often sufficient to treat biliary leaks from the cystic duct stump or small accessory ducts. Incomplete transections may be bridged by endobiliary stents, with the need for subsequent operative intervention determined over time. In cases of common bile duct ligation, or in instances where a segment of the extrahepatic duct is excised with the gallbladder leaving an open proximal and distal extrahepatic bile duct, ERCP may not be adequate to provide anatomic detail of the proximal biliary tree, nor be able to facilitate crossing the injury. In these cases, percutaneous transhepatic cholangiogram (PTC) with placement of transhepatic biliary drains is typically necessary.

PTC in a patient with a decompressed biliary system is very difficult and requires sophisticated interventional radiology resources and expertise. It is not uncommon for these procedures to take repeated attempts at access and then advancement of transhepatic catheters over a series of days. It is often necessary to place additional percutaneous drains to control bile leakage and drain infected bilomas until the biliary drainage is adequately diverted. These patients truly require multidisciplinary management to ensure that procedures are coordinated with the goals of improving the patient's condition, defining the relevant anatomy, and facilitating eventual definitive repair. For this reason, the hepatobiliary surgeon needs to be involved in all decisions about placement of drains and transhepatic catheters and the timing of these procedures.

As with any surgical procedure, associated injuries from electrocautery, lysis of adhesions, or passing of instruments to the bowel or solid organs should be considered. Wound complications, though uncommon following laparoscopic cholecystectomy, should be managed appropriately. Bleeding complications after cholecystectomy are fortunately rare, but can be seen more commonly in patients on systemic anticoagulation, patients with chronic liver disease, or patients with thrombocytopenia due to hematologic disease. One clinical scenario that does arise occasionally is the postcholecystectomy patient with abdominal pain who is found to have a collection in the former gall bladder fossa. These collections do not typically need specific intervention, though may need further evaluation primarily to determine whether or not they contain bile and thus represent the manifestation of a biliary injury. If no biliary leak is demonstrated by HIDA and/or cholangiogram, gall bladder fossa fluid collections do not usually require drainage. Hematomas should preferably not be instrumented and will resolve over time. Infected fluid collections are unusual, but can occur in the context of acute or gangrenous cholecystitis (56) or as a consequence of spilled stones at the time of cholecystectomy (57,58). Image-guided percutaneous drainage is typically adequate in such cases to distinguish a subhepatic abscess from a biloma and resolve any associated septic complications.

Late presentations of bile duct injury may be more subtle. Studies from large referral centers suggest that up to 50% of biliary injuries not recognized in the operating room will present in a delayed fashion (i.e., >30 days postoperatively) (54,59,60). Patients may present with jaundice and abdominal pain, or cholangitis may be the initial presenting symptom. Some segmental injuries may be diagnosed incidentally, either by a mildly abnormal liver profile on routine laboratories or with segmental ductal dilatation or atrophy on imaging. Biliary stricture is typically the etiology of all these delayed presentations of occult bile duct injury during cholecystectomy, though rare delayed leaks with contained bilomas or biliary fistulas may occur (54). In these cases, the evaluation of the patient typically proceeds more methodically in a subacute or elective fashion, although the development of cholangitis may require more urgent procedures to improve biliary drainage. MRI with MRCP can be a very informative study in these patients, as it gives excellent segmental biliary anatomy as well as the opportunity to investigate associated vascular injuries. MRCP has the advantage of delineating excluded biliary segments that may not be apparent by ERCP or PTC. MRCP thus often facilitates decision-making about what route is most appropriate for direct cholangiography.

Classification of Bile Duct Injury

Effective management of biliary injury following cholecystectomy relies upon understanding of the anatomic details of the injured biliary tract and applying the appropriate percutaneous, endoscopic, and surgical interventions catered to the severity of injury. To assist with these decisions and to provide accurate communication among providers, the Bismuth–Strasberg classification system has been adopted (Fig. 35.2) (10). These injuries vary in their presentation and require specific considerations in their diagnosis.

Type A—Type A injuries present as a bile leak, either from the cystic duct stump or from small accessory ducts in the cystic plate (ducts of Luschka). The extrahepatic biliary system is intact and not compromised. These injuries typically present in the first week after surgery, although they have been reported as late as 2 to 3 weeks postoperatively. They are rarely discovered intraoperatively. Patients present with signs and symptoms of a biliary leak or biloma, with abdominal pain, fever, anorexia, and nausea. Jaundice is rare, though mild hyperbilirubinemia in the range of 2 to 3 mg/dL may occur due to absorption of bile from the peritoneum. Cystic duct stump leaks may occur due to inaccurate clip placement, perforation proximal to the clip, cystic duct necrosis, or clip dislodgment due to increased intraductal pressure secondary to a retained common bile duct stone. These leaks are often readily demonstrated by ERCP. Accessory duct leaks are distinct from the aberrant segmental duct injuries classified as Type B or C, as accessory leaks imply that they are not the only route of biliary drainage for the involved liver segment. These leaks may be of relatively low volume and sometimes hard to see on ERCP. They may present as a biloma without significant ongoing demonstrated leak. Type A injuries are the most common bile duct injuries following cholecystectomy, with the vast majority being cystic duct stump leaks (10).

Type B—Type B injuries are defined as ligation and division of an aberrant segmental hepatic duct, typically the duct draining the right posterior section (segments 6 and 7) or the segmental duct to segment 6 alone. This injury is often facilitated by the associated anomaly where the cystic duct drains into this aberrant right posterior duct, an anatomic variant well described by Couinaud (61). The proximal and distal ends of the aberrant duct are clipped and divided during control of the cystic duct. Type B injuries are often asymptomatic or present late with abdominal pain or cholangitis involving the occluded liver segment. Normally, the liver behind a Type B injury will atrophy and the remaining liver will hypertrophy.

Type C—Type C injuries are defined as division of an aberrant right posterior segmental duct without ligation. They arise due to the same anatomic variant as Type B injuries but vary in their presentation as they cause spillage of bile into the peritoneal cavity with the development of bile peritonitis or a biloma. Their initial presentation may be very similar to Type A injuries, and it will often appear on initial cholangiograms that the entire biliary system is intact. Careful inspection of a good-quality ERCP will allow detection of the lack of filling of the posterior segment(s). PTC may also miss this injury if either the left ductal or right anterior system is entered. Persistent biliary leak in the presence of an intact cystic duct ligature should prompt investigation for a Type C injury. Injection into a subhepatic biloma drain (drain sinogram) may opacify the transected and leaking segmental duct. PTC via the right posterior segment can confirm the diagnosis and gain control of the biliary fistula.

Type D—Type D injuries are defined as lateral injury, typical incomplete transaction or cautery injury, to an extrahepatic bile duct. As in Type A injuries, all hepatic segments remain in continuity with the distal biliary tree and duodenum, though the severity of the leak may be significant depending on the size and location of the injury. These injuries may be generated in protean ways, including sharp lateral injury during dissection, thermal injury to the lateral aspect of the right or common hepatic duct during dissection, or partial occlusion or laceration of a hepatic duct during clip placement. These injuries may present early, with bile leak and sepsis. However, Type D injuries due to thermal trauma or clip placement may present late with the development of a biliary stricture without extravasation of bile. Given their central nature, Type D injuries are readily seen on ERCP or PTC.

Type E—Type E injuries are defined by complete disruption of biliary–enteric continuity due to transection, excision, and/or ligation of the extrahepatic biliary tree. Injuries that include a free biliary leak will present early with bile peritonitis and sepsis. Injuries with occlusion of the proximal hepatic drainage may present in a delayed fashion with jaundice and/or cholangitis, although still typically within 2 weeks of cholecystectomy as all biliary drainage is blocked. Type E injuries are further subclassified according to the Bismuth classification, with important implications about the complexity of establishing biliary drainage and obtaining ultimate definitive repair.

Type E1: Circumferential injury to the common duct >2 cm from the bifurcation.

Type E2: Circumferential injury to the common duct <2 cm from the bifurcation.

Type E3: Circumferential injury to the common duct at the bifurcation.

Type E4: Injury to the right or left hepatic duct.

Type E5: Combined injury to the common duct and an aberrant right hepatic duct.

The majority of Type E injuries will require PTC to definitively reveal the anatomic details of the injury and to establish stable biliary drainage.

Management of bile duct injury

Bile duct injuries may be diverse in their presentation, and the management should always be catered to the patient's clinical condition and the anatomic details of the injury. Principles that apply in all cases include control of sepsis, drainage of all bile collections, and establishment of secure biliary drainage. Vigilant reassessment of the patient's clinical condition, with frequent reimaging to detect undrained sources of intraabdominal sepsis, will get even the frailest patients through what can be tenuous early stages of their injury, allowing definitive repair to be performed typically in an elective fashion on a healthy patient. Timing of definitive repair for those patients who require biliary reconstruction is an individualized decision that requires careful surgical judgment and patience. While pressure may exist from the patient, the patient's family, referring physicians, and colleagues to get the patient to the operating room soon after injury, it is critically important that the patient be physiologically appropriate for what can be a prolonged operation and recovery period and that the surgeon has a full understanding of the degree of the patient's injury. Once biliary drainage is established and infection is controlled, there is no need to rush, and these repairs can be quite straightforward when performed in an elective fashion after acute inflammation subsides.

As with their diagnosis and presentation, management of bile duct injuries can be derived from their Strasberg classification.

Type A—Type A injuries can typically be addressed definitively with percutaneous drainage of bile collections and endoscopic therapy. Endoscopic sphincterotomy will decompress the distal biliary tree, allowing diversion of bile away from the leaking cystic duct stump or accessory hepatic duct. Placement of an endobiliary stent is typically performed at this procedure and will usually promptly stop any ongoing leak. ERCP has the additional advantage of surveying the bile duct for choledocholithiasis, which may be associated with Type A biliary leaks (62). Removal of the stent in 4 to 6 weeks is usually all that is required in this setting. As the extrahepatic biliary drainage was not directly compromised, the risk of subsequent stricture or associated problem is minimal.

Type B—Type B injuries may not require specific intervention, especially when the injury is diagnosed late in patients without cholangitis. If significant atrophy of the affected segment(s) has already occurred, or the segment(s) involved is(are) small in volume, the value of an intervention is probably low. In fact, instrumenting the occluded segment(s) is(are) inevitably associated with the introduction of bacteria and subsequent risk of cholangitis. In patients who are symptomatic, access to the affected segment(s) is performed via PTC. If the involved segmental duct may be identified and is >2 to 3 mm, it can be reconstructed with a Roux-en-Y hepaticojejunostomy. An indwelling PTC catheter at the time of surgery can be helpful in locating the involved duct and may be placed across the anastomosis to lessen the risk of postoperative leak. A follow-up cholangiogram at 3 to 6 weeks postoperatively may be performed with removal of the biliary catheter if the segmental drainage is appropriate. In cases where reconstruction of a small segmental biliary duct is not possible, hepatic resection of the involved segment(s) will eliminate the problem of cholangitis and segmental biliary stasis. Outcomes from reconstruction of right segmental hepatic ducts are noted to be less durable than repairs of larger ducts, with more frequent need for repeat intervention (63).

Type C—Type C injuries may be managed exactly like Type B injuries, although in a more urgent fashion due to the associated biliary leak. Access to the involved segmental duct may be difficult and may require atypical methods such as opacifying the involved segmental biliary radicles by injection of a biloma drain or a combined ERCP–PTC "rendezvous" procedure to facilitate placement of a percutaneous biliary catheter across the injury (64). As in Type A injuries, percutaneous drainage of bile collections is typically necessary to alleviate symptoms and control infection. While it may be possible to restore biliary continuity via placement of a percutaneous biliary catheter, the risk of stricture across the healed injury is high. In the acute setting, experts have recommended ligation of small segmental ducts <2 mm, but this is an option only in ducts that have not been instrumented due to the risk of cholangitis. Therefore, appropriate options include segmental Roux-en-Y hepaticojejunostomy, or hepatic resection. Hepatic resection may be most appropriate with a small involved segmental duct, especially when the stricture or injury is at or above the portal plate or previous attempts at repair have failed (Fig. 35.3) (23).

Type D—Type D injuries may be diagnosed either intraoperatively or in the early or late postoperative period. When recognized intraoperatively, the extent and mechanism (sharp vs. thermal) must be considered in choosing the appropriate repair. A true partial transection performed sharply is likely the only reasonable indication for a primary repair in the setting of bile duct injury during cholecystectomy. Placement of a T-tube, either through the injury or via a separate choledochotomy, would be the classic method for repairing this type of partial injury. In the case of larger injuries, or injuries sustained with a thermal mechanism with devitalized tissue, it may be necessary to debride back the duct to healthy tissue. A primary end to end repair either over an internal catheter placed across the ampulla (such as an endobiliary stent, double J ureteral stent, or trimmed silastic pediatric feeding tube) or a T-tube may be performed. Unfortunately, what data exist about primary bile duct repair suggests a high rate of early failure and a stricture rate of up to 50% typically requiring a future

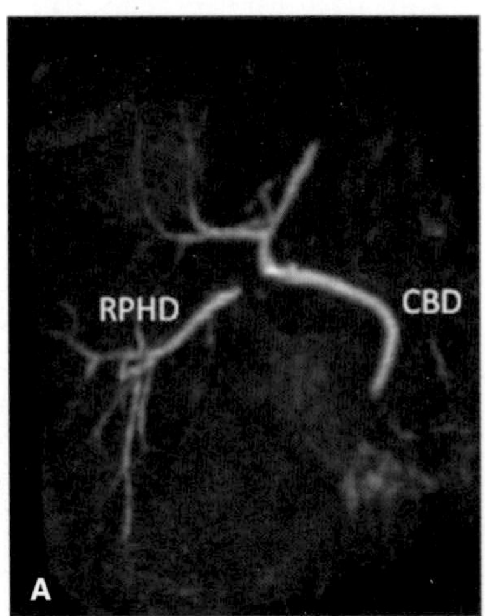

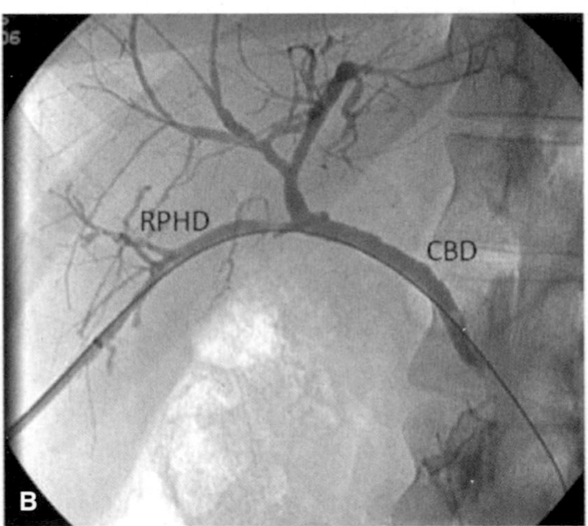

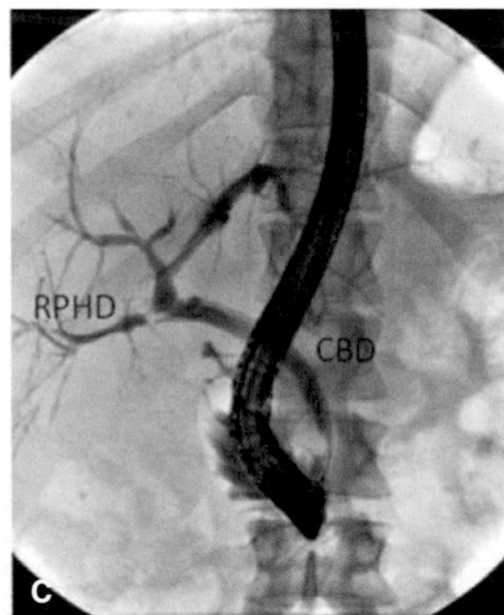

FIGURE 35.3. Type C biliary injury. The patient, a 33-year-old woman, developed bile peritonitis following a laparoscopic cholecystectomy. Percutaneous drains were placed, but the source of the leak was erroneously assumed to be cystic duct stump leak. She eventually developed abdominal pain and fever; magnetic resonance cholangiopancreatography (Panel **A**) revealed a disruption between her aberrant right posterior hepatic duct (RPHD) and common bile duct (CBD). This disruption and subsequent stricture were studied further with percutaneous transhepatic cholangiography (Panel **B**) and eventually dilated. However, the stricture recurred as documented by endoscopic retrograde cholangiopancreatography (Panel **C**), and the patient suffered recurrent bouts of cholangitis. She was eventually treated with a laparoscopic liver resection of segments 6 and 7 and is now clinically well.

revision (51). Thus, in cases where the injury appears more substantial, either due to involvement of more than half the ductal circumference or due to associated tissue devitalization, or in cases with associated vascular injury, Roux-en-Y hepaticojejunostomy to healthy ductal tissue above the injury should be performed.

Type E—Management of Type E injuries requires command of a spectrum of hepatobiliary surgical techniques and expertise (11,51,52). Repairs are typically done at or above the level of the hepatic duct bifurcation, with dissection into the portal plate necessary for exposure. Decisions about the timing and technique for the repair requires a full understanding of the anatomy involved, and thus proceeding with immediate repair should be done cautiously. In the situation where an experienced surgeon is available at the time of injury or a patient is transferred immediately after intraoperative recognition of an injury, early repair has been shown to be safe with acceptable long-term outcomes (54,59,60). In the case of patients transferred early after their injury, the question of when is too late to attempt immediate repair is controversial. Patients must be physiologically well without evidence of intraabdominal sepsis and should not have evidence of significant liver injury, suggesting associated vascular injury, and the extent of the injury should be understood either from IOC and discussion with the primary surgeon or via preoperative cholangiography. Repair beyond 72 hours from injury is probably ill-advised, particularly if there is a substantial biliary leak with associated perihepatic inflammation and staining.

In patients who present beyond 72 hours from their injury and have ongoing sepsis and/or a poorly managed biliary leak, initial interventions should be focused at draining bile collections and establishing control of biliary drainage. This rarely if ever should require operative intervention and can be accomplished by a combination of percutaneous and endoscopic means. Some hepatobiliary surgeons advocate an attempt at ERCP for delineation and control of the injury, before moving to a percutaneous transhepatic approach (60). However, the majority of injuries will require transhepatic control from above the level of the injury, an approach that promptly controls the biliary output and facilitates the eventual repair (20,54,55). In rare cases where the extrahepatic biliary tree is partially intact or at least the proximal and distal ends of the injury are adjacent to each other, a combined endoscopic and transhepatic approach can be used to bring a biliary catheter across the injury into the duodenum (65–68). In rare cases, particularly in patients with comorbid disease that delays or prevents definitive repair, this rendezvous approach may prove to facilitate healing of the injury over the percutaneous catheter (Fig. 35.4).

The preferred method for repairing most injuries is a Roux-en-Y hepaticojejunostomy, and the key principles include creation of a tension-free anastomosis to healthy

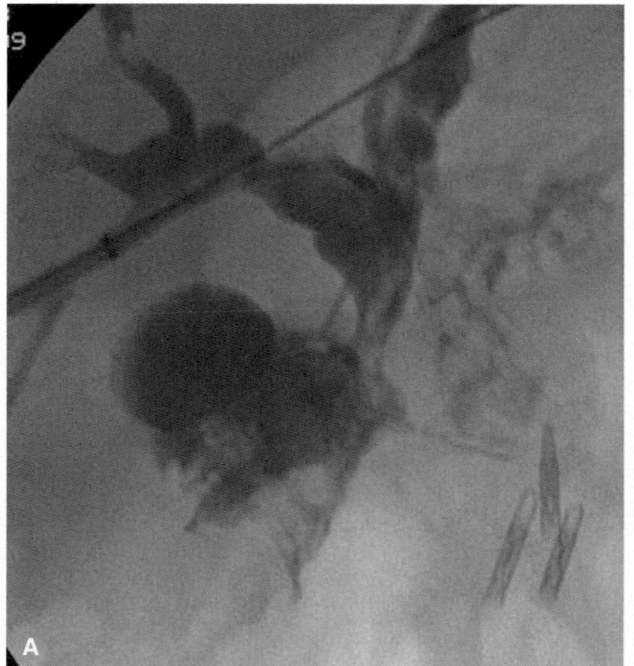

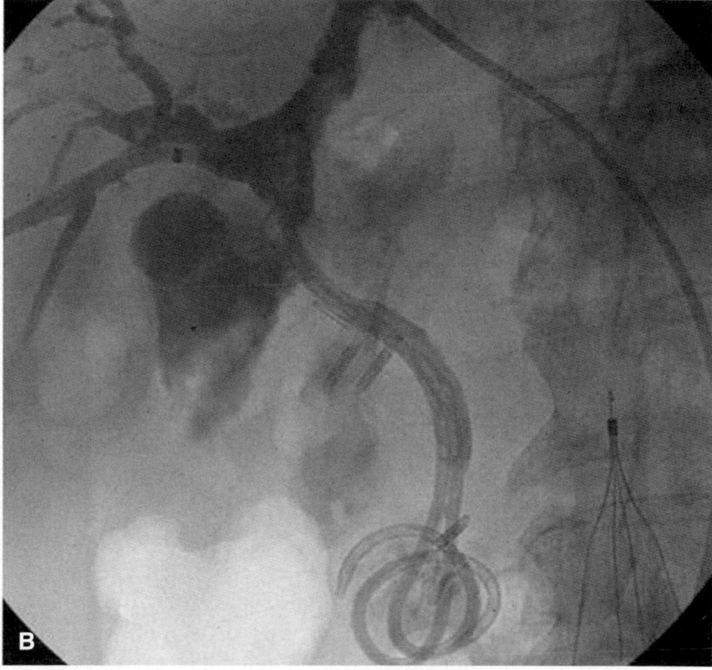

FIGURE 35.4. Type E2 biliary injury managed with combined endoscopic retrograde cholangiopancreatography–percutaneous transhepatic cholangiography (ERCP–PTC) "rendezvous" procedure. Panel A displays PTC images of a large volume biliary leak from an injury within 2 cm of the hepatic duct bifurcation, with no visible filling of the distal common bile duct. ERCP was performed introducing a wire into the subhepatic space through the transected distal common bile duct. The wire was snared via the transhepatic catheter, allowing introduction of bilateral percutaneous biliary catheters across this complex injury, as seen in Panel B. This biliary injury was managed with the percutaneous catheters alone; the biliary leak sealed and the tubes were left in place.

hepatic ducts that drain all biliary segments. Stewart and Way analyzed the treatment of 88 patients who sustained a major bile duct injury during laparoscopic cholecystectomy (51). Four factors were found to play a major role in the success or failure of treatment: performance of preoperative cholangiography in order to define the site of injury and biliary anatomy, the choice of surgical repair, details of the operative technique, and the experience of the surgeon performing the repair. The importance of delineation of the biliary anatomy preoperatively is clear: 96% of procedures that were performed in which cholangiograms were not obtained prior to surgery were not successful and 69% of the procedures in which the cholangiographic data was incomplete prior to operation were unsuccessful. In contrast, with preoperative cholangiographic data, repairs were successful in 84% of cases (51). This study and others documented the inadequacy of primary repair for these high Type E injuries; a primary end-to-end ductal repair was never successful when there was a complete bile duct transection (51,52).

The necessity of transhepatic biliary stents for repair of Type E injuries has been debated among hepatobiliary surgeons (19,23,54,55,69). Clearly obtaining PTC preoperatively can offer anatomic detail that may be difficult to determine intraoperatively due to associated injury and the challenges of IOC in high ductal injuries. If PTC access can be established, many surgeons and interventional radiologists argue that a stent should be placed and used as a bridge across the eventual hepaticojejunostomy. Clearly, in the setting of a patient not undergoing an early definitive repair, transhepatic biliary stents are necessary for maintenance of biliary drainage and can be used during the eventual repair to assist in identification of the ductal anatomy and for temporary stenting of the hepaticojejunostomy. Large series describe the use of transhepatic stents for as long as 12 months after definitive repair, allowing access for cholangiography and percutaneous interventions such as anastomotic dilatation when necessary (55,70). However, recent trends suggest that these catheters can be removed early in the postoperative period if no anastomotic complications are suspected (54,60,69).

The utility of transhepatic stents in early repairs is less well defined. Historically, silastic catheters were placed retrograde over Bakes dilators or other instruments passed out of the ductal system and through the hepatic parenchyma (21,71). This technique is not in the armamentarium of most active hepatobiliary surgeons, and these catheters are far more commonly placed percutaneously in modern practice. Given the potential difficulty in placing percutaneous transhepatic catheters into a decompressed biliary system after an early recognized bile duct injury (and therefore the potential delays implied), some surgeons will go to the operating room without a transhepatic catheter if the decision is made to attempt early repair.

The construction of an effective Roux-en-Y hepaticojejunostomy is critical to the long-term results of all patients with Type E injuries. Care should be taken to choose a part of the proximal jejunum that reaches easily to the right upper quadrant. In patients with previous abdominal surgery, time should be taken to meticulously lyse any adhesions that tether the small bowel mesentery. In cases where patients have a foreshortened mesentery, either due to previous surgery, radiation or due to other conditions, a medial visceral rotation of the right colon will expose the root of the small bowel mesentery that can be mobilized up to the level of the duodenum and neck of the pancreas. The small bowel should be divided at an appropriate place with a stapler, and the mesentery should be divided to allow the Roux limb maximum mobility. Division of the first vascular arcade of the small bowel mesentery can usually be done safely, though the end of the Roux limb should always be inspected for sufficient perfusion. A retrocolic Roux-en-Y hepaticojejunostomy, brought to the right upper quadrant through a defect made in the mesocolon to the right of the middle colic vessels and above the duodenum, provides the most direct route to the porta and can avoid any undue tension created by draping the Roux limb over the colon.

A few important principles apply to the dissection of the porta in these complex Type E injuries. The mechanism of bile duct injury in these cases often arises from unintentional dissection of a long segment of the bile duct, which can strip the duct of its blood supply, which runs through the periductal adventitial tissue. In early repair cases, it is therefore important to identify a portion of the duct that has not been completely dissected and carefully expose or shorten the hepatic duct in a location that is amenable to construction of the biliary anastomosis. In Type E1 or E2 injuries, it may be possible therefore to stay below the true hepatic duct bifurcation, but care should be taken not to sew to a traumatized end of the hepatic duct. Opening the duct on its anterior surface, with a ductotomy extended toward the long extrahepatic portion of the left hepatic duct, can expose healthy tissue, hold suture, and avoid further dissection behind the duct, which can further compromise ductal blood supply. In later repair cases, avoiding dissection behind the hepatic duct is really essential, as this allows preservation of any collateralized blood supply that has been created at the site of the injury. This principle of "anterior-only" dissection also avoids creating additional vascular injury, as the right hepatic artery is often directly behind the hepatic duct at this level and can be obscured or difficult to identify in a chronically inflamed or scarred field.

For Type E3 injuries or higher, the hepatic duct bifurcation needs to be exposed, by lowering the portal plate. This involves incising into the liver parenchyma to get above the hepatic duct bifurcation, beginning above the left hepatic duct in the technique described by Hepp and Couinaud (Fig. 35.5) (72). This can often be done with a blunt technique and through judicious use of electrocautery but can be facilitated in difficult cases by the use of an ultrasonic or hydrojet dissector. Bleeding may be

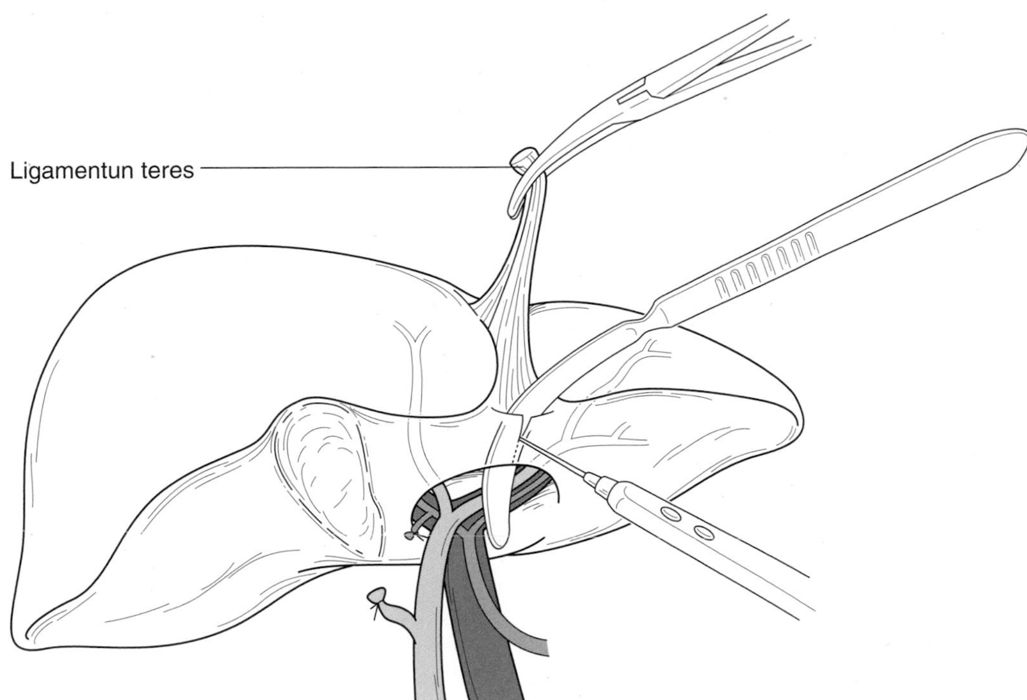

FIGURE 35.5. Hepp–Couinaud method to expose the left portal plate and the extrahepatic portion of the left hepatic duct.

encountered during this technique, but can be stopped by packing gauze or other hemostatic material into the hepatotomy for a period of time. Returning to this area after completing other tasks, such as creating the enteroenterostomy of the Roux limb, allows performance of the biliary anastomosis in a dry and controlled field.

Though perhaps counterintuitive to surgeons not experienced with these complex repairs, creation of a long ductotomy that crosses the hepatic duct bifurcation and incorporates exposure of all major hepatic ducts is essential to a durable repair. Mistakes can be made in Type E2 or E3 injury repairs by exposing only the scarred confluence of the hepatic duct at or below the bifurcation, reasoning that a "single-barrel" anastomosis would be technically simpler to perform. This approach ignores the importance of identifying healthy ductal tissue with preserved blood supply, by dissecting carefully above the level of injury. Winslow et al. (60) described this approach nicely as the "sideways" technique, allowing a long "side-to-side" hepaticojejunostomy that could be adapted to variations in the sectoral biliary drainage (Fig. 35.6). Use of the left hepatic duct to extend the length of the hepaticojejunostomy is a key element, as described by Couinaud (73), Hepp (74), and Voyles and Blumgart (75).

The management of Type E4 and E5 injuries can be even more challenging. Separate anastomoses to right and left ducts are often required, although sometimes a central portion of the former hepatic duct bifurcation can be used to bridge a long "double-barreled"-type anastomosis. Exposure to the left hepatic duct is often straightforward, as described earlier, but reaching a healthy portion of the right hepatic duct or its proximal branches can require significant intrahepatic dissection. Mercado et al. (59,76) have described a limited resection of liver segment 5 and sometimes 4B to facilitate exposure of the right hepatic duct within the parenchyma. These anastomoses may be facilitated by the presence of bilateral transhepatic biliary stents. In the case of injuries managed in a delayed fashion, a U tube (transhepatic biliary stent entering the right ductal system, crossing the bifurcation, and exiting the left ductal system) offers an effective and stable method of extrahepatic drainage (Fig. 35.7). The U tube can then be exchanged for separate bilateral silastic catheters at the time of repair, with an individual tube across each of the right and left ductal anastomoses.

All biliary anastomoses of these complex injuries should be performed under loupe magnification, using fine monofilament absorbable suture, typically in an interrupted fashion. Placement of subhepatic drains to monitor for biliary leak is typically performed. After completion of the biliary anastomosis, the Roux limb can be further anchored to relieve tension by taking seromuscular bites of the jejunum and tacking it to the former gallbladder fossa, portal plate, or umbilical fissure.

Associated vascular injury

Associated vascular injury is not uncommon in bile duct injury and may be associated with both acute liver injury and delayed biliary stricture due to ischemia. Significant vascular injury associated with a measurable rise in liver enzymes and systemic inflammatory response is a relative contraindication to early repair of bile duct injury, as not only may the patient not be optimized for what may

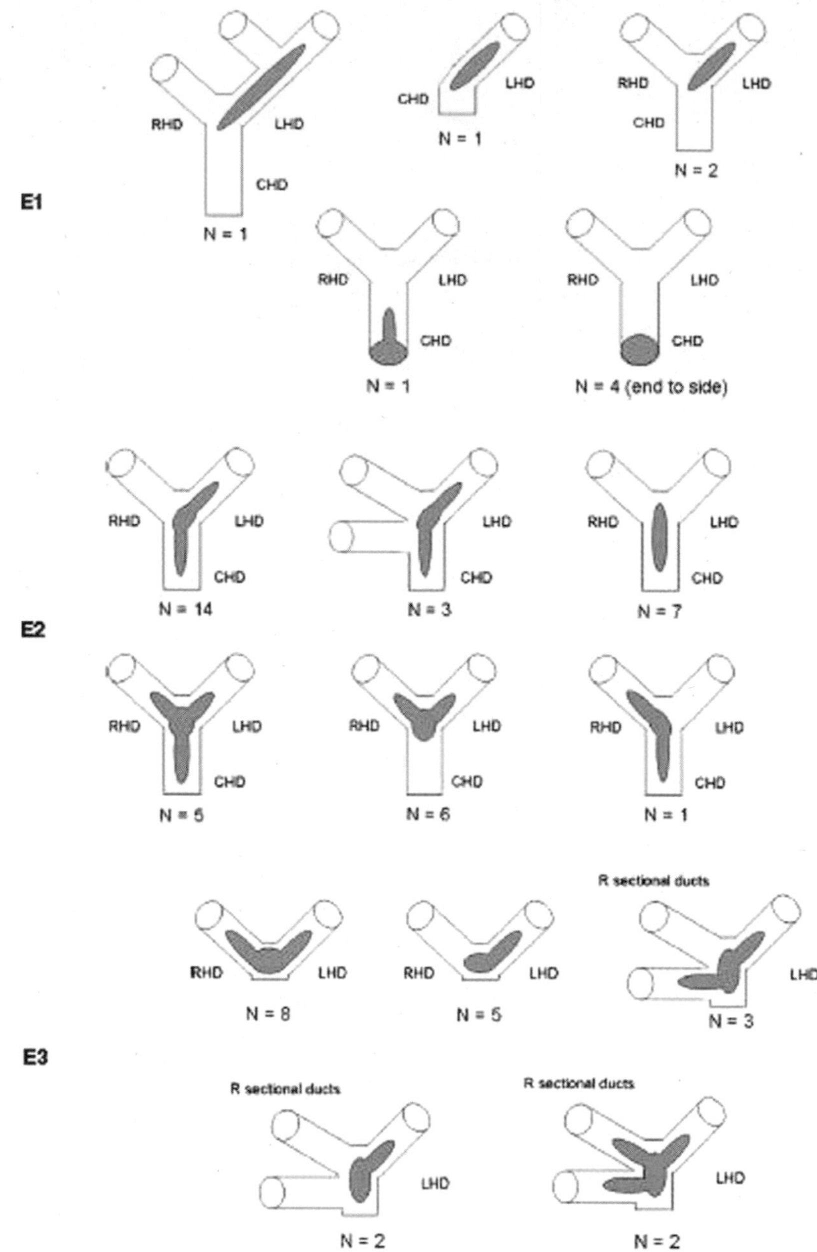

FIGURE 35.6. Longitudinal ductotomies performed to facilitate side-to-side hepaticojejunostomy for Type E1, Type E2, and Type E3 biliary injuries. (Reproduced with permission from Winslow ER, Fialkowski EA, Linehan DC, et al. "Sideways": results of repair of biliary injuries using a policy of side-to-side hepaticojejunostomy. *Ann Surg* 2009;249(3):426–434) (60).

be a complex operation, but will also not allow for collateral blood flow to involved biliary segments to mature over time prior to definitive repair. Fortunately, segmental hepatic vascular injuries do not typically require reconstruction due to the redundant blood flow to the liver (77). Exceptions to this general rule would include ligation or severe stenotic injury to the main portal vein or proper hepatic artery. Unrecognized vascular injury, particularly to the right hepatic artery, may be more common than appreciated and appears to be associated with a high rate of biliary stricture following repair (78,79). Vascular injuries appear to be associated with high bile duct injuries of Types E3 to E5 and should be suspected in cholecystectomies were excessive bleeding was reported or multiple (>6) surgical clips are visualized on postoperative radiologic studies. Strictures secondary to arterial insufficiency may develop over a longer period of time than technical failures resulting from a suboptimal anastomosis or other mechanisms of injury, such as a thermal injury (79).

Long-term outcomes following repair of bile duct injury

In experienced hands, repair of bile duct injury should be associated with excellent short-term results and restoration of patients to a good quality of life (23,54,60,80,81).

However, the rate of delayed stricture formation is probably as high as 15% to 20% (54,81). Risk factors for delayed stricture formation include associated vascular injuries,

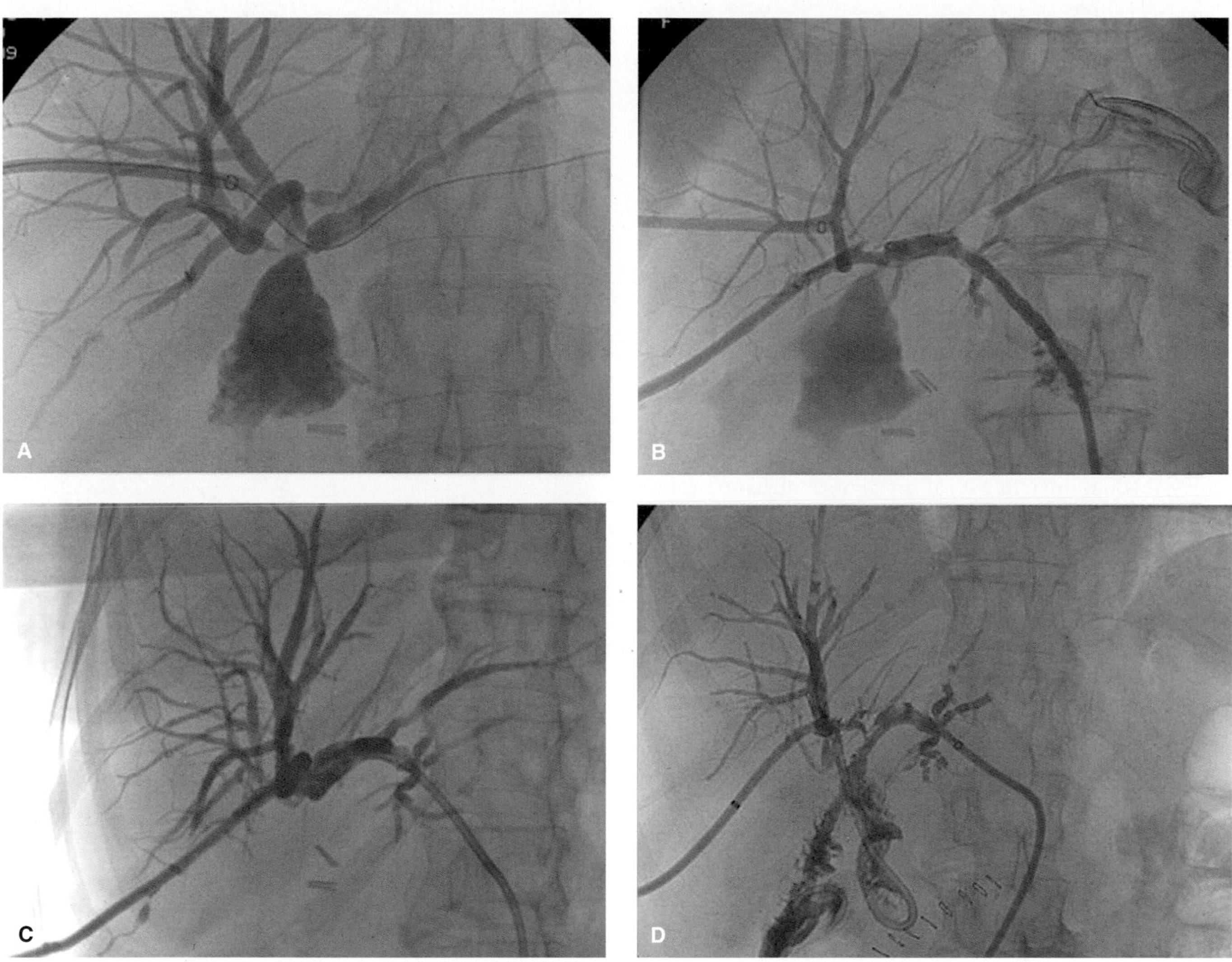

FIGURE 35.7. Type E3 biliary injury managed with U tube percutaneous biliary drainage and delayed Roux-en-Y hepaticojejunostomy. Percutaneous transhepatic cholangiography on POD 5 following laparoscopic cholecystectomy reveals Type E3 injury with biliary leak (Panel **A**). A wire was able to be passed from percutaneous access to the right hepatic duct, across the hepatic duct bifurcation and retrieved from percutaneous access to the left hepatic duct, allowing placement of a U tube for external biliary drainage (Panel **B**). The patient recovered over the ensuing 12 weeks, during which time the biliary leak resolved with stable U tube drainage (Panel **C**). At the time of hepaticojejunostomy, the U tube was exchanged for individual bilateral biliary catheters placed across the anastomosis. The catheters were removed 3 weeks after repair when cholangiogram revealed a well-healed patent hepaticojejunostomy (Panel **D**).

Type E3 to E5 injuries, and the need for revision of an initial attempt at primary repair. Strictures appear to present most commonly in the first 2 years after definitive repair, but can present in a more delayed fashion, emphasizing the need for longitudinal follow-up of these patients (55,82). When biliary strictures do occur, the vast majority can be managed without operative intervention, relying on percutaneous stenting and cholangioplasty (54,60). In patients refractory to conventional balloon cholangioplasty, internal metallic stents have been proposed as effective interventions with a high rate of success in strictured hepaticojejunostomies (83). Covered metallic stents offer a seemingly attractive option as they do not foster ingrowth and can be removed after temporary placement (84). However, these interventions are likely best reserved for patients that cannot undergo operative revision, as placement of metallic stents may eliminate later surgical options. In refractory cases of biliary stricture, associated secondary biliary cirrhosis and liver dysfunction may occur. While liver transplantation has been reported for severe and unreconstructable bile duct injuries, this should be an option rarely employed given modern surgical and interventional techniques to establish adequate biliary drainage (23).

RETAINED COMMON BILE DUCT STONES AFTER CHOLECYSTECTOMY

It is estimated that 10% to 18% of patients presenting for cholecystectomy with an indication of cholelithiasis will have common bile duct stones (85–89). When suspected preoperatively, endoscopic and surgical approaches to management of choledocholithiasis are available, with recent results suggesting that the strategies may be equivalent in efficacy and should be selected based upon local expertise and individual patient considerations (90). The use of IOC, as discussed earlier, may be guided by the suspicion of choledocholithiasis at the time of cholecystectomy. In ~1% of patients, choledocholithiasis will present following cholecystectomy (56). This delay in presentation is due to a lack of appropriate suspicion of the diagnosis preoperatively, due to failure to demonstrate common duct stones at cholangiography performed either intraoperatively or endoscopically, or due to stone migration that occurs at the time of cholecystectomy.

Clinical presentation with retained common bile duct stones following cholecystectomy typically occurs in the first 2 weeks postoperatively. Symptoms may include abdominal pain, jaundice, fever, nausea, and emesis. Laboratory evaluation will reveal an abnormal liver profile, particularly with elevation of the total bilirubin and alkaline phosphatase. Concomitant elevation of amylase and lipase should raise high suspicion of this diagnosis, suggesting a distal biliary or ampullary obstruction, as opposed to more proximal biliary obstruction following cholecystectomy that would not typically cause pancreatitis and should raise concern about bile duct injury. Because bile duct injury is the other major diagnosis in the differential of retained bile duct stones, the diagnostic evaluation should proceed in a similar manner. Right upper quadrant ultrasound is a reasonable initial diagnostic test and can sometimes visualize distal bile duct stones. HIDA scan can be a useful adjunct in cases where obstruction or biliary dilatation is not clear, as this test can document any associated biliary leak or obstruction. However, as with the diagnosis of bile duct injury, cholangiography is the definitive test to diagnose retained common bile duct stones.

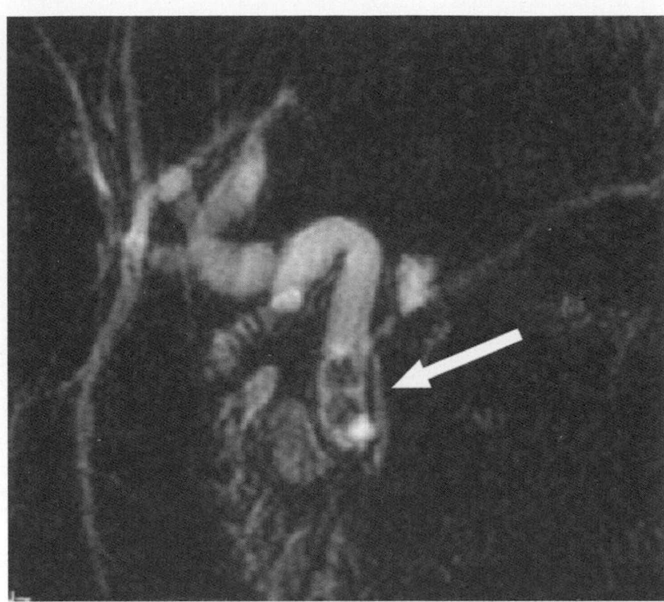

FIGURE 35.8. Magnetic resonance cholangiopancreatography demonstrating common bile duct stones. Arrow points to two stones in the distal common bile duct.

Endoscopic therapy of common bile duct stones

In the postoperative setting, ERCP is the preferred method for managing choledocholithiasis (91). Though past studies debated the role for ERCP and surgical methods of common bile duct stone extraction (92,93), more recent data suggest that ERCP is a safe and effective approach, particularly in the postoperative setting (94). Complications of ERCP include pancreatitis, duodenal perforation, and bleeding, though life-threatening complications should occur in <1% of cases (95,96). Risk factors for complications following ERCP include comorbid disease, obesity, or lengthy or complicated procedures (95). Recent prospective studies document that ERCP is effective in clearing the bile duct of retained stones in >93% to 96% of cases (92,97–99).

Given the rare but notable incidence of post-ERCP complications, efforts have been made to avoid biliary cannulation and sphincterotomy unless absolutely necessary. The use of EUS has provided an additional diagnostic modality to diagnose choledocholithiasis and appears to be most appropriate in clinical scenarios where choledocholithiasis is suspected but not confirmed by conventional imaging studies. In addition, EUS may be appropriate in patients who have an abnormal but improving liver profile, as a method to confirm that any common duct stones have passed spontaneously. This allows such "intermediate-risk" patients to avoid biliary cannulation and sphincterotomy unless the EUS confirms choledocholithiasis, an algorithm that appears to be accurate and safe (99). A recent meta-analysis suggests that performing EUS first could allow avoidance of ERCP in up to 67% of patients with suspected choledocholithiasis (100). A similar principle of "EUS-first" has been demonstrated in other studies, including the investigation of patients with suspected biliary pancreatitis (101,102). An obvious advantage of EUS over other noninvasive studies, namely MRCP, is that ERCP can immediately be used in the same endoscopic procedure if EUS findings confirm choledocholithiasis. Of course, EUS requires a skilled endoscopist that may not be available in all centers. Thus, MRCP might be equally appropriate to aid in the diagnosis of patients with suspected but not confirmed choledocholithiasis (Fig. 35.8), as a way of avoiding unnecessary ERCP (103).

Acute cholangitis due to choledocholithiasis is a relatively rare but serious problem, occurring in 6% to 9% of patients with symptomatic gallstone disease (92). Prior to the advent of endoscopic approaches, open common bile duct exploration was the standard of care for this problem, with a mortality rate of 10% to 40% (92). The use of ERCP in this setting has significantly decreased the mortality rate to the range of 0.4% to 7%. For patients who are acutely ill with cholangitis due to common bile duct stones, the overall success rate for ERCP cannulation is 95%. In this setting,

84% of patients have been noted to have stones, and biliary decompression was achieved in all patients (92). Transhepatic percutaneous routes to biliary decompression can be considered in patients who fail endoscopic biliary decompression for cholangitis, with little role for surgical approaches in the acute setting.

Surgical management of common bile duct stones

Surgical common bile duct procedures for stone disease are becoming increasingly less common with the advancing efficacy and versatility of endoscopic therapies. However, these techniques will always have a place in select circumstances where either endoscopic or percutaneous procedures fail to relieve biliary obstruction, or when ERCP is not feasible due to anatomic constraints (e.g., gastric bypass). In addition, choledocholithiasis recognized preoperatively can be safely managed in experienced hands either by sequential ERCP and cholecystectomy, or with concomitant cholecystectomy and common bile duct exploration (91,92). When performed laparoscopically by experienced operators, common bile duct exploration appears effective in >80% of cases in extracting common bile duct stones, with ERCP reserved for cases where stone extraction was unsuccessful or choledocholithiasis was not recognized until the postoperative period (91,104).

Common bile duct exploration can be performed using either a transcystic technique or choledochotomy. If stones are >15 mm, a transcystic approach may be employed (104). Stones >15 mm are an indication for choledochotomy, and stones >25 mm may require conversion to an open procedure. If the initial transcystic approach does not allow satisfactory removal of large stones or fragments, a choledochotomy is indicated. Choledochoscopy allows direct visualization of the duct system. A completion cholangiogram should always be performed after all stone extraction is complete. If there are concerns about the possibility of retained stones, a T-tube may be inserted either via the cystic duct stump or via the choledochotomy, although postoperative ERCP is also a reasonable approach. Observation in equivocal cases could be considered as most small stones pass spontaneously, though no prospective data support a policy of expectant management of retained common bile duct stones.

Patients with refractory stone disease or associated distal bile duct inflammatory strictures can be definitively treated with either choledochoduodenostomy or Roux-en-Y choledochojejunostomy. Both procedures have been advocated for patients with a high probability of stone retention and recurrent stone formation. Indications include difficulty in extracting stones; the presence of soft friable stones; retained, recurrent, or impacted stones; a dilated common bile duct with or without associated ampullary stenosis; multiple intrahepatic stones; or multiple common duct stones. Choledochoduodenostomy is easier to perform and is amenable to minimally invasive approaches (105–107). Roux-en-Y choledochojejunostomy is typically more involved to perform and precludes later endoscopic evaluation and treatment. Both short-term and long-term risks of cholangitis are similar for choledochoduodenostomy and choledochojejunostomy. The mortality rates for both procedures are similar, approximating 1.5% to 6% (107). Choledochoduodenostomy has a long-term risk of cholangitis that ranges from 0% to 12%; this complication is usually associated with stricture formation at the anastomosis (Fig. 35.9) (107). Stricture may be minimized by performing a mucosa-to-mucosa anastomosis of at least 14 mm length. Following Roux-en-Y choledochojejunostomy, a similar rate of cholangitis is seen, most commonly due to residual intrahepatic stones (107). Choledochojejunostomy is recommended when there has been a prior bile duct repair, when there is a difficult or recurrent biliary stricture, or when the duodenum is scarred, obstructed, or cannot be safely mobilized for an anastomosis.

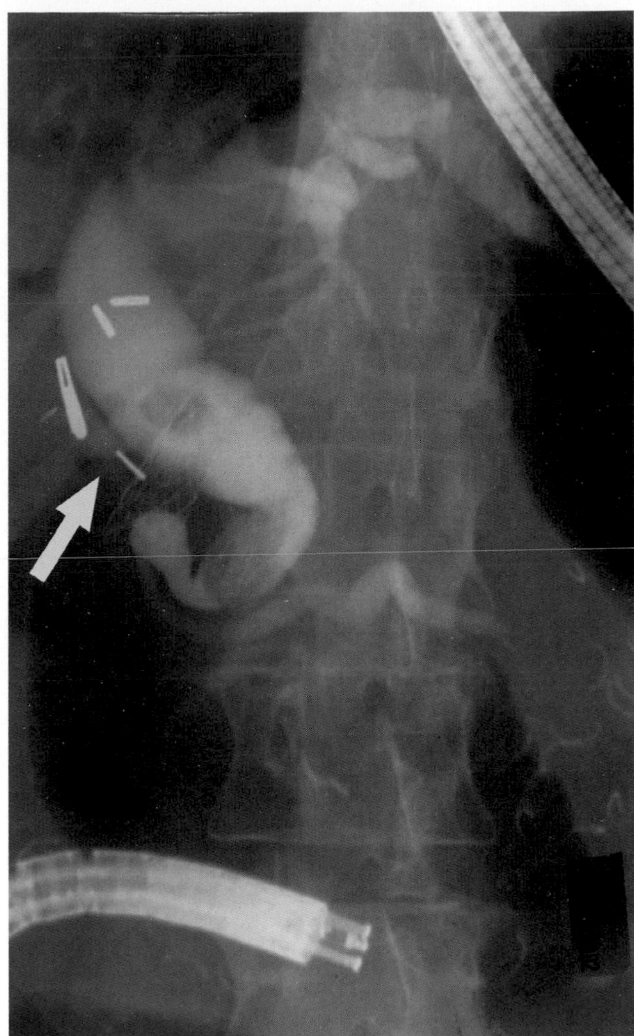

FIGURE 35.9. Endoscopic retrograde cholangiopancreatography of a strictured choledochoduodenostomy with a stone above the stricture. Arrow points to stone.

UNRECOGNIZED GALLBLADDER CANCER

Postoperative diagnosis of gallbladder cancer following cholecystectomy (i.e., on pathology of the gallbladder specimen) is a rare but vexing clinical problem. Gallbladder cancer is an uncommon disease, with <10,000 cases annually in the United States (108). Long-term survival is poor (5-year survival 5% to 10%), with nonincidental cases of the disease presenting nearly universally at advanced stages with fatal outcomes (108). Recent data suggest that an increasing proportion of gallbladder cancer patients are being diagnosed incidentally (109). Although several reports initially suggested an increased rate of port site or peritoneal seeding after laparoscopic cholecystectomy in the setting of gallbladder cancer (110,111), a multicenter evaluation demonstrated that the prognosis of unsuspected gallbladder cancer was no worse after laparoscopic than after open cholecystectomy (112–114). Survival correlates with stage of disease and with bile spillage during the first operation. Release of tumor cells inevitably occurs during cholecystectomy if the tumor is located on the hepatic surface during resection of the gallbladder from the liver bed. This factor may explain peritoneal tumor seeding that is sometimes seen in the absence of bile spillage.

During laparoscopic cholecystectomy, the gallbladder should be opened immediately after extraction to detect a possible malignancy. If a malignancy is suspected, a frozen section should be obtained. If gallbladder cancer is pathologically confirmed, the abdomen should be irrigated with a large volume of saline in an attempt to prevent implantation of malignant cells. Additional surgery is not recommended until the final pathology report to obtain accurate staging, as it is often difficult to determine depth of invasion based on frozen section. Delay of definitive surgical therapy does not have an adverse effect on prognosis (114).

Surgical treatment of incidental gallbladder cancer

Decision-making about the role of additional surgery for patients with incidentally diagnosed gallbladder cancer is primarily based upon the pathologic T stage of the tumor, as detailed in the sixth edition of the AJCC staging guidelines and outlined in Table 35.2 (115). Recommendations for appropriate surgical therapy are detailed in Table 35.3. Patients with T2 and T3 tumors who are good surgical candidates should undergo resection of segments 5 and 4B of the liver, with associated portal lymphadenectomy. For patients who have undergone laparoscopic cholecystectomy prior to radical resection, port site excision is also recommended. Resection of the extrahepatic biliary tree is also sometimes indicated if there is direct involvement of this area, or if the cystic duct stump margin is positive. More radical resections may be undertaken in order to achieve microscopically negative margins, which significantly improve prognosis. In patients with T2 disease, radical resection appears to significantly improve survival (61% 5-year survival with radical resection vs. 19% with simple cholecystectomy) (116) and is associated with a high yield of additional residual disease (57% of patients) (117). In patients with T3 disease, ~80% of patients will have residual disease in either the portal nodes or liver parenchyma (117), and 5-year survival is notably worse at ~25% (116).

The management of patients with T1 incidental gallbladder cancer is more challenging. Patients with T1a disease, that is, disease that invades the mucosa only to the

Table 35.2 AJCC staging for gallbladder cancer, 6th ed. (115)

T Classification	
Tis	Carcinoma in situ
T1a	Tumor invades mucosa to lamina propria only
T1b	Tumor invades muscle layer
T2	Tumor invades perimuscular connective tissue; not beyond serosa
T3	Tumor perforates serosa and/or invades liver to any depth and/or one other adjacent organ or structure
T4	Tumor invades main portal vein or hepatic artery or invades multiple extrahepatic organs or structures
N Classification	
N1	Regional lymph node metastases (cystic, pericholedochal, and/or hilar nodes)
M Classification	
M1	Metastasis to distant organs and/or to peripancreatic, periduodenal, celiac, superior mesenteric nodes
Stage	
Stage 0	Tis N0 M0
Stage IA	T1 N0 M0
Stage IB	T2 N0 M0
Stage IIA	T3 N0 M0
Stage IIB	T1–3 N1 M0
Stage III	T4 NX M0
Stage IV	TX NX M1

Table 35.3 Recommended surgical treatment for gallbladder cancer

Pathologic T Stage	Recommended Surgical Therapy
Tis	Simple cholecystectomy
T1a	Simple cholecystectomy
T1b	Segment 4B/5 hepatic resection + portal lymphadenectomy
T2	Segment 4B/5 hepatic resection + portal lymphadenectomy
T3	Segment 4B/5 hepatic resection + portal lymphadenectomy
T4	Surgical therapy not indicated

layer of the lamina propria, have excellent outcomes with simple cholecystectomy alone. In patients with T1b disease invading the muscular layer of the gallbladder, the incidence of associated nodal disease upon portal lymphadenectomy is ~12% to 15% (117,118). Despite this reasonable likelihood of residual disease, the survival for T1b gallbladder cancer with simple cholecystectomy is 85% to 96% (119,120). As the morbidity of radical resection for gallbladder cancer should be low in experienced hands (117), current recommendations support resection for T1b disease, though acknowledging this approach may overtreat a majority of patients in hopes of improving the survival of a few (121).

COMPLICATIONS OF BILIARY–ENTERIC ANASTOMOSIS

Other standard biliary operations for which complications can be considered are those procedures that include a biliary–enteric anastomosis. Biliary–enteric anastomoses can be included in resection or bypass procedures, or as part of the liver transplant operation. They can vary in complexity from the relatively straightforward, such as a choledochoduodenostomy on a large chronically obstructed distal common bile duct, to the highly technical, such as segmental or multiple duct anastomoses as a hepaticojejunostomy following a complicated hepatobiliary resection. Biliary–enteric anastomoses can be included as part of the operation for both benign and malignant disease of the hepatobiliary tract. Despite these protean applications, the important complications following these biliary procedures generally present as either leak or stricture, and their management principles are similar regardless of the patient and indication for the procedure. Control of infection and maintenance of adequate biliary drainage are paramount to their effective management.

The incidence of complications following biliary–enteric anastomosis is variable and dependent in large part on the indication and clinical setting. Biliary leak and stricture may be seen in up to 20% of patients following liver transplantation (122), likely due to the added impact of associated ischemia–reperfusion injury of the allograft, but should be relatively uncommon in other circumstances even after a complex hepaticojejunostomy (54,60). In more routine biliary anastomoses, leak or stricture should be rare occurrences in <3% to 5% of patients (107,123).

As with bile duct injury after cholecystectomy, understanding complications following the biliary–enteric anastomosis is derived from comprehension of their etiology and prevention. The principles inherent to a successful biliary–enteric anastomosis include exposure of a healthy and well-vascularized bile duct, a well-apposed epithelial to mucosa anastomosis free of tension, use of absorbable suture, and a healthy and unobstructed portion of the enteric tract as the distal target. Early complications after a biliary–enteric anastomosis are most often technical in nature and can be avoided by meticulous attention to technique. Handling of the biliary duct prior to the anastomosis is important, with attention paid to avoiding excessive dissection that strips the periductal blood supply. The bile duct should be cut sharply, with bleeding controlled by pressure or fine absorbable suture, rather than using thermal energy that may damage the most distal extent of the duct. Exposure is critical to being able to visualize every stitch, and techniques used to present the duct such that each suture may be placed accurately should be employed (21,124).

Early complications following biliary–enteric anastomosis

Early postoperative complications of these procedures include external biliary fistula and bile peritonitis, usually related to an anastomotic leak. If this complication occurs, percutaneous drainage of bile collections is the preferred approach, avoiding reoperation. If reoperation is required, it should not typically be combined with any immediate attempts at biliary repair, as the biliary tissue quality is often quite friable and prone to further complications with another attempt at anastomosis. Broad spectrum antibiotic therapy should be utilized and catered to cultures of drained peritoneal collections. Control of sepsis is the first and most urgent priority.

Many biliary anastomotic leaks will require establishing control of biliary drainage to achieve resolution. ERCP with endobiliary stenting and PTC with placement of a percutaneous transhepatic biliary drain are the options for gaining control and diverting biliary flow away from a biliary leak. Decisions between these two procedures should be made based upon anatomic considerations, as ERCP is likely only applicable to choledochoduodenostomies or more proximal jejunal anastomoses that can be reached by double-balloon techniques (125). In some cases of segmental biliary anastomoses—such as those performed following an extended hepatic resection with biliary reconstruction, or living donor liver transplantation—surgeons may elect not to percutaneously access the biliary tree for control of a small or well-controlled biliary leak. In these cases, the difficulty of the PTC may be greater than the morbidity of a modest biliary leak, and generally, these leaks will resolve over time as long as the anastomosis is not completely disrupted. Biliary–enteric stents, whether placed endoscopically or percutaneously, should be left in place until any associated sepsis is resolved, the leak has been demonstrated to be sealed by repeat cholangiography, and the patency of the biliary–enteric anastomosis is established. Replacement of stents left for >4 to 6 weeks is necessary to prevent stent occlusion and subsequent biliary obstruction or cholangitis.

Biliary leak, particularly following hepatic resection or liver transplantation, is a risk factor for the development of hemobilia, a rare but highly morbid complication (126). The etiology of this complication appears to arise from the traumatic nature of biliary drainage on adjacent vessels, particularly if the vessels themselves have been injured or surgically ligated. Branches of the hepatic artery are typically involved, though portal fistulas can also occur. These injuries can probably at times develop secondary to procedures to address an associated biliary leak, as both ERCP and PTC-placed stents have been associated with adjacent artery erosion or pseudoaneurysm formation (127–129). Arterial pseudoaneurysms typically present with a herald bleed that may be followed by more catastrophic hemorrhage. When hemobilia is suspected, visceral angiography should be performed emergently. Embolization of identified pseudoaneurysms can be definitive, though hepatic artery reconstruction may be necessary in some circumstances when percutaneous embolization either is not feasible or would be associated with occlusion of hepatic inflow.

Late complications of biliary–enteric anastomoses

Anastomotic stricture is the most commonly delayed complication of the biliary–enteric anastomosis, and it may present with jaundice or cholestasis, cholangitis, obstruction, and/or stone formation. When suspected, cholangiography should be performed. MRCP offers a noninvasive means of documenting anastomotic stricture, and associated contrast-enhanced MRI can assess for associated vascular injury or other anatomic concerns that may be associated with biliary stricture formation. Once documented, direct cholangiography by either ERCP or PTC—as anatomically appropriate—can be definitive and therapeutic (Fig. 35.10). Operative revision of a biliary–enteric anastomosis should be reserved for appropriate surgical candidates that fail percutaneous or endoscopic attempts at cholangioplasty and stenting. Multiple studies document the efficacy of percutaneous techniques in managing biliary–enteric strictures in >75% of patients (128,130–132). While some patients required two to four procedures, the long-term ability to avoid surgical revision is notable (Fig. 35.11).

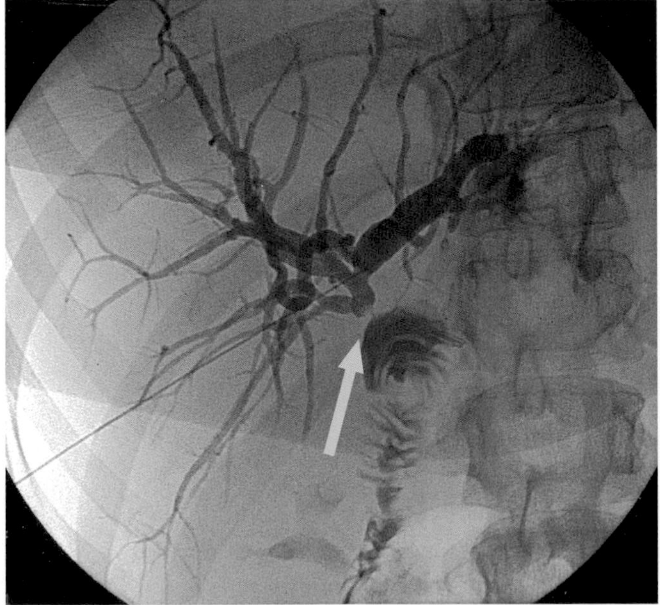

FIGURE 35.10. Percutaneous transhepatic cholangiography of a strictured hepaticojejunostomy, originally performed to treat a Type E2 bile duct injury. Arrow illustrates the strictured biliary–enteric anastomosis.

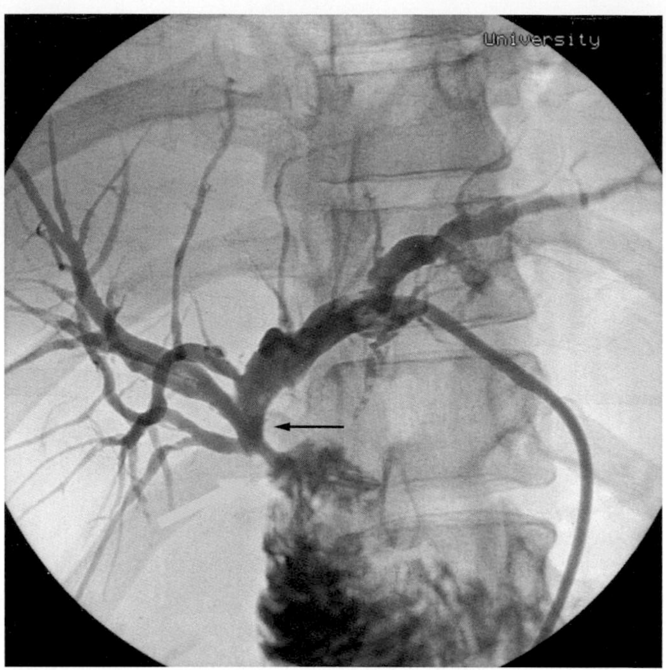

FIGURE 35.11 Percutaneous transhepatic cholangiography of the strictured biliary–enteric anastomosis illustrated in Figure 35.10 following successful balloon dilatation. Arrow indicates the area of prior stricture.

Although self-expanding metallic stents are quite useful in the treatment of inoperable malignant biliary strictures (133,134), their use in the treatment of benign strictures is controversial. Studies have examined the results of the use of self-expanding metallic stents for the treatment of benign biliary strictures with reasonable follow-up periods (83,135). The authors concluded that surgical repair should remain the mainstay of treatment for benign biliary strictures, with metallic stents reserved for patients who are poor surgical candidates, have intrahepatic biliary strictures or after multiple unsuccessful attempts at operative repair. Most of these patients eventually develop recurrent cholangitis and stent obstruction and required repeat intervention. Ductal mucosal hyperplasia develops in res ponse to stents and is a contributing factor to stent obstruction. The incorporation of the stent into the biliary wall can cause severe inflammation, which can complicate stent removal if this becomes necessary. The mean stent patency interval in published series was 30.6 months (83,135). In addition, there are concerns that chronic inflammation and obstruction may predispose to the development of cholangiocarcinoma. Although the risk of cholangiocarcinoma is well documented in association with primary sclerosing cholangitis, it has not been previously documented in the context of other benign strictures. The recent introduction of covered metallic biliary stents may expand their application, as these stents may stimulate less associated tissue ingrowth and inflammation and may be removed in a delayed fashion (84). More recently, degradable biliary stents have been proposed and may be applied more commonly in future applications (136).

CONCLUSIONS

Biliary procedures are common operations in general surgery, and complications may generate considerable patient morbidity and risk of mortality. Complications after cholecystectomy include bile duct injury, the management of which is predicated upon early recognition and expert management. Retained common bile duct stones can be dealt with through endoscopic, percutaneous, or surgical techniques with good results. Incidental gallbladder cancer diagnosed after cholecystectomy should be managed based upon pathologic T staging, with T1b, T2, and T3 cancer outcomes improved by subsequent hepatic resection and portal lymphadenopathy.

Complications following biliary–enteric anastomosis include leak and stricture. Both these complications require accurate and prompt diagnosis to limit patient morbidity, but can typically be managed without the need for reoperation. The effective management of all biliary complications is dependent on control of associated intraabdominal sepsis and establishment of definitive biliary drainage.

REFERENCES

1. Shaffer EA. Gallstone disease: epidemiology of gallbladder stone disease. *Best Pract Res Clin Gastroenterol* 2006;20(6):981–996.
2. Russo MW, Wei JT, Thiny MT, et al. Digestive and liver diseases statistics, 2004 *Gastroenterology* 2004;126(5):1448–1453.
3. McMahon AJ, Russell IT, Baxter JN, et al. Laparoscopic versus minilaparotomy cholecystectomy: a randomised trial. *Lancet* 1994;343(8890):135–138.
4. Jackson H, Granger S, Price R, et al. Diagnosis and laparoscopic treatment of surgical diseases during pregnancy: an evidence-based review. *Surg Endosc* 2008;22(9):1917–1927.
5. Brunt LM, Quasebarth MA, Dunnegan DL, et al. Outcomes analysis of laparoscopic cholecystectomy in the extremely elderly. *Surg Endosc* 2001;15(7):700–705.
6. Poggio JL, Rowland CM, Gores GJ, et al. A comparison of laparoscopic and open cholecystectomy in patients with compensated cirrhosis and symptomatic gallstone disease. *Surgery* 2000;127(4):405–411.
7. Polychronidis A, Botaitis S, Tsaroucha A, et al. Laparoscopic cholecystectomy in elderly patients. *J Gastrointestin Liver Dis* 2008;17(3):309–313.
8. Puggioni A, Wong LL. A metaanalysis of laparoscopic cholecystectomy in patients with cirrhosis. *J Am Coll Surg* 2003;197(6):921–926.
9. Roslyn JJ, Binns GS, Hughes EF, et al. Open cholecystectomy. A contemporary analysis of 42,474 patients. *Ann Surg* 1993;218(2):129–137.
10. Strasberg SM, Hertl M, Soper NJ. An analysis of the problem of biliary injury during laparoscopic cholecystectomy. *J Am Coll Surg* 1995;180(1):101–125.
11. Flum DR, Cheadle A, Prela C, et al. Bile duct injury during cholecystectomy and survival in medicare beneficiaries. *JAMA* 2003;290(16):2168–2173.
12. Nuzzo G, Giuliante F, Giovannini I, et al. Bile duct injury during laparoscopic cholecystectomy: results of an Italian national survey on 56 591 cholecystectomies. *Arch Surg* 2005;140(10):986–992.
13. Waage A, Nilsson M. Iatrogenic bile duct injury: a population-based study of 152 776 cholecystectomies in the Swedish Inpatient Registry. *Arch Surg* 2006;141(12):1207–1213.
14. Archer SB, Brown DW, Smith CD, et al. Bile duct injury during laparoscopic cholecystectomy: results of a national survey. *Ann Surg* 2001;234(4):549–558; discussion 558–559.
15. Strasberg SM. Biliary injury in laparoscopic surgery: part 2. Changing the culture of cholecystectomy. *J Am Coll Surg* 2005;201(4):604–611.
16. Strasberg SM. Biliary injury in laparoscopic surgery: part 1. Processes used in determination of standard of care in misidentification injuries. *J Am Coll Surg* 2005;201(4):598–603.
17. Way LW, Stewart L, Gantert W, et al. Causes and prevention of laparoscopic bile duct injuries: analysis of 252 cases from a human factors and cognitive psychology perspective. *Ann Surg* 2003;237(4):460–469.
18. Strasberg SM, Eagon CJ, Drebin JA. The "hidden cystic duct" syndrome and the infundibular technique of laparoscopic cholecystectomy—the danger of the false infundibulum. *J Am Coll Surg* 2000; 191(6):661–667.
19. Davidoff AM, Pappas TN, Murray EA, et al. Mechanisms of major biliary injury during laparoscopic cholecystectomy. *Ann Surg* 1992; 215(3):196–202.
20. Branum G, Schmitt C, Baillie J, et al. Management of major biliary complications after laparoscopic cholecystectomy. *Ann Surg* 1993;217(5): 532–540; discussion 540–541.
21. Cameron JL, Sandone C. *Atlas of gastrointestinal surgery*, 2nd ed. Hamilton: BC Decker; 2007.
22. Souba WW, Fink MP, Jurkovich GJ, et al.; for American College of Surgeons. *ACS surgery: principles & practice 2004*. New York, NY: WebMD Professional Pub; 2004, xxiii, 1505.
23. Chapman WC, Abecassis M, Jarnagin W, et al. Bile duct injuries 12 years after the introduction of laparoscopic cholecystectomy. *J Gastrointest Surg* 2003;7(3):412–416.
24. Strasberg SM, Brunt LM. Rationale and use of the critical view of safety in laparoscopic cholecystectomy. *J Am Coll Surg* 2010;211(1): 132–138.
25. Yegiyants S, Collins JC. Operative strategy can reduce the incidence of major bile duct injury in laparoscopic cholecystectomy. *Am Surg* 2008;74(10):985–987.
26. Avgerinos C, Kelgiorgi D, Touloumis Z, et al. One thousand laparoscopic cholecystectomies in a single surgical unit using the "critical view of safety" technique. *J Gastrointest Surg* 2009;13(3):498–503.
27. Heistermann HP, Tobusch A, Palmes D. Prevention of bile duct injuries after laparoscopic cholecystectomy. "The critical view of safety" [in German]. *Zentralbl Chir* 2006;131(6):460–465.
28. Wauben LS, Goossens RH, van Eijk DJ, et al. Evaluation of protocol uniformity concerning laparoscopic cholecystectomy in the Netherlands. *World J Surg* 2008;32(4):613–620.
29. Plaisier PW, Pauwels MM, Lange JF. Quality control in laparoscopic cholecystectomy: operation notes, video or photo print? *HPB (Oxford)* 2001;3(3):197–199.
30. Flum DR, Dellinger EP, Cheadle A, et al. Intraoperative cholangiography and risk of common bile duct injury during cholecystectomy. *JAMA* 2003;289(13):1639–1644.
31. Richardson MC, Bell G, Fullarton GM; for West of Scotland Laparoscopic Cholecystectomy Audit Group. Incidence and nature of bile duct injuries following laparoscopic cholecystectomy: an audit of 5913 cases. *Br J Surg* 1996;83(10):1356–1360.
32. Wright KD, Wellwood JM. Bile duct injury during laparoscopic cholecystectomy without operative cholangiography. *Br J Surg* 1998;85(2): 191–194.
33. Flum DR, Flowers C, Veenstra DL. A cost-effectiveness analysis of intraoperative cholangiography in the prevention of bile duct injury during laparoscopic cholecystectomy. *J Am Coll Surg* 2003;196(3): 385–393.
34. Ohtani T, Kawai C, Shirai Y, et al. Intraoperative ultrasonography versus cholangiography during laparoscopic cholecystectomy: a prospective comparative study. *J Am Coll Surg* 1997;185(3):274–282.
35. Barkun JS, Barkun AN, Meakins JL; for The McGill Gallstone Treatment Group. Laparoscopic versus open cholecystectomy: the Canadian experience. *Am J Surg* 1993;165(4):455–458.
36. Barkun JS, Fried GM, Barkun AN, et al. Cholecystectomy without operative cholangiography. Implications for common bile duct injury and retained common bile duct stones. *Ann Surg* 1993;218(3):371–377; discussion 377–379.
37. Holmin T, Jönsson B, Lingren B, et al. Selective or routine intraoperative cholangiography: a cost-effectiveness analysis. *World J Surg* 1980; 4(3):315–322.
38. Livingston EH. Intraoperative cholangiography and risk of common bile duct injury. *JAMA* 2003;290(4):459; author reply 459–460.

39. Livingston EH, Miller JA, Coan B, et al. Costs and utilization of intraoperative cholangiography. *J Gastrointest Surg* 2007;11(9):1162–1167.
40. Sanjay P, Fulke JL, Exon DJ. 'Critical view of safety' as an alternative to routine intraoperative cholangiography during laparoscopic cholecystectomy for acute biliary pathology. *J Gastrointest Surg* 2010;14(8):1280–1284.
41. Sanjay P, Kulli C, Polignano FM, et al. Optimal surgical technique, use of intra-operative cholangiography (IOC), and management of acute gallbladder disease: the results of a nation-wide survey in the UK and Ireland. *Ann R Coll Surg Engl* 2010;92(4):302–306.
42. Massarweh NN, Devlin A, Elrod JA, et al. Surgeon knowledge, behavior, and opinions regarding intraoperative cholangiography. *J Am Coll Surg* 2008;207(6):821–830.
43. De Waele E, Op de Beeck B, De Waele B, et al. Magnetic resonance cholangiopancreatography in the preoperative assessment of patients with biliary pancreatitis. *Pancreatology* 2007;7(4):347–351.
44. Mofidi R, Lee AC, Madhavan KK, et al. The selective use of magnetic resonance cholangiopancreatography in the imaging of the axial biliary tree in patients with acute gallstone pancreatitis. *Pancreatology* 2008;8(1):55–60
45. Biffl WL, Moore EE, Offner PJ, et al. Routine intraoperative laparoscopic ultrasonography with selective cholangiography reduces bile duct complications during laparoscopic cholecystectomy. *J Am Coll Surg* 2001;193(3):272–280.
46. Hublet A, Dili A, Lemaire J, et al. Laparoscopic ultrasonography as a good alternative to intraoperative cholangiography (IOC) during laparoscopic cholecystectomy: results of prospective study. *Acta Chir Belg* 2009;109(3):312–316.
47. Machi J, Johnson JO, Deziel DJ, et al. The routine use of laparoscopic ultrasound decreases bile duct injury: a multicenter study. *Surg Endosc* 2009;23(2):384–388.
48. Machi J, Oishi AJ, Tajiri T, et al. Routine laparoscopic ultrasound can significantly reduce the need for selective intraoperative cholangiography during cholecystectomy. *Surg Endosc* 2007;21(2):270–274.
49. Tranter SE, Thompson MH. A prospective single-blinded controlled study comparing laparoscopic ultrasound of the common bile duct with operative cholangiography. *Surg Endosc* 2003;17(2):216–219.
50. Machi J, Tateishi T, Oishi AJ, et al. Laparoscopic ultrasonography versus operative cholangiography during laparoscopic cholecystectomy: review of the literature and a comparison with open intraoperative ultrasonography. *J Am Coll Surg* 1999;188(4):360–367.
51. Stewart L, Way LW. Bile duct injuries during laparoscopic cholecystectomy. Factors that influence the results of treatment. *Arch Surg* 1995;130(10):1123–1128; discussion 1129.
52. Woods MS, Traverso LW, Kozarek RA, et al. Characteristics of biliary tract complications during laparoscopic cholecystectomy: a multi-institutional study. *Am J Surg* 1994;167(1):27–33; discussion 33–34.
53. Mercado MA, Chan C, Jacinto JC, et al. Voluntary and involuntary ligature of the bile duct in iatrogenic injuries: a nonadvisable approach. *J Gastrointest Surg* 2008;12(6):1029–1032.
54. Sicklick JK, Camp MS, Lillemoe KD, et al. Surgical management of bile duct injuries sustained during laparoscopic cholecystectomy: perioperative results in 200 patients. *Ann Surg* 2005;241(5):786–792; discussion 793–795.
55. Lillemoe KD, Martin SA, Cameron JL, et al. Major bile duct injuries during laparoscopic cholecystectomy. Follow-up after combined surgical and radiologic management. *Ann Surg* 1997;225(5):459–468; discussion 468–471.
56. Duca S, Bălă O, Al-Hajjar N, et al. Laparoscopic cholecystectomy: incidents and complications. A retrospective analysis of 9542 consecutive laparoscopic operations. *HPB (Oxford)* 2003;5(3):152–158.
57. Horton M, Florence MG. Unusual abscess patterns following dropped gallstones during laparoscopic cholecystectomy. *Am J Surg* 1998;175(5):375–379.
58. Khalid M, Rashid M. Gallstone abscess: a delayed complication of spilled gallstone after laparoscopic cholecystectomy. *Emerg Radiol* 2009;16(3):227–229.
59. Mercado MA, Chan C, Salgado-Nesme N, et al. Intrahepatic repair of bile duct injuries. A comparative study. *J Gastrointest Surg* 2008;12(2):364–368.
60. Winslow ER, Fialkowski EA, Linehan DC, et al. "Sideways": results of repair of biliary injuries using a policy of side-to-side hepaticojejunostomy. *Ann Surg* 2009;249(3):426–434.
61. Couinaud C. Studies on intrahepatic bile ducts. *J Chir (Paris)* 1954;70(4):310–328.
62. Christoforidis E, Goulimaris I, Tsalis K, et al. The endoscopic management of persistent bile leakage after laparoscopic cholecystectomy. *Surg Endosc* 2002;16(5):843–846.
63. Lillemoe KD, Petrofski JA, Choti MA, et al. Isolated right segmental hepatic duct injury: a diagnostic and therapeutic challenge. *J Gastrointest Surg* 2000;4(2):168–177.
64. Gronroos JM. Unsuccessful endoscopic stenting in iatrogenic bile duct injury: remember rendezvous procedure. *Surg Laparosc Endosc Percutan Tech* 2007;17(3):186–189.
65. Agarwal N, Sharma BC, Garg S, et al. Endoscopic management of postoperative bile leaks. *Hepatobiliary Pancreat Dis Int* 2006;5(2):273–277.
66. Dowsett JF, Vaira D, Hatfield AR, et al. Endoscopic biliary therapy using the combined percutaneous and endoscopic technique. *Gastroenterology* 1989;96(4):1180–1186.
67. Wallace M, Middlebrook M. Percutaneous biliary reconstruction: a report of two cases utilizing "blunt" recanalization and "rendezvous" techniques. *Cardiovasc Intervent Radiol* 2001;24(5):339–342.
68. Wayman J, Mansfield JC, Matthewson K, et al. Combined percutaneous and endoscopic procedures for bile duct obstruction: simultaneous and delayed techniques compared. *Hepatogastroenterology* 2003;50(52):915–918.
69. Mercado MA, Chan C, Orozco H, et al. To stent or not to stent bilioenteric anastomosis after iatrogenic injury: a dilemma not answered? *Arch Surg* 2002;137(1):60–63.
70. Johnson SR, Koehler A, Pennington LK, et al. Long-term results of surgical repair of bile duct injuries following laparoscopic cholecystectomy. *Surgery* 2000;128(4):668–677.
71. Cameron JL, Gayler BW, Zuidema GD. The use of silastic transhepatic stents in benign and malignant biliary strictures. *Ann Surg* 1978;188(4):552–561.
72. Hepp J, Couinaud C. Approach to and use of the left hepatic duct in reparation of the common bile duct [in French]. *Presse Med* 1956;64(41):947–948.
73. Couinaud C. Exposure of the left hepatic duct through the hilum or in the umbilical of the liver: anatomic limitations. *Surgery* 1989;105(1):21–27.
74. Hepp J. Hepaticojejunostomy using the left biliary trunk for iatrogenic biliary lesions: the French connection. *World J Surg* 1985;9(3):507–511.
75. Voyles CR, Blumgart LH. A technique for the construction of high biliary–enteric anastomoses. *Surg Gynecol Obstet* 1982;154(6):885–887.
76. Mercado MA, Orozco H, de la Garza L, et al. Biliary duct injury: partial segment IV resection for intrahepatic reconstruction of biliary lesions. *Arch Surg* 1999;134(9):1008–1010.
77. Schmidt SC, Settmacher U, Langrehr JM, et al. Management and outcome of patients with combined bile duct and hepatic arterial injuries after laparoscopic cholecystectomy. *Surgery* 2004;135(6):613–618.
78. Gupta N, Solomon H, Fairchild R, et al. Management and outcome of patients with combined bile duct and hepatic artery injuries. *Arch Surg* 1998;133(2):176–181.
79. Koffron A, Ferrario M, Parsons W, et al. Failed primary management of iatrogenic biliary injury: incidence and significance of concomitant hepatic arterial disruption. *Surgery* 2001;130(4):722–728; discussion 728–731.
80. Melton GB, Lillemoe KD, Cameron JL, et al. Major bile duct injuries associated with laparoscopic cholecystectomy: effect of surgical repair on quality of life. *Ann Surg* 2002;235(6):888–895.
81. Schmidt SC, Langrehr JM, Hintze RE, et al. Long-term results and risk factors influencing outcome of major bile duct injuries following cholecystectomy. *Br J Surg* 2005;92(1):76–82.
82. Moraca RJ, Lee FT, Ryan JA Jr, et al. Long-term biliary function after reconstruction of major bile duct injuries with hepaticoduodenostomy or hepaticojejunostomy. *Arch Surg* 2002;137(8):889–893; discussion 893–894.
83. Bonnel DH, Liguory CL, Lefebvre JF, et al. Placement of metallic stents for treatment of postoperative biliary strictures: long-term outcome in 25 patients. *AJR Am J Roentgenol* 1997;169(6):1517–1522.
84. van Boeckel PG, Vleggaar FP, Siersema PD. Plastic or metal stents for benign extrahepatic biliary strictures: a systematic review. *BMC Gastroenterol* 2009;9:96.
85. Lezoche E, Paganini AM. Technical considerations and laparoscopic bile duct exploration: transcystic and choledochotomy. *Semin Laparosc Surg* 2000;7(4):262–278.
86. Soltan HM, Kow L, Toouli J. A simple scoring system for predicting bile duct stones in patients with cholelithiasis. *J Gastrointest Surg* 2001;5(4):434–437.

87. Heili MJ, Wintz NK, Fowler DL. Choledocholithiasis: endoscopic versus laparoscopic management. *Am Surg* 1999;65(2):135–138.
88. Hermann RE. The spectrum of biliary stone disease. *Am J Surg* 1989; 158(3):171–173.
89. Houdart R, Perniceni T, Darne B, et al. Predicting common bile duct lithiasis: determination and prospective validation of a model predicting low risk. *Am J Surg* 1995;170(1):38–43.
90. Martin DJ, Vernon DR, Toouli J. Surgical versus endoscopic treatment of bile duct stones. *Cochrane Database Syst Rev* 2006;(2):CD003327.
91. Cuschieri A, Croce E, Faggioni A, et al. EAES ductal stone study. Preliminary findings of multi-center prospective randomized trial comparing two-stage vs single-stage management. *Surg Endosc* 1996;10(12): 1130–1135.
92. Poon RT, Liu CL, Lo CM, et al. Management of gallstone cholangitis in the era of laparoscopic cholecystectomy. *Arch Surg* 2001;136(1):11–16.
93. Suc B, Escat J, Cherqui D, et al. Surgery vs endoscopy as primary treatment in symptomatic patients with suspected common bile duct stones: a multicenter randomized trial. French Associations for Surgical Research. *Arch Surg* 1998;133(7):702–708.
94. Byrne MF, McLoughlin MT, Mitchell RM, et al. For patients with predicted low risk for choledocholithiasis undergoing laparoscopic cholecystectomy, selective intraoperative cholangiography and postoperative endoscopic retrograde cholangiopancreatography is an effective strategy to limit unnecessary procedures. *Surg Endosc* 2009; 23(9):1933–1937.
95. Cotton PB, Garrow DA, Gallagher J, et al. Risk factors for complications after ERCP: a multivariate analysis of 11,497 procedures over 12 years. *Gastrointest Endosc* 2009;70(1):80–88.
96. Ryan ME. ERCP complication rates: how low can we go? *Gastrointest Endosc* 2009;70(1):89–91.
97. Nathanson LK, O'Rourke NA, Martin IJ, et al. Postoperative ERCP versus laparoscopic choledochotomy for clearance of selected bile duct calculi: a randomized trial. *Ann Surg* 2005;242(2):188–192.
98. Rhodes M, Sussman L, Cohen L, et al. Randomised trial of laparoscopic exploration of common bile duct versus postoperative endoscopic retrograde cholangiography for common bile duct stones. *Lancet* 1998;351(9097):159–161.
99. Berdah SV, Orsoni P, Bege T, et al. Follow-up of selective endoscopic ultrasonography and/or endoscopic retrograde cholangiography prior to laparoscopic cholecystectomy: a prospective study of 300 patients. *Endoscopy* 2001;33(3):216–220.
100. Petrov MS, Savides TJ. Systematic review of endoscopic ultrasonography versus endoscopic retrograde cholangiopancreatography for suspected choledocholithiasis. *Br J Surg* 2009;96(9):967–974.
101. Lee YT, Chan FK, Leung WK, et al. Comparison of EUS and ERCP in the investigation with suspected biliary obstruction caused by choledocholithiasis: a randomized study. *Gastrointest Endosc* 2008;67(4): 660–668.
102. Liu CL, Fan ST, Lo CM, et al. Comparison of early endoscopic ultrasonography and endoscopic retrograde cholangiopancreatography in the management of acute biliary pancreatitis: a prospective randomized study. *Clin Gastroenterol Hepatol* 2005;3(12):1238–1244.
103. Ledro-Cano D. Suspected choledocholithiasis: endoscopic ultrasound or magnetic resonance cholangio-pancreatography? A systematic review. *Eur J Gastroenterol Hepatol* 2007;19(11):1007–1011.
104. Snow LL, Weinstein LS, Hannon JK, et al. Management of bile duct stones in 1572 patients undergoing laparoscopic cholecystectomy. *Am Surg* 1999;65(6):530–545; discussion 546–547.
105. Cuschieri A, Adamson GD. Multimedia article. Laparoscopic transection choledochoduodenostomy. *Surg Endosc* 2005;19(5):728.
106. Khalid K, Shafi M, Dar HM, et al. Choledochoduodenostomy: reappraisal in the laparoscopic era. *ANZ J Surg* 2008;78(6):495–500.
107. Panis Y, Fagniez PL, Brisset D, et al.; for The French Association for Surgical Research. Long term results of choledochoduodenostomy versus choledochojejunostomy for choledocholithiasis. *Surg Gynecol Obstet* 1993;177(1):33–37.
108. Jemal A, Siegel R, Ward E, et al. Cancer statistics, 2008. *CA Cancer J Clin* 2008;58(2):71–96.
109. Steinert R, Nestler G, Sagynaliev E, et al. Laparoscopic cholecystectomy and gallbladder cancer. *J Surg Oncol* 2006;93(8):682–689.
110. Paolucci V, Schaeff B, Schneider M et al. Tumor seeding following laparoscopy: international survey. *World J Surg* 1999;23(10):989–995; discussion 996–967.
111. Z'Graggen K, Birrer S, Maurer CA, et al. Incidence of port site recurrence after laparoscopic cholecystectomy for preoperatively unsuspected gallbladder carcinoma. *Surgery* 1998;124(5):831–838.
112. Sarli L, Contini S, Sansebastiano G, et al. Does laparoscopic cholecystectomy worsen the prognosis of unsuspected gallbladder cancer? *Arch Surg* 2000;135(11):1340–1344.
113. Suzuki K, Kimura T, Ogawa H. Is laparoscopic cholecystectomy hazardous for gallbladder cancer? *Surgery* 1998;123(3):311–314.
114. Suzuki K, Kimura T, Ogawa H. Long-term prognosis of gallbladder cancer diagnosed after laparoscopic cholecystectomy. *Surg Endosc* 2000;14(8):712–716.
115. Greene FL, Page DL, Fleming ID, et al. *AJCC cancer staging manual*, 6th ed. New York: Springer; 2002:xiv, 421.
116. Fong Y, Jarnagin W, Blumgart LH. Gallbladder cancer: comparison of patients presenting initially for definitive operation with those presenting after prior noncurative intervention. *Ann Surg* 2000;232(4): 557–569.
117. Pawlik TM, Gleisner AL, Vigano L, et al. Incidence of finding residual disease for incidental gallbladder carcinoma: implications for re-resection. *J Gastrointest Surg* 2007;11(11):1478–1486; discussion 1486–1487.
118. de Aretxabala X, Roa I, Burgos L, et al. Gallbladder cancer in Chile. A report on 54 potentially resectable tumors. *Cancer* 1992;69(1):60–65.
119. Wakai T, Shirai Y, Yokoyama N, et al. Early gallbladder carcinoma does not warrant radical resection. *Br J Surg* 2001;88(5):675–678.
120. You DD, Lee HG, Paik KY, et al. What is an adequate extent of resection for T1 gallbladder cancers? *Ann Surg* 2008;247(5):835–838.
121. Hueman MT, Vollmer CM Jr, Pawlik TM. Evolving treatment strategies for gallbladder cancer. *Ann Surg Oncol* 2009;16(8):2101–2115.
122. Welling TH, Heidt DG, Englesbe MJ, et al. Biliary complications following liver transplantation in the model for end-stage liver disease era: effect of donor, recipient, and technical factors. *Liver Transpl* 2008; 14(1):73–80.
123. Nealon WH, Urrutia F. Long-term follow-up after bilioenteric anastomosis for benign bile duct stricture. *Ann Surg* 1996;223(6):639–645; discussion 645–648.
124. Ammori JB, Mulholland MW. Adult type I choledochal cyst resection. *J Gastrointest Surg* 2009;13(2):363–367.
125. Koornstra JJ, Fry L, Mönkemüller K. ERCP with the balloon-assisted enteroscopy technique: a systematic review. *Dig Dis* 2008;26(4): 324–329.
126. Finley DS, Hinojosa MW, Paya M, et al. Hepatic artery pseudoaneurysm: a report of seven cases and a review of the literature. *Surg Today* 2005;35(7):543–547.
127. al-Jeroudi A, Belli AM, Shorvon PJ. False aneurysm of the pancreaticoduodenal artery complicating therapeutic endoscopic retrograde cholangiopancreatography. *Br J Radiol* 2001;74(880):375–377.
128. Cantwell CP, Pena CS, Gervais DA, et al. Thirty years' experience with balloon dilation of benign postoperative biliary strictures: long-term outcomes. *Radiology* 2008;249(3):1050–1057.
129. Savader SJ, Trerotola SO, Merine DS, et al. Hemobilia after percutaneous transhepatic biliary drainage: treatment with transcatheter embolotherapy. *J Vasc Interv Radiol* 1992;3(2):345–352.
130. Kocher M, Cerná M, Havlík R, et al. Percutaneous treatment of benign bile duct strictures. *Eur J Radiol* 2007;62(2):170–174.
131. Millis JM, Tompkins RK, Zinner MJ, et al. Management of bile duct strictures. An evolving strategy. *Arch Surg* 1992;127(9):1077–1082; discussion 1082–1084.
132. Saad WE, Saad NE, Davies MG, et al. Transhepatic balloon dilation of anastomotic biliary strictures in liver transplant recipients: the significance of a patent hepatic artery. *J Vasc Interv Radiol* 2005;16(9): 1221–1228.
133. Lee BH, Choe DH, Lee JH, et al. Metallic stents in malignant biliary obstruction: prospective long-term clinical results. *AJR Am J Roentgenol* 1997;168(3):741–745.
134. Neuhaus H, Hagenmüller F, Griebel M, et al. Percutaneous cholangioscopic or transpapillary insertion of self-expanding biliary metal stents. *Gastrointest Endosc* 1991;37(1):31–37.
135. Lopez RR Jr, Cosenza CA, Lois J, et al. Long-term results of metallic stents for benign biliary strictures. *Arch Surg* 2001;136(6):664–669.
136. Petrtyl J, Brfůha R, Horák L, et al. Management of benign intrahepatic bile duct strictures: initial experience with polydioxanone biodegradable stents. *Endoscopy* 42(Suppl 2):E89–E90.

demonstrates resolution of the pseudocyst. While the reported success rates with both approaches are favorable, there is a relatively high bleeding and perforation rate (15,16).

Complications of Surgical Drainage

Mortality. The mortality rate following internal drainage procedure ranges from 0% to 13% with several recent series reporting a 0% mortality rate (12–14).

Recurrence

The recurrence rate following internal drainage of pseudocysts ranges from 0% to 15% (12–14). Pseudocysts might recur following internal drainage owing to several reasons. If an inadequately sized opening (<4 cm) has been created between the stomach, jejunum, or duodenum and the pseudocyst cavity, a pseudocyst may recur. This is a technical complication that can be easily avoided. Inadequate drainage of multiple pseudocysts may be a cause of persistent abdominal pain or recurrence. Additionally, a cyst may recur if it is a cystic neoplasm that was mistaken for a pseudocyst, highlighting the need to send a frozen section of the pseudocyst wall to confirm the absence of an epithelial lining.

Bleeding. Hemorrhage occurs following internal drainage of pancreatic pseudocysts in 2% to 16% of patients (2,12,13). Hemorrhage following an internal drainage procedure may be due to bleeding at a suture line, and if bleeding occurs in the immediate postoperative period, it should be treated by re-exploration. Alternatively, patients may have erosion of a pancreatic pseudocyst into adjacent vessels, which can result in massive hemorrhage. The splenic artery is most commonly involved (45%), followed by the gastroduodenal (18%) and pancreaticoduodenal (18%) arteries (17). In this setting, selective visceral angiography should be performed, with angiographic embolization using coils or pledgets usually resulting in definitive therapy (18,19) (Fig. 36.2). Surgery should be reserved for patients who are hemodynamically unstable or have failed embolization procedures. Peripancreatic inflammation and postoperative changes may make operative control difficult. Initial control of bleeding may be obtained by digital compression of the bleeding vessel or packing of the pseudocyst. Surgical approaches for definitive treatment include proximal and distal arterial ligation combined with intracystic suture ligation, distal pancreatectomy, and splenectomy for bleeding arising from the body and tail of the pancreas, or in rare cases, pancreaticoduodenectomy (18–20).

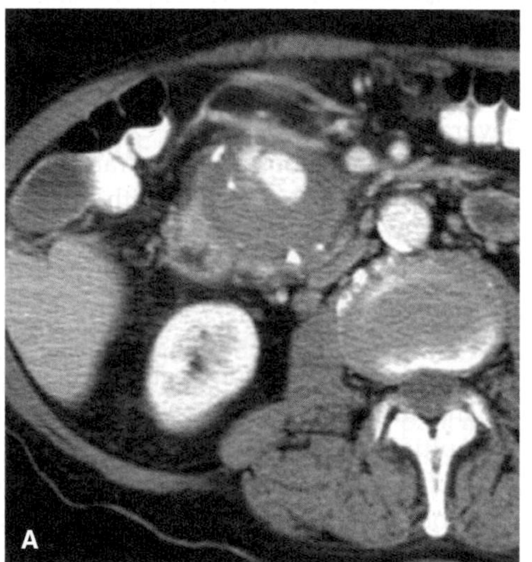

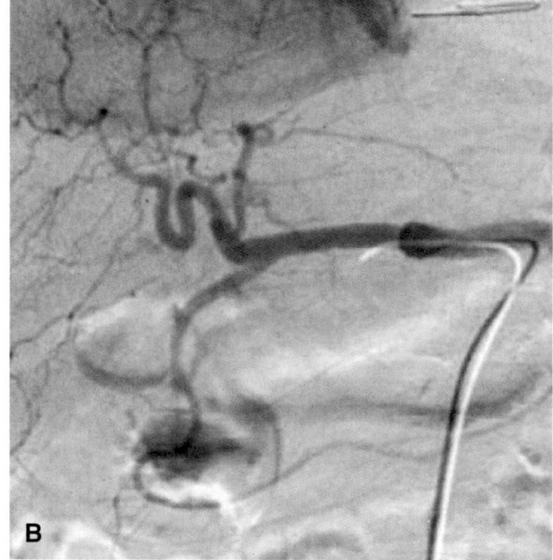

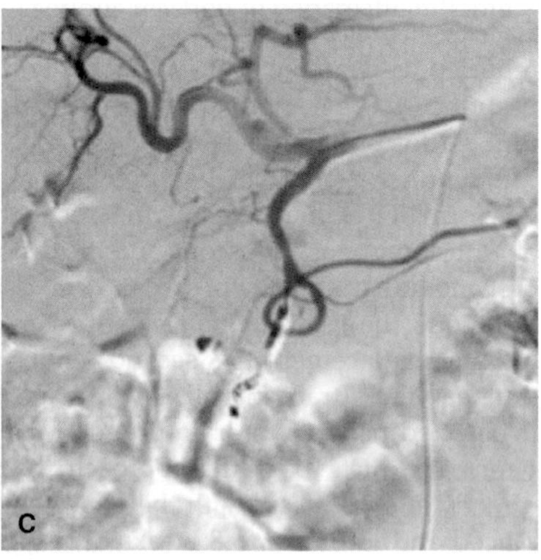

FIGURE 36.2. A: CT scan of a pancreatic pseudocyst with intravenous contrast within the pseudocyst, demonstrating active hemorrhage. **B:** Visceral angiogram documenting a pseudoaneurysm of the gastroduodenal artery. **C:** Postembolization angiogram depicting successful coil embolization of the pseudoaneurysm.

External Drainage

External drainage of pancreatic pseudocysts is indicated for pseudocysts that are found to be grossly infected or that do not have a mature wall sufficient for anastomosis at the time of exploration. External drainage is performed by opening the pseudocyst, evacuating its contents, and inserting a soft, silastic catheter into the pseudocyst cavity. A pancreaticocutaneous fistula may develop following the external drainage procedure. In most cases, these fistulas will close spontaneously.

Special Consideration—Multiple Pseudocysts

Multiple pseudocysts that require treatment may occasionally be present. While pancreatic resection is an option (especially if the pseudocysts are located in the tail of the gland), the preferred treatment is internal drainage. This can performed by converting multiple cysts into one large cyst to be used for a single anastomosis cystjejunostomy or combined treatment with cystgastrostomy and cystjejunostomy. In all cases, the surgeon should ensure that all cysts have been drained, using intraoperative ultrasound if needed.

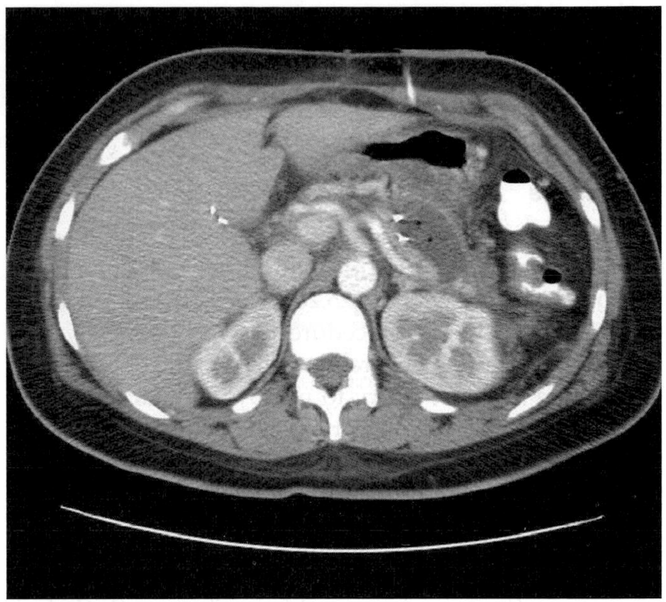

FIGURE 36.3. A CT scan of a patient with necrotizing pancreatitis with evidence of extraluminal gas.

DRAINAGE OF INFECTED PANCREATIC NECROSIS

Introduction

While the majority of cases of acute pancreatitis are mild and self-limiting, necrotizing pancreatitis develops in about 15% of patients, with infection of pancreatic and peripancreatic necrosis representing the most important risk factor for a fatal outcome. Infection of pancreatic necrosis typically occurs in the second or third week after the onset of the disease and should be suspected in any patient with a particularly severe bout of acute pancreatitis who develops multisystem organ dysfunction and/or systemic signs of sepsis. In such patients, a dynamic CT scan with intravenous contrast should be obtained to determine if there is evidence of pancreatic necrosis, represented by areas of nonperfusion. If there are obvious signs of infection, such as presence of extraluminal gas, surgical exploration and debridement are indicated (Fig. 36.3). Otherwise, patients should undergo CT-guided fine needle aspiration (FNA) with Gram stain and bacteriological cultures if infection of necrosis is clinically suspected. Infection of pancreatic necrosis as proven by FNA is regarded as an indication for surgical debridement. The indications for surgical debridement of sterile pancreatic necrosis remain controversial (21–23).

Operative technique

Infected pancreatic necrosis is an indication for operative necrosectomy. Several approaches have been advocated, including debridement with immediate closure over drains (with or without continuous lavage of the lesser sac), debridement with open or semi-open packing, and staged debridement with closure over drains. (21–25). We favor the technique of repeated operative necrosectomy with closure over drains (26). A recent CT scan is used to guide surgical exploration to ensure that all areas of necrosis or fluid are explored. Upon entering the abdomen, the lesser sac may be entered through the gastrocolic ligament or through the transverse mesocolon. Peripancreatic necrotic tissue should be removed bluntly. Forceful or sharp dissection should be avoided, as this may result in bleeding or injury to the bowel. A sample of the necrotic tissue should be sent for bacteriologic analysis. If fluid collections or necrosis extend to the pararenal or retrocolic spaces, these should be opened and debrided. Extensive irrigation is then performed. If all necrotic debris has been removed, then the abdomen may be closed over drains. If necrotic or questionably viable tissue remains adherent, then repeated operative evaluation should be performed in 48 hours, and further necrosectomy should be performed as outlined. This process is repeated as necessary until all necrotic tissue is removed, and the abdomen is closed over drains. Soft silastic drains rather than firm sump drains should be used to minimize the risk of pressure injury to blood vessels and the bowel. Repeated exploration may be facilitated by use of zipper placement, which allows easy, rapid entry into the abdomen and prevents loss of abdominal domain (26).

Complications

Mortality

In patients with infected pancreatic necrosis managed without intervention, the mortality rate approaches 100%. The mortality rate in several recent series for patients who undergo operative treatment of infected pancreatic necrosis ranges from 6% to 25% (24–26), morbidity rates remain high. The management of patients with infected pancreatic necrosis is challenging, as these patients often requiring

($n = 72$) (49). Pancreaticojejunostomy was performed in two layers without stents in either an end-to-side or end-to-end fashion at the surgeon's discretion. Pancreaticogastrostomy was performed by anastomosing the pancreatic remnant to the posterior gastric wall. The incidence of pancreatic fistula was 11% for pancreaticojejunostomy and 12% for pancreaticogastrostomy reconstructions. This trial demonstrated that pancreaticogastrostomy is a safe and viable option for pancreatic-enteric reconstruction with similar perioperative morbidity and mortality.

The effectiveness of perioperative octreotide in patients undergoing elective pancreatic resection was initially investigated in several prospective, randomized European trials (50–53). A subsequent meta-analysis of the European trials found that the use of octreotide significantly reduced the rate of pancreatic fistula formation (10.7% for octreotide vs. 23.4% for placebo) (54). However, there were inherent limitations in extrapolating the data from these studies to validate the use of prophylactic octreotide in patients undergoing pancreaticoduodenectomy. First, the trials examined all types of pancreatic resections including pancreaticoduodenectomy, distal pancreatectomy, and enucleation. It is possible that the fistula rates vary based on the type of resection, and therefore, this result may not be applicable for pancreaticoduodenectomy. Second, the rates of pancreatic fistula reported in these studies were much higher than rates reported at major institutions in the United States, which might amplify the benefit of octreotide observed in these studies (55). To address these issues, Lowy et al. (56) evaluated the use of perioperative octreotide specifically in patients undergoing pancreaticoduodenectomy for malignant disease. No significant differences were found in pancreatic fistula rates, mortality, or length of hospitalization between the two groups. In a similar study on pancreatic cancer patients by Yeo et al., no differences were found in pancreatic fistula rate in patients treated with octreotide versus placebo (39). Multivariate analysis revealed that soft pancreatic gland consistency was an independent predictor of the development of a pancreatic fistula. Overall, these studies demonstrate that routine use of perioperative octreotide for patients undergoing pancreaticoduodenectomy cannot be justified based on the available data. Further studies are needed to determine if perioperative octreotide is of benefit in specific patient groups who undergo pancreaticoduodenectomy, i.e., soft versus firm glands, or in patients with malignant versus benign disease. The use of fibrin glue has not been found to provide any benefit in decreasing pancreatic fistula formation.

Pancreatic fistulae that develop following pancreaticoduodenectomy can usually be managed conservatively if there is no evidence of abdominal sepsis. The presence of a pancreatic fistula should be suspected in a postoperative patient who develops clinical evidence of intra-abdominal sepsis. Isolated fluid collections should be drained, percutaneously if possible, and usually heal spontaneously if adequately drained. Octreotide is often used to treat established pancreatic anastomotic leaks that require percutaneous drainage.

Anastomotic Leak at Biliary-Enteric Anastomosis

Development of an anastomotic leak at the biliary-enteric anastomosis is reported to occur in 1% to 8% of pancreaticoduodenectomies from several large series (41–43,57). Diagnosis of a biliary leak may be evident if an intraoperatively placed drain develops bilious output, or may require evaluation with a cholangiogram or fistulogram. A small bile leak that is adequately drained often seals spontaneously. In more persistent cases, biliary anastomotic leaks may require a transhepatic catheter to allow for external biliary drainage.

Delayed Gastric Emptying

Delayed gastric emptying is a frequent and significant postoperative problem following pancreaticoduodenectomy. In most series, delayed gastric emptying, which is defined as the need for postoperative nasogastric decompression for more than 10 days, has a reported incidence ranging from 20% to 40% (58,59). Although not life-threatening, delayed gastric emptying results in a significant prolongation of hospital stay and contributes to increased hospitalization costs. The etiology of delayed gastric emptying following pancreaticoduodenectomy is uncertain; possible etiologies include decreased motilin levels, removal of the duodenal pacemaker and disruption of gastroduodenal neural connections. Erythromycin, a motilin agonist, has been found to improve gastric emptying of both solids and liquids when administered intravenously during the postoperative period. To test the potential role of erythromycin in gastric emptying following pancreaticoduodenectomy, a prospective, randomized trial was performed in which patients received either 200 mg of intravenous erythromycin or placebo from the third to tenth postoperative days, and on the tenth postoperative day, dual phase gastric emptying studies were performed (58). The erythromycin group had a significantly reduced incidence of delayed gastric emptying (19% vs. 30%), with measurable improvements in gastric emptying studies, supporting the use of erythromycin to decrease early delayed gastric emptying after pancreaticoduodenectomy.

Other factors influencing morbidity and mortality following pancreaticoduodenectomy

Hyperbilirubinemia and Preoperative Biliary Drainage

The effect of preoperative hyperbilirubinemia on mortality risk with pancreaticoduodenectomy remains controversial. While quite a few studies examining various other surgical procedures have shown that preoperative jaundice is associated with increased mortality risk, the literature describing the effect of preoperative hyperbilirubinemia on mortality following pancreaticoduodenectomy is unclear. While several studies have not reported an effect of preoperative hyperbilirubinemia on perioperative mortality (60–63), other studies have identified hyperbilirubinemia as a risk factor for mortality after pancreaticoduodenectomy (64–67). In a retrospective analysis of 279 patients by Braasch et al., patients with serum bilirubin >20 mg/100 ml had significant higher mortality rates (6/28, 22%) than patients with lower bilirubin levels (29/251, 11.5%), suggesting that the mortality rate may well be associated with the severity of hyperbilirubinemia.

While there does remain some controversy as to whether preoperative hyperbilirubinemia contributes to mortality, it is not clear whether risk can be decreased by preoperative biliary drainage. Results from a number of prospective trials and retrospective analyses have not shown a reduction in operative mortality by preoperative biliary drainage (67–71). A number of studies have sought to address the issue of whether preoperative biliary drainage impacts outcomes following pancreaticoduodenectomy. Patients who had preoperative biliary stents placed clearly experienced significantly increased rates of wound infection (increased from average of 4% to 10%), with mixed results regarding the effect of preoperative stenting on pancreatic fistula formation. No differences were observed between stented and unstented groups in incidence of intra-abdominal abscess or other major complications. Overall, the preponderance of data does not suggest benefit or detriment for preoperative biliary drainage procedures with regard to perioperative mortality. Preoperative biliary drainage demonstrates an increased risk of wound infection and may increase the risk of pancreatic fistula formation. In general, preoperative biliary drainage is relatively safe but should be reserved for patients with intolerable jaundice in which definitive surgical treatment is delayed.

Surgical Technique: Pylorus-Preserving Pancreaticoduodenectomy Versus Standard Pancreaticoduodenectomy

In the classic pancreaticoduodenectomy, as described by Whipple (72), an antrectomy is performed, whereas in the pylorus-preserving modification, the duodenum is transected 2 to 3 cm distal to the pylorus. The rationale for the more extensive gastric resection in the standard Whipple procedure was that it was a better oncologic operation, and it would reduce the acid burden and subsequent incidence of marginal ulceration. Pylorus preservation, on the other hand, has been touted as maintaining more normal gastrointestinal physiology, specifically in terms of acid production, gastric reservoir and emptying functions, and hormone secretion.

A number of studies have been performed to compare the outcomes of the standard versus pylorus-preserving procedure. Several reports have shown no difference in survival between patients with periampullary tumors treated with pylorus-preserving pancreaticoduodenectomy (PPPD) versus standard pancreaticoduodenectomy (73–75). In one of the reports (73), a randomized clinical trial of 77 patients compared the clinical results of classic pancreaticoduodenectomy versus PPPD. The PPPD group had a significantly shorter operative time and reduced blood loss. The incidence of delayed gastric emptying was identical in both groups. A similar incidence of delayed gastric emptying with standard versus PPPD has been verified in other studies (76,77). Postoperative nutritional parameters remain normal in most patients regardless of which procedure is performed. There were no differences in tumor recurrence or long-term survival (59,74). The published data do not indicate a significant advantage of the PPPD over standard pancreaticoduodenectomy, and the procedure chosen can be at the surgeon's discretion.

COMPLICATIONS OF DISTAL AND SUBTOTAL PANCREATECTOMY

Introduction

Distal pancreatectomy (50%–60% of the gland) is performed for a variety of benign and malignant conditions. They include chronic pancreatitis, cystic neoplasms, intraductal papillary mucinous tumors, pancreatic adenocarcinoma, neuroendocrine tumors, pancreatic pseudocysts, and resection en bloc for management of tumors arising from nearby organs such as the stomach or kidney. Subtotal pancreatectomy (80%–95% of the gland) may be required for neoplastic disease processes requiring a more extensive resection. Although commonly performed in the past, subtotal resection of the pancreas is rarely indicated for the treatment of intractable pain caused by diffuse chronic pancreatitis when the pancreatic duct is not dilated. In both distal and subtotal pancreatectomy, the spleen is typically removed because of the extensive collaterals that exist between the splenic vessels and the body and tail of the pancreas. If transection of the pancreas is carried out to the left of the portal and superior mesenteric vessels, this constitutes a less than 60% resection, whereas resection at the level of the portal vein and superior mesenteric vessels is a 60% to 70% resection, and resection to the right of the vessels is an 80% or greater resection (Fig. 36.7). In a large, multicenter report in which laparoscopic distal pancreatectomy was compared to open distal pancreatectomy in a matched cohort of patients, laparoscopic distal pancreatectomy was associated with less morbidity and a shorter hospital stay than open distal pancreatectomy. Consequently, it should be considered in appropriate patients (78). Currently, the indications for laparoscopic distal pancreatectomy and the learning curve for competency are being defined.

Complications

Pancreatic Fistula Formation

The pancreatic fistula rate in patients undergoing distal pancreatectomy is reported to be 5% to 25% (41,79–81). Surgeons have tried to determine the optimal management strategy for the residual transected pancreatic parenchyma

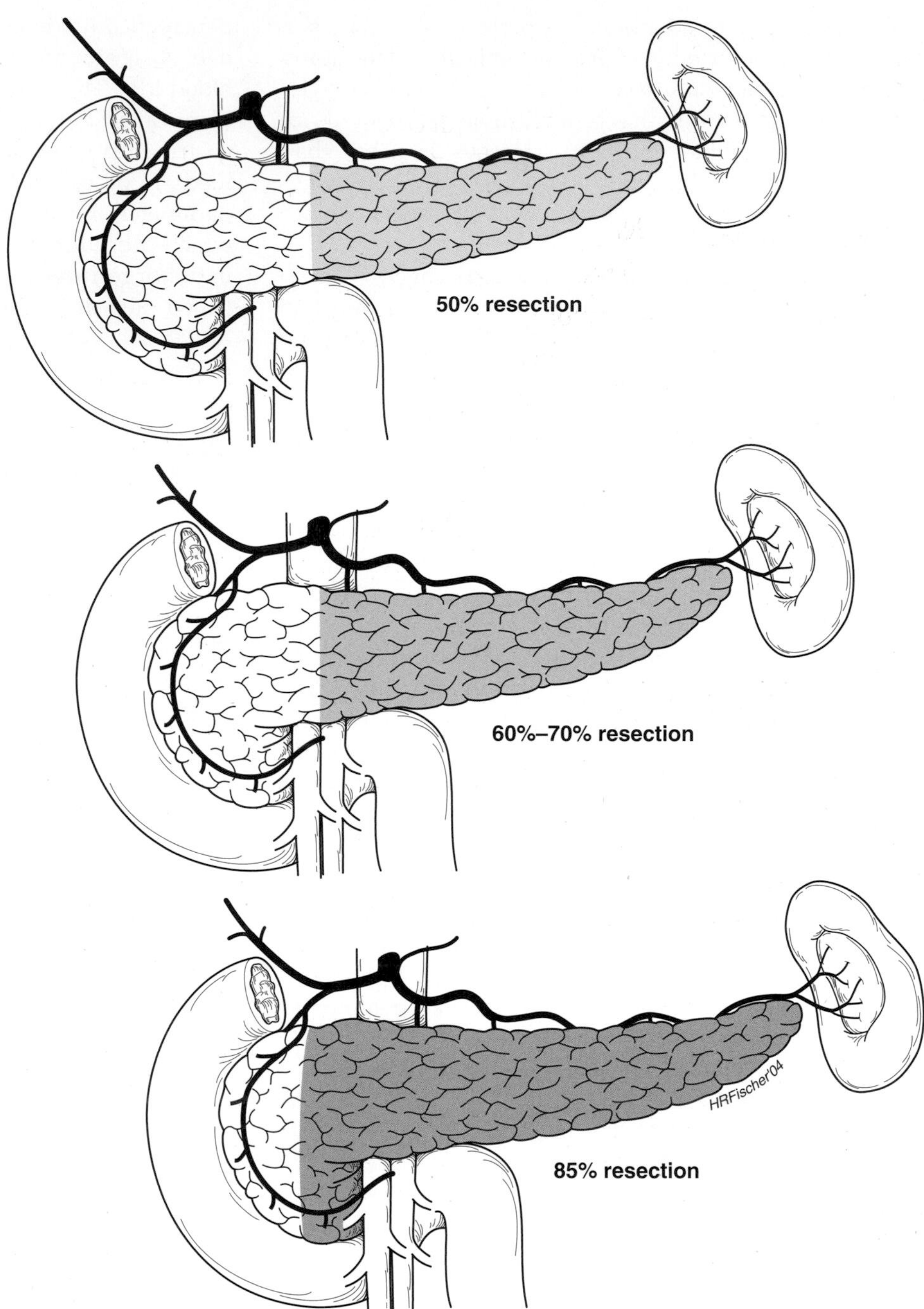

FIGURE 36.7. Level of parenchymal transection for 50%, 60%–70%, and 85% distal pancreatectomy.

and the divided pancreatic duct. Commonly used techniques for management of the transected parenchyma include oversewing of the remnant or staple closure, with or without direct ductal ligation. In two large series, there were no differences in pancreatic leak rates between patients whose stumps were sutured versus those whose stumps were stapled (79,81). However, in a study by Bilimoria et al., the incidence of pancreatic leak was found to be significantly decreased (9.6% versus 34%, $p < 0.001$) when the pancreatic duct was identified and ligated, independent of whether the remnant was sutured or stapled closed. Based on these data, every effort should be made to directly ligate the pancreatic duct following parenchymal transection, irrespective of the technique employed for stump closure. There are no studies currently that have adequately addressed the role for routine use of octreotide after elective distal pancreatectomy.

Endocrine Insufficiency

Diabetes may be a complication of distal pancreatectomy or subtotal pancreatectomy in patients operated upon for chronic pancreatitis if a major portion of the gland is removed. In an otherwise normal pancreas, as much as 80% of the pancreas may be removed without the development of diabetes. However, in the setting of diffuse parenchymal disease, as in chronic pancreatitis, resection of as little as 50% of the gland may cause diabetes or may worsen diabetes in chronic pancreatitis patients who have antecedent diabetes before surgical resection. In several large series, the overall reported incidence of new onset, insulin-dependent diabetes mellitus following distal pancreatectomy is approximately 8% (80,81). However, in patients with chronic pancreatitis, the risk is reported to range from 12% to 46% (82–85).

Exocrine Insufficiency

Like diabetes, exocrine insufficiency following distal or subtotal pancreatectomy is predominantly a complication that occurs in patients with chronic pancreatitis. Exocrine insufficiency occurs in about one-third of patients with a diagnosis of chronic pancreatitis before surgical intervention and has been reported to be present in 55% of postsurgical patients (83). Exocrine insufficiency is not considered a serious complication of pancreatic surgery and can usually be easily treated by oral pancreatic enzyme supplementation.

COMPLICATIONS OF TOTAL PANCREATECTOMY

Introduction

Total pancreatectomy has been used to treat both benign and malignant disease of the pancreas, but its use has been limited by concerns about management of the apancreatic state with its attendant total endocrine and exocrine insufficiency. Total pancreatectomy is a viable option for the treatment of patients with chronic pancreatitis complicated by diffuse gland involvement and severe, unremitting pain, multicentric or extensive neuroendocrine tumors, patients with familial pancreatic cancer with premalignant lesions, and in patients with intraductal papillary mucinous neoplasia with diffuse main duct involvement or invasive disease. Total pancreatectomy was a popular operation for adenocarcinoma of the pancreas in the 1970s because the long-term survival following pancreaticoduodenectomy was relatively poor. However, the results from total pancreatectomy in this group of patients were not improved (86), and there is currently little data to support the routine use of total pancreatectomy in this setting.

Complications

Mortality

The mortality rate for total pancreatectomy has demonstrated the same improvement over time as that observed with pancreaticoduodenectomy. While it was not uncommon for mortality rates following total pancreatectomy to be as high as 26% to 28% in older series, reports from several series over the last decade list operative mortality rates ranging from 3% to 5% (86,87).

Endocrine Insufficiency

The most significant complication encountered in patients who undergo total pancreatectomy is endocrine insufficiency. Pancreatogenic diabetes is characterized by (a) absence of the major glucoregulatory hormones insulin and glucagon, (b) instability, and (c) frequent hypoglycemia, with the latter parameters improving with rigorous home glucose monitoring. Dresler et al. (88) reported on the metabolic consequences of total pancreatectomy in 49 patients, with one-third of the patients being followed for more than 48 months. Although patients became diabetic and experienced alterations in lifestyle, most patients were able to resume a reasonable functional status and level of activity. Only one of the 49 patients died from metabolic complications due to the surgical procedure, while no other patients had serious sequelae from their diabetes. At the time of the report, no patient had developed clinically overt diabetic micro- or macrovascular disease. Other reports have demonstrated good performance status in patients following total pancreatectomy, with intermittent hypoglycemia being the most frequent complication (89). The use of different insulin formulations with varying half-lives as well as the development of an effective subcutaneous insulin infusion pump has improved postoperative glucose control (90). For patients with severe, unremitting pain due to chronic pancreatitis, an alternative approach is total pancreatectomy with either autologous islet cell transplantation or transplantation of a pancreatic allograft. In highly specialized centers, this approach has demonstrated promising results (91,92).

REFERENCES

1. Yeo CJ, Bastidas JA, Lynch-Nyhan A, et al. The natural history of pancreatic pseudocysts documented by computed tomography. *Surg Gynecol Obstet* 1990;170:411–417.
2. Vitas GJ, Sarr MG. Selected management of pancreatic pseudocysts: operative versus expectant management. *Surgery* 1992;111:123–130.
3. Tanaka M, Chari S, Adsay V, et al. International consensus guidelines for management of intraductal papillary mucinous neoplasms and mucinous cystic neoplasms of the pancreas. *Pancreatology* 2006;6:17–32.
4. Johnson LB, Rattner DW, Warshaw AL. The effect of size of giant pancreatic pseudocysts on the outcome of internal drainage procedures. *Surg Gynecol Obstet* 1991;173:171–174.
5. Siperstein A. Laparoendoscopic approach to pancreatic pseudocysts. *Semin Laparosc Surg* 2001;8:218–222.
6. Mori T, Abe N, Sugiyama M. Laparoscopic pancreatic cystogastrostomy. *J Hepatobiliary Pancreat Surg* 2002;9:548–554.
7. Bhattacharya D, Ammori BJ. Minimally invasive approaches to management of pancreatic pseudocyst: review of the literature. *Surg Laparosc Endosc Percutan Tech* 2003;13:141–148.
8. von Sonnenberg E, Wittich G, Casola G. Percutaneous drainage of infected and noninfected pancreatic pseudocysts: experience in 101 cases. *Radiology* 1989;170:757–761.
9. Adams D, Anderson M. Percutaneous catheter drainage compared with internal drainage in the management of pancreatic pseudocysts. *Ann Surg* 1992;215:571–578.
10. D'Egidio A, Schein M. Percutaneous drainage of pancreatic pseudocysts: a prospective study. *World J Surg* 1991;16:141–146.
11. Criado E, DeStefano AA, Weiner TM, et al. Long term result of percutaneous catheter drainage of pancreatic pseudocysts. *Surg Gynecol Obstet* 1992;175:293–298.
12. Spivak H, Galloway JR, Amerson JR, et al. Management of pancreatic pseudocysts. *J Am Coll Surg* 1998;186:507–511.
13. Heider R, Meyer AA, Galanko JA, et al. Percutaneous drainage of pancreatic pseudocysts is associated with a higher failure rate than surgical treatment in unselected patients. *Ann Surg* 1999;229:781.
14. Nealon WH, Walser E. Main pancreatic ductal anatomy can direct choice of modality for treating pancreatic pseudocysts (surgery versus percutaneous drainage). *Ann Surg* 2002;235:751–758.

15. De Palma GD, Galloro G, Puzziello A, et al. Endoscopic drainage of pancreatic pseudocysts: a long-term follow-up study of 49 patients. *Hepatogastroenterology* 2002;49:1113–1115.
16. Binmoeller KF, Seifert H, Walter A, et al. Transpapillary and transmural drainage of pancreatic pseudocysts. *Gastrointest Endosc* 1995;42:219.
17. Lillemoe K, Yeo CJ. Management of complications of pancreatitis. *Curr Prob Surg* 1998;35:33–51.
18. Carr JA, Cho JS, Shepard AD, et al. Visceral pseudoaneurysms due to pancreatic pseudocysts: rare but lethal complications of pancreatitis. *J Vasc Surg* 2000;32:722–730.
19. Steckman ML, Dooley MC, Jaques PF, et al. Major gastrointestinal hemorrhage from peripancreatic blood vessels in pancreatitis: treatment by embolotherapy. *Dig Dis Sci* 1984;29:486–497.
20. Bresler L, Boissel P, Grosdidier J. Major hemorrhage from pancreatic pseudocysts and pseudoaneurysms caused by chronic pancreatitis: surgical therapy. *World J Surg* 1991;15:649–653.
21. Bradley EL, Allen K. A prospective longitudinal study of observation versus surgical intervention in the management of necrotizing pancreatitis. *Am J Surg* 1991;161:19–25.
22. Buchler MW, Gloor B, Muller CA, et al. Acute necrotizing pancreatitis: treatment strategy according to status of infection. *Ann Surg* 2000;232: 619–626.
23. Warshaw AL. Pancreatic necrosis: to debride or not to debride—that is the question. *Ann Surg* 2000;232:627–629.
24. Branum G, Galloway J, Hirchowitz W, et al. Pancreatic necrosis: results of necrosectomy, packing, and ultimate closure over drains. *Ann Surg* 1998;227:870–877.
25. Fernandez-del Castillo C, Rattner DW, Makary MA, et al. Debridement and closed packing for the treatment of necrotizing pancreatitis. *Ann Surg* 1998;228:676–684.
26. Tsiotos GG, Luque-de Leon E, Soreide JA, et al. Management of necrotizing pancreatitis by repeated operative necrosectomy using a zipper technique. *Am J Surg* 1998;175:91–98.
27. Broome AH, Eisen GM, Harland RC, et al. Quality of life after treatment for pancreatitis. *Ann Surg* 1996;223:665–672.
28. Tsiotos GG, Smith CD, Sarr MG. Incidence and management of pancreatic and enteric fistulas after surgical management of severe necrotizing pancreatitis. *Arch Surg* 1995;130:48–52.
29. Bradley EL. Long-term results of pancreaticojejunostomy in patients with chronic pancreatitis. *Am J Surg* 1987;153:207–213.
30. Ihse I, Borch K, Larsson J. Chronic pancreatitis: results of operation for relief of pain. *World J Surg* 1990;14:53–58.
31. Prinz RA, Greelee HB. Pancreatic duct drainage in 100 patients with chronic pancreatitis. *Ann Surg* 1981;194:313–320.
32. Prinz RA, Aranha GV, Greenlee HB. Redrainage of the pancreatic duct in chronic pancreatitis. *Am J Surg* 1986;151:150–156.
33. Taylor RH, Bagley FH, Braasch JW, et al. Ductal drainage or resection for chronic pancreatitis. *Am J Surg* 1981;141:28.
34. Nealon WH, Thompson JC. Progressive loss of pancreatic function in chronic pancreatitis is delayed by main duct decompression: a longitudinal prospective analysis of the modified Puestow procedure. *Ann Surg* 1993;217:458–468.
35. Yeo CJ, Cameron JL, Sohn TA, et al. Six hundred fifty consecutive pancreaticoduodenectomies in the 1990's: pathology, complications, outcomes. *Ann Surg* 1997;226:248–260.
36. Trede M, Schwall G, Saeger H-D. Survival after pancreaticoduodenectomy: 118 consecutive resections without a mortality. *Ann Surg* 1990; 211:447–458.
37. Cameron JL, Pitt HA, Yeo CJ, et al. One hundred and forty five consecutive pancreaticoduodenectomies without mortality. *Ann Surg* 1993;217: 430–438.
38. Birkmeyer JD, Siewers AE, Finlayson EV, et al. Hospital volume and surgical mortality in the United States. *New Engl J Med* 2002;346(15): 1128–1137.
39. Yeo CJ, Cameron JL, Lillemoe KD, et al. Does prophylactic octreotide decrease the rates of pancreatic fistula and other complications after pancreaticoduodenectomy? Results of a prospective randomized placebo-controlled trial. *Ann Surg* 2000;232:419–429.
40. Bassi C, Dervenis C, Butturini G, et al. Post-operative pancreatic fistula: An International Study Group (ISGPF) definition. *Surgery* 2005;138: 8–13.
41. Balcom JH, Rattner DW, Warshaw AL, et al. Ten-year experience with 733 pancreatic resections. *Arch Surg* 2001;136:391–398.
42. Gouma DJ, van Geenen RCI, van Gulik TM, et al. Rates of complications and death after pancreaticoduodenectomy: risk factors and the impact of hospital volume. *Ann Surg* 2000;232:786–795.
43. Sohn TA, Yeo CJ, Cameron JL. Resected adenocarcinoma of the pancreas- 616 patients: results, outcomes, and prognostic indicators. *J Gastrointest Surg* 2000;4:567–579.
44. Bartoli FG, Arnone GB, Ravera G, et al. Pancreatic fistula and relative mortality in malignant disease after pancreaticoduodenectomy. Review and statistical meta-analysis regarding 15 years of literature. *Anticancer Res* 1991;11:1831–1848.
45. Tran K, van Eijck C, Di Carlo V, et al. Occlusion of the pancreatic duct versus pancreaticoduodenectomy: a prospective randomized trial. *Ann Surg* 2002;236:422–428.
46. Chou FF, Sheen-Chen SM, Chen YS, et al. Postoperative morbidity and mortality of pancreaticoduodenectomy for periampullary cancer. *Eur J Surg* 1996;162:477–481.
47. Winter JM, Cameron JL, Campbell KA, et al. Does pancreatic duct stenting decrease the rate of pancreatic fistula following pancreaticoduodenectomy? Results of a prospective randomized trial. *J Gastrointest Surg* 2006;10:1280–1290.
48. Poon RTP, Fan ST, Lo CM, et al. External drainage of pancreatic duct with stent to reduce leakage rate of pancreatectomy after pancreaticoduodenectomy: a prospective randomized trial. *Ann Surg* 2007;246: 425–435.
49. Yeo CJ, Cameron JL, Maher MM, et al. A prospective randomized trial of pancreatico-gastrostomy and pancreatico-jejunostomy after pancreaticoduodenectomy. *Ann Surg* 1995;225:580–588.
50. Buchler M, Friess H, Klempa I, et al. Role of octreotide in the prevention of postoperative complications following pancreatic resection. *Am J Surg* 1992;163:125–130.
51. Pederzoli P, Bassi C, Falconi M, et al. Efficacy of octreotide in the prevention of complications following pancreatic resection: Italian Study Group. *Br J Surg* 1994;81:265–269.
52. Montorsi M, Zago M, Mosca F, et al. Efficacy of octreotide in the prevention of pancreatic fistula after elective pancreatic resections: a prospective, controlled, randomized clinical trial. *Surgery* 1995;117:26–31.
53. Friess H, Beger HG, Sulkowski U, et al. Randomized controlled multicentre study of the prevention of complications by octreotide in patients undergoing surgery for chronic pancreatitis. *Br J Surg* 1995;82:1270–1273.
54. Rosenberg L, MacNeil P, Turcotte L. Economic evaluation of the use of octreotide for prevention of complications following pancreatic resection. *J Gastrointest Surg* 1999;3:225–232.
55. Yeo CJ. Does prophylactic octreotide benefit patients undergoing elective pancreatic resection? *J Gastrointest Surg* 1999;3:223–224.
56. Lowy AM, Lee JE, Pisters PWT, et al. Prospective randomized trial of octreotide to prevent pancreatic fistula after pancreaticoduodenectomy for malignant disease. *Ann Surg* 1997;226:632–641.
57. Miedema BW, Sarr MG, Van Heerden JA, et al. Complications following pancreaticoduodenectomy. Current management. *Arch Surg* 1992; 127:945–949.
58. Yeo CJ, Barry MK, Sauter PK, et al. Erythromycin accelerates gastric emptying after pancreaticoduodenectomy. A prospective randomized placebo-controlled trial. *Ann Surg* 1993;218:229–238.
59. Spanknebel K, Conlon K. Advances in the surgical management of pancreatic cancer. *Cancer J* 2001;7:312–323.
60. Sohn TA, Yeo CJ, Cameron JL, et al. Do preoperative biliary stents increase postpancreaticoduodenectomy complications? *J Gastrointest Surg* 2000;4:258–268.
61. Pisters PW, Hudec WA, Hess KR, et al. Effect of preoperative biliary decompression on pancreaticoduodenectomy-associated mortality in 300 consecutive patients. *Ann Surg* 2001;234:47–55.
62. Bakkevold KE, Kambestad B. Morbidity and mortality after radical and palliative pancreatic cancer surgery. Risk factors influencing short-term results. *Ann Surg* 1993;217(4):356–368.
63. Hodul P, Creech S, Pickleman J, et al. The effect of preoperative biliary stenting on postoperative complications after pancreaticoduodenectomy. *Am J Surg* 2003;186:420–425.
64. Braasch JW, Gray BN. Considerations that lower pancreaticoduodenectomy mortality. *Am J Surg* 1977;133:480–484.
65. Andren-Sandberg A, Ihse I. Factors influencing survival after total pancreatectomy in patients with pancreatic cancer. *Ann Surg* 1983;198: 605–610.
66. Bottger TC, Junginger T. Factors influencing morbidity and mortality after pancreaticoduodenectomy: critical analysis of 221 resections. *World J Surg* 1999;23:164–171.
67. Povoski SP, Karpeh MS, Conlon KC, et al. Preoperative biliary drainage: impact on intraoperative bile cultures and infectious morbidity and mortality after pancreaticoduodenectomy. *J Gastrointest Surg* 1999;3: 496–505.

68. Pitt HA, Gomes AS, Lois JF, et al. Does preoperative percutaneous biliary drainage reduce operative risk or increase hospital cost? *Ann Surg* 1985;201:545–553.
69. Trede M, Schwall G. The complications of pancreatectomy. *Ann Surg* 1988;207:39–47.
70. Heslin MJ, Brooks AD, Hochwald SN, et al. A preoperative biliary stent is associated with increased complications after pancreatoduodenectomy. *Arch Surg* 1998;133:149–154.
71. Ceuterick M, Gelin M, Rickaert F, et al. Pancreaticoduodenal resection for pancreatic or periampullary tumors- a ten year experience. *Hepatogastroenterology* 1989;36:467–473.
72. Whipple A. Present day surgery of the pancreas. *N Engl J Med* 1942;226: 515–518.
73. Seiler CA, Wagner M, Sadowski C, et al. Randomized prospective trial of pylorus-preserving vs. classic duodenopancreatectomy (Whipple procedure): initial clinical results. *J Gastrointest Surg* 2000;4:443–452.
74. Mosca F, Giulianotti PC, Balestracci T, et al. Long-term survival in pancreatic cancer: pylorus preserving versus Whipple pancreaticoduodenectomy. *Surgery* 1997;122:553–566.
75. Patel AG, Toyama MT, Kusske AM, et al. Pylorus-preserving Whipple resection for pancreatic cancer: is it any better? *Arch Surg* 1995;130:838–843.
76. Crist DW, Sitzmann JV, Cameron JL. Improved hospital morbidity, mortality, and survival after the Whipple procedure. *Ann Surg* 1987;206: 358–365.
77. van Berge Henegouwen MI, van Gulik TM, DeWit LT, et al. Delayed gastric emptying after standard pancreaticoduodenectomy versus pylorus-preserving pancreaticoduodenectomy: an analysis of 200 consecutive patients. *J Am Coll Surg* 1997;185:373–379.
78. Kooby DA, Gillespie T, Bentrem D, et al. Left-sided pancreatectomy: a multicenter comparison of laparoscopic and open approaches. *Ann Surg* 2008;248:438–446.
79. Bilimoria MM, Cormier JN, Mun JE, et al. Pancreatic leak after left pancreatectomy following main pancreatic duct ligation. *Br J Surg* 2003;90: 190–196.
80. Fahy BN, Frey CF, Ho HS, et al. Morbidity, mortality, and technical factors of distal pancreatectomy. *Am J Surg* 2002;183:237–241.
81. Lillemoe KD, Kaushal S, Cameron JL, et al. Distal pancreatectomy: indications and outcomes in 235 patients. *Ann Surg* 1999;229: 693–700.
82. Cogbill TH, Moore EE, Morris JA, et al. Distal pancreatectomy for trauma: a multicenter experience. *J Trauma* 1991;31:1600–1606.
83. Sohn TA, Campbell KA, Pitt HA, et al. Quality of life and long-term survival after surgery for chronic pancreatitis. *J Gastrointest Surg* 2000; 4:355–365.
84. Hutchins RR, Hart RS, Pacifico M, et al. Long-term results of distal pancreatectomy for chronic pancreatitis in 90 patients. *Ann Surg* 2002;236: 612–618.
85. Slezak LA, Anderson DK. Pancreatic resection: effects on glucose metabolism. *World J Surg* 2001;25:452–460.
86. Karpoff HM, Klimstra DS, Brennan MF, et al. Results of total pancreatectomy for adenocarcinoma of the pancreas. *Arch Surg* 2001;136:44–47.
87. Fleming WR, Williamson RC. Role of total pancreatectomy in the treatment of patients with end-stage chronic pancreatitis. *Br J Surg* 1995;82: 1409–1412.
88. Dresler CM, Fortner JG, McDermott K, et al. Metabolic consequences of (regional) total pancreatectomy. *Ann Surg* 1991;214:131–140.
89. Assan R, Alexandre JH, Tiengo A, et al. Survival and rehabilitation after total pancreatectomy: a follow-up of 36 patients. *Diabete Metab* 1985;11: 303–309.
90. Heidt DG, Burant C, Simeone DM. Total pancreatectomy: indications, operative technique, and post-operative sequelae. *J Gastrointest Surg* 2007;11:209–216.
91. Rilo R, Ahmad SA, D'Alessio SA, et al. Total pancreatectomy and autologous islet transplantation a means to treat severe chronic pancreatitis. *J Gastrointest Surg* 2003;7:978–989.
92. Gruessner RW, Sutherland DE, Dunn DL, et al. Transplant options for patients undergoing total pancreatectomy for chronic pancreatitis. *J Am Coll Surg* 2004;198:559–567.

CHAPTER

37

Complications of Intestinal Surgery: Small Bowel

Arden M. Morris

The small bowel integrates digestive and barrier functions resulting in a metabolic engine that is the body's largest barrier to the outside world. Yet it remains remarkably resistant to infection, toxins, and neoplasm growth. Digestive functions—such as secretion of hormones, enzymes, and electrolytes into the bowel lumen—confer resistance to infection and injury. Physical, immunologic, and physiologic barriers provide key defenses against infection and malignant transformation of cells. In fact, although it comprises 90% of the entire gastrointestinal surface area, the small intestine produces fewer than 5% of gut tumors (1). Thus, the need for operative intervention for intestinal failure is frequently the result of a previous operation rather than treatment of an intrinsic small bowel issue.

INTESTINAL FAILURE

Intestinal failure is "the reduction in functioning gut mass below the amount necessary for adequate digestion and absorption of food" (2). This simple definition focuses on the functional role of the intestine, clarifying the pathophysiology of numerous possible underlying mechanisms of failure, resulting from even more numerous possible disease states (Table 37.1).

Subacute or chronic failure results in slowly escalating debilitation due to the associated malnutrition. Wound healing slows and stops without adequate amino acid, carbohydrate, fat, and vitamin and mineral substrates. Immunity is broadly suppressed, including neutrophil, T-cell, and antibody function. Longer-term markers like serum albumin are more useful for prognostication, while shorter-term markers such as prealbumin or retinol-binding protein can assist with day-to-day assessment of nutritional repletion. Patients with unintentional weight loss of more than 10% to 15% of baseline body weight or with a serum albumin level <3.0 are severely malnourished. Prior to elective surgery, the most severely malnourished patients may benefit from preoperative parenteral nutritional supplementation to reduce the perioperative risk of infection or nonhealing (3,4).

Medical therapy for intestinal failure aims to reduce the severity of malnutrition, avoid complications, and maximize quality of life (5). Prevention of bowel edema due to excessive saline administration, limitation of intestinal electrolyte losses due to ingestion of hypotonic fluids, and monitoring serum and urine electrolytes frequently are important steps in management. An elemental or low residue diet and pharmacological agents to slow intestinal transit time can be helpful. The value of exogenous trophic factors has not yet been adequately defined in human studies (6).

If nonoperative management fails, operative intervention can sometimes re-establish nutritional function and relieve underlying pathology (Table 37.2). Restoration of the intestine's nutritional role may be an anatomic, physiologic, or combined effort. For example, placement of a colon interposition graft to interrupt peristalsis for patients with rapid small bowel transit uses an anatomic alteration to correct a physiologic problem. Surgical tradition holds that avoidable perioperative complications arise as a result of technical or, more commonly, judgment errors. Errors are prevented or limited by clear goals, careful technique, and appropriate alternative strategies. In addition, many less controllable factors can have an impact on short- and long-term complications, such as age, functional status, underlying disease, and severity of illness. Therefore, consideration of specific preoperative and intraoperative measures to reduce risk is critical.

Previous surgical treatment plays a major role in the development of intestinal failure. In an extensive review of the literature, Tera and Aberg (7) determined that 1.6% of abdominal operations result in a reoperation and 34% to 43% of reoperations result in mortality, a number confirmed by more recent studies (8–11). The two most common reasons for return to the operating room are peritonitis (32% of reoperative cases) and ileus or obstruction (25% of cases). Other series (12,13) determined that adhesions after a previous operation accounted for more than half of episodes of small bowel obstruction; however, most episodes were successfully managed with nasogastric tube decompression. Thirteen percent to 38% of obstructed patients ultimately returned to the operating room after 6 to 8 days of unsuccessful decompression, and risk increased with each subsequent operation.

PREOPERATIVE RISK MODIFICATION

Prudent planning for operation must include maximizing preoperative care designed to prevent complications. For

Arden M. Morris: Associate Professor of Surgery Chief, Colon and Rectal Surgery University of Michigan

Table **37.1** **Underlying etiologies of intestinal failure**

Etiology of Failure	Mechanism	Specific Disease Examples
Mechanical obstruction		
	Extrinsic compression	Peritoneal adhesions, incarcerated hernia, extra-luminal mass
	Stricture	Crohn's disease, ischemia
	Torsion	Postoperative, congenital malrotation
	Obstruction	Tumor, stool, gallstone, bezoar
Dysmotility		
	Ileus	Postoperative, Narcotic use, Inflammation, Distal obstruction
	Neuromuscular	Acquired or congenital visceral myopathy, enteric neuropathy, disorder
Hemorrhage		
	Vascular	Arteriovenous malformations, vascular-enteric fistula formation, ulceration
	Tumor erosion	Adenocarcinoma, carcinoid, lymphoma, gastrointestinal stromal tumor
	Other erosion	Meckel's diverticulum
Necrosis		
	Chronic ischemia	Atherosclerotic disease, radiation enteritis
	Acute ischemia	Thromboembolic disease, mesenteric torsion
Leak of intestinal contents (fistula, abscess, peritonitis)		
	Iatrogenic injury	Unrecognized intraoperative injury, technical failure during anastomosis, ischemia
	Anastomotic breakdown	Inflammation, infection, malnutrition, immunosuppression
	Spontaneous	Ischemia, Crohn's disease, postradiation, distal obstruction, tumor erosion, ischemia, foreign body
Nutritional deficits		
	Malabsorption	Previous ileal resection, Crohn's disease, radiation enteritis, sprue, infectious diarrhea, bacterial overgrowth
	Short bowel syndrome	Postoperative, Crohn's disease, radiation enteritis, ischemic bowel

example, preoperative optimization of respiratory and hemodynamic parameters may limit perioperative morbidity and mortality. In a randomized trial of normal preparation versus preoperative breathing exercises among upper abdominal surgery patients at significant risk, postoperative pulmonary complication rate decreased from 60% to 19% (14). Subsequent work demonstrated even better results among abdominal surgery patients with preoperative incentive spirometry training and chest physiotherapy (15). By contrast, a recent meta-analysis did not demonstrate significantly improved prevention of postoperative pulmonary complications with the use of incentive spirometry (16). These data underscore the urgent need for well-designed clinical trials—and we continue to recommend preoperative incentive spirometry training with consideration for preoperative physiotherapy among high-risk abdominal surgery patients.

Table **37.2** **Therapeutic goals of intestinal surgery**

Restore nutritional role of small bowel
Adequate length
Adequate lumen
Adequate absorption
Relieve pathology
Obstruction
Bleeding
Infection
Ischemia
Prevent postoperative complications
Sepsis
Obstruction

Timely intervention for previously unrecognized cardiac arrhythmias or poorly controlled hypertension has been shown to reduce perioperative risk of circulatory embarrassment (17,18). A recent meta-analysis demonstrated significant mortality reduction among high-risk patients who received early optimization of hemodynamic parameters and oxygen delivery, but no such benefit after organ failure had occurred (19).

Recognition of barriers to healing is another part of the preoperative risk management process. The association between severe malnutrition and increased risk for postoperative complications or death are well established (Table 37.3) (20,21). The severely nutritionally depleted patient can benefit substantially from 7 to 10 days of preoperative hyperalimentation. Comorbid diseases associated with impaired microcirculation, such as renal failure and diabetes, also inhibit mechanisms of healing and merit scrupulous preoperative medical control. Glucocorticoids interfere with virtually every step in the phases of wound healing. A multivariate analysis of a large retrospective cohort reported

Table 37.3 Impact of nutritional status on postoperative complications among intestinal failure patients

Degree of Malnutrition	Weight Loss Over 3 Months (%)	Serum Albumin	Postoperative Complication Risk (%)
Mild	5–10	2.8–3.4	20–30
Moderate	10–20	2.1–2.7	30–45
Severe	20	≤2.0	40–60

that long-term steroid use was the only variable associated with a significantly higher rate of serious complications after anastomosis among Crohn's patients (22). Cumulative data suggest retinoids and transforming growth factor beta counter the steroid effect on collagen metabolism, (23–25) but, in the absence of adequate translational studies, neither has been incorporated effectively into clinical practice. There has been considerable debate regarding the operative risk associated with other immuno-suppressive medications such as infliximab, a recombinant anti-TNF alpha antibody. An early prospective study funded by the manufacturer indicated minimal operative risks beyond those already faced by Crohn's disease patients (26). A larger retrospective study demonstrated significantly increased risk of postoperative sepsis, abscess, and readmissions in Crohn's patients treated with infliximab within 3 months prior to operation, as compared with infliximab naïve patients (27). These results are in contrast to another retrospective study (28). Given the potential for selection bias among even carefully conducted retrospective studies, prospective data would be especially useful to address the question of best practice with regard to avoiding infliximab preoperatively.

INTRAOPERATIVE TECHNICAL ISSUES

Evidence-based recommendations for intraoperative technique to prevent postoperative complications largely rest upon Halsted's early tenets to handle tissue gently, employ aseptic technique, avoid closing under tension, and close wounds completely whenever possible. Limiting intra-abdominal dissection to that required for adequate exposure and handling tissue gently will help to prevent serosal injury and limit blood loss, thereby restricting adhesion formation (29,30). Massive adhesions and herniations can lead to loss of abdominal domain, a vexing intraoperative problem that may require use of mesh or relaxing incisions to close without tension.

Exploration

During exploratory laparotomy of a nonhostile abdomen, initial evaluation of the small bowel consists of examination from the ligament of Treitz to the cecum. Serosal injuries should be repaired when identified. Other incidental lesions may be addressed after correcting the preoperative issue. Incidentally identified tumors should be excised. Frozen section examination can be useful to determine benign versus malignant features and to ascertain clear margins. Meckel's diverticula should be excised except in moribund patients, according to long-term population-based data from the Mayo clinic (31). Anecdotally, incidental appendectomy has fallen into disfavor. While cumulative data suggest prohibitive risk among patients who are more than 50 years old, immunosuppressed, medically unstable, having prosthetic material or previous diagnosis of Crohn's disease, many studies support performing incidental appendectomy on patients less than 30 years old (32–35). Resisting the urge to "tidy up" the abdomen is generally appropriate, limiting the operation to the problem at hand.

Anastomosis

Much has been written and little resolved about anastomotic technique; stapled versus sutured, single layer versus double layer, type of suture material, and impact of diversion are all controversies still under discussion. The goal of enteric anastomosis is to prevent leakage, promote healing, preserve bowel length, and prevent stricture formation. An effective anastomosis requires adequate mobilization, perfusion, apposition, and inversion of the mucosal edges into the bowel lumen. Healing depends on approximation of the collagen-containing submucosal layer. Inadequate perfusion or tension across the anastomosis may cause early leakage or late stricture formation.

Anastomotic leakage is a potentially disastrous complication, running the gamut from a contained self-limited event to sepsis and abdominal catastrophe (9–11). Covering the anastomosis with omentum may contribute to prevention or containment of leakage. Investigations into the frequency of leakage after stapled versus sewn anastomoses are contradictory; available data support the superiority of each and of neither (36,37). Current American College of Surgeons-sponsored efforts to record, analyze, and improve postoperative outcomes may shed further light on these difficult analyses. It is also plausible, however, that national registries may be limited by inadequate data capture in the traditional 30-day postoperative window. An important recent study of anastomotic leaks revealed that 12% were diagnosed after the 30(th) postoperative day and 42% were diagnosed only after readmission to the hospital (38).

Anastomotic strictures form as a result of ischemia, tension, or infection due to previous anastomotic failure. Technical choices are fairly forgiving but may also play a role. In a randomized controlled trial of esophagogastrostomy anastomoses, a double-layer closure led to significantly more stricture formation than single layer (39). Much of the remaining research addressing anastomosis is limited to the colon and rectal literature, which has limited application to small bowel issues. The principles of a safe anastomosis can be observed using a variety of techniques.

Mesenteric defects

Literature addressing closure of mesenteric defects is also scarce. Customarily, an absorbable suture incorporating only the peritoneal leaves of divided mesentery is run from the apex of the defect toward the bowel. With the advent of laparoscopic colon resection, the utility of mesenteric closure has been questioned and the technique simply abandoned by some. However, many surgeons elect to close defects small enough to potentially incarcerate bowel.

Adhesion prevention

Placement of a bioresorbable adhesion barrier over abdominal contents prior to anterior wall closure can limit or even prevent postoperative abdominal wall adhesion formation (40–42). This is an especially useful exercise for patients with temporary ileostomy or other anticipated future laparotomy. Wrapping a fresh anastomosis in such an adhesion barrier results in a higher leak rate and is discouraged (43). Additionally, several case report studies describe a rare, intense, nonseptic peritonitis reaction following application of Seprafilm (44–46). This manifests as a high fever with severe diffuse abdominal pain in the early postoperative period, necessitating return to the operating room and most frequently resulting in a negative exploratory laparotomy. The etiology of this process remains unclear but anecdotally it arises most commonly among Crohn's disease patients. No data are available from the manufacturer with regard to this phenomenon.

Ileus

Postoperative ileus is a predictable but poorly understood phenomenon, which generally lasts 3 to 5 days and is managed expectantly. A recent review (47) has identified laparoscopy, thoracic epidural anesthesia, avoidance of opioids, and early feeding as potential interventions to limit ileus duration. Nasogastric decompression does not reduce ileus duration. Effectiveness of the selective opioid antagonist alvimopan remains uncertain but will likely be clarified with larger multi-center trials. If the ileus is prolonged more than 7 days in a patient with previously normal motility, an early mechanical obstruction or possible enteric leak should be considered (48–50). Timing of reoperation becomes especially relevant during the 2 to 6 week postoperative window, when extensive adhesions and inflammation create a significant technical challenge increasing the risk of bleeding, fistula, abscess, and abdominal sepsis (8).

SPECIFIC INTESTINAL DISORDERS REQUIRING INTERVENTION

Although the potential complications of intestinal surgery are myriad, they tend to be closely related and even overlapping (Fig. 37.1). Many underlying diseases predispose to particular postoperative issues. This section examines the complications that arise most frequently after operative intervention for specific underlying diseases or conditions.

Short bowel syndrome

Short bowel syndrome describes a constellation of symptoms including malnutrition, weight loss, steatorrhea, and diarrhea, resulting from inadequate absorptive gut surface area. The disorder may follow massive intestinal resection for ischemia, infection, mesenteric desmoid tumors, or other diseases. Short bowel syndrome may be the cumulative effect of sequential excisions or the functional result of proximal fistula formation. Although individual variation and adaptation can occur, most patients with less than 100 cm total bowel or less than 150 cm without the ileocecal valve will not survive with enteric nutrition alone.

In addition to the expected complications of malnutrition, other associated complications include cholelithiasis, nephrolithiasis, and gastric hypersecretion. Symptomatic cholelithiasis develops in 20% to 40% of patients, and is most frequent in those dependent on parenteral nutrition. In reviews of the topic, Thompson recommends considering

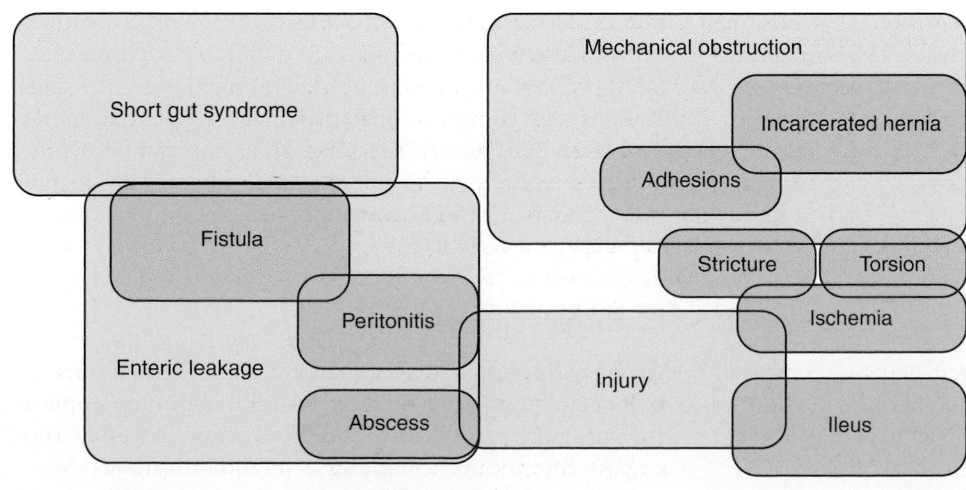

FIGURE 37.1. Schematic association of common postoperative complications.

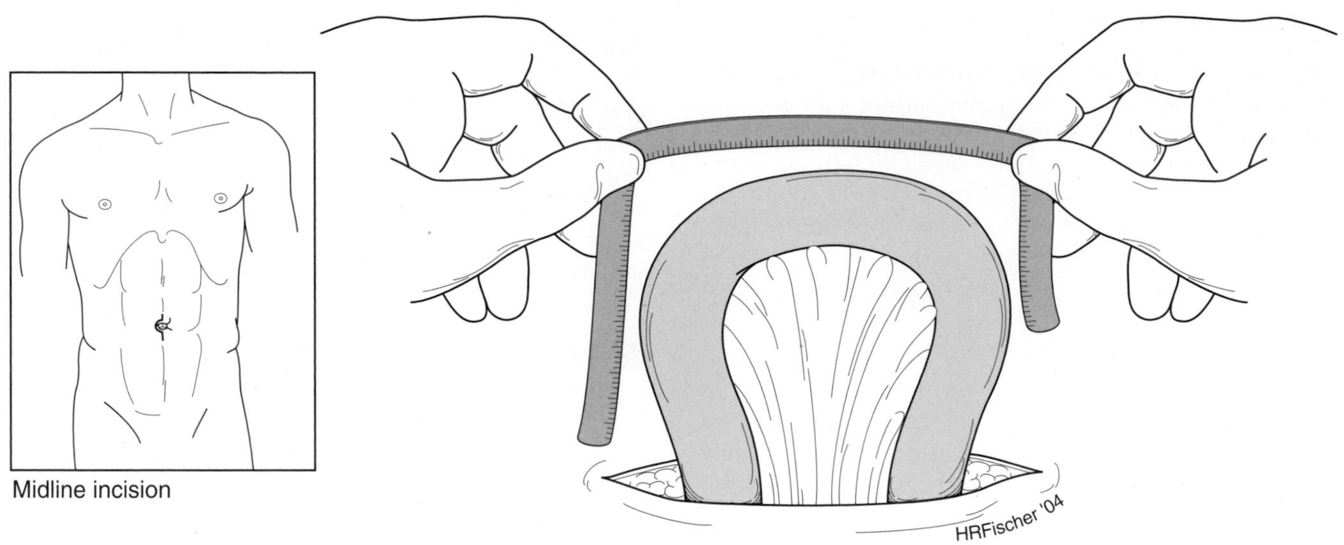

FIGURE 37.2. Measuring the small bowel (short gut).

prophylactic gall bladder excision prior to the development of hepatic changes, dense adhesion formation, and medical complications of malnutrition (51,52). Nephrolithiasis arises in about 25% of patients with some retained colon, due to increased colonic oxalate absorption and excretion through the urinary system. Calcium oxalate stone formation may be prevented by careful diet management and cholesterol binding medication (53). Gastric hypersecretion after massive bowel resection is poorly understood and usually temporary, but can lead to peptic ulcer disease requiring use of proton pump inhibitors (54).

Efforts to prevent and manage short bowel syndrome have advanced substantially in the past two decades. Prevention is the foremost treatment strategy, especially when future abdominal operations are anticipated. In cases of viable but obstructed bowel, limiting the extent of resection and performing stricturoplasty have become standards of care. Measurement of remaining bowel is easily performed before closing the abdomen (Fig. 37.2), and facilitates diagnosis of related disorders and planning of future therapy.

Effective medical treatment for short bowel syndrome improves absorption of nutrients and slows intestinal transit time. Postoperative mucosal hyperplasia occurs over a period of 6 to 12 months. Early reports suggested that glutamine and growth hormones enhance mucosal adaptation, but these data have not been replicated in well-designed subsequent studies (55–57). An elemental, high-carbohydrate, low-fat diet may have a trophic effect and improve absorption (56). Agents that slow bowel transit are staples of therapy. Loperamide decreases intestinal motility and secretion and has been shown to increase sphincter pressure; (58). In the sufficiently impaired patient, codeine or tincture of opium may be necessary. Octreotide may prove useful if transit is too rapid or the intestine is too short for absorption of oral antisecretory medication.

Operative treatment of short bowel syndrome consists of procedures to relieve obstruction, increase bowel surface area, and slow transit time. Relief of obstruction is usually achieved by stricturoplasty and is most relevant in the Crohn's disease patient. The most useful method for increasing the absorptive surface is reconstruction of defunctionalized bowel. Although reapproximation of the small intestine and colon increases surface area and provides a trophic effect, it can also exacerbate diarrhea and stone formation. Tapering and lengthening procedures improve absorption and motility, and have been most extensively used in pediatric patients (59,60). Transit slowing procedures have been less successful. Creation of an antiperistaltic segment has had variable efficacy. Interposition of a colonic segment has shown promising results in some reports but led to obstruction and failure in others (51,52,61).

Refractory short bowel disease, whether anatomic or physiologic, requires nutritional support and consideration of transplantation (62). Hyperalimentation has become increasingly sophisticated since its introduction in 1968, but is associated with many inherent potential complications. These will be addressed in detail in a separate chapter. For patients in whom hyperalimentation has been fraught with complications, intestinal transplantation may be an option. Several studies now indicate outcomes approximating those of lifelong total parenteral nutrition, if the transplant can be accomplished prior to the onset of hepatic cirrhosis (63–65).

Crohn's disease

Crohn's disease is a chronic, segmental, transmural, T helper cell-mediated disease that can arise anywhere in the gastrointestinal tract and various extraintestinal organs. Symptomatic hallmarks include diarrhea, weight loss, and abdominal pain. Seventy percent of Crohn's patients overall and 84% of those with ileocecal disease require surgical intervention at some time (66). Solid data is limited regarding the impact of preoperative immunosuppressive medication on postoperative complication rates among Crohn's patients. Steroid use has been associated with greater risk in some large retrospective series (22,67) but not others (68,69). Preoperative treatment with nonsteroid immunosuppressives has actually been associated with better postoperative outcomes (26,69).

Acute or chronic obstruction, fistula or abscess formation, and complications of previous operations are the most common indications for operation. Short bowel syndrome, fistula formation, and development of an abdomen so rife with adhesions that it must be considered frankly hostile are among the many potential complications of operating in this setting.

Malabsorption

Malabsorption and diarrhea, intimately related manifestations of Crohn's disease, may result in a functional short bowel syndrome but are also caused by an anatomically short gut due to multiple resections. Micronutrient malnutrition depends on the anatomic site and length of bowel resection. Cyanocobalamin (vitamin B12) is the most common deficiency and occurs predictably after resection of 50 to 60 cm of terminal ileum. Folate deficiency results from resection or disease of the proximal jejunum. Diminished absorption of fat soluble vitamins (A, D, E, and K) may occur with reduced absorption of bile salts, contributing to a host of sequelae including calcium deficiency, osteoporosis, bleeding diatheses, and others.

Iatrogenic short bowel syndrome is one of the most notorious and challenging complications of operating for Crohn's disease. Short bowel syndrome is of particular concern among Crohn's patients due to their common presentation with terminal ileal disease, necessitating ileocecal valve resection. Patients are subject to dehydration, exacerbation of diarrhea, and inadequate nutrition for healing and health maintenance. Stricturoplasty for preserving bowel length in Crohn's disease patients is essential to long-term outcome and is reviewed in detail below.

Fistula Formation

Spontaneous intra-abdominal abscesses and fistulae form in 20% to 40% of Crohn's patients and are a fundamental characteristic of the disease. Postoperative fistula formation occurs in about 10% to 15% of patients in the 30-day perioperative period, (22,67) but in more than 20% over the ensuing 5 years (70). Either may be identified preoperatively based on symptoms and radiologic studies, or identified incidentally while examining the bowel during laparotomy. Appropriate therapy is based on the clinical situation. Lichtenstein's review of medical therapy reports encouraging early results with use of infliximab, but acknowledges frequent need for surgical intervention (71). Treatment of symptomatic fistulae includes resection of the fistulizing bowel and tract, with simple closure of the involved nondiseased viscus. No intervention is warranted for spontaneous, asymptomatic enteroenteric fistula formation (72).

Management of an enterocutaneous fistula is based on symptoms, duration, and, most importantly, output (Table 37.4). Preliminary therapeutic goals are treatment of sepsis, skin protection, accurate output measurement, and ascertainment of adequate nutrition. Spontaneous closure is possible depending primarily on the cause, location, related

Table 37.4 Management of enterocutaneous fistulae

		Management		Likelihood of Spontaneous Resolution	Mortality (%)
	Quantity/24 hr	Early	Late		
Low output	<200 cc	Bowel rest, Nutrition repletion, Skin protection, Appropriate drainage	After 30–40 days: Consider curettage of tract, Instillation of noxious substance or fibrin glue, or Resection of tract with primary closure.	Moderate	5
Medium output	200–500 cc	Bowel rest, TPN, Skin or wound protection, Drainage of sepsis	After 40–90 days or resolution of sepsis: Consider diversion with delayed repair versus resection.	Low	30
High output	>500 cc	Diversion, TPN, Skin or wound protection including consideration of vacuum-assisted closure, Drainage of sepsis	After 40–90 days or resolution of sepsis: Resection with temporary diversion	None	35–50

Table 37.5 Factors preventing spontaneous fistula closure
Sepsis
Distal obstruction
Radiation injury
Mucosal eversion at the skin level
High output/proximal fistula
Poor nutrition

infection, and nutritional status (Table 37.5). Proximal fistulae are associated with a higher daily output and nutritional deficiency (a functional short gut); distal fistulae are more likely to have a lower output and to heal spontaneously. Low to moderate output enterocutaneous fistulae (<200 cc/day and 200 to 400 cc/day, respectively) may be managed by observation, consideration of bowel rest, and parenteral nutrition if indicated. Some authors advocate curettage of the fistula tract, with or without fibrin glue insertion, or instillation of a noxious substance to facilitate scar formation, such as phenol. Reported outcomes are highly variable and largely based on small series with poorly quantified follow-up.

Obstruction

Intestinal obstruction in the Crohn's patient generally begins as an acute inflammatory process, best controlled by immunosuppressive medication if possible. If medical therapy is ineffective after 7 to 10 days or if acute obstruction repeatedly recurs, operative resection or bypass should be considered (73,74). There is no need to resect beyond macroscopically non-involved bowel, and a conservative approach to resection has decreased the incidence of postoperative short bowel syndrome in recent years. Recording the measured bowel length in the operative note will help with future treatment planning.

In contrast to the inflammation, adhesions, and abscesses observed in an acute Crohn's disease obstruction, chronic obstruction is primarily a fibrotic process. Strictures may be detected preoperatively based on computed tomography (CT) or small bowel contrast studies. Fibrosis may be identified during intraoperative bowel examination. At these sites, the small bowel appears and feels thickened and firm. Proximal bowel may appear distended with a smooth edematous or thickened wall. If access to the lumen has already been obtained, a balloon catheter distended to 2.5 cm may be pulled from the ligament of Treitz to the cecum to assess the luminal diameter. Sometimes even areas of intestine that appear normal externally will reveal a narrow lumen with extensive internal fibrotic strands.

Short strictures can be dilated with the catheter balloon. Longer strictures or those with extensive fibrosis are best managed by resection or stricturoplasty (Fig. 37.3). The judgment for resection versus preservation with stricturoplasty is based upon the length, proximity, and overall number of strictures, and on the length of remaining short bowel. The risk of stricture recurrence is high. At least 30% of Crohn's patients operated on for acute disease will require at least one additional operation for obstruction.

Recurrence

Perhaps the most common complication of operating for Crohn's disease is Crohn's recurrence. Asymptomatic endoscopic evidence of disease has been reported as early as 3 months postoperatively and in up to 75% of patients within the first postoperative year (75,76). Data regarding the influence of endoscopically identified disease on development of symptoms requiring operation are inconclusive. The extent of resection does not appear to have an impact on recurrence; while macroscopic disease should be removed, the presence of residual microscopic disease has no correlation with symptomatic recurrence. Inconsistent data have made clear identification of risk factors difficult (70,77) (Table 37.6). Prophylaxis against recurrence using medical therapy has been disappointing overall, but several well-designed studies of newer medication are currently underway.

Irradiated bowel

Many of the complications resulting from radiation injury to the small bowel are reminiscent of Crohn's disease,

Table 37.6 Risk factors for postoperative recurrence of Crohn's disease

	Factor	Impact on Clinical Recurrence
Patient-related factors	Age Gender Smoking	Mild increase in recurrence. No impact on recurrence. Independent risk factor for recurrence with odds ratio = 2–4 compared to nonsmokers. Odds are especially high among women who smoke.
Disease-related factors	Location of disease Duration of disease	Data have suggested increased recurrence with ileocolonic disease, but are inconclusive. No impact on recurrence.
Surgical factors	Margin	Histologic evidence of residual Crohn's has no impact on recurrence.
	Anastomotic method Diversion of the fecal stream	No impact on recurrence. Specific toxins or antigens the feces have not been identified, but lack of diversion and reversal of diversion appear associated with higher recurrence rates.

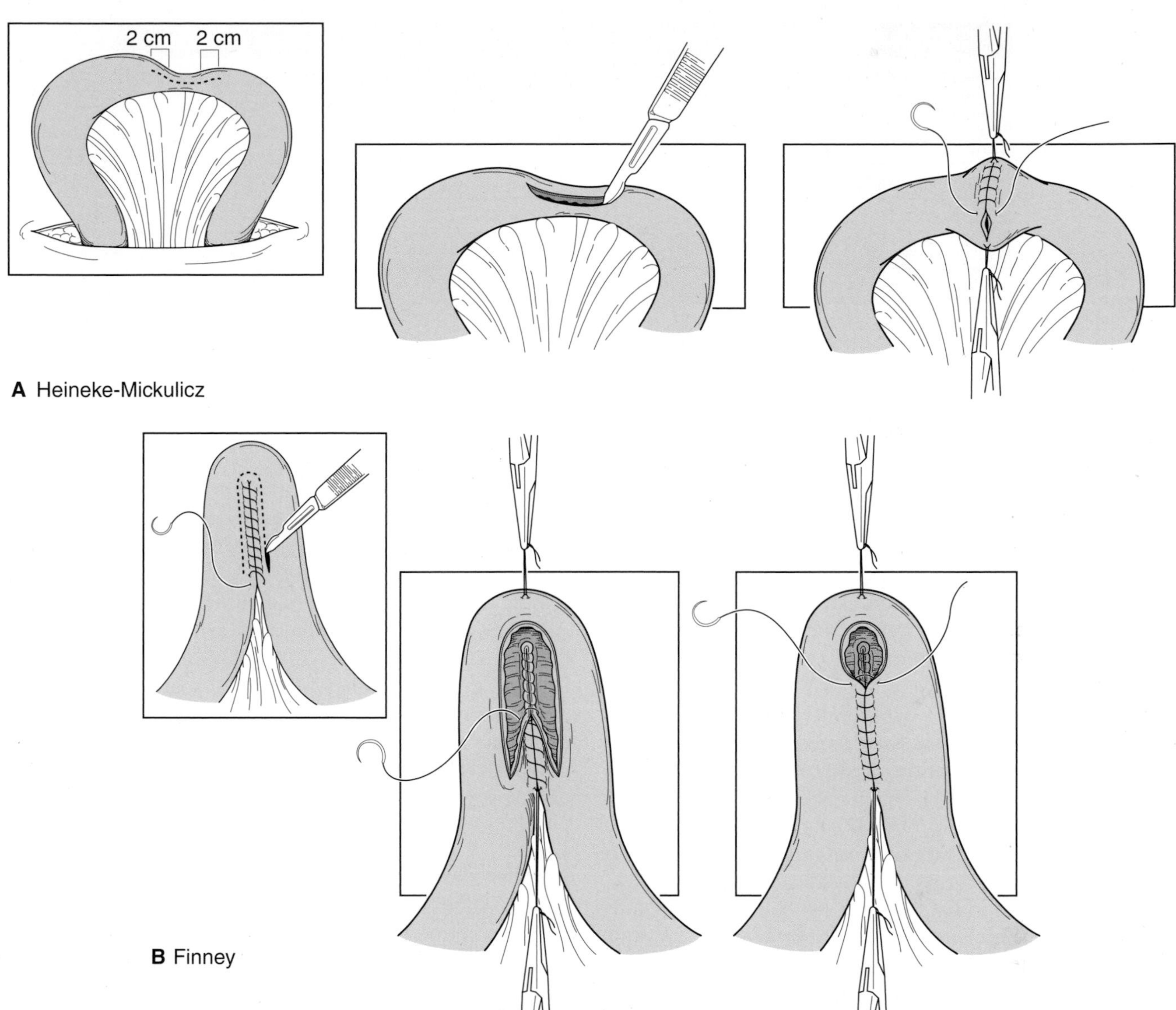

FIGURE 37.3. Bowel-preserving techniques for management of intestinal strictures. **A:** Heineke-Mickulicz stricturoplasty. A longitudinal incision is created sharply in the antimesenteric wall to 2 cm beyond the proximal and distal boundaries of the stricture. Two 3–0 silk stay sutures are placed on either side of the incision at the midpoint and retracted to reorient the incision to transverse. A single layer of full-thickness 3–0 silk interrupted sutures is placed to reapproximate the bowel edges in the new transverse orientation. **B:** Finney stricturoplasty. The Finney technique is advised for very long (≥25 cm) strictures of the small bowel. A longitudinal incision is created sharply in the antimesenteric wall. A stay suture placed at the apical midpoint is retraced to facilitate an upside-down U orientation. The inner edge is sutured to itself longitudinally from the luminal side to become a new posterior wall, with the previous distal-most bowel now abutting the proximal-most bowel. Similarly, the outer edge of the U is closed with simple interrupted full-thickness suture to become the new anterior wall.

such as stricture (obstruction), chronic bleeding, diarrhea, malabsorption, fistula formation, and abdominal pain. One may infer from the broad variety of interventions designed to slow motility and enhance absorption that surgical therapy has limited efficacy. However, a symptom–directed operation may be unavoidable and in this setting the extreme fragility of irradiated bowel must be respected. Resection and bypass are the foundations of surgical therapy. Complication rates are high, with anastomotic leakage rates up to nearly 60%, probably due to compromised perfusion (78). Although the value of resection versus bypass has been debated, bypass is associated with lower short-term complication and mortality rates (Table 37.7). Longer-term issues arising from bypass include ongoing fibrotic stricture formation, bacterial overgrowth, and issues of chronic mucosal damage (79). One small series reported encouraging results using stricturoplasty for long-segment radiation-associated obstruction (80). The importance of cautious consideration of operative goals and alternative strategies is widely recognized. Because radiation damage and obstructive symptoms can continue to manifest sometimes over decades, preserving bowel length even in the initial operation is recommended.

Table 37.7 Postoperative mortality after intervention for irradiated intestine

Source	Bypass *n*	Mortality (%)	Resection *n*	Mortality (%)
Joelsson and Raf (108)	—	—	19	16
Swan et al. (109)	28	7	17	53
Schmitt and Symmonds (110)	20	0	65	9
Lillemoe et al. (111)	11	0	6	17
Wobbes et al. (78)	20	10	7	57
Galland and Spencer (112)	2	0	18	44
Total	81	5	132	23

Intussusception

Intussusception, or telescoping of the bowel, is a rare event usually identified by a symptoms of bowel obstruction and a CT scan revealing an asymmetrical target sign (Fig. 37.4). In contrast to the pediatric patient, intussusception in the adult is more frequently due to an anatomic leadpoint abnormality, such as a tumor, thus traditionally treated by exploratory celiotomy and probable resection (81). Potential complications of such intervention are the usual postoperative ileus, bleeding, infection, damage to nearby structures, and adhesion formation. Delay in operation for incarcerated intussuscepted bowel can lead to ischemic necrosis. However, an interesting artifact of improved CT technology has led to a new possible complication of surgery for diagnosis of intussusception: unnecessary exploratory laparotomy. High resolution circular CT has become so rapid and images are so clear that bowel seen end-on may be captured during peristalsis, potentially resulting in a diagnosis of intussusception that does not actually require intervention. A large single institution review identified intussusception length of less than 3.5 cm to be a reliable predictor of a self-limiting process (82). Thus far, no prospective test of criteria for nonoperative intussusception has been performed.

Neoplasms of the small bowel

Tumors of the small bowel are rare and tend to be diagnosed at advanced stages due to nonspecific symptoms and difficult access. The most common presenting symptoms are pain, anemia, and weight loss. About half of tumors are found in the jejunum; the remainders are evenly split between the duodenum and the ileum. The resectability rate is high; however, 1- and 5-year survival rates are less encouraging (Table 37.8). In a 10-year series, Naef and others reported that 71% of all small bowel tumors were malignant and 62% had already metastasized at the time of diagnosis (83). Major postoperative complications occurred in 24% of patients; 4% required reoperation for anastomotic leaks, and 4% died.

Benign Neoplasms

Benign neoplasms of the small bowel are uncommon and typically discovered incidentally during laparotomy for another purpose. Although all may occur sporadically, many are associated with specific underlying diseases. For example, hamartomas are associated with Peutz-Jaegers syndrome and Cronkite-Canada syndrome; hemangiomas are associated with Osler-Weber-Rendu syndrome; and adenomas are associated with familial adenomatous polyposis syndrome. Resection of symptomatic tumors or tumors

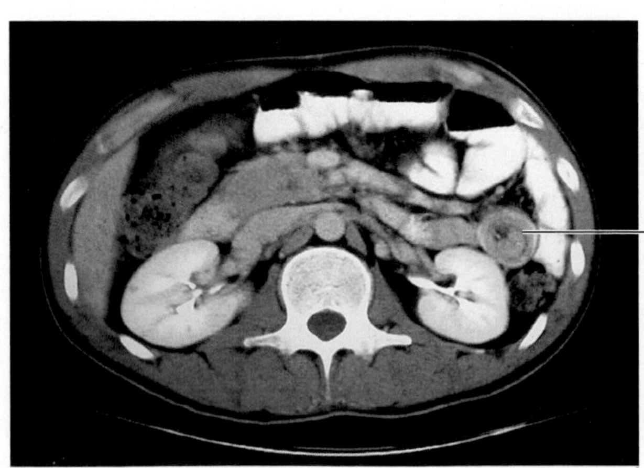

FIGURE 37.4. Computed tomography scan revealing an asymmetrical target sign previously considered the sine qua non of small bowel intussusception. This asymptomatic patient was referred for further evaluation of incidentally identified "intussusception."

Table **37.8** **Neoplasms of the small intestine: incidence and prognosis**

Tumor Type	Incidence	Examples of Associated Syndromes	1-Year Survival	5-Year Survival
Leiomyoma	75%	Spontaneous		
Adenoma	17%	Familial adenomatous polyposis		
Hamartoma	8%	Peutz-Jaegers, Cronkite-Canada		
Hemangioma	<1%	Osler-Webber-Rendu		
Lymphangioma	<1%	Spontaneous		
Other	<1%			
Total benign	12/54 (22%)		67%	50%
Adenocarcinoma	33%	Familial adenomatous polyposis		
Carcinoid tumor	17%	Multiple Endocrine Neoplasia I, Von Hippel-Lindau, Neurofibromatosis-1		
Gastrointestinal stromal tumor	17%	Spontaneous		
Non-Hodgkins Lymphoma	12%	Spontaneous		
Melanoma	9%	Dysplastic Naevus syndrome		
Other	12%			
Total malignant	42/54 (78%)		43%	21%

Adapted from Naef M, Buhlmann M, Baer HU. Small bowel tumors: diagnosis, therapy and prognostic factors. *Langenbecks Arch Surg* 1999;384(2):176–180.

which are dysplastic can be performed endoscopically, through an enterotomy which should then be closed transversely, or by limited local excision with end-to-end anastomosis. Resection of isolated asymptomatic benign lesions is reasonable in the setting of intra-abdominal examination. However, resection of numerous asymptomatic benign tumors is not warranted, due to the limited benefit and additive complication risk of each enterotomy.

Adenocarcinoma

Adenocarcinoma is the most common malignancy of the small intestine, accounting for about one-third of cases. Adenocarcinoma may occur sporadically or in association with a defined polyposis syndrome. Adenomas and adenocarcinomas of the small bowel are not associated with particularly high complication rates; however, lesions due to underlying Gardner's syndrome may have associated desmoid tissue. Desmoid tumors, a histologically benign but behaviorally malignant process, are a cause for grave concern. They are composed of fibroblasts growing in thick, white plaques which gradually surround, contract, and compress viscera and vessels. Desmoid tumors are akin to biological cement, inexorably filling the peritoneal cavities of these unfortunate patients. No real cure or prevention has been identified, although estrogen and nonsteroidal anti-inflammatory medications have shown limited efficacy. Operative intervention should be undertaken cautiously.

Carcinoid Tumor

Carcinoid tumors originate from neuroendocrine tissue and can be sporadic or associated with a number of family cancer syndromes. Patients typically present with complaints of vague abdominal pain and weight loss. Carcinoid tumors generally produce symptoms due to ischemia from mesenteric microvascular invasion, desmoplasia, and lymphedema from metastases to draining lymph nodes. Fibrosis can extend to the root of the mesenteric vessels creating a major technical challenge to resection, and potentially mandating bypass to avoid massive intestinal ischemia.

Carcinoid syndrome occurs in about 10% of patients with midgut carcinoids, and frequently indicates hepatic involvement. A carcinoid syndrome "attack" is mediated by neurotransmitters, hormones, and peptides released by the tumor cells. The humoral products stimulate vasomotor changes, bronchospasm, gastrointestinal hypermotility, and hypotension.

Carcinoid crisis is a potentially fatal carcinoid syndrome attack, with pronounced changes in blood pressure, diarrhea, confusion, bronchoconstriction, cardiac arrhythmia, and hyperthermia. Carcinoid crisis may occur spontaneously, during induction of anesthesia, while handling tumor in the operating room, or during hepatic arterial embolization or chemotherapy treatment. Octreotide, and histamine blockers as well as supportive care must be administered immediately.

Gastrointestinal Stromal Tumor

Gastrointestinal stromal tumors (GISTs) have captured scientific and clinical attention in recent years due to major advances in understanding of pathophysiology and treatment. These tumors were often miscategorized as sarcomas previously, but now are believed to derive from the interstitial cells of Cajal, the intrinsic pacemakers cells of the gut. Complications arising from resection are predictable: anastomotic leakage, stricture formation, adhesions. When malignant, these cells tend to metastasize hematogenously and to recur either locally (possibly due to inadequate margins) or in the liver.

Exogenous Tumors

Endometriomas are benign collections of endometrial tissue which have spread outside of the female reproductive anatomy. They can result in adhesion formation, ill-defined abdominal pain, obstruction, and can even erode through the bowel wall resulting in bleeding into the lumen. In general, endometriomas can be treated medically and tend to recede during the postmenopausal period.

Intraperitoneal metastases from nonintestinal sites are reminiscent of desmoid tumors, and are best diagnosed by CT or positive emission tomography scan. Such lesions portend a dismal prognosis; operation for minimal gain that confers substantial risk should be avoided. However, palliative intervention such as enteroenteric bypass or simply gastrostomy drainage may be indicated.

Hemorrhage

Intestinal hemorrhage between the duodenal bulb and the ileocecal valve accounts for 3% to 5% of bleeding from the gastrointestinal tract, (84) but may be caused by a greater variety of lesions than in the entire remaining bowel (Table 37.9). Prevention of complications of surgery for intestinal hemorrhage is based upon timely diagnosis, appropriate diagnostic testing, and judgment regarding the advantages of resection versus observation.

Identification of an intestinal bleeding source can be difficult due to its infrequent and usually intermittent occurrence, the length of the small intestine, and the paucity of sensitive tests. Traditionally, after upper and lower endoscopy, evaluation of a suspected small intestine bleeding source begins with a small bowel X-ray, which is only diagnostic in 5% to 10% of cases (85,86). The technetium-99 labeled red blood cell scan is a more sensitive diagnostic test and carries few risks beyond time delay. Additionally, as long as no transfusion is required, the tagged cells will remain positive for 12 to 24 hours, permitting delayed testing. Although this test can help to diagnose blood loss within the small intestine, pooled blood can be deceptive. Localization of the exact bleeding site is difficult unless the site has specific anatomic features, as in the duodenum or terminal ileum. Angiography can help to localize a lesion bleeding at ≥0.5 mL/min but is less than 50% sensitive if bleeding has slowed or stopped. Moreover, a major advantage of angiography, its therapeutic value, is limited in the small, branching arcades of the small intestine. For slower or more obscure sources of small bowel blood loss, capsule endoscopy has become the standard localizing test. A small wireless endoscopic capsule is swallowed and takes two pictures of the lumen per second. Recording devices worn by the patient capture images and track the route of the capsule for localization, with generally acceptable sensitivity and specificity (87,88).

Table 37.9 Etiologies of small intestinal bleeding

Causes of Intestinal Bleeding	Location	Features
Vascular lesions		
Angiodysplasias or vascular ectasias	Throughout, but most concentrated in the right colon	Mucosal and submucosal dilated arterial vessels
Telangiectasias	Throughout the intestine	Full thickness dilated vessels, diffuse
Arteriovenous malformations	Throughout	Thick-walled arteries and veins without intervening capillaries
Vascular anomalies		
Small bowel varices	Duodenum, proximal jejunum	Associated with prehepatic portal hypertension
Aortoenteric fistula	Duodenum, ileum	Herald bleeding followed by massive hemorrhage.
Dieulafoy lesion	Fundus, duodenum, jejunum	Painless, massive bleeding
Vasculidities		
Collagen-vascular diseases		Large and small arterial compromise
Venulitis		Mucosal edema, malabsorption, ulcerations
Radiation damage		Mucosal edema and ulcerations
Ulcerations		
Crohn's disease	Throughout	Transmural ulceration, bleeding is usually indolent
Gastrinomas	Duodenum, jejunum	
Infection associated	Throughout	
Medication induced	Throughout	
Meckel's diverticulum	100 cm proximal to the ileocecal valve	Ulceration and brisk bleeding due to ectopic gastric mucosa within the diverticulum.
Pseudo-diverticula	Jejunum	Mesenteric border of the intestine, unlikely to be a source of blood loss but may bleed massively
Small bowel tumors (see above)		

Exploratory surgery may be excessively invasive but has both diagnostic and therapeutic value. Because many of the causative lesions are flat or small and thus hard to palpate, exploration is best accompanied by diagnostic endoscopy of the small bowel. Intraoperative enteroscopy, termed "push enteroscopy," requires advancement of a colonoscope or sometimes a specialized enteroscope under direct visualization with mechanical assistance. Localization of the bleeding site occurs in 38% to 75% of cases and many lesions can be treated endoscopically (89).

Timing of an operation requires judicious planning. After the initial presentation, many vascular lesions demonstrate no further bleeding. Angioectasias represent 80% of bleeding lesions in patients over age 60, but only rebleed in 10% of cases (90). In contrast, small bowel tumors, the most common source of small intestinal bleeding in patients younger than age 50, are best resected unless too numerous or diffusely distributed. Briskly bleeding lesions also must be addressed, preferably before extensive transfusion is required.

Ischemia

Intestinal ischemia in adults is generally the result of thromboembolic disease, small vessel disease such as collagen-vascular disorders, or a complication of previous operation. Diagnosis of intestinal ischemia can be difficult, and is based on symptoms and an examination consistent with impending peritonitis. The traditional admonition of "pain out of proportion to physical examination" is most easily appreciated with hindsight. Useful serology studies include the leukocyte count, lactate level, and bicarbonate level. Thromboembolic disease, chronic mesenteric ischemia, and small vessel disease are explored in a separate chapter. Nonvascular reasons for a low flow state, such as reduced cardiac output, usually compromise "watershed" areas of the colon prior to affecting the small bowel.

The most common etiology of postoperative intestinal ischemia is an incarcerated or strangulated small bowel hernia. The diagnosis is relatively straightforward among nonobese patients with a ventral hernia. Ultrasound or CT scan can help to make the diagnosis in the patient whose examination is obscured by a thicker abdominal wall. An incarcerated intraperitoneal hernia can sometimes be appreciated on CT scan, particularly if a clear transition point in the small bowel lumen is seen. Mesenteric torsion is another source of intestinal ischemia. In adults, mesenteric torsion may be a complication of the anastomotic alignment and is easily avoided by purposefully orienting the mesenteric edges during anastomosis or stoma formation.

Intraoperatively, questions regarding viability of bowel or an anastomosis can be resolved by obtaining a Doppler signal at the antimesenteric border. Alternatively, intravenous injection of 1 mg of fluorescein dye followed by use of a Wood's lamp can delineate inadequately perfused bowel. In addition, prudent use of a follow-up second look operation will reveal ongoing ischemia or nonviable resection margins.

Small intestinal bypass

Defunctionalization of some portion of the small intestine can occur due to enteroenteric fistula, but is more commonly the result of operative intervention. Surgical bypass is categorized as therapeutic for weight loss or palliative for obstruction. While intestinal bypass for either purpose carries similar operative risks, the underlying disease process has a major impact on long term outcome. Several late complications of defunctionalized bowel or "blind loops" have been identified. Bacterial overgrowth due to reduced or absent peristalsis and diversion of digestive juices can lead to formation of metabolites toxic to the intestinal mucosa, poor nutrient absorption, intractable diarrhea and resultant mechanical trauma. Diagnosis is usually based on symptoms of diarrhea, bloating, fever, and malaise and a positive hydrogen breath test (91). Intermittent treatment with metronidazole helps to re-establish normal flora and control symptoms. Micronutrient malnutrition can lead to osteoporosis, night blindness, skin rashes, calculi formation, anemia, and immunopathy. Prevention is effected by careful attention to vitamin, mineral, and electrolyte replacement.

Therapeutic Intestinal Bypass for Weight Loss

While intestinal surgery generally is founded on improving the availability of nutrition, the unique aim of a bariatric intestinal bypass is to reduce nutritional volume. In the United States, bariatric surgery is enjoying renewed popularity and is now the most common electively performed abdominal operation (92,93). Early complications of bariatric surgery generally fall within the same categories as complications of palliative bypass, and anastomotic leak is independently predictive of postoperative mortality (94). In previous decades, profound late complications of jejunoileal bypass, especially hepatic cirrhosis, led to a moratorium on the procedure (95–97). More recently, creation of a common intestinal channel >50 cm in length has helped to mitigate protein-calorie malnutrition (97). Flow of bile and pancreatic fluid through the defunctionalized limb has reduced bacterial overgrowth, and resultant diarrhea, fever, and malaise. Close postoperative attention to vitamin supplementation, prevention of electrolyte disturbances, and adequate protein intake have helped to ameliorate sequelae of micronutrient depletion and malnutrition.

Palliative Bypass for Obstruction

Intestinal bypass is an important alternative strategy when resection is not feasible, for example in the setting of short bowel, previous radiation, matted bowel or mesenteric fibrosis, or widely disseminated tumor. The primary goal of palliative surgical bypass is relief of obstructive pain. Secondary goals are prevention of perforation and peritonitis, and re-establishment of anatomic continuity. The patient's preferences and a realistic assessment of the prognosis must be carefully considered preoperatively. For example, a patient with slowly advancing obstruction due to mesenteric fibrosis or longstanding radiation damage potentially could have many remaining years with a satisfactory quality of life. Alternatively, a moribund patient who is not expected to recover may be best served by a less invasive procedure for decompression. The underlying disease process affects tissue quality and perfusion, which have a direct impact on intraoperative risks of unplanned enterotomy and anastomotic leakage. Late complications include malnutrition, bacterial overgrowth, and renal and biliary calculi formation.

Hypomotility

Intestinal motility is mediated by an assortment of peptides, hormones, and extrinsic and intrinsic neural pathways. Transient hypomotility secondary to postoperative ileus, narcotic use, bowel edema, or systemic inflammation is best managed supportively, with decompression, fluid replacement, and removal of the offending source if possible. Longer-term hypomotility can be iatrogenic as a result of surgically disrupted pathways, for example post-vagotomy or intestinal bypass, or intrinsic as in the setting of connective tissue disorders, or visceral neuropathy or myopathy.

Chronic Intestinal Pseudoobstruction

Intestinal pseudo-obstruction is manifested by abdominal distension, nausea, vomiting, and pain, and can be difficult to distinguish clinically from mechanical obstruction. An incorrect presumption of mechanical obstruction leading to operation can result in combined functional and mechanical obstruction, an even more challenging clinical situation. The etiology of pseudo-obstruction is generally an underlying autoimmune connective tissue disorder, such as systemic lupus erythematosus, scleroderma, or amyloidosis. The prognosis is directly related to progress of the underlying disease. Treatment is based on avoidance of laparotomy, use of promotility agents, and supportive care (98). Anaerobic bacterial overgrowth can lead to steatorrhea and may require treatment with antibiotics. Chronic pain due to distension may become severe enough to warrant creation of a venting enterostomy. Correcting derangements of electrolytes, especially magnesium, can also ameliorate symptoms.

Visceral Myopathy/Neuropathy

Pseudo-obstruction patients with no clear underlying connective tissue abnormality are thought to have an abnormality of the enteric smooth muscle or (less frequently) intrinsic nervous system (99). Numerous case series report such ill-defined syndromes, which tend to be familial, progressive, and to extend to other visceral or even skeletal muscle systems. Supportive care includes hyperalimentation and medication for vague but frequently severe pain. Promotility agents have not proven useful. Surgical intervention is generally ineffective, leaving patients vulnerable to all of the risks but no advantages of laparotomy. However, patients unable to tolerate long-term hyperalimentation may benefit from consideration of small intestinal transplantation.

Table **37.10** **Complications of ileostomy formation and closure**

	Early Complications	Late Complications
Both loop and end ileostomies	Poor location Poor orifice size Ischemic necrosis Dehydration Bowel obstruction Parastomal abscess Dermatitis	Prolapse Parastomal herniation Peristomal fistula formation Bowel obstruction Dermatitis
End ileostomy		Retraction Stenosis Variceal bleeding
Loop ileostomy	Erroneous closure of the proximal end	Closure-related: Bowel obstruction Anastomotic leakage Stricture formation

Ileostomy complications

Ileostomies are usually created at the end of an operative case, after the abdomen has been closed and the senior surgeon may have stepped back from the table. Although ileostomy formation seems simple enough, the technical complication rate is not trivial. In 1952, Brooke made a major contribution to reduction of ileostomy complications by proposing immediate maturation (eversion) of the ileostomy end (100). However, in an actuarial analysis with a decade of yearly follow-up, Leong and colleagues found that ileostomy complications still approached 76% among ulcerative colitis patients (101). Complications of end or loop ileostomy formation can be immediately obvious or can continue to accrue over years (Table 37.10). Although much of the surgical dogma is now disputed, specific technical issues merit special attention. Additionally, volume replacement and treatment with a bulking agent and anti-diarrheal medication can prevent the numerous sequelae of dehydration.

Brooke Ileostomy

The most important initial steps in stoma creation, and prevention of complications, are appropriate siting, aligning the abdominal wall tunnel through the rectus abdominus muscle, and eversion of an adequate length of intestine (Fig. 37.5).

The proposed area should be flat, within the patient's view, and away from scars, skin folds, or bony prominences. Optimally this site is located through the rectus sheath, at 1/3 of the distance between the umbilicus and the anterior superior iliac spine. In obese patients, the stoma site should be shifted upward for visualization. An inappropriate site may lead to poor appliance fit, leakage, and sometimes profound dermatitis.

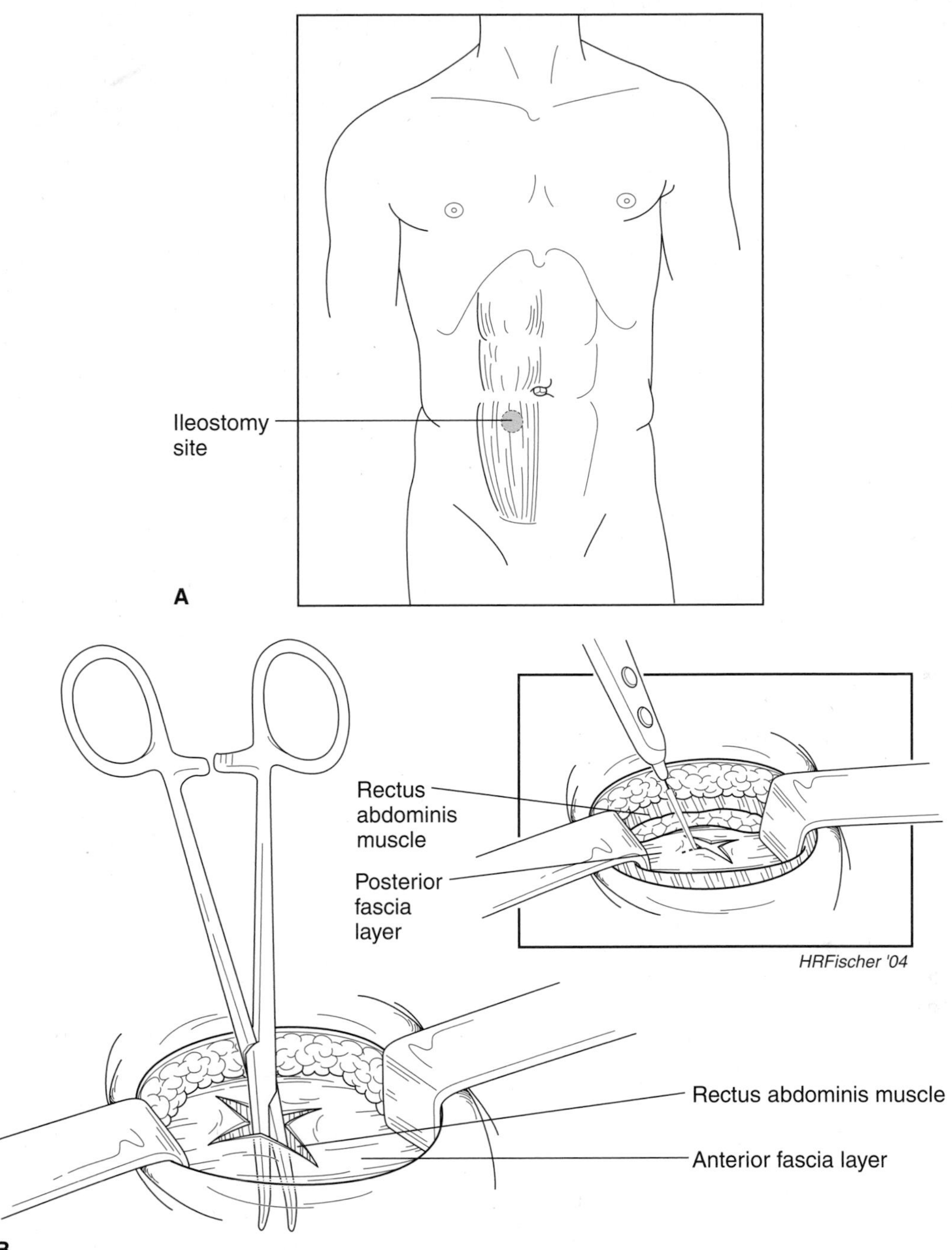

FIGURE 37.5. Brooke ileostomy formation. **A:** Ileostomy site, **B:** Muscle splitting incision (*continued*)

A circular incision of 2 cm diameter is created sharply and fat is divided to the anterior fascial sheath. The tract should be aligned by retracting the skin and fascia to the midline intraoperatively. A poorly aligned tract can cause obstruction, edema, and ischemia. A cruciate incision is created in the anterior rectus muscle sheath using Bovie electrocautery. A muscle splitting incision through the rectus muscle should preserve the epigastric vessels and expose the posterior fascia for the next cruciate incision. The tract should be bluntly dilated to about a 2 finger width, for withdrawal of the mobilized terminal ileum.

Vigorous clearing of mesentery from the ileal end can result in ischemia and is generally unnecessary. Adequate mobilization for eversion is crucial at this step, especially if weight gain is anticipated. Inadequate mobilization can lead to tension on the mesentery and ischemia. Additionally, a poorly everted stoma may retract and stenose, resulting in poor appliance fit, leakage, dermatitis, skin ulcerations, and obstruction. Repair of a retracted, stenotic stoma frequently requires laparotomy.

Small bowel obstruction, the most common complication of ileostomy formation after skin breakdown, is most

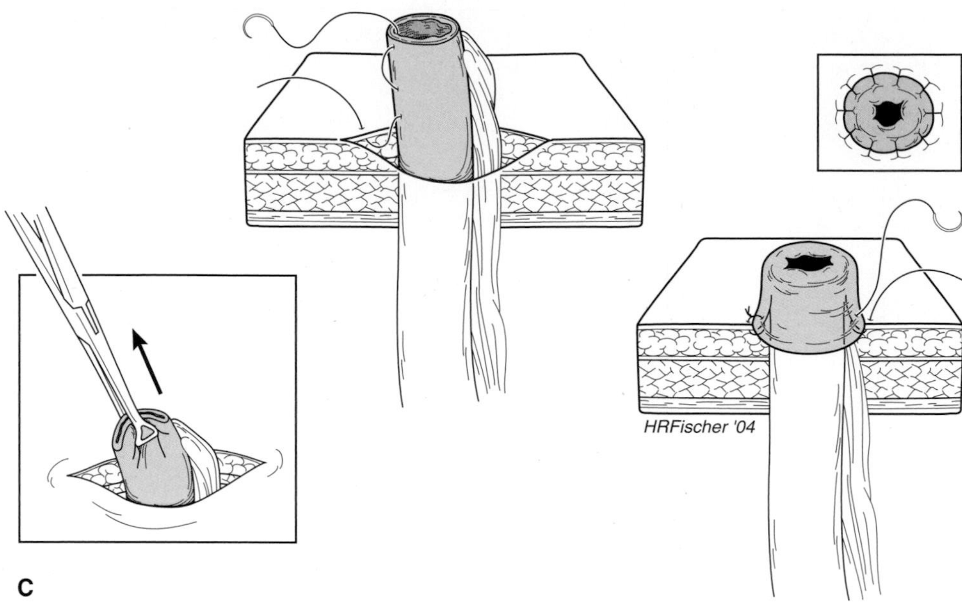

FIGURE 37.5. (*Continued*) **C:** Eversion.

often caused by intra-abdominal adhesions. Other reasons for bowel obstruction include fibrinous food bolus, parastomal herniation, intra-abdominal torsion, and recurrent Crohn's disease. Closing the lateral space or sewing the mesentery to the abdominal wall appears to have no impact on the long-term obstruction rate (101).

Parastomal herniation is essentially a ventral herniation. The actuarial risk is about 16% and risk factors are identical to those of other incisional hernias: age, obesity, pulmonary disease, steroid dependence, and a history of hernias. Symptom relief can be provided by a customized truss. Rubin and others reported a 76% recurrence rate with primary fascia repair, 33% recurrence rate with stoma translocation, and an overall operative complication rate of 62% (102). Based on these data, the authors recommended translocation as the initial repair strategy, followed by mesh placement for recurrent herniation.

Peristomal fistulae develop in about 7% of patients, most of whom have Crohn's disease. Tacking suture through the dermis only, thus avoiding a tract through the epidermis, and a well-fitted stoma appliance that limits skin pressure may help to minimize this problem.

Ileostomy provides an additional communication between the portal and systemic venous systems. Bleeding varices can potentially develop in cirrhotic patients. Temporizing measures include oversewing the bleeding site, cauterization or sclerosis, or even disconnecting and reanastomosing the mucocutaneous junction. Longer term management requires changing the portal flow or curing the cirrhosis with a liver transplant.

Loop Ileostomy

A loop ileostomy is intended to be temporary. Although the loop ileostomy is associated with many of the same short-term complications as the end ileostomy, a few notable differences exist. Furthermore, closure of the ileostomy summons a whole different group of potential complications.

Loop ileostomy formation begins with the same principles as an end ileostomy (Fig. 37.6). Ascertainment of no twist in the bowel and mesentery is essential prior to orientation of the stoma limbs. Placing the distal limb in the dependent position is standard technique and can be helpful for future operative planning. In the event that the loop ileostomy is to be converted to an end ileostomy, appropriate orientation can help to prevent closing the wrong (proximal) limb. Wrapping the intestinal loop in an adhesion barrier prior to delivery through the fascia can greatly facilitate future stoma closure.

Loop ileostomies are more prone to prolapse, which can be quite distressing to the patient. Fortunately, adverse sequelae are rare. Data are inconclusive regarding effectiveness of fixing the mesentery to prevent prolapse.

Complications of ileostomy closure center on obstruction and leakage. Because the distal limb may be substantially narrowed, a side-to-side closure is best. In a randomized trial of stapled versus sutured closure, Hasegawa and colleagues determined that a stapled closure was associated with 80% fewer postoperative bowel obstructions (37). However, hospital stay, readmission rates, and reoperative rates were the same.

Jejunostomy tube complications

Feeding jejunostomy tube placement has been an adjunct to a variety of abdominal operations, but is associated with respective major complication and mortality rates of 4% to 10% and 1.4% to 3.2% (103–106). The classic method for jejunostomy placement has been a sizeable tube through an imbricated tract (Fig. 37.7) at least 30 cm beyond the ligament

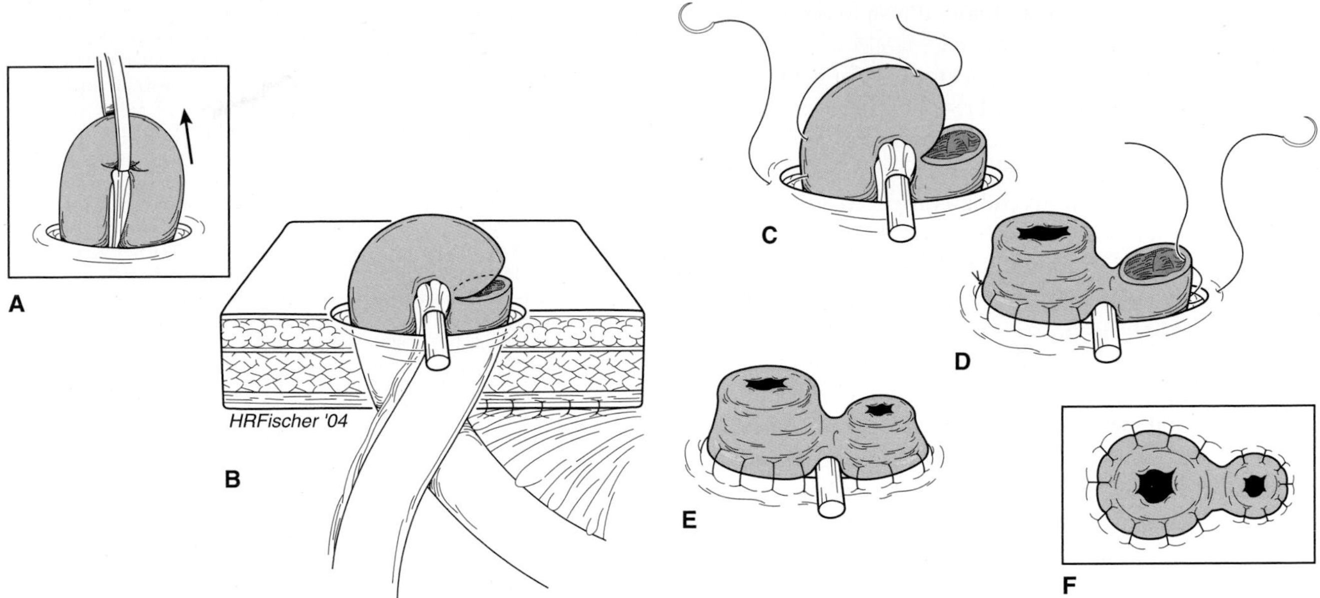

FIGURE 37.6. Loop ileostomy formation. **A:** Delivery of intestine through the stoma incision, **B:** Proper orientation of the bowel: no bowel torsion and distal limb inferior, **C:** Mechanical prevention of reduction prior to healing, **D:** Eversion of both limbs in a Brooke fashion, **E** and **F:** Final loop ileostomy appearance.

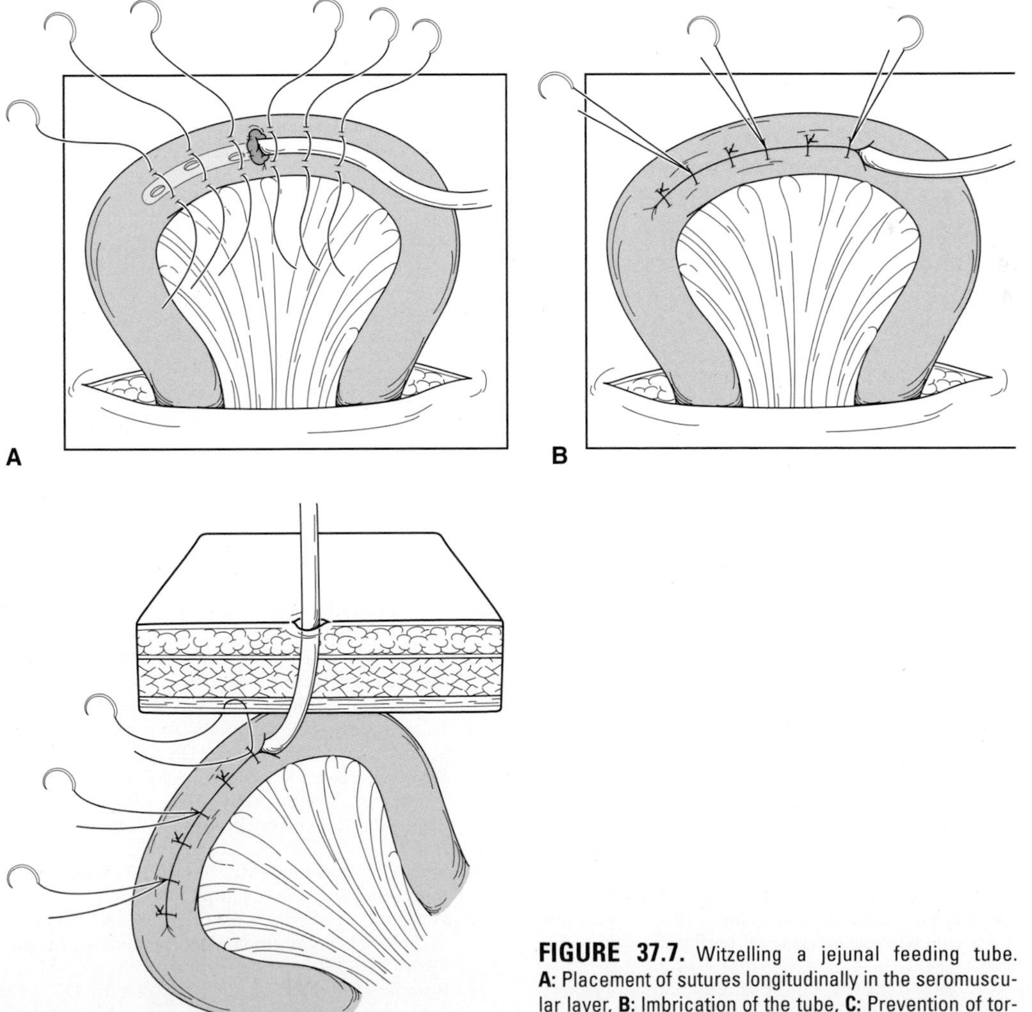

FIGURE 37.7. Witzelling a jejunal feeding tube. **A:** Placement of sutures longitudinally in the seromuscular layer, **B:** Imbrication of the tube, **C:** Prevention of torsion or kinking by fixing the bowel to the abdominal wall.

of Treitz, with sutures to the abdominal wall to prevent kinking or torsion.

A primary indication for jejunostomy over gastrostomy has been a perception of reduced risk of aspiration. Fox and others retrospectively reviewed gastrostomy and jejunostomy tube placements and reported aspiration in 4 of 69 patients with a gastrostomy tube compared with 2 of 86 patients with a jejunostomy tube (107). In contrast, Weltz and others found a substantially reduced rate of aspiration with feeding by jejunostomy tube compared with feeding by nasogastric tube (105).

Leakage, torsion, and erosion with perforation of viscera occur infrequently but consistently. The traditional jejunostomy tube may soon be outmoded by newer enthusiasm for percutaneous, laparoscopic, and needle catheter placement. However, no clearly superior method has been established thus far.

SUMMARY

In summary, intestinal surgery is performed for an enormous variety of underlying diseases. Complications that arise as a result of technical errors can be associated broadly with obstruction or anastomotic leakage. Careful postoperative attention to the patient will permit an earlier diagnosis, which usually allows more effective intervention. Complications that arise as a result of errors of judgment may be more specific to the underlying disease or operation. Prevention of errors of judgment rests on a timely and thorough preoperative evaluation, and a treatment plan based on specific features of the underlying disease. Optimization of the patient's preoperative nutritional status, appropriate timing of surgery, and appreciation of alternative treatment strategies are keys to the prevention and management of complications.

REFERENCES

1. Ashley SW, Wells SA Jr. Tumors of the small intestine. *Semin Oncol* 1988;15(2):116–128.
2. Fleming CR, Remington M. Intestinal Failure. In: Hill GL, ed. *Nutrition and the Surgical Patient*. New York: Churchill Livingstone; 1981:219–235.
3. Perioperative total parenteral nutrition in surgical patients. The Veterans Affairs Total Parenteral Nutrition Cooperative Study Group. *N Engl J Med* 1991;325(8):525–532.
4. Buzby GP. Overview of randomized clinical trials of total parenteral nutrition for malnourished surgical patients. *World J Surg* 1993;17(2): 173–177.
5. Nightingale JM. The medical management of intestinal failure: methods to reduce the severity. *Proc Nutr Soc* 2003;62(3):703–710.
6. Ziegler TR, Evans ME, Fernandez-Estivariz C, et al. Trophic and cytoprotective nutrition for intestinal adaptation, mucosal repair, and barrier function. *Annu Rev Nutr* 2003;23:229–261.
7. Tera H, Aberg C. Relaparotomy. A ten-year series. *Acta Chir Scand* 1975;141(7):637–644.
8. Zer M, Dux S, Dintsman M. The timing of relaparotomy and its influence on prognosis. A 10 year survey. *Am J Surg* 1980;139(3):338–343.
9. van Goor H, Hulsebos RG, Bleichrodt RP. Complications of planned relaparotomy in patients with severe general peritonitis. *Eur J Surg* 1997;163(1):61–66.
10. Golub R, Golub RW, Cantu R Jr, et al. A multivariate analysis of factors contributing to leakage of intestinal anastomoses. *J Am Coll Surg* 1997; 184(4):364–372.
11. Ching SS, Muralikrishnan VP, Whiteley GS. Relaparotomy: a five-year review of indications and outcome. *Int J Clin Pract* 2003;57(4):333–337.
12. Ellozy SH, Harris MT, Bauer JJ, et al. Early postoperative small-bowel obstruction: a prospective evaluation in 242 consecutive abdominal operations. *Dis Colon Rectum* 2002;45(9):1214–1217.
13. Fraser SA, Shrier I, Miller G, et al. Immediate postlaparotomy small bowel obstruction: a 16-year retrospective analysis. *Am Surg* 2002;68(9): 780–782.
14. Roukema JA, Carol EJ, Prins JG. The prevention of pulmonary complications after upper abdominal surgery in patients with noncompromised pulmonary status. *Arch Surg* 1988;123(1):30–34.
15. Hall JC, Tarala RA, Tapper J, et al. Prevention of respiratory complications after abdominal surgery: a randomised clinical trial. *BMJ* 1996; 312(7024):148–152; discussion 152–143.
16. Guimaraes MM, El Dib R, Smith AF, et al. Incentive spirometry for prevention of postoperative pulmonary complications in upper abdominal surgery. *Cochrane Database Syst Rev* 2009;(3):CD006058.
17. Eagle KA, Berger PB, Calkins H, et al. ACC/AHA guideline update for perioperative cardiovascular evaluation for noncardiac surgery–executive summary: a report of the American College of Cardiology/American Heart Association Task Force on Practice Guidelines (Committee to Update the 1996 Guidelines on Perioperative Cardiovascular Evaluation for Noncardiac Surgery). *J Am Coll Cardiol* 2002; 39(3):542–553.
18. Potyk D, Raudaskoski P. Preoperative cardiac evaluation for elective noncardiac surgery. *Arch Fam Med* 1998;7(2):164–173.
19. Kern JW, Shoemaker WC. Meta-analysis of hemodynamic optimization in high-risk patients. *Crit Care Med* 2002;30(8):1686–1692.
20. Giner M, Laviano A, Meguid MM, et al. In 1995 a correlation between malnutrition and poor outcome in critically ill patients still exists. *Nutrition* 1996;12(1):23–29.
21. Middleton MH, Nazarenko G, Nivison-Smith I, et al. Prevalence of malnutrition and 12-month incidence of mortality in two Sydney teaching hospitals. *Intern Med J* 2001;31(8):455–461.
22. Post S, Betzler M, von Ditfurth B, et al. Risks of intestinal anastomoses in Crohn's disease. *Ann Surg* 1991;213(1):37–42.
23. Wicke C, Halliday B, Allen D, et al. Effects of steroids and retinoids on wound healing. *Arch Surg* 2000;135(11):1265–1270.
24. Anstead GM. Steroids, retinoids, and wound healing. *Adv Wound Care* 1998;11(6):277–285.
25. Slavin J, Unemori E, Hunt TK, et al. Transforming growth factor beta (TGF-beta) and dexamethasone have direct opposing effects on collagen metabolism in low passage human dermal fibroblasts in vitro. *Growth Factors* 1994;11(3):205–213.
26. Marchal L, D'haens G, Van Aasche G, et al. The risk of post-operative complications associated with infliximab therapy for Crohn's disease: a controlled cohort study. *Aliment Pharmacol Ther* 2004;19:749–754.
27. Appau KA, Fazio VW, Shen B, et al. Use of infliximab within 3 months of ileocolonic resection is associated with adverse postoperative outcomes in Crohn's patients. *J Gastrointest Surg* 2008;12(10):1738–1744.
28. Kunitake H, Hodin R, Shellito PC, et al. Perioperative treatment with infliximab in patients with Crohn's disease and ulcerative colitis is not associated with an increased rate of postoperative complications. *J Gastrointest Surg* 2008;12(10):1730–1736; discussion 1736–1737.
29. Holmdahl L, Risberg B, Beck DE, et al. Adhesions: pathogenesis and prevention-panel discussion and summary. *Eur J Surg Suppl* 1997(577): 56–62.
30. Thompson J. Pathogenesis and prevention of adhesion formation. *Dig Surg* 1998;15(2):153–157.
31. Cullen JJ, Kelly KA, Moir CR, et al. Surgical management of Meckel's diverticulum. An epidemiologic, population-based study. *Ann Surg* 1994;220(4):564–568; discussion 568–569.
32. Fisher KS, Ross DS. Guidelines for therapeutic decision in incidental appendectomy. *Surg Gynecol Obstet* 1990;171(1):95–98.
33. Snyder TE, Selanders JR, Strom PR, et al. Incidental appendectomy—yes or no? A retrospective case study and review of the literature Safety of incidental appendectomy. *Infect Dis Obstet Gynecol* 1998;6(1): 30–37.
34. Strom PR, Turkleson ML, Stone HH. Safety of incidental appendectomy. *Am J Surg* 1983;145(6):819–822.
35. Warren JL, Penberthy LT, Addiss DG, et al. Appendectomy incidental to cholecystectomy among elderly Medicare beneficiaries. *Surg Gynecol Obstet* 1993;177(3):288–294.
36. Brundage SI, Jurkovich GJ, Grossman DC, et al. Stapled versus sutured gastrointestinal anastomoses in the trauma patient. *J Trauma* 1999;47(3):500–507; discussion 507–508.

37. Hasegawa H, Radley S, Morton DG, et al. Stapled versus sutured closure of loop ileostomy: a randomized controlled trial. *Ann Surg* 2000; 231(2):202–204.
38. Hyman N, Manchester TL, Osler T, et al. Anastomotic leaks after intestinal anastomosis: it's later than you think. *Ann Surg* 2007;245(2): 254–258.
39. Zieren HU, Muller JM, Pichlmaier H. Prospective randomized study of one- or two-layer anastomosis following oesophageal resection and cervical oesophagogastrostomy. *Br J Surg* 1993;80(5):608–611.
40. Kumar S, Wong PF, Leaper DJ. Intra-peritoneal prophylactic agents for preventing adhesions and adhesive intestinal obstruction after non-gynaecological abdominal surgery. *Cochrane Database Syst Rev* 2009;(1):CD005080.
41. Vrijland WW, Tseng LN, Eijkman HJ, et al. Fewer intraperitoneal adhesions with use of hyaluronic acid-carboxymethylcellulose membrane: a randomized clinical trial. *Ann Surg* 2002;235(2):193–199.
42. Becker JM, Dayton MT, Fazio VW, et al. Prevention of postoperative abdominal adhesions by a sodium hyaluronate-based bioresorbable membrane: a prospective, randomized, double-blind multicenter study. *J Am Coll Surg* 1996;183(4):297–306.
43. Beck DE, Cohen Z, Fleshman JW, et al. A prospective, randomized, multicenter, controlled study of the safety of Seprafilm adhesion barrier in abdominopelvic surgery of the intestine. *Dis Colon Rectum* 2003;46(10):1310–1319.
44. Remzi FH, Oncel M, Church JM, et al. An unusual complication after hyaluronate-based bioresorbable membrane (Seprafilm) application. *Am Surg* 2003;69(4):356–357.
45. Klingler PJ, Floch NR, Seelig MH, et al. Seprafilm-induced peritoneal inflammation: a previously unknown complication. Report of a case. *Dis Colon Rectum* 1999;42(12):1639–1643.
46. David M, Sarani B, Moid F, et al. Paradoxical inflammatory reaction to Seprafilm: case report and review of the literature. *South Med J* 2005;98(10):1039–1041.
47. Carroll J, Alavi K. Pathogenesis and management of postoperative ileus. *Clin Colon Rectal Surg* 2009;22(1):47–50.
48. Seror D, Feigin E, Szold A, et al. How conservatively can postoperative small bowel obstruction be treated? *Am J Surg* 1993;165(1): 121–125; discussion 125–126.
49. Shih SC, Jeng KS, Lin SC, et al. Adhesive small bowel obstruction: how long can patients tolerate conservative treatment? *World J Gastroenterol* 2003;9(3):603–605.
50. Fevang BT, Jensen D, Svanes K, et al. Early operation or conservative management of patients with small bowel obstruction? *Eur J Surg* 2002;168(8–9):475–481.
51. Thompson JS. Surgical considerations in the short bowel syndrome. *Surg Gynecol Obstet* 1993;176(1):89–101.
52. Thompson JS. Edgar J. Poth Memorial Lecture. Surgical aspects of the short-bowel syndrome. *Am J Surg* 1995;170(6):532–536.
53. Nightingale JM, Lennard-Jones JE, Gertner DJ, et al. Colonic preservation reduces need for parenteral therapy, increases incidence of renal stones, but does not change high prevalence of gall stones in patients with a short bowel. *Gut* 1992;33(11):1493–1497.
54. Tang SJ, Nieto JM, Jensen DM, et al. The novel use of an intravenous proton pump inhibitor in a patient with short bowel syndrome. *J Clin Gastroenterol* 2002;34(1):62–63.
55. Scolapio JS, Camilleri M, Fleming CR, et al. Effect of growth hormone, glutamine, and diet on adaptation in short-bowel syndrome: a randomized, controlled study. *Gastroenterology* 1997;113(4):1074–1081.
56. Scolapio JS. Effect of growth hormone and glutamine on the short bowel: five years later. *Gut* 2000;47(2):164.
57. Szkudlarek J, Jeppesen PB, Mortensen PB. Effect of high dose growth hormone with glutamine and no change in diet on intestinal absorption in short bowel patients: a randomised, double blind, crossover, placebo controlled study. *Gut* 2000;47(2):199–205.
58. Hallgren T, Fasth S, Delbro DS, et al. Loperamide improves anal sphincter function and continence after restorative proctocolectomy. *Dig Dis Sci* 1994;39(12):2612–2618.
59. Bianchi A. Intestinal loop lengthening—a technique for increasing small intestinal length. *J Pediatr Surg* 1980;15(2):145–151.
60. Bianchi A. Experience with longitudinal intestinal lengthening and tailoring. *Eur J Pediatr Surg* 1999;9(4):256–259.
61. Thompson JS. Strategies for preserving intestinal length in the short-bowel syndrome. *Dis Colon Rectum* 1987;30(3):208–213.
62. Fishbein TM, Matsumoto CS. Intestinal replacement therapy: timing and indications for referral of patients to an intestinal rehabilitation and transplant program. *Gastroenterology* 2006;130(2 Suppl 1):S147–S151.
63. Sudan DL, Kaufman SS, Shaw BW Jr, et al. Isolated intestinal transplantation for intestinal failure. *Am J Gastroenterol* 2000;95(6):1506–1515.
64. Abu-Elmagd K, Reyes J, Bond G, et al. Clinical intestinal transplantation: a decade of experience at a single center. *Ann Surg* 2001;234(3): 404–416; discussion 416–407.
65. Abu-Elmagd K, Bond G. Gut failure and abdominal visceral transplantation. *Proc Nutr Soc* 2003;62(3):727–737.
66. Bernell O, Lapidus A, Hellers G. Risk factors for surgery and recurrence in 907 patients with primary ileocaecal Crohn's disease. *Br J Surg* 2000;87(12):1697–1701.
67. Yamamoto T, Allan RN, Keighley MR. Risk factors for intra-abdominal sepsis after surgery in Crohn's disease. *Dis Colon Rectum* 2000; 43(8):1141–1145.
68. Bruewer M, Utech M, Rijcken EJ, et al. Preoperative steroid administration: effect on morbidity among patients undergoing intestinal bowel resection for Crohn's disease. *World J Surg* 2003;27(12):1306–1310.
69. Tay GS, Binion DG, Eastwood D, et al. Multivariate analysis suggests improved perioperative outcome in Crohn's disease patients receiving immunomodulator therapy after segmental resection and/or strictureplasty. *Surgery* 2003;134(4):565–572; discussion 572–563.
70. Borley NR, Mortensen NJ, Jewell DP. Preventing postoperative recurrence of Crohn's disease. *Br J Surg* 1997;84(11):1493–1502.
71. Lichtenstein GR. Treatment of fistulizing Crohn's disease. *Gastroenterology* 2000;119(4):1132–1147.
72. Broe PJ, Bayless TM, Cameron JL. Crohn's disease: are enteroenteral fistulas an indication for surgery? *Surgery* 1982;91(3):249–253.
73. Wullstein C, Gross E. Laparoscopic compared with conventional treatment of acute adhesive small bowel obstruction. *Br J Surg* 2003; 90(9):1147–1151.
74. Yamamoto T, Keighley MR. Long-term results of strictureplasty for ileocolonic anastomotic recurrence in Crohn's disease. *J Gastrointest Surg* 1999;3(5):555–560.
75. de Jong E, van Dullemen HM, Slors JF, et al. Correlation between early recurrence and reoperation after ileocolonic resection in Crohn's disease: a prospective study. *J Am Coll Surg* 1996;182(6):503–508.
76. Tytgat GN, Mulder CJ, Brummelkamp WH. Endoscopic lesions in Crohn's disease early after ileocecal resection. *Endoscopy* 1988;20(5): 260–262.
77. Williams JG, Wong WD, Rothenberger DA, et al. Recurrence of Crohn's disease after resection. *Br J Surg* 1991;78(1):10–19.
78. Wobbes T, Verschueren RC, Lubbers EJ, et al. Surgical aspects of radiation enteritis of the small bowel. *Dis Colon Rectum* 1984;27(2):89–92.
79. Swan RW. Stagnant loop syndrome resulting from small-bowel irradiation injury and intestinal by-pass. *Gynecol Oncol* 1974;2(4):441–445.
80. Dietz DW, Remzi FH, Fazio VW. Strictureplasty for obstructing small-bowel lesions in diffuse radiation enteritis–successful outcome in five patients. *Dis Colon Rectum* 2001;44(12):1772–1777.
81. Agha FP. Intussusception in adults. *AJR Am J Roentgenol* 1986;146(3): 527–531.
82. Lvoff N, Breiman RS, Coakley FV, et al. Distinguishing features of self-limiting adult small-bowel intussusception identified at CT. *Radiology* 2003;227(1):68–72.
83. Naef M, Buhlmann M, Baer HU. Small bowel tumors: diagnosis, therapy and prognostic factors. *Langenbecks Arch Surg* 1999;384(2):176–180.
84. Netterville RE, Hardy JD, Martin RS Jr. Small bowel hemorrhage. *Ann Surg* 1968;167(6):949–957.
85. Rabe FE, Becker GJ, Besozzi MJ, et al. Efficacy study of the small-bowel examination. *Radiology* 1981;140(1):47–50.
86. Lewis BS. Small intestinal bleeding. *Gastroenterol Clin North Am* 2000; 29(1):67–95, vi.
87. Mata A, Bordas JM, Feu F, et al. Wireless capsule endoscopy in patients with obscure gastrointestinal bleeding: a comparative study with push enteroscopy. *Aliment Pharmacol Ther* 2004;20(2):189–194.
88. Mylonaki M, Fritscher-Ravens A, Swain P. Wireless capsule endoscopy: a comparison with push enteroscopy in patients with gastroscopy and colonoscopy negative gastrointestinal bleeding. *Gut* 2003;52(8): 1122–1126.
89. Zuckerman GR, Prakash C, Askin MP, et al. AGA technical review on the evaluation and management of occult and obscure gastrointestinal bleeding. *Gastroenterology* 2000;118(1):201–221.
90. Lewis B, Goldfarb N. Review article: The advent of capsule endoscopy–a not-so-futuristic approach to obscure gastrointestinal bleeding. *Aliment Pharmacol Ther* 2003;17(9):1085–1096.
91. Riordan SM, McIver CJ, Walker BM, et al. The lactulose breath hydrogen test and small intestinal bacterial overgrowth. *Am J Gastroenterol* 1996;91(9):1795–1803.

92. Livingston EH. Procedure incidence and in-hospital complication rates of bariatric surgery in the United States. *Am J Surg* 2004;188(2): 105–110.
93. Pope GD, Birkmeyer JD, Finlayson SR. National trends in utilization and in-hospital outcomes of bariatric surgery. *J Gastrointest Surg* 2002;6(6):855–860; discussion 861.
94. Fernandez AZ Jr, Demaria EJ, Tichansky DS, et al. Multivariate analysis of risk factors for death following gastric bypass for treatment of morbid obesity. *Ann Surg* 2004;239(5):698–702; discussion 702–693.
95. Backman L, Hallberg D. Some somatic complications after small intestinal bypass operations for obesity. Possible factors of significance in the incidence. *Acta Chir Scand* 1975;141(8):790–800.
96. Dean P, Joshi S, Kaminski DL. Long-term outcome of reversal of small intestinal bypass operations. *Am J Surg* 1990;159(1):118–123; discussion 123–114.
97. Sugerman HJ, Kellum JM, DeMaria EJ. Conversion of Proximal to Distal Gastric Bypass for Failed Gastric Bypass for Superobesity. *J Gastrointest Surg* 1997;1(6):517–525.
98. Hirsh EH, Brandenburg D, Hersh T, et al. Chronic intestinal pseudo-obstruction. *J Clin Gastroenterol* 1981;3(3):247–254.
99. Mann SD, Debinski HS, Kamm MA. Clinical characteristics of chronic idiopathic intestinal pseudo-obstruction in adults. *Gut* 1997;41(5): 675–681.
100. Brooke BN. The management of an ileostomy, including its complications. *Lancet* 1952;2(3):102–104.
101. Leong AP, Londono-Schimmer EE, Phillips RK. Life-table analysis of stomal complications following ileostomy. *Br J Surg* 1994;81(5):727–729.
102. Rubin MS, Schoetz DJ Jr, Matthews JB. Parastomal hernia. Is stoma relocation superior to fascial repair? *Arch Surg* 1994;129(4):413–418; discussion 418–419.
103. Holmes JH IV, Brundage SI, Yuen P, et al. Complications of surgical feeding jejunostomy in trauma patients. *J Trauma* 1999;47(6):1009–1012.
104. Sonawane RN, Thombare MM, Kumar A, et al. Technical complications of feeding jejunostomy: a critical analysis. *Trop Gastroenterol* 1997;18(3):127–128.
105. Weltz CR, Morris JB, Mullen JL. Surgical jejunostomy in aspiration risk patients. *Ann Surg* 1992;215(2):140–145.
106. Simon T, Fink AS. Recent experience with percutaneous endoscopic gastrostomy/jejunostomy (PEG/J) for enteral nutrition. *Surg Endosc* 2000;14(5):436–438.
107. Fox KA, Mularski RA, Sarfati MR, et al. Aspiration pneumonia following surgically placed feeding tubes. *Am J Surg* 1995;170(6): 564–566; discussion 566–567.
108. Joelsson I, Raf L. Late injuries of the small intestine following radiotherapy for uterine carcinoma. *Acta Chir Scand* 1973;139(2): 194–200.
109. Swan RW, Fowler WC Jr, Boronow RC. Surgical management of radiation injury to the small intestine. *Surg Gynecol Obstet* 1976;142(3): 325–327.
110. Schmitt EH III, Symmonds RE. Surgical treatment of radiation induced injuries of the intestine. *Surg Gynecol Obstet* 1981;153(6):896–900.
111. Lillemoe KD, Brigham RA, Harmon JW, et al. Surgical management of small-bowel radiation enteritis. *Arch Surg* 1983;118(8):905–907.
112. Galland RB, Spencer J. Natural history and surgical management of radiation enteritis. *Br J Surg* 1987;74(8):742–747.

CHAPTER

38

Complications of Appendectomy and Colon and Rectal Surgery

Emily Finlayson

Appendicitis is the most common cause of acute pain in the abdomen requiring surgical intervention and must be considered in any patient complaining of abdominal pain. The lifetime incidence of acute appendicitis is 6.7% to 20%, with the lifetime incidence of appendectomy of 12% for men and 23% for women (1). The presentation of appendicitis is often confusing and may cause delayed diagnosis, especially in patient populations in which other changes in physiology, such as pregnancy or extremes in age, may exist. The accepted pathophysiology of appendicitis contributes directly to presentation, diagnosis, and complications.

The classic history of pain—first diffuse, then localizing to the right lower quadrant of the abdomen—associated with fever is obtained in only half of patients (2). Associated symptoms of anorexia and vomiting may be absent. Therefore, clinical suspicion must be maintained in patients still possessing an appendix when history or physical examination is atypical. Diagnosis can be particularly difficult in small children, who are unable to give a history, and in the elderly. Ultrasound or computed tomography (CT) can often clarify an atypical clinical picture. The radiologic literature reports diagnostic sensitivities as high as 92% (3) when these studies are used as adjuncts to history and physical examination. Radiographic studies are helpful in confirming the diagnosis of appendicitis, and they decrease the incidence of negative appendectomy. In addition, abdominal imaging can identify patients with perforated appendicitis with a well-defined periappendiceal abscess collection who would benefit from percutaneous drainage followed by interval appendectomy.

COMPLICATIONS AT PRESENTATION

Peritonitis is a common complication of appendicitis, and it implies that the disease process has progressed, with associated ischemia, mucosal ulceration, transmural necrosis, and leakage of bacteria and fecal material. Peritonitis may be localized if the surrounding organs—the small bowel, colon, omentum, or colonic epiploicae—contain the perforation. In the absence of this protective host response, generalized peritonitis may occur. Generalized peritonitis is more common in children, who possess a less generous omentum. Although localized peritonitis may occur in patients with a periappendiceal abscess due to perforated appendicitis, generalized peritonitis may also occur if the abscess loses its containment. Associated sepsis is due to mixed colonic flora, including anaerobic *Bacteroides*, aerobic *Escherichia coli*, and streptococci. Antimicrobial treatment should be targeted to these organisms.

When a patient presents several days after the onset of symptoms, a contained perforation with abscess is common. In this setting, operative drainage with or without appendectomy is associated with a high morbidity of 18% to 50% (4,5). Radiologic imaging in the form of ultrasound or CT scan can confirm the diagnosis and facilitates nonoperative management. Small (<3 cm) abscesses respond to bowel rest and intravenous antibiotics, whereas larger abscesses require percutaneous drainage. With this approach, an initial failure rate of 12% necessitates urgent appendectomy, which has a complication rate of 12% (6). Because recurrent appendicitis occurs with an incidence of 8% to 14% following resolution of the acute episode, the practice of routine interval appendectomy after the resolution of symptoms is controversial (7). Although the risk of recurrence is low, additional pathology may be identified in the appendix or cecum. A barium enema or colonoscopy can be performed to determine whether other pathology exists.

POSTOPERATIVE COMPLICATIONS

The most common postoperative complication of appendicitis is wound infection. Similar to much of the morbidity of appendicitis, this complication's incidence is correlated with the pathology's severity. In patients with nonperforated appendicitis, the incidence of wound infection is <10%; wound infection increases with perforated appendicitis to 15% to 20% and is highest with diffuse peritonitis (35%) (8). Wound infection is significantly less common after appendectomy performed laparoscopically (9). The offending organisms are colonic bacteria, especially *Bacteroides fragilis* and *E. coli.*

If the patient does not resolve fever postoperatively and the wound is excluded as a source of infection, an intraabdominal abscess should be suspected. The most common

Emily Finlayson: Department of Surgery, University of California, San Francisco locations for abscesses are the iliac fossa, the pericecal area, and the pelvis. Both CT scan and ultrasound are useful imaging techniques for diagnosis, and both provide a guide for drainage.

Continued feculent drainage raises concern for a fecal fistula. Usually, a fecal fistula is the result of a necrotic appendiceal stump or cecum. A fecal fistula may also suggest a new diagnosis of Crohn disease. Imaging studies should be used to ensure that drainage is adequate and to determine the source of the fistula. A low-output fistula should close in the absence of distal obstruction, neoplasia, radiation, or inflammatory bowel disease.

Special considerations

Pregnancy

The gravid uterus alters both the presentation and the morbidity of appendicitis. The increasing size of the uterus displaces the appendix out of its usual pelvic position, into the mid and upper abdomen. Nausea and vomiting, which often accompany early pregnancy, further confuse the picture. Ultrasound is key to determine the viability of the pregnancy and to diagnose appendicitis. CT scan and magnetic resonance imaging (MRI) have been used, but fear of radiation to a fetus and unknown effects of MRI have made these modalities less popular.

Since miscarriage is associated with appendicitis, early diagnosis and therapy are critical. The incidence of miscarriage is 10% in the absence of perforation, but it increases to 30% in the presence of perforation (10). Concerns about the laparoscopic approach, including decreased uterine blood flow, fetal hypotension and hypoxia, and acidosis due to CO_2, do not seem to be major issues; however, current information is retrospective in nature. In addition, the complications that have been reported with laparoscopy have been associated also with appendicitis, general anesthesia, and the open surgical procedure (11).

Elderly

Although people older than 70 years constitute only 5% to 10% of patients with appendicitis, morbidity and mortality in this age group is high. These patients may have significant comorbidities, which, with atypical and delayed presentations, contribute to an incidence of perforation as high as 70% (12,13). Often, elderly patients with appendicitis are incorrectly diagnosed with diverticulitis and bowel obstruction, and operative intervention may be delayed (14). Recent advances in imaging and laparoscopy have facilitated the diagnosis and treatment of appendicitis. However, adoption of these modalities has not yet influenced results in the elderly, with consistently elevated rates of perforation and morbidity (15).

Tumors of the Appendix

Carcinoid tumor is the most common neoplasm of the appendix. Many carcinoid tumors are discovered incidentally and often only as a histopathologic finding. Therapy depends on size and histologic features. Right hemicolectomy is indicated for tumors >2 cm, for those with evidence of lymphovascular invasion, and for tumors of intermediate size in younger patients.

Mucocele of the appendix is caused by either benign or malignant disease. In the benign form, mucus accumulates distal to an obstruction of the appendiceal lumen. The malignant form is due to mucous cystadenocarcinoma, a tumor that usually does not metastasize but that produces mucus. If the malignant form ruptures, intraperitoneal tumor causes pseudomyxoma peritonei. The large amounts of gelatinous material may cause mechanical obstruction, with debulking and chemotherapy necessary for symptomatic relief. For the benign form of disease, appendectomy is sufficient. For the malignant form, right hemicolectomy is recommended.

Adenocarcinoma of the appendix is rare and presents either as appendicitis or as ruptured, disseminated disease. Right hemicolectomy is recommended to remove the associated lymph nodes.

COLORECTAL SURGERY

Surgical procedures for diseases of the colon and rectum are among the most common procedures performed. Brief summaries of disease processes for which colorectal resection is necessary follow, with discussion of the complications that are common to all the disease processes for which colon or rectal resection is required. Unique complications of the ileal pouch–anal anastomosis will then be outlined, followed by complications distinct to procedures in which an anastomosis is not created—that is, to permanent stoma formation.

INDICATIONS FOR SURGERY

Diverticular disease

Although initial reports early in the 20th century described an incidence of diverticulosis in the 5% to 10% range (16), current estimates describe an occurrence as high as 65% in those older than 85 years. Although diverticulosis is quite common, only 10% to 30% of patients will become symptomatic (17) from inflammation, obstruction, or bleeding.

Multiple classification schemes have been developed to categorize acute inflammatory episodes. The most quoted is the Hinchey classification (18). In the absence of generalized peritonitis, stage I and II presentations may be treated with antimicrobial agents and percutaneous drainage as needed, allowing a delayed, elective procedure. However, the more severe presentations of purulent peritonitis (stage III) or fecal peritonitis (stage IV) mandate emergent resection of the perforated sigmoid colon.

Lower gastrointestinal tract hemorrhage due to diverticula will often cease spontaneously (19) and presents one of the most difficult diagnostic dilemmas within surgery. Angiodysplasia is more common on the right side of the colon. Exclusion of both an anorectal source of bleeding and an upper gastrointestinal cause is necessary. Once these sources have been excluded, colonoscopy is the next step. The opportunity for therapeutic embolization and localization exists with angiography. Prior to operative resection, localization is required to ensure a successful segmental resection.

Ulcerative Colitis

In the United States, this enigmatic disease has an incidence of 5 to 15 per 100,000 (20). The causative agent or provoking elements for ulcerative colitis have not been identified. Familial tendencies do exist. Indications for surgery include toxic megacolon, perforation, bleeding, growth retardation in children and, most commonly, intractability to medical therapy. One of the most serious complications of extensive or long-standing ulcerative colitis is the development of colon or rectal carcinoma. Early in the disease process, the risk is <5%. With an increased duration of the disease, the risk rises to 50% and 75%, respectively, after 30 and 40 years (21).

Total proctocolectomy with ileostomy is the standard against which other operations are measured. The ileal pouch–anal anastomosis was first described in 1978 and has become the most popular curative reconstruction. Usually created with a diverting loop ileostomy, which may itself become the source of complication, this procedure removes the diseased tissue and allows for maintenance of continence. Total abdominal colectomy with ileostomy and the Hartmann procedure or mucus fistula may be performed in the emergent setting.

Crohn Disease

In the United States, the incidence of Crohn disease is approximately 5 per 100,000. The etiology is unknown. Crohn disease is not limited to the colorectum and may involve the gastrointestinal tract anywhere from mouth to anus. Ileocolic disease is the most common, but Crohn colitis may be the only manifestation in up to 45% of patients (22). Disease limited to the anorectum occurs in 5% of patients.

For intractable Crohn colitis, proctocolectomy with ileostomy is the standard of treatment. For limited disease, segmental colectomy or total abdominal colectomy is possible, provided that grossly normal bowel is available for anastomosis.

Familial Adenomatous Polyposis

Familial adenomatous polyposis is an autosomal dominant disease characterized by the development of multiple polyps in the colon. The disease is caused by a deletion mutation in chromosome 5q21 at the adenomatous polyposis coli gene, which normally acts as a tumor suppressor. Relatively common, with an incidence of 1 in 7,000 to 10,000, spontaneous mutations do occur and represent 15% to 20% of patients. Since transformation to malignancy is ensured by the age of 40 years, total proctocolectomy is recommended. Total proctocolectomy has been combined with ileostomy, ileal pouch reconstruction, or ileorectal anastomosis.

Rectal Prolapse

Rectal prolapse is an intussusception of the full thickness of the rectal wall through the anal sphincter. The other disease process that may be confused with rectal prolapse is rectal mucosal or hemorrhoidal prolapse. In contrast to rectal prolapse, where mucosal folds are circular, in hemorrhoidal prolapse, these folds are orientated radially.

Since pathophysiology is poorly understood, a variety of procedures are available for treating this entity. The most popular perineal approaches include those of Altemeier and Delorme, whereas the choices for the abdominal approaches include sutured rectopexy, the Ripstein procedure, anterior resection, abdominal rectopexy, and sigmoid resection, with laparoscopic options available for the abdominal approaches. Variations in recurrence rates have been reported and may influence the choice of procedure.

Ischemic Colitis

The most common form of gastrointestinal ischemia is ischemic colitis. The etiology is believed to be "watershed" areas of colonic blood supply, including the splenic flexure and the rectosigmoid. Treatment of ischemic colitis depends on the degree of injury. With early diagnosis of mild cases, bowel rest with adjunctive intravenous antibiotics is beneficial. Optimization of blood flow to prevent further ischemia is mandatory. More severe cases, with peritonitis, perforation, sepsis, clinical deterioration despite medical therapy, or gangrene, require colectomy.

Colorectal Carcinoma

Recent cancer statistics show that colorectal cancer remains the third most common cause of cancer death in the United States (23). In 2003, approximately 147,000 new cases of colorectal cancer were diagnosed, with approximately 55,100 deaths. In North America, there is a 6% lifetime risk. Since surgical resection is the only curative treatment for colon cancer, colectomy, including the tumor, adequate margins, segmented blood supply, and draining lymph nodes, is the mainstay of treatment.

POSTOPERATIVE COMPLICATIONS OF COLORECTAL SURGERY

Ileus

Postoperative ileus is a form of temporary bowel motor dysfunction that follows operative procedures in the abdomen. This reflex is caused by excitation of the splanchnic sympathetic nerves that occurs during manipulation of the bowel, but it may also be associated with surgery or trauma to other organs. The stomach recovers from this state within several hours, whereas the small bowel requires 1 to 2 days and the colon 2 to 3 days. Recovery that includes coordinated motor function may require up to 5 days. Although the auscultation of bowel sounds or resumption of appetite have been used to herald the resolution of ileus, the passage of flatus is the only true indicator that colonic ileus has resolved. An ileus lasting for longer periods may be associated with peritonitis or hematoma.

Prolonged ileus may be difficult to distinguish from mechanical small bowel obstruction. CT scan is helpful in assessing the possibility of intraabdominal abscess and to determine whether the patient has an ileus or a mechanical small bowel obstruction (24). In the absence of other pathology, supportive care with nasogastric decompression is all that is necessary. Most partial mechanical small bowel obstructions resolve within 1 week with this plan. Because adhesions may be very dense in the perioperative period, reoperation for partial small bowel obstruction should be avoided in the absence of signs of intestinal ischemia. For prolonged postoperative ileus, an alternative is continued bowel rest and nutritional support in the outpatient environment.

Leak

Anastomotic healing occurs as a function of the patient's general condition, and, importantly, of local factors such as blood supply, tension, and the health of the bowel utilized. The mesentery should provide appropriate vasculature to the bowel, with clearance of <5 mm from the cut edge. Tension on the anastomosis may cause disruption and compromise of the blood supply. Thin, healthy bowel is preferred to thickened, inflamed, or edematous bowel.

The risk of operative mortality increases 10-fold with an anastomotic leak. Among the most significant risk factors for anastomotic leak is the location of the anastomosis. In large series, intraabdominal leak rates range from 1% to 5% and pelvic leak rates range from 5% to 30%. The closer the anastomosis is to the anal verge, the higher the probability of leakage. Several studies have noted that anastomoses distal to 7 cm from the anal verge are at the highest risk for leakage (25). Historically, leakage occurred in >30% of low pelvic anastomoses. Contemporary rates are <10%. The improvement may be due to the practice of air insufflation at the time of creation of the anastomosis to verify the absence of a leak and due to improved stapling devices. Diversion of stool in the form of an ostomy does not prevent leak.

Typically, anastomotic leak is discovered 5 to 7 days after surgery (Fig. 38.1). Hindsight usually reveals earlier signs that should make the surgeon more suspicious of a leak, including fever, leukocytosis, localized or generalized tenderness, generalized ileus with abdominal distention, and tachycardia. CT scan is helpful to determine whether there is an associated abscess. In cases where leak is suspected, a gentle Gastrografin enema may assist the diagnosis.

Once recognized, aggressive management of the anastomotic leak is mandatory. Patients with generalized peritonitis require exploration. At exploration, dismantling of the intraabdominal anastomosis and fecal diversion is the goal. In the case of a distal left-sided anastomosis, the inflammatory response may be so intense as to impair safe

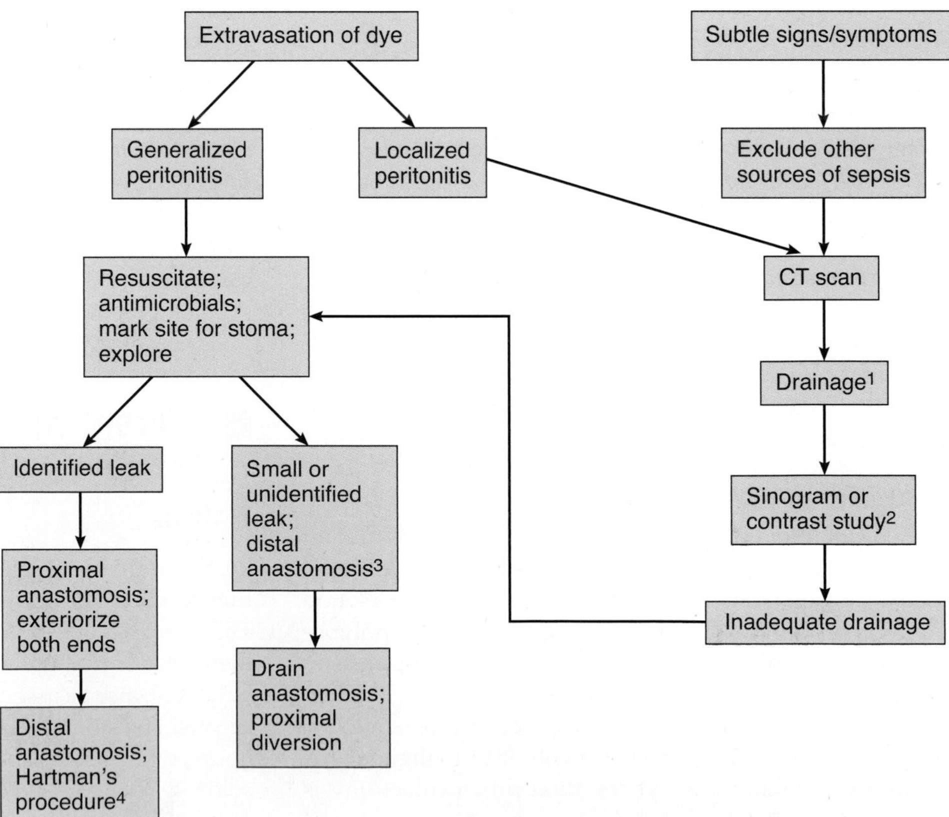

FIGURE 38.1. Algorithm for anastomotic leak. [1]Drainage may usually be accomplished percutaneously, but it may be accomplished either transrectally or by open laparotomy if necessary. [2]If the abscess is associated with an anastomotic leak, a fistulogram or contrast study may be helpful to determine the location, size, and so on, which may be helpful to determine subsequent management. [3,4]In the case of low or distal anastomoses, the inflammatory response may be so intense that dismantling the anastomosis may be difficult. In this situation, lavage, wide drainage, and proximal diversion is the most appropriate operative approach.

recognition of the anastomosis. In these cases, prudent management includes proximal diversion with lavage of the peritoneal cavity and placement of drains near the anastomosis.

If the patient has low-grade sepsis and the leak is subtle enough to require a contrast study to demonstrate and if there is no concurrent abscess, close observation with intravenous antibiotics and bowel rest is initiated. If there is failure of improvement, exploration is necessary.

Abscess

An intraabdominal abscess may be the presenting sign of acute inflammatory conditions such as appendicitis, diverticulitis, perforated colon cancer, or Crohn disease. In the case of elective colorectal surgery, postoperative intraabdominal abscess may be due to a break in technique—spillage of enteric or colonic contents, especially into a hematoma or other devitalized tissues. It may also be the result an anastomotic leak. CT scan is the surest means to determine the presence of an abscess. Although ultrasound may document the amount and the location of fluid, there are no specific sonographic characteristics to distinguish free postoperative fluid from an abscess cavity. Abscesses are usually identified at a time when reentry into the abdomen may be difficult or hazardous, and thus percutaneous drain placement is often a safer and less morbid option for abscess drainage. To treat bacteremia, antibiotics are indicated.

Fistula

Fecal fistula may be the expression of an intraabdominal leak or abscess. CT scanning is necessary to identify the abscess and to direct appropriate drain placement. Antibiotics and supportive care are initiated. In the absence of distal obstruction, foreign body, radiation, or inflammatory bowel disease, many fistulas resolve. Low-output distal colonic fistulas do not routinely require parenteral nutrition. Fistulas originating from proximal small bowel or proximal colonic sources may require this additional supportive care. Fistulas that do not resolve or recur may require surgical correction once the acute inflammation has subsided (Fig. 38.1).

Presacral Hemorrhage

Preservation of the presacral fascia is paramount to preventing this complication, which occurs during rectal mobilization. If a presacral vein is torn, bleeding is brisk but may be controlled with tacks, bone wax, or cautery. Massive hemorrhage occurs in patients who have basivertebral connections to the presacral vein. This anatomy is encountered in approximately 15% of individuals (26). Occlusion with the direct pressure is necessary for temporary arrest of the hemorrhage; permanent hemostasis is possible by inserting a thumbtack into the sacrum over the area of bleeding.

Anastomotic Hemorrhage

The incidence of anastomotic hemorrhage is low, with an incidence of 0.5% to 1% (27). Many anastomotic bleeds are self-limited and do not require intervention. Gastrointestinal hemorrhage in the early postoperative period can be challenging to manage. An upper gastrointestinal source should be excluded. Distal anastomoses may be viewed endoscopically and controlled with injections of dilute epinephrine or short bursts of cautery. The manipulation may increase the incidence of anastomotic leakage. More proximal anastomoses may require exploration for control. If suture reinforcement is not effective or if the bleeding point is not obvious, dismantling the anastomosis with resection and reanastomosis may be required.

Splenic Injury

Splenic injury may occur during operations in which the splenic flexure is mobilized (3%) (28). The injury is usually small, involving a capsular tear at the anterior or medial surface of the spleen's inferior pole. The injury is caused by disrupting the normal splenic attachments or by traction on the omentum. In the case of injury caused by traction on the omentum, the injury may extend to the splenic hilum. To avoid such injuries, the distal omentum should be mobilized prior to the initiation of splenic flexure mobilization.

There are several techniques to preserve the spleen (Fig. 38.2). Pressure, topical hemostatic agents, and cautery can be used for hemostasis for small injuries. For larger injuries, the spleen must be mobilized so that it becomes nearly a midline organ. For larger parenchymatous injuries, an absorbable mesh may be used to wrap the spleen to facilitate tamponade.

Should these measures fail, splenectomy is indicated. The lifelong risk of postsplenectomy infection is nontrivial. Protective vaccination should include encapsulated bacteria such as *Streptococcus pneumoniae* (pneumococcus),

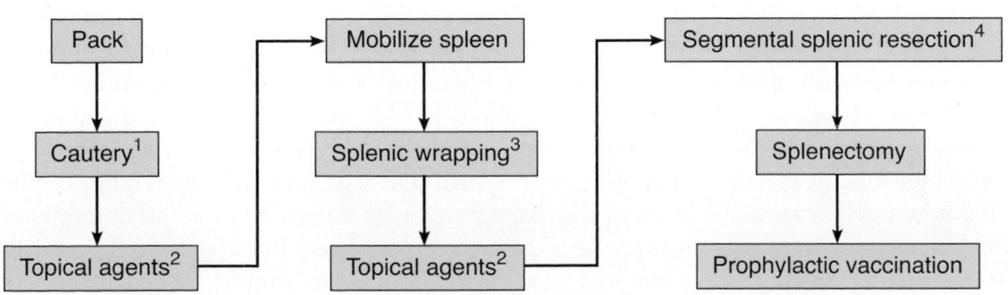

FIGURE 38.2. Algorithm for intraoperative splenic capsular tear. [1]Cautery placed on a high setting may be used to achieve hemostasis. [2]Topical agents such as thrombin with Gelfoam may be used in addition to the above measures. [3]Use of the omentum or polyglycolic mesh may facilitate hemostasis. [4]Preservation of a portion of the spleen in the absence of central arterial supply may not maintain immunocompetency.

Haemophilus influenzae (type B), and *Neisseria meningitidis*. Pneumococcus is the most common and is associated with a mortality rate of 60%. The vaccination for pneumococcus (Pneumovax, Merck, Sharp & Dohme, West Point, New York) utilizes a 23-valent polysaccharide capsular vaccine, which is 90% effective in adults older than 55 years. The reimmunization schedule is every 5 to 10 years. Vaccination for *H. influenzae* is now administered to most children. Immunity from the initial vaccination series may not be sufficient in the asplenic host, and repeat vaccination or determination of effective titers may be necessary. Vaccination for meningococcus is unnecessary for the asplenic patient, except when traveling to an area with increased risk.

Ureteral Injury

Inflammation, radiation, previous surgery, or malignancy alter the anatomic relationship of the colorectum and the ureter and is associated with iatrogenic ureteral injury. For colorectal surgery, an incidence of 0.3% to 10% has been reported (29). Recognition of injury is critical, since immediate repair results in improved healing. Delayed recognition is associated with significant morbidity, and it increases the incidence of nephrectomy sevenfold (30).

In colonic operations, the left ureter is more commonly injured than the right ureter. The abdominal ureter originates at the renal pelvis and travels superficial to the psoas muscle. As the ureter enters the pelvis, it crosses the bifurcation of the iliac arteries, passing posteriorly and inferiorly along the pelvis to the levator muscles before entering the posterior bladder. In women, the distal ureter passes in the ureterosacral ligament behind the ovary and continues inferiorly in the broad ligament. In colorectal procedures several types of injuries may occur: crush, partial or complete transaction, ligation, or devascularization.

These injuries occur in association with ligation of the inferior mesenteric vessels, division of the lateral rectal stalks, and surgery in the cul-de-sac or sacral promontory or during reperitonealization. Intraoperatively, if the surgeon is suspicious of ureteral injury or is unable to identify the ureter, administration of indigo carmine or methylene blue may be helpful (Fig. 38.3). Unfortunately, these maneuvers do not aid in the identification of a ureteral ligation but only of a transection injury. If transection is suspected, a retrograde study, either with contrast or via cystoscopy with stent placement, may identify the injury (Fig. 38.3).

If an injury is identified, a urologist should be consulted to perform the repair. The principles involved in repair include debridement of devitalized tissues, a tension-free anastomosis that is spatulated and repaired with fine, absorbable, monofilament sutures over a stent, with drainage. For most injuries, ureteroureterostomy is sufficient. With significant tissue loss, the kidney, bladder, and ureter may require additional mobilization and advanced reconstruction, including a psoas hitch, Boari flap, ureteroneocystostomy, or transureteroureterostomy (Fig. 38.4).

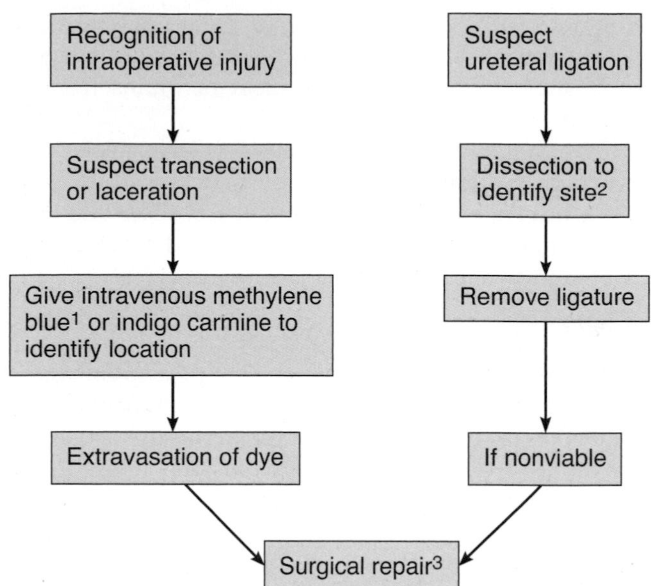

FIGURE 38.3. Algorithm for intraoperative ureteral injury. If the ureteral injury is confirmed urologic consultation is indicated. [1]Administration of methylene blue causes the urine to have a blue color and may transiently decrease oxygenation as measured by pulse oximetry. Indigo carmine is not associated with this transient decrement. [2]If the ureter is not able to be clearly delineated, cystotomy with passage of a ureteral catheter proximally may aid in the identification. [3]Proper surgical repair depends on the injury's area and extent. Proximal to the pelvic rim, a ureteroureterostomy may be used. To facilitate a tension-free repair, not only is the ureter mobilized but also both the bladder and the kidney may be mobilized. The repair should be spatulated, sutured with absorbable monofilament suture over a stent, and drained. Injuries to the ureter within 5 cm of the bladder may be repaired with a ureteroneocystostomy. To minimize the tension on this repair, a psoas hitch or Boari flap may be indicated.

Although preoperative ureteral stenting in situations in which a difficult dissection is anticipated has not been shown to decrease the incidence of injury, stenting may facilitate identification of injuries (31). A small number of complications have been documented, including failure to pass the stents, hematuria, and reflex anuria upon stent removal.

Bladder Dysfunction

This complication of procedures on the rectum is multifactorial. Injury to the parasympathetic nerves that innervate the detrusor muscle or to the sympathetic nerves that innervate the bladder neck, trigone, and urethra during the pelvic dissection may be contributory. Postoperative bladder distension, prostatic hypertrophy, medication, and pain may all contribute.

Bladder dysfunction occurs in 20% to 30% of patients following rectal dissection (32). Leaving the Foley catheter in place for several days after surgery may allow for some of the immediate operative edema, pain, and diuresis to resolve. The patient who is maintained on medication for prostatic hypertrophy should reinitiate this medication for 48 hours prior to an attempt at spontaneous voiding. If the patient develops frequency, especially of small amounts of urine, the catheter is replaced and the trial of void is reinitiated in a few days. Urinalysis should be performed to

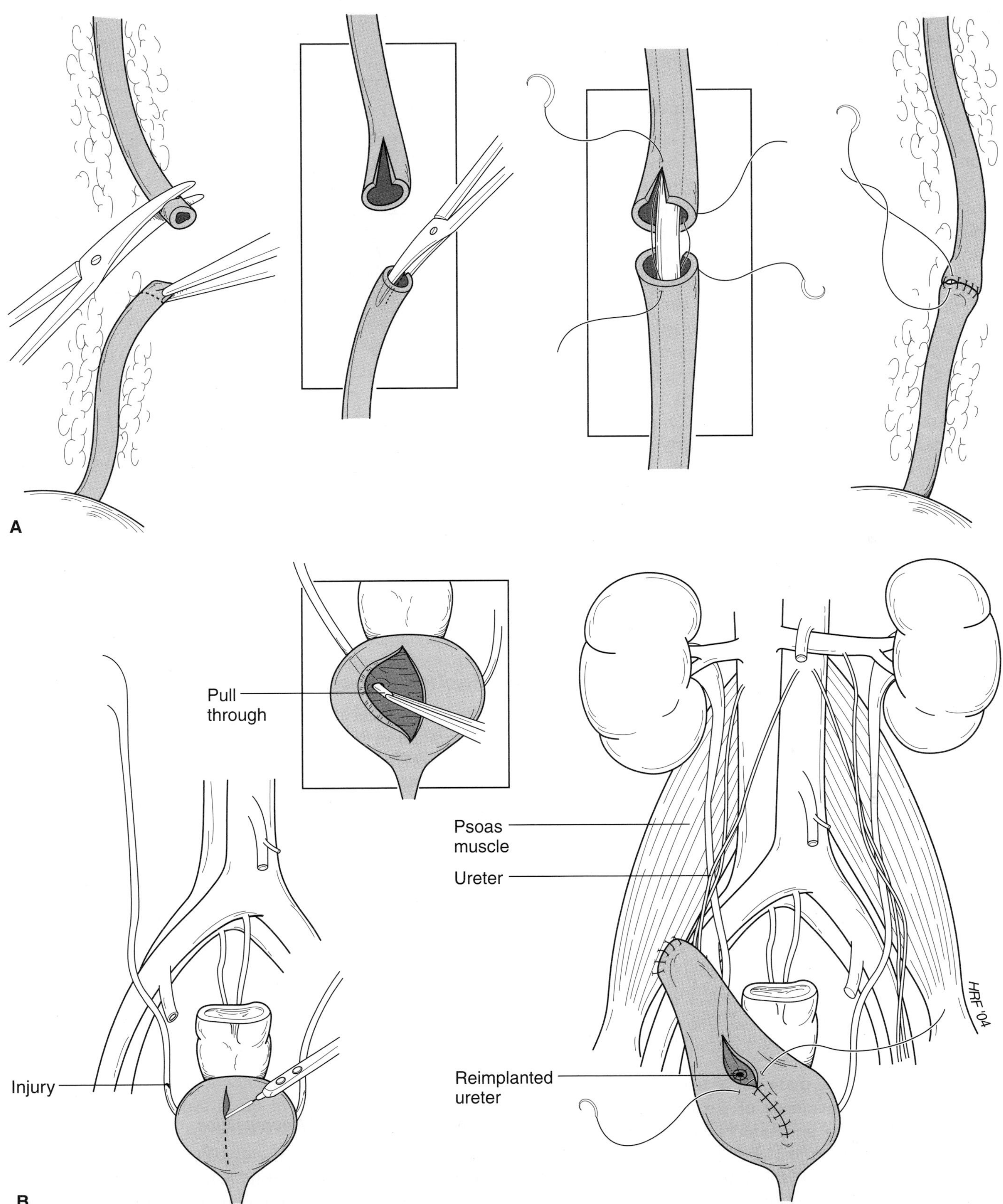

FIGURE 38.4. Surgical options for repair of ureteral injury. **A:** Ureteroureterostomy. The repair is completed in a tension-free manner. The ends are spatulated, and monofilament absorbable suture is used to affect the repair over a stent. The area is drained. **B:** Psoas hitch. In the pelvis, if the ureter is injured, the ureter may be reimplanted into the bladder and tension on the repair alleviated by approximation of the superior bladder to the psoas tendon. (*continued*)

Pouchitis

Pouchitis represents acute or chronic inflammation of the ileal reservoir. Although it is common in patients with ulcerative colitis, pouchitis is essentially absent in those who have had restorative proctocolectomy for polyposis. Pathogenesis is poorly understood and includes bacterial stasis, ischemia, recurrent ulcerative colitis, and fatty acid deficiency. Other theories include overproduction of nitric oxide and free radical production (51). The incidence of pouchitis is not related to the type of pouch created. The prevalence of acute pouchitis varies from 10% to 60% (52). However, 5% to 15% of patients suffer from chronic pouchitis, although only 1% to 3% of the patients require pouch excision (53).

Symptoms of pouchitis include bleeding, increased stool frequency, abdominal discomfort, and fever. In addition to these clinical symptoms, endoscopic findings include mucosal edema, granularity, friability, loss of vascular pattern, mucous exudates, and ulceration, with histologic evidence of acute leukocyte infiltration and ulceration. Initial treatment includes administration of metronidazole. Alternatives include ciprofloxacin, erythromycin, and tetracycline. Topical anti-inflammatory agents, including steroid enemas, mesalamine enemas, and suppositories, may be attempted. If there is no response, oral agents may be used to supplement local measures. Unfortunately, this strategy returns patients to the regimens they so wanted to leave behind. Oral bismuth or other immunosuppressants, including azathioprine, may be successful in aborting symptoms. Ultimately, if the condition persists, pouchitis may necessitate pouch excision.

Poor Pouch Function

Although >85% of patients are pleased with pouch activity, a minority will have poor pouch function. The incidence of total failure requiring pouch excision, with the establishment of permanent ileostomy, is 3% to 10% (54). The most common causes leading to pouch failure include pelvic sepsis, pouch fistulization, and Crohn disease (55).

Stoma complications

Although many complications are avoidable with careful creation and siting of the stoma and enterostomal nursing, a significant number of patients will have problems ranging from a mild skin irritation to parastomal hernia.

Dermatitis

Dermatitis is very common (>30%), with most cases occurring during the first year after stoma formation (56). Contact dermatitis may take two forms: due to the stomal effluent or due to the pouch, its solvents, or adhesives. Effluent dermatitis is an inflammation or excoriation of the skin due to leakage of the stoma output. More common in patients with an ileostomy or urostomy, approximately 20% of colostomy patients will have this type of dermatitis (57). Gut enzymes and bile are irritating to the skin and damage the keratinized surface. Some aspects may be corrected with patient education by teaching patients to cut a correctly sized aperture to avoid improper placement or pancaking. *Pancaking* refers to lack of air in the appliance, which creates negative pressure and causes the appliance's plastic sides to stick together, thus preventing stool from passing freely into the appliance. Other causes of effluent dermatitis include an overfull appliance, an appliance that is left on too long, or an excessively liquid output.

Other etiologies relate to preoperative and intraoperative management. For example, a poor stoma site leading to poor visualization of the appliance or an inadequate seal may contribute to leakage. Similarly, the creation of a stoma that lacks an adequate spout will cause leakage deep to the appliance. Ideally, ileostomies should be created with a 2- to 3-cm spout and should be everted. Techniques to enhance eversion include circumferential suture placement before tying down. The mesentery of the end of the ileum must provide good blood supply without tension; lack of these factors contributes to retraction.

Allergic contact dermatitis is caused by an antigenic response to a stomal product. A systematic review of possible etiologic agents is necessary so that a nonoffending substitute product may be identified.

Enterostomal nurses are instrumental for the preoperative siting, education, and continued support of these patients. Their input has been documented to improve the lives of ostomates (58,59).

Prolapse

Although alarming to the patient when prolapse initially occurs, there is usually no functional significance (Fig. 38.5). An overly large fascial defect contributes to the pathophysiology. Prolapse is more common with loop than with end stomas and is more common with colostomies than with ileostomies. In the acute setting, osmotic therapy with table sugar may shrink an incarcerated prolapse sufficiently to allow reduction (60). The

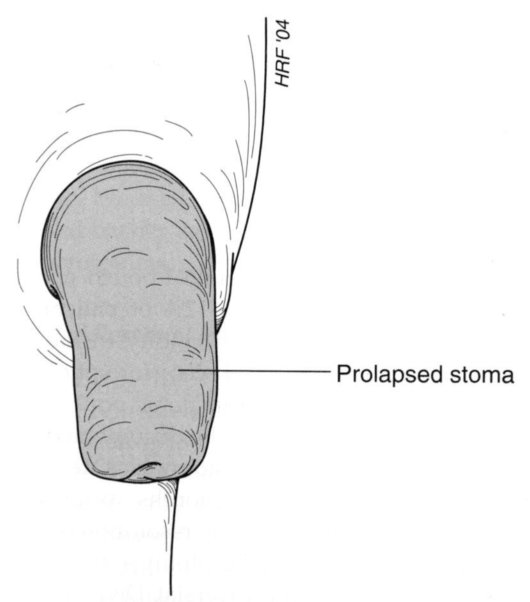

FIGURE 38.5. Stomal prolapse.

long-term prolapse rate for all types of stomas is approximately 11% to 12% (61,62).

Simple prolapse may be repaired by mobilizing the mucocutaneous junction and resecting the redundant bowel through a local incision. Recurrence may require laparotomy and resiting of the stoma. For patients in whom a full laparotomy is ill-advised with prolapse from either a loop or transverse colostomy, a procedure that strips the redundant mucosa with plication of the bowel from the apex to the mucocutaneous junction may be performed (63).

Retraction

Stomal retraction occurs as a result of the failure to mobilize sufficient bowel and its mesentery to avoid tension. Retraction occurs in 1% to 6% of colostomies (64,65) and 3% to 17% of ileostomies (62). Retraction permits the stomal effluent to seep underneath the appliance and may result in pouch loosening.

Although local procedures may be sufficient for the management of retraction, laparotomy is often necessary. For left-sided end colostomies, mobilization of the splenic flexure may be required to produce a tension-free mucocutaneous apposition. If the mesentery is providing tension, the use of the "end-loop" or "divided loop" stoma, in which the stapled ends are left in place, with opening and maturation of only the stapled proximal end, may provide additional length.

Necrosis

Early postoperative necrosis is secondary to vascular insufficiency at the distal edge of the stoma, either due to arterial insufficiency or venous congestion. This complication is caused by mesenteric ischemia with overtrimming of the mesentery from the end of the bowel, inadequate proximal mobilization, or too tight a fascial opening. Immediately postoperatively, a normal stoma may appear dusky due to venous engorgement or stomal edema; this appearance should evolve to a bright pink color as these processes resolve. Necrosis is more likely in patients who are obese and in those who have undergone an emergent procedure, encompassing 1% to 10% of colostomies and 1% to 5% of ileostomies (66).

If necrosis is suspected, the immediate question relates to the depth and extent of necrosis. This determination is facilitated by the placement of a clear glass or plastic tube inside the stoma and shining a pen flashlight down the barrel. If necrosis extends to the level of the fascia, reoperation is necessary to prevent tension, retraction, stricture, or passage of fecal material into the peritoneal cavity.

Stenosis

Stomal stenosis occurs in 2% to 10% of end ileostomies and colostomies (58). The stricturing of Crohn disease may increase stomal stenosis (62). At the minimum, stenosis may cause loud passage of air and bowel content into the appliance, and at worst, it may cause obstruction.

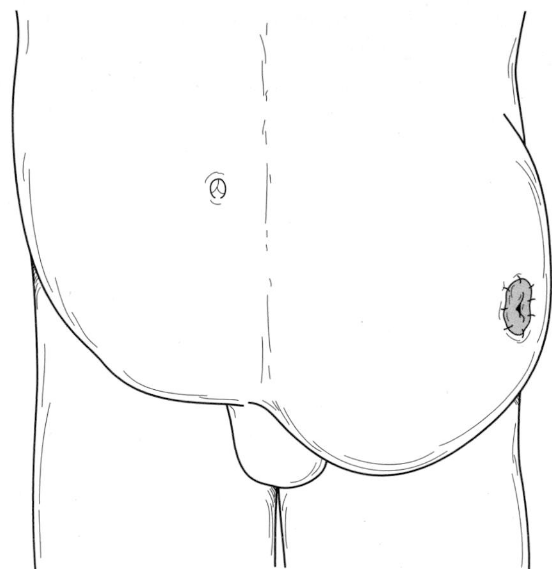

FIGURE 38.6. Parastoma hernia associated with nonprotruding stoma may be associated with obstruction, peristomal skin care, and pouching difficulty.

For colostomies, stricture almost always occurs at the skin level. Since most colostomies are now matured at the time of creation, stricture is the result of necrosis of the distal stoma. Minor stricture may be managed by daily manual dilation. Long length narrowing, especially when due to ischemia, tension, or Crohn disease, requires laparotomy for complete mobilization.

Parastomal Hernia

Parastomal hernias are challenging problems, occurring in up to 37% of colostomies and 16% of ileostomies (58). Similar to other types of incisional hernias, parastomal hernias are more common in patients with obesity, malnutrition, steroid dependency, or wound infection (Fig. 38.6).

Indications for repair include difficulty with appliance adherence, pain, incarceration or strangulation, poor location, or an association with other stoma-related problems such as stricture. Options to repair the hernia locally include application of mesh. Newer options for mesh repair or reinforcement include porcine collagen, which is resistant to absorption, permitting a scaffold for native collagen, resisting infection and an inflammatory response.

The recurrence rate of parastomal hernia is quite high, ranging from 33% to 50% after relocation (67), 50% to 100% after fascial repair, and 50% after prosthetic repair. In addition, after relocation nearly half of patients will develop an incisional hernia.

ANORECTAL SURGERY

Hemorrhoidectomy

Vascular "cushions" consisting of bundles of submucosa with an arteriovenous network, smooth muscle, and elastic and connective tissues are present in every patient. The term *hemorrhoids* usually refers to pathologic conditions associated with these "cushions." Primary internal hemorrhoids lie in constant positions: right anterior, right posterior, and left lateral. External hemorrhoids are distal to the dentate line, whereas internal hemorrhoids are proximal to the dentate line.

Early complications of hemorrhoidectomy

Bleeding

Bleeding that occurs in the recovery room is due to technical error, most commonly the result of inadequate ligation of the vascular pedicle. To control significant hemorrhage, a Foley catheter with the balloon inflated can be inserted to tamponade the hemorrhage as the operating room is prepared.

Pain

The moderate degree of anal pain and rectal spasm is common after hemorrhoidectomy. Pain not only is challenging to manage but also contributes to urinary retention and fecal impaction. Multiple approaches have been used to minimize this expected outcome. Ketorolac tromethamine has been given intravenously, with subsequent recommendations for the outpatient intake of anti-inflammatory agents. In the belief that low-grade infection may contribute to pain, metronidazole has been given intravenously, with follow-up outpatient dosing for 3 to 7 days. Although initially noted to have positive responses, later studies reveal no efficacy (68). Perioperative application of 0.2% glyceryl trinitrate ointment, in an effort to increase blood flow and relax the sphincter muscles, has also been attempted, with mixed success (69). Even postoperative pain pumps placed directly into the anal canal have received some attention (69).

Severe anal pain may be a sign of a perianal hematoma. The dressing should be removed and the wound inspected. Undue tension in the closure is the most likely cause of discomfort; it is better to leave a wound open than to close it with excessive tension.

Urinary Retention

Urinary retention occurs with an incidence from 3% to 20% (70,71). This complication's etiology is multifactorial. Contributing factors include prostatic hypertrophy fluid overload, rectal pain and spasm, high ligation of the hemorrhoidal pedicle, heavy suture material, tight packing, bulky dressings, anticholinergics, and narcotics (70). Anorectal surgery may decrease parasympathetic input to the detrusor muscle, whereas pain may increase sympathetic input to the urethral sphincter, both contributing to spasm.

Intraoperative fluids should be limited to avoid perioperative bladder distension. Patients are asked to void prior to entry into the operating room, where intravenous fluids are limited to 500 mL or less. Patients who receive a local anesthetic with sedation have a decreased incidence of this complication.

If the patient is unable to void, the subject should undergo catheterization. If residual is >500 cc, the catheter should be left in place, with a trial of voiding in 24 hours. With a residual <500 cc, the catheter should be removed, and a trial of voiding reinitiated. Urinary retention may also be an early sign of severe perineal infection—a rare complication of hemorrhoidectomy.

Fecal Impaction

Fecal impaction is serious, although rare, occurring in 0.4% of patients after hemorrhoidectomy (72). Most patients dread their first posthemorrhoidectomy bowel movement due to the anticipated discomfort. They must be warned that constipation that evolves into impaction is even more uncomfortable. Constipation should be prevented with laxatives, stool softeners, oral fiber, adequate hydration, and activity.

Impaction may be difficult to diagnose postoperatively. Perineal discomfort, lack of bowel function, and overflow diarrhea are dominant symptoms. Discomfort out of proportion to operative trauma is a common finding. If rectal examination is possible, the fecal bolus is palpable. A high enema given with a red rubber catheter may be all that is required to allow stool egress. In cases when discomfort is severe and disimpaction is not possible, evacuation in the operating room with the assistance of anesthesia may be necessary.

Late Complications of Hemorrhoidectomy

Anal Tags. After hemorrhoidectomy, the anal area becomes edematous. Occasionally, external thrombosed hemorrhoids may occur, and in the resolution, a skin tag is left. Tags may also simply be a manifestation of wound healing. Nuisance skin tags may cause discomfort to the patient if they impair local hygiene.

Stricture. Removal of an excessive amount of mucosa, especially anoderm, is responsible for anal stricture. Acute management of hemorrhoids with extirpation of all the edematous, inflamed, or thrombosed tissue may lead to inadequate elastic anal tissue, which, as healing progresses, leads to a fibrous scar. This complication may result in the elective setting as well, and adequate anodermal bridges are necessary to preserve sufficient tissue to prevent its occurrence. Indicators to help prevent this complication include tension-free placement of a large-sized Hill–Ferguson retractor and at least 1-cm bridges between each excised area.

If stricture is a long-term outcome of the procedure, postoperative dilation, ensuring the passage of stool, and maintained physician observation is necessary. If stricturing ensues and is epithelialized and fixed, anoplasty is indicated.

Anoplasty involves mobilization of perianal skin to cover a defect in the anal canal. If the stricturing process involves the sphincter, a careful lateral sphincterotomy may be indicated as well. Anoplasty flaps take many shapes, including V–Y, Y–V, house, and rotational flaps. The stricture's length and depth, along with the local tissue availability, dictate which flap is preferred (Fig. 38.7).

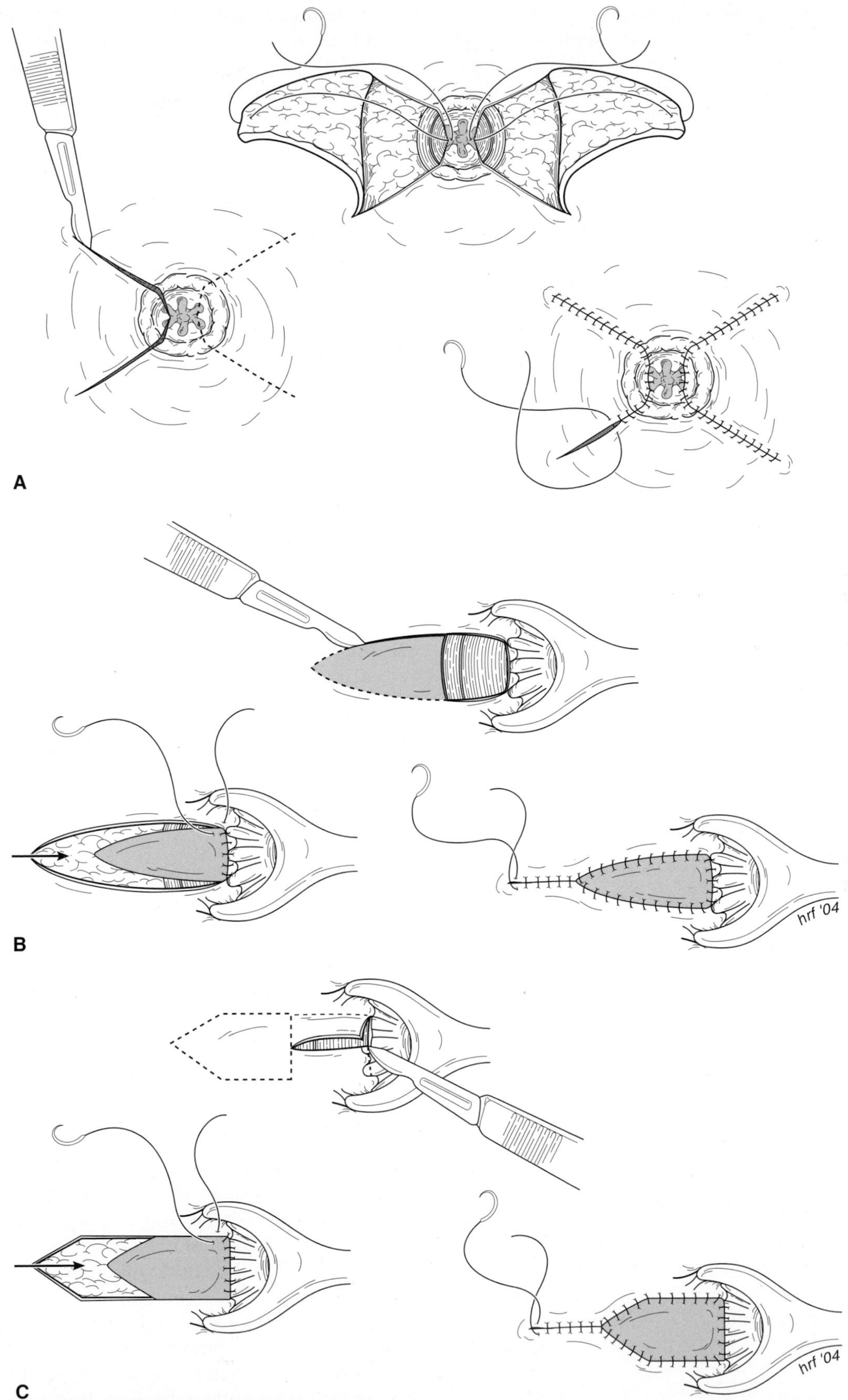

FIGURE 38.7. Anoplasty for stricture/stenosis. **A:** Bilateral V-flaps advance into the anal canal. **B:** V–Y flap may be repeated bilaterally. **C:** House flaps are a modification of the V–Y flap, may be repeated on the contralateral side, and may advance additional anoderm into the canal.

Mucosal Prolapse and Ectropion. Inadequate removal of redundant mucosa at the time of hemorrhoidectomy contributes to prolapsing mucosa. Patients will report a wet lump of tissue discharging mucus that requires manual reduction. The wet perianal tissue contributes to local pruritus. Rubber band ligation may effectively deal with this complication.

An ectropion results when rectal mucosa descends and heals outside the anal canal. Ectropion may result from mobilization of the rectal mucosa and fixing the mucosa to the anoderm. Similar to mucosal prolapse, the "wet anus" produces mucus that contributes to discomfort and pruritus.

If the ectropion is evident in a limited area, the mucosa may be excised, with suture fixation of the remaining distal rectal edge to the proximal sphincter. If the ectropion is more pronounced, an anoplasty may be indicated.

Incontinence. Anal sensation may be impaired in up to 50% of patients after hemorrhoidectomy, but by 6 weeks, the majority resolve their symptoms (73). Classically, hemorrhoidectomy removes vascular tissue superficial to the sphincter muscles. The elderly are especially at risk for this complication. Careful preoperative questioning is necessary to discern preexisting incontinence, although the symptoms may be mild.

Anal fissure

A fissure is a painful linear tear or ulcer in the anal canal, distal to the dentate line that may extend to the anal margin. Primary fissures are most often due to a change in bowel habits and are located posteriorly, with 10% in women and 1% in men located anteriorly. Secondary fissures are due to inflammatory bowel disease, sexually transmitted diseases, neoplasms, or trauma and are located laterally.

At least 85% of acute fissures will respond to medical management (74,75). Relief of constipation and management of spasm with a high-fiber diet, stool softeners, sitz baths, and mild analgesics are foremost in the nonoperative approach. "Chemical sphincterotomy" with nitroglycerin or nifedipine ointment or botulinum toxin can decrease anal resting pressure and increase blood flow to facilitate healing. When medical management fails, lateral internal sphincterotomy should be considered.

Complications of Internal Sphincterotomy

Abscess. The incidence of abscess following the closed internal sphincterotomy is <1%, nearly always associated with an anal fistula (76). As with other abscesses and fistulas related to cryptoglandular disease, principles of treatment include drainage of the abscess and management of the fistula.

Recurrence/Nonhealing Wound. Following lateral internal sphincterotomy, the recurrence rate ranges from 0% to 12% (77,78). Recent literature suggests a failure rate of <5%. When failure of sphincterotomy is documented, an ultrasound and anal manometry are indicated prior to performance of a second lateral sphincterotomy on the opposite side. If the initial sphincterotomy is anatomically correct and fears of incontinence are present, treatment with botulinum toxin is indicated. The possibility of another process, particularly Crohn disease, must be explored.

Incontinence. The length of internal sphincter that may be safely divided to treat patients with anal fissure and the closed versus open approach to sphincterotomy continue to be debated. Although most symptoms are due to incontinence to flatus, which usually resolves, there is persistence of fecal incontinence of 1% to 2%. When the length of sphincter divided is examined by ultrasound, more sphincter may have been transected than was intended (79). With short follow-up, a 0.5-cm open sphincterotomy yielded only a 3% incidence of postprocedural incontinence to fluid and flatus (80). Others have suggested tailoring the length of sphincter divided, depending on the length of the fissure, with no incidence of incontinence of feces or stool leakage (81). Preoperative assessment of continence of gas and stool is essential for appropriate patient selection.

Anorectal abscesses

Anorectal abscess is a common surgical emergency. In the acute phase the abscess produces signs of inflammation: erythema, pain, heat, and loss of function, seen at or near the anal verge. However, an intersphincteric abscess may not be visible at this level and may require examination under anesthesia both for diagnosis and management. Likewise, a deep ischiorectal abscess may be difficult to detect on preliminary physical examination, especially in the immunocompromised host.

The presence of an abscess mandates surgical drainage. Although drainage may often be accomplished in the office, large abscesses, pain without an appreciable source, significant cellulitis, or an uncooperative patient may require examination and drainage in the operating room. The drainage site is selected over the area of greatest fluctuance, close to, but not into, the sphincter complex.

Complications of Abscess Drainage

Incomplete Drainage. The major cause of recurrent anorectal abscesses is inadequate drainage. Most causes are due to cryptoglandular disease, and drainage is necessary. If the origin cannot be ascribed to an anorectal source, extra-anal sources include hidradenitis suppurativa or pilonidal disease. Chrabot et al. (82) reported that >70% of patients with recurrent abscesses have fistula, with 30% of these patients having undergone a prior procedure.

Horseshoe abscesses present a special challenge and can present recurrently if the opposite arm of the abscess is incompletely drained. Horseshoe abscesses may occur in three planes: the intersphincteric plane, the ischioanal plane, or the supralevator plane. Classically, the horseshoe originates from the posterior midline and enters the deep postanal space with arms extending anteriorly. The opposite configuration may also occur. Entrance into the deep postanal space and drainage, consisting of counterincisions placed radially, allow drainage of pus and rapid healing of the tracts.

Intersphincteric abscess may present without external signs of inflammation in patients who have symptoms of an abscess. These patients often will not permit digital rectal examination and will require an examination under anesthesia. Once the abscess is identified, it is unroofed to the level of the dentate line, allowing drainage of the offending crypt. The edges of the wound are sutured for hemostasis, which also permits continued drainage.

Necrotizing Perineal Infections. In fewer than 1% of cases, anorectal suppuration may be the cause of necrotizing perineal infection (83). Patients particularly at risk include those with immunocompromise, including diabetes, renal insufficiency, and inflammatory bowel disease. In these high-risk groups, necrosis can occur in the absence of an obvious source of infection, and systemic toxicity can be severe.

Aggressive resuscitation is required with parenteral antibiotics and extensive debridement. Return trips to the operating room may be necessary to remove devitalized tissue. The anorectal fistulous origin must be identified and appropriately managed.

Fistula. Although not truly a complication, a fistula remains in 30% to 70% of patients presenting with an abscess. The abscess is the distal expression of the fistula.

Fistula-in-Ano

An abscess is usually due to a cryptoglandular infection from anal duct obstruction. Approximately half do not heal but eventuate into a fistula. A fistula is an abnormal connection between two epithelial structures—in this case, the mucosa of the anal canal and the skin. Other causes of fistulas include inflammatory bowel disease, anorectal malignancy, actinomycosis, trauma, sexually transmitted diseases, and pelvic sepsis.

Although most fistulas stem from an original intersphincteric source (56%), other fistulas are transsphincteric (21%), suprasphincteric (4%), or extrasphincteric (3%). Patients present with intermittent pain, which may herald bloody or purulent discharge. An external opening is usually identified, but the internal opening may not be obvious on routine office anoscopy.

Intraoperative techniques for identification of the internal opening include the instillation of methylene blue or hydrogen peroxide. Complex fistulas may require ultrasound, CT, or MRI to determine the pathway of the tract and the possible source.

Management is individualized, but the goals are to eradicate the infection and the source, prevent recurrence, and maintain continence. Although the surest method for abolishing the infection is to perform a fistulotomy, this technique also divides the most muscle and may contribute to incontinence. Anterior fistulas, especially in women, may require alternative management, including seton placement, mucosal advancement flaps, or ligation of intersphincteric fistula tract, to achieve the goals outlined earlier.

Complications of Surgery for Fistula-in-Ano

Recurrence after Fistulotomy. After fistulotomy, recurrence is noted in 4% to 10% of cases (84). The most common cause of recurrence is failure to identify the primary internal opening. Other factors include complex fistulas with horseshoe or upward extensions, prior surgery, and failure of adequate fistulotomy for fear of causing incontinence. Crohn disease may also contribute to recurrence. Management of acute suppuration, followed by adjunctive imaging, by using ultrasound or MRI, is helpful to define the tract and the offending anal gland.

Incontinence after Fistulotomy. The reported rates for incontinence following fistulotomy range from 10% to 50% (85). Although most agree that severance of the anorectal ring results in incontinence, the question of how much muscle may be safely divided is still unanswered and may depend on age, gender, previous anorectal or local procedures (e.g., an episiotomy), and location (anterior vs. posterior). When decreased continence is a consideration, staged management of the tract is most prudent.

REFERENCES

1. Addiss DG, Shaffer N, Fowler BS, et al. The epidemiology of appendicitis and appendectomy in the United States. *Am J Epidemiol* 1990;132:920–925.
2. Lewis FR, Holcroft JW, Boey J, et al. Appendicitis: a critical review of the diagnosis and treatment in 1000 cases. *Arch Surg* 1975;110:677–684.
3. Peck J, Peck A, Peck C, et al. The clinical role of noncontrast helical computed tomography in the diagnosis of acute appendicitis. *Am J Surg* 2000;180:133–136.
4. Gale ME, Birnbaum S, Stephen GG, et al. CT appearance of appendicitis and its local complications. *J Comput Assist Tomogr* 1985;9:34–37.
5. Oliak D, Yamini D, Udani VM, et al. Initial nonoperative management for periappendiceal abscess. *Dis Colon Rectum* 2001;44(7):936–941.
6. Bagi P, Dueholm S. Nonoperative management of the ultrasonically evaluated appendiceal mass. *Surgery* 1987;101:602–605.
7. Deakin DE, Ahmed I. Interval appendectomy after resolution of adult inflammatory appendix mass—is it necessary? *Surgeon* 2007;5(1):45–50.
8. Lemieur TP, Rodriguez JL, Jacobs DM, et al. Wound management in perforated appendicitis. *Am Surg* 1999;65:339–443.
9. Sauerland S, Lefering R, Neugebauer EA. Laparoscopic versus open surgery for suspected appendicitis. *Cochrane Database Syst Rev* 2004;(4):CD001546.
10. Fisher KS, Ross DS. Guidelines for therapeutic decision in incidental appendectomy. *Surg Gynecol Obstet* 1990;171:95–98.
11. Fatum M, Rojansky N. Laparoscopic surgery during pregnancy. *Obstet Gynecol Surv* 2001;56(1):50–59.
12. Hardin D. Acute appendicitis: review and update. *Am Fam Physician* 1999;60:2027–2036.
13. Yamini D, Hernan V, Bongard F, et al. Perforated appendicitis: is it truly a surgical urgency? *Am Surg* 1998;64:970–975.
14. Storm-Dickerson TL, Horattas MC. What have we learned over the past 20 years about appendicitis in the elderly? *Am J Surg* 2003;185:198–201.

15. Hui TT, Major KM, Avital I, et al. Outcome of elderly patients with appendicitis. *Arch Surg* 2002;137:995–1000.
16. Painter NS, Burkitt DP. Diverticular disease of the colon: a 20th century problem. *Clin Gastroenterol* 1975;4:3.
17. Ryan P. Two kinds of diverticular disease. *Ann R Coll Surg Engl* 1991;73: 73–79.
18. Hinchey EJ, Schaal PGH, Richards GK. Treatment of perforated disease of the colon. *Adv Surg* 1978;12:86–109.
19. Forde KA, Treat MR. Colonoscopy for lower gastrointestinal bleeding. In: Dent TL, Strudel SF, Turcotte JG, et al., eds. *Surgical endoscopy*. Chicago, IL: Yearbook Medical Publishers; 1988:261–275.
20. Garland CF, Lilienfeld AM, Mendeloff AI, et al. Incidence rates of ulcerative colitis and Crohn's disease in fifteen areas of the United States. *Gastroenterology* 1981;81:1115–1124.
21. Devroede G. Risk of cancer in inflammatory bowel disease. In: Winawer SJ, Schottenfeld D, Sherlock P, eds. *Colorectal cancer: prevention, epidemiology and screening*. New York, NY: Raven; 1980: 325–334.
22. Ritchie JK. The results of surgery for large bowel Crohn's disease. *Ann R Coll Surg Engl* 1990;72:155–157.
23. Jemal A, Murray T, Samuels A, et al. Cancer statistics. *CA Cancer J Clin* 2003;53(1):5–26.
24. Frager DH, Baer JW, Rothpearl A, et al. Distinction between postoperative ileus and mechanical small-bowel obstruction: value of CT compared with clinical and other radiographic findings. *AJR Am J Roentgenol* 1995;164(4):891–894.
25. Vignali A, Fazio VW, Lavery IC, et al. Factors associated with the occurrence of leaks in stapled rectal anastomoses: a review of 1014 patients. *J Am Coll Surg* 1997;185:105–113.
26. Wang O, Shi W, Zhaw Y, et al. New concepts in severe presacral hemorrhage during proctectomy. *Arch Surg* 1985;120:1015–1020.
27. Dochetry JG, McGregor JR, Akyol AM, et al. Comparison of manually constructed and stapled anastomoses in colorectal surgery. *Ann Surg* 1995;221:176–184.
28. Langevin JM, Rothenberger DA, Goldberg SM. Accidental splenic injury during surgical treatment of the colon and rectum. *Surg Gynecol Obstet* 1984;159:139–144.
29. Fry DE, Milhalen L, Harbeecht R. Iatrogenic ureteral injury. *Arch Surg* 1983;118:454.
30. McGinty DM, Mendez R. Traumatic ureteral injuries with delayed recognition. *Urology* 1977;10:115–117.
31. Bothwell WN, Bleicher RJ, Dent TL. Prophylactic ureteral catheterization in colon surgery: a five-year review. *Dis Colon Rectum* 1994;37: 330–334.
32. Janu NC, Bokey EL, Chapuis PH, et al. Bladder dysfunction following anterior resection for carcinoma of the rectum. *Dis Colon Rectum* 1986;29: 182–183.
33. Walsh PC, Schlegel PN. Radical pelvic surgery with preservation of sexual function. *Ann Surg* 1988;208:391–400.
34. Hojo K, Sawada T, Moriya Y. An analysis of survival and voiding, sexual function after wide iliopelvic lymphadenectomy in patients with carcinoma of the rectum, compared with conventional lymphadenectomy. *Dis Colon Rectum* 1989;32:128–133.
35. Lindsay I, George B, Kettlewell M, et al. Randomised, double-blind, placebo-controlled trial of sildenafil (Viagra) for erectile dysfunction after rectal excision for cancer and inflammatory bowel disease. *Dis Colon Rectum* 2002;45(6):727–732.
36. Rasmussen OO, Peterson IK, Christianson J. Anorectal function following low anterior resection. *Colorectal Dis* 2003;5(3):258–261.
37. Ikeuchi H, Kasunoki M, Shoji Y, et al. Clinicophysiological results after sphincter-preserving resection for rectal carcinoma. *Int J Colorectal Dis* 1996;11:172–176.
38. Brasch RC, Bufo AJ, Kreienberg PF, et al. Femoral neuropathy secondary to the use of self-retaining retractor. Report of three cases and review of the literature. *Dis Colon Rectum* 1995;38:1115–1118.
39. Goldman JA, Feldberg D, Dicker D, et al. Femoral neuropathy subsequent to abdominal hysterectomy: a comprehensive study. *Eur J Obstet Gynecol Reprod Biol* 1985;20:385–392.
40. Dillavou ED, Anderson LR, Bernert RA, et al. Lower extremity iatrogenic nerve injury due to compression during intraabdominal surgery. *Am J Surg* 1997;173(6):504–508.
41. Smith RL, Bohl JK, McElearney ST, et al. Wound infection after elective colorectal resection. *Ann Surg* 2004;239(5):599–605.
42. Pineda CE, Shelton AA, Hernandez-Boussard T, et al. Mechanical bowel preparation in intestinal surgery: a meta-analysis and review of the literature. *Gastrointest Surg* 2008;12(11):2037–2044.
43. Slim K, Vicaut E, Launay-Savary MV, et al. Updated systematic review and meta-analysis of randomized clinical trials on the role of mechanical bowel preparation before colorectal surgery. *Ann Surg* 2009;249(2): 203–209.
44. Fazio VW, Ziv Y, Church JM, et al. Ileal pouch-anal anastomosis complications and function in 1005 patients. *Ann Surg* 1995;222(2):120–127.
45. Grobler SP, Hosie KB, Keighley MR. Randomized trial of loop ileostomy in restorative proctocolectomy. *Br J Surg* 1992;79:903–906.
46. Shah NS, Remzi F, Massmann A, et al. Management and treatment outcome of pouch-vaginal fistulas following restorative proctocolectomy. *Dis Colon Rectum* 2003;46(7):911–917.
47. Fazio VW, Wu JS, Lavery IC. Repeat ileal pouch-anal anastomosis to salvage septic complications of pelvic pouches. *Ann Surg* 1998;228(4): 588–597.
48. Senapati A, Tibbs CJ, Ritchie JK, et al. Stenosis of the pouch anal anastomosis following restorative proctocolectomy. *Int J Colorectal Dis* 1996; 11:57–59.
49. Lewis WG, Kuzu A, Sagar PM, et al. Stricture at the pouch-anal anastomosis after restorative proctocolectomy. *Dis Colon Rectum* 1994;37: 120–125.
50. Fazio VW, Tjandra JJ. Pouch advancement and neoileoanal anastomosis for anastomotic stricture and anovaginal fistula complicating restorative proctocolectomy. *Br J Surg* 1992;79:694–696.
51. Kuhbacher T, Schreiber S, Runkel N. Pouchitis: pathophysiology and treatment. *Int J Colorectal Dis* 1998;13:196–207.
52. Stein RB, Lichtenstein GR. Complications after ileal pouch-anal anastomosis. *Semin Gastrointest Dis* 2000;11(1):2–9.
53. Stahlberg D, Gullberg K, Liljeqvist L, et al. Pouchitis following pelvic pouch operation for ulcerative colitis: incidence, cumulative risk, and risk factors. *Dis Colon Rectum* 1996;39:1012–1018.
54. MacRae HM, McLeod RS, Cohen Z, et al. Risk factors for pelvic pouch failure. *Dis Colon Rectum* 1997;40:257–262.
55. Breen EM, Schoetz DJ, Marcello PW, et al. Functional results after perineal complications of ileal pouch-anal anastomosis. *Dis Colon Rectum* 1998;41(6):691–695.
56. Leong APK, Londono-Schimmer EE, Phillips RKS. Life-table analysis of stomal complications following ileostomy. *Br J Surg* 1994;81: 727–729.
57. Collett K. Practical aspects of stoma management. *Nurs Stand* 2002;17(8): 45–52.
58. Duchesne JC, Wang YZ, Weintraub SL, et al. Stoma complications: a multivariate analysis. *Am Surg* 2002;68(11):961–966.
59. Bass EM, Del Pino A, Tao A, et al. Does preoperative stoma marking and education by the enterostomal therapist affect outcome? *Dis Colon Rectum* 1997;40(4):440–442.
60. Myers JO, Rothenberger DA. Sugar in the reduction of incarcerated prolapsed bowel: report of two cases. *Dis Colon Rectum* 1991;34:416–418.
61. Williams NS, Nasmyth DG, Jones D, et al. Defunctioning stomas: a prospective controlled trial comparing loop ileostomy with loop transverse colostomy. *Br J Surg* 1986;72:566–570.
62. Carlsen E, Bergen A. Technical aspects and complication of end ileostomies. *World J Surg* 1995;19:632–636.
63. Abulafi AM, Sherman JW, Fiddian RV. Delorme operation for prolapsed colostomy. *Br J Surg* 1989;76:1321–1322.
64. Shellito PC. Complications of abdominal stoma surgery. *Dis Colon Rectum* 1998;41(12):1562–1572.
65. Doberneck RC. Revision and closure of the colostomy. *Surg Clin North Am* 1991;71(1):193–201.
66. Leenan LP, Kyuypers JH. Some factors influencing the outcome of stoma surgery. *Dis Colon Rectum* 1989;32:500–504.
67. Rubin MS, Schoetz DJ, Matthew JB. Parastomal hernia: is stoma relocation superior to fascial repair? *Arch Surg* 1994;129:413–418.
68. Balfour L, Stojkovic SG, Botterill ID, et al. A randomized, double-blind trial of the effect of metronidazole on pain after closed hemorrhoidectomy. *Dis Colon Rectum* 2002;45:1186–1190.
69. Goldstein ET, Williamson PR, Lach SW. Subcutaneous morphine pump for postoperative hemorrhoidectomy pain management. *Dis Colon Rectum* 1993;36(5):439–446.
70. Bailey HR, Ferguson JA. Prevention of urinary retention by fluid restriction following anorectal operations. *Dis Colon Rectum* 1976;19: 250–252.
71. Bleday R, Pena JP, Rothenberger DA. Symptomatic hemorrhoids, current incidence and complications of operative therapy. *Dis Colon Rectum* 1992;35:477.
72. Buls JG, Goldberg SM. Modern management of hemorrhoids. *Surg Clin North Am* 1978;58:469–478.

73. Roe AM, Bartolo DCC, Vellacort KD, et al. Submucosal versus ligation excision hemorrhoidectomy: a comparison of anal sensation, anal sphincter manometry, and postoperative pain and function. *Br J Surg* 1987;74:948–951.
74. Jensen SL. Treatment of first episodes of acute anal fissure: prospective randomized study of lignocaine ointment versus hydrocortisone ointment or warm sitz baths plus bran. *Br Med J* 1986;292:1167–1169.
75. Lund JN, Armitage NC, Scholefield JH. Use of glyceryl trinitrate ointment in the treatment of anal fissure. *Br J Surg* 1996;83:776–777.
76. Oh C, Divino CM, Steinhagen RM. Anal fissure: 20-year experience. *Dis Colon Rectum* 1995;38(4):378–382.
77. Romano G, Rotondano G, Santangelo M, et al. A critical appraisal of pathogenesis and morbidity of surgical treatment of chronic anal fissure. *J Am Coll Surg* 1994;178:600–604.
78. Hiltunen KM, Metikainen M. Closed lateral subcutaneous sphincterotomy under local anesthesia in the treatment of chronic anal fissure. *Ann Chir Gynaecol* 1991;80:353–356.
79. Sultan AH, Kamm MA, Nicholls RJ, et al. Prospective study of the extent of internal anal sphincter division during lateral sphincterotomy. *Dis Colon Rectum* 1994;37(10):1031–1033.
80. Garcia G, Sutton C, Mansoori S, et al. Results following conservative lateral sphincterotomy for the treatment of chronic anal fissures. *Colorectal Dis* 2003;5:311–314.
81. Littlejohn DR, Newstead GL. Tailored lateral sphincterotomy for anal fissure. *Dis Colon Rectum* 1997;40(12):1439–1442.
82. Chrabot CM, Prasad ML, Abcarian H. Recurrent anorectal abscesses. *Dis Colon Rectum* 1983;24:105–108.
83. Huber J, Kissack AS, Simonton CT. Necrotizing soft tissue infection from rectal abscess. *Dis Colon Rectum* 1983;26:507–511.
84. Lilius HG. Fistula-in-ano, an investigation of human fetal anal ducts and intramuscular glands and a clinical study of 150 patients. *Acta Chir Scand Suppl* 1968;383:1–88.
85. Joy H, Williams JG. The outcome of surgery for high anal fistulas. *Colorectal Dis* 2002;4(4):254–261.

majority of incision hernias are derived from undetected or occult fascial dehiscences. The preponderance of data supports the use of a running, mass closure with a SL:WL ratio of 4:1 or greater (6).

Suture tension that raises the interstitial pressure in the center of the incision above capillary perfusion pressure (30 to 40 mm Hg) may cause fascial necrosis. In animal studies, this situation has increased the risk of acute wound failure. Ideal suture tension should approximate fascia while maintaining the perfusion of healing tissue. A short, 1-cm stitch interval with a moderate tension load should prevent omentum or intestine from protruding through the suture line.

Unplanned Visceral Injury

Abdominal organs may be injured when the peritoneum is opened. The risk of visceral injury during laparotomy is increased by the presence of previous abdominal wall scars, adhesions, and distended organs. The risk of visceral injury can be reduced by incising the abdominal wall in layers, carefully identifying component structures and layers, retracting as needed, and identifying the peritoneum. In the presence of dense scars or adhesions, sharp dissection is usually recommended until potential planes between organs and the peritoneum are identified. This may avoid uncontrolled heat injury from electrocautery. Often, a lateral dissection must be pursued away from the midline scar until the uninjured peritoneum is identified and more safely and easily opened. The introduction of synthetic mesh prostheses to repair incisional ventral hernias has led to an increased incidence of unplanned bowel injury and bowel resection during a later abdominal operation (8,9). This is a significant development in the safety of mesh prostheses, since some estimate that at least 12% of all abdominal surgery patients will be reoperated in their lifetime, with >25% of incisional hernia patients repaired with a synthetic mesh (3,10).

Retractors may also cause unintended organ injury. Great vigilance must be used in the safe application of handheld and self-retaining abdominal retractors. In a normal peritoneum, each retractor should be placed under direct vision and the deep edge palpated to ensure safe placement without undue tension on organs. In a reoperative peritoneum with dense adhesions, great care must be used to prevent torque injuries caused by retractors pulling on adhered structures. Following removal of retractors, abdominal organs should routinely be examined for injury. Retractor injury is not always obvious at the time of abdominal wall closure, and the first sign of injury may be delayed hemorrhage or intestinal perforation during the convalescent period.

Sutures may penetrate the intestines during closure of the abdominal wall and can result in bowel obstruction and fistulization. This is most easily avoided by maintaining careful anatomic identification of abdominal wall and visceral structures at the end of the case. Communication with the anesthesiologist is helpful to maintain adequate levels of abdominal wall relaxation to complete the optimum closure. Prospective studies of abdominal wall closure techniques suggest that the optimum depth of a fascial stitch is 1 cm into normal fascia (7). Deeper fascial stitches, such as those placed as retention sutures, increase the risk of bowel injury. Distended organs also increase the risk for injury.

Retained Instrument

A retained instrument, sponge, or needle is a technical error that can occur during laparotomy. The complication occurs most often during emergency procedures or when operating in two or more widely separated fields and when using packs for hemostasis (11). Retained gauze causes abscess formation. Retained instruments or needles may penetrate viscera and cause an abscess, fistula, or obstruction. The retention of needles is best avoided by the compulsive reapplication of needles to needle drivers and by accounting for every needle when an empty driver is returned. In most hospitals, all instruments and needles are counted.

The incidence of retained gauze sponges may be reduced when restricted to using only large laparotomy pads when operating in the abdomen. Sponge stick or peanut dissectors should be avoided. Large gauze pads are more easily palpated during a careful manual search of the peritoneal cavity. The surgeons should vigilantly account for the placement and removal of all laparotomy pads. Surgeons should routinely examine all locations where gauze pads might have been placed, such as behind the liver or spleen. The nursing sponge count needs to be correct. An incomplete closing count requires a reexamination of the peritoneal cavity and retrieval of the missing sponge. If the final count remains incomplete, an intraoperative radiograph should be performed to prove without any doubt that no radiopaque marker remains in the abdomen.

Despite systematic approaches and a correct count, a gauze pad or even an instrument might be left. If this situation is detected in the postoperative period, the surgeon should first inform the patient or the patient's family, or both, of the presence of the foreign body and then recommend its removal at the safest interval.

Incisional Pain

Clinical experience suggests that some abdominal wall incisions are more painful than others in the perioperative period. Methods for measuring incisional pain include the use of pain analog scales and narcotic analgesic requirements. Respiratory splinting due to abdominal wall incisional pain and narcotic therapy both predispose to reduced pulmonary tidal volumes and atelectasis. Urinary retention and delayed gastrointestinal function may also follow increased narcotic usage due to abdominal wall pain. It is generally believed that pain is greatest following vertical midline and paramedian incisions because they are subject to the greatest distractive forces during recovery. Abdominal wall flexion and extension and lateral traction from the oblique musculature are the primary sources of vertical laparotomy wound motion. Less pain is reported following transverse and oblique abdominal wall incisions, especially retroperitoneal flank incisions. In these incisions, the normal abdominal wall load forces are distributed parallel to the abdominal wall wounds, thereby minimizing distractive wound-load vectors. Many surgeons believe that a transverse incision minimizes respiratory dysfunction in patients with pulmonary disease. A definitive study of pain associated with abdominal wall incisions is difficult to control and has not been done.

Abdominal Wall Wound Infections

Abdominal wall wound infections may be categorized as superficial, deep, or organ space, depending on the anatomic location of the infected wounded tissue. Most serious are deep laparotomy wound infections. The best-characterized invasive organisms include hemolytic streptococci, staphylococci, clostridia, and synergistic combinations of gram-negative rods and anaerobes (streptococci or bacteroides). The invasive infections frequently cause intense pain and tenderness. Patients developing these signs and symptoms as early as the second postoperative day must be followed closely for progression to abdominal wall crepitus and signs of toxemia. The primary therapy for abdominal wall wound infections is to open the wound, begin moist dressing changes, and allow healing by secondary intent. Gram-positive cellulitis may respond to β-lactam antibiotics. All other invasive infections require urgent surgical debridement of destroyed tissue and intravenous antibiotics directed toward the offending organism or organisms. Resistant *Staphylococcus aureus* is increasingly the cause of wound infection following hernia repair, especially in the presence of a synthetic mesh implant. Repeated debridements may be required until the infection is controlled, including mesh explantation.

Debridement of abdominal wall infections may result in full-thickness defects exposing the peritoneum. These are difficult surgical circumstances requiring a variety of approaches to effect successful abdominal wall wound management. Traditionally, a temporary alloplastic implant like polypropylene mesh has been used to bridge the myofascial defect. Alloplastic materials may, however, behave as foreign bodies within a contaminated field and become chronically infected. In addition, a high incidence of bowel fistulization has been reported using meshed alloplastics. It is ideal if a large omentum or existing preperitoneal tissue protects peritoneal organs before alloplastic implantation of a contaminated or infected field. Microporous alloplastics like extruded polytetrafluoroethylene (ePTFE) have also been successfully used for serial temporary closure of the abdominal wall. This approach involves intensive care unit level sedation or a return to the operating room every 2 to 3 days for wound debridement and "reefing" of the alloplastic bridge closure to reduce the implant surface area. Ultimately, closure with autologous ventral abdominal wall myofascia is achieved. Newer, lighter-weight and larger pore size synthetic mesh implants may incorporate into the abdominal wall better and be more likely to clear a mesh-associated infection.

Another approach to temporary closure of infected and/or contaminated abdominal wall defects has been the use of absorbable implants such as polyglycolic acid polymer mesh. These materials may also fistulize to bowel and always result in a large incisional hernia that presents a set of significant secondary surgical problems and complications. Large series and a growing experience demonstrate the successful management of infected or contaminated abdominal wall defects using collagen-based biological soft-tissue implants (12–14). Biological mesh sheets are derived from porcine dermis, porcine submucosa (xenografts), or cadaveric dermis (allografts) following the removal of all cells. Ideally, biological meshes act as an extracellular matrix scaffold. The grafts are repopulated with host abdominal wall cells like repair fibroblasts and become vascularized so that wound infections may clear and long-term abdominal wall wound mechanical integrity is maintained. Prospective, randomized studies are required to determine the safety and efficacy of newer abdominal wall implants.

Most abdominal wall wound infections are confined to the subcutaneous fat as cellulitis. There infections manifest as increasing wound pain and tenderness on postoperative days 5 to 7 when a normal wound inflammatory response should be resolving. Subcutaneous tissue necrosis also predisposes to abscess formation following cautery, mass ligature, or creation of ischemic suture lines. The incidence of subcutaneous abscesses appears to be higher in obese patients.

Once diagnosed, especially in the presence of fever and an elevated white blood cell count, a superficial wound should be opened through the skin and all pus should be drained. Antibiotics are usually not necessary unless the abscess is associated with an invasive soft-tissue infection or an adjacent prosthesis, or both. These wounds should be lightly packed with moistened gauze two to three times a day until normal granulation tissue appears and wound contraction begins.

Multifilament, nonabsorbable sutures may harbor bacteria and predispose a wound to stitch abscess and sinuses. A recurrent stitch abscess diagnosed months or years after an operation should be treated by excision of the offending stitch. Waiting may result in spontaneous expulsion of the stitch, or the wound may be operatively reexplored under controlled conditions.

Myofascial dehiscence and evisceration

The reported incidence of fascial dehiscence (acute laparotomy wound failure) ranges from 0.2% to 10% (4,6). The Veterans Affairs National Surgical Quality Improvement Program (NSQIP) maintains the largest prospective database of perioperative surgical risk factors and outcomes in the United States (15). An analysis of 34,809 laparotomies performed between 1996 and 2000 revealed a 3.3% incidence of fascial dehiscence. This rate is in agreement with

likely to occur in men with symptoms of prostatism or bladder outlet obstruction and in patients with a history of an abdominal aortic aneurysm (4,5). Presumably, prostatism contributes to the higher rate of hernia recurrence because of repetitive Valsalva maneuvers or loading of the repaired abdominal wall that occurs with urination. Patients who develop abdominal aortic aneurysms express abnormal tissue collagen isoforms and metalloproteinase levels. The aberrant structural collagen and increased turnover catalyzed by tissue proteinases result in defective wound repair (22,23).

Another established risk factor for recurrent herniation is operating upon an already recurrent hernia. The incidence of recurrent herniation following repair increases with each subsequent repair (3). A prospective, randomized, controlled trial of incisional hernia repair established a 24% recurrence rate with the use of a polypropylene synthetic mesh implant and a 54% recurrence rate following a primary repair using in situ local autologous tissues after the initial hernia repair (4,5). Many less well- controlled studies and large clinical experiences report hernia recurrence rate of ≥50% after the second hernia repair and 60% after the third. Preclinical wound healing data suggest that part of the explanation for increased recurrent hernia rates following each repair is the selection of a defective, chronic wound.

Since incisional hernias are iatrogenic, they are associated with a unique set of preoperative risk factors. It was long held in the surgical wound healing literature that incisional hernias were a late event, developing years after celiotomy closure. Small series and class II data suggested that abnormal progression through all the phases of wound healing (inflammation, fibroplasia, and scar maturation) ultimately resulted in wound breakdown and herniation (24). Biochemical measurements suggested defects in collagen isoform structure and tissue proteinase expression as a late phenomenon.

A more recent and provocative hypothesis suggests that most incisional hernias occur as the result of very early occult abdominal wall wound dehiscence (16,18). Prospectively, at the time of celiotomy closure in 149 patients, metal clips were placed along the border of the myofascial incision and the skin closed as usual. Plain film abdominal x-rays were then performed on postoperative day 30. Eighteen (12%) of the patients developed clinically obvious incisional hernias during the 43-month follow-up, as demonstrated by separation of the metallic markers on postoperative x-ray. Of the 18 patients who developed incisional hernias, 17 (94%) demonstrated 12 mm or greater fascial clip separation by postoperative day 30. By contrast, only one of the remaining 131 patients who did not develop 12-mm fascial separation by postoperative day 30 developed a hernia. This simple, but well-done study indicates a much higher rate of occult primary celiotomy wound failure—in the vicinity of 11% to 15%. The high incidence appears to be due to the lag phase in the recovery of wound tensile strength following injury. It appears that obesity increases this already high baseline rate of primary fascial dehiscence (17).

The wound infection rate appears to be higher following abdominal wall hernia repair than for other clean cases, although the mechanism is unclear (25,26). One possibility is that patients with significant comorbid conditions are at risk for both hernia formation and wound infection. A Veterans Administration NSQIP study found a 4.3% wound infection rate and 15.1% hernia recurrence rate. Another study reported a 16% wound infection rate following incisional ventral hernia repair (26). The expected clean surgical wound infection rate for nonhernia cases is closer to 1%. Multiple logistic and linear regression analyses have documented that coronary artery disease, chronic obstructive pulmonary disease, low serum albumin, and steroid use are independent risk factors for wound infection and prolonged hospital stay.

Modification of preoperative risk factors

On the basis of prospective, randomized, controlled trials of hernia repair, it is prudent to screen prospective hernia repair patients for signs and symptoms of prostatism (4,5). By logical extension, questions should be asked during the preoperative evaluation about other symptoms leading to chronic Valsalva maneuvers or loading of the abdominal wall. Increased difficulties having bowel movements or a chronic cough are common examples. Important colorectal pathology is often diagnosed during workups for hernias. When time permits, a urologic or gastrointestinal evaluation may be indicated prior to hernia surgery to diagnose and treat occult processes and to potentially improve the results of repair.

Most biological risk factors are more difficult to correct. Clearly, when there is an infection of the abdominal wall, all effort must be made to reduce bacterial bioburden prior to repair or reconstruction. Common clinical scenarios are an existing mesh infection or associated enterocutaneous fistula. Patients with abdominal aortic aneurysms express defective tissue repair pathways that cannot be treated today (27,28). Operating during periods of profound shock is often unavoidable when a life is at stake. All efforts should be directed toward correcting hemodynamics and using optimum surgical technique. Cessation of cigarette smoking has been shown to improve skin healing, but it is not clear that cessation affects rates of abdominal wall wound failure (29). It is likely that cigarette smoking impedes tissue repair pathways dependent on oxygen delivery and that associated chronic coughs overload abdominal wall closure. Obesity has never been shown to cause a wound healing defect. However, increased mechanical forces are likely to contribute to abdominal wall wound failure. Class I data show an increased incidence of incisional hernia formation in obese patients (17). Efforts to lose weight prior to hernia repair surgery should improve outcomes, although this belief has never been definitively proven. Reduced weight reduces fascial wound load forces and also provides locally mobile skin to assure fascial wound coverage.

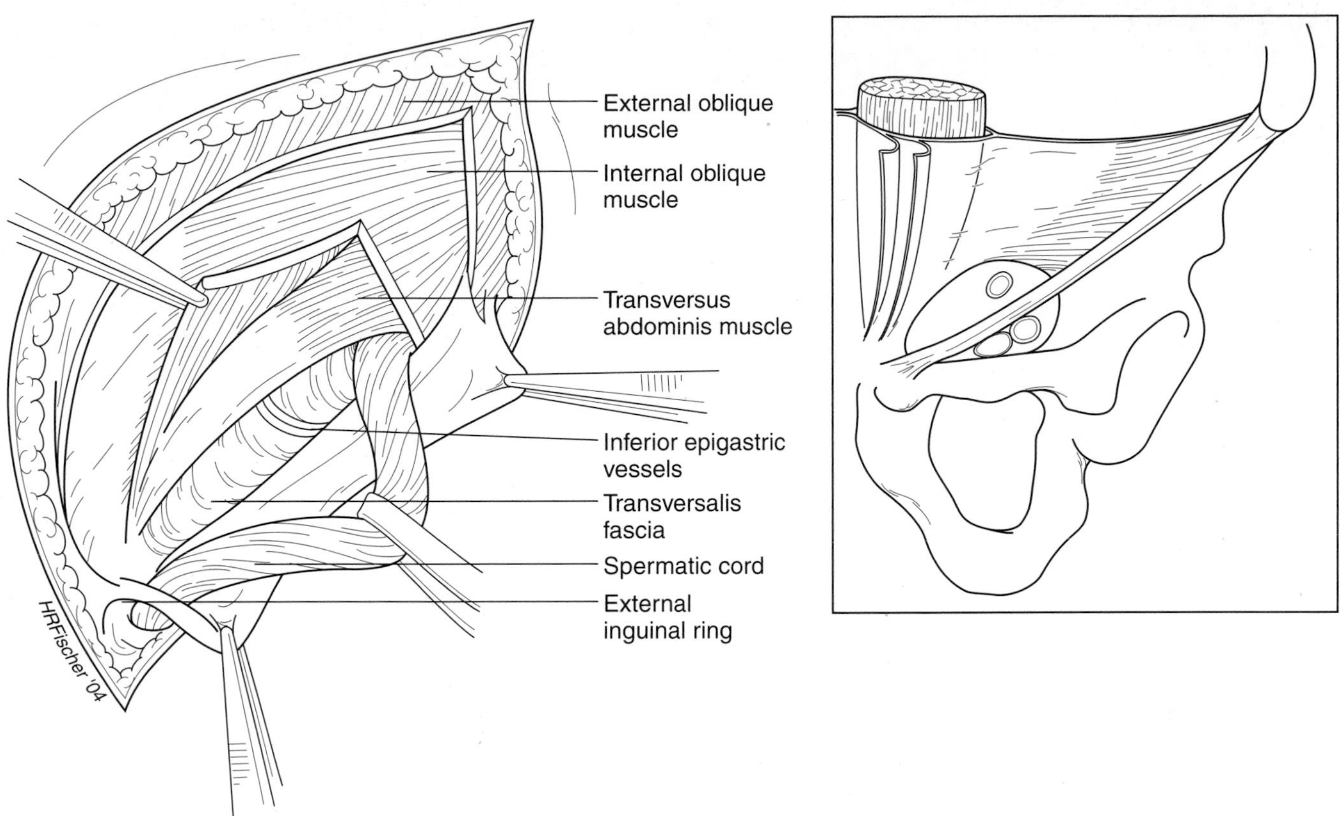

FIGURE 39.3. Normal anatomy of the left inguinal canal.

Inguinal Hernias

Inguinal hernia repair is the most common abdominal wall operation and the most frequent elective procedure performed by general surgeons (Fig. 39.3). Comparing the results of different operative approaches to hernia repair is difficult. There is no agreed-upon definition of hernia recurrence, typically the most cited outcome measure. Most hernia surgeons support the appearance of any new hernia on the operative side as the definition of a recurrence. Distinguishing a new hernia from a recurrent hernia through an existing repair is often inexact. The other possibility is that an adjacent defect went undetected and a persistent hernia manifests in the postoperative period. The length of follow-up also affects the quality of hernia repair outcome databases. Recurrence rates increase with increased length of follow-up. Recurrence rates also increase when dedicated, expert postoperative examinations are used for assessment (30).

The original operations designed for inguinal hernia repair all depended on locoregional tissue transfers, usually based on repairing and reinforcing the posterior wall of the inguinal canal, or the transversalis muscle and fascia (Bassini and Shouldice repairs). The advantages of these approaches include simple operations without the need for prostheses and the reliable healing of well-vascularized tissues. The problems associated with local tissue repairs include biomechanical limitations (closing "under tension") and the use of abnormal tissue that already demonstrates a tendency to herniate. Although proponents of each technique report very low personal recurrence rates, prospectively controlled series report recurrence rates of 6% to 11% when general surgeons use these techniques outside of dedicated centers (31).

The posterior wall of the inguinal canal is composed of the transversalis muscle, its aponeurosis, and the transversalis fascia that together insert on Cooper ligament. In the inferior abdominal wall, there is a weak area in the groin where overlying myofascia do not reinforce this posterior layer. This area of the posterior, inferior abdominal wall is often referred to as the myopectineal orifice. The area is defined by the rectus muscle medially, the internal oblique and transversalis muscles superiorly, the iliopsoas muscle laterally, and the pubis inferiorly. The myopectineal orifice is crossed by the inguinal ligament and traversed by the spermatic cord and femoral vessels. All groin hernias begin as weaknesses within the myopectineal orifice. The transversalis fascia deteriorates, resulting in peritoneal protrusion. Inguinal hernias are surgically treated by repairing all or part of the myopectineal orifice directly using autologous tissue or by implanting a prosthesis to augment or replace the defective transversalis fascia.

A method of classifying inguinal hernias helps to standardize the operations performed and to quantify surgical outcomes. One frequently used classification system for inguinal hernias was devised by Nyhus (Table 39.2). Type I inguinal hernias occur most commonly in infants and children where the internal ring is normal in size and structure

Table 39.2 Nyhus classification of inguinal hernias

Type I indirect inguinal hernia Internal ring is normal
Type II indirect inguinal hernia Internal ring is dilated, but the posterior inguinal wall is intact
Type III posterior inguinal wall defects Direct inguinal hernia Indirect inguinal hernia with dilated internal ring and attenuated medial transversalis fascia of the Hesselbach triangle Femoral hernias
Type IV recurrent inguinal hernias Direct Indirect Femoral Combined

and the Hesselbach triangle is normal as well. The mechanism of herniation is a patent processus vaginalis of variable length from the internal ring. Type II inguinal hernias are indirect defects where the internal ring is now enlarged with some impingement on the deep inferior epigastric vessels but without defects within the Hesselbach triangle. Examination of the inguinal canal's medial floor may be performed through the dilated internal ring, confirming its integrity. Type III inguinal hernias involve defects in the posterior wall (floor) of the inguinal canal and have been classified into three subtypes: direct, indirect, and femoral. Type IIIA defects are direct inguinal hernias without protrusion through the internal ring. Type IIIB defects are indirect and occur through a much-dilated internal ring with significant impingement and deterioration of the inguinal floor medial to the inferior epigastric vessels with or without a scrotal component to the hernia. The distortion of the internal ring may occur without displacement of the inferior epigastric vessels. The hernia may have both direct and indirect components, resulting in a pantaloon hernia surrounding the inferior epigastric vessels. Femoral hernias are classified as type IIIC. Type IV inguinal hernias are recurrent.

Prospective nonrandomized data and many large reviews suggest that recurrence rates should be lower for type I and type II inguinal hernia repairs. These include simple and complex internal ring plasties following high ligation of an indirect hernia sac. Surgical experience supports the concept that the most difficult inguinal hernias to repair are types III and IV. These include indirect and direct hernias with significant posterior inguinal canal wall deterioration, femoral hernias, and recurrent inguinal hernias.

Autologous tissue repairs

Shouldice Repair

The principles of the Shouldice repair are a paradigm for the use of autologous tissues during inguinal hernia operations. The results of the Shouldice technique are also widely reported in the surgical literature and maintained in a large database. As performed at The Shouldice Clinic, the Shouldice repair promotes an integrated concept of hernia surgery that includes preoperative preparation and education, an extensive inguinal floor dissection, and closely supervised early postoperative convalescence. It is generally considered a complex technical operation, with wide variation in results reported. The Shouldice Clinic itself continues to report long-term total hernia recurrence rates of 1% (31). These outstanding results are rarely duplicated outside of the Shouldice Clinic or in a controlled and powered, prospective, randomized trial of inguinal hernia repair.

Shouldice pioneered early postoperative ambulation without increased complications, a fundamental principle of modern surgery. Hospital stays following inguinal herniorrhaphy were reduced from 21 to 3 days. General or spinal anesthetics were converted to local infiltration of anesthetic to promote earlier ambulation and return to usual activity. Fine silk sutures were found to be associated with an increased risk of suture abscess and were exchanged for less reactive monofilaments like fine wire, and now polypropylene or PDS. Groin wound infection rates were also reduced by staging bilateral inguinal hernia repairs 2 days apart, which also facilitates the use of local anesthetics.

The successful multifaceted approach of the Shouldice Clinic and the Shouldice technique may be extended to all types of management for inguinal hernias. In addition to an open technique using local anesthetics and encouraging early ambulation, the Shouldice Clinic applies other general principles to its management of inguinal hernias. Weight reduction is a frequently overlooked preoperative preparation that may make hernia repair technically more successful. Most series of herniorrhaphy outcomes now show that increased weight increases the risk of hernia recurrence. Weight loss improves the effectiveness of the local anesthetic technique and improves anatomic dissections for bilateral and recurrent hernias. They also believe that the postoperative load placed across the repair is more conducive for hernia repair scar formation, treating the abdominal wall like an orthopedic structure. A 3-day supervised convalescence is followed by a return to normal activity as comfort permits. The maximum convalescence period is 4 weeks for patients involved in strenuous activity (Table 39.3).

Table 39.3 Shouldice clinic principles of inguinal herniorrhaphy

Weight reduction
Open technique with complete anatomic dissection
Use of local anesthetics
Autologous tissue repairs
Early return to usual activity

Local anesthetic infiltration is used in association with conscious sedation (diazepam and meperidine). Awake procedures using local anesthesia may reduce cardiac and pulmonary complications, especially in elderly patient populations. The incidence of deep venous thrombosis, pulmonary embolism, and pulmonary atelectasis is well below 1%. The Shouldice series mortality is reported as 0.01%.

A complete dissection of all groin anatomy, normal and abnormal, is performed. Prior to opening the external oblique fascia, the inferior edge of the inguinal ligament is examined in the thigh to rule out a femoral hernia component. The external oblique aponeurosis is incised and opened from the external ring to 3 cm lateral to the internal ring. The lateral dissection rules out an unsuspected Spigelian or interstitial hernia. The ilioinguinal and iliohypogastric nerves are identified, isolated, and preserved without injury if possible. The cremasteric muscle fibers are then incised longitudinally, and the spermatic cord with any associated indirect hernia is freed from its sheath. Unique to the Shouldice technique, cremasteric fibers are then excised to facilitate accurate transversalis fascia to fascia repair. Part of the proximal stump of the cremasteric fibers is used during reconstruction of the internal ring. The inferomedial stump of the excised cremasteric fiber is included in the repair of the inguinal floor in order to suspend the testicle. Concern has been raised about testicular dependency or even ischemia following the extensive cremasteric dissection and excision.

The internal ring is thoroughly dissected. The peritoneum is identified and completely dissected back along the spermatic cord. Most males have protrusion of preperitoneal fat at the superolateral quadrant of the internal ring, which is usually not the source of hernia symptoms unless it extends significantly (2 cm) down the spermatic cord. The incidence of sliding hernias in the Shouldice series is ~1%. Great care should be used to recognize a sliding viscous component at the internal ring, to work distally to proximally to separate it from the spermatic cord and to protect the sliding organ's blood supply. If the indirect hernia sac is transected at the internal ring, some authors recommend leaving the distal end of the sac in situ to avoid spermatic cord injury and to reduce the risk of an ischemic testicle or testicular atrophy. Others advocate dissection of the remnant sac from the spermatic cord to eliminate the possibility of hydrocele. Most series report an incidence of testicular atrophy of <0.1%. The Shouldice experience also suggests that ligation of indirect hernia sacs is not mandatory. In their view, complete reduction of the hernia sac with meticulous reconstruction of the internal ring minimizes recurrence rates.

The Shouldice technique requires incision and opening of the posterior wall of the inguinal canal (the inguinal floor), which is composed mainly of transversalis fascia. Any direct hernias thus encountered are carefully reduced. If opening of a direct hernia sac is required, it is performed from the lateral edge to avoid injury to potential medial wall bladder components. Finally, the inferior preperitoneal space is explored beneath the inferolateral transversalis flap to again rule out a femoral hernia component.

The Shouldice repair incorporates an indirect and direct reconstruction in all instances, overlapping inguinal floor muscle and fascia in what is described as their natural sequence. Continuous monofilament permanent sutures are used on the posterior wall. A continuous suturing technique is advocated to evenly distribute tension and to leave no gaps. The Shouldice Clinic preference has been 34- or 32-gauge stainless steel wire because it is inert in tissues and provides maximum breaking strength for its caliber (tensile strength) and well-placed knots maintain integrity. Two disadvantages of steel wire include a tendency to kink and break if mishandled and the risk of laceration to surgeons and assistants. One continuous suture with two opposing lines of repair is then used to repair the inguinal floor. The first layers approximate transversalis fascia and peritoneum running from medially to laterally, and the second layer approximates muscle and aponeurotic fibers from the internal oblique and transversalis muscles down to the inguinal ligament. Relaxing incisions on the ipsilateral rectus sheath are seldom required, but are recommended if necessary prior to the initiation of the first half of the suture line. Two more lines of running suture are then placed to reinforce the repair. This time, starting just medial to the internal ring, the external oblique aponeurosis is plicated toward the pubic crest and then reversed back to the internal ring. The external oblique aponeurosis is then closed in a continuous manner, recreating the external ring.

Femoral hernias may be a cause of recurrence following hernia repair, which is the reason for advocating that the femoral sheath be routinely examined and even explored during suprainguinal herniorrhaphy. In the Shouldice series, 1 in 400 inguinal hernia repairs recurred as a femoral hernia. Most operative modifications applied to reduce the incidence of recurrent femoral hernias involve opening of the posterior wall of the inguinal canal (transversalis fascia) and closing the space medial to the femoral outlet (the femoral ring) using Cooper ligament. Conversely, when only a femoral hernia was suspected on clinical grounds, simultaneous significant suprainguinal pathology was detected at operation in 87% of males and 63% of females in the Shouldice series (31). This observation reinforces the need for careful and complete suprainguinal and infrainguinal examination during all inguinal hernia repairs in order to minimize recurrence rates.

The incidence of recurrent hernia increases with each subsequent repair, most likely due to tissue loss and scarring (32,33). Highest recurrence rates (12%) are reported following repairs of multiply recurrent inguinal hernias. Because recurrent wound failure appears to select abnormal scar and fascia expressing a tissue repair defect, the implantation of prosthetic material has been advocated. The interval between the first and second operations should be at least 6 months to allow optimum recovery of the tissue to be used again for repair. When the inguinal ligament was intact, an autologous tissue repair was possible in 91% of the cases of recurrent hernia repair in the Shouldice experience. For the remaining 9% of patients, the groin defect was described as too extensive or the groin tissue as too friable and inelastic to allow autologous tissue repair. In these cases, an alloplastic prosthetic implant in the preperitoneal space was used. When the bowel was covered with peritoneum, polypropylene mesh was used. When the bowel was exposed, a microporous PTFE patch was used. With a minimum follow-up of 18 months, the reported recurrence rate was 2.2% (31).

Cooper Ligament Repair

The first reported use of the Cooper ligament (the superior pubic ligament) in hernia repair was to treat femoral hernias by suturing the inguinal ligament down to it, obliterating the femoral sheath space (30). Later, McVay popularized the technique by recommending a rectus sheath-relaxing incision and transfer of the transversalis abdominus aponeurosis and muscle and transversalis fascia down to the Cooper ligament in order to repair the inguinal canal's posterior wall. This maneuver requires opening the floor of the inguinal canal and exploring the preperitoneal space. This added dissection is also believed to reduce the incidence of missed hernias, especially femoral hernias.

In most descriptions, the ilioinguinal nerve is preserved. If the nerve is traumatized during groin dissection, many experts recommend ligation and division of the nerve to reduce the incidence of postoperative chronic pain syndromes. The spermatic cord is fully mobilized in the inguinal canal. No dissection is performed medial to the pubic tubercle in order to avoid injury to the external pudendal blood supply and to preserve collateral circulation to the testicles. Starting laterally, the anterior surfaces of the femoral artery and vein are cleared and the anterior femoral fascia is identified. Working medial to the femoral vein, fat and lymphatics are dissected free from the femoral canal and any femoral sac is reduced. The tendinous portion of the transversus abdominis aponeurotic arch is then identified, and a relaxing incision is placed at the point of fusion of the external oblique muscles and the rectus sheath. This starts at the pubic tubercle and then extends superiorly by 6 to 8 cm. The remainder of the repair can be performed with the patient in the Trendelenburg position to minimize intestinal injuries. In independent, noncontrolled, or randomized series, recurrence rates of 2% have been reported by high-volume surgeons who limit their practice to herniorrhaphy (30).

The disadvantages of the Copper ligament (McVay) repair include the more extensive dissection and reported prolonged recovery period. Some authors have argued that the tension placed on the posterior wall repair is suboptimal as well and that vascular injuries are more common with the McVay repair. Proponents of this procedure recommend relaxing incisions and careful dissections around the femoral vessels to achieve a reliable procedure with low recurrence rates and minimal morbidity.

Synthetic Tissue Implants (Mesh)

Billroth wrote in 1878, "If we could artificially produce tissues of the density and toughness of fascia and tendon, the secret of the radical cure of hernia would be discovered" (34). In addition to replacing defective soft tissue, synthetic mesh implants are believed to reduce the chance for "missed" hernia. Recurrent hernias often result from simultaneous inguinal defects that were missed at the time of the initial herniorrhaphy. Covering the entire myopectineal orifice with a prosthesis should reduce the incidence of missed simultaneous hernia. Finally, replacing or augmenting abnormal inguinal soft tissue may prevent the development of future hernias.

Today, various prosthetic meshes are available for hernia repair. Knitted polypropylene mesh is used most commonly. This material induces a rapid and reliable fibroblastic response and is efficiently incorporated into the abdominal wall. Synthetic meshes, however, tend to stiffen and shrink over time, inducing disorganized scar tissue. Polyethylene meshes are hydrophilic and more pliable than most heavyweight or small-pore polypropylene meshes. PTFE meshes are extruded with a microporous surface to allow abdominal wall fibroblast and macrophage ingrowth for abdominal wall incorporation and immune surveillance, while at the same time minimizing adherence to the bowel and other intraabdominal viscera.

The term "tension-free" hernioplasty was first published by Lichtenstein et al. in 1986 (35,36). That report described an onlay technique using sutured polypropylene mesh. What was most significant about this approach was that the mesh was not used as reinforcement to an antecedent autologous tissue reconstruction, but defined the repair itself. No attempt is made to use abnormal autologous groin tissues in the reconstruction. The initial report from this noncontrolled or randomized, single experience cited 1,000 consecutive repairs with no recurrences over 5 years.

Mesh Plugs

Another surgical concept developed to replace or augment biologically defective groin tissue and achieve tension-appropriate repairs was mesh-plugging herniorrhaphy (Fig. 39.4). This was first described by Lichtenstein and Shore in 1974 for the treatment of recurrent or femoral hernias (37). In this operation, the hernia sac is dissected and reduced to the level of the myofascial hernia ring. The sac neck is then dissected from the hernia ring, and the hernia is invaginated without ligation or excision. A sheet of synthetic mesh (usually knitted polypropylene) of dimensions of approximately 2 cm × 20 cm is rolled into a cylindrical shape that best fits the defect. The plug is inserted into the preperitoneal space until the outer edge is flush with the hernia defect margin and secured into place with circumferential interrupted sutures. Single institution series with minimum follow-up of 1 year reports recurrence rates of <5%. Proponents of the technique argue that it is simple to learn and safe. The minimum dissection required lowers

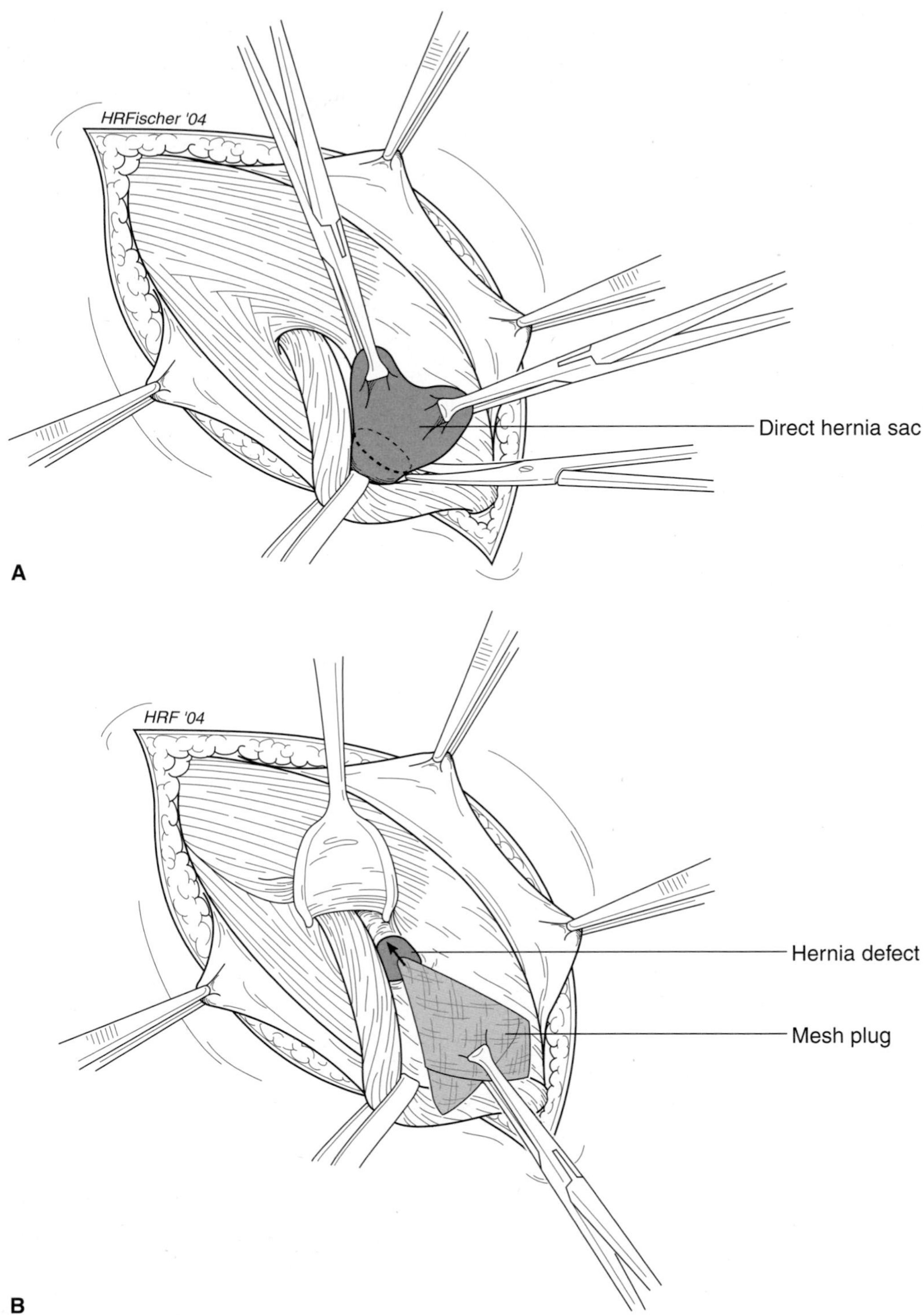

FIGURE 39.4. Mesh-plug inguinal herniorrhaphy starts with a careful dissection of the limits of the hernia sac (**A**), reduction of the hernia sac to the preperitoneal space and the sizing of a cone-shaped mesh plug (**B**), and anchoring of the seated mesh plug to the surrounding transversalis fascia or mature hernia ring with several interrupted sutures. (*continued*)

the incidence of inguinal nerve and adjacent organ injury. In addition, the absence of extensive groin dissection and opening of the inguinal floor prevents iatrogenic injury to the structures of the inguinal canal. A common modification of the mesh-plug technique includes the addition of a sheet mesh onlay onto the floor of the inguinal canal following implantation of the mesh plug. Proponents of this technique believe this repair can be done without suture anchors, again lowering the risk of inguinal nerve and adjacent organ injury, with equal medium-term results. The mesh plug and mesh plug combined with a mesh sheet onlay appear most amenable to Nyhus types I and II (indirect) inguinal hernia repairs and to easily definable recurrent inguinal hernias.

Preperitoneal Inguinal Hernia Repair

The posterior approach to the inguinal canal and iliopubic tract repair using a prosthetic buttress has reported success

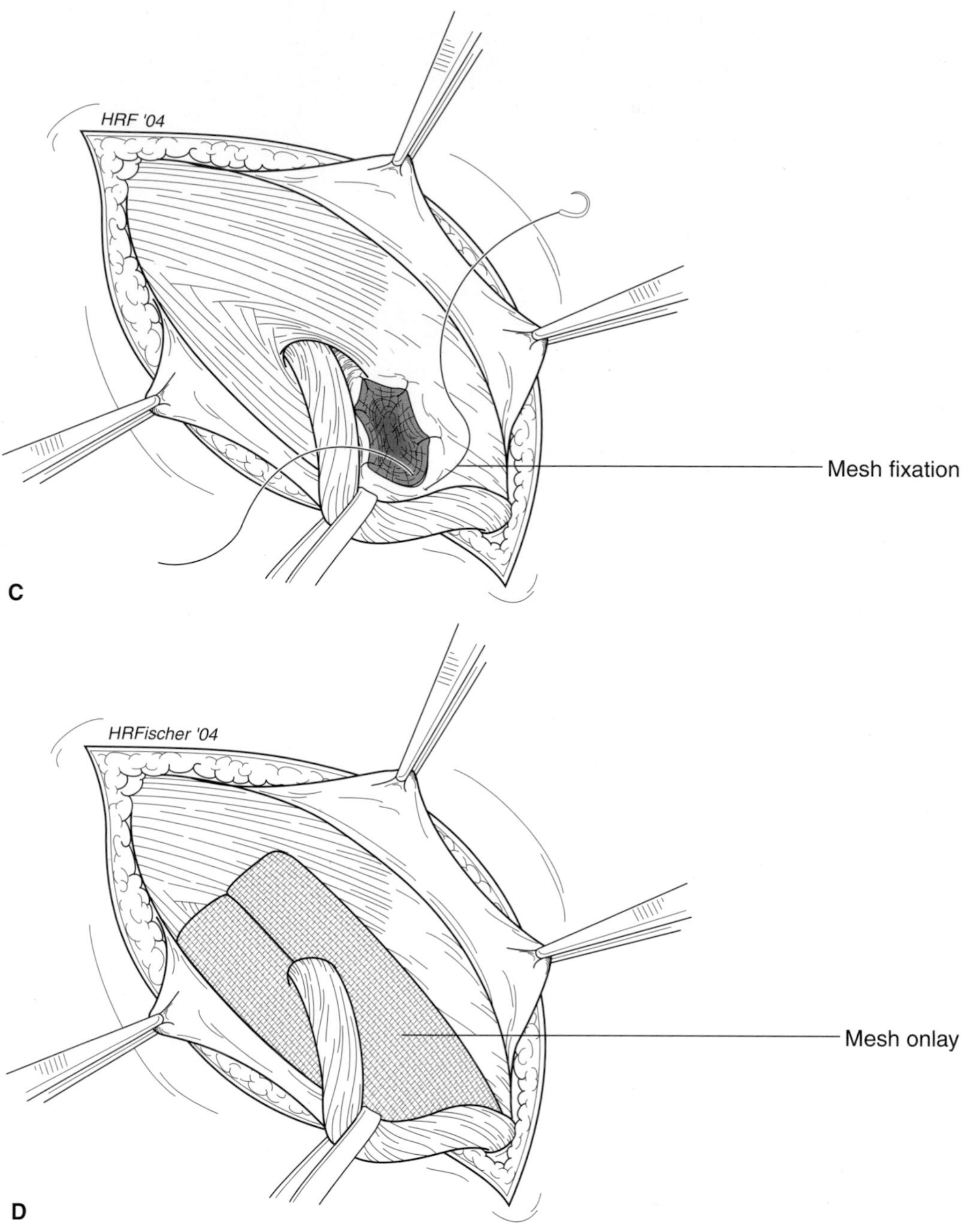

FIGURE 39.4. (*Continued*) Some surgeons advocate the addition of a mesh onlay, often without sutures or tacks, to reinforce the plug and to protect against herniation through adjacent tissue within the floor of the inguinal canal (**C** and **D**).

in both complicated primary and recurrent inguinal hernias (Nyhus types III and IV) (38,39). Procedures to repair the iliopubic tract using a posterior approach have several immediate advantages. Primary among these is operation for recurrent hernia, where dissection can be carried out through unscarred and undistorted preperitoneal tissue planes. All defects within the myopectineal orifice can be reduced and repaired via the same incision. These principles have now been adapted to minimally invasive technologies. The preperitoneal space can be entered and developed using two or three 5- or 10-mm incisions and an identical repair completed laparoscopically.

An open approach to the preperitoneal space is typically completed using a transverse lower abdominal wall incision placed ~4 cm superior to the pubic symphysis. The incision is slightly higher than that used for anterior inguinal herniorrhaphies. The external ring is identified so that an estimation of the location of the internal ring may be made. The posterior approach to the floor of the inguinal canal requires that the abdominal wall incision be fashioned above the internal ring. The transversalis fascia is incised transversely, and the preperitoneal space is carefully developed with blunt dissection. It is usually unnecessary to ligate and divide the deep inferior epigastric vessels in order to achieve adequate exposure. The inferior epigastric vessels can be inadvertently injured at the lateral margin of this incision. Care must be used to avoid unintended opening of the peritoneum and entry into the peritoneal cavity. Examination of the posterior wall of the inguinal canal allows for diagnosis and reduction of hernia defects. Most direct hernia sacs are easily reduced and inverted. A large direct hernia sac may be invaginated using a purse-string suture carefully placed in the transversalis fascia or aponeurosis. Injury to the adjacent bladder should be avoided, especially if a decision is made to excise a direct hernia sac. In performing an autologous tissue repair, the superior transversalis fascia and aponeurosis of the transversalis arch are typically sewn to the iliopubic tract to close the direct defect. Medially, the suture may also be passed through both the Cooper ligament and the medial iliopubic tract for reinforcement.

If there is an indirect hernia, the sac is reduced with careful traction and a high ligation is performed. If dissection of a large indirect hernia sac is difficult, abdominal organs are reduced and the sac may be transected at its neck and closed with a purse-string suture. The distal sac is left open to minimize the incidence of postoperative hydrocele. An internal ring plasty is then performed.

Femoral hernias may also be gently reduced via the preperitoneal approach. If there is an incarcerated femoral hernia, it might be released by incising the insertion of the iliopubic tract to the Cooper ligament at the medial border of the femoral ring. Once reduced, the femoral sheath defect is obliterated using sutures between the iliopubic tract and the Cooper ligament. On rare occasion, a counter incision in the upper thigh over an incarcerated femoral hernia may be necessary to affect a safe release from restricting fascia. This should, however, be an uncommon maneuver.

Hemostasis is especially important during the preperitoneal approach. A relatively larger potential space exists for hematoma accumulation following the preperitoneal dissection. However, the tamponading effect of the peritoneal sac and preperitoneum once it is returned to its normal anatomic location makes the incidence of significant postoperative bleeding very low following the preperitoneal approach. Investigators have reported a lower incidence of testicular atrophy and chronic neuropathic pain following the posterior preperitoneal approach to inguinal hernias (39), believed to be the result of sparing injury to the inguinal nerve supply that courses lateral and anterior to this operative field. Reported hernia recurrence rates average 3% to 6%.

The preperitoneal posterior repair of recurrent inguinal hernias is usually "buttressed" with an approximately 5 cm × 12 cm polypropylene mesh that is anchored to the Cooper ligament and the transversalis fascia superior to the previous repair. The preperitoneal position of the mesh implant imparts a mechanical advantage to the radial load forces of the abdominal wall.

Laparoscopic Inguinal Herniorrhaphy

Various laparoscopic techniques for repairing inguinal hernia are the newest developments in the long history of hernia surgery. Proponents of laparoscopic approaches to inguinal herniorrhaphy argue that they are the most anatomically appropriate. The advantages are a clear, upclose videoscopic examination of the posterior inguinal floor and myopectineal orifice, simultaneous examination of the three major sites of inguinal herniation (internal ring, Hesselbach triangle, and femoral triangle), and the most mechanically advantageous repair. Following reduction of hernia contents, reinforcement of all myopectineal defects is completed in the preperitoneal position. Placement of a mesh prosthesis posterior to the inguinal floor is such that distractive forces originating in the peritoneum tend to secure the prosthesis in place.

The most commonly reported technique for laparoscopic inguinal hernia repair today is the totally extraperitoneal preperitoneal approach (TEPPA) (Fig. 39.5). Like

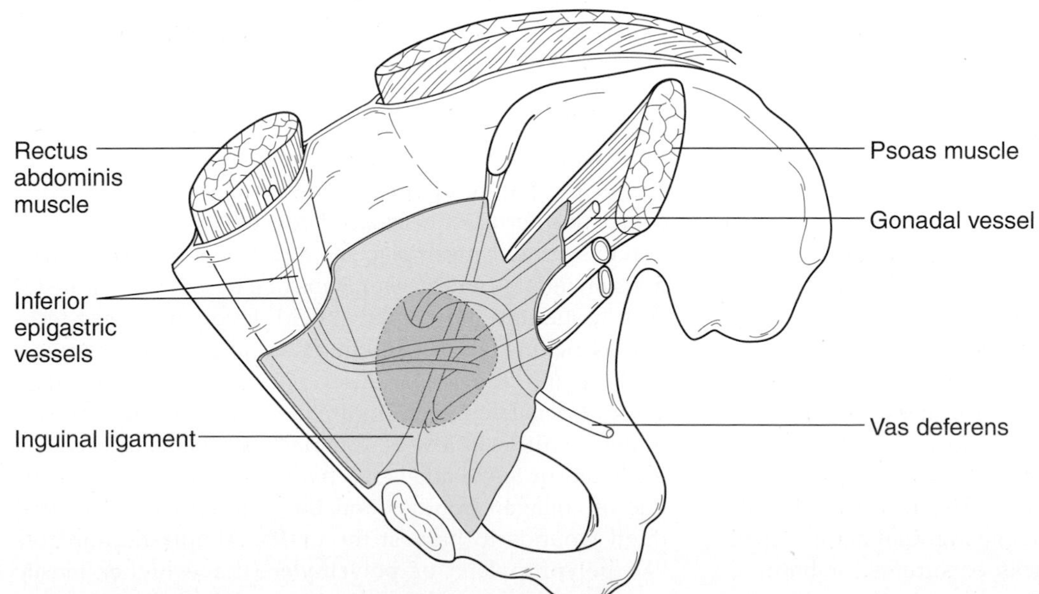

FIGURE 39.5. The TEPPA during laparoscopic inguinal hernia repair requires the development of the preperitoneal space of the lower abdominal wall. This allows a posterior approach to the potential and real defects of the inguinal canal. Important nearby structures are illustrated, including the vas deferens, iliac vessels, inferior epigastric vessels, rectus muscle, and inguinal ligament. Mesh delivered into this preperitoneal space may be secured in place by the radial pressure of the peritoneal sac following desufflation. This finding has led to the successful development of TEPPA inguinal hernia repairs without the need for suture or tack fixation. It is believed that this modification lowers the incidence of chronic pain syndromes due to nerve injuries.

most laparoscopy, TEPPA herniorrhaphy requires a general anesthetic. The operation begins with dissection and development of a preperitoneal space. This dissection is typically achieved through an infraumbilical incision with subsequent incision of the anterior rectus sheath and lateral retraction of the rectus muscle. A balloon dissector may be directed toward the pubic symphysis and inflated slowly to create this operating space. Some surgeons omit using a balloon dissector and create the preperitoneal space using finger or hemostat dissection.

Great care must be exercised to avoid inadvertent entry into the peritoneal space, which obviates the advantages of the TEPPA approach. The most obvious advantage of the TEPPA approach is the ability to stay out of the peritoneal cavity and reduce the chance of injury to abdominal organs. The preperitoneal space is fairly avascular, with occasional small vessels traversing between the transversalis fascia and the reflected peritoneum. If a balloon dissector is used, it may remain inflated for several minutes to tamponade these crossing vessels. Significant hematomas can form in the preperitoneal space, especially in older patients with more areolar tissue planes.

An adequate dissection should extend just beyond the midline, below the Cooper ligament (6 to 8 cm below the inguinal ligament), well above the transversus abdominis aponeurotic arch, and widely beyond the internal ring. Experts report that an inadequate dissection of the peritoneum away from the posterior inguinal wall is the most common reason for recurrent hernias following TEPPA repairs.

An appropriately sized piece of synthetic mesh (~12 cm × 6 cm) is delivered via the endoscopic port site into the preperitoneal space to reinforce the posterior wall of the inguinal canal. Debate exists on whether it is necessary to secure this mesh in place with either sutures or tacks. It is also unclear whether it is necessary to split the mesh and encircle the spermatic cord through a "keyhole." Proponents argue that a minimum of mesh anchors placed into the transversalis fascia and encircling of the spermatic cord through a slit mesh results in lower hernia recurrence rates. Opponents suggest that anchoring the mesh and the additional dissection of the spermatic cord increases the incidence of postoperative chronic pain. No definitive reports have resolved these technical issues.

The TEPPA repair can result in recurrence rates equivalent to open herniorrhaphy, without significant wounding of the anterior abdominal wall and, therefore, with a lower wound complication rate. Recurrences tend to occur medially where the iliac vessels pass beneath the mesh or laterally, especially when there is dilated internal ring. For these reasons, the medial and lateral mesh edges are often held in place during desufflation after unilateral TEPPA repairs. There is a slightly earlier return to usual activities following TEPPA inguinal herniorrhaphy. The incidence of neuropathic pain following laparoscopic inguinal hernia repairs is minimized if anchoring tacks or sutures, or both, are placed above the inguinal ligament and away from the course of the ilioinguinal, iliofemoral, and hypogastric nerves (40).

The transabdominal preperitoneal (TAPP) approach for laparoscopic inguinal hernia repair was described before the TEPPA technique was developed. The TAPP approach is intraabdominal and has a higher risk of abdominal organ injury. The hernia dissection is somewhat easier because the space is greater. The preperitoneal space is ultimately exposed with this approach as well. It is important to incise completely through the peritoneum and preperitoneum posterior to the inguinal floor until the areolar space of Bogros is entered between the transversalis fascia and the peritoneum. If not, dissection in the amorphous preperitoneal fat and fascia may lead to bleeding and confusion about inguinal anatomy.

Complications unique to the laparoscopic approach to inguinal herniorrhaphy include trocar injuries and problems with insufflation. The operating space for the TEPPA procedure is a much smaller volume than for intraperitoneal laparoscopic operations. Operating ports should always be placed under direct vision so that injury to adjacent structures and organs may be avoided. Injury to the inferior epigastric vessels can cause significant bleeding. Blunt, radially dilating ports have lower incidences of adjacent organ injury and lower abdominal wall complications than bladed laparoscopic ports. Occasionally, insufflation of the preperitoneal space will result in unexpected pneumoperitoneum. This occurrence suggests the presence of a defect in the peritoneum. If a defect in the peritoneum is identified, the hole should be closed with sutures or clips, taking care to protect against injury to intraabdominal organs. Preperitoneal insufflation may induce the same hemodynamic changes observed during intraabdominal laparoscopic procedures, usually the result of reduced venous return. One distressing effect of preperitoneal insufflation is the appearance of scrotal dissection and pneumoscrotum. This development is almost uniformly self-limiting, and patients should be reassured. With experience, TEPPA repairs may be performed at lower insufflation pressures to minimize subcutaneous emphysema.

Autologous Tissue Transfers

Recurrent hernias often occur because of local tissue loss and or the failure of collagenous tissues to obliterate the course of a hernia or because of infection and contraindication to synthetic mesh placement. When sufficient collagenous material is not present, it may be necessary to transfer such tissue into the operative field. Frequently used techniques include harvest and implantation of free tensor fascia lata and the tensor fascia lata myocutaneous flap. Tensor fascia lata free grafts are ideal for small area defects under medium to low abdominal wall loads. The risk of using tensor fascia lata is mechanical failure parallel to the line of collagen bundles and the requirement for lateral thigh wounds to harvest the grafts. Alloplastic implants like polypropylene or polyethylene have higher tensile strengths, but have a higher incidence of bowel fistulization and foreign body infections. Collagen-based biological mesh implants offer a potential alternative without the need for the wounding of autologous donor sites.

Strangulated Hernias

If the preoperative evaluation raises any concern for a strangulated viscus, a transperitoneal approach to the involved bowel should be strongly considered. Transperitoneal exposure of the unaffected intestine at the hernia ring improves the control of the gangrenous bowel segment. The posterior iliopubic tract repair may follow intestinal resection and anastomosis. In the obese patient, it may be difficult to diagnose impending strangulation due to hernia incarceration. A high index of suspicion must be maintained. Imaging studies may show soft-tissue gas, bowel wall thickening, or free air. The skin overlying the strangulation may be firm, erythematous, and tender.

Table **39.4** Risk factors for wound infection following incisional hernia repair
Operative time
Devascularized tissue
Obesity
Hematoma formation
Foreign material (mesh)
Bowel or bladder injury
Malnutrition
Advanced age
Chronic disease
Polypharmacy

Incisional hernias

Incisional hernia is the most common indication for reoperation in abdominal surgery patients (3). Many recurrent inguinal hernias are also incisional hernias. Incisional hernias are unique because they are the only abdominal wall hernias considered iatrogenic. Because the reported incidence of acute fascial dehiscence is 0.5% and the incidence of primary incisional hernia formation is 11%, it is clear that many incisional hernias go unrecognized in the early postoperative period (16,18). It appears that the incidence of incisional hernia approached one in three in patients with a BMI >35 (obese).

Fascial wound healing achieves only 60% to 80% of unwounded fascial strength after 6 weeks (29). Collagen deposition and fiber orientation along lines of stress occur during this interval. Nine to 12 months pass before fascial scar approaches uninjured breaking strength. For this reason, most patients should be cautioned to avoid overloading their abdominal wall for at least 6 weeks following celiotomy. A common practice is to resume near-normal activity and abdominal wall loads 2 weeks following fascial closure, with great care to load the abdominal wound only as comfort permits. Patients should be educated about the biology of wound repair and the need to restrict sudden loads of their ventral wounds, as with coughing or sneezing.

Success of incisional hernia repair depends on basic surgical principles. These precepts include the incorporation of normal fascial tissue brought together under a physiologic abdominal wall load and the avoidance of the risk factors for recurrent herniation.

Autologous tissue repairs

At first, incisional hernia repairs made use of local, autologous abdominal wall tissue to correct abdominal wall defects. Most often, this amounted to no more than reclosure of a laparotomy incision or mature incisional hernia ring. The reoperative nature of incisional herniorrhaphy increases the risk of unplanned visceral injuries due to the requirement for adhesiolysis and enterolysis. Blood loss may also be increased, depending on the extent of the adhesiolysis. Many prospective series have documented the extremely high incisional hernia recurrence rate following repair with local, autologous tissue (24% to 54%) (3–5).

Recent large reviews have also found an increased risk of wound infection following incisional hernia repair (25,26). The risk factors for incisional hernia formation and the risk factors for wound infections are often the same. These risks include obesity, malnutrition, advanced age, chronic pulmonary disease, and polypharmacy. Wounds following incisional hernia repair are at increased risk for infection due to technical factors like prolonged operations, hematoma formation, devascularized or ischemic tissue, bowel injury, and the presence of foreign material such as previously placed mesh (Table 39.4).

A prospective, randomized, and controlled study of incisional hernia repair concluded that mesh implantation is required to achieve the lowest recurrent hernia rate (4,5). In practice, synthetic mesh implantation is not always a clinical option or the patient's preference, and even with mesh implantation, the recurrent incisional hernia rate was still 24%. For all these reasons, autologous tissue closures are still occasionally recommended and undertaken.

The size of the fascial defect and the quality of the fascia should guide the selection of the hernia repair. The skin and subcutaneous tissue are dissected away from the hernia sac, but great care should be used to preserve the blood supply to the overlying skin. Viable skin provides the most important coverage for the underlying hernia repair, by whatever method. Normal-appearing fascia should be identified back from the fascial hernia ring on both ventral and peritoneal surfaces. A minimum of 3 cm of fascial exposure for suture placement is the published expert consensus (41).

If a fascial defect is so large as to preclude incisional hernia repair by simple reclosure, a number of other repairs using autologous tissue have been described. Simplest among these is the use of internal retention sutures. Other variations of local myofascial relaxing incisions are used. During the Keel procedure, vertical relaxing incisions are placed along the lateral edge of the anterior rectus sheath, allowing medial advancement of the medial edge of the anterior rectus sheath. This approach is especially useful in upper midline abdominal wall hernias, where a stout posterior rectus sheath protects against further iatrogenic injury (42). For midline defects in the lower abdomen, mobilization of the lower section of rectus muscle and enveloping fascia and reapproximation to the contralateral side has been described.

Abdominal wall component separation techniques have gained in popularity in an effort to reconstruct large abdominal wall defects, restore abdominal wall function, and minimize the use of synthetic mesh implants in contaminated or infected operative fields (43). Fundamentally, these operations include the elevation of wide, lateral skin flaps to identify the underlying myofascial anatomy and to release the fascia from its dermal attachments. Next, the full length of the external oblique muscle is incised, usually from the costal margin to the pubis. Great care is used to preserve the integrity of the underlying internal oblique and transversalis muscles. The subcostal and lateral segmental nerve supply to the anterior abdominal wall run in the plane between the internal oblique and transversalis muscles. Inadvertent entry into this plane and nerve injury may cause anterior eventration due to denervation. The external oblique incision is typically placed ~1 cm lateral to the lateral edge of the rectus sheath (linea semilunaris). This maneuver provides on average 4 to 6 cm of medial advancement of the rectus sheath. Anterior rectus sheath or posterior rectus sheath relaxing incisions may be added to increase the advancement distance of the midline, although this may compromise the integrity of the rectus sheath. All variations of abdominal wall component separations increase the risk for bleeding and hematoma/seroma formation. Prolonged subcutaneous drainage is frequently indicated and recommended. The risk for overlying skin necrosis is increased because of the necessity for wide skin flaps. Wound ischemia is minimized by the preservation of periumbilical vascular stalks traveling from the myofascial of the rectus component to the ventral skin.

Synthetic Abdominal Wall Meshes

The implantation of synthetic tissue prostheses was introduced to incisional herniorrhaphy in an attempt to reduce the unacceptably high incisional hernia recurrence rates when using only local, autologous tissue for reclosure (Fig. 39.6) (44). Prospective, randomized studies found that an independent risk factor for recurrent incisional hernia is the technique of primary tissue repair without the use of a mesh implant (4,5). Synthetic implants are, however, associated with a characteristic set of complications. First among these complications is mesh-associated infection and foreign body inflammatory reaction. The risk of mesh infection and prolonged inflammation is greatest following incisional ventral hernia repair (26). Other series report a significant incidence of chronic pain following mesh implantation (45–47).

The most commonly used mesh materials are knitted monofilament polypropylene (Marlex), woven polypropylene (Prolene), woven polyester (Mersilene, Parietex), expanded or extruded polytetrafluoroethylene (ePTFE, Gore-Tex), knitted polyglycolic acid (Vicryl), and knitted polygalactic acid (Dexon) (48–50). Newer fabric designs for the woven meshes suggest that lighter polymer weights

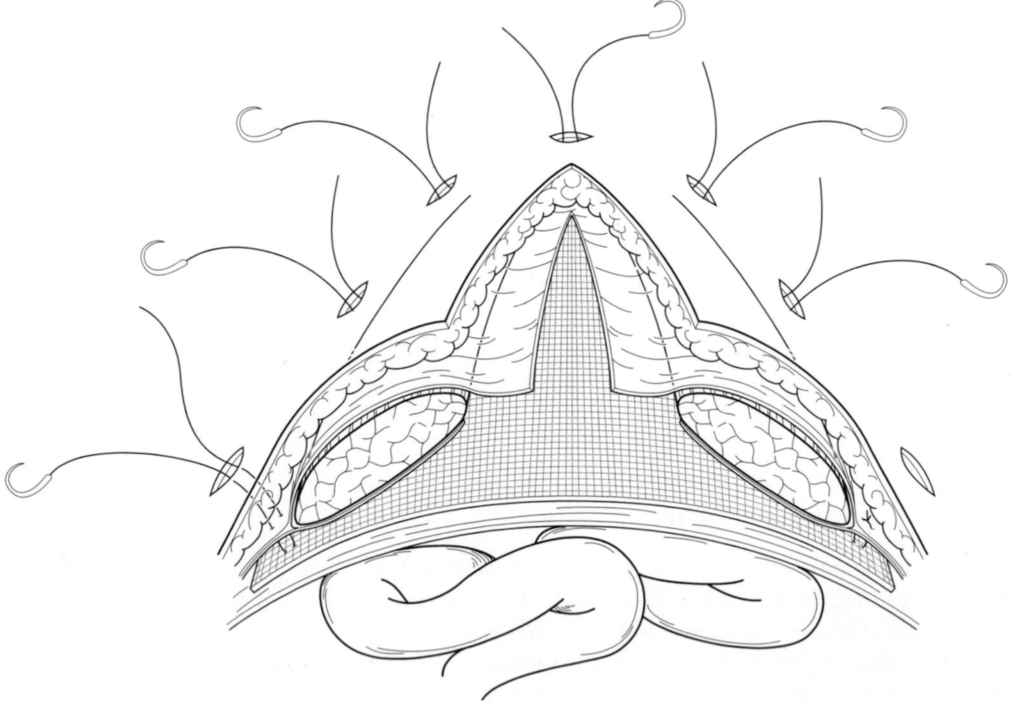

FIGURE 39.6. The best available evidence suggests that a mesh "underlay" technique results in the lowest recurrence rates following incisional hernia repairs. Anatomically, retrofascial/retromuscular, preperitoneal, and intraperitoneal mesh fixation is described. Circumferential, transfascial, or transabdominal fixation sutures are frequently used following the repair of large incisional hernias or when using the laparoscopic technique.

and large weave pore size lowers the foreign body inflammatory response and improves incorporation. PTFE gained popularity because of its reported reduced tissue reactivity and adhesion formation, although concerns have been raised about seroma formation and mesh infection rates. Most authors conclude that absorbable mesh should not be used for permanent abdominal wall reconstruction because of the universal development of recurrent incisional hernias and an increased risk for bowel fistulization (Fig. 39.6).

Serious complications have been observed in patients after incisional hernia repairs with synthetic mesh implantation. The most important serious problems are mesh-associated infection, chronic skin sinus tract formation, erosion into adjacent structures, including bowel, and chronically exposed or extruded mesh (51,52). Mesh placement in the presence of heavy contamination was reported to be associated with a >50% acute wound failure rate (dehiscence) and 22% enteric fistulization rate. Administrative databases now report that the presence of a synthetic mesh in the intraperitoneal position increases the risk of an unplanned enterotomy or bowel resection from 3% to 23% during subsequent abdominal operations (8,9).

Recurrent Hernia

A prospective, randomized study of incisional hernia repair found that risk factors for recurrent hernias included primary reclosure without the use of mesh, postoperative prostatism, and a history of abdominal aortic aneurysm (4). These findings point to potential mechanisms for recurrent incisional herniation. The first two conditions highlight the importance of increased mechanical loads on abdominal wall hernia recurrence. The history of aortic aneurysm disease suggests biological risk factors for hernia recurrence, such as the elevated expression of tissue metalloproteinase. Typically, recurrent incisional hernias are small in area or volume as the result of a limited disruption, usually between the synthetic mesh and the fascia. Often, a simple repair can be undertaken, directed to the area of this defect (Fig. 39.7). When mesh failure occurs, it is almost always at the mesh:fascia interface rather than mesh material central failure.

Infection increases the risk of hernia recurrence. Deep wound infections prolong inflammation and impede collagen deposition. Elective repair should therefore not be attempted if any signs of infection exist, such as a stitch abscess or sinus or overlying skin excoriation. Foreign materials associated with infections should be removed and the overlying skin healed prior to hernia repairs.

The use of autologous local tissues is sometimes preferred during ventral hernia repair. A common situation occurs when infected synthetic mesh is removed. The autologous tissues may be mobilized using component separation of the abdominal wall. One or both sides of the

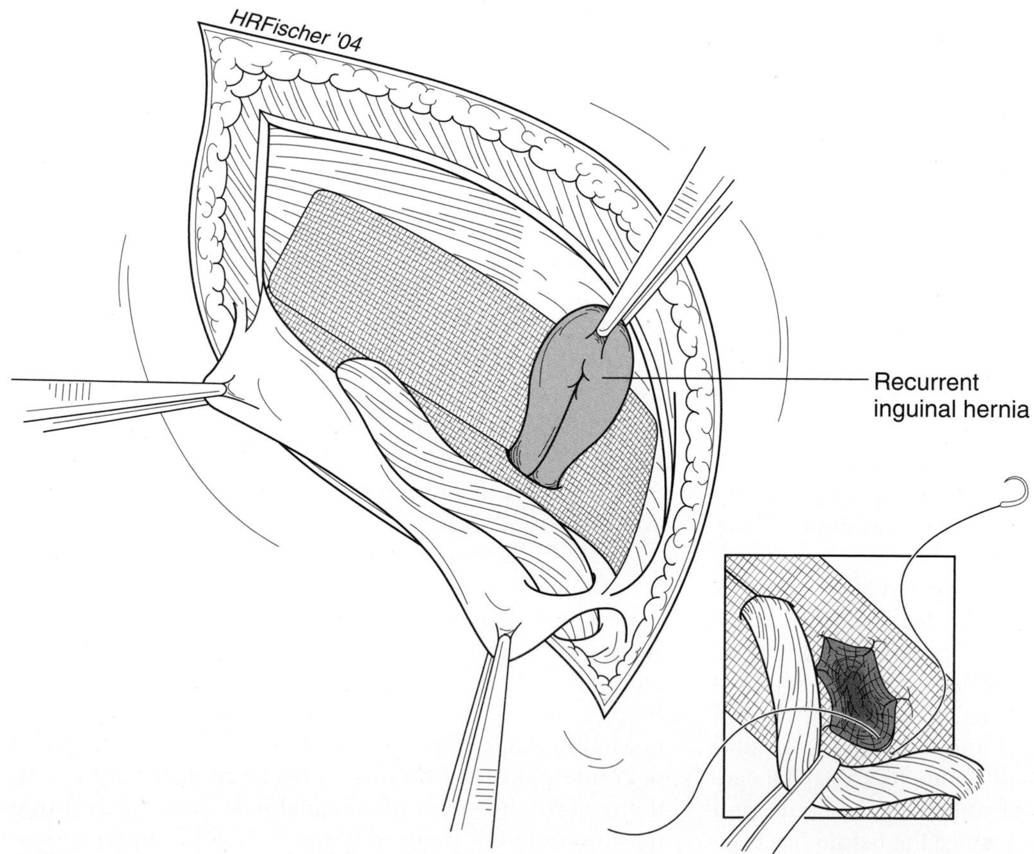

FIGURE 39.7. When detected early, recurrent incisional hernias are usually of a small area or volume as a result of a limited disruption. The mechanism of recurrent incisional hernia formation includes a failure of tissue repair at the interface between the mesh implant and the native fascia. Often, a limited salvage repair can be undertaken, directed to the area of this defect.

abdominal wall may not be amenable to component separation because of previous existing defects such as stoma sites.

Giant Ventral Hernias

Patients with massive incisional hernias usually present with functional loss of the abdominal wall and substantial protrusion of abdominal viscera. Such hernias are frequently associated with chronic abdominal pain, chronic back pain, and erosion of overlying skin. Severe skin lymphedema may ensue. Peritoneal volume (abdominal domain) is gradually lost as abdominal viscera remain herniated. Massive ventral hernias with significant loss of abdominal domain also can cause diaphragmatic dysfunction and intestinal circulatory congestion (38).

The technique of serial preoperative therapeutic pneumoperitoneum to reestablish abdominal domain offers one approach to the problem of peritoneal volume loss (38). This method has lost popularity with the increased use of "tension-free" mesh-based repairs. Because the incidence of primary and recurrent incisional hernias remains so high and the complications associated with synthetic mesh implantation have not been solved, there is renewed interest in tissue expansion and other techniques for the development of autologous tissue sources to repair these difficult wounds (53,54).

Compulsive preparation for operation is mandatory in patients with giant incisional hernias. All skin erosions should be treated prior to elective repair in order to reduce the risk of subsequent infection. Pulmonary function should be optimized, including smoking cessation. Smoking is also a recognized impediment to wound healing. Weight loss is encouraged and medically supported. A multidisciplinary plan involving both general and plastic surgeons is often applied.

Visceral Injuries

The bowel may be injured during the opening or high ligation of an indirect hernia sac. The complication is minimized by careful dissection and the identification of groin structures and by inspection for sliding components. The bladder may be injured during opening of a lower midline incisional hernia or the medial extent of a direct inguinal hernia. The preoperative placement of a urinary drainage catheter (Foley) may reduce the risk of bladder injury. If the bladder is injured, it should be repaired and continuously drained with an indwelling catheter until a cystogram provides proof of healing.

Enterocutaneous fistulas are associated with complex abdominal wall defects and large hernias. The presence of knitted or woven polypropylene or polyethylene meshes appears to increase the risk for delayed enteric fistulization. The presence of mesh during reoperative incisional hernia repair increases the risk of unintended bowel injury due to the presence of dense adhesions (8,9,51). Management should be directed toward control of the fistula and metabolic support of the patient. Once the fistula has been controlled, 6 to 8 weeks of bowel rest should be allowed to pass to permit spontaneous closure. This is most likely in the setting of low or medium output fistulae. If closure does not occur, this period of time will allow surrounding tissue inflammation and infection to improve in anticipation of definitive repair. When operative closure of an enteric fistula is planned in association with a recurrent hernia repair, preoperative diagnostic staging should be done to precisely identify the fistula's anatomy, and especially identify and manage distal gastrointestinal strictures causing obstruction. Every effort should be made to repair the abdominal wall defect with autologous tissue, such as a local advancement flap or free tensor fascia lata. Commercially available biological collagen prostheses offer an alternative to the added wounding of autologous tissue harvesting and the unpredictability of the mechanical integrity of tensor fascia lata, for example.

Vascular Injuries

Inadvertent injury to an aberrant inferior epigastric or obturator artery may occur during lower abdominal wall hernia repairs. Inferior epigastric injuries may result in significant hemorrhage. Another source of inferior epigastric artery injury is the placement of lower abdominal wall ports for laparoscopic hernia operations. Open inguinal floor repairs, such as the Cooper ligament repair and laparoscopic inguinal hernia repairs, place the iliac and femoral vessels at risk for major injury.

Nerve Injuries

Three nerves are exposed to injury during inguinal hernia repairs—the ilioinguinal, genitofemoral, and iliohypogastric nerves (Fig. 39.8). The ilioinguinal and genitofemoral nerves are adjacent to the spermatic cord and the iliohypogastric runs within the internal oblique muscle of the lower abdominal wall. Nerve transection usually results in self-limiting groin or inner thigh anesthesia. Nerve injury is presumably the mechanism for cases of disabling postoperative pain. Recent prospective studies report a 29% incidence of chronic pain following inguinal herniorrhaphy (45–47). For these reasons, great care should be exercised during dissections and repairs to not include the nerves in suture lines or at mesh or tack sites. If pain develops after an initial recovery period, a deep space abscess or dehiscence should be considered. Without either of these two complications, most pain resolves with supportive measures only.

Postherniorrhaphy neuralgia can become a disabling condition. It is important to determine whether the patient had pain prior to hernia repair, whether postoperative pain is the same in character as the preoperative pain, and when inguinodynia began. Most postherniorrhaphy neuralgia is the result of perineural fibrosis, a normal biological process following operation. Delayed neuroma pain may be due to nerve contact with a synthetic mesh; however, the available studies suggest that mesh-associated inguinodynia is not an independent

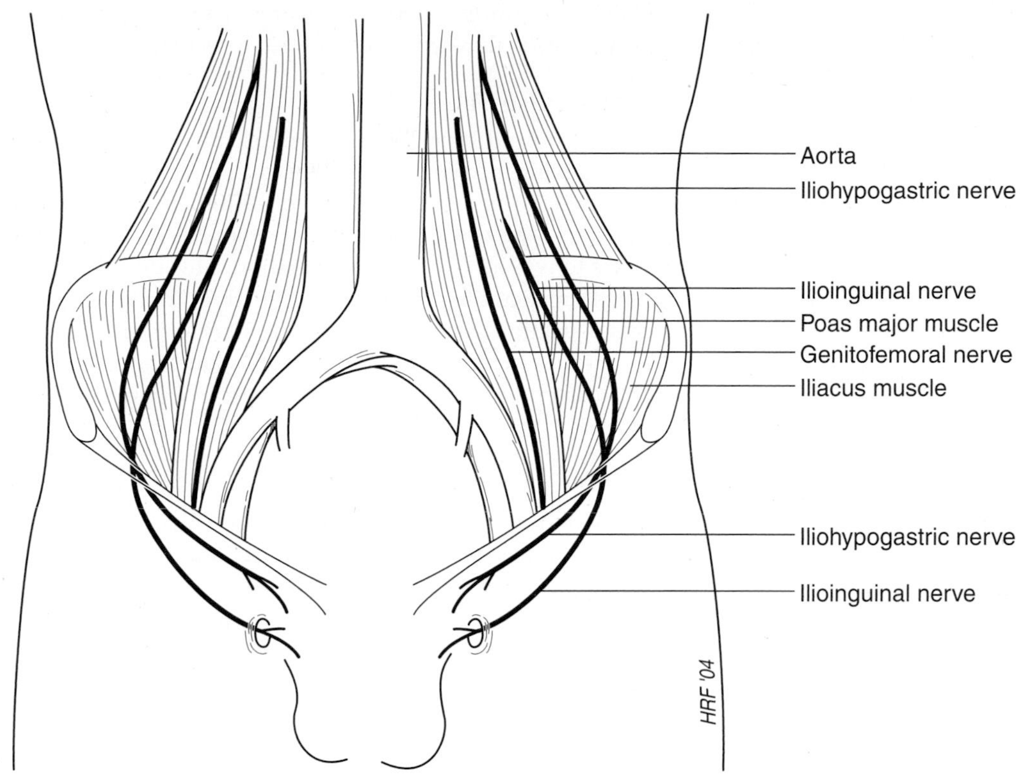

FIGURE 39.8. The ilioinguinal, genitofemoral, and iliohypogastric nerves are exposed to injury during inguinal hernia repairs. The ilioinguinal and genitofemoral nerves are encountered posteriorly during a preperitoneal inguinal hernia repair or within the spermatic cord. The iliohypogastric nerve courses within the internal oblique muscle of the lower abdominal wall and is especially at risk for injury when tacks are placed below the inguinal ligament during a laparoscopic inguinal hernia repair.

entity and the evidence does not support clinical references to mesh-induced chronic pain syndrome. Apparent neuromas associated with mesh explants have been observed in patients with no pain syndrome when reoperated for another reason, such as recurrence.

The most common mechanism of inguinal nerve injury is failure to identify and protect the three major groin nerves exposed during herniorrhaphy. Limited dissection without the identification of all major structures of the inguinal canal increases the risk of nerve injury and therefore of chronic inguinodynia. The external ring should not be closed too tightly to prevent exposure of the ilioinguinal nerve to the suture line of the external oblique fascial closure. The ilioinguinal nerve should not be extensively mobilized from the cremasteric layer in order to minimize injury to its neurolemmal sheath. During the dissection of the subcutaneous adipose tissue, early surface branches of the ilioinguinal and/or iliohypogastric nerves should be spared. Deep stapling or tacking should be avoided during laparoscopic inguinal hernia repair in order to prevent entrapment of the iliohypogastric, genital (medial to the internal ring), and ilioinguinal (lateral to the internal ring) nerves.

When conservative measures fail for at least 6 months, surgical therapy of neuralgia may be considered. Surgery is usually required for perineural fibrosis, nerve entrapment by suture, staple, or prosthetic device, and neuroma formation. The triggering or aggravation of neuropathic pain by walking or during hyperextension of the hip and alleviation by rest and flexion of the thigh suggest that traction of the involved nerve due to its adherence to the aponeurotic tissue of the groin is an important mechanism. Surgical therapy of postherniorrhaphy inguinodynia is most likely to be successful if the three involved nerves are resected. Neurolysis is not recommended. The approach to the lower abdominal wall is preperitoneal via a lower midline or high inguinal incision. The entire lengths of the nerves should be resected as proximally as possible to include the involved segment and the numerous neural communications that exist between the three nerves. The transected proximal nerve ends are ligated and embedded into the internal oblique muscle layer to reduce the incidence of neuroma formation. Any suture, staple, or alloplastic mesh material encountered along the length of the nerves is also excised. The complete removal of mesh does not appear to be necessary.

Testicular Infarct

Severe testicular pain, swelling, and tenderness may occur after inguinal hernia repair, especially if the spermatic cord is skeletonized of muscle and fat or divided. The risk is increased following a reoperation using an open technique through the scarred inguinal canal. Orchiectomy is sometimes required to resolve this complication. If obliteration of the internal ring is anticipated, such as during the repair of a multiply recurrent inguinal hernia, consent for orchiectomy may be obtained. During the dissection of fat and muscle from the spermatic cord, great care should be used in preserving the testicular artery and vein.

Scrotal Hematoma

Hematoma in the scrotum arises from small vessels within the cremasteric muscles. In the loose, areolar tissue of the scrotum, tamponade is minimal. This complication may be avoided by minimizing dissection of indirect sacs off the spermatic cord. Only the high point of the indirect sac is mobilized for ligation of the internal ring. When a long indirect sac must be mobilized, as in a sliding hernia, the risk for a scrotal hematoma may be reduced by the use of a scrotal support after operation. Prophylactic drainage does not prevent scrotal hematoma formation.

When a scrotal hematoma occurs, it is usually dispersed between several layers of the repair and the spermatic cord. Needle aspiration is therefore usually not helpful. Effective evacuation would require reopening of the wound and is necessary only for very large and tense hematomas that occur immediately following surgery. Stable or delayed hematomas may be managed with rest, warm and cold compresses, and close observation for continued bleeding or infection, or both.

Chronic Abdominal Wall Wounds

Abdominal wall wounds may lead to chronic clinical complaints, including incisional pain, protrusion, numbness, or unappealing appearance. An underlying visceral abnormality must first be excluded. Questions may be raised about secondary gain, especially in cases of chronic pain and disability claims (55,56). It is often helpful to educate patients about the expected course of surgical recovery, especially as it relates to the phases of wound healing. For example, patients are often concerned about the color or mass of scars. This anxiety may be reduced by explaining that the inflammatory and proliferative phases of tissue repair may last weeks to months. Laparotomy patients may develop a prominent "healing ridge" as fascial scar proliferation maximizes 2 to 6 weeks postoperatively. Some patients complain of numbness below transverse or oblique incisions. This occurs as the result of transected distal spinal nerves and usually becomes unnoticeable after several months.

Chronic pain in a scar may be difficult to explain and treat. Prior to any intervention, an incisional hernia should be excluded by careful examination and noninvasive imaging. An intraperitoneal disorder is unlikely if the symptom is reproduced or aggravated by straining the muscles of the abdominal wall. Rarely, incisional pain is caused by ossification of the scar and relieved by excision of bony tissue, although heterotopic ossification notoriously recurs. Chronic pain at the epigastrium may be due to injury to the xiphoid process during wound closure. Rarely, excision of the xiphoid process relieves this source of discomfort. Underlying fascial sutures that came close to the skin surface may cause chronic pain, especially in thin patients. Ultimately, suture removal may be required.

Eccentric bulging of the abdominal wall may occur when nerve or arterial supply is severed during surgical incision. Examples include division of the 12th intercostal nerve during flank incision with rib resection.

Wound Hematoma

During ventral hernia repair, the fascia is widely exposed and relaxing incisions are made to minimize the hernia ring area and to maximize the use of autologous local tissue transfers. The broad subcutaneous skin dissection predisposes to wound hematoma formation. This potential mandates meticulous hemostasis during operation and closed-suction drainage until discharge stops. Surgical techniques to reduce tissue dead space and the application of pressure dressings may also help reduce hematoma formation.

Pulmonary Complications

Reduction and repair of large hernias may impair pulmonary function by inhibiting coughing due to the incisional pain and by mechanically restricting diaphragmatic excursion. The repair of a giant hernia with the loss of abdominal domain may require prolonged ventilator dependence until incisional pain improves and the peritoneal cavity accommodates its restored contents. The implantation of an allograft mesh is often required to minimize abdominal cavity pressures. Peak airway pressure intraoperatively may be used as a surrogate marker for elevated intraabdominal pressure during abdominal wall reconstruction. There is growing evidence that abdominal wall reconstructive procedures like component separation increase abdominal volume following the repair of large abdominal wall defects with the protection of pulmonary function (57,58).

REFERENCES

1. Dubay DA, Franz MG. Acute wound healing: the biology of acute wound failure. *Surg Clin North Am* 2003;83(3):463–481.
2. National Center for Health Statistics. *Detailed diagnoses and procedures, National Hospital Discharge Survey, 1995.* Hyattsville, MD: National Center for Health Statistics; 1997.
3. Flum DR, Horvath K, Koepsell T. Have outcomes of incisional hernia repair improved with time? A population-based analysis. *Ann Surg* 2003;237(1):129–135.
4. Luijendijk RW, Hop WCJ, van den Tol P, et al. A comparison of suture repair with mesh repair for incisional hernia. *N Engl J Med* 2000;343(6): 392–398.
5. Burger JW, Luijendijk RW, Hop WC, et al. Long-term follow-up of a randomized controlled trial of suture versus mesh repair of incisional hernia. *Ann Surg* 2004;240(4):578–583.
6. Carlson MA. Acute wound failure. *Surg Clin North Am* 1997;77(3): 607–636.
7. Jenkins TPN. The burst abdominal wound: a mechanical approach. *Br J Surg* 1976;63:873.
8. Gray SH, Vick CC, Graham LA, et al. Risk of complications from enterotomy or unplanned bowel resection during elective hernia repair. *Arch Surg* 2008;143(6):582–586.
9. Halm JA, de Wall LL, Steyerberg EW, et al. Intraperitoneal polypropylene mesh hernia repair complicates subsequent abdominal surgery. *World J Surg* 2007;31(2):423–429.
10. Webster C, Neumayer L, Smout R, et al. Prognostic models of abdominal wound dehiscence after laparotomy. *J Surg Res* 2003;109:130–137.
11. Etchells E, O'Neill C, Bernstein M. Patient safety in surgery: error detection and prevention. *World J Surg* 2003;27(8):936–941.

12. Diaz JJ Jr, Guy J, Berkes MB, et al. Acellular dermal allograft for ventral hernia repair in the compromised surgical field. *Am Surg* 2006;72(12): 1181–1187.
13. Diaz JJ Jr, Conquest AM, Ferzoco SJ, et al. Multi-institutional experience using human acellular dermal matrix for ventral hernia repair in a compromised surgical field. *Arch Surg* 2009;144(3):209–215.
14. Kim H, Bruen K, Vargo D. Acellular dermal matrix in the management of high-risk abdominal wall defects. *Am J Surg* 2006;192(6):705–709.
15. Best WR, Khuri SF, Phelan M. Identifying patient preoperative risk factors and postoperative adverse events in administrative databases: results from the Department of Veterans Affairs National Surgical Quality Improvement Program. *J Am Coll Surg* 2002;194(3):257–266.
16. Burger JW, Lange JF, Halm JA, et al. Incisional hernia: early complication of abdominal surgery. *World J Surg* 2005;29(12):1608–1613.
17. Merkow RP, Bilimoria KY, McCarter MD, et al. Effect of body mass index on short-term outcomes after colectomy for cancer. *J Am Coll Surg* 2009;208:53–61.
18. Pollock AV, Evans M. Early prediction of late incisional hernias. *Br J Surg* 1989;76:953–954.
19. Franz MG. The biology of hernia formation. *Surg Clin North Am* 2008; 88(1):1–15, vii.
20. Smith PD, Kuhn MA, Franz MG, et al. Initiating the inflammatory phase of incisional healing prior to tissue injury. *J Surg Res* 2000;92(1): 11–17.
21. Banda MJ, Dwyer KS, Beckmann A. Wound fluid angiogenesis factor stimulates the directed migration of capillary endothelial cells. *J Cell Biochem* 1985;29:183–193.
22. Ayde B, Luna G. Incidence of abdominal wall hernia in aortic surgery. *Am J Surg* 1998;175:400–402.
23. Hall KA, Peters B, Smyth SH. Abdominal wall hernias in patients with abdominal aortic aneurysm versus aortoiliac occlusive disease. *Am J Surg* 1995;170:572.
24. Peacock J. Fascia and muscle. In: Peacock J, ed. *Wound repair*, 3rd ed. Philadelphia, PA: W.B. Saunders; 1984:332–362.
25. Dunne JR, Malone DL, Tracy JK, et al. Abdominal wall hernias: risk factors for infection and resource utilization. *J Surg Res* 2003;111(1):78–84.
26. Houck JP, Rypins EB, Sarfeh IJ, et al. Repair of incisional hernia. *Surg Gynecol Obstet* 1989;169(5):397–399.
27. Tilson MD, Seashore MR. Human genetics of the abdominal aortic aneurysm. *Surg Gynecol Obstet* 1984;158:129–132.
28. Lehnert B, Wadouh F. High coincidence of inguinal hernias and abdominal aortic aneurysms. *Ann Vasc Surg* 1992;6:134–137.
29. Leaper DJ, Gottrup F. Surgical wounds. In: Leaper DJ, Harding KG, eds. *Wounds: biology and management*, 1st ed. Oxford: Oxford University Press; 1998:23–40.
30. Rutledge RH. The Cooper ligament repair. *Surg Clin North Am* 1993; 73(3):471–485.
31. Welsh DRJ, Alexander MAJ. The Shouldice repair. *Surg Clin North Am* 1993;73(3):451–469.
32. Nilsson E, Kald A, Anderberg B, et al. Hernia surgery in a defined population. A prospective three year audit. *Eur J Surg* 1997;163:823–829.
33. Kald A, Nilsson E, Anderberg B, et al. Reoperation as surrogate endpoint in hernia surgery: a three year follow-up of 1565 herniorrhaphies. *Eur J Surg* 1998;164:45–50.
34. Halstead WS. *Surgical papers by William Stewart Halstead*. Baltimore, MD: Johns Hopkins Press; 1924. Report No. 1.
35. Lichtenstein IL, Shulman AG. Ambulatory outpatient hernia surgery, including a new concept. *Int Surg* 1986;71:1.
36. Lichtenstein IL, Shulman AG, Anderberg B. The tension-free hernioplasty. *Am J Surg* 1989;157:188.
37. Lichtenstein IL, Shore JM. Simplified repair of femoral and recurrent inguinal hernias by a "plug" technique. *Am J Surg* 1974;128:439–444.
38. Stoppa RE. The treatment of complicated groin and incisional hernias. *World J Surg* 1989;13(5):545–554.
39. Nyhus LM, Condon RE, Harkins HN. Clinical experience with preperitoneal hernia repair for all types of hernia of the groin. *Am J Surg* 1960; 100:234.
40. Ferzli GS, Frezza EE, Pecoraro AM, et al. Prospective randomized study of stapled versus unstapled mesh in laparoscopic preperitoneal inguinal hernia repair. *J Am Coll Surg* 1999;188(5):461–465.
41. Franz MG. The biological treatment of the hernia disease. In: Schumpelick V, Fitzgibbons RJ, eds. *Recurrent hernia*. Heidelberg: Springer; 2007:401–410.
42. Pollock AV, Nyhus LM. Incisional hernias. In: Schwartz SI, Ellis H, eds. *Maingot's abdominal operations*, 8th ed. Norwalk: Appleton-Century-Crofts; 1985:335–350.
43. Ramirez OM, Ruas E, Dellon AL. Components separation method for closure of abdominal wall defects: an anatomic and clinical study. *Plast Reconstr Surg* 1990;86(3):519–526.
44. Usher FC, Ochsner J, Tuttle LL Jr. Use of Marlex mesh in the repair of incisional hernias. *Am Surg* 1958;24(12):969–974.
45. Bay-Nielsen M, Perkins FM, Kehlet H. Pain and functional impairment 1 year after inguinal herniorrhaphy: a nationwide questionnaire study. *Ann Surg* 2001;233(1):1–7.
46. Evans DS. Value of herniography in the management of occult hernia and chronic groin pain in adults. *Br J Surg* 2001;88(1):153–154.
47. Hair A, Paterson C, Wright D, et al. What effect does the duration of an inguinal hernia have on patient symptoms? *J Am Coll Surg* 2001;193(2): 125–129.
48. Chan STF, Esufali ST. Extended indications for polypropylene mesh closure of the abdominal wall. *Br J Surg* 1986;73:3–6.
49. Molloy RG, Moran KT, Waldron RP, et al. Massive incisional hernia: abdominal wall replacement with Marlex mesh. *Br J Surg* 1991;78(2): 242–244.
50. Klinge U, Klosterhalfen B, Muller M, et al. Foreign body reaction to meshes used for the repair of abdominal wall hernias. *Eur J Surg* 1999; 165(7):665–673.
51. Kaufman Z, Engelberg M, Zager M. Fecal fistula: a late complication of Marlex mesh repair. *Dis Colon Rectum* 1981;24(7):543–544.
52. Voyles CR, Richardson JD, Bland KI, et al. Emergency abdominal wall reconstruction with polypropylene mesh: short-term benefits versus long-term complications. *Ann Surg* 1981;194(2):219–223.
53. Caldirone MW, Romano M, Bozza F. Progressive pneumoperitoneum in management of giant incisional hernias. *Br J Surg* 1990;77:306–308.
54. Raynor RW, Del Geurcio LRM. The place for pneumoperitoneum in the repair of massive hernia. *World J Surg* 1989;13:581–585.
55. Salcedo-Wasicek MC, Thirlby RC. Postoperative course after inguinal herniorrhaphy. A case-controlled comparison of patients receiving worker's compensation versus patients with commercial insurance. *Arch Surg* 1995;103(1):29–32.
56. Barkun JS, Keyser EJ, Wexler MJ, et al. Short-term outcomes in open versus laparoscopic herniorrhaphy: confounding impact of worker's compensation on convalescence. *J Gastrointest Surg* 1999;3(6):575–582.
57. Reilingh TSD, van Goor H, Rosman C, et al. "Components separation technique" for the repair of large abdominal wall hernias. *J Am Coll Surg* 2003;196(1):32–37.
58. O'Mara MS, Papasavas PK, Newton ED, et al. Modified separation of parts as an intervention for intraabdominal hypertension and the abdominal compartment syndrome in a swine model. *Plast Reconstr Surg* 2004;114(7):1842–1845.

CHAPTER

40

Complications of Laparoscopic Surgery

Jonathan F. Finks

INTRODUCTION

The origins of modern laparoscopic surgery reach back over a century. In 1902, Kelling performed celioscopy to examine the abdominal organs of dogs using a cystoscope with a heated light source at its distal end. Since that time, tremendous advances in optics, video imaging, equipment, and techniques have made laparoscopic surgery applicable to a broad array of abdominal procedures. With the increased use of laparoscopy has come an awareness of significant complications associated with these techniques. Understanding how to prevent, recognize, and manage these complications is critical to safe practice in laparoscopic surgery.

EARLY COMPLICATIONS

Early complications during laparoscopic surgery include events that occur while obtaining access to the abdominal cavity and those related to the effects of pneumoperitoneum.

Access-related injuries

Access-related injuries are those that occur during establishment of pneumoperitoneum or during trocar placement and include injuries to blood vessels of the abdominal wall, mesentery, or retroperitoneum as well as bowel, bladder, and other visceral structures. Reported rates of access-related bowel injury range from 0.07% to 0.18%, while rates of major vascular injury range from 0.04% to 0.09%. Although rare, access injuries account for up to half of all complications occurring during laparoscopic surgery and can have devastating consequences, including hemorrhage, sepsis, multisystem organ failure, and death. Furthermore, these injuries account for a disproportionate amount of medical liability claims (1). Understanding how these injuries occur and identifying strategies to optimize safety at entry is essential to safe practice in laparoscopic surgery. Measures for avoiding access-related complications are summarized in Table 40.1.

Jonathan F. Finks: University of Michigan, Ann Arbor, MI 48109.

The most commonly injured blood vessels are the inferior epigastrics, usually during placement of a lateral trocar. Injury to these vessels has been reported in 0.2% to 2% of cases (1). While the superficial epigastric vessels can be seen with transillumination in nonobese patients, the deeper epigastrics cannot. One should attempt to visualize these vessels laparoscopically and follow their course from the level of the inguinal ligament cephalad along the abdominal wall (2). Anatomic studies suggest that these vessels are typically located in an area between 4 and 8 cm from the midline and ports should be placed lateral to this zone to prevent injury. Minor bleeding from the epigastrics can sometimes be controlled with direct pressure. More significant bleeding can be managed with tamponade by inserting the balloon from a Foley catheter directly into the trocar site. Alternatively, bleeding can be controlled using full-thickness abdominal wall suture ligation of the vessels. In cases of persistent bleeding, wound exploration may be required. Care should be taken to control even minor bleeding from a port site, as postoperative abdominal wall hematoma can lead to a significant drop in hematocrit. Observation of all lateral ports during removal from the abdominal wall at the end of a procedure remains an important step in preventing this complication.

Major vascular injury is associated with a mortality rate of 9% to 17% (3) and typically occurs during placement of the initial trocar (54%) or at insertion of the Veress needle (46%), most commonly at the umbilicus (3,4). Very thin patients are at particular risk for this complication, as the distance between the abdominal wall and the retroperitoneal vessels at the level of the umbilicus may be as little as 2 cm in the anesthetized patient with muscle relaxation (4). The vessels most at risk for injury include the aorta (usually at its bifurcation), the iliac vessels (especially on the right), and the vena cava, although injury to mesenteric, omental, splenic, and liver vasculature has also been reported (2). The position of the aortic bifurcation relative to the umbilicus is quite variable, ranging from 5 cm cephalad to 3 cm caudal to the umbilicus in the supine position (5), and does not correlate with body mass index. The umbilicus is therefore an unreliable landmark for determining its location.

There are several measures that may be utilized to reduce the risk for major vascular injury. First, patients must be completely relaxed prior to insertion of the Veress needle and primary trocar, as contraction of the abdominal

Table 40.1 Measures for avoiding access-related complications

Setup phase
- Maintain table height at waist level of the operating surgeon
- Keep patient in a neutral position
- Employ nasogastric decompression
- Ensure adequate abdominal wall relaxation
- Increase intra-abdominal pressure between 20 and 25 mm Hg prior to initial access

Initial access and placement of first trocar
- Use left upper quadrant (Palmer's point) for initial entry in
  - Very thin patients
  - Obese patients
  - Patients with previous laparotomy
- Elevate abdominal wall anteriorly before insertion of the Veress needle and first trocar (may grasp fascia or umbilical stalk)
- Insert laparoscope as soon as insufflation is sufficient to allow visualization
- Inspect the area beneath the initial entry site for vascular or visceral injury
- Immediate conversion to open for
  - Blood on aspiration of the Veress needle
  - Evidence of retroperitoneal hematoma

Placement of secondary trocars
- Transilluminate abdominal wall to identify superficial epigastric vessels
- Visualize the deep epigastric vessels laparoscopically
- Insert trocars in the midline or at least 8 cm lateral to the midline
- Avoid angling lateral trocars toward the midline
- Laparoscopically, visualize each port during placement

Procedure end
- Laparoscopically, visualize each lateral port during removal and inspect port site for bleeding
- Close the fascia of all ports with diameter ≥10 mm

musculature will bring the abdominal wall in closer contact to the retroperitoneal structures. Also, it is generally recommended to keep the patient in the supine position during placement of the Veress needle and/or trocars, as placement into the Trendelenburg position often rotates the sacral promontory and aorta closer to the umbilicus. When entering the abdomen at the umbilicus, the abdominal wall should be lifted anteriorly. An effective way to accomplish this is to grasp and elevate the fascia or umbilical stalk after the initial skin incision has been made (6). Elevation of the abdominal wall has been shown to substantially increase the distance between the abdominal wall and the retroperitoneal structures (7,8). Increasing intraabdominal pressure (IAP) to between 20 and 25 mm Hg prior to placement of the first trocar has also been shown to increase the distance between the abdominal wall and abdominal contents without significant hemodynamic effects (9,10). Finally, the area beneath the initial entry site should be inspected and all secondary trocars should be placed under direct vision to reduce the risk for vascular or visceral injury.

The risk for bowel injury is highest in those with abdominal wall adhesions from prior surgery, particularly in patients whose postoperative course was complicated by infection, intraabdominal abscess, or bowel obstruction, all of which increase the likelihood of adhesions. Over half of these injuries are not detected at the time of operation and typically present within 48 to 72 hours postoperatively (6,7), often with abdominal sepsis. Bowel injuries lead to laparotomy in >60% of patients and are associated with a 2.5% to 5% risk for mortality, mostly due to delayed presentation (3).

There is no fool-proof method to eliminate the risk for bowel injury. In patients at high risk for midline adhesions, however, one should consider left upper quadrant access by placement of a Veress needle at Palmer's point, 3 cm below the left costal margin in the midclavicular line (7). There are several advantages to left upper quadrant access. First, this area is typically free from small bowel adhesions (7). Additionally, the abdominal wall is thinner here than at the umbilicus, making access easier in obese patients (8). Furthermore, entry at this site also carries less risk for major vascular injury than does an umbilical approach. For these reasons, entry at Palmer's point is recommended for obese patients, very thin patients, and those with high risk for adhesions. Complete abdominal wall relaxation and gastric decompression are mandatory prior to left upper quadrant access, and this approach should be avoided in patients with hepatomegaly or splenomegaly due to the added risk for injury to these structures.

There is no convincing evidence to recommend one access technique over another. In a recent meta-analysis, there was no difference in rates of major vascular or visceral injury between open (Hasson) and closed (Veress) techniques (4). The study acknowledged, however, that the examined studies had small numbers and often excluded high-risk patients. Furthermore, earlier meta-analyses suggested that open entry was associated with a higher rate of bowel injury, while the closed technique was associated with a higher rate of vascular injury. Given the rarity of the primary outcomes, a definitive randomized trial to compare the various access techniques would require >10,000 patients in each study arm and is unlikely to occur (10,11).

Recent advances in trocars have been touted to increase operative safety. These include radially expanding trocars with blunt tips, as well as optical trocars that allow for direct visualization of entry into the peritoneal cavity. While radially dilating trocars have been shown to reduce port site bleeding, neither these nor the optical trocars have been shown to reduce the risk for significant vascular or visceral injury (2,4,11,12). Reports of major injury have been associated with both types of trocars.

A basic principle of abdominal access is to maintain controlled insertion of the trocar. An essential but often overlooked aspect of controlled entry is attention to ergonomic principles. As the table height increases relative to the operating surgeon, the surgeon tends to compensate for the height by abducting his or her arms; this is associated with a loss of control of arm movement. The table should be placed at a height that is comfortable for the surgeon and that allows the arms and shoulders to remain relaxed with elbows close to the body. This will allow for a smoother, more controlled trocar placement, with better control of the depth of insertion, stopping the thrust when the peritoneum is entered.

Effects of pneumoperitoneum

Laparoscopic surgery requires insufflation of the abdomen with gas, typically carbon dioxide (CO_2), to facilitate exposure of the surgical field. Creation of the pneumoperitoneum results in increased IAP and absorption of large amounts of CO_2, both of which can have a significant impact on hemodynamics, pulmonary mechanics, and acid–base status. Although pneumoperitoneum is well-tolerated by most healthy patients, it can have a markedly detrimental effect on those with underlying cardiopulmonary disease. The effects associated with pneumoperitoneum are summarized in Table 40.2.

Cardiovascular Effects

The effect of pneumoperitoneum on hemodynamics depends on several factors, including degree of IAP, patient position, intravascular volume status, degree of hypercarbia, ventilation strategy, and underlying cardiopulmonary status. Most studies suggest that pneumoperitoneum, with an IAP ≥15 mm Hg, leads to elevations in systemic vascular resistance (SVR) and mean arterial pressure (MAP) with a concomitant drop in cardiac output, largely dependent on the patient position (13–15). The combined effects of anesthesia, pneumoperitoneum and the reverse Trendelenburg position can reduce cardiac output by as much as 30% to 50% (16–18). In otherwise healthy patients, this effect is usually only significant in the setting of hypovolemia, as the reduction in venous return associated with the head-up position is compensated by the pneumoperitoneum in normovolemic patients. When combined with the Trendelenburg position, pneumoperitoneum results in a marked increase in venous return, which could lead to congestive heart failure in patients with underlying heart disease (12).

SVR can increase by as much as 65% (11) and is related to a number of factors, including catecholamine release (9), compression of splanchnic capillary beds (10), and elevations in production of antidiuretic hormone and circulating levels of plasma renin and aldosterone (12). One study identified a four-fold increase in the levels of renin and aldosterone following pneumoperitoneum and head-up positioning. Furthermore, the authors found that changes in MAP were linearly correlated with changes in levels of these neurohormones (19). Whatever the cause, the substantial elevation in afterload can lead to increased myocardial oxygen demand. In patients with underlying cardiac disease, this could lead to myocardial ischemia or even infarction (20).

There are several measures that may mitigate the hemodynamic effects of pneumoperitoneum. First, surgeons should apply the least possible IAP necessary to provide adequate exposure. Hemodynamic effects are directly proportional to IAP and are minimal when IAP is kept <12 mm Hg (21–23). In addition, preoperative volume loading to achieve normovolemia may help to maintain cardiac output, particularly when the reverse Trendelenburg position is anticipated (24,25). Finally, upward displacement of the diaphragm during pneumoperitoneum leads to elevated intrathoracic pressures and a rise in central venous pressure (CVP), particularly when positive end-expiratory pressure is used. CVP measurements do not correlate well with cardiac filling status. For that reason, patients with significant underlying cardiac compromise may benefit from more invasive hemodynamic monitoring with a pulmonary artery catheter and/or transesophageal echocardiogram can help to optimize volume status (15,24).

Cardiac arrhythmias are another common complication of pneumoperitoneum, reported in up to 47% of patients undergoing laparoscopic surgery (16,17). Some arrhythmias, such as sinus tachycardia, are benign and occur as a result of an increase in circulating catecholamines. Others can occur as a result of myocardial irritability related to hypercarbia (12). The most common and more dangerous arrhythmias are bradyarrhythmias, which include sinus

Table 40.2 Effects of carbon dioxide pneumoperitoneum

Cardiovascular
- Heart rate
  - Bradycardia most common at insufflation
  - Sinus tachycardia secondary to catecholamine release
- Cardiac contractility decreased
- Cardiac output decreased
- Systemic vascular resistance increased
- Mean arterial pressure increased
- Central venous pressure increased

Respiratory
- Hypercarbia/acidosis
- Elevation of the diaphragm
  - Peak airway pressure increased
  - Functional residual capacity decreased
  - Respiratory compliance decreased
  - Intrapulmonary shunting increased
    - Alveolar–arterial gradient increased

Vascular
- Splanchnic bed compressed
- Common femoral venous flow reduced
  - Lower extremity venous pooling

Neurohormonal
- Catecholamine release
- Aldosterone production increased
- Elevation in plasma concentrations of
  - Renin
  - Cortisol
  - Vasopressin

Somatosensory
- Peritoneal/diaphragmatic irritation
  - Abdominal wall pain
  - Shoulder-tip pain

bradycardia, atrioventricular dissociation, and asystole. These result from vagal stimulation during peritoneal distension, usually during initial insufflation, and have been reported in up to 28% of patients (18). Fortunately, most of these arrhythmias can be successfully managed with release of pneumoperitoneum and hyperventilation with a FiO_2 of 1.0, although vagolytics are sometimes required (12,13). They rarely recur with reinsufflation.

Respiratory System Effects

CO_2 is widely used for abdominal insufflation because it is inexpensive, highly soluble, rapidly eliminated by the lungs, and noncombustible (13). During laparoscopic surgery, CO_2 is rapidly absorbed by the peritoneal membrane, resulting in a nearly 50% increase in CO_2 output (14). Some CO_2 will be absorbed by intracellular and plasma buffers. Once these are saturated, progressive hypercapnia and acidosis can develop.

Hypercapnia is exacerbated by the impairment of respiratory mechanics that result from elevated IAP from insufflation and by the Trendelenburg position. Both of these factors serve to reduce pulmonary compliance and functional residual capacity, while elevating airway pressures (15). To overcome these changes and restore eucapnia, minute ventilation must be increased by 12% to 16% (17,18). In obese patients, respiratory compliance is further reduced (26–28) and minute ventilation may need to be increased by up to 21% to avoid acidosis (29).

While the excess CO_2 burden is usually well-tolerated in healthy patients, those with underlying cardiopulmonary disease (American Society of Anesthesiologists Class III or IV) may develop persistent hypercapnia and acidosis despite an increase in minute ventilation. At particular risk are patients with respiratory compromise (e.g., severe chronic obstructive pulmonary disease), diminished cardiac function, or an elevated metabolic rate (e.g., patients with sepsis) (9). In a study of patients undergoing laparoscopic cholecystectomy, preoperative pulmonary function tests revealing forced expiratory volumes <70% of predicted values and diffusion defects <80% of predicted values were risk factors for development of hypercapnia and acidosis (24). In these high-risk patients, intraoperative arterial blood gas monitoring of CO_2 levels is recommended, as the end-tidal CO_2 ($ETCO_2$) will often underestimate the arterial partial pressure of CO_2 ($PaCO_2$), particularly when the $PaCO_2$ is >41 mm Hg (18). Strategies for improving gas exchange in these patients include minimizing IAP, using the head-up position where possible to improve pulmonary compliance, and employing positive end-expiratory pressure (29,30). In some patients, conversion to an open procedure may be required.

Despite the negative effects of abdominal insufflation on pulmonary mechanics and hypercapnia, hypoxemia during laparoscopic surgery is relatively uncommon, particularly in otherwise healthy patients (15,21,31), and its presence should prompt an immediate search for its cause. The major causes of acute hypoxia during laparoscopic surgery are listed in Table 40.3 (31). This differential diagnosis applies to sudden changes in hemodynamics and $ETCO_2$ as well.

Table 40.3 Causes of acute hypoxia and hemodynamic instability during laparoscopic surgery

Comorbid conditions
• Respiratory disease (chronic obstructive pulmonary disease)
• Morbid obesity
Ineffective ventilation
• Endotracheal tube obstruction
• Massive subcutaneous emphysema
• Anesthesia circuit disconnect
• Excessive intra-abdominal pressure/Trendelenburg position
Intrapulmonary shunt
• Endotracheal tube displacement (mainstem intubation)
• Pneumothorax/carbothorax
• Aspiration of gastric contents
Diminished cardiac output
• Myocardial depression/ischemia/infarction
• Arrhythmia
• Venous gas embolism
• Hemorrhage
• Hypovolemia
Pericardial tamponade

INTRAOPERATIVE COMPLICATIONS

This section consists of an overview of intraoperative complications, including vascular, gastrointestinal tract and urinary tract injuries, as well as cardiopulmonary complications such as venous CO_2 embolism, pneumothorax, pneumomediastinum, and subcutaneous emphysema. A large proportion of intraoperative injuries are related to instrumentation, often in association with the use of electrocautery. A discussion of complications related to surgical staplers and electrocautery are also included in this section.

Urinary tract injury

Bladder Injury

The incidence of bladder injuries during laparoscopy surgery is estimated to be 0.02% to 8.3%, with injuries to the dome accounting for 90% of these injuries (21). In a large single-center series of bladder injuries, gynecologic operations accounted for 62% of all injuries, with 26% occurring during general surgery procedures and 12% during urologic procedures (16). Laparoscopically assisted vaginal hysterectomy is the most common operation leading to bladder injuries, followed by procedures for endometriosis (3,17,21). The most common cause of bladder injuries is sharp dissection with electrocautery (21). Risk factors for bladder injury include adhesions from previous pelvic operations and pelvic inflammatory processes. These processes can be acute, as seen with infection, or chronic, as seen with endometriosis, malignant infiltrative disease, and previous radiation (18,21).

There are several measures that may help prevent bladder injuries. Placement of a Foley catheter during pelvic procedures will keep the bladder decompressed, minimizing the chances for a trocar injury. Direct visualization of the bladder dome is recommended prior to placement of secondary trocars, although bladder identification is possible only in about 45% of patients, and visibility of the dome diminishes with increasing BMI (18). In cases where the bladder must be dissected off the anterior cervix and vagina or off the anterior abdominal wall, insufflation of the bladder with saline or even CO_2 can facilitate the dissection (29).

Intraoperative hematuria or pneumaturia noted in the Foley bag should raise suspicion for a bladder injury. Intravesical instillation of betadyne, methylene blue, or indigo carmine can facilitate inspection for leaks. Delayed presentation of bladder injury may be accompanied by fever, ileus, abdominal pain, oliguria, azotemia, and urinary ascites (30). CT cystography can aid in the diagnosis. Pelvic fluid collections should be percutaneously drained, and the fluid should be sent for creatinine measurement.

Most bladder injuries are recognized intraoperatively (16,17,32). These can often be repaired laparoscopically, with a layered closure using absorbable suture (21). Although there are reports of laparoscopic closure using staples, this is not currently recommended, both because of the lack of clinical trials attesting to its effectiveness and because of the risk of permanent foreign bodies in the bladder wall, which can act as a nidus for calculus formation or recurrent urinary tract infections or may interfere with normal contraction of the bladder. Following repair, a Foley catheter is left in place for 7 to 10 days. Cystography to confirm closure of the leak should be performed prior to catheter removal. Long-term success rates from bladder repair are approximately 98% (16).

Ureteral Injury

The incidence of ureteral injuries reported during laparoscopic gynecologic surgery ranges from 0% to 3.4% (32) and during general surgery procedures ranges between 0% and 1.5% (22,23,25,33). As with bladder injuries, the majority of ureteral injuries (64%) result from gynecologic procedures, with 25% from general surgery operations and 11% following urologic procedures (34). The majority of ureteral injuries occur through the use of electrocautery, followed by ligation, although injuries also occur through crushing and devascularization (26,32,35). Most ureteral injuries in general surgery follow colorectal resection. Injuries often occur during mobilization of the sigmoid colon, ligation of the inferior mesenteric vessels, or division of the lateral rectal ligaments (27). Lower in the pelvis, the ureter courses medially at the base of the broad ligament, passing below the uterine vessels and entering the bladder on its posterolateral aspect, approximately 2.3 cm from the edge of the cervix. This region, near the ureterovesical junction, is the most common location for injury during gynecologic laparoscopic procedures (28). As with bladder injuries, a common associated risk factor is inflammatory adhesions limiting visualization during the operation.

Unlike bladder injuries, most ureteral injuries (75% to 88%) are discovered postoperatively (32,34,36) and can present between 3 days and 2 months from the date of surgery. These delayed injuries typically present as fistulas (ureterovaginal, ureterorectal, and ureterocutaneous) with associated fever, hematuria, flank pain, and/or peritonitis (32). Diagnosis is made by excretory urography. If suspected intraoperatively, the integrity of the ureter should be confirmed by retrograde ureterocystography.

Most ureteral injuries, whether discovered late or at the time of surgery, will require operative repair, as most studies have found simple stenting of ureteral lacerations to be inadequate. By contrast, success rates from ureteral repair top 94% (37). Distal injuries are best managed by reimplantation of the ureter into the bladder. A psoas hitch can be used for injuries involving the entire lower third of the ureter. The addition of an anterior bladder flap may be required for injuries involving the distal two-thirds of the ureter. Another option for extensive injuries to the distal half of the ureter is a transureteroureterostomy, whereby the injured ureter is anastomosed to the contralateral ureter (or renal pelvis). Lacerations to the proximal or midureter are best repaired by primary ureteroureterostomy, performed over a ureteral stent (16,38).

Gastrointestinal injury

The incidence of bowel injury during laparoscopic surgery is estimated to be between 0.07% and 0.9% (39–41). Most of these involve the small bowel (56%), including the duodenum, or colon (39%) (42). The majority of bowel injuries not related to abdominal access result from the use of electrocautery (39,42,43). Most visceral injuries are not detected at the time of operation (39,43,44). Injuries associated with direct perforation or blunt force typically present within 12 to 36 hours, while those resulting from electrothermal injury present between 4 and 10 days after surgery (44). Although some patients will present with frank peritonitis and sepsis, many will present with vague complaints of discomfort, low-grade fevers, and often only mild laboratory abnormalities (39). For that reason, surgeons should have a high index of suspicion for the presence of bowel injury in patients with abdominal discomfort following laparoscopic procedures, even in the absence of frank peritonitis and sepsis.

While injuries identified intraoperatively can often be managed laparoscopically, >80% of delayed injuries require laparotomy (39,45). If recognized at the time of surgery, minor lacerations can be repaired by oversewing the defect, either laparoscopically or open, depending upon the surgeon's comfort level. Electrocautery injuries create a larger area of coagulative necrosis, often well beyond what is apparent initially. Anything beyond superficial electrothermal injuries should be treated with excision well beyond the area of injury in order to prevent late perforation (44).

A key principle in avoidance of gastrointestinal tract injuries during laparoscopic surgery is to keep sharp (e.g., scissors) or "hot" (e.g., electrocautery and ultrasonic dissectors) instruments within the visual field at all times. In addition, bowel should be handled gently without excessive traction or torsion. Adhesions should always be divided sharply with scissors, and hemostasis should be achieved with hemoclips instead of electrocautery, unless the bowel is well away from the area of dissection. Finally, when using staplers or clip appliers, both sides of the device should be clearly visualized to prevent inadvertent injury to nearby structures.

Vascular injury

Reported rates of vascular injury during laparoscopic surgery range from 0.04% to 3.3%, with rates of major vascular injury between 0.04% and 0.1% (3,46–48). Although uncommon, vascular injuries are the second leading cause for mortality following laparoscopic procedures and one of the primary causes for conversion to laparotomy (49,50). Despite several decades of experience with minimally invasive techniques, hemorrhage remains a significant complication of laparoscopic procedures. This is due, at least in part, to the expanding indications for laparoscopic surgery, which now include more complex and high-risk procedures (51).

In most series, access-related injuries account for the greatest proportion of major vascular injuries, although a substantial proportion of these injuries, and most minor vascular injuries, result from misuse of surgical instruments, usually in association with electrocautery (2,47,48, 51,52). Movement of an electrosurgical instrument outside the visual field and inadvertent activation of the monopolar electrode were commonly cited causes for injury in one series from a large nationwide Swiss registry (51). The vessels most commonly injured include the iliac vessels, aorta, inferior vena cava, and mesenteric vessels (52). Injuries to hepatic, splenic, gastric, and omental vessels have also been reported.

Most significant vascular injuries are identified intraoperatively. Vascular injuries beneath a thick omentum or in the retroperitoneum, however, may not be immediately apparent. Any sudden deterioration in the patient's condition (i.e., hypoxia, tachycardia, and hypotension) should be assumed to represent an occult vascular injury until proven otherwise. Careful examination of the entire abdomen, including the mesentery, as well as the retroperitoneum is warranted. The same is true for blood seen on entry into the abdomen.

Minor vascular injuries can be managed laparoscopically in most cases. Injuries to major retroperitoneal vessels, however, should prompt conversion to laparotomy. The first step is to apply pressure to the bleeding area with a laparoscopic instrument or a sponge, which can be inserted through a 10-mm trocar. A midline laparotomy is then performed, while pressure is held via a lateral trocar. In general, the retroperitoneum should not be opened until the team (preferably including a vascular surgeon) is prepared to gain proximal and distal control of the injured vessel. Good communication with the anesthesiologist and the operating room staff is critical to ensure that the patient is adequately resuscitated, blood products are called for, and the necessary equipment and personnel are made available in an expeditious manner.

Pneumothorax, pneumomediastinum, and subcutaneous emphysema

Subcutaneous emphysema refers to the extravasation of CO_2 into the subcutaneous tissues. This can result from misplacement of the Veress needle during initial insufflation or from defects in the peritoneum. Subcutaneous emphysema is also significantly more common in cases of extraperitoneal or retroperitoneal laparoscopy than in transabdominal cases (53,54). Extraperitoneal gas can extend along fascial planes from the abdomen up to the chest wall and neck, resulting in palpable crepitus. From the neck, gas can track down into the chest and mediastinum, resulting in pneumothorax and pneumomediastinum. Gas can also reach the thorax and mediastinum through congenital defects or lacerations in the diaphragm or during procedures involving the esophageal hiatus, such as hiatal hernia repairs. While subcutaneous emphysema is usually of little consequence, extensive buildup can significantly increase airway pressure and impair ventilation. The increased surface area available for absorption of CO_2 can also lead to hypercapnia and acidosis. Generally, these sequelae resolve with desufflation of the abdomen. Reinsufflation at lower pressure may be required (12).

CO_2 pneumothorax can also result from inadvertent injury to the mediastinal pleura and usually occurs during cases involving mediastinal dissection, such as operations for hiatal hernia, gastroesophageal reflux, and achalasia. Such defects can lead to tension pneumothorax with an associated increase in airway pressures, $ETCO_2$, hypoxia, and hemodynamic instability. Evidence of pneumothorax includes an acute elevation in airway pressures and $ETCO_2$, visualization of the lung parenchyma, and bulging of the ipsilateral diaphragm. When pneumothorax occurs in this setting, the pleural defect should be enlarged to help prevent tension pneumothorax. To prevent sealing of the defect during inspiration, an 18-Fr red rubber catheter with side holes at its distal end should be placed across the defect. This will help equalize pressures across the diaphragm. At the end of the procedure, the proximal end of the tube is pulled out through a 10-mm

procedures (77). Furthermore, 86% of hernias and 80% of wound infections in the laparoscopic group occurred at the specimen extraction site. This highlights the importance of wound protection and meticulous closure technique at sites of specimen extraction.

Port site recurrence

Early reports of high rates of port site metastasis following oncologic resection raised concerns about the safety of laparoscopic oncologic procedures (78,79). Since that time, numerous investigators have sought to determine what effect the laparoscopic approach has on tumor biology and specifically on the incidence of port site recurrence. There are several proposed mechanisms for port site recurrence: (a) increased exfoliation of tumor cells during laparoscopic manipulation with subsequent aerosolization of tumor cells, which can leak around trocars along with escaping gas in what has been described as a "chimney effect;" (b) direct contact between tumor cells and the abdominal wall due to the small size of the incisions; (c) tissue trauma at port sites; (d) tumor contamination of instruments, which then come in contact with the port site wounds, and (e) detrimental effects of CO_2 pneumoperitoneum on immune function (78,80,81).

The results from in vivo and in vitro studies have been conflicting, as some studies have suggested that aerosolization is not the mechanism for port site recurrence and that port site metastasis does not require CO_2 pneumoperitoneum (78,82–84). This latter point is supported by the finding that port site recurrence has been reported in thoracoscopic cancer resections, where CO_2 is not used (85). Furthermore, more recent clinical studies have demonstrated that port site recurrence after laparoscopic cancer resection is comparable to wound recurrence after open surgery, particularly in the setting of colon cancer (86–89). Laparoscopy is also considered safe in cases of early ovarian cancer, as the vast majority of port site metastases with ovarian cancer occur in the setting of advanced disease and carcinomatosis (90,91). With regard to gallbladder cancer, however, the general consensus is that an open approach is warranted, given high rates of port site metastasis and concerns about perforation during laparoscopic resection. If a gallbladder cancer is diagnosed after the completion of a laparoscopic cholecystectomy, the port sites should be excised (92,93).

Despite the lack of conclusive evidence regarding the etiology of port site recurrence during laparoscopic surgery, there are several steps one should take to minimize the risk of this serious complication. First desufflation episodes should be kept to a minimum during the procedure. Consideration should be given to leaving all of the ports in the abdomen until the pneumoperitoneum has been released at the end of the procedure, although this step may increase the risk for missed port site hemorrhage. Tumor manipulation should be minimized, and surgeons should avoid direct contact between contaminated instruments, which have touched malignant tissue, and the abdominal wall.

Conclusion

The application of laparoscopic techniques to a wide variety of complex procedures has provided significant benefits to patients in terms of reduced postoperative pain, shorter recovery periods, improved cosmesis, and lower rates of wound complications. However, there are also numerous complications unique to laparoscopic surgery. Surgeons and other members of the healthcare team should have a thorough understanding of the physiologic changes and adverse effects associated with CO_2 pneumoperitoneum. Surgeons must also be mindful of some of the pitfalls of the laparoscopic approach. Excellent visualization is always required, and instruments, particularly those associated with energy sources, must be kept in the visual field at all times. Finally, the surgeon should always be willing to convert to an open approach whenever the safety of proceeding laparoscopically is in doubt. Conversion to an open procedure should not be considered a complication of the procedure, but rather an exercise of sound judgment.

REFERENCES

1. Saber AA, Meslemani AM, Davis R, et al. Safety zones for anterior abdominal wall entry during laparoscopy: a CT scan mapping of epigastric vessels. *Ann Surg* 2004;239(2):182–185.
2. Makai G, Isaacson K. Complications of gynecologic laparoscopy. *Clin Obstet Gynecol* 2009;52(3):401–411.
3. Magrina JF. Complications of laparoscopic surgery. *Clin Obstet Gynecol* 2002;45(2):469–480.
4. Ahmad G, Duffy JM, Phillips K, et al. Laparoscopic entry techniques. *Cochrane Database Syst Rev* 2008(2):CD006583.
5. Nezhat F, Brill AI, Nezhat CH, et al. Laparoscopic appraisal of the anatomic relationship of the umbilicus to the aortic bifurcation. *J Am Assoc Gynecol Laparosc* 1998;5(2):135–140.
6. Philosophe R. Avoiding complications of laparoscopic surgery. *Fertil Steril* 2003;80(Suppl 4):30–39; quiz 54–56.
7. Molloy D, Kaloo PD, Cooper M, et al. Laparoscopic entry: a literature review and analysis of techniques and complications of primary port entry. *Aust N Z J Obstet Gynaecol* 2002;42(3):246–254.
8. Tulikangas PK, Nicklas A, Falcone T, et al. Anatomy of the left upper quadrant for cannula insertion. *J Am Assoc Gynecol Laparosc* 2000;7(2): 211–214.
9. Grabowski JE, Talamini MA. Physiological effects of pneumoperitoneum. *J Gastrointest Surg* 2009;13(5):1009–1016.
10. Ishizaki Y, Bandai Y, Shimomura K, et al. Changes in splanchnic blood flow and cardiovascular effects following peritoneal insufflation of carbon dioxide. *Surg Endosc* 1993;7(5):420–423.
11. Joris JL, Noirot DP, Legrand MJ, et al. Hemodynamic changes during laparoscopic cholecystectomy. *Anesth Analg* 1993;76(5):1067–1071.
12. Henny CP, Hofland J. Laparoscopic surgery: pitfalls due to anesthesia, positioning, and pneumoperitoneum. *Surg Endosc* 2005;19(9):1163–1171.
13. Tsereteli Z, Terry ML, Bowers SP, et al. Prospective randomized clinical trial comparing nitrous oxide and carbon dioxide pneumoperitoneum for laparoscopic surgery. *J Am Coll Surg* 2002;195(2):173–179; discussion 9–80.
14. Kazama T, Ikeda K, Kato T, et al. Carbon dioxide output in laparoscopic cholecystectomy. *Br J Anaesth* 1996;76(4):530–535.
15. Sharma KC, Brandstetter RD, Brensilver JM, et al. Cardiopulmonary physiology and pathophysiology as a consequence of laparoscopic surgery. *Chest* 1996;110(3):810–815.
16. Armenakas NA, Pareek G, Fracchia JA. Iatrogenic bladder perforations: longterm followup of 65 patients. *J Am Coll Surg* 2004;198(1):78–82.

17. Saidi MH, Sadler RK, Vancaillie TG, et al. Diagnosis and management of serious urinary complications after major operative laparoscopy. *Obstet Gynecol* 1996;87(2):272–276.
18. Hurd WW, Amesse LS, Gruber JS, et al. Visualization of the epigastric vessels and bladder before laparoscopic trocar placement. *Fertil Steril* 2003;80(1):209–212.
19. O'Leary E, Hubbard K, Tormey W, et al. Laparoscopic cholecystectomy: haemodynamic and neuroendocrine responses after pneumoperitoneum and changes in position. *Br J Anaesth* 1996;76(5):640–644.
20. Westerband A, Van De Water J, Amzallag M, et al. Cardiovascular changes during laparoscopic cholecystectomy. *Surg Gynecol Obstet* 1992; 175(6):535–538.
21. Ostrzenski A, Ostrzenska KM. Bladder injury during laparoscopic surgery. *Obstet Gynecol Surv* 1998;53(3):175–180.
22. Chahin F, Dwivedi AJ, Paramesh A, et al. The implications of lighted ureteral stenting in laparoscopic colectomy. *JSLS* 2002;6(1):49–52.
23. Kockerling F, Rose J, Schneider C, et al. Laparoscopic colorectal anastomosis: risk of postoperative leakage. Results of a multicenter study. Laparoscopic Colorectal Surgery Study Group (LCSSG). *Surg Endosc* 1999;13(7):639–644.
24. Wittgen CM, Naunheim KS, Andrus CH, et al. Preoperative pulmonary function evaluation for laparoscopic cholecystectomy. *Arch Surg* 1993; 128(8):880–885; discussion 5–6.
25. Larach SW, Patankar SK, Ferrara A, et al. Complications of laparoscopic colorectal surgery. Analysis and comparison of early vs. latter experience. *Dis Colon Rectum* 1997;40(5):592–596.
26. Oh BR, Kwon DD, Park KS, et al. Late presentation of ureteral injury after laparoscopic surgery. Obstet Gynecol 2000;95(3):337–339.
27. Cass AS, Bubrick MP. Ureteral injuries in colonic surgery. *Urology* 1981; 18(4):359–364.
28. Kalisvaart JF, Finley DS, Ornstein DK. Robotic-assisted repair of iatrogenic ureteral ligation following robotic-assisted hysterectomy. *JSLS* 2008;12(4):414–416.
29. O'Hanlan KA. Cystosufflation to prevent bladder injury. *J Minim Invasive Gynecol* 2009;16(2):195–197.
30. Tai CK, Li SK, Hou SM, et al. Bladder injury mimicking acute renal failure after cesarean section: a diagnostic challenge and minimally invasive management. *Surg Laparosc Endosc Percutan Tech* 2008;18(3):301–303.
31. O'Malley C, Cunningham AJ. Physiologic changes during laparoscopy. *Anesthesiol Clin North America* 2001;19(1):1–19.
32. Leonard F, Fotso A, Borghese B, et al. Ureteral complications from laparoscopic hysterectomy indicated for benign uterine pathologies: a 13-year experience in a continuous series of 1300 patients. *Hum Reprod* 2007;22(7):2006–2011.
33. Regadas FS, Rodrigues LV, Nicodemo AM, et al. Complications in laparoscopic colorectal resection: main types and prevention. *Surg Laparosc Endosc* 1998;8(3):189–192.
34. Parpala-Sparman T, Paananen I, Santala M, et al. Increasing numbers of ureteric injuries after the introduction of laparoscopic surgery. *Scand J Urol Nephrol* 2008;42(5):422–427.
35. Tsujinaka S, Wexner SD, DaSilva G, et al. Prophylactic ureteric catheters in laparoscopic colorectal surgery. *Tech Coloproctol* 2008;12(1):45–50.
36. Hove LD, Bock J, Christoffersen JK, et al. Analysis of 136 ureteral injuries in gynecological and obstetrical surgery from completed insurance claims. *Acta Obstet Gynecol Scand* 2010;89(1):82–86.
37. De Cicco C, Ret Davalos ML, Van Cleynenbreugel B, et al. Iatrogenic ureteral lesions and repair: a review for gynecologists. *J Minim Invasive Gynecol* 2007;14(4):428–435.
38. Tamussino KF, Lang PF, Breinl E. Ureteral complications with operative gynecologic laparoscopy. *Am J Obstet Gynecol* 1998;178(5):967–970.
39. Bishoff JT, Allaf ME, Kirkels W, et al. Laparoscopic bowel injury: incidence and clinical presentation. *J Urol* 1999;161(3):887–890.
40. Kwon AH, Inui H, Kamiyama Y. Laparoscopic management of bile duct and bowel injury during laparoscopic cholecystectomy. *World J Surg* 2001;25(7):856–861.
41. Schrenk P, Woisetschlager R, Rieger R, et al. Mechanism, management, and prevention of laparoscopic bowel injuries. *Gastrointest Endosc* 1996; 43(6):572–574.
42. van der Voort M, Heijnsdijk EA, Gouma DJ. Bowel injury as a complication of laparoscopy. *Br J Surg* 2004;91(10):1253–1258.
43. El-Banna M, Abdel-Atty M, El-Meteini M, et al. Management of laparoscopic-related bowel injuries. *Surg Endosc* 2000;14(9):779–782.
44. Wu MP, Ou CS, Chen SL, et al. Complications and recommended practices for electrosurgery in laparoscopy. *Am J Surg* 2000;179(1):67–73.
45. Chapron C, Pierre F, Harchaoui Y, et al. Gastrointestinal injuries during gynaecological laparoscopy. *Hum Reprod* 1999;14(2):333–337.
46. Larobina M, Nottle P. Complete evidence regarding major vascular injuries during laparoscopic access. *Surg Laparosc Endosc Percutan Tech* 2005;15(3):119–123.
47. Opitz I, Gantert W, Giger U, et al. Bleeding remains a major complication during laparoscopic surgery: analysis of the SALTS database. *Langenbecks Arch Surg* 2005;390(2):128–133.
48. Roviaro GC, Varoli F, Saguatti L, et al. Major vascular injuries in laparoscopic surgery. *Surg Endosc* 2002;16(8):1192–1166.
49. Breda A, Veale J, Liao J, et al. Complications of laparoscopic living donor nephrectomy and their management: the UCLA experience. *Urology* 2007;69(1):49–52.
50. Richstone L, Seideman C, Baldinger L, et al. Conversion during laparoscopic surgery: frequency, indications and risk factors. *J Urol* 2008;180(3): 855–859.
51. Schafer M, Lauper M, Krahenbuhl L. A nation's experience of bleeding complications during laparoscopy. *Am J Surg* 2000;180(1):73–77.
52. Chapron CM, Pierre F, Lacroix S, et al. Major vascular injuries during gynecologic laparoscopy. *J Am Coll Surg* 1997;185(5):461–465.
53. Saggar VR, Singhal A, Singh K, et al. Factors influencing development of subcutaneous carbon dioxide emphysema in laparoscopic totally extraperitoneal inguinal hernia repair. *J Laparoendosc Adv Surg Tech A* 2008;18(2):213–216.
54. Zhao LC, Han JS, Loeb S, et al. Thoracic complications of urologic laparoscopy: correlation between radiographic findings and clinical manifestations. *J Endourol* 2008;22(4):607–614.
55. Hunter JG, Jobe BA. Minimally invasive surgery, robotics and natural orifice transluminal endoscopic surgery. In: Brunicardi FC, Andersen DK, Billiar TR, et al., eds. *Schwartz's principles of surgery*, 9th ed. New York, NY: McGraw Hill; 2009. Available at http://www.accesssurgery.com/content.aspx?aID = 5014248, accessed January, 2010.
56. Derouin M, Couture P, Boudreault D, et al. Detection of gas embolism by transesophageal echocardiography during laparoscopic cholecystectomy. *Anesth Analg* 1996;82(1):119–124.
57. Kim CS, Kim JY, Kwon JY, et al. Venous air embolism during total laparoscopic hysterectomy: comparison to total abdominal hysterectomy. *Anesthesiology* 2009;111(1):50–54.
58. Joshi GP. Complications of laparoscopy. *Anesthesiol Clin North America* 2001;19(1):89–105.
59. Abut YC, Eryilmaz R, Okan I, et al. Venous air embolism during laparoscopic cholecystectomy. *Minim Invasive Ther Allied Technol* 2009;18(6): 366–368.
60. Ikegami T, Shimada M, Imura S, et al. Argon gas embolism in the application of laparoscopic microwave coagulation therapy. *J Hepatobiliary Pancreat Surg* 2009;16(3):394–398.
61. Min SK, Kim JH, Lee SY. Carbon dioxide and argon gas embolism during laparoscopic hepatic resection. *Acta Anaesthesiol Scand* 2007;51(7):949–953.
62. Simper SC, Erzinger JM, Smith SC. Comparison of laparoscopic linear staplers in clinical practice. *Surg Obes Relat Dis* 2007;3(4):446–450; discussion 50–51.
63. Chan D, Bishoff JT, Ratner L, et al. Endovascular gastrointestinal stapler device malfunction during laparoscopic nephrectomy: early recognition and management. *J Urol* 2000;164(2):319–321.
64. Deng DY, Meng MV, Nguyen HT, et al. Laparoscopic linear cutting stapler failure. *Urology* 2002;60(3):415–419; discussion 9–20.
65. Bradshaw WA, Gregory BC, Finley CR, et al. Frequency of postoperative nausea and vomiting in patients undergoing laparoscopic foregut surgery. *Surg Endosc* 2002;16(5):777–780.
66. Apfel CC, Laara E, Koivuranta M, et al. A simplified risk score for predicting postoperative nausea and vomiting: conclusions from cross-validations between two centers. *Anesthesiology* 1999;91(3):693–700.
67. Koivuranta M, Laara E, Snare L, et al. A survey of postoperative nausea and vomiting. *Anaesthesia* 1997;52(5):443–449.
68. Apfel CC, Korttila K, Abdalla M, et al. A factorial trial of six interventions for the prevention of postoperative nausea and vomiting. *N Engl J Med* 2004;350(24):2441–2451.
69. Smith I. Anesthesia for laparoscopy with emphasis on outpatient laparoscopy. *Anesthesiol Clin North America* 2001;19(1):21–41.
70. White PF, Sacan O, Nuangchamnong N, et al. The relationship between patient risk factors and early versus late postoperative emetic symptoms. *Anesth Analg* 2008;107(2):459–463.
71. Cunniffe MG, McAnena OJ, Dar MA, et al. A prospective randomized trial of intraoperative bupivacaine irrigation for management of shoulder-tip pain following laparoscopy. *Am J Surg* 1998;176(3):258–261.
72. Gurusamy KS, Samraj K, Davidson BR. Low pressure versus standard pressure pneumoperitoneum in laparoscopic cholecystectomy. *Cochrane Database Syst Rev* 2009;(2):CD006930.

PART

VI

Complications of Endocrine and Oncologic Surgery

CHAPTER 41

Complications of Adrenal Surgery

Paul G. Gauger

INTRODUCTION

Surgically remediable adrenal diseases define a fascinating spectrum from small tumors with large physiologic consequences to physiologically silent large tumors with major surgical consequences. Adrenalectomy is an example of a procedure that has been transformed from an invasive and temporarily disabling operation to one that gives many patients a minimally invasive and less morbid alternative. Yet diverse complications can still ensue. Some complications relate to the disease process being treated and some relate to the specific surgical approach. With proper vigilance and preparation, most complications can be either avoided or managed.

THERAPEUTIC GOALS OF ADRENALECTOMY

Appropriate utilization of adrenalectomy conceptually applies to (a) patients with clinically or biochemically apparent hormonal hyperfunction, (b) patients with a probable or certain malignant adrenal mass, and (c) patients with an adrenal mass of uncertain significance. Patients with hormonal syndromes for whom adrenalectomy is a consideration commonly include those with primary hyperaldosteronism, primary or secondary hypercortisolism, and pheochromocytoma. For hormonal excess, the goal of adrenalectomy—whether unilateral or bilateral—is to provide long-term relief of the hormonal syndrome. Resection of an adrenocortical carcinoma (ACC) is offered in the hope (rarely realized) of providing long-term disease-free survival. Resection of a metastasis from another malignancy to the adrenal gland is occasionally indicated if histologic proof is required to determine the type and intensity of adjuvant therapy for the primary cancer, or if the adrenal mass is the only identifiable residual tumor in a patient for whom removal would be expected to be of benefit. Finally, adrenalectomy may be offered to patients for whom workup of an incidentally noted adrenal mass has failed to yield a conclusive etiology and in whom the risk of observation is determined to exceed the risk of removal.

Paul G. Gauger: University of Michigan Department of Surgery, Division of Endocrine Surgery.

EXPECTED OUTCOMES

For most benign conditions, the disease-related outcomes may be relatively independent of the specific surgical approach. This is not true for primary adrenal malignancies where the surgical approach for locally aggressive tumors can more directly affect outcomes. Complications and other outcomes important to the patient may be associated with the particular surgical approach. For example, the open transabdominal approaches may be complicated by pancreatitis, incidental splenectomy, pneumonia, longer hospitalization, and more prolonged recovery. Laparoscopic approaches have been shown to be superior to open approaches in terms of length of stay and pain control as well as complication rates (1,2). Many long-term outcomes are determined by the specific adrenal disorder being treated.

Primary hyperaldosteronism

This chapter will discuss only surgically remediable hyperaldosteronism, which affects approximately two-thirds of all patients with primary hyperaldosteronism. The characterization of primary hyperaldosteronism, as caused by an adrenocortical adenoma, is commonly attributed to Jerome Conn (3). Awareness of primary hyperaldosteronism has increased over time—and perhaps along with an increase in incidental adrenal imaging. Because of variability in screening practices and diagnostic criteria, Conn syndrome is likely more common than prevalence statistics would suggest. There is large variability between series, but perhaps 5% to 7% of patients evaluated in hypertension clinics have primary hyperaldosteronism. Although most patients (69%) have hypokalemia accompanying hypertension, the diagnosis is often more subtle and conventional diagnostic criteria have been expanded.

Primary hyperaldosteronism most often affects patients between 30 and 60 years of age (mean 47 years) and is more common in women by a ratio of 2:1 (4). The severity and duration of hypertension are often indistinguishable from essential hypertension. Polyuria and nocturia are common. Symptoms of hypokalemia such as muscle weakness or cramps may be present. Rarely, periodic paralysis can occur as hypokalemia acutely worsens following increased sodium intake or administration of potassium-wasting diuretics.

Evaluation of metabolic and hormonal disturbances is most accurate if the patient has a diet with normal sodium intake (6 to 9 g/day) and is not taking diuretics, β-blocker agents, angiotensin-converting enzyme inhibitors, or angiotensin II receptor blockers. In this setting, relative hypokalemia, with a potassium of <3.9 mEq/L, and a metabolic alkalosis, with HCO_3^- of >32 mEq/L, are both consistent with the diagnosis. Twenty-four-hour urinary aldosterone secretion is often elevated. Plasma aldosterone levels are more commonly obtained. Isolated plasma aldosterone levels may not be remarkably elevated above the upper end of normal, but patients with primary hyperaldosteronism typically have plasma aldosterone concentrations 15 ng/dL. However, in the context of a suppressed plasma renin activity, a ratio of plasma aldosterone/plasma renin activity >25 is highly suggestive of primary hyperaldosteronism, while a ratio of >20 is used in screening to increase the ability to detect patients with mild primary hyperaldosteronism. The aldosterone/ renin ratio is a nonstandardized test with little published data to suggest appropriate diagnostic thresholds. However, most groups use cutoffs of 20 to 40 for the ratio (5).

Primary hyperaldosteronism is generally caused by either an adenoma (Conn syndrome) or bilateral hyperplasia of the zona glomerulosa of the adrenal glands. The classification of primary hyperaldosteronism has expanded to include (a) multiple or bilateral adenomas, or adenomas arising in hyperplastic glands; (b) familial dexamethasone-suppressible hyperaldosteronism; and (c) unilateral hyperplasia (somewhat controversial). Not all these entities are surgically remediable. As the specific pathophysiology influences the indications for operation and, ultimately, the expected outcomes, it is important to identify the specific condition responsible for primary hyperaldosteronism.

Clinical features may be somewhat helpful in this regard. The degree of hypertension and hypokalemia is often relatively more severe in Conn syndrome than in idiopathic hyperaldosteronism. In response to an upright position for 2 hours, plasma aldosterone increases in patients with idiopathic hyperaldosteronism, but does not increase in patients with Conn syndrome. Idiopathic hyperaldosteronism is suggested if plasma aldosterone levels are reduced in response to saline loading or captopril administration. Serum 18-OH-corticosterone levels are often elevated in Conn syndrome, but they are not elevated in idiopathic hyperaldosteronism.

Differentiation of Conn syndrome from idiopathic hyperaldosteronism is an imperfect process. The dichotomous concept of the unilateral adrenal mass amenable to surgery versus the bilateral adrenal enlargement amenable to medical therapy is oversimplified and does not account for the full spectrum of disease. Apart from the suggestive clinical factors noted earlier, anatomic and functional imaging tests are necessary. Cross-sectional imaging performed under appropriate specific adrenal protocols is quite sensitive in determining the presence of an adrenal mass. The most practical initial imaging test is a computed tomography (CT) scan (Fig. 41.1). Magnetic resonance imaging (MRI) scanning is usually more expensive and yields equivalent information.

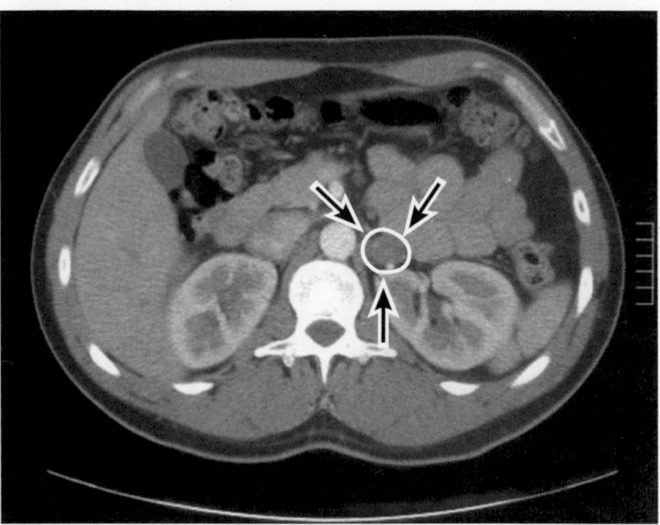

FIGURE 41.1. Arrows indicate a 2.1-cm left adrenal mass seen on CT scan of a 38-year-old male with primary hyperaldosteronism as determined by hypertension, hypokalemia, and an aldosterone/PRA ratio of 48.

If a unilateral mass is evident on cross-sectional imaging, it may be nonsecreting in the presence of a contralateral microaldosteronoma or a background of bilateral hyperplasia. A unilateral aldosteronoma may arise in the background of microscopic hyperplasia, and yet the patient will be cured by unilateral adrenalectomy (6,7). Bilateral adrenal adenomatous changes may be relatively hypersecreting on one side only. These variable possibilities become important during the preoperative workup and patient selection.

If CT scan detects a unilateral adrenal mass and the contralateral adrenal appears normal, the presumption that this represents unilateral disease, curable by unilateral adrenalectomy, is correct >90% of the time. If there is bilateral enlargement, it is necessary to corroborate anatomic data with functional information from selective adrenal venous sampling.

Some investigators utilize selective venous sampling in an individualized or selective manner while others employ the test routinely for functional confirmation of anatomic information. In a recent series, compared to patient selection based on CT results alone, adrenal vein sampling changed management in 36% of patients when employed routinely (7). Adrenal venous sampling for aldosterone levels provides the most specific confirmation of a unilateral or bilateral hypersecretory process. Adrenal venous sampling is technically demanding, related to the challenge of catheterizing the right central adrenal vein (Fig. 41.2). In addition to aldosterone levels, cortisol levels are sampled to assure proper catheter position. Adrenocorticotropic hormone (ACTH) is infused to equalize stress-induced fluctuations in adrenal output. Although ACTH is usually

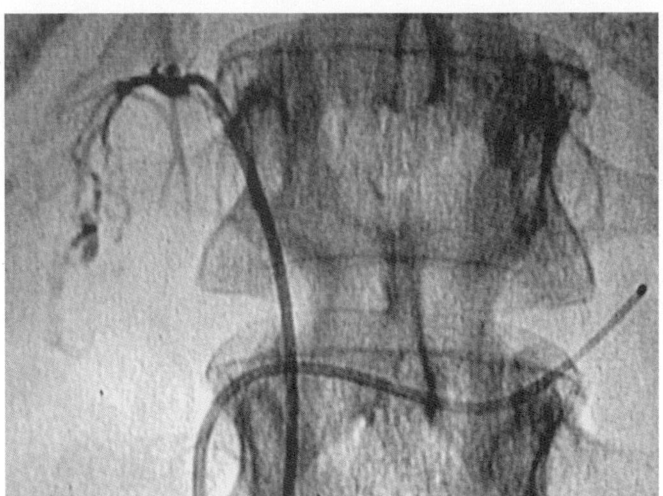

FIGURE 41.2. Bilateral adrenal vein catheterization (with contrast injection into right central adrenal vein) that was done in the course of selective adrenal venous sampling in a patient with primary hyperaldosteronism.

Table 41.2 Criteria for interpretation of selective adrenal vein sampling data

Ratio	Number
Evidence of Catheter Placement in Adrenal Vein	
Pre-ACTH adrenal vein cortisol:IVC cortisol	>3
Lateralization	
Primary Evidence	
Dominant aldosterone/cortisol:nondominant aldosterone/cortisol	>4, preferably >6
Supporting Evidence	
Dominant aldosterone:nondominant aldosterone	>3
Dominant aldosterone/cortisol:IVC aldosterone/cortisol	>1.5
Nondominant aldosterone/cortisol:IVC aldosterone/cortisol	<1

ACTH, adrenocorticotropic hormone; IVC, inferior vena cava.

thought of as a stimulatory hormone for glucocorticoid secretion, it is typical to also observe a brisk response in aldosterone secretion in the abnormal gland (Table 41.1).

Thoughtful patient selection and a thorough preoperative workup are necessary to ensure excellent outcomes. As a general rule, primary hyperaldosteronism caused by an adrenocortical adenoma responds to surgical resection while idiopathic hyperaldosteronism does not. However, some patients with idiopathic hyperaldosteronism who have asymmetric hypersecretion of excess aldosterone respond well to surgical resection of the dominant gland. Selective venous sampling can be very helpful in identifying these patients. Criteria for interpretation of data are shown in Table 41.2. Most patients with idiopathic hyperaldosteronism and bilateral hypersecretion are treated without operation. Both hypertension and hypokalemia can be controlled with chronic spironolactone or eplerenone therapy. In the spectrum of disease between these two entities are cortical adenomas arising in a background of hyperplasia. Hyperplasia can occur as an asymmetric (unilaterally dominant) disease. If this condition can be determined by preoperative workup, these patients can be offered unilateral adrenalectomy with the expectation of excellent outcomes (7).

Unilateral adrenalectomy for primary hyperaldosteronism caused by a cortical adenoma nearly always provides rapid resolution of hypokalemia. The residual need for potassium supplements is approximately 1.5% in surgically treated patients versus approximately 80% in medically treated patients (7). The response of hypertension can be more variable, from complete response to continued reliance on antihypertensive medications. However, it is common for most properly selected patients to decrease the number and dose of antihypertensive medications. Definitions of cure are inconsistent, but of patients successfully treated, 65% to 70% may become normotensive while most of the remainder will improve with some residual degree of hypertension. With the assistance of adrenal vein sampling in patient selection, approximately 70% of patients with prototypical Conn syndrome are normotensive postoperatively while 67% of patients with unilaterally dominant bilateral disease are normotensive postoperatively. In properly selected, surgically treated patients, only approximately 5% will have residual Stage 2 hypertension while 25% of medically treated patients will have Stage 2 hypertension. Disease-related outcomes are largely independent of specific

Table 41.1 Selective adrenal venous sampling for aldosterone and cortisol levels indicating oversecretion of aldosterone from the right adrenal gland

Aldosterone R/L/IVC (1–16 ng/dL)	R/L Aldo Ratio	Cortisol R/L/IVC (7–22 μg/dL)	A/C Ratio R/L/IVC	Ratio of A/C R/L
3,860/53/39	72	89/25/22	43/2.1/1.7	20
10-, 20-, and 30-min post-ACTH				
17,344/504/46	34	486/390/24	36/1.3/1.9	28
20,018/714/87	28	526/401/22	38/1.8/3.9	21
17,984/540/96	33	569/437/28	31/1.2/3.3	25

ACTH, adrenocorticotropic hormone; **A/C Ratio, Aldosterone/Cortisol Ratio;** R/L/IVC, Right/Left/Inferior Vena Cava.

operative approach, such as anterior adrenalectomy, posterior adrenalectomy, or laparoscopic adrenalectomy.

Hypercortisolism

All conditions resulting from excess glucocorticoid are commonly known as Cushing's syndrome. (Cushing's disease is Cushing's syndrome because of an ACTH-producing pituitary adenoma.) Hypercortisolism can be classified as either corticotropin dependent or corticotropin independent. The former is responsible for >80% of patients with hypercortisolism. Chronic corticotropin (ACTH) stimulation results in adrenocortical hyperplasia with overproduction of cortisol and other adrenal hormones. The pituitary-dependent form (Cushing's disease) accounts for 70% of corticotropin-dependent hypercortisolism, while the ectopic ACTH syndrome accounts for 10%, usually from small cell carcinoma of the lung, carcinoid tumor, medullary thyroid carcinoma, or malignant tumors of the pancreas or thymus. With the exception of iatrogenic steroid excess, corticotropin-independent hypercortisolism implies primary overproduction of cortisol from the adrenal gland(s). This condition usually occurs as a function of a unilateral cortical adenoma, accounting for 10% of patients with hypercortisolism overall, but it may be caused by primary hyperplasia of both adrenal glands. Primary ACC can also present as an adrenal mass accompanied by hypercortisolism.

An adrenocortical adenoma is best treated by unilateral adrenalectomy. Cushing's syndrome caused by primary or secondary adrenal hyperplasia can often be managed medically, but when this fails, bilateral adrenalectomy is indicated. In these situations, delayed referral is common and perioperative morbidity will increase as the ravages of hypercortisolism progress. Although many patients with ectopic ACTH syndrome have advanced malignancies and, accordingly, a poor prognosis, operation is often indicated to remove the source of ACTH overproduction and to simplify medical management. If the source of ectopic ACTH syndrome can be localized and safely resected, this is the most appropriate treatment. Because of the small size of some tumors, such as bronchial tumors or carcinoid tumors, localization is not always possible. In that case, palliative pharmacologic treatment with ketoconazole, mitotane, or octreotide is indicated. If this therapy is not effective in controlling hypercortisolemia, bilateral adrenalectomy is indicated. Palliative operation may involve bilateral adrenal resection to treat refractory Cushing's syndrome if the secretion of ACTH cannot be adequately controlled. In general, long-term prognosis of patients with ectopic ACTH syndrome is poor. Some patients (bronchial carcinoid or medullary thyroid carcinoma) may live for years with residual neoplasm while others (e.g., with pancreatic carcinoid or lung carcinomas) have short survival.

The clinical presentation of Cushing's syndrome usually includes insidious onset of weakness, increased appetite, weight gain, and oligomenorrhea in females. As the syndrome develops, patients develop centripetal obesity with rounded facies, gradual obscuration of the ears in the frontal profile, fullness of the supraclavicular fat pads, and a "buffalo hump." Skin fragility and bruising are common, as are purple striae on the flanks, abdomen, and limbs. Hirsutism, acne, and facial plethora, as well as hypertension and diabetes, may occur.

Diagnosis of Cushing's syndrome requires biochemical confirmation. An effective way to establish that hypercortisolism exists is a 24-hour urinary free cortisol level. Alternatively, a low-dose dexamethasone suppression test can be obtained by administering 1 mg oral dexamethasone at 11 PM followed by serum cortisol determination at 8 AM the next morning. Classically, patients without hypercortisolism should have cortisol value <5 μg/dL with this test. However, about 15% of patients with Cushing's disease can suppress with dexamethasone. If the goal of screening is to enhance sensitivity of the test, increasing the stringency of this threshold to <1.8 μg/dL will increase sensitivity to 95% (8). However, the resultant clinical benefit of detection of mild cortisol excess is not yet proven, and data regarding outcomes of early identification and treatment of subclinical disease are not conclusive.

To establish whether the corticotropin-dependent or corticotropin-independent form is present, it is necessary to measure plasma ACTH at basal levels. If ACTH is normal or elevated, this implies corticotropin-dependent pathophysiology. A high-dose (8 mg) dexamethasone suppression test typically reveals that patients with Cushing's disease suppress cortisol production, while those with ectopic ACTH syndrome do not. Selective venous catheterization of bilateral petrosal venous sinuses during corticotropin-releasing hormone stimulation can confirm pituitary hypersecretion of ACTH. Patients with ectopic ACTH secretion usually have markedly elevated corticotropin levels, often >200 pg/mL. If corticotropin levels are low or undetectable, the suppression of the hypothalamic–pituitary axis is usually caused by a cortisol-secreting adrenal tumor.

Adrenal imaging is useful in the setting of hypercortisolism. Since secondary adrenal stimulation caused by ACTH excess predictably affects both adrenals, imaging is most helpful in the setting of corticotropin-independent Cushing's syndrome. CT and MRI scanning of the adrenals can document unilateral or bilateral enlargement.

The treatment of Cushing's disease is usually accomplished by (a) transsphenoidal microsurgery to remove pituitary tumor; (b) external or interstitial pituitary irradiation; or (c) pharmacologic therapy. Bilateral adrenalectomy for control of hypercortisolism is occasionally indicated: (a) if transsphenoidal resection is not possible or not successful; (b) if hypercortisolism is rapidly progressive and particularly severe; (c) if palliation of ectopic ACTH syndrome is required; or (d) if the patient has primary adrenal hyperplasia. Up to 50% of patients with pituitary Cushing's disease ultimately require bilateral adrenalectomy (9). Adrenalectomy can often be accomplished by a laparoscopic or retroperitoneoscopic approach, and an associated increased quality of life has been documented (10). However, recovery is often prolonged and incomplete. Approximately 30% of patients remain hypertensive, 20% continue to have diabetes, and 20% remain obese (11).

Until the last two decades, adrenalectomy in patients with hypercortisolism was associated with significant morbidity (about 30%) and mortality (5% to 10%). In recent series, the outcomes have improved appreciably to a range that approaches that of treatment of other adrenal diseases. Approximately 10% of patients will have a complication such as hemorrhage, deep venous thrombosis, pulmonary embolus, respiratory failure, coagulopathy, pneumonia, or wound infection. Complication rates are lowest in patients requiring unilateral adrenalectomy (approximately 10% morbidity and 1% mortality) and are improved by minimally invasive approaches. In general, patients requiring unilateral adrenalectomy for a hypersecreting cortical adenoma have better long-term outcomes than those requiring bilateral adrenalectomy for medically refractory disease. Patients undergoing unilateral adrenalectomy have gradual disappearance of the signs and symptoms of hypercortisolism and have excellent long-term survival. Although the metabolic derangements tend to improve in the months following operation, it may take up to 12 months for some of the physical changes, such as hirsutism, obesity, and acne, to reverse.

Pheochromocytoma

Pheochromocytoma is a tumor derived from the adrenal medulla. This tumor's physiologic effects demand accurate and early preoperative diagnosis to benefit the patient. Although pheochromocytoma is present in only 0.1% to 1% of hypertensive patients, the overall incidence is approximately 1 to 2 per 100,000. Despite improved clinical understanding of the syndrome, many patients still go undiagnosed. For patients with pheochromocytoma discovered at autopsy, most have died suddenly from myocardial infarction or cerebrovascular accident, and pheochromocytoma remains a cause of sudden death.

The clinical presentation of pheochromocytoma includes a wide array of symptoms. The most typical are headache, sweating, palpitations, and episodic hypertension. Less common symptoms include nausea, anxiety, abdominal pain, pallor, and exacerbation of hyperglycemia. Hypertension is sustained in approximately 50%. The presentation can occasionally be acute and severe, involving massive catecholamine release from tumor hemorrhage or necrosis and leading to critical hypertension and subsequent cardiovascular collapse. Pheochromocytoma must always be considered in the gravid patient with a hypertensive crisis during pregnancy or labor.

The diagnosis requires discriminating clinical suspicion and biochemical confirmation. Serum or urine catecholamine levels are often inaccurate and difficult to interpret. Metabolites of catecholamines (metanephrines, normetanephrines, and vanillylmandelic acid) can be measured in the urine

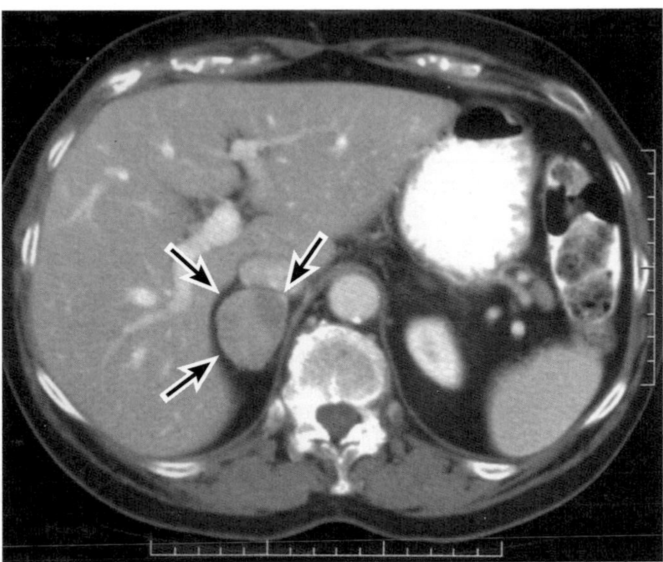

FIGURE 41.3. CT scan of a 71-year-old woman with intermittent hypertension, pounding chest sensations, headaches, and elevation of plasma metanephrine levels. The arrows indicate a 3.8-cm right adrenal pheochromocytoma.

with acceptable sensitivity and specificity. Plasma fractionated metanephrines involve an assay with very high sensitivity (up to 99%) but limited specificity (90%). For that reason, the test performs best in patients with a higher pretest probability of pheochromocytoma (e.g., familial patients). If plasma metanephrines are used for routine screening due to logistical convenience, one must be aware of the potential for false-positive tests and the need to follow up with a less sensitive (75%), but more specific (95%), test (95%) such as 24-hour urinary metanephrine measurements, if clinical uncertainty remains.

When biochemical testing supports the diagnosis of pheochromocytoma, evidence of an adrenal tumor is sought, typically, by abdominal CT or MRI scanning (Fig. 41.3). Since 10% of pheochromocytomas are extra-adrenal, additional anatomic and functional imaging may be required. ^{123}I or ^{131}I metaiodobenzylguanidine (MIBG) is a radionuclide that concentrates in abnormal adrenergic tissue. MIBG can be very useful in defining the presence of metastatic or extraadrenal disease. In the patient with clear-cut clinical and biochemical evidence of pheochromocytoma and a unilateral adrenal mass on CT scan, MIBG scanning adds little additional preoperative information (Fig. 41.4) (12,13). However, MIBG scanning may still add critical information for the management of patients with bilateral, extra-adrenal, familial, or malignant disease.

Although the first resection of a pheochromocytoma was performed in 1926, adrenalectomy remained an operation that was associated with high rates of morbidity and mortality until the introduction of phentolamine for α-receptor blockade and norepinephrine for postresection hypotension. Outcomes have improved substantially in the last decades. In large part, complications are related to the hemodynamic pathophysiology associated with the tumor and its removal. The specific surgical approach does not seem to influence

pancreatic tail or in the case of large tumors. In that case, an alternative approach involves dividing the superior and lateral splenic attachments to mobilize the spleen and distal pancreas en bloc via partial medial visceral rotation. It is often possible to expose and divide the central adrenal vein early in the dissection where it joins with the left renal vein. It is helpful to divide the inferior phrenic pedicle early in the dissection as well to allow some caudad retraction of the tumor. With large tumors, splenectomy may be necessary due to tumor invasion or to provide adequate exposure. An en bloc distal pancreatectomy may also be necessary because of local invasion. Nephrectomy may be required for renal parenchymal invasion or hilar vessel involvement.

Open posterior adrenalectomy

A direct route to the retroperitoneum can avoid the morbidity associated with major laparotomy. A hockey stick–type incision is carried down to the level of the ipsilateral paraspinous muscle and carried obliquely over the course of the 12th rib (Fig. 41.6). The latissimus dorsi fibers are divided, and the paraspinous muscle is mobilized medially but not divided. The 12th rib is resected subperiosteally, avoiding the intercostal bundle. It is easy to violate the pleura here and enter the costophrenic sulcus—especially in the medial portion of the field. If pleural entry occurs, it is straightforward to evacuate the resultant air from the pleura and close this again. A tube thoracostomy is unnecessary if no pulmonary injury is incurred. When the retroperitoneum is entered, the kidney is palpated in the deep medial aspect of the wound and gently pulled caudad to allow the adrenal mass to be exposed. Because the right adrenal gland is anatomically posterior to the inferior vena cava, the central adrenal vein is the last major structure seen and divided when removing the right adrenal gland by this approach. This effect is less pronounced on the left side where the central adrenal vein may be encountered and divided earlier in the dissection. Overall, this approach is rarely used and its place in the surgical armamentarium has largely been supplanted by the posterior retroperitoneoscopic approach.

Open thoracoabdominal adrenalectomy

Because of the associated pulmonary morbidity of this approach, it is used only for very large malignant adrenal masses. Although occasionally necessary on the left side, a thoracoabdominal incision is most relevant to large right-sided ACCs when venous involvement is present. The patient is positioned intermediate between supine and flank orientation with the table flexed (Fig. 41.6). A single incision is made over the 10th rib (11th on the left) and carried obliquely onto the abdomen. The rib is resected subperiosteally. The diaphragm is divided curvilinearly to limit denervation of fibers that are distributed from the central aspect. Superior retraction of the lung and anterior retraction of the right hepatic lobe provides wide exposure for adrenalectomy. Occasionally, this approach on the left may be accomplished without pleural entry. After adrenalectomy, the diaphragm and peritoneum are repaired. A tube thoracostomy is necessary if the pleural cavity is entered.

Laparoscopic transperitoneal adrenalectomy

The patient is secured with a padded beanbag in flank position with the table flexed. The arms must be padded and secured in gentle anterior flexion. Typical port placement is along the line of a subcostal incision with the exception of the camera port (for a 30-degree surgical telescope). It is often useful to triangulate that port out of line with the others toward the umbilicus, which decreases intracorporeal instrument collisions. For right adrenalectomy, an additional port is usually necessary for retraction of the right lobe of the liver after it is mobilized. The right lobe of the liver is mobilized by dividing the triangular ligament with an ultrasonic shears. This is done progressively to open the space anterolateral to the adrenal gland until the vena cava is seen. After division of Gerota fascia, blunt dissection between the vena cava and the medial margin of the gland will define the central adrenal vein. This vein is taken between endoscopic clips and divided. If the vein is particularly broad, division may require application of an endoscopic linear stapler. The inferior phrenic pedicle is divided after controlling small vessels with endoscopic clips or the ultrasonic shears. The remaining attachments include small arterial branches from the renal artery or aorta, which can be easily controlled with the ultrasonic shears. The gland is removed in an endoscopic specimen bag.

For left-sided lesions, the port placement is similar, and a fourth port is only necessary when the spleen is difficult to reflect adequately. After introduction of the 30-degree scope and instruments, the lateral attachments of the spleen are divided with ultrasonic shears. To begin this dissection, it may be necessary to take down the splenic flexure of the colon by dividing the lienocolic ligament in a limited fashion. As the plane is developed, the spleen will begin to fall medially. The plane must be developed posterior to the pancreatic tail to locate the adrenal gland without injuring the pancreas. This dissection must be continued until the adrenal gland is seen, which will be nearly adjacent to the aorta. Small glands may be obscured in retroperitoneal fat, especially in males and in patients with Cushing's syndrome. Laparoscopic ultrasound can help identify the gland and indicate the proper target for exposure. Once the gland is located, it is circumferentially mobilized with ultrasonic shears. The inferior phrenic pedicle and the central adrenal vein are exposed with blunt dissection. These structures are controlled with endoscopic clips and divided. On the left, there is often an anastomotic vein between these two vessels, and it is important to divide these main veins away from the anastamotic complex to prevent bleeding. The central adrenal vein is often short, but it is usually not necessary to expose the left renal vein in order to safely divide it.

Posterior retroperitoneoscopic adrenalectomy

An anatomically direct videoscopic approach to the adrenal, which minimized dissection and afforded early access to the central adrenal vein, has been popularized by Walz et al. (32). After initial description as a three-port technique (33), it has evolved into a single-port alternative (34). Yet, many surgeons have been slow to adopt this approach due to perceived concerns of limited exposure and operating space, as well as lack of traditional familiar anatomic landmarks. As with the open posterior approach, the retroperitoneoscopic approach allows access to the adrenal gland without traversal of the peritoneal space but adds the patient benefits of minimally invasive techniques. With the patient in prone position, the approach usually uses three or fewer trocar sites, and the retroperitoneal space is created and maintained by high-pressure pneumoretroperitoneum (20 to 24 mm Hg), which is well tolerated by patients compared to similar degrees of pneumoperitoneum. Because of the excellent visualization via this approach, partial adrenalectomy is also possible if a cortical-sparing procedure is indicated (35). This approach is not appropriate for primary ACC, but isolated metastases have been successfully removed in this fashion (36).

IDENTIFICATION AND MANAGEMENT OF POSTOPERATIVE COMPLICATIONS

Bleeding

Although usually avoided with careful and patient application of surgical technique, significant bleeding can occur with any approach to the adrenal gland. Hemorrhage is often from injury to the renal vein, inferior vena cava, or liver on the right or to the renal vein, splenic vein, or spleen on the left. Major bleeding during right adrenalectomy may be caused by failure to recognize the right hepatic vein or an aberrant central adrenal vein that drains into the right hepatic vein. Often, a hole in the inferior vena cava can be primarily repaired with suture venorrhaphy, but occasionally a patch of bovine pericardium or PTFE may be required to prevent iatrogenic inferior vena cava stenosis.

Glucocorticoid insufficiency

This problem may occur if hypercortisolism with suppression of the hypophyseal–pituitary–adrenal axis is not recognized preoperatively and the patient is not adequately supplemented with corticosteroids perioperatively. Insufficiency will also occur after bilateral adrenalectomy if not actively prevented and appropriately treated. Glucocorticoid insufficiency should be considered after adrenalectomy in any patient who develops hypotension, hyponatremia, hyperkalemia, hypoglycemia, and acidosis. If suspected, the problem should be treated immediately with intravenous hydrocortisone. Patients at risk should receive 100 mg IV hydrocortisone every 6 hours on the day of the operation. Usually, 200 mg hydrocortisone distributed over postoperative day 1 and 100 mg over postoperative day 2 is adequate. When oral alimentation is established, the dose is converted and weaned to a maintenance dose of approximately 15 to 37.5 mg hydrocortisone per day, divided into three doses. Following unilateral adrenalectomy, the recovery of the hypophyseal–pituitary–adrenal axis can be determined with a Cosyntropin stimulation test no earlier than approximately 3 to 6 months. However, it should be understood that average time to recovery of the HPA axis is usually >1 year. An alternative strategy may apply to patients in whom the suppression of the hypophyseal–pituitary–adrenal axis is conceivable, but not likely. In this case, a Cosyntropin stimulation test may be performed on the morning of postoperative day 1. This is done by administering 250 μg Cortrosyn IV. Cortisol measurements are obtained at 0, 30, and 60 minutes after administration. A cortisol level ≥18 μg/dL indicates sufficient function. If the hypophyseal–pituitary–adrenal axis is intact, the patient will not need supplemental steroids but will still need to be counseled about the critical symptoms and signs of adrenal insufficiency.

Hernia

Incisional hernia can be a long-term complication of any approach to the adrenal gland. Hernia must be distinguished from segmental abdominal muscle relaxation due to denervation resulting from approaches such as the posterior or thoracoabdominal incisions that require rib resection. Although incisional hernia may be related to operative choices and techniques, it also appears to be more likely to occur in patients with hypercortisolism due to poor tissue integrity at the time of port site closure.

Hypertension

Hypertension can be an indication of incomplete resection of a hormonally active tumor. Especially with hyperaldosteronism, the patient may also be left with underlying essential hypertension even after excess aldosterone secretion is addressed. An occasional cause of postoperative hypertension may be inadvertent injury to a renal artery. This injury may not have been an obvious intraoperative event if only a superior polar vessel was ligated.

Hypotension

This complication can follow resection of pheochromocytoma. Overall lability including hypotension is minimized by adequate preoperative pharmacologic preparation to decrease vasoconstriction and cardiac afterload while volume expansion occurs. Adequate intraoperative resuscitation is also critical. Decisions about ongoing postoperative invasive blood pressure monitoring can be made in the

CHAPTER

42

Complications of Thyroid and Parathyroid Surgery

Gerard Doherty

INTRODUCTION

Thyroid and parathyroid operations are generally safe procedures with rare life-threatening complications. While the complications common to any operation, such as bleeding, infection, and anesthetic reactions can occur, they are all quite unusual. Bleeding during the procedures is limited, and almost never is sufficient blood lost to require transfusion. Bleeding following the procedure can cause dangerous local effects, but still rarely requires blood replacement. The neck is a privileged site for wound healing, with a robust blood supply to the skin and soft tissue that can withstand substantial contamination without clinical infection. These procedures are typically performed as ambulatory or overnight hospitalizations, with short (1–3 hours) general, or regional, anesthetic techniques, thus limiting the risk of anesthetic or pulmonary complications, and deep venous thrombotic events.

In spite of these features, cervical endocrine surgery is considered a delicate, somewhat risky area of clinical practice. Significant technical complications can occur that can create permanent, life-altering changes to patient function. The most common of these are hypoparathyroidism and nerve injury. Other less frequent complications include cervical hematoma and aerodigestive tract damage. Finally, failure of the operative strategy to fulfill its goals, as with persistent hyperparathyroidism, can complicate overall patient care.

THYROID SURGERY

Thyroid operations are performed to manage actual or potential malignancy, thyroid hyperfunction, or thyromegaly producing local symptoms from compression of surrounding structures. The indications and strategies for these procedures are considered in their clinical contexts.

Diagnostic thyroid evaluation

The diagnostic evaluation of a thyroid nodule addresses two issues: (1) Is the nodule or the remaining thyroid hyperfunctional? and (2) Is the nodule malignant? All patients have a thorough history and physical examination, with a focus on the personal history of thyroid disease and radiation exposure, the family history of thyroid diseases, and the physical features in the neck including regional adenopathy. An ultrasound evaluation of the thyroid is a part of the physical examination and should accompany all thyroid nodule evaluations. Patients with personal history of therapeutic or accidental (but not apparently diagnostic) doses of radiation exposure (>2,500 cGy) to the thyroid have an increased risk of both thyroid nodules and thyroid cancer, with a latency of two to four decades; this information can change the diagnostic scheme and in particular leads most surgeons to remove the entire thyroid if any operative procedure is necessary (1–3). A family history of thyroid disease is very common and may include a variety of benign or malignant diagnoses within one family. Often, different family members have multinodular goiter, papillary thyroid cancer, Graves disease, or Hashimoto thyroiditis in a variety of first-degree relatives. These families seem to have a predilection to develop any one of several thyroid conditions. In addition, there are specific heritable genetic defects that can predispose to papillary (Familial Adenomatous Polyposis—*APC* gene) or medullary (Multiple Endocrine Neoplasia Type 2 syndromes—*Ret* proto-oncogene) thyroid cancers. Evidence of these abnormalities should prompt further evaluation and genetic counseling.

Thyroid ultrasound adds very useful information in the evaluation of thyroid nodules (4–6). It can accurately characterize the size, nature (solid vs. cystic), and texture (homogeneous, macro- or microcalcifications, smooth or irregular margins) of the index nodule, as well as the remainder of the thyroid gland. As the thyroid gland can be difficult to reproducibly and accurately investigate on physical examination alone, ultrasound is critical. Ultrasound can also be used to guide tissue sampling. Thyroid function tests, specifically including thyroid-stimulating hormone (TSH) and tetraiodothyronine (T4) levels, demonstrate the status of the pituitary–thyroid axis and the physiologic appropriateness of thyroid hormone production. Notably, the only clinical situation in which thyroid scintigraphy (nuclear medicine scanning) is currently useful in the diagnostic evaluation of a thyroid nodule is when the patient is

Gerard Doherty: N.W. Thompson Professor of Surgery; Vice-Chair, Department of Surgery; University of Michigan, Ann Arbor, Michigan

hyperthyroid (6–8). It allows distinction between a hyperfunctioning nodule with suppressed surrounding thyroid parenchyma and a neoplastic nodule in Graves disease.

For the most typical patient, who is euthyroid with a dominant solitary nodule, the mainstay of the diagnostic evaluation is fine-needle aspiration cytology (6–10). This procedure is done in the clinic, often under ultrasound guidance, and provides the best information to address whether the nodule is malignant. The potential results are (a) malignant, prompting specific therapy; (b) benign, prompting interval follow-up evaluation for most patients; (c) insufficient sample, prompting repeat needle aspiration cytology; and (d) indeterminate. Indeterminate aspirations imply that there is adequate cellular material for assessment, but that the diagnosis is uncertain because of the nature of the lesion. This frequently occurs with follicular lesions of the thyroid gland. In this clinical situation, the best next step is typically a diagnostic thyroid resection.

The minimum appropriate procedure for assessing the nature of a potentially malignant thyroid lesion is lobectomy and isthmusectomy (11–14). This should include some gross margin of normal thyroid gland between the line of division and the lesion in question. The complications of removing one side of the thyroid gland are similar to the complications of total thyroidectomy, with some important distinctions. First, as a single functional parathyroid gland is sufficient to maintain normal parathyroid control of calcium flux and there are parathyroid glands on each side of the larynx, it is not possible to produce permanent hypoparathyroidism by thyroid lobectomy. Second, while injury to the ipsilateral recurrent laryngeal nerve (RLN) can produce permanent voice changes, thyroid lobectomy does not carry a risk of bilateral recurrent nerve injury and consequent airway occlusion. Finally, for most patients who require only unilateral thyroidectomy, there is no need for thyroid hormone replacement therapy, thus eliminating the possibility of iatrogenic hyper- or hypothyroidism.

Therapeutic thyroidectomy

Thyroidectomy has a major role in the therapy of several thyroid processes (Table 42.1). For patients with unilateral,

Table 42.1 Therapeutic thyroidectomy indications

Thyroid lobectomy
Solitary toxic nodule
Unilateral benign adenoma or cyst producing local symptoms
Best-prognosis thyroid cancers
Total thyroidectomy
Most thyroid carcinoma
Graves disease
Hashimoto's thyroiditis
Toxic multinodular goiter
Symptomatic multinodular goiter
Substernal goiter (most)

Table 42.2 Classification of thyroid carcinoma

Cell of Origin	Tumor Type	Subtypes
Follicular cell	Papillary	Classic
		Follicular variant
		Tall cell
		Diffuse sclerosing
	Follicular	Minimally invasive
		Hürthle cell
		Insular
	Anaplastic	
C-cell	Medullary	
Lymphocyte	Lymphoma	

symptomatic lesions, thyroid lobectomy can be the therapeutic procedure of choice and carries risks similar to diagnostic lobectomy. For most patients requiring therapeutic thyroidectomy, however, the procedure involves resection of both lobes of the thyroid gland (total thyroidectomy).

Thyroid Carcinoma

Thyroid carcinoma can be categorized based upon the cell of origin and the growth pattern of the tumor (Table 42.2). The follicular cell–derived thyroid cancers are by far the most common, and the bulk of these (≥75%) are well-differentiated papillary thyroid cancers with an excellent long-term survival. A variety of prognostic scoring systems are available to categorize the probable patient outcome. One of the most used, and easiest to apply because the information is available soon after resection, is the MACIS system (Table 42.3) (15). There is a subgroup of patients that comprise the very best prognosis lesions: women <45 years of age, with tumors that measure (≤10 mm in diameter and that are confined entirely to the thyroid gland, with no thyroid capsule invasion or lymph node metastasis. All investigators agree that this group of people does not benefit from the additional dissection done for a total thyroidectomy and can be treated by thyroid lobectomy (12,16–18). For most patients, however, there is some advantage to total thyroidectomy, mainly in improved disease-free survival though there are also data to support an overall mortality advantage (18). Improved disease-free survival releases the patient from the need for additional episodes of care and the associated potential side effects, complications, and time lost. The magnitude of the advantage is more substantial for some groups than others. In general, being older, male, having a larger tumor, and having spread of disease outside of the thyroid gland, each individually correlate with having a greater risk of recurrence and/or death. These patients benefit from total thyroidectomy, and further adjuvant therapy with radioiodine and thyroid hormone suppression of TSH (6,12,16).

For anaplastic cancer and lymphoma, the role of operative intervention is mainly for diagnosis, although

facial muscle contraction due to increased nerve irritability. This sign is present in some minority of people with a normal serum level of calcium and so is not entirely reliable in the diagnosis of hypocalcemia, but can be helpful in following levels in some people. Trousseau sign is elicited by placing a sphygmomanometer cuff on the upper arm and inflating to systolic pressure. Within a few minutes, the patient develops severe carpal spasm, with flexion of the wrist and fingers and abduction of the thumb. This sign is very uncomfortable for the patient and should not be used clinically. In general, the symptoms of hypocalcemia are much more reliable and useful for patient assessment than the signs.

The acute management of hypocalcemia in the postoperative patient depends upon the severity of the hypocalcemia and symptoms. Total serum calcium levels correlate roughly with symptoms, but are quite variable between individuals. Some patients can have extremely low total serum levels of calcium with no symptoms, while others can have severe symptoms and signs, with nearly normal calcium levels. Ionized calcium measurements correlate better than total serum calcium levels, but there is still variability. Replacement is generally guided by symptoms. For mild hypocalcemia with tingling, oral calcium supplements (calcium carbonate, 500 to 1,500 mg p.o., two to four times daily) are often sufficient to resolve the hypocalcemia. Daily doses of calcium >3,000 mg provide little incremental benefit, however, because of the limits of gastrointestinal absorption of calcium. If supplementation beyond this level is necessary (as it is for most patients with severe hypocalcemia), then the addition of supplemental vitamin D (calcitriol 0.25 to 1.0 μg daily) increases the gastrointestinal absorption of calcium. Vitamin D requires 48–72 hours to have its effect, however, and so intravenous calcium supplementation may be needed until then. Anticipation of the need for vitamin D can smooth the patient management considerably by starting it early.

Hypocalcemia not controlled by oral supplements, or accompanied by severe symptoms such as muscle cramping, is best managed by intravenous calcium administration. Intravenous calcium gluconate is the only option for calcium supplementation. Calcium chloride can cause severe tissue damage if accidental tissue infiltration occurs and should never be used outside of an acute, life-threatening cardiac emergency. Bolus administration of calcium gluconate (supplied in 1,000-mg ampules containing 90 mEq calcium) corrects serum levels of calcium rapidly and safely, though the effect is short-lived. An alternative is to use a calcium gluconate solution (six ampules of calcium gluconate = 6 g calcium gluconate = 540 mEq calcium in 500 mL D5W) infused at 1 mL/kg/h. This provides a steady calcium supplement and can be adjusted to maintain the calcium in the normal range while oral supplements are absorbed.

Temporary hypocalcemia occurs in about 10% of patients after total thyroidectomy, and permanent hypocalcemia in about 1% (Table 42.5) (31–37). The temporary hypocalcemia can be severe and requires intravenous and oral supplementation for the duration of the effect. Permanent hypoparathyroidism requires lifelong support with calcium supplements and vitamin D analogs. Missing doses of the supplements will usually produce symptoms of varying severity and which, while manageable, are often quite bothersome for patients. In addition to the discomfort and inconvenience of the supplements, patients develop low-turnover bone disease, which resembles osteomalacia. Though dysmorphic, bone mass is generally preserved or increased in hypoparathyroidism, and fracture risk is not apparently increased (38). Finally, the calcium and vitamin D supplements with low PTH lead to an increased daily urinary excretion of calcium and significant risk or nephrolithiasis.

The recent availability of pharmacologic PTH for exogenous administration has opened the opportunity to replace PTH in patients with postoperative hypoparathyroidism. The experience with this to date is limited, but early results demonstrate that PTH delivered subcutaneously twice daily can maintain serum calcium levels in the same range as oral calcium and vitamin D supplements and decreases the amount of hypercalciuria (39,40). Further experience

Table 42.5 Incidence of complications after total thyroidectomy

Authors, Year	Number of Patients	Transient Nerve Paresis, *N* (%)	Permanent Nerve Paresis, *N* (%)	Transient Hypoparathyroidism, *N* (%)	Permanent Hypoparathyroidism, *N* (%)
Thompson et al., 1978 (32)	165	NR	0	NR	<2%
Farrar et al., 1980 (31)	29	NR	1 (3%)	2 (7%)	4 (14%)
Schroder et al., 1986 (33)	56	1 (2%)	0	9 (17%)	3 (6%)
Clark et al., 1988 (34)	160	4 (2.5%)	3 (2%)[a]	NR	1 (0.6%)
Ley et al., 1993 (35)	124	1 (0.8%)	1 (0.8%)	13 (10%)	2 (1.6%)
Tartaglia et al., 2003 (36)	1,636	31 (1.9%)	15 (0.9%)	NR	14 (0.9%)
Rosato et al., 2004 (37)	9,599	195 (2%)	94 (1%)	797 (8.3%)	163 (1.7%)

NR, not reported.

[a]Each from deliberate sacrifice of the recurrent laryngeal nerve due to tumor involvement.

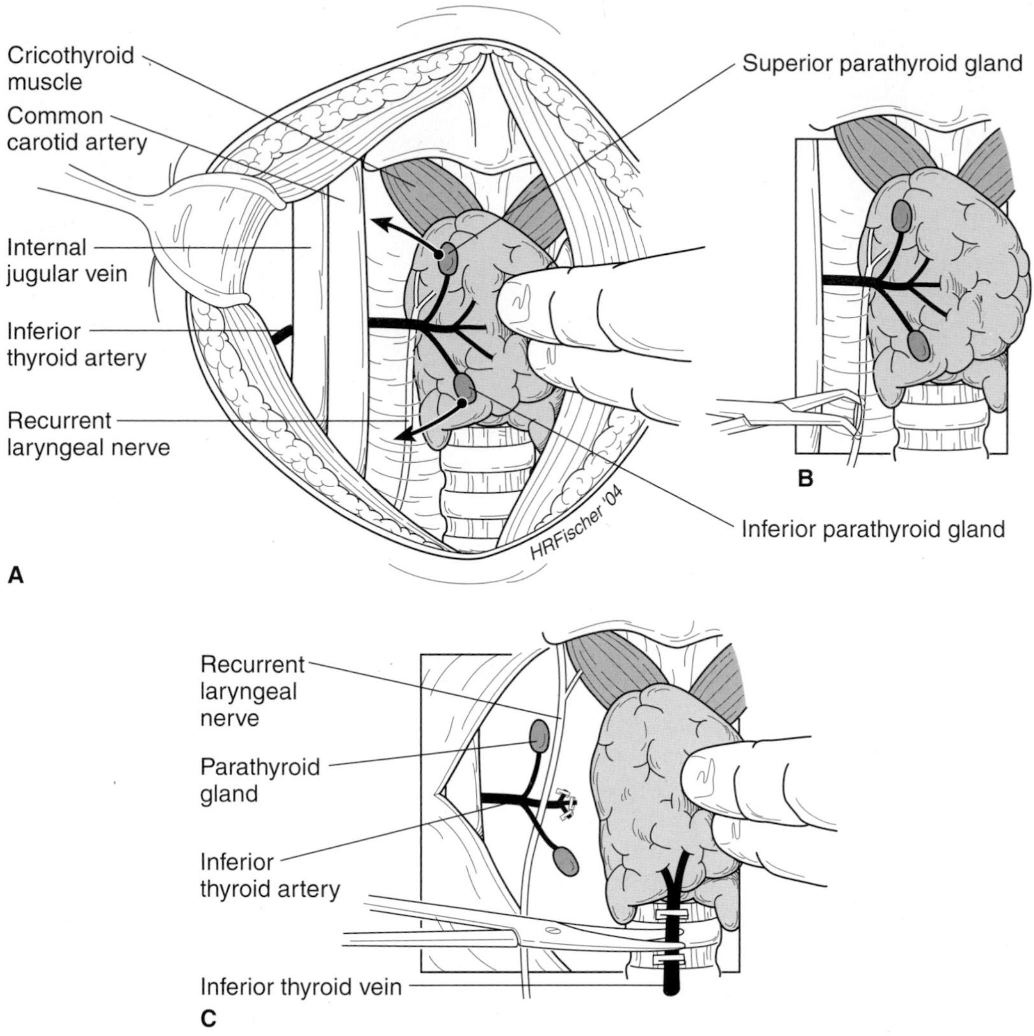

FIGURE 42.1. Relationship and dissection of the parathyroid gland blood supply and the recurrent laryngeal nerve (RLN). **A:** Once the upper pole vessels have been divided and the thyroid lobe has been reflected anteriorly, dissection of the tracheoesophageal groove exposes the blood supply to the parathyroid glands. The glands are usually entrapped under adherent soft tissue stretched across the surface of the thyroid gland. The parathyroid dissection begins along the edge away from its blood supply, and the parathyroid glands are released back toward the carotid artery (arrows). **B:** The RLN is identified below the inferior thyroid artery, at or below the level of the lower pole of the thyroid gland. The nerve is predictable in its position at this level, in the groove between the trachea and esophagus (easily identified if a stethoscope or temperature probe is in the lumen). The RLN is not tethered by any attachments at this level and so can be dissected with less danger of injury. The nerve dissection then continues superiorly to the inferior thyroid artery. The inferior thyroid artery branches can then be divided with the nerve in full view, to ensure the safety of the dissection. **C:** Once the inferior thyroid artery branches have been divided and the thyroid separated from the dense attachments to the trachea near the level of the RLN insertion under the cricopharyngeal muscle, the lower pole vessels can be divided safely.

with this strategy will be necessary before the full long-term effects are clear.

Avoidance of permanent hypoparathyroidism is far more desirable than treatment of it. This can be accomplished by preservation of the parathyroid glands on their native blood supply, or autografting of parathyroid tissue to a muscular bed (41). During thyroidectomy, the blood supply to each parathyroid gland should be identified and specifically considered during dissection. Every parathyroid gland should be treated as though it were the only remaining gland. The parathyroid glands receive their blood supply via the inferior thyroid artery (Fig. 42.1). During dissection of the thyroid, the inferior thyroid artery branches should be divided distal to the branching of the parathyroid end arteries. The parathyroid glands can then be moved posteriorly in the neck away from the thyroid, to allow safe dissection of the RLN and thyroid attachments to the trachea.

If the parathyroid glands cannot be preserved on their native blood supply, then transfer of the gland to a convenient grafting site can maintain function (25,41). For normal parathyroid glands, transfer to the sternocleidomastoid muscle provides a convenient vascular bed for transplant (Fig. 42.2). The parathyroid gland must be reduced to pieces that can survive on the diffusion of nutrients temporarily, while neovascular ingrowth occurs

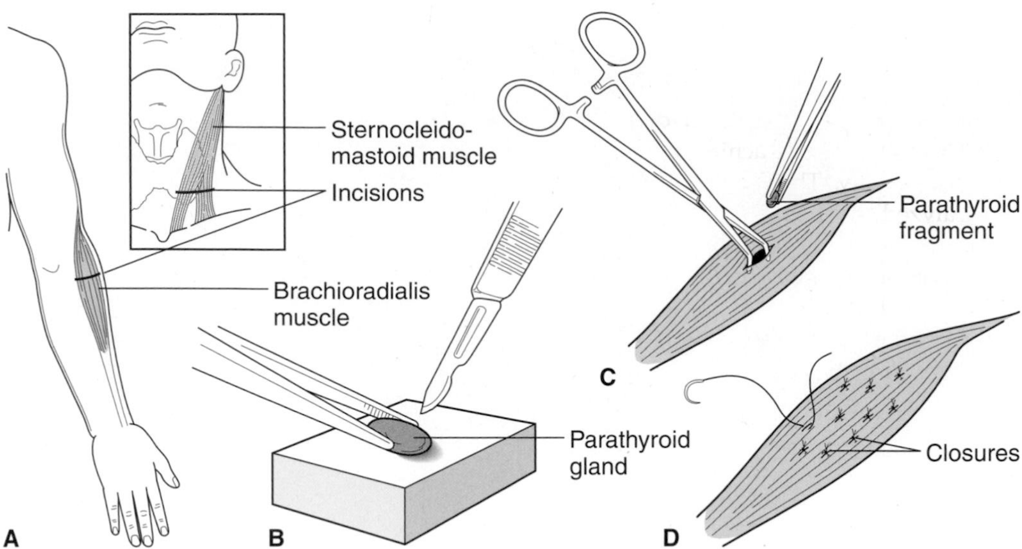

FIGURE 42.2. Parathyroid autograft: If a parathyroid gland has been devascularized during dissection, then the best management is to autograft the gland. In addition, there are certain conditions (e.g., familial parathyroid multiple gland disease or renal osteodystrophy) for which it may be advantageous to remove the parathyroid glands from the native site and autograft them elsewhere. **A:** Normal parathyroid glands can be grafted into the sternocleidomastoid muscle. As a rule, abnormal parathyroid glands should not be autografted back into the neck, but rather grafted to a distant location, such as the nondominant forearm. Transverse incisions over the brachioradialis muscle heal much better than longitudinal incisions. **B:** The parathyroid gland is sliced cleanly into pieces 1–2 mm in maximum dimension. **C:** Each piece to be grafted is placed into an individual pocket in the selected muscle. **D:** Each pocket is closed with a suture to prevent extrusion of the graft. For abnormal parathyroid glands grafted into the arm, the sites may be marked by using permanent sutures; however, for normal glands grafted in the neck, resorbable sutures are preferable.

over several weeks. This strategy is effective as is clear from operative series in which all parathyroid glands were autografted in order to try to optimize the long-term outcome of normal parathyroid function. All patients became temporarily hypoparathyroid, but all recovered to become dependent fully on their autografts. While this strategy is effective, it leads to significant short-term morbidity due to the uniform, severe hypocalcemia that occurs before graft function begins. A selective strategy of autografting only the parathyroid glands that are devascularized during dissection is equally effective and more comfortable for the majority of the patients.

Nerve injuries

There are several nerves adjacent to the thyroid gland that can be deliberately or inadvertently affected during thyroidectomy. These include the RLN immediately adjacent to the thyroid and the vagus nerve, which is slightly more removed, but causes the same symptoms when damaged. The external branch of the superior laryngeal nerve can be injured during dissection of the upper pole of the thyroid gland, and the sympathetic chain and stellate ganglion can be injured near the posterior aspect of the upper pole of the gland as well.

Recurrent Laryngeal Nerve

The RLN fibers are a part of the vagus nerve on each side, until they branch off in the upper chest, course around the ligamentum arteriosum (left RLN) or the subclavian artery (right RLN), and back along the tracheoesophageal groove on each side. They pass between the thyroid and the larynx and insert in the larynx at the inferior border of the cricopharyngeal muscle. The nerve often branches at about the level of the lower pole of the thyroid and inserts to the larynx as two or more adjacent fibers; there is also an esophageal branch that extends posteriorly from about the level of the thyroid lower pole.

Damage to the RLN causes unilateral paralysis of the muscles that control ipsilateral vocal cord tension. Unilateral RLN injury changes the voice substantially in most patients and also significantly affects the swallowing mechanism. The voice can range from a soft, whispery voice, with the inability to increase the volume at all, to a nearly normal sounding voice, which cannot be raised to a yell. The difference between these is based on the ability of the contralateral vocal cord to cross the midline and appose the affected cord. If the cords cannot meet, then the voice will be soft and breathy. If the cords can meet, then the speaking voice will be more normal in timbre, but the affected cord prolapses with increased airway pressure, and the ability to yell is lost. Swallowing is also affected, and the aspiration of liquids is a mark of severe RLN paresis. This improves with time and can be helped by swallowing training.

Bilateral RLN injury causes paralysis of both cords and usually results in a very limited airway lumen at the cords. These patients usually have a normal-sounding speaking voice, but severe limitations on inhalation velocity because of upper airway obstruction. They often require reintubation to maintain ventilation.

RLN paresis is usually temporary and resolves over days to months (Table 42.5) (31–37). There is no known method of aiding or speeding recovery. If a unilateral paresis proves to be permanent, then palliation of the cord immobility and voice changes can be achieved with vocal cord injection or laryngoplasty. These procedures stiffen and medialize the paralyzed cord, in order to allow the contralateral cord to appose the paralyzed cord during speech. If both cords are affected, then the palliative procedures are more limited and involve creating an adequate airway for ventilation; improvements in voice quality are not likely as there is no muscular control of the cord function.

Avoidance of RLN injury is far superior to palliation. Great care must be taken during the dissection of the nerve, in order to protect it. In some clinical situations, the RLN is sacrificed to allow an adequate tumor resection. Absent this unusual circumstance, though, careful dissection can generally preserve cord function. The principles of the dissection are as follows:

1. **Avoid dividing any structures in the tracheoesophageal groove until the nerve is definitively identified.** Small branches of the inferior thyroid artery may seem like they can clearly be safely transected; however, the distortion of tumor, retraction, or previous scar may lead the surgeon to mistakenly divide a branch of the RLN. The identifying feature of the RLN is that the more it is dissected, the more it looks like the correct structure. This is based upon the morphologic appearance and the anatomic course. The nerve can tolerate manipulation, but not cutting. Once cut, repair of the nerve is of unproven benefit.
2. **Identify the nerve low in the neck, well below the inferior thyroid artery, at the level of the lower pole of the thyroid gland, or below** (Fig. 42.1). This allows dissection of the nerve at a site where it is not tethered by its attachments to the larynx or its relation to the inferior thyroid artery. Traction injuries to the nerve can occur when the nerve is manipulated near a site of fixation.
3. **Keep the nerve in view during the subsequent dissection of the thyroid away from the larynx.** Once the nerve is identified, the dissection can generally proceed from inferior to superior along the nerve, dividing the inferior thyroid artery branches and preserving the parathyroid glands. This allows careful dissection of the tissues with minimal manipulation of the RLN.
4. **Minimize the use of powered dissection posterior to the thyroid.** Although the electrocautery and high-frequency ultrasonic scalpel are useful tools in dissection, they have some risk of lateral thermal spread, which can damage adjacent tissues. Careful cold dissection and hemostasis with ligatures or clips will avoid this risk. This is particularly important at the entry of the RLN to the larynx, immediately adjacent to the ligament of Berry and its vessels.

The use of nerve stimulators and laryngeal muscle potential monitors has recently been investigated as a tool to try to limit or avoid nerve injuries (42,43). The data do not currently support the mandatory use of these devices, as the risk of nerve injury is related to several factors (44–46). However, many experienced surgeons now routinely use a nerve-monitoring system intraoperatively. This may be because they merely help to identify the nerve, while the portion of the operation most likely to produce damage in experienced hands is the dissection of the RLN at the fixed point of the cricopharyngeus.

About 10% of patients have some evidence of RLN paresis after thyroidectomy; however, this resolves in most patients. About 1% or fewer patients have permanent nerve injury when total thyroidectomy is performed by experienced surgeons (Table 42.5).

External Branch of the Superior Laryngeal Nerve

This nerve courses adjacent to the superior pole vessels of the thyroid gland before separating to penetrate the cricopharyngeus muscle fascia at its superoposterior aspect (Fig. 42.3). The nerve supplies motor innervation of the inferior constrictor muscles of the larynx. Damage to this nerve changes the ability of the larynx to control high-pressure phonation, such as high-pitched singing (soprano/falsetto) or yelling (37,47).

To avoid damaging this nerve, the dissection of the upper pole vessels should proceed from a space where the nerve is safely sequestered under the cricopharyngeal fascia to the superior vessels themselves, thus safely separating the nerve from the tissue to be divided (Fig. 42.3).

Sympathetic chain

Although it is separated from the posterior aspect of the thyroid, the sympathetic chain and stellate ganglion can be damaged during thyroidectomy, producing a Horner's syndrome (ipsilateral ptosis, miosis, and anhidrosis). This is probably due to retractor-induced injury, as the sympathetic chain and ganglion itself are out of the operative field. These injuries are nearly always temporary.

Airway management

As the thyroid lies directly anterior to the trachea, enlargement of the thyroid or direct invasion of the trachea by tumor can cause airway compromise that can become critical during the induction of anesthesia (48–51). Compression of the trachea can cause loss of airway patency in the supine patient under anesthesia. Once the negative intrathoracic pressure needed to lift the thyroid and keep the trachea patent is lost, it may be difficult or impossible to ventilate the patient with positive pressure. This can be avoided by awake intubation, to maintain airway patency.

Compression of the trachea in the neck can narrow the lumen substantially and require placement of a smaller endotracheal tube at intubation. However, the more difficult management issue can be significant lateral deviation of the trachea. Although these patients can usually be ventilated by positive pressure mask ventilation, the shift of

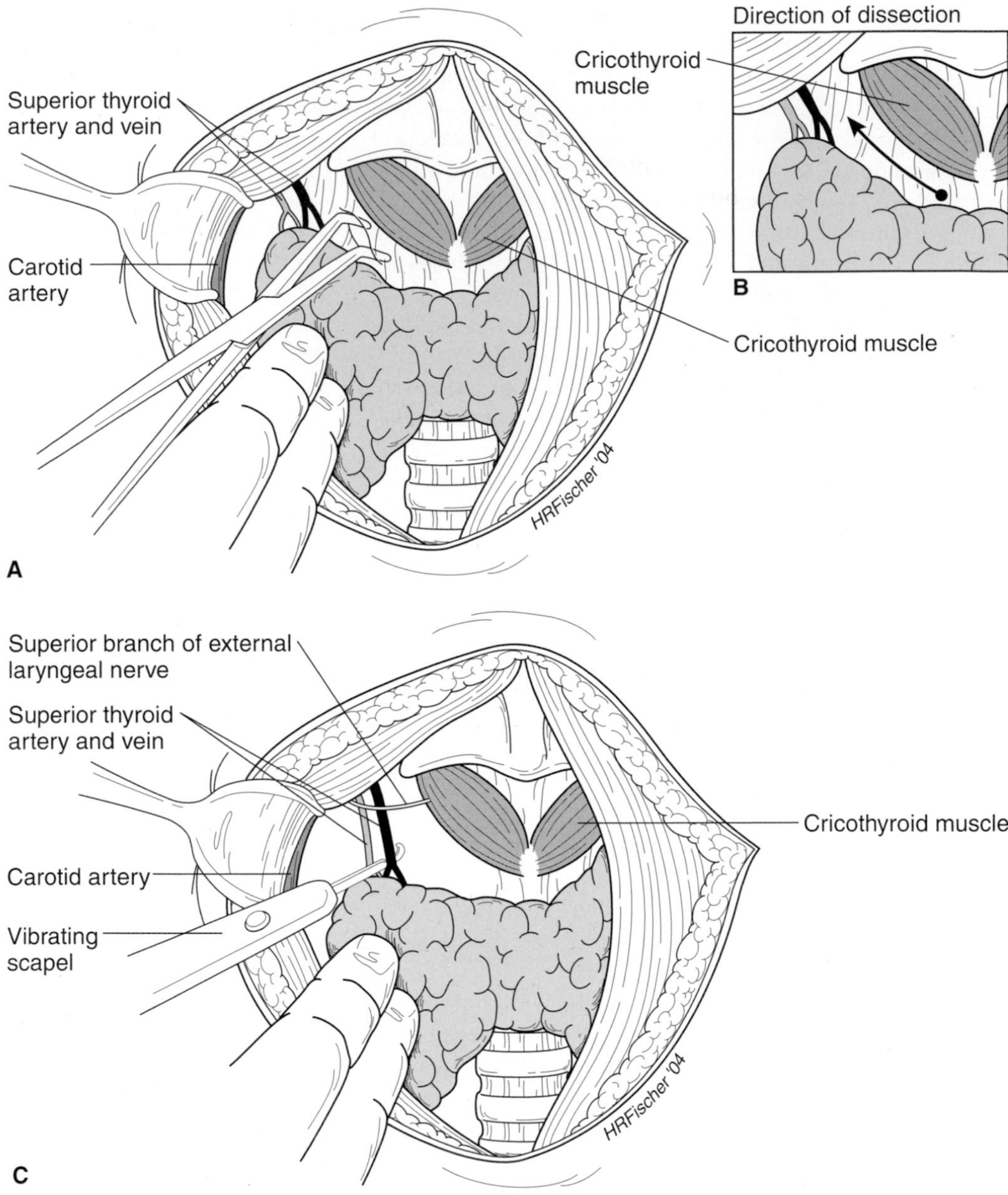

FIGURE 42.3. Protection of the external branch of the superior laryngeal nerve. **A:** After separation of the lateral border of the thyroid gland from the carotid sheath to expose the lateral portion of the upper pole vessels, the medial aspect of the upper pole is exposed by bluntly entering the avascular space between the thyroid gland and the cricothyroid muscle. This space is safe if dissected directly posteriorly to the anterior surface of the spine. **B:** The dissection is then carried superolaterally between the surfaces of the thyroid gland and the cricothyroid muscle (arrow). **C:** This maneuver clears the medial aspect of the superior thyroid vessels, and traction on the thyroid gland inferiorly separates the external branch of the superior laryngeal nerve from these vessels. The vessels can then be safely divided using any technique, including the high-frequency ultrasonic dissector (depicted).

the larynx can make it difficult or impossible to access the vocal cords for placement of an endotracheal tube. Intubation over a fiberoptic laryngobronchoscope can be helpful in most patients. However, there are patients who cannot be intubated in spite of all attempts, who require tracheostomy at the outset of the thyroidectomy, in order to safely perform the operation. Anticipation of the difficulties that may be faced, the assembly of a team expert in airway management, and the readiness of an experienced surgeon prepared to access the airway operatively is critical to the safe outcome of these occasionally extremely challenging and dangerous situations.

Injury to other cervical structures

There are a variety of other structures in the neck that are vulnerable to injury during operation, particularly if there are large tumors that extend out of the usual confines of the thyroid gland. The thoracic duct empties into the left internal jugular vein, posterior to the clavicular insertion of the sternocleidomastoid muscle. Damage to the thoracic duct can cause a large collection of lymph or chyle in the operative bed. This can heal spontaneously after drainage if the leak is small; however, frequently, the leak continues in spite of attempts to allow healing by decreasing output (NPO, total parenteral nutrition, and octreotide injections). If the leak persists for >3 weeks, then the thoracic duct can be divided in the left hemithorax using thoracoscopic techniques. This will nearly always allow the leak to heal.

Tracheal injuries can occur, particularly during removal of large invasive tumors. Most tracheal injuries can be repaired primarily with resorbable suture. For defects >10 mm, it may be preferable to patch the trachea with a pedicle of the sternocleidomastoid muscle, or to perform a sleeve resection of the affected area. If resected, the cut ends of the trachea are reapproximated with absorbable suture. A drain should be placed to evacuate any air that escapes through the repair. This is less of an issue if the patient is extubated at the completion of the operation, avoiding the effects of positive pressure ventilation on the repair. A tracheostomy is rarely necessary, although if there are other issues concerning airway safety, then placement of a temporary tracheostomy may be preferable to prolonged intubation.

Esophageal injuries rarely occur during thyroidectomy. If the esophageal lumen is entered, then the operative options include primary repair or closure of the distal lumen and construction of a cervical esophagostomy. Primary repair is generally preferable, unless there is extensive tissue loss or damage.

Iatrogenic hyperthyroidism or hypothyroidism

After total thyroidectomy, and as a part of the therapy for most thyroid carcinoma, patients receive thyroid hormone replacement therapy (12). As a chronic medication, thyroid hormone is among the most well-tolerated. It has a long half-life, which makes daily dosing adequate and which means that patients do not develop symptoms if they miss or change the timing of doses. The problems with thyroid hormone administration, however, are as follows: (a) its long half-life allows adjustment of dosage only once per month or so, making the titration of the proper dose a slow process; (b) its narrow therapeutic window means that small changes in dosing or medication preparation can change the physiologic effect; and (c) it is largely protein-bound, and so other protein-bound drugs or changes in the proteins themselves can change the effects of a given dose of the drug. Once patients understand that the process of titration can take time, they are usually accepting. Trying to speed the process by making more frequent changes often delays the identification of the appropriate dose by overcorrecting the dose.

The narrow therapeutic window of thyroid hormone efficacy is another aspect that patients should understand. In particular, the effect of changing thyroid hormone preparations, from one brand to another, or to generic preparations, may change the patient's response to the drug. Patients should be encouraged to be consistent about the preparation that they use or, if a change is unavoidable, to recheck their TSH levels a month after a change, to document the effect. This has been well-documented in the medical and lay literature, and most pharmacists are also sensitive to this issue (52–60).

A more frequent problem is the addition or subtraction of some other chronic medication, such as oral contraceptive pills or estrogen replacement therapy that changes the serum protein binding of the thyroid hormone dose. Patients should be informed of this potential effect and the need to redocument and adjust thyroid hormone dosing after these changes in other medications.

PARATHYROID SURGERY

Parathyroidectomy is performed frequently for primary hyperparathyroidism and less frequently for secondary or tertiary hyperparathyroidism. The indications for intervention vary with the clinical situation. Although some recent changes in operative strategy have made the operation simpler for many patients, this procedure can still be difficult and surgeons undertaking it must be skilled at recognizing the pathology and correcting it, while avoiding the complications of persistent hyperparathyroidism and hypoparathyroidism.

Indications for operation in patients with primary hyperparathyroidism

Patients with primary hyperparathyroidism can be separated into symptomatic and asymptomatic groups (61). Barring other life-limiting illness, all patients with symptomatic hyperparathyroidism should have operative correction of the disease. The symptoms that can occur include fractures, particularly vertebral compression fractures, renal stones, severe neuromuscular weakness, easy fatigability and loss of stamina, sleep disturbance, depression, memory loss, and pancreatitis. All these issues improve with correction of hyperparathyroidism. The hypertension that occurs more frequently in the hyperparathyroid population probably stops worsening with correction of the disease, but does not reliably improve.

Patients with asymptomatic disease can present more complex decision-making (61–63). Management guidelines for patients with asymptomatic hyperparathyroidism from the National Institutes of Health recognize risk factors for long duration of disease (age), rate of calcium loss (serum calcium and urine calcium), and end-organ effects (serum creatinine and bone density) (Table 42.6). The patient's risk for the operation and concurrent illnesses must be considered to determine whether the patient is likely to gain benefit from the procedure. These guidelines were designed in an NIH Consensus Conference in 1991 and then revisited and revised in an NIH-sponsored meeting in 2002 (61,63) and have been since revisited again (62). The most significant change was from *Z* score for bone density that was used in 1991 to *T* score in 2002. *Z* score compares patient bone density to age, gender, and race-matched controls, whereas *T* score compares patient bone density to ideal bone mass. *T* score correlates better with fracture risk and so is more appropriate in judging the patient's personal risk.

Once the decision to operate is clear, then the best strategy for resolution of the hyperparathyroidism can be considered, including decisions regarding preoperative imaging. Imaging should not be used to determine the diagnosis of hyperparathyroidism, nor the decision for operation.

4% of patients after operation in experienced hands. Proper performance of the neck exploration and use of the intraoperative PTH assay should minimize the occurrence of this problem (70,71).

To maximize the therapeutic value and minimize the operative risks of parathyroidectomy, the most important factor is thorough and precise dissection technique. The operation, whether performed as a focused exploration beginning at one site or performed as a full parathyroid exploration, must proceed in an organized way. The parathyroid glands are exposed by dissecting the superficial structures of the neck (from the strap muscles out) away from the underlying structures that derive their blood supply from the laryngeal system (Fig. 42.4). Thus, all the tissues attached to the larynx remain attached at the end of the mobilization so that the parathyroid glands and their blood supply are not separated and dropped into an "acquired ectopic" position. Once the tissues have been mobilized, then the normal sites for parathyroid glands can be easily explored. Most missed parathyroid adenomas that cause persistent hyperparathyroidism are in normal anatomic sites and were missed at initial operation.

If no parathyroid gland is identified in a corresponding normal site, then knowledge of the ectopic sites where parathyroid glands can be guides further exploration (Fig. 42.5). While ectopic parathyroid adenomas

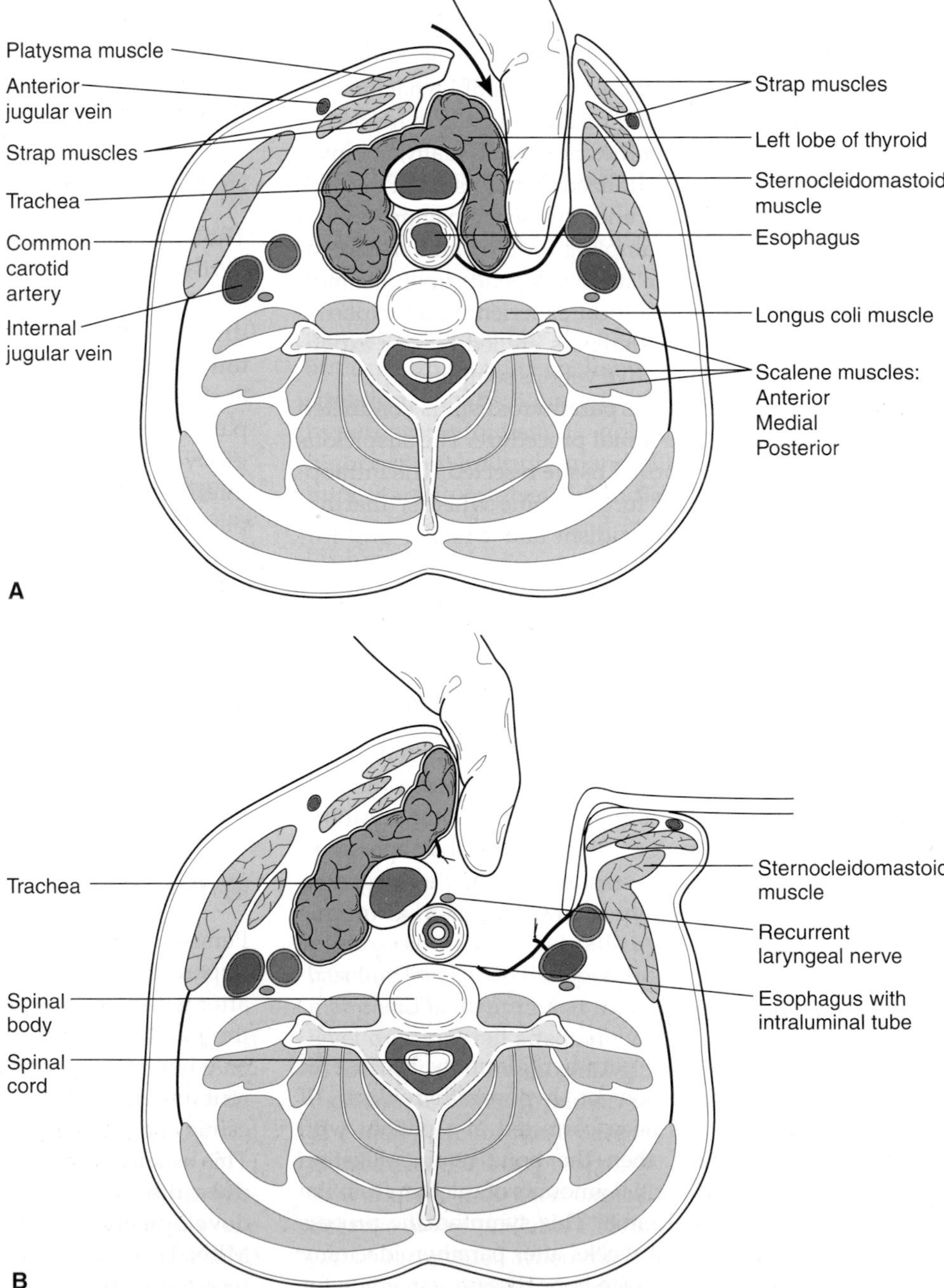

FIGURE 42.4. Exposure and identification of the parathyroid glands in their normal anatomic positions. **A:** After making subplatysmal flaps and separating the strap muscles in the midline, the elevation of the strap muscle proceeds immediately along the strap muscles and the carotid sheath directly posteriorly to the longus coli muscle. Only after the anterior surface of the longus coli muscle has been exposed medial to the carotid sheath along the length of the thyroid gland, is the dissection turned medially. This plane leaves all of the tissues likely to contain the parathyroid glands attached to the larynx. **B:** The thyroid gland is rolled anteriorly, rotating the larynx and upper trachea to bring the tracheoesophageal tissues into view. The middle thyroid vein, if it is placed on tension by this maneuver, is divided.

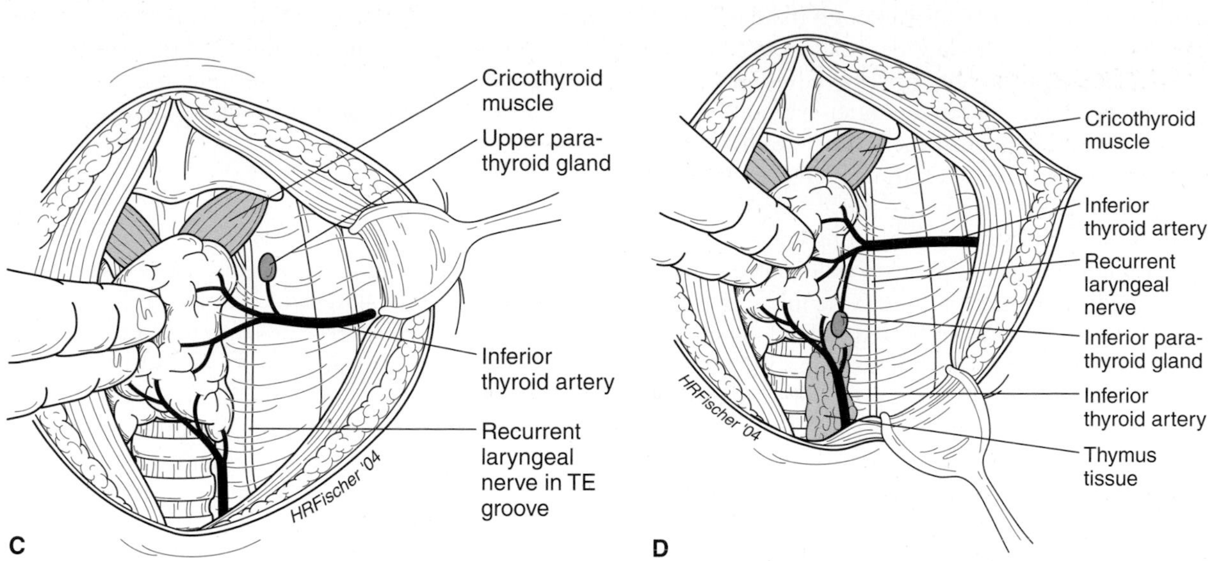

FIGURE 42.4. (*Continued*) **C:** The upper parathyroid gland is most often identified immediately adjacent to the thyroid gland, posterior to the recurrent laryngeal nerve (RLN), and superior to the inferior thyroid artery. However, when enlarged, the gland often grows inferiorly, with the bulk lying deep to, and extending inferior to, the inferior thyroid artery, still posterior to the RLN. The blood supply remains from the upper branches of the inferior thyroid artery, however, and can be identified in the normal position. **D:** The lower pole of the thyroid gland is retracted superiorly to identify the lower parathyroid gland. This is most often immediately adjacent to the thyroid gland, though it can "slide down" within the sheath of the thymus and often resides there. To uncover the parathyroid in this area, the sheath overlying the thymus is opened, but the attachments to the thyroid gland are not divided as they provide important traction superiorly.

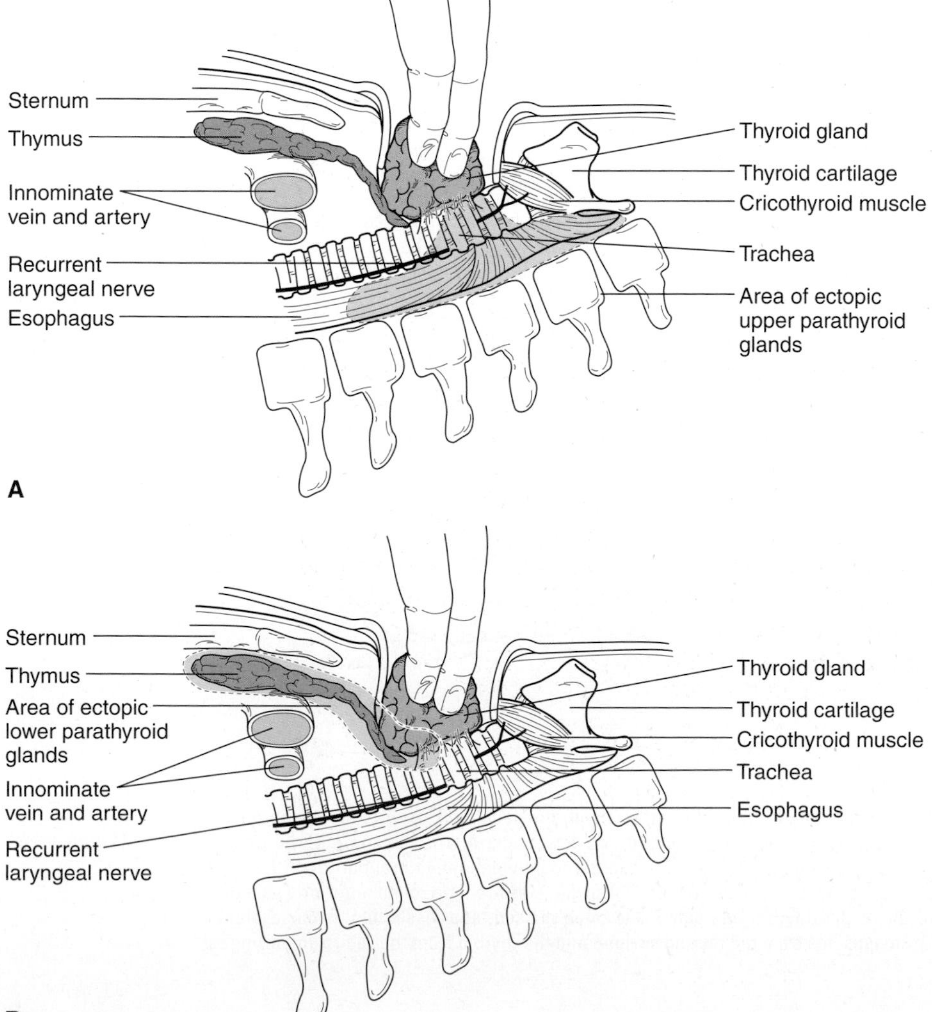

FIGURE 42.5. Identification of the parathyroid glands in ectopic sites. **A:** The upper parathyroid glands usually remain close to the thyroid, however, if the gland is not present there, then it is most likely posterior to the recurrent laryngeal nerve along the esophagus or pharynx (shaded area). **B:** The lower parathyroid gland is usually near the lower pole of the thyroid gland; however, it can slide down into the anterior mediastinum within the thymus (shaded area). More rarely, the lower parathyroid gland can be in the upper neck along the carotid artery, often with a bit of residual thymus attached there as well.

are unusual, they occur frequently enough that no surgeon should undertake this operation without complete familiarity with this anatomy. If no abnormal parathyroid tissue is found after full neck exploration and after exploration of all cervically accessible ectopic sites, then most parathyroid surgeons would close the wound, terminate the operation, and re-evaluate the patient postoperatively. This should include reconfirmation of the diagnosis and imaging to try to identify the abnormal gland. Most surgeons would not perform a trans-sternal mediastinal exploration at the initial operation without localizing studies that indicated a gland there.

Operative strategy at reoperation should include consideration of alternative anatomic approaches that might avoid operating through previous scar. The most common alternative approach is most useful for a posteriorly placed (usually upper) parathyroid adenoma (Fig. 42.6). This lateral approach takes the operation through fresh tissue lateral to the strap muscles, along the anterior border of the sternocleidomastoid muscle, and only then to the previously operated area medial to the carotid sheath. This sheath is quite durable and tolerates dissection easily, even in reoperation. In addition, this area posteriorly has often been left undissected, thus leaving the posteriorly placed gland unidentified at the initial attempt. This avoids the tedious and sometimes bloody dissection of the strap muscles from the anterior surface of the thyroid gland.

SUMMARY

In conclusion, operations for diseases of the thyroid and parathyroid glands are quite common. Most of the complications of these procedures are technical in nature, and the risk in these procedures can be minimized by proper understanding of the indications for operation, the anatomy and pathology of the area, and the proper dissection approach. The management of the complications depends upon the severity and temporal nature of the complication. For many temporary issues, reassurance alone and explanation of the natural history of the recovery is all that is necessary. The permanent, life-altering nature of some of the complications makes it mandatory, as with all invasive procedures, that the indications for the intervention be very clear.

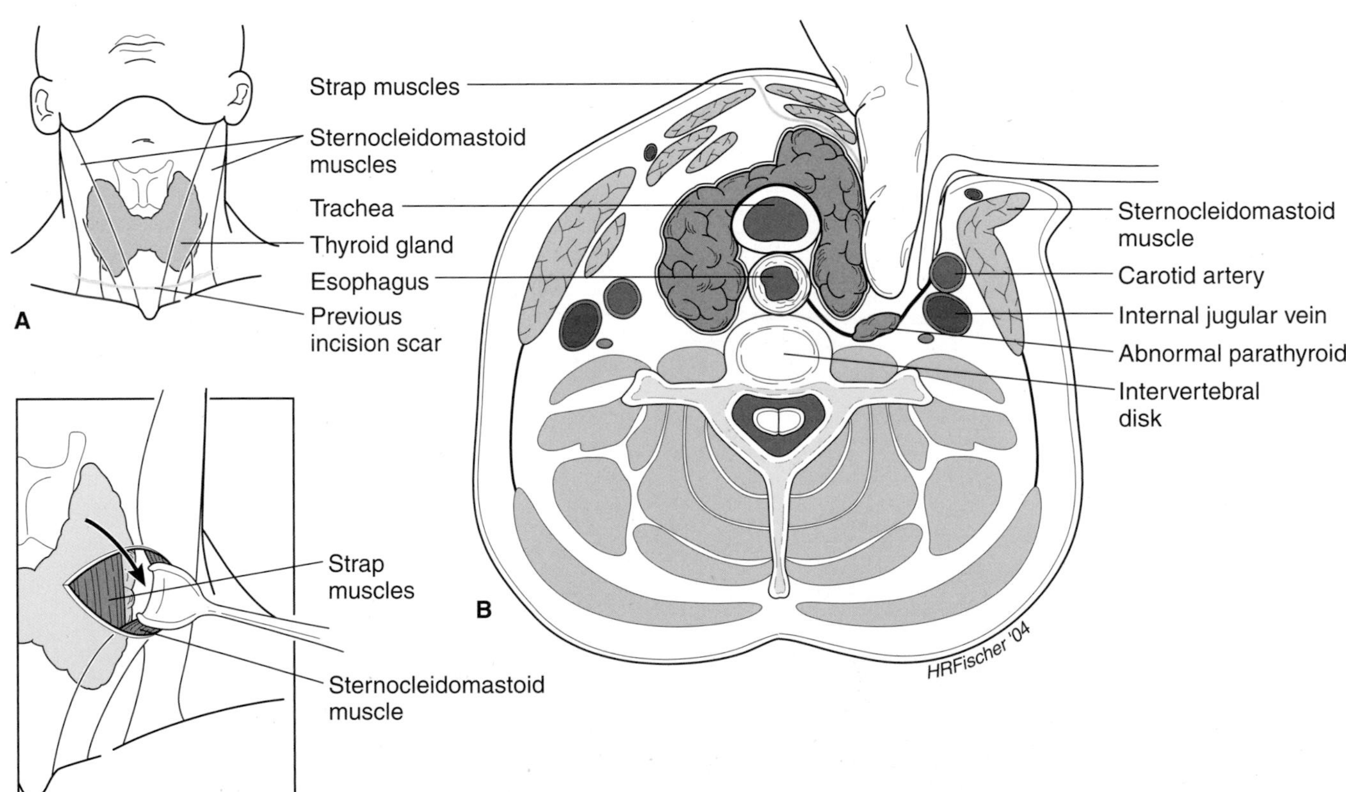

FIGURE 42.6. The lateral approach to the tracheoesophageal groove. For patients with previous neck explorations, who have a posteriorly placed parathyroid gland, a lateral approach can avoid some treacherous dissection. **A:** The neck is entered usually through the old incision, or a new more laterally placed incision. **B:** A fresh plane is entered between the lateral border of the strap muscles and the medial border of the sternocleidomastoid muscle. The thyroid and strap muscles are then rolled anteriorly as a unit, exposing the esophagus. This is the area where upper parathyroid adenomas are often missed, and dissection in these planes avoids the area of the previous dissection of the strap muscles from the thyroid surface and the thyroid from the recurrent laryngeal nerve.

REFERENCES

1. Schneider AB, Ron E, Lubin J, et al. Dose–response relationships for radiation-induced thyroid cancer and thyroid nodules: evidence for the prolonged effects of radiation on the thyroid. *J Clin Endocrinol Metab* 1993;77:362–369.
2. Antonelli A, Silvano G, Bianchi F, et al. Risk of thyroid nodules in subjects occupationally exposed to radiation: a cross sectional study. *Occup Environ Med* 1995;52:500–504.
3. Williams D. Radiation carcinogenesis: lessons from Chernobyl. *Oncogene* 2008;27(Suppl 2):S9–S18.
4. Kouvaraki MA, Shapiro SE, Fornage BD, et al. Role of preoperative ultrasonography in the surgical management of patients with thyroid cancer. *Surgery* 2003;134:946–954; discussion 954–945.
5. Ito M, Yamashita S, Ashizawa K, et al. Childhood thyroid disease around Chernobyl evaluated ultrasound examination and fine needle aspiration cytology. *Thyroid* 1995;5:365–368.
6. Cooper DS, Doherty GM, Haugen BR, et al. Revised American Thyroid Association management guidelines for patients with thyroid nodules and differentiated thyroid cancer [see comment]. *Thyroid* 2009;19: 1167–1214.
7. Jones AJ, Aitman TJ, Edmonds CJ, et al. Comparison of fine needle aspiration cytology, radioisotopic and ultrasound scanning in the management of thyroid nodules. *Postgrad Med J* 1990;66:914–917.
8. Belfiore A, La Rosa GL, La Porta GA, et al. Cancer risk in patients with cold thyroid nodules: relevance of iodine intake, sex, age, and multinodularity. *Am J Med* 1992;93:363–369.
9. Layfield LJ, Mohrmann RL, Kopald KH, et al. Use of aspiration cytology and frozen section examination for management of benign and malignant thyroid nodules. *Cancer* 1991;68:130–134.
10. Gharib H. Fine-needle aspiration biopsy of thyroid nodules: advantages, limitations, and effect. *Mayo Clin Proc* 1994;69:44–49.
11. Udelsman R, Westra WH, Donovan PI, et al. Randomized prospective evaluation of frozen-section analysis for follicular neoplasms of the thyroid. *Ann Surg* 2001;233:716–722.
12. Mazzaferri EL. An overview of the management of papillary and follicular thyroid carcinoma. *Thyroid* 1999;9:421–427.
13. Hay ID, Grant CS, Bergstralh EJ, et al. Unilateral total lobectomy: is it sufficient surgical treatment for patients with AMES low-risk papillary thyroid carcinoma? *Surgery* 1998;124:958–964; discussion 964–956.
14. Chen H, Nicol TL, Zeiger MA, et al. Hurthle cell neoplasms of the thyroid: are there factors predictive of malignancy? *Ann Surg* 1998;227: 542–546.
15. Hay ID, Bergstralh EJ, Goellner JR, et al. Predicting outcome in papillary thyroid carcinoma: development of a reliable prognostic scoring system in a cohort of 1779 patients surgically treated at one institution during 1940 through 1989. *Surgery* 1993;114:1050–1057; discussion 1057–1058.
16. Hay ID, Thompson GB, Grant CS, et al. Papillary thyroid carcinoma managed at the Mayo Clinic during six decades (1940–1999): temporal trends in initial therapy and long-term outcome in 2444 consecutively treated patients. *World J Surg* 2002;26:879–885.
17. Yim JH, Doherty GM. Papillary thyroid cancer. *Curr Treat Options Oncol* 2000;1:329–338.
18. Bilimoria KY, Bentrem DJ, Ko CY, et al. Extent of surgery affects survival for papillary thyroid cancer [see comment]. *Ann Surg* 2007;246: 375–381; discussion 381–374.
19. McIver B, Hay ID, Giuffrida DF, et al. Anaplastic thyroid carcinoma: a 50-year experience at a single institution. *Surgery* 2001;130:1028–1034.
20. Sweeney PJ, Haraf DJ, Recant W, et al. Anaplastic carcinoma of the thyroid. *Ann Oncol* 1996;7:739–744.
21. Kobayashi T, Asakawa H, Umeshita K, et al. Treatment of 37 patients with anaplastic carcinoma of the thyroid. *Head Neck* 1996;18:36–41.
22. Shimizu K, Kumita S, Kitamura Y, et al. Trial of autotransplantation of cryopreserved thyroid tissue for postoperative hypothyroidism in patients with Graves' disease [see comment]. *J Am Coll Surg* 2002;194: 14–22.
23. Thomusch O, Machens A, Sekulla C, et al. Multivariate analysis of risk factors for postoperative complications in benign goiter surgery: prospective multicenter study in Germany. *World J Surg* 2000;24:1335–1341.
24. Cobin RH. Thyroid carcinoma and Graves' disease. *Endocr Pract* 2000; 6:264–267.
25. Thomusch O, Machens A, Sekulla C, et al. The impact of surgical technique on postoperative hypoparathyroidism in bilateral thyroid surgery: a multivariate analysis of 5846 consecutive patients. *Surgery* 2003; 133:180–185.
26. Burkey SH, van Heerden JA, Thompson GB, et al. Reexploration for symptomatic hematomas after cervical exploration. *Surgery* 2001;130: 914–920.
27. Adler JT, Sippel RS, Schaefer S, et al. Preserving function and quality of life after thyroid and parathyroid surgery. *Lancet Oncol* 2008;9:1069–1075.
28. Leyre P, Desurmont T, Lacoste L, et al. Does the risk of compressive hematoma after thyroidectomy authorize 1-day surgery? *Langenbecks Arch Surg* 2008;393:733–737.
29. Rosenbaum MA, Haridas M, McHenry CR. Life-threatening neck hematoma complicating thyroid and parathyroid surgery. *Am J Surg* 2008;195:339–343; discussion 343.
30. Harding J, Sebag F, Sierra M, et al. Thyroid surgery: postoperative hematoma—prevention and treatment. *Langenbecks Arch Surg* 2006;391: 169–173.
31. Farrar WB, Cooperman M, James AG. Surgical management of papillary and follicular carcinoma of the thyroid. *Ann Surg* 1980;192:701–704.
32. Thompson NW, Nishiyama RH, Harness JK. Thyroid carcinoma: current controversies. *Curr Probl Surg* 1978;15:1–67.
33. Schroder DM, Chambous A, France CJ. Operative strategy for thyroid cancer, is total thyroidectomy worth the price? *Cancer* 1986;58:2320.
34. Clark OH, Levin K, Zeng QH, et al. Thyroid cancer: the case for total thyroidectomy. *Eur J Cancer Clin Oncol* 1988;24:305–313.
35. Ley PB, Roberts JW, Symmonds RE Jr, et al. Safety and efficacy of total thyroidectomy for differentiated thyroid carcinoma: a 20-year review. *Am Surg* 1993;59:110–114.
36. Tartaglia F, Sgueglia M, Muhaya A, et al. Complications in total thyroidectomy: our experience and a number of considerations. *Chir Ital* 2003;55:499–510.
37. Rosato L, Avenia N, Bernante P, et al. Complications of thyroid surgery: analysis of a multicentric study on 14,934 patients operated on in Italy over 5 years. *World J Surg* 2004;28:271–276.
38. Rubin MR, Dempster DW, Zhou H, et al. Dynamic and structural properties of the skeleton in hypoparathyroidism. *J Bone Miner Res* 2008;23: 2018–2024.
39. Winer KK, Ko CW, Reynolds JC, et al. Long-term treatment of hypoparathyroidism: a randomized controlled study comparing parathyroid hormone-(1–34) versus calcitriol and calcium. *J Clin Endocrinol Metab* 2003;88:4214–4220.
40. Winer KK, Sinaii N, Peterson D, et al. Effects of once versus twice-daily parathyroid hormone 1–34 therapy in children with hypoparathyroidism. *J Clin Endocrinol Metab* 2008;93:3389–3395.
41. Olson JA Jr, DeBenedetti MK, Baumann DS, et al. Parathyroid autotransplantation during thyroidectomy. Results of long-term follow-up [see comment]. *Ann Surg* 1996;223:472–478; discussion 478–480.
42. Rea JL, Khan A. Clinical evoked electromyography for recurrent laryngeal nerve preservation: use of an endotracheal tube electrode and a postcricoid surface electrode. *Laryngoscope* 1998;108:1418–1420.
43. Otto RA, Cochran CS. Sensitivity and specificity of intraoperative recurrent laryngeal nerve stimulation in predicting postoperative nerve paralysis. *Ann Otol Rhinol Laryngol* 2002;111:1005–1007.
44. Dralle H, Sekulla C, Lorenz K, et al. Intraoperative monitoring of the recurrent laryngeal nerve in thyroid surgery. *World J Surg* 2008;32: 1358–1366.
45. Dralle H, Sekulla C, Haerting J, et al. Risk factors of paralysis and functional outcome after recurrent laryngeal nerve monitoring in thyroid surgery. *Surgery* 2004;136:1310–1322.
46. Thomusch O, Sekulla C, Machens A, et al. Validity of intra-operative neuromonitoring signals in thyroid surgery. *Langenbecks Arch Surg* 2004;389:499–503.
47. Stojadinovic A, Shaha AR, Orlikoff RF, et al. Prospective functional voice assessment in patients undergoing thyroid surgery. *Ann Surg* 2002;236:823–832 [see comment].
48. Kitamura Y, Shimizu K, Nagahama M, et al. Immediate causes of death in thyroid carcinoma: clinicopathological analysis of 161 fatal cases. *J Clin Endocrinol Metab* 1999;84:4043–4049.
49. Rudow M, Hill AB, Thompson NW, et al. Helium–oxygen mixtures in airway obstruction due to thyroid carcinoma. *Can Anaesth Soc J* 1986;33: 498–501.
50. Allo MD, Thompson NW. Rationale for the operative management of substernal goiters. *Surgery* 1983;94:969–977.
51. Sippel RS, Gauger PG, Angelos P, et al. Palliative thyroidectomy for malignant lymphoma of the thyroid. *Ann Surg Oncol* 2002;9:907–911.
52. Mikosch P, Obermayer-Pietsch B, Jost R, et al. Bone metabolism in patients with differentiated thyroid carcinoma receiving suppressive levothyroxine treatment. *Thyroid* 2003;13:347–356.

Table 43.3 Complication rates related to type of resection of pancreatic endocrine tumors

		All Complications			Pancreatic/Biliary Fistula			
Author(s) (Year)	***n***	**E (%)**	**DP (%)**	**PD (%)**	**E (%)**	**DP (%)**	**PD (%)**	**Other (%)**
Lairmore et al. (2000) (1)	21	80	27.3	100	0	9.1	40	
Guo et al. (2004) (46)	41	33	9.1	20	33	9	10	
Fernández-Cruz et al. (2008) (9)	49	42.8	22		38	8.7		
Nikfarjam et al. (2008) (10)	61				23.8	12.5	20.0	16.7
You et al. (2009) (11)	90	4	11	44				
Luo et al. (2009) (12)	29				22.2	0		
Average		40.0	17.4	54.7	23.4	7.9	23.3	16.7

E, enucleation; DP, distal pancreatectomy; PD, pancreaticoduodenectomy; Other, other pancreatic resections.

As a group, patients with endocrine pancreatic tumors have significant anatomic and physiologic differences compared to patients with pancreatic adenocarcinoma. Patients with pancreatic NETs occurring in the setting of one of the hereditary endocrine neoplasia syndromes (MEN 1 and von Hippel-Lindau) are often diagnosed early as a result of prospective screening. Sporadic pancreatic NETs are relatively rare entities that are frequently diagnosed in young patients. These patients are more likely to have soft pancreatic tissue without fibrosis or calcification and nondilated pancreatic and biliary ducts. Soft pancreatic parenchyma and a small pancreatic duct (<3 mm) increase the overall incidence of pancreatic fistula (21,42–44) but do not increase the incidence of clinically significant (grades B and C) fistulae (21). Importantly, these patients are also more likely to have fewer medical comorbidities and greater physiologic reserve to overcome potential surgical complications. These clinical features significantly affect operative decision-making, technical concerns, and postoperative outcome. It is interesting to note that the overall rate of postoperative pancreatic fistula rate in studies of patients undergoing pancreaticoduodenectomy for malignant disease is similar or even lower than fistula rates in patients with NETs undergoing a variety of, often less-invasive, pancreatic procedures (enucleation, distal pancreatectomy, and pancreaticoduodenectomy) with or without construction of a pancreatic–enteric anastomosis (1,2,23–29,45,46). As mentioned earlier, patients with pancreatic NETs are likely to be younger, with fewer medical comorbidities, nondilated pancreatic/biliary ducts, and normal, soft, nonfibrosed pancreatic parenchyma. In addition to these characteristics, NETs are more likely to be treated by enucleation than more formal resections, resulting in the slightly higher fistula rates associated with enucleation (Table 43.3). Although fistula rates are higher for enucleation, most resolve spontaneously with little morbidity (19). Therefore, even though only a subset of patients with NETs requires major pancreatic resection or construction of a pancreatic–enteric anastomosis to adequately excise the tumor, perhaps the slightly higher overall fistula rates are due to the combination of enucleation on a soft, normal pancreas. Patients undergoing major pancreatic resection or enucleation of pancreaticoduodenal NETs develop the expected postoperative complications, including pancreatic or biliary fistulas, peripancreatic abscess, wound complications, bleeding, and cardiopulmonary complications, at rates ranging from 17% to 67% (9–19,30,31) (Table 43.2). However, as a group, these patients are more likely to have the attributes of younger age, fewer associated medical conditions, and greater physiologic reserve to overcome these complications. Nonoperative management of pancreas-associated complications is nearly always successful in these patients, and overall outcomes are excellent.

Intra-abdominal abscess/peripancreatic fluid collection

Approximately 80% of patients with pancreatic fistula following pancreatic resections heal with nonoperative management (23,32). Nonoperative management may include bowel rest, total parenteral nutrition, pharmacologic intervention (octreotide, H_2-receptor antagonists, etc.) where indicated, local wound and skin care, infection control, and continued closed-suction external drainage until the fistula output decreases to a minimal volume. Approximately 10% to 30% of patients may require image-guided placement of percutaneous drainage catheters, to remove undrained or loculated peripancreatic fluid collections (32). Approximately 5% to 13% of patients develop severe sequelae, including sepsis, bleeding, or development of a pancreatic abscess, that require operative intervention (32).

Pancreatic ductal disruption and anastomotic failure result in leakage of pancreatic exocrine secretions, including pancreatic proteases and lipase, that result in severe inflammatory changes, fistula formation, and tissue necrosis surrounding the pancreas. The result may be a loculated peripancreatic fluid collection or, with the addition of bacterial superinfection, intra-abdominal abscess, or sepsis. The treatment of intra-abdominal abscess requires appropriate intravenous antibiotics, in combination with adequate percutaneous or operative drainage.

The development of a postoperative intra-abdominal abscess following pancreatic resection is associated with increased mortality and is clearly associated with the occurrence of a leak from the pancreatic or biliary anastomosis. Following pancreaticoduodenectomy for malignant disease, approximately 50% of intra-abdominal abscesses are associated with leakage from the pancreatic anastomosis (23). Less frequently, abscess formation results from anastomotic failure of the hepaticojejunostomy or the gastrojejunostomy. Peripancreatic fluid collections may also occur after enucleation and may develop as an area of loculated fluid that does not communicate effectively with the surgically placed closed-suction drain. Small fluid collections are commonly seen on computed tomography (CT) scans following pancreatic surgery, and most are clinically insignificant in the absence of systemic signs of toxicity or sepsis.

In series of patients undergoing a variety of procedures for resection of neuroendocrine pancreatic or duodenal tumors (1,2,9,10,15,30,45,46), the incidence of intra-abdominal abscess formation is approximately 2% to 14% and is related to, but somewhat less frequent than, the occurrence of pancreatic or biliary fistula due to anastomotic failure (Table 43.2).

Metabolic disorders

Operative procedures involving the pancreas carry the potential for adverse sequelae relating to exocrine or endocrine pancreatic function. Postoperative pancreatic function is determined by the extent of organ resection, the underlying disease process, and any preexisting abnormalities of endocrine and exocrine function (47). Few scientific studies available in the literature specifically address preoperative risk factors, the relative risk related to the extent of pancreatic resection, and a rigorous review of surgical outcomes.

In general physiologic terms, the pancreas has digestive functions (exocrine secretion in the postprandial state), endocrine function centered on glucose homeostasis and tight regulatory control of insulin secretion and counterregulatory hormones, and the interdigestive phase of pancreatic secretion. Both the digestive and interdigestive phases of exocrine and endocrine pancreatic function are affected by major pancreatic resection and are related to the extent of resection as well as the presence of underlying deficiencies.

Exocrine or endocrine pancreatic insufficiency occurs following operative intervention for either chronic pancreatitis or excision of pancreatic malignancies. Varying degrees of pancreatic dysfunction exist in patients with chronic pancreatitis prior to any surgical intervention. Resection of pancreatic tumors may be required in patients with either normal or altered preoperative pancreatic function. Postoperative deficits in exocrine or endocrine secretion are due to a combination of preexisting disease and sequelae that are procedure-related. The specific type of surgical procedure and the magnitude of pancreatic resection have a direct relationship to postoperative impairment of exocrine or endocrine function. The degree of impairment is related to both the extent of pancreatic parenchyma resected and the functional state of the residual pancreas. Enucleations or limited pancreatic resections would be predicted to carry minimal risk for disturbance of digestive or endocrine pancreatic function, although related procedures that affect gastric or biliary secretion may also cause dysfunction due to alterations in the intricate balance of the hormonal and electrolyte physiology of the upper gastrointestinal tract. For instance, the addition of partial gastrectomy to a pancreatic resection results in further impairment in the release of gastrin, pancreatic polypeptide, and cholecystokinin, with resultant effects on overall exocrine digestive function.

The influence of different surgical procedures on pancreatic exocrine function has been investigated in a few clinical studies. In patients undergoing a pylorus-preserving pancreaticoduodenectomy, results following pancreaticojejunostomy versus pancreaticogastrostomy were compared by Jang et al. (48). A significant deterioration of pancreatic exocrine function was seen in patients who were treated with pancreaticogastrostomy compared to patients undergoing pancreaticojejunostomy. The proposed mechanism was early deactivation of pancreatic enzymes by gastric acid. Tran et al. (49) demonstrated that the extent of postoperative exocrine pancreatic insufficiency strongly correlated with preoperative fibrosis. In patients requiring oral supplementation with pancreatic exocrine enzymes following pancreatic surgery, treatment with proton-pump inhibitors is indicated to avoid enzyme degradation by gastric acid.

Disturbances of endocrine secretion may also occur following operative procedures on the pancreas. Diabetes mellitus may occur after resection of >60% to 75% of the pancreatic parenchyma, especially in patients with preexisting impairment of glucose homeostasis. The most challenging sequela of major pancreatic resection is recurrent hypoglycemia, which may result from increased postoperative insulin sensitivity due to concomitant decrease in glucagon secretion (47).

General complications

General postoperative complications occur following operation for endocrine pancreatic tumors with a frequency that is expected for similar open, upper-abdominal procedures for either malignant or benign processes. Not surprisingly, these general operative risks are related to the patient's overall health and the existence of associated medical conditions. Because these general surgical risks are not unique to either the decision-making or specific techniques employed for resection of endocrine pancreatic neoplasms, these risks will be acknowledged but not discussed in detail.

Bleeding may occur with either an early or a late time course following pancreatic surgery. Early bleeding may be associated with technical failure of the suture ligation of a small venous or arterial vessel, technical failure of any of several tissue coagulation methods currently used to divide surrounding soft tissues containing an intricate vascular supply, or bleeding related to construction of a surgical anastomosis. Anastomotic bleeding may be manifested as hematobilia, intraluminal gastrointestinal bleeding, or intra-abdominal bleeding. Late bleeding (after postoperative day 5) is more likely to result from complications relating to the development of a pancreatic fistula, such as rupture of an arterial pseudoaneurysm, or erosion of a large vessel. Alternatively, late gastrointestinal bleeding may be associated with marginal ulceration following construction of a gastrojejunostomy. It is reasonable to assume that the risk of postoperative bleeding relating directly to a technical failure should be associated with the magnitude of the required dissection and the need to secure multiple small vessels, the need to perform a major regional pancreatic resection with division of the pancreatic parenchyma, or the requirement for the construction of multiple surgical anastomoses. Because resection of pancreaticoduodenal NETs may frequently be successfully performed without major pancreatic resection, the risk of major postoperative bleeding would be expected to be low. Indeed, in the collected series of 775 patients undergoing resection of NETs reported in Table 43.2, the incidence of significant bleeding requiring transfusion was only 3.9%.

Delayed gastric emptying is a very frequent cause of morbidity following pancreaticoduodenectomy for adenocarcinoma of the pancreas, occurring in up to one-third of patients (23,50). Park et al. (50) demonstrated two independent factors for delayed gastric emptying: clinically relevant pancreatic fistulae (grade B/C) and benign pathology. Delayed gastric emptying may be defined as the need for gastric decompression for >10 days postoperatively. Patients undergoing resection of endocrine pancreatic tumors develop delayed gastric emptying with reduced frequency (approximately 6.4%) (Table 43.2). Most patients present with persistent nausea, abdominal fullness, early satiety, or the need for nasogastric tube reinsertion in the first week postoperatively. Poor gastric emptying may occur following any pancreatic procedure, but is frequently seen when a gastrojejunostomy has been constructed. Inadequate gastric emptying is multifactorial and may occur even when a water-soluble contrast study demonstrates a patent gastrojejunostomy, with or without associated anastomotic edema. Adequate treatment usually involves continued gastric decompression, judicious use of prokinetic agents, enteral or parenteral feeding as indicated, and patience until oral feeding can be reinitiated.

Other complications, including wound infections, DVT, and significant cardiac or pulmonary events, may also occur following endocrine pancreatic surgery. Wound infections following operation for pancreatic endocrine tumors occur with rates similar to other patients undergoing upper-abdominal operation with or without division of the gastrointestinal tract. Coexistent disorders, including morbid obesity, diabetes, collagen vascular disease, and immunosuppression secondary to underlying medical conditions or steroid use, increase the risk of wound infection. Superficial or deep wound infection occurred in an average of 8.5% of 775 patients undergoing resection of pancreatic endocrine tumors in the collected series summarized in Table 43.2. Wound infection rates ranged from approximately 1% to 24%, with the highest rates in studies involving more complex resections (pancreaticoduodenectomy) (2). The incidence of DVT was not consistently addressed in the available series of patients undergoing resection of pancreatic endocrine neoplasms; however, these patients appear to be at lower risk than patients with adenocarcinoma of the pancreas. Finally, the frequency of cardiopulmonary or other major complications in the collected series of patients with endocrine pancreatic tumors averaged 10%, with an average mortality of 0.9% (Table 43.2). In the reviewed series of 775 patients there were four deaths, three following pancreaticoduodenectomy and one due to pulmonary embolism. All four cases were also associated with severe preoperative medical limitations.

SUMMARY

NETs of the pancreas are infrequent neoplasms that may occur sporadically or in association with one of several hereditary endocrine neoplasia syndromes. Many patients with NETs, especially in the familial setting, are diagnosed at a young age in the absence of significant medical comorbidities. Furthermore, neuroendocrine pancreatic tumors are more likely to occur in association with soft, nonfibrotic pancreatic parenchyma and without associated dilation of the pancreatic or biliary ducts compared to patients with adenocarcinoma. The unique features of familial endocrine pancreatic tumors, such as those occurring in the MEN 1 syndrome, include multifocal involvement within a target tissue and the development of tumors in multiple target organs. As a general rule, many pancreatic NETs pursue a relatively indolent course, although a subset may metastasize and result in significant morbidity and mortality. Surgical decision-making in these patients should be based on the unique features of these uncommon neoplasms, the expected natural history, and the most significant operative risks. The most important of these are the risks of postoperative pancreatic fistula formation and the development of peripancreatic abscess and subsequent sepsis. The ideal surgical treatment of pancreatic NETs relieves the patient of significant risk of malignant progression while preserving pancreatic endocrine and exocrine function and minimizing morbidity from either surgery or the underlying disease process.

REFERENCES

1. Lairmore TC, Chen VY, DeBenedetti MK, et al. Duodenopancreatic resections in patients with multiple endocrine neoplasia type 1. *Ann Surg* 2000;231:909–918.
2. Phan GQ, Yeo CJ, Cameron JL, et al. Pancreaticoduodenectomy for selected periampullary neuroendocrine tumors: fifty patients. *Surgery* 1997;122:989–997.

3. Ekeblad S, Skogseid B, Dunder K, et al. Prognostic factors and survival in 324 patients with pancreatic endocrine tumor treated at a single institution. *Clin Cancer Res* 2008;14(23):7798–7803.
4. Moley JF, Lairmore TC, Phay J. Hereditary endocrinopathies. *Curr Probl Surg* 1999;36:653–764.
5. Knudson AG Jr, Hethcote HW, Brown BW. Mutation and childhood cancer: a probabilistic model for the incidence of retinoblastoma. *Proc Natl Acad Sci USA* 1975;72:5116–5120.
6. Lairmore TC, Piersall LD, DeBenedetti MK, et al. Clinical genetic testing and early surgical intervention in patients with multiple endocrine neoplasia type 1 (MEN 1). *Ann Surg* 2004;239:637–647.
7. Akerstrom G, Hessman O, Skogseid B. Timing and extent of surgery in symptomatic and asymptomatic neuroendocrine tumors of the pancreas in MEN 1. *Langenbecks Arch Surg* 2002;386(8):558–569.
8. Dralle H, Krohn SL, Karges W, et al. Surgery of resectable nonfunctioning neuroendocrine pancreatic tumors. *World J Surg* 2004;28(12):1248–1260.
9. Fernández-Cruz L, Blanco L, Cosa R, et al. Is laparoscopic resection adequate in patients with neuroendocrine pancreatic tumors? *World J Surg* 2008;32:904–917.
10. Nikfarjam M, Warshaw AL, Axelrod L, et al. Improved contemporary surgical management of insulinomas: a 25-year experience at the Massachusetts General Hospital. *Ann Surg* 2008;247(1):165–172.
11. You DD, Lee HG, Paik KY, et al. The outcomes after surgical resection in pancreatic endocrine tumors: an institutional experience. *Eur J Surg Oncol* 2009;35:728–733.
12. Luo Y, Liu R, Hu M, et al. Laparoscopic surgery for pancreatic insulinomas: a single-institution experience of 29 cases. *J Gastrointest Surg* 2009;13:945–950.
13. Liu H, Peng C, Zhang S, et al. Strategy for the surgical management of insulinomas: analysis of 52 cases. *Dig Surg* 2007;24:463–470.
14. Gumbs A, Grès P, Madureira F, et al. Laparoscopic vs open resection of pancreatic endocrine neoplasm's: single institution's experience over 14 years. *Langenbecks Arch Surg* 2008;393:391–395.
15. Roland CL, Lo C, Miller BS, et al. Surgical approach and perioperative complications determine short-term outcomes in patients with insulinoma: results of a bi-institutional study. *Ann Surg Oncol* 2008;15(12): 3532–3537.
16. España-Gómez MN, Velázquez-Fernández D, Bezaury P, et al. Pancreatic insulinoma: a surgical experience. *World J Surg* 2009;33:1966–1970.
17. Arbuckle JD, Kekis PB, Lim A, et al. Laparoscopic management of insulinomas. *Br J Surg* 2009;96:185–190.
18. Toniato A, Meduri F, Foletto M, et al. Laparoscopic treatment of benign insulinomas localized in the body and tail of the pancreas: a single-center experience. *World J Surg* 2006;20:1916–1919.
19. Sweet MP, Izumisato Y, Way LW, et al. Laparoscopic enucleation of insulinomas. *Arch Surg* 2007;142(12):1202–1204.
20. Bassi C, Dervenis C, Butturini G, et al. Postoperative pancreatic fistula: an international study group (ISGPF) definition. *Surgery* 2005;138(1): 8–13.
21. Kawai M, Tani M, Hirono S, et al. How do we predict the clinically relevant pancreatic fistula after pancreaticoduodenectomy?—an analysis in 244 consecutive patients. *World J Surg* 2009;33(12):2670–2678.
22. Ferrone CR, Warshaw AL, Rattner DW, et al. Pancreatic fistula rates after 462 distal pancreatectomies: staplers do not decrease fistula rates. *J Gastrointest Surg* 2008;12(10):1691–1697.
23. Yeo CJ. Management of complications following pancreaticoduodenectomy. *Surg Clin North Am* 1995;75(5):913–924.
24. Braasch JW, Gray BN. Considerations that lower pancreatoduodenectomy mortality. *Am J Surg* 1977;133(4):480–484.
25. Edis AJ, Kiernan PD, Taylor WF. Attempted curative resection of ductal carcinoma of the pancreas: review of Mayo Clinic experience, 1951–1975. *Mayo Clin Proc* 1980;55(9):531–536.
26. Grace PA, Pitt HA, Tompkins RK, et al. Decreased morbidity and mortality after pancreatoduodenectomy. *Am J Surg* 1986;151(1):141–149.
27. Trede M, Schwall G. The complications of pancreatectomy. *Ann Surg* 1988;207(1):39–47.
28. Cameron JL, Pitt HA, Yeo CJ, et al. One hundred and forty-five consecutive pancreaticoduodenectomies without mortality. *Ann Surg* 1993; 217(5):430–435; discussion 435–438.
29. Cullen JJ, Sarr MG, Ilstrup DM. Pancreatic anastomotic leak after pancreaticoduodenectomy: incidence, significance, and management. *Am J Surg* 1994;168(4):295–298.
30. Vagefi PA, Razo O, Deshpande V, et al. Evolving patterns in the detection and outcomes of pancreatic neuroendocrine neoplasms. *Arch Surg* 2007;142:347–354.
31. Liu H, Zhang S, Wu Y, et al. Diagnosis and surgical treatment of pancreatic endocrine tumors in 36 patients: a single-center report. *Chin Med J* 2007;120(17):1487–1490.
32. Munoz-Bongrand N, Sauvanet A, Denys A, et al. Conservative management of pancreatic fistula after pancreaticoduodenectomy with pancreaticogastrostomy. *J Am Coll Surg* 2004;199:198–203.
33. Shrikhande SV, D'Souza MA. Pancreatic fistula after pancreatectomy: evolving definitions, preventive strategies and modern management. *World J Gastroenterol* 2008;14(38):5789–5796.
34. Winter JM, Cameron JL, Campbell KA, et al. Does pancreatic duct stenting decrease the rate of pancreatic fistula following pancreaticoduodenectomy? Results of a prospective randomized trial. *J Gastrointest Surg* 2006;10(9):1280–1290.
35. Lillemoe KD, Cameron JL, Kim MP, et al. Does fibrin glue sealant decrease the rate of pancreatic fistula after pancreaticoduodenectomy? Results of a prospective randomized trial. *J Gastrointest Surg* 2004;8(7): 766–772.
36. Suc B, Mskia S, Fingerhut A, et al. Temporary fibrin glue occlusion of the main pancreatic duct in the prevention of intra-abdominal complications after pancreatic resection: prospective randomized trial. *Ann Surg* 2003;237(1):57–65.
37. Schulick RD, Yoshimura K. Stents, glue, etc.: is anything proven to help prevent pancreatic leaks/fistulae? *J Gastrointest Surg* 2009;13:1184–1186.
38. Fisher WE, Chai C, Hodges SE, et al. Effect of BioGlue® on the incidence of pancreatic fistula following pancreas resection. *J Gastrointest Surg* 2008;12:882–890.
39. Kollmar O, Moussavian MR, Richter S, et al. Prophylactic octreotide and delayed gastric emptying after pancreaticoduodenectomy: results of a prospective randomized double-blinded placebo-controlled trial. *Eur J Surg Oncol* 2008;34:868–875.
40. Ramos-De la Medina A, Sarr MG. Somatostatin analogues in the prevention of pancreas-related complications after pancreatic resection. *J Hepatobiliary Pancreat Surg* 2006;13:190–193.
41. Zeng Q, Zhang Q, Han S, et al. Efficacy of somatostatin and its analogues in prevention of postoperative complications after pancreaticoduodenectomy: a meta-analysis of randomized controlled trials. *Pancreas* 2008;36(1):18–25.
42. Yang YM, Tian XD, Zhuang Y, et al. Risk factors of pancreatic leakage after pancreaticoduodenectomy. *World J Gastroenterol* 2005;11(16):2456–2461.
43. DeOliveira ML, Winter JM, Schafer M, et al. Assessment of complications after pancreatic surgery: a novel grading system applied to 633 patients undergoing pancreaticoduodenectomy. *Ann Surg* 2006;244(6):931–939.
44. Butturini G, Daskalaki D, Molinari E, et al. Pancreatic fistula: definition and current problems. *J Hepatobiliary Pancreat Surg* 2008;15:247–251.
45. Park BJ, Alexander HR, Libutti SK, et al. Operative management of islet-cell tumors arising in the head of the pancreas. *Surgery* 1998;124(6): 1056–1061; discussion 1061–1062.
46. Guo KJ, Liao HH, Tian YL, et al. Surgical treatment of nonfunctioning islet cell tumor: report of 41 cases. *Hepatobiliary Pancreat Dis Int* 2004; 3(3):469–472.
47. Kahl S, Malfertheiner P. Exocrine and endocrine pancreatic insufficiency after pancreatic surgery. *Best Pract Res Clin Gastroenterol* 2004; 18(5):947–955.
48. Jang JY, Kim SW, Park SJ, et al. Comparison of the functional outcome after pylorus-preserving pancreaticoduodenectomy: pancreaticogastrostomy and pancreaticojejunostomy. *World J Surg* 2002;26:366–371.
49. Tran TC, van't Hof G, Kazemeir G, et al. Pancreatic fibrosis correlates with exocrine pancreatic insufficiency after pancreaticoduodenectomy. *Dig Surg* 2008;25(4):311–318.
50. Park JS, Hwang HK, Kim JK, et al. Clinical validation and risk factors for delayed gastric emptying based on the International Study Group of Pancreatic Surgery (ISGPS) Classification. *Surgery* 2009;146(5): 882–887.

CHAPTER

44

Complications in Breast Surgery

Alicia Growney, Ahmad Azari, and Lisa A. Newman

INTRODUCTION

The breast is a relatively clean organ, comprised of skin, fatty tissue, and mammary glandular elements that have no direct connection to any major body cavity or visceral structures. In the absence of concurrent major reconstruction being performed, breast surgery is generally not accompanied by large-scale fluid shifts, infectious complications, or hemorrhage. Thus, the breast is largely perceived as being associated with relatively low risk for surgical morbidity. The breast is, however, the site of the most common cancer afflicting American women, and a myriad of complications can occur in association with the procedures designed to detect and treat breast cancer. Some of these complications are related to the breast itself, and others are associated with axillary staging procedures. This chapter will address some general nonspecific complications first (wound infections, seroma formation, and hematoma), followed by discussions of complications that are specific to particular breast-related procedures: lumpectomy (including both diagnostic open biopsy and breast conservation therapy for cancer); mastectomy; axillary lymph node dissection (ALND); lymphatic mapping/sentinel lymph node biopsy; and reconstruction. Finally, a few conditions requiring special surgical considerations such as immediate breast reconstruction (IBR) and neoadjuvant chemotherapy will be presented.

General wound complications related to breast and axillary surgery

As a peripheral soft-tissue organ, many wound complications related to breast procedures are relatively minor and frequently managed on an outpatient basis. It is therefore difficult to establish accurate incidence rates for these events. As discussed below however, reported studies document that surgical morbidity from breast and/or axillary wound infections, seromas, and hematomas occur in up to 30% of cases. Very few of these require a prolongation of hospital stay or a readmission for inpatient care. A fourth complication, chronic incisional pain, can also occur in conjunction with various surgical breast procedures.

Rare complications can also occur in conjunction with various breast procedures and will not be discussed in depth. For example, pneumothorax can be related either to inadvertent pleural puncture during wire localization or to inadvertently deep dissection within an intercostal space. Also, patients can develop brachial plexopathy related to stretch injury from positioning in the operating room (1). The American Society of Anesthesiology recommends upper extremity positioning such that maximal abduction at the shoulder is 90 degrees, with neutral forearm position, and use of padded armboards (2).

Mondor's disease, or thrombosis of the thoracoepigastric vein, can occur spontaneously, or following any breast procedure such as lumpectomy or even percutaneous needle biopsy (3–7). While Mondor's disease is not an established breast cancer risk factor, there are case reports of patients who have presented with this condition at the time of their breast cancer diagnosis (4). This condition typically presents as a palpable, sometimes tender cord running vertically from the mid-lower hemisphere of the breast toward the abdominal wall. It is usually a self-limited condition, and resolution can be expedited by soft-tissue massage.

Wound Infections

Rates of postoperative infections in breast and axillary incisions have ranged from <1% of cases and to nearly 20%, as shown in Table 44.1 (8–21). In 2007, El-Tamer et al. (22) reported a study based upon the National Surgical Quality Improvement Program Patient Safety in Surgery. They prospectively collected inpatient and outpatient 30-day postoperative morbidity and mortality data on patients undergoing surgery (mastectomy or lumpectomy with an axillary procedure) at 14 university and 4 community centers. In a 30-day follow-up of 3,107 patients, the most frequent morbid complication found was wound infection, which more commonly occurs in the mastectomy (4.34%) group versus the lumpectomy group (1.97%). A meta-analysis by Platt et al. (23), in 1993, analyzed data on 2,587 surgical breast procedures and found an overall wound infection rate of 3.8% of cases. Staphylococcal organisms are usually implicated in these infections (8,17), introduced via skin flora. Obesity, older age, smoking, diabetes mellitus, malignancy, and amount of tissue removal have been some of the most consistently identified risk factors for breast wound sepsis. Several investigators (11,14,21) have

Alicia Growney, Ahmad Azari, Lisa A. Newman: University of Michigan, Ann Arbor, MI 48109.

Table 44.1 Selected studies evaluating wound infection rates following breast surgery

Study	No. of Cases	Type of Procedures Analyzed	Type of Study	Wound Infection Rate	Study Findings/Risk Factors for Infection
Platt et al., 1990 (8)	606	Lumpectomy Mastectomy ALND Reduction mammoplasty	Phase 3 study of preoperative antibiotics	9.4%	Preoperative antibiotic coverage reduced wound infection rate (6.6% vs. 12.2%)
Hoefer et al., 1990 (9)	101	Mastectomy	Retrospective review	8.9%	*Risk factor:* • Cautery
Wagman et al., 1990 (10)	118	Mastectomy	Phase 3 study of preoperative antibiotics	6.8%	Preoperative antibiotics had no effect on wound infection rates (5% vs. 8%)
Chen et al., 1991 (11)		Mastectomy Lumpectomy	Retrospective review	2.6%–11.1%	*Risk factors:* • Older age; • Surgery performed in 1970s versus 1980s; • Prior open diagnostic biopsy versus single-stage surgery
Vinton et al., 1991 (12)	560	Mastectomy Lumpectomy ALND	Retrospective review	15% (mastectomy) 13% (lumpectomy)	*Risk factors:* • Older age; • Mastectomy versus lumpectomy; • Tobacco smoking; • Obesity
Platt et al., 1992 (13)	1,981	Mastectomy Lumpectomy ALND Reduction mammoplasty	Retrospective review	3.4%	Preoperative antibiotic coverage reduced wound infection rate (OR 0.59; 95% confidence interval 0.35–0.99)
Lipshy et al., 1996 (14)	289	Mastectomy	Retrospective review	5.3%	*Risk factor:* Prior open diagnostic biopsy versus diagnostic needle biopsy (6.9% vs. 1.6%) Preoperative antibiotic coverage reduced wound infection rate
Bertin et al., 1998 (15)	18 Cases 37 Controls	Mastectomy Lumpectomy	Case–control	NA	*Risk factors:* • Obesity; • Older age
Thomas et al., 1999 (16)	1,766	Mastectomy Lumpectomy ALND	Phase 3 study of preoperative antibiotics	0.6%	Short-acting versus long-acting preoperative cephalosporin (0.91% vs. 0.45%)
Gupta et al., 2000 (17)	334	Mastectomy Lumpectomy ALND	Phase 3 study of preoperative antibiotics	18.3%	Preoperative antibiotics had no effect on wound infection rates (17.7% vs. 18.8%)
Nieto et al., 2002 (18)	107	Mastectomy Lumpectomy ALND	Prospective observational study	7% (mastectomy) 17% (lumpectomy)	*Risk factors:* • Lumpectomy versus mastectomy; • Older age; • Obesity
Sorensen et al., 2002 (19)	425	Mastectomy Lumpectomy ALND	Retrospective review	10.5%	*Risk factors:* • Tobacco smoking; • Diabetes mellitus; • Obesity; • Heavy ethanol consumption

(*continued*)

Table **44.1** **Selected studies evaluating wound infection rates following breast surgery (*Continued*)**

Study	No. of Cases	Type of Procedures Analyzed	Type of Study	Wound Infection Rate	Study Findings/Risk Factors for Infection
Witt et al., 2003 (20)	326	Mastectomy Lumpectomy ALND	Prospective observational study	15.3%	*Risk factors:* • Older age; • Obesity; • Diabetes mellitus; • Prior diagnostic core-needle biopsy versus open diagnostic biopsy • Preoperative antibiotic coverage reduced wound infection rate
Tran et al., 2003 (21)	320	Mastectomy Lumpectomy	Retrospective review	6.1%	*Risk factors:* • Prior open diagnostic biopsy versus diagnostic needle biopsy (11.1% vs. 9.7%)
Felippe et al., 2007 (3)	354	Breast cancer	Prospective cohort study	17%	*Risk factors:* • Drain in place • Older age • Skin flap necrosis
Gravante et al., 2008 (2)	87	Breast reduction	Retrospective review	27.9%	*Risk factors:* Smoking (OR 2.04) Amount of removed tissue (OR: 4.7)
Olsen et al., 2008 (8)	325	Mastectomy Reconstruction Reduction	Retrospective case–control study	17.5%	*Risk factors:* Implant or tissue expander placement Suboptimal prophylactic antibiotic dosing

ALND, axillary lymph node dissection; NA, not applicable; OR, odds ratio.

found that patients undergoing definitive surgery for cancer had a lower risk for wound infection if their diagnosis had been established by prior needle biopsy rather than an open surgical biopsy, yet one investigator found the opposite effect (20). Nicotine and other components of tobacco cigarettes have well-known adverse effects on small vessels of the skin, resulting in a nearly fourfold increase in risk of wound infection following breast surgery (19). As demonstrated by the various studies summarized in Table 44.1, there is no consistent correlation between wound infection risk and mastectomy versus lumpectomy as definitive breast cancer surgery.

Use of preoperative antibiotic coverage to minimize infection rates has been evaluated in multiple retrospective as well as prospective, randomized controlled trials. These studies have yielded disparate results; many have shown that a single dose of a preoperative antibiotic (usually a cephalosporin, administered approximately 30 minutes prior to incision) effectively reduces wound infection rates by ≥40% (8,13,21,23), and the Platt et al. (23) meta-analysis revealed that antibiotic prophylaxis reduced wound infection rates by 38%, despite the selection bias of antibiotics being predominantly utilized in higher-risk cases. Furthermore, the lowest reported rates of breast wound infections occurred in a phase 3 study (16) of a long-acting versus a short-acting cephalosporin, revealing greatest risk reduction with the former (0.45% vs. 0.91%). In contrast, Wagman et al. (10) found no effect of perioperative cephalosporin in a placebo-controlled phase 3 trial involving 118 breast cancer patients (5% vs. 8%); however, the infections among the antibiotic arm were delayed in onset (17.7 vs. 9.6 days). Gupta et al. (17) reported similar wound infection rates in a phase 3 study of prophylactic amoxicillin/clavulanic acid (17.7%) versus placebo (18.8%) and concluded that perioperative antibiotics are unnecessary in elective breast surgery. Hall et al. (24) in a randomized clinical trial showed that administration of a single dose of flucloxacillin failed to reduce the rate of wound infection after nonreconstructive breast surgery. However, in a systematic review and meta-analysis by Tejirian et al. (25) regarding use of prophylactic antibiotics for prevention of wound infection after breast surgery, it was concluded that prophylactic antibiotics did reduce postoperative wound infections in breast operations. Because of these disparate results, and in an attempt to avoid excessive cost as well as risk of promoting resistant organisms, many clinicians have adopted the practice of limiting antibiotic prophylaxis to high-risk patients and to cases involving foreign bodies, such as wire localization biopsies. Penel et al. (26) conducted a prospective observational cohort study and reported an 81% reduction in frequency of surgical site infection (3.5% vs. 0.8%) by using prophylactic cefuroxime in high-risk/selected patients. Despite this common practice, it should be noted that wire localization procedures have not been specifically identified as a wound infection (21) risk factor.

Mild incisional cellulitis can be treated with oral antibiotics, but nonresponding or extensive soft-tissue infection requires intravenous therapy. Indelicato et al. (27) described and reported the clinical entity of delayed breast cellulites (occurring >3 months after breast conservation surgery) in 8% of their population of patients and believed that it was primarily related to bacterial infection in the setting of impaired lymphatic drainage. A minority of breast wound infections progress into a fully developed abscess. The pointing, fluctuant, and exquisitely tender mass of a breast abscess usually becomes apparent 1 to 2 weeks postoperatively and occur at a lumpectomy, mastectomy, or axillary incision site. When there is uncertainty regarding the diagnosis (as may be the case with deep-seated abscesses following lumpectomy), ultrasound imaging is occasionally helpful, but the complex mass visualized can appear identical to a consolidating seroma or hematoma. Aspiration can also confirm the diagnosis, but the possibility of sampling error can mislead the clinician as well. Definitive management of an abscess requires incision and drainage; curative aspiration of purulent material is rarely successful, and the abscess generally reaccumulates. Usually, the incision and drainage can be accomplished by reopening the original surgical wound, and the resulting cavity must be left open to heal by secondary intention. When recurrent cancer is a concern, biopsy of the abscess cavity wall is prudent.

Chronic recurrent periareolar abscess formation (also known as Zuska's disease) does not necessarily develop as a consequence of primary breast surgical procedures, but this condition is notable for its high risk of complications following surgical treatment attempts. This condition has been associated with cigarette smoking, and afflicted patients should also be checked for tuberculosis as a factor in their recurrent superficial soft-tissue infections. Resection of the involved subareolar ductal system(s) is frequently offered in an attempt to break the cycle of repeated abscesses, but these procedures are frequently complicated by wound infections themselves and chronically draining sinus tracts. Some patients with the most refractory cases have even resorted to complete resection of the entire nipple-areolar complex, but this strategy should certainly be reserved as a last-ditch effort.

Seroma

The rich lymphatic drainage of the breast from intramammary lymphatics to the axillary, supraclavicular, and internal mammary nodal basins establishes the tendency for seroma formation within any closed space that results from breast surgery. Seroma occurs at rates ranging from 3% to 85% after breast or axillary surgery (28). It has been proposed (29,30) that the low fibrinogen levels and net fibrinolytic activity within lymphatic fluid collections account for seroma formation. The closed spaces of lumpectomy cavities, axillary wounds, and the anterior chest wall cavity left under mastectomy skin flaps all harbor seroma. After a lumpectomy, this seroma is advantageous to the patient, as it usually preserves the normal breast contour even after a large-volume resection, eventually replaced by scar formation as the cavity consolidates. Occasionally, the lumpectomy seroma is overly exuberant, and if the patient experiences discomfort from a bulging fluid collection, simple aspiration of the excess is usually adequate management.

Seroma formation under the skin flaps of axillary or mastectomy wounds impairs the healing process, and drains are therefore usually left in place to evacuate postoperative fluid collections. Most breast cancer surgery is performed in the outpatient setting, and patients must be instructed about proper drainage catheter care. After 1 to 3 weeks, the skin flaps heal and adhere to the chest wall, as evidenced by diminished drain output. Seroma collections that develop after drain removal can be managed by percutaneous aspiration. Aspiration is usually well tolerated because the mastectomy and axillary incisions tend to be insensate; these procedures can be repeated as frequently as necessary in order to ensure that the skin flaps are densely adherent to the chest wall. Seroma aspiration is necessary in 10% to 80% of ALND and mastectomy cases according to reported series and as reviewed in detail by Pogson et al. (29). As per a retrospective review, performed on 324 consecutive breast cancer patients who underwent of 561 breast and axillary procedure, by Boostrom et al. (28) in 2009, seroma requiring intervention occurs in 2% to 16% of patients after breast or axillary operations and was more frequent after mastectomy than breast-conserving surgery. In addition, seroma appeared to be significantly associated with development of a surgical site infection. Axillary surgery limited to the sentinel lymph node biopsy appears to confer a lower risk of seroma formation, but this procedure is usually performed without drain insertion, and therefore, occasional patients will require subsequent seroma aspiration (31).

Several investigators have studied strategies that might minimize seroma formation in order to decrease the duration that drainage catheters are needed, or to obviate their need altogether. Talbot et al. (32) subjected ninety consecutive breast cancer patients undergoing ALND to (a) conventional, prolonged closed suction drainage; (b) 2-day short-term drainage; or (c) no drainage. There were no differences in infectious wound complication rates between the three groups, and at a minimum follow-up of 1 year, there were no differences in lymphedema risk. In group 1, the drain was removed at a median of nearly 10 days, with 73% of cases requiring subsequent seroma aspiration. As expected, the short-term and no-drain groups required more frequent seroma aspirations (86% and 97%, respectively). The mean duration of suction drainage and/or aspiration drainages was similar for all three groups (25 to 27 days). In all groups, fluid accumulation had mostly

their mastectomy incisions, commonly known as "dog-ears." Frequently, the incisional dog-ear will not be readily apparent while the patient is lying supine on the operating room table, but when he/she sits or stands upright postoperatively, these unsightly protrusions of axillary fat become obvious and create significant discomfort to the patient because they are irritating to the ipsilateral upper extremity. Similar to the inframammary fold prior to mastectomy, these dog-ears can sometimes be the site for recurrent candidal/yeast infections.

Numerous surgical approaches have been recommended to either prevent or eliminate the dog-ear problem. One option is to bring the redundant axillary tissue forward and create a "T" or "Y" configuration at the lateral aspect of the transverse mastectomy incision (73). Alternatively, the redundant axillary skin and fatty tissue can be resected either by elongating the standard elliptical mastectomy wound or by utilizing a broad "tear-drop" incision, with the point of the tear-drop oriented medially (74,75).

Complications specific to lumpectomy procedures

Breast fibrosis, breast lymphedema, arm lymphedema, breast asymmetry, and chronic/recurrent breast cellulitis: The presence of long-term adverse sequelae related to breast conservation therapy for cancer is being increasingly acknowledged and reported (76,77). These complications are secondary to the combined tissue effects of surgery and radiation therapy. Collette et al. (78) evaluated 10-year follow-up of EORTC trial 22881–10882 in 5,178 conservatively treated early breast cancer patients and showed that a 16-Gy boost dose significantly improved local control, but increased the risk of breast fibrosis. Risk of fibrosis significantly increased (p <0.01) with increasing maximum whole breast irradiation dose and with concomitant chemotherapy, but was independent of age. In the boost arm of the study, the risk further increased if patients had postoperative breast edema or hematoma, but it decreased if whole breast radiation was given with more than 6 MV photons. The European Organization for Research and Treatment and the Radiation Therapy Oncology Group have proposed that late effects of breast conservation therapy (including breast edema, fibrosis, and atrophy/retraction) be graded according to the Late Effects of Normal Tissue-Subjective, Objective, Management, and Analytic (LENT-SOMA) scales (79). The LENT-SOMA system stratifies breast symptoms on the basis of pain magnitude as reported by the patient, measurable differences in breast appearance, intervention requirements for control of pain and/or lymphedema, and presence of image-documented breast sequelae (e.g., photos, mammography, CT/MRI, etc.).

Using the LENT-SOMA four-point grading system, Fehlauer et al. (77) reported grade 3–4 toxicity in 4% to 18% of breast cancer patients treated between 1983 and 1984 (external beam radiotherapy [XRT] fractionation schedule 2.5 Gy 4×/week to 60 Gy, with median follow-up of 171 months), and these rates declined to ≤2% for patients treated between 1994 and 1995 (XRT fractionation schedule 2.0 Gy 5×/week to 55 Gy, with median follow-up of 75 months). These findings suggest that extent of side effects is a function of both follow-up duration and radiation delivery technique. Similarly, Meric et al. (76) reported chronic breast symptoms in 9.9% of breast cancer patients treated by lumpectomy and radiation from 1990 to 1992 and followed for at least 1 year posttreatment.

Arm lymphedema after breast surgery has been studied by many investigators. Tsai et al. (80) conducted a 2009 meta-analysis, which covered for 98 independent studies, and found that the risk ratio for arm lymphedema was increased after mastectomy compared to lumpectomy. The estimated relative risk was reported 1.4.

Moyer et al. (81) utilized three-dimensional, digital imaging and documented a positive correlation between percentage of breast parenchyma excised (during breast conservation therapy) and asymmetry. The location of the cancer, age of the patient, and need for multiple operations did not influence cosmetic results. These women are candidates for various surgical techniques with either immediate or delayed breast reconstruction that can restore breast symmetry. Options include local tissue rearrangement, therapeutic reduction mammaplasty, and various flap reconstruction procedures. Each technique has advantages and disadvantages. Immediate reconstruction (at the time of breast conservation surgery) is preferred over delayed reconstruction. Patients tend to be satisfied with the cosmetic outcome of these procedures, but thorough patient counseling and preoperative or immediate planning is critical to a good result.

Recurrent episodes of breast cellulitis occurring several months to years after lumpectomy and/or breast radiation therapy is reported to afflict <5% of patients, but this unusual and delayed complication causes significant concern because of the need to rule out an inflammatory breast cancer recurrence (82–86). This condition can present as a myriad of scenarios: acutely inflamed seroma formation; localized mastitis; or diffuse breast pain and swelling. Repeat breast imaging is indicated to look for parenchymal features suggesting recurrence, such as an underlying speculated mass, calcifications, etc., and if present, an image-guided biopsy should be pursued. Otherwise benign-appearing cases that are refractory to a standard course of antibiotics should undergo punch biopsy for further evaluation. Occasionally, patients who ultimately request mastectomy because of intractable pain and inflammation are encountered.

The cause of delayed breast edema and cellulitis is incompletely understood, but is presumed to be related to lymphatic obstruction affecting intramammary drainage. Risk factors for this condition include history of early postoperative complications such as hematoma and seroma; upper extremity lymphedema; and large-volume lumpectomies (83). Most cases have followed resection of upper outer quadrant tumors. Rarely is a causative bacterial pathogen identified in these cases, but the conventional management includes antibiotic coverage for skin flora nonetheless. Indelicato et al. (27) conducted a retrospective study involving 601 patients with breast cancer undergoing breast conservation therapy and reported an overall incidence of 8% for delayed. Median time of onset was 226 days. More than 90% of all effected patients were treated empirically with antibiotics. Twenty-two percent had recurrent episodes of delayed breast cellulitis (DBC) and 4% underwent mastectomy for intractable breast pain related to DBC. They concluded DBC is primarily related to a bacterial infection in the setting of impaired lymphatic drainage and may appear months after completion of radiotherapy. The development of this complication does not appear to carry any cancer-related prognostic significance.

Lumpectomy and Brachytherapy-Related Complications

Several breast programs are currently exploring strategies of partial breast irradiation that allow for shortening of the conventional 5- to 6-week external beam program. One such strategy involves insertion of a balloon-type catheter (the MammoSite applicator) into the lumpectomy cavity for delivery of brachytherapy. This device is typically inserted in the operating room at the time of lumpectomy, with the expectation that margin control will be achieved; if this is not the case, then additional surgery and a second implantation is required. While investigations of the long-term efficacy of these accelerated breast irradiation programs are being conducted, experience with catheter-related risks is accumulating. CT imaging is subsequently performed to ensure adequate balloon placement, as defined by a minimum applicator–skin distance of 5 mm, and appropriate conformance, with uniform contact between the balloon and lumpectomy walls. Optimal positioning can be challenging, but is essential for delivery of therapy with minimal risk of local complications.

Breast radiation therapy (especially for left-sided disease) has been implicated in risk for cardiac disease. A retrospective study by Gutt et al. (87) in 2008 evaluated cardiac morbidity and mortality after breast conservation treatment in patients with early staged breast cancer and preexisting cardiac disease. These investigators found a higher incidence of cardiac death in patients with left breast cancer. This finding was presumed to be related to secondary cardiac effects of irradiation. Whole breast radiation techniques and tangent/field planning has evolved substantially over the past several decades, and extent of cardiac effects in contemporary breast cancer treatment is therefore less clear. It is likely that use of CT planning and other advances has resulted in minimized scatter effects to intrathoracic organs, rendering adverse impact to be primarily experienced by patients with underlying cardiac and/or pulmonary disease.

Results from a prospective, multicenter study of the MammoSite device (88) revealed that of seventy patients enrolled, 21 (30%) could not complete the study because of lumpectomy-related issues (cavity size, skin spacing, or conformance). Of the 54 patients who had a balloon inserted, 57% experienced overlying skin erythema and two patients developed wound infections, including one abscess.

Breast Conservation Therapy-Related Angiosarcoma

Reviewed in detail by Monroe et al. (89), angiosarcomas of the breast following lumpectomy and XRT for breast cancer are very rare, but are being reported with increasing infrequency. These secondary angiosarcomas are to be distinguished from primary breast angiosarcomas, which occur in relatively younger-aged women and which have no well-defined risk factors. Secondary angiosarcomas occur 4 to 10 years after primary breast cancer treatment (89–91). Hodgson et al. (92) conducted a retrospective study of 70 women with breast angiosarcoma and reported the mean time to diagnosis of the angiosarcoma as 5.2 years after breast cancer irradiation. He concluded secondary breast angiosarcoma patients present with more advanced disease and surgical resection is the primary therapy. Lymphedema-related extremity angiosarcoma (Stewart–Treves syndrome, discussed below) has a longer latency period from time of breast cancer treatment. Furthermore, the occurrence of breast angiosarcomas in the irradiated field, coupled with the implications for genetic predisposition to radiation-induced tumorigenesis (e.g., ataxia-telangiectasia) have prompted speculation that these lesions have a different etiology compared to Stewart–Treves syndrome. Median survival, however, is similarly poor, at 1 to 3 years (89).

Complications specific to diagnostic open biopsy procedures

Sampling Error

The primary potential risk specifically associated with a diagnostic open biopsy is related to missing a cancerous lesion and resecting adjacent fibrocystic tissue, thereby misdiagnosing the patient. This complication exists with palpable masses as well as with screen-detected nonpalpable lesions.

The risk of misdiagnosis with palpable breast masses can be minimized by complete preoperative breast imaging, including mammography and ultrasonography. Palpable lesions that have a suspicious-appearing imaging correlate should have an initial attempt at percutaneous core-needle biopsy to establish a diagnosis. If malignancy is confirmed, then cancer-directed management options can be promptly addressed. Neoadjuvant chemotherapy is one such option for eligible patients while the patient has measurable disease in the breast, and the potential benefits of tumor downstaging to improve breast conservation therapy success as well as to monitor chemosensitivity then remain available to the patient (93). If the percutaneous biopsy was performed freehand and returns nondiagnostic, an image-guided (either by ultrasound or stereotactic/mammographic) needle biopsy can be attempted. Alternatively

Table **44.3** **Selected studies of allergic reactions to blue dye in breast cancer cases**

Study, Year	Blue Dye Type	No. of Cases (Type)	Incidence (%)	No. of Second Reactions
Lyew et al., 2000 (153)	Isosulfan blue	1 (anaphylactic)	NR	No
Mullan et al., 2001 (154)	Patent blue			
Cimmino et al., 2001 (135)	Isosulfan blue	5 (3 anaphylactic[a]; 2 blue urticaria)	2	No
Albo et al., 2001 (155)	Isosulfan blue	7 (all anaphylactic)	1.1	2/7 (%)
Montgomery et al., 2002 (156)	Isosulfan blue	39 (27 blue hives; 12 anaphylactic)	1.6	NR
Efron et al., 2002 (133)	Isosulfan blue	1 (anaphylactic)	NR	No
Laurie et al., 2002 (132)	Isosulfan blue	2 (anaphylactic)	NR	No
Stefanutto, 2002 (157)	Isosulfan blue	1 (anaphylactic)	NR	No
Crivellaro et al., 2003 (158)	Patent blue	1 (anaphylactic)	NR	No
Sprung et al., 2003 (159)	Isosulfan blue	1 (anaphylactic)	NR	Possibly; protracted hypotension noted

[a]Series includes two cases of lymphatic mapping performed for breast cancer.

surgical procedure have been resumed and completed uneventfully after the patient has been stabilized. Some surgeons, however, have elected to abort the surgical procedure (132) and reschedule the mapping without blue dye, and in one reported case (133), a planned lumpectomy was converted to a mastectomy so that the allergen focus would be completely resected. Many other patients have proceeded to undergo successful lumpectomies, but they should be monitored closely for 24 hours because continued uptake of the blue dye from skin and soft tissue can result in protracted or delayed secondary (biphasic) reactions.

"Blue urticaria," a less severe form of blue dye allergy characterized by blue-tinged hives, is another pattern that has been reported (134,135). There is no correlation with past allergy history, and preoperative skin testing is unreliable in identifying highest-risk patients. One hypothesis is that many individuals have prior sensitization from exposure to industrial dyes in cosmetics, textiles, detergents, etc. Routine premedication of all mapping cases with steroids, antihistamines, and/or histamine receptor blockade has been proposed, but the added expense and risks of this approach for a low-incidence allergic reaction has not been documented. Known allergy to triphenylmethane is a contraindication to blue dye use. Thus far, methylene blue appears to be less allergenic (136), but caution must be exercised to avoid skin necrosis from dermal injections of this agent.

Blue dyes can also cause a spurious decline in pulse oximetry measurements, related to intravascular uptake and interference with spectroscopy; arterial blood gas measurement in these circumstances reveals normal oxygenation. Additionally, it should be noted that blue dyes are contraindicated during pregnancy because the risk of teratogenicity is unknown.

Complications specific to immediate breast reconstruction

A detailed discussion of breast reconstruction options and their complication risks is beyond the scope of this chapter, but a few particular issues warrant mention. The risk of wound complications associated with any type of reconstruction will be increased by smoking history, obesity, and chest wall irradiation.

Skin-Sparing Mastectomy

The skin-sparing mastectomy technique has become increasingly popular as a means of improving the cosmetic results achieved by IBR, but the surgeon should take particular caution in raising the elongated skin flaps so that risk of retained breast tissue and increased local recurrence rates is minimized. When the oncologic principles of the mastectomy are upheld, breast cancer outcome is equivalent for patients undergoing skin-sparing and conventional mastectomy with IBR (137–139). Localized wound problems such as minor infections, focal epidermolysis, and fat necrosis are usually managed successfully without need for additional surgery. When fat necrosis associated with a mass is equivocal for local recurrence, then a needle or excisional biopsy may become necessary.

Nipple-Sparing Mastectomy

The nipple-sparing mastectomy (also known as total skin-sparing mastectomy) is occasionally performed to improve cosmesis in a select subset of patients undergoing a mastectomy. Controversy exists regarding the oncologic implications of this procedure, as it potentially can be associated with excessive retained breast ductal tissue in the nipple-areolar skin, or it can compromise the adequacy of the mastectomy related to residual breast tissue left in the elongated skin flaps remote from the mastectomy incision. These risks are problematic regardless of whether the mastectomy is being performed therapeutically for a cancer diagnosis or for prophylaxis. A literature review by Chung and Sacchini (140) reported complications specific to preservation of the nipple-areolar complex. They found that nipple or areola loss from ischemia or necrosis occurred in 2% to 20% of cases. Nipple-areolar necrosis can be associated with devastating effects on the reconstructed breast; in one study, the underlying implant/tissue expander had to be sacrificed in 3 of 51 procedures or 5.8% (141).

IBR and Chest Wall Irradiation

Chest wall irradiation can compromise reconstruction outcome regardless of whether the mastectomy and IBR are performed before or after the radiation exposure. Mastectomy and IBR performed on a previously irradiated chest wall (as in the setting of patients undergoing surgery for local recurrence after prior BCT, or in breast cancer patients with a history of therapeutic chest wall irradiation for Hodgkin's disease) is more challenging because of the stiffer, less compliant chest wall skin. Autogenous tissue reconstructions are usually preferred in this setting because of difficulties in expanding the chest wall to accommodate an implant.

Mastectomy and IBR are performed prior to irradiation in cases requiring postmastectomy irradiation (extensive nodal disease, locally advanced breast cancer, or cases mastectomy flaps with inadequate margin control). In this setting, irradiation of the reconstructed breast increases risk of fat necrosis and wound infection. Implant reconstructions are particularly sensitive to this effect, and up to one half will require ultimate explantation because of contractures and/or recurrent infections (142). Some investigators have reported that transverse rectus abdominus muscle (TRAM) flap reconstructions tolerate irradiation with acceptable early results (143), but more recent studies have indicated that on long-term follow-up, there is increased morbidity, including high rates of fibrosis/shrinkage and progressive deformity (144). Therefore, when there is a significant likelihood that postmastectomy irradiation will be required, patients should be informed of the risks associated with IBR and delayed reconstruction should be encouraged. An alternative approach that has been proposed is the insertion of a tissue expander at the time of mastectomy for the sole purpose of skin expansion and with the plan for final surgery upon completion of chest wall irradiation, by either autogenous tissue reconstruction or exchange to the final implant. While this strategy may be reasonable in concept, the long-term results and rates of attendant-infectious morbidity remain to be defined.

Other issues related to breast surgery complication rates

Neoadjuvant Chemotherapy

The benefits of increased breast preservation rates (because of primary tumor downstaging) and monitoring of chemosensitivity have led to broadened applications for induction chemotherapy regimens. Numerous studies have demonstrated the oncologic and medical safety of this approach. However, patients should have their surgery timed with the last chemotherapy cycle so that adequate bone marrow recovery has occurred (usually by 3 to 4 weeks), as evidenced by a platelet count >75,000 and an absolute neutrophil count >1,500.

Patients with unifocal breast cancers and no mammographically suspicious calcifications who are receiving induction chemotherapy in order to improve eligibility for breast preservation should have radio-opaque clips inserted into the tumor bed by the first or second cycle of treatment. If no markers are inserted and the patient has a complete clinical response, then she will be committed to a mastectomy because of inability to localize the tumor bed at time of lumpectomy. Alternatively, patients with diffuse suspicious microcalcifications associated with their cancers and patients with multicentric disease should be informed at the time of diagnosis that mastectomy will be required regardless of the magnitude of response to induction chemotherapy because of limited ability to accurately monitor significance of response in these clinical scenarios (145).

The optimal strategy for integrating lymphatic mapping technology into neoadjuvant chemotherapy protocols also remains to be defined. As shown in Table 44.4, numerous investigators have reported on the accuracy of sentinel lymph node biopsies performed after the delivery of neoadjuvant chemotherapy, and the success rates have been quite varied. Identification rates range from 70% to 100% and false-negative rates range from 0% to 33%, with averages approximating 90% and 9%, respectively. Nonetheless, many of these series reveal axillary metastases limited to the sentinel node, comparable to the primary surgery cases, and supporting the validity of the technology from a biologic perspective. An alternative strategy is to perform the axillary staging via sentinel lymph node biopsy prior to delivery of the neoadjuvant chemotherapy. Unfortunately, this sequence commits many patients to an "unnecessary" completion axillary dissection, as the sentinel node(s) is the isolated site of metastases in a significant proportion of patients, and chemotherapy can sterilize axillary metastases in approximately one-quarter of cases. This issue remains to be further evaluated in prospective clinical trials.

83. Brewer VH, Hahn KA, Rohrbach BW, et al. Risk factor analysis for breast cellulitis complicating breast conservation therapy. *Clin Infect Dis* 2000;31:654–659.
84. Staren ED, Klepac S, Smith AP, et al. The dilemma of delayed cellulitis after breast conservation therapy. *Arch Surg* 1996;131:651–654.
85. Rescigno J, McCormick B, Brown AE, et al. Breast cellulitis after conservative surgery and radiotherapy. *Int J Radiat Oncol Biol Phys* 1994;29: 163–168.
86. Miller SR, Mondry T, Reed JS, et al. Delayed cellulitis associated with conservative therapy for breast cancer. *J Surg Oncol* 1998;67: 242–245.
87. Gutt R, Correa CR, Hwang WT, et al. Cardiac morbidity and mortality after breast conservation treatment in patients with early-stage breast cancer and preexisting cardiac disease. *Clin Breast Cancer* 2008;8: 443–448.
88. Keisch M, Vicini F, Kuske RR, et al. Initial clinical experience with the MammoSite breast brachytherapy applicator in women with early-stage breast cancer treated with breast-conserving therapy. *Int J Radiat Oncol Biol Phys* 2003;55:289–293.
89. Monroe AT, Feigenberg SJ, Mendenhall NP. Angiosarcoma after breast-conserving therapy. *Cancer* 2003;97:1832–1840.
90. Edeiken S, Russo DP, Knecht J, et al. Angiosarcoma after tylectomy and radiation therapy for carcinoma of the breast. *Cancer* 1992;70: 644–647.
91. Feigenberg SJ, Mendenhall NP, Reith JD, et al. Angiosarcoma after breast-conserving therapy: experience with hyperfractionated radiotherapy. *Int J Radiat Oncol Biol Phys* 2002;52:620–626.
92. Hodgson NC, Bowen-Wells C, Moffat F, et al. Angiosarcomas of the breast: a review of 70 cases. *Am J Clin Oncol* 2007;30:570–573.
93. Fisher B, Brown A, Mamounas E, et al. Effect of preoperative chemotherapy on local-regional disease in women with operable breast cancer: findings from National Surgical Adjuvant Breast and Bowel Project B-18. *J Clin Oncol* 1997;15:2483–2493.
94. Liberman L, Goodstone S, Dershaw D. One operation after percutaneous diagnosis of nonpalpable breast cancer: frequency and associated factors. *AJR Am J Roentgenol* 2002;178:673–679.
95. Singletary SE, Dowlatshahi K, Dooley W et al. Minimally invasive operation for breast cancer. *Curr Prob Surg* 2004;41:394–447.
96. Montrey JS, Levy JA, Brenner RJ. Wire fragments after needle localization. *AJR Am J Roentgenol* 1996;167:1267–1269.
97. Petrasek AJ, Semple JL, McCready DR. The surgical and oncologic significance of the axillary arch during axillary lymphadenectomy. *Can J Surg* 1997;40:44–47.
98. Wright FC, Walker J, Law CH, et al. Outcomes after localized axillary node recurrence in breast cancer. *Ann Surg Oncol* 2003;10:1054–1058.
99. Erickson VS, Pearson ML, Ganz PA, et al. Arm edema in breast cancer patients. *J Natl Cancer Inst* 2001;93:96–111.
100. Beaulac SM, McNair LA, Scott TE, et al. Lymphedema and quality of life in survivors of early-stage breast cancer. *Arch Surg* 2002;137: 1253–1257.
101. Sener SF, Winchester DJ, Martz CH, et al. Lymphedema after sentinel lymphadenectomy for breast carcinoma. *Cancer* 2001;92:748–752.
102. Roses DF, Brooks AD, Harris MN, et al. Complications of level I and II axillary dissection in the treatment of carcinoma of the breast. *Ann Surg* 1999;230:194–201.
103. Thompson M, Korourian S, Henry-Tillman R, et al. Axillary reverse mapping (ARM): a new concept to identify and enhance lymphatic preservation. *Ann Surg Oncol* 2007;14:1890–1895.
104. Grobmyer SR, Daly JM, Glotzbach RE, et al. Role of surgery in the management of postmastectomy extremity angiosarcoma (Stewart–Treves syndrome). *J Surg Oncol* 2000;73:182–188.
105. Janse AJ, van Coevorden F, Peterse H, et al. Lymphedema-induced lymphangiosarcoma. *Eur J Surg Oncol* 1995;21:155–158.
106. Stewart FW, Treves N. Classics in oncology: lymphangiosarcoma in postmastectomy lymphedema: a report of six cases in elephantiasis chirurgica. *CA Cancer J Clin* 1981;31:284–299.
107. Moskovitz AH, Anderson BO, Yeung RS, et al. Axillary web syndrome after axillary dissection. *Am J Surg* 2001;181:434–439.
108. Caluwe GL, Christiaens MR. Chylous leak: a rare complication after axillary lymph node dissection. *Acta Chir Belg* 2003;103:217–218.
109. Carcoforo P, Soliani G, Maestroni U, et al. Octreotide in the treatment of lymphorrhea after axillary node dissection: a prospective randomized controlled trial. *J Am Coll Surg* 2003;196:365–369.
110. Krag DN, Weaver DL, Alex JC, et al. Surgical resection and radiolocalization of the sentinel lymph node in breast cancer using a gamma probe. *Surg Oncol* 1993;2:335–339; discussion 340.
111. Giuliano AE, Kirgan DM, Guenther JM, et al. Lymphatic mapping and sentinel lymphadenectomy for breast cancer. *Ann Surg* 1994;220: 391–398; discussion 398–401.
112. Kim T, Agboola O, Lyman G. Lymphatic mapping and sentinel lymph node sampling in breast cancer. In: *Proceedings of the American Society of Clinical Oncology 2002 Annual Symposium, Orlando, FL*. Chicago: American Society of Clinical Oncology; 2002.
113. Cox CE, Bass SS, Boulware D, et al. Implementation of new surgical technology: outcome measures for lymphatic mapping of breast carcinoma. *Ann Surg Oncol* 1999;6:553–561.
114. Derossis AM, Fey J, Yeung H, et al. A trend analysis of the relative value of blue dye and isotope localization in 2,000 consecutive cases of sentinel node biopsy for breast cancer. *J Am Coll Surg* 2001;193: 473–478.
115. Haigh PI, Hansen NM, Qi K, et al. Biopsy method and excision volume do not affect success rate of subsequent sentinel lymph node dissection in breast cancer. *Ann Surg Oncol* 2000;7:21–27.
116. Wong SL, Edwards MJ, Chao C, et al. The effect of prior breast biopsy method and concurrent definitive breast procedure on success and accuracy of sentinel lymph node biopsy. *Ann Surg Oncol* 2002;9: 272–277.
117. Linehan DC, Hill AD, Akhurst T, et al. Intradermal radiocolloid and intraparenchymal blue dye injection optimize sentinel node identification in breast cancer patients. *Ann Surg Oncol* 1999;6:450–454.
118. Chao C, Wong SL, Woo C, et al. Reliable lymphatic drainage to axillary sentinel lymph nodes regardless of tumor location within the breast. *Am J Surg* 2001;182:307–311.
119. Veronesi U, Paganelli G, Galimberti V, et al. Sentinel-node biopsy to avoid axillary dissection in breast cancer with clinically negative lymph-nodes. *Lancet* 1997;349:1864–1867.
120. Veronesi U, Paganelli G, Viale G, et al. Sentinel lymph node biopsy and axillary dissection in breast cancer: results in a large series. *J Natl Cancer Inst* 1999;91:368–373.
121. Bedrosian I, Reynolds C, Mick R, et al. Accuracy of sentinel lymph node biopsy in patients with large primary tumors. *Cancer* 2000;88: 2540–2545.
122. Chung MH, Ye W, Giuliano AE. Role for sentinel lymph node dissection in the management of large (>or = 5 cm) invasive breast cancer. *Ann Surg Oncol* 2001;8:688–692.
123. Klimberg VS, Rubio IT, Henry R, et al. Subareolar versus peritumoral injection for location of the sentinel lymph node. *Ann Surg* 1999; 229:860–864; discussion 864–865.
124. Bauer TW, Spitz FR, Callans LS, et al. Subareolar and peritumoral injection identify similar sentinel nodes for breast cancer. *Ann Surg Oncol* 2002;9:169–176.
125. Kern KA. Breast lymphatic mapping using subareolar injections of blue dye and radiocolloid: illustrated technique. *J Am Coll Surg* 2001; 192:545–550.
126. Jin Kim H, Heerdt AS, Cody HS, et al. Sentinel lymph node drainage in multicentric breast cancers. *Breast J* 2002;8:356–361.
127. Kumar R, Jana S, Heiba S, et al. Retrospective analysis of sentinel node localization in multifocal, multicentric, palpable, or nonpalpable breast cancer. *J Nucl Med* 2003;2003:7–10.
128. Tousimis E, van Zee K, Fey J, et al. The accuracy of sentinel lymph node biopsy in multicentric and multifocal invasive breast cancers. *J Am Coll Surg* 2003;197:529–535.
129. Zavagno G, Meggiolaro F, Rossi C, et al. Subareolar injection for sentinel lymph node location in breast cancer. *Eur J Surg Oncol* 2002;28: 701–704.
130. Schrenk P, Wayand W. Sentinel node biopsy in axillary lymph node staging for patients with multicentric breast cancer. *Lancet* 2001; 357:122.
131. Leidenius M, Leppanen E, Krogerus L, et al. Motion restriction and axillary web syndrome after sentinel node biopsy and axillary clearance in breast cancer. *Am J Surg* 2003;185:127–130.
132. Laurie SA, Khan DA, Gruchalla RS, et al. Anaphylaxis to isosulfan blue. *Ann Allergy Asthma Immunol* 2002;88:64–66.
133. Efron P, Knudsen E, Hirshorn S, et al. Anaphylactic reaction to isosulfan blue used for sentinel node biopsy: case report and literature review. *Breast J* 2002;8:396–399.
134. Sadiq TS, Burns WW III, Taber DJ, et al. Blue urticaria: a previously unreported adverse event associated with isosulfan blue. *Arch Surg* 2001;136:1433–1435.
135. Cimmino VM, Brown AC, Szocik JF, et al. Allergic reactions to isosulfan blue during sentinel node biopsy—a common event. *Surgery* 2001;130:439–442.

136. Mostafa A, Carpenter R. Re: Anaphylaxis to patent blue dye during sentinel lymph node biopsy for breast cancer. *Eur J Surg Oncol* 2001;27:610.
137. Newman LA, Kuerer HM, Hunt KK, et al. Presentation, treatment, and outcome of local recurrence afterskin-sparing mastectomy and immediate breast reconstruction. *Ann Surg Oncol* 1998;5:620–626.
138. Medina-Franco H, Vasconez LO, Fix RJ, et al. Factors associated with local recurrence after skin-sparing mastectomy and immediate breast reconstruction for invasive breast cancer. *Ann Surg* 2002;235:814–819.
139. Rivadeneira DE, Simmons RM, Fish SK, et al. Skin-sparing mastectomy with immediate breast reconstruction: a critical analysis of local recurrence. *Cancer J* 2000;6:331–335.
140. Chung AP, Sacchini V. Nipple-sparing mastectomy: where are we now? *Surg Oncol* 2008;17:261–266.
141. Caruso F, Ferrara M, Castiglione G, et al. Nipple sparing subcutaneous mastectomy: sixty-six months follow-up. *Eur J Surg Oncol* 2006;32: 937–940.
142. Newman LA, Kuerer HM, Hunt KK, et al. Feasibility of immediate breast reconstruction for locally advanced breast cancer. *Ann Surg Oncol* 1999;6:671–675.
143. Hunt KK, Baldwin BJ, Strom EA, et al. Feasibility of postmastectomy radiation therapy after TRAM flap breast reconstruction. *Ann Surg Oncol* 1997;4:377–384.
144. Tran NV, Evans GR, Kroll SS, et al. Postoperative adjuvant irradiation: effects on transverse rectus abdominis muscle flap breast reconstruction. *Plast Reconstr Surg* 2000;106:313–317; discussion 318–320.
145. Newman LA, Buzdar AU, Singletary SE, et al. A prospective trial of preoperative chemotherapy in resectable breast cancer: predictors of breast-conservation therapy feasibility. *Ann Surg Oncol* 2002;9: 228–234.
146. Canavese G, Gipponi M, Catturich A et al. Technical issues and pathologic implications of sentinel lymph node biopsy in early-stage breast cancer patients. *J Surg Oncol* 2001; 77:81–87.
147. Albertini JJ, Lyman GH, Cox C, et al. Lymphatic mapping and sentinel node biopsy in the patient with breast cancer. *JAMA* 1996;276: 1818–1822.
148. McMasters KM, Tuttle TM, Carlson DJ, et al. Sentinel lymph node biopsy for breast cancer: a suitable alternative to routine axillary dissection in multi-institutional practice when optimal technique is used. *J Clin Oncol* 2000;18:2560–2566.
149. Cox CE, Pendas S, Cox JM, et al. Guidelines for sentinel node biopsy and lymphatic mapping of patients with breast cancer. *Ann Surg* 1998;227:645–651; discussion 651–653.
150. Krag D, Weaver D, Ashikaga T, et al. The sentinel node in breast cancer—a multicenter validation study. *N Engl J Med* 1998;339:941–946.
151. O'Hea BJ, Hill AD, El-Shirbiny AM, et al. Sentinel lymph node biopsy in breast cancer: initial experience at Memorial Sloan-Kettering Cancer Center. *J Am Coll Surg* 1998;186:423–427.
152. Guenther JM. Axillary dissection after unsuccessful sentinel lymphadenectomy for breast cancer. *Am Surg* 1999;65:991–994.
153. Lyew MA, Gamblin TC, Ayoub M. Systemic anaphylaxis associated with intramammary isosulfan blue injection used for sentinel node detection under general anesthesia. *Anesthesiology* 2000;93:1145–1146.
154. Mullan MH, Deacock SJ, Quiney NF, et al. Anaphylaxis to patent blue dye during sentinel lymph node biopsy for breast cancer. *Eur J Surg Oncol* 2001;27:218–219.
155. Albo D, Wayne JD, Hunt KK, et al. Anaphylactic reactions to isosulfan blue dye during sentinel lymph node biopsy for breast cancer. *Am J Surg* 2001;182:393–398.
156. Montgomery LL, Thorne AC, Van Zee KJ, et al. Isosulfan blue dye reactions during sentinel lymph node mapping for breast cancer. *Anesth Analg* 2002;95:385–388, table of contents.
157. Stefanutto TB, Shapiro WA, Wright PM. Anaphylactic reaction to isosulfan blue. *Br J Anaesth* 2002;89:527–528.
158. Crivellaro M, Senna G, Dama A, et al. Anaphylaxis due to patent blue dye during lymphography, with negative skin prick test. *J Investig Allergol Clin Immunol* 2003;13:71–72.
159. Sprung J, Tully MJ, Ziser A. Anaphylactic reactions to isosulfan blue dye during sentinel node lymphadenectomy for breast cancer. *Anesth Analg* 2003;96:1051–1053, table of contents.
160. Breslin TM, Cohen L, Sahin A, et al. Sentinel lymph node biopsy is accurate after neoadjuvant chemotherapy for breast cancer. *J Clin Oncol* 2000;18:3480–3486.
161. Nason KS, Anderson BO, Byrd DR, et al. Increased false negative sentinel node biopsy rates after preoperative chemotherapy for invasive breast carcinoma. *Cancer* 2000;89:2187–2194.
162. Haid A, Tausch C, Lang A, et al. Is sentinel lymph node biopsy reliable and indicated after preoperative chemotherapy in patients with breast carcinoma? *Cancer* 2001;92:1080–1084.
163. Fernandez A, Cortes M, Benito E, et al. Gamma probe sentinel node localization and biopsy in breast cancer patients treated with a neoadjuvant chemotherapy scheme. *Nucl Med Commun* 2001;22:361–366.
164. Tafra L, Verbanac KM, Lannin DR. Preoperative chemotherapy and sentinel lymphadenectomy for breast cancer. *Am J Surg* 2001;182:312–315.
165. Stearns V, Ewing CA, Slack R, et al. Sentinel lymphadenectomy after neoadjuvant chemotherapy for breast cancer may reliably represent the axilla except for inflammatory breast cancer. *Ann Surg Oncol* 2002;9:235–242.
166. Julian TB, Dusi D, Wolmark N. Sentinel node biopsy after neoadjuvant chemotherapy for breast cancer. *Am J Surg* 2002;184:315–317.
167. Miller AR, Thomason VE, Yeh IT, et al. Analysis of sentinel lymph node mapping with immediate pathologic review in patients receiving preoperative chemotherapy for breast carcinoma. *Ann Surg Oncol* 2002;9:243–247.
168. Brady EW. Sentinel lymph node mapping following neoadjuvant chemotherapy for breast cancer. *Breast J* 2002;8:97–100.
169. Piato JR, Barros AC, Pincerato KM, et al. Sentinel lymph node biopsy in breast cancer after neoadjuvant chemotherapy. A pilot study. *Eur J Surg Oncol* 2003;29:118–120.
170. Balch GC, Mithani SK, Richards KR, et al. Lymphatic mapping and sentinel lymphadenectomy after preoperative therapy for stage II and III breast cancer. *Ann Surg Oncol* 2003;10:616–621.
171. Schwartz GF, Meltzer AJ. Accuracy of axillary sentinel lymph node biopsy following neoadjuvant (induction) chemotherapy for carcinoma of the breast. *Breast J* 2003;9:374–379.
172. Reitsamer R, Peintinger F, Rettenbacher L, et al. Sentinel lymph node biopsy in breast cancer patients after neoadjuvant chemotherapy. *J Surg Oncol* 2003;84:63–67.
173. Mamounas EP, Brown A, Anderson S, et al. Sentinel node biopsy after neoadjuvant chemotherapy in breast cancer: results from National Surgical Adjuvant Breast and Bowel Project Protocol B-27. *J Clin Oncol* 2005;23:2694–2702.
174. Mamounas E, Brown A, Smith R, et al. Accuracy of sentinel lymph node biopsy after neoadjuvant chemotherapy in breast cancer: updated results from NSABP B-27 (abstract #140), Presented at the American Society of Clinical Oncology 38th Annual Meeting, Orlando, FL, 2002.

CHAPTER

45

Complications of Soft-Tissue Tumor Surgery

Sandra L. Wong

INTRODUCTION

Surgical procedures done for soft-tissue tumors include biopsies for diagnosis, resections of the primary site with en bloc structures as necessary, and sentinel node biopsies/completion lymph node dissections. The surgical management of cutaneous melanoma, soft-tissue sarcoma, and several other types of soft-tissue neoplasms can be associated with many potential, although rarely life-threatening, complications. Meticulous attention to detail throughout all aspects of soft-tissue surgery will minimize adverse outcomes. A thorough discussion with patients should include the possible risks of any operation, such as postoperative bleeding, infection, hematoma and/or seroma formation, damage to surrounding structures, inability to completely resect, recurrence despite resection, and other complications associated with anesthesia and hospitalization (e.g., thromboembolism, myocardial infarction, and pneumonia). Specific risks with soft-tissue tumors are usually related to the tumor's location and extent of resection.

MELANOMA

Surgical management of a cutaneous melanoma usually begins with the identification of the primary lesion, which presents as a suspicious nevus. The spectrum of necessary treatment and prognosis associated with a diagnosis of melanoma is largely dependent on stage at presentation, and this can be grouped as localized, regional, or metastatic disease. Surgical resection and surgical staging are important components of treatment for localized melanoma. Nodal metastases, either microscopic or bulky, should be resected when possible for regional disease control. Because of the lack of effective adjuvant therapies for melanoma, there is a lack of consensus about standard surgical therapies for advanced or metastatic melanoma, although resection could be considered for selected patients.

Biopsy of the primary lesion

Principles of a good biopsy must be adhered to in order to provide an accurate diagnosis and to prevent downstream complications from the definitive operation. If the primary lesion is sufficiently broad based and variegated in appearance, punch biopsy is a preferred method of sampling. Selection of the site of biopsy should be based on the location most likely to represent the thickest portion of the lesion so that an accurate Breslow depth can be rendered on histopathologic examination. Since intermediate-thickness (1 to 4 mm Breslow depth) and thick (>4 mm) melanomas can be considered for regional staging with sentinel lymph node biopsy (SLNB), it is important to obtain representative sampling.

If an incisional biopsy is performed instead, it is important to ensure that incisions are oriented such that a definitive resection can be performed with minimal morbidity. Specifically, in cases of extremity lesions, incisions must be made along the vertical axis rather than transversely. The approach for definitive resection is dependent on the initial incision and surgical procedures carry additional morbidity if improperly oriented incisions preclude primary closure, leading to use of skin grafting. (Fig. 45.1).

Excision of the primary and complex closures

The surgical treatment of melanoma begins with the proper management of the primary lesion. An excess of 90% of all thin primary melanomas (<1 mm Breslow depth) can be cured with surgical excision alone, using 1-cm margins circumferentially and soft-tissue resection down to the fascial layer. Generally, 2-cm margins are used for thicker lesions (>1 to 2 mm). Straightforward elliptical excisions followed by primary closure are commonly used. The length of the long axis of the ellipse can be measured in a 3:1 or 4:1 manner to ensure adequate full-thickness closure without undue tension or cosmetically unappealing "dog-ears" at the periphery. Alternatively, dog-ears can be trimmed following resection of the primary with adequate margins. Sensitive sites such as the face or digits require special attention and modified surgical techniques for resection and closure.

Large transverse incisions along the extremities and trunk with extensive undermining of the surrounding skin flaps are at high risk of seroma and/or hematoma formation in the postoperative period. Cutaneous nerves are necessarily transected during soft-tissue tumor excision, often resulting in transient sensory deficits and numbness surrounding the incision. This is especially true for excisions of

Sandra L. Wong: Division of Surgical Oncology, Department of Surgery, University of Michigan, Ann Arbor, MI.

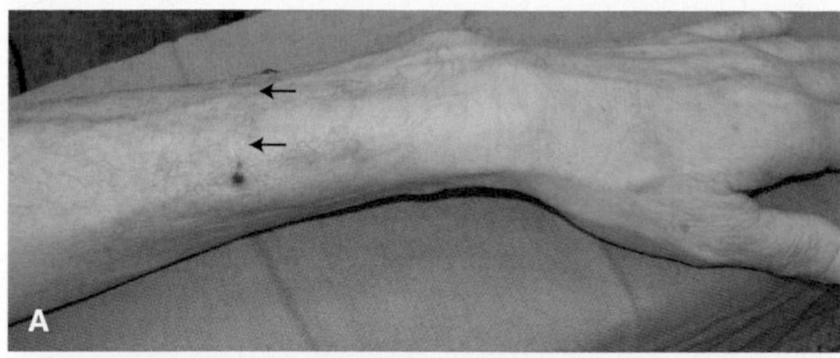

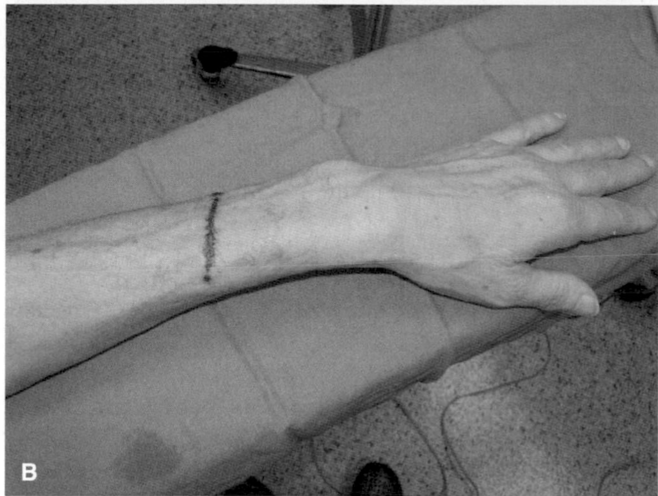

FIGURE 45.1. Transversely oriented incisions for extremity melanomas should be avoided. An incisional biopsy done with a transversely oriented incision (*arrows*) resulted in two complications: **(A)** residual disease/local recurrences at the extremes of the incision, and **(B)** a subsequent wide excision with 2 cm margins resulted in a defect requiring skin graft closure as opposed to primary closure.

melanomas on the face, head, and neck, with the possibility of inadvertent damage to many important structures, such as the facial, spinal accessory, vagus, and hypoglossal nerves, and vascular structures, such as the external and internal jugular vein and internal carotid artery. Tumor location may dictate other areas sensitive to tumor involvement (requiring intentional sacrifice) or inadvertent injury, such as adjacent nerves, arteries, veins, and vital structures. Wound infections can occur as soon as 12 to 24 hours after an operation, and special attention should be given to rare, but potentially morbid and even lethal necrotizing infections, such as necrotizing fasciitis or clostridial infections.

In general, attempts should be made to adequately excise the primary lesion while minimizing scar formation and the need for skin grafts. For locations such as the distal extremities, joints, head and neck, hands, and feet, primary closure is often not possible and other reconstructive options must be considered. Soft-tissue coverage with adjacent tissue rearrangement or skin graft is often the preferred method of closure.

Skin grafts are associated with a higher surgical morbidity, cosmetic disfigurement, and overall cost compared with primary closure. Possibility of skin graft failure or poor healing of the graft should be fully explained to the patient prior to surgery and known risk factors such as excessive shear forces and infection should be minimized in the early postoperative period. In the era of SLNB, many surgeons have increasingly used full-thickness skin grafts harvested from the node biopsy site to close defects that would otherwise require split-thickness skin grafting from a third surgical site (1). However, decisions about thickness of skin grafts should take recipient sites into consideration, since contractile properties of the graft are directly related to the quantity of elastic fibers in the graft used. Split-thickness grafts have fewer elastic fibers and ultimately have more contraction over time. Full-thickness grafts are usually better able to resist wound contraction and can result in better aesthetic and functional outcomes for anatomic sites such as the face and hands.

Tissue rearrangement can provide excellent soft-tissue coverage through the use of local, regional, or distant (pedicled or free tissue transfer) flaps. Flaps are tissue that are transplanted with vascular supply. Complex rearrangements can be time consuming and often necessitate expertise with microvascular surgery. Flap loss is often associated with arterial insufficiency or poor venous outflow and can be a devastating complication, requiring long-term wound management. Optimal healing occurs when blood supply is ample and tissue quality is not compromised by factors that presage poor wound healing, such as poor nutritional status, use of corticosteroids, diabetes, or prior radiation to the site.

Occasionally, skin grafts or other complex reconstruction options should be planned as staged procedures if there is any concern about involvement of surgical margins. A temporary covering can be used over the site, giving pathologists several days to determine a final histopathologic diagnosis with margin status. It is important to understand that removal of the appropriate surgical margins with the excision of a primary melanoma is instrumental in minimizing the risk of local tumor recurrence prior to definitive closure.

Diagnosis and management of regional disease

Historically, the elective lymph node dissection was the main operation performed for the staging of patients presenting with localized melanoma. This involved the removal of clinically nonpalpable lymph nodes, in contrast to palpable adenopathy that would be removed by a therapeutic lymph node dissection. For patients without clinically apparent disease, the evaluation and management of the draining lymph node basins in patients with intermediate-thickness (or thick) melanomas has evolved from discussions regarding elective lymph node dissection to more routine use of SLNB. SLNB is a minimally invasive procedure, which typically uses a combination of radioactive tracer agents and isosulfan blue dye to reliably identify the first draining nodes, leading to accurate pathological nodal staging of the entire nodal basin. Currently accepted recommendations following findings of nodal metastases include completion lymphadenectomy (2), and so SLNB incisions should be planned accordingly in order to allow en bloc resection of the biopsy incision with the main specimen at time of the definitive procedure.

While the SLNB procedure itself utilizes a much smaller incision and a small field of dissection than a full lymph node dissection, there are several well-described complications specific to the SLNB procedure. Complications specifically associated with SLNB (3) have been reported. In patients who underwent an SLNB alone, common complications included wound infection, hematoma/seroma formation, and sensory nerve injury. Other less common complications that were noted included hemorrhage, motor nerve injury, deep venous thrombosis, lymphedema, and even thrombophlebitis. Complication rates vary from study to study, ranging from 0.7% to 9% in reports of consecutive sentinel node biopsies for melanoma, all of which were considered minor in nature (3–5).

Isosulfan blue is a rosaniline dye of the triphenylmethane type, that is, a 2,5-disulfonated isomer of patent blue dye. Isosulfan blue dye is the only dye approved by the Food and Drug Administration in the United States for the visualization of lymphatics. Adverse reactions to blue dye have been reported within a few minutes or up to an hour after injection. Reactions range from mild allergic reactions with hives (so-called "blue hives") and erythema to angioneurotic edema with or without laryngospasm and cardiovascular collapse. Other reported symptoms include angioedema, rash, gastrointestinal distress, pulmonary edema, and cardiac arrhythmias. Additionally, patients may appear to be cyanotic, having a slight ashen and/or pale blue color to their skin as dye drains from the lymphatics into the venous system and capillary beds. The true incidence of reactions to this blue dye is unknown, but is generally reported to be in the range of 0% to 2.0% (3,5–9).

The patient should be made aware of this rare but serious complication of blue dye injection, which is attributable to an immunoglobulin E–mediated reaction. It is important to have clear communication with the anesthesiology team about possible symptoms. The anesthesiologist should establish a preinjection Spo_2 baseline and verify adequate oxygenation and hemodynamic stability prior to blue dye injection. Immediate changes in respiratory or cardiac status can then be directly correlated to the injection itself and so careful monitoring of the patient during and after the blue dye injection is critical. Management is supportive, and patients usually respond to oxygenation and fluid resuscitation. Certainly, rapid changes in the patient's status should not be falsely attributed to the blue dye injection, and other possible causative factors that may decrease oxygenation or cause tachycardia and/or hypotension should be kept in the differential diagnosis with such episodes. Some have considered the use of prophylactic histamine blockade prior to intraoperative mapping, but this is not currently routine practice (9).

There are some surgeons who have substituted the use of methylene blue dye for isosulfan blue dye as the mapping agent. A recent nationwide shortage of isosulfan blue dye as well as concerns about its relatively high cost, have driven the use of methylene blue dye as an alternative agent for SLNB. The side effect profile of methylene blue differs from that of methylene blue and warrants separate consideration. Anaphylactic reactions are not reported, but cross-reactivity between blue dyes is possible (7). There have been reports of cutaneous reactions such as skin erythema, ulcers, and necrosis associated with the site of intradermal injection in up to 21% of patients (10,11). More subtle inflammatory cutaneous adverse effects such as cellulitis or fat necrosis may be noted even when frank skin necrosis is not present (12). Deeper (subcutaneous) injections or use of either a lower total volume or diluted methylene blue solution have been reported to ameliorate such reactions and are recommended if using methylene blue during a SLNB procedure.

It is noteworthy that a significantly higher rate of total number of complications occurs in those patients who underwent a complete lymph node dissection (23.2%) after SLNB. There is a higher risk of complications associated with inguinal node site (51.2%) compared to neck or axillary sites (10% and 20%, respectively). After a sentinel node biopsy alone in the axilla or groin, a total of 14 (0.7%) of 2,083 patients developed some degree of lymphedema. Lymphedema was also more common for patients who underwent a complete inguinal lymph node dissection compared to a complete axillary lymph node dissection (ALND; 31.5% vs. 4.6%, $p < 0.0001$) (3).

Nevertheless, lymph node dissection provides durable regional control for most patients with lymph node metastases. Extrapolating from historic data comparing therapeutic lymph node dissection, performed for patients with clinically evident regional lymphadenopathy, to elective lymph node dissection provides rationale for surgical management of regional lymph node involvement when there is occult, rather than grossly evident, disease. Bulky adenopathy often grows to the point where large lymph nodes coalesce into a matted mass that may become fixed to surrounding structures, such as the thoracodorsal neurovascular bundle, long thoracic nerve, axillary vein, and even the brachial plexus. While attention to anatomic localization and preservation of nerves and vessels is essential, sacrifice of the thoracodorsal neurovascular bundle or long thoracic nerve may be necessarily for complete extirpation. Complications associated with therapeutic lymphadenectomy far outweigh those seen with elective lymphadenectomy: 61% compared to 39% (13). Local wound complications were most common although the incidence of lymphedema was higher in the therapeutic group (23%) than in the elective group (10%) as well.

The overall complication rate with regional lymphadenectomy is relatively high, but major and life-threatening problems are rare. Surgical morbidity after lymphadenectomy is well described (14–17). Commonly reported rates of overall complications are in the 25% range. Most patients experience wound-related, short-term issues common to all sites of nodal dissection. Meticulous surgical technique may ameliorate some superficial surgical site infections: careful placement of surgical incisions, avoidance of nonviable skin flaps, and prevention of wound contamination/infection.

There are specific complications associated with the various sites of lymph node dissection. ALND performed for melanoma is somewhat different from the procedure done for breast cancer, although reported complications are similar. Because the procedure usually includes dissection of level III nodes in addition to levels I and II, additional morbidity may be ascribed to a deeper dissection and transection of the pectoralis minor muscle in some patients. However, adjuvant radiation therapy is rarely prescribed for melanoma while its use is somewhat more common, even if only directed to the breast/chest wall field, for breast cancer, potentially changing the profile of postoperative complications. Overall complication rates, including incidence of wound infection, seroma, numbness, and lymphedema, range from 20% to 47% (3,18). The incidence of lymphedema ranges from 10% to more than 50% (19,20).

Sentinel node biopsy for head and neck melanomas have been associated with mapping to multiple nodal basins and with a higher rate of false-negative results (21–23). With modified radical neck dissections, often including superficial parotidectomy, postoperative complications are seen in approximately 10% of patients (3,18). SLNB or completion lymphadenectomy in this area carries an overall lower risk of infection, skin necrosis/dehiscence, skin necrosis, and lymphedema, but risk of injury to cranial nerves, particularly the facial nerve when operating in the periparotid area, must be remembered (24). Familiarity with unusual, or less common, drainage patterns is important since lymphatic flow patterns include accessible nodal basins such as the popliteal (25) and the epitrochlear (26) nodal basins.

Described techniques and surgeon preferences for superficial (and deep) inguinal lymph node dissection vary widely. Deep inguinal dissection, in addition to superficial inguinal dissection, is used selectively and most commonly performed in the setting of enlarged iliac nodes on preoperative cross-sectional imaging and in cases in which Cloquet's node is found to contain metastatic disease. Incisions range from obliquely oriented incisions to those that cross the inguinal crease in a "lazy-S" or inverted hockey stick fashion, though the oblique incisions are thought to be more prone to complication. Some surgeons employ discontiguous incisions for the deep (iliac/obturator) dissection to allow for preservation of the inguinal ligament and decrease the risk of hernia development. Drains are routinely employed, though a sartorius muscle flap for coverage of the exposed femoral vessels is used on a more selective basis. Classically, the saphenous vein is ligated during the course of dissection, though there are some surgeons who preserve the structure because they believe that doing so decreases the risk of lymphedema (27).

Most surgeons use routine perioperative antibiotics, though a small prospective randomized trial did not demonstrate improved results (complications of any kind) with cefazolin compared to placebo for inguinal lymph node dissection (69% compared to 62%, respectively) (28). In a contemporary series, 19% of patients had a significant wound complication, either dehiscence or infection, requiring IV antibiotics or operative management. Risk factors for wound complication included obesity and lymphadenectomy done for palpable disease (16).

Seromas are commonly seen postoperatively and can usually be managed expectantly. Drainage is appropriate if the seroma is infected. Postoperative groin lymphoceles are largely caused by the transection of lymphatic channels without adequate ligation during lymphadenectomy. As a result, the potential space from the site of dissection fills with protein-rich lymphatic fluid, which is devoid of clotting factors. Lymphoceles are at risk for infection or spontaneous drainage. The management of groin lymphoceles is difficult since recurrence rates are reported to be as high as 50%. Treatment options range from expectant management (observation), antibiotics, aspiration with compression, sclerotherapy (instillation of tetracycline or doxycycline or bleomycin), and argon cauterization, to surgical resection of the lymphocele cavity, followed by suture closure/coverage with local flaps. While lymphoceles are seen around the femoral vessels following any procedures, they are much more common following lymphadenectomy than arterial reconstruction procedures (up to 49% compared to up to 8%). Immunosuppression, malnutrition, diabetes mellitus, and underlying chronic illness have been found to be highly associated with complicated wound healing (29). The use of intraoperative lymphatic mapping with isosulfan blue dye to specifically identify damaged lymphatic channels has been described and found to be helpful in select cases when an operative approach is deemed necessary. Injection of blue dye into the distal extremity (i.e., near circumferential injection of dye at the ankle) is made following exposure of the lymphocele cavity; identification of lymphatics for ligation is typically made 10 to 15 minutes postinjection. Obliteration of dead space with multiple layers of absorbable monofilament suture or local muscle flap is an important adjunct (30).

Lymphedema represents one of the most common long-term complications following radical lymphadenopathy and is seen in approximately 30% of patients, though it is noted to be more common following groin dissection than axillary lymphadenectomy. Older age and obesity are often cited as risk factors for lymphedema. While some cases of lymphedema are mild or subclinical, lymphedema with associated intradermal fibrosis leads to prominent skin and soft-tissue changes. Measurements of girth and volume of the affected limb are conducted, and classically, a maximum girth difference of 2 cm or more or a volume difference of 200 mL or more, when compared to the contralateral limb, is considered diagnostic of lymphedema (31). Prevention of lower extremity lymphedema is empiric and, most importantly, includes measures taken to prevent wound infection. With wound infection, there can be increased fibrosis of the soft tissues in the groin and subsequent obliteration of microscopic lymphatics, leading to lymphedema. Because lymphedema itself predisposes to infection, a vicious cycle of infection (usually in the form of cellulitis) and worsening lymphedema can ensue.

Postoperative management with elevation and compression is routine. Patients undergoing groin dissection are measured preoperatively for fitted compression garments (25 to 40 mm Hg) as a pre-emptive treatment measure. For patients with established lymphedema, decongestive therapies such as manual lymph drainage techniques are employed with reasonable results (59% and 68% reduction in lymphedema volume for upper and lower extremities, respectively) (32). Several components make up the treatment phase: skin and nail care, manual lymph drainage, compression bandaging, and therapeutic exercise (20). Sequential compression devices as well as massage therapy, thought to work by mimicking the natural pumping action of musculature, are controversial since evidence from a Cochrane systematic review suggests no benefit above the use of compression (33). There are little data to support the use of diuretics for the treatment or prevention of lymphedema.

SOFT-TISSUE SARCOMAS

Introduction

Like melanoma, soft-tissue sarcomas can occur anywhere in the body and the complications associated with their surgical treatment vary with their anatomic site. Any and all of the complications associated with soft-tissue surgery for other malignancies can occur during and after resection of sarcoma as well. Multimodality therapy is frequently used in the management of sarcomas. Combining surgical resection with other treatments—usually radiation, and occasionally cytotoxic chemotherapy or other systemic agents—has the potential to improve outcomes compared to resection alone but can also lead to increased complications as well. Minimizing the complications associated with sarcoma surgery starts by appropriate selection of candidates for multimodality therapy, but it also depends on meticulous technique during the procedure.

Complications of surgical resection for truncal or extremity sarcomas

Most soft-tissue sarcomas are primarily treated with surgical resection. Extremity sarcomas should be approached with a limb-sparing approach to achieve local control with minimal morbidity, though amputation should be considered in cases with major neurovascular involvement, bony involvement, or extensive soft-tissue/skin involvement. Although some small or superficial high-grade sarcomas in favorable locations can be treated successfully with resection alone, most soft tissue sarcomas of the extremity are treated with a limb-sparing approach using a combination of surgical resection and radiation therapy. Although radiation lowers recurrence rates, it can increase the complications of surgery. Radiation can be administered either before or after resection, and the complication profile varies according to the timing of radiation. In a randomized trial, patients who received preoperative radiation were statistically significantly more likely to have wound complications than those received radiation after surgery (35% vs. 17%, $p = 0.01$) (34) (Table 45.1). Overall survival was not significantly different between the two groups. Other modalities used have included postoperative brachytherapy

Table 45.1 Wound complications in a randomized trial of preoperative versus postoperative radiation for patients with resectable extremity sarcomas

	Preoperative ($n = 88$)	Postoperative ($n = 94$)
Wound complications		
Yes[a]	31 (35%)	16 (17%)
Secondary operation for wound repair	14 (45%)	5 (31%)
Invasive procedure for wound management[b]	5 (16%)	4 (25%)
Deep wound packing deep to dermis in area of wound at least 2 cm with or without prolonged dressings >6 weeks from wound breakdown[c]	11 (35%)	7 (44%)
Readmission for wound care[d]	1 (3%)	0
No complications	57 (65%)	78 (83%)

[a]$p = 0.01$ for yes versus no.
[b]Without secondary operation.
[c]Without secondary operation or invasive procedure.
[d]Without secondary operation, invasive procedure, deep wound packing, or prolonged dressing.
From O'Sullivan B, Davis AM, Turcotte R, et al. Preoperative versus postoperative radiotherapy in soft-tissue sarcoma of the limbs: a randomised trial. *Lancet* 2002;359(9325):2235–2241, with permission.

as a means of delivering radiation via afterloading catheters placed into the operative field. In selected patients, there was a demonstrated improved local disease-free survival (compared to resection alone) with a shorter course of well-tolerated treatments. The entire radiation dose could be administered in 4 to 6 days, compared to a typical 6-week course for external beam radiation, but wound healing was impaired if loading was done too early in the postoperative period (35). Recurrences following prior limb-sparing procedures often require amputation for local control.

Complications can adversely affect the cosmetic, functional, and quality-of-life outcomes after sarcoma surgery (36). One significant long-term complication of radiation is pathologic fracture of the underlying bone since this complication is difficult to treat and associated with a very high risk of subsequent amputation (37,38). The risk of pathologic fracture increases with the radiation dose delivered to the bone and with extensive stripping of the periosteum of the bone (if done as part of the surgical resection). Prophylactic placement of intramedullary nails in weight-bearing long bones has been advocated by some to prevent this complication. Irradiated areas of the trunk can present a major challenge for reconstruction since large soft-tissue defects are associated with delayed healing and may require complex myocutaneous flaps for closure.

Patients who undergo neoadjuvant (preoperative) chemotherapy may be more likely to have surgical complications. This appears to be particularly true if both chemotherapy and radiation are given together prior to resection (39). Combined, chemotherapy and radiation present both acute and chronic wound-healing problems that must be considered in the surgical planning, both for resection and for reconstruction (40). Even in the era of molecularly targeted agents, which are generally better tolerated than cytotoxic chemotherapy agents, due consideration must be given to potential complications of treatment, which can lead to an urgent need for surgical intervention (41). The use of imatinib (Gleevec™) for the treatment of gastrointestinal stromal tumors (GISTs) has become a paradigm of targeted therapies. Current indications for use include metastatic tumors and adjuvant treatment of high-risk GISTs (42). Serious adverse events reported with the use of imatinib and other tyrosine kinase inhibitors include hemorrhage, and less commonly, bowel perforation and tumor rupture. Its use is associated with anastomotic leaks and delayed would healing following surgical resection and may be due to hematologic changes and immunosuppression with long-term use of such drugs.

Complications of amputation

With proper selection of patients for limb-salvage therapy, amputation is infrequently necessary. Although it seems obvious that amputation is associated with a greater disruption of function and quality of life than limb-sparing procedures, quality-of-life studies are sparse (43,44). With proper support and work with a rehabilitation medicine specialist, patients can have good function, especially with modern prosthetic devices and extensive rehabilitation and training. Unfortunately, amputation leads to immobility and a severe decline in function for many patients. A problematic complication of amputation is the so-called phantom pain, a series of painful sensations emanating from the extremity's transected nerves and perceived as if the extremity were still in place. Remarkably little is known about how to prevent or treat this complication. Phantom pain is more frequent and severe with more proximal amputations but tends to subside over time. In view of that consideration, most management strategies aim at providing short-term relief through the use of gabapentin, tricyclic antidepressants, and anxiolytics. One randomized trial suggested that dextromethorphan in high doses could minimize the development and intensity of phantom pain (45).

Complications of resections for retroperitoneal sarcomas

Management of retroperitoneal and intra-abdominal sarcomas is dependent on complete surgical resection, though location and proximity to visceral organs can frequently preclude wide margins or microscopically clear margins. Differential diagnosis of retroperitoneal masses includes lymphoma, metastatic testes cancer (lymphadenopathy), or neuroendocrine cancers. Appropriate preoperative workup should be undertaken when diagnosis is in question to avoid unexpected intraoperative findings. To avoid precipitating a hypertensive crisis if a retroperitoneal tumor proves to be a functional extra-adrenal pheochromocytoma rather than sarcoma, a high index of suspicion needs to be maintained if preoperative diagnosis is not established and complete endocrine workup is not done.

Since en bloc resection of one or more visceral organs is often necessary for complete resection, careful examination of cross-sectional imaging is of paramount importance. Even when there is no obvious involvement of bowel itself, extensive tumor involvement of the mesentery and vascular supply to the bowel may necessitate resection. Complication rates after resection are high, especially if there is concomitant resection of spleen, pancreas, and/or colon, all adding to the likelihood of site-specific morbidity. Commonly, nephrectomy is required due to encasement of the kidney or renal vessels by tumor or because of dense adherence to the renal capsule. Radiographic evidence of bilateral renal function should be ensured prior to resection, but concomitant nephrectomy is usually well tolerated (46). Partial resection of retroperitoneal sarcomas is associated with survival outcomes that are little or no better than no resection at all (47). Thus, partial resection conveys all the morbidity without any of the therapeutic benefit and should only be considered in select cases for palliation when bulk of disease results in bowel obstruction or end-organ failure.

Radiation to the retroperitoneum places viscera at risk, and adequate doses of external beam radiation for treatment are frequently accompanied by unacceptable acute and late toxicities. Effects of radiation on small bowel include fistula formation, stricture, ulceration with hemorrhage, and intractable obstruction, all of which can be particularly morbid and even potentially fatal. Use of conformal techniques and/or preoperative radiation have been used to decrease the risks of morbidity since nearby structures are protected, but have not met with improved outcomes in terms of local control (48) or overall survival (49).

CONCLUSION

Complications of soft-tissue tumor surgery can be minimized by good technique and preoperative preparation. Specific operative risks with soft-tissue tumors are usually related to the tumor's location and extent of resection. Postoperative issues can range from superficial surgical site infections to more serious and chronic complications. Judicious use of multimodality therapy, combined with appropriately but not excessively radical surgery, strikes the proper balance between tumor control and avoidance of complications and highlights the important role the surgical oncologist plays in the management of soft-tissue malignancies.

REFERENCES

1. Dresel A, Kuhn JA, McCarty TM. Sentinel node biopsy site used as full thickness skin graft donor for cutaneous melanoma. *Am J Surg* 2002; 184(2):176–178.
2. Morton DL, Thompson JF, Cochran AJ, et al. Sentinel-node biopsy or nodal observation in melanoma. *N Engl J Med* 2006;355(13):1307–1317.
3. Wrightson WR, Wong SL, Edwards MJ, et al. Complications associated with sentinel lymph node biopsy for melanoma. *Ann Surg Oncol* 2003;10(6):676–680.
4. Jansen L, Nieweg OE, Peterse JL, et al. Reliability of sentinel lymph node biopsy for staging melanoma. *Br J Surg* 2000;87(4):484–489.
5. Wrone DA, Tanabe KK, Cosimi AB, et al. Lymphedema after sentinel lymph node biopsy for cutaneous melanoma: a report of 5 cases. *Arch Dermatol* 2000;136(4):511–514.
6. Leong SP, Donegan E, Heffernon W, et al. Adverse reactions to isosulfan blue during selective sentinel lymph node dissection in melanoma. *Ann Surg Oncol* 2000;7(5):361–366.
7. Keller B, Yawalkar N, Pichler C, et al. Hypersensitivity reaction against patent blue during sentinel lymph node removal in three melanoma patients. *Am J Surg* 2007;193(1):122–124.
8. Morton DL, Cochran AJ, Thompson JF, et al. Sentinel node biopsy for early-stage melanoma: accuracy and morbidity in MSLT-I, an international multicenter trial. *Ann Surg* 2005;242(3):302–311; discussion 311–313.
9. Cimmino VM, Brown AC, Szocik JF, et al. Allergic reactions to isosulfan blue during sentinel node biopsy—a common event. *Surgery* 2001; 130(3):439–442.
10. Stradling B, Aranha G, Gabram S. Adverse skin lesions after methylene blue injections for sentinel lymph node localization. *Am J Surg* 2002;184(4):350–352.
11. Zakaria S, Hoskin TL, Degnim AC. Safety and technical success of methylene blue dye for lymphatic mapping in breast cancer. *Am J Surg* 2008;196(2):228–233.
12. Bleicher RJ, Kloth DD, Robinson D, et al. Inflammatory cutaneous adverse effects of methylene blue dye injection for lymphatic mapping/sentinel lymphadenectomy. *J Surg Oncol* 2009;99(6):356–360.
13. Ingvar C, Erichsen C, Jonsson PE. Morbidity following prophylactic and therapeutic lymph node dissection for melanoma—a comparison. *Tumori* 1984;70(6):529–533.
14. Urist MM, Maddox WA, Kennedy JE, et al. Patient risk factors and surgical morbidity after regional lymphadenectomy in 204 melanoma patients. *Cancer* 1983;51(11):2152–2156.
15. Tonouchi H, Ohmori Y, Kobayashi M, et al. Operative morbidity associated with groin dissections. *Surg Today* 2004;34(5):413–418.
16. Sabel MS, Griffith KA, Arora A, et al. Inguinal node dissection for melanoma in the era of sentinel lymph node biopsy. *Surgery* 2007;141(6):728–735.
17. Meyer T, Merkel S, Gohl J, et al. Lymph node dissection for clinically evident lymph node metastases of malignant melanoma. *Eur J Surg Oncol* 2002;28(4):424–430.
18. Serpell JW, Carne PW, Bailey M. Radical lymph node dissection for melanoma. *ANZ J Surg* 2003;73(5):294–299.
19. Starritt EC, Joseph D, McKinnon JG, et al. Lymphedema after complete axillary node dissection for melanoma: assessment using a new, objective definition. *Ann Surg* 2004;240(5):866–874.
20. Lawenda BD, Mondry TE, Johnstone PA. Lymphedema: a primer on the identification and management of a chronic condition in oncologic treatment. *CA Cancer J Clin* 2009;59(1):8–24.
21. Carlson GW, Page AJ, Cohen C, et al. Regional recurrence after negative sentinel lymph node biopsy for melanoma. *Ann Surg* 2008;248(3):378–386.
22. Fincher TR, O'Brien JC, McCarty TM, et al. Patterns of drainage and recurrence following sentinel lymph node biopsy for cutaneous melanoma of the head and neck. *Arch Otolaryngol Head Neck Surg* 2004; 130(7):844–848.
23. de Wilt JH, Thompson JF, Uren RF, et al. Correlation between preoperative lymphoscintigraphy and metastatic nodal disease sites in 362 patients with cutaneous melanomas of the head and neck. *Ann Surg* 2004;239(4):544–552.
24. Picon AI, Coit DG, Shaha AR, et al. Sentinel lymph node biopsy for cutaneous head and neck melanoma: mapping the parotid gland. *Ann Surg Oncol* 2006.
25. Sholar A, Martin RC II, McMasters KM. Popliteal lymph node dissection. *Ann Surg Oncol* 2005;12(2):189–193.
26. Tanabe KK. Lymphatic mapping and epitrochlear lymph node dissection for melanoma. *Surgery* 1997;121(1):102–104.
27. Zhang SH, Sood AK, Sorosky JI, et al. Preservation of the saphenous vein during inguinal lymphadenectomy decreases morbidity in patients with carcinoma of the vulva. *Cancer* 2000;89(7):1520–1525.
28. Coit DG, Peters M, Brennan MF. A prospective randomized trial of perioperative cefazolin treatment in axillary and groin dissection. *Arch Surg* 1991;126(11):1366–1371; discussion 1371–1372.
29. Stadelmann WK, Digenis AG, Tobin GR. Impediments to wound healing. *Am J Surg* 1998;176(2A Suppl):39S–47S.
30. Stadelmann WK, Tobin GR. Successful treatment of 19 consecutive groin lymphoceles with the assistance of intraoperative lymphatic mapping. *Plast Reconstr Surg* 2002;109(4):1274–1280.
31. Armer JM, Stewart BR. A comparison of four diagnostic criteria for lymphedema in a post-breast cancer population. *Lymphat Res Biol* 2005;3(4):208–217.
32. Ko DS, Lerner R, Klose G, et al. Effective treatment of lymphedema of the extremities. *Arch Surg* 1998;133(4):452–458.
33. Badger C, Preston N, Seers K, et al. Physical therapies for reducing and controlling lymphoedema of the limbs. *Cochrane Database Syst Rev* 2004;(4):CD003141.
34. O'Sullivan B, Davis AM, Turcotte R, et al. Preoperative versus postoperative radiotherapy in soft-tissue sarcoma of the limbs: a randomised trial. *Lancet* 2002;359(9325):2235–2241.
35. Pisters PW, Harrison LB, Leung DH, et al. Long-term results of a prospective randomized trial of adjuvant brachytherapy in soft tissue sarcoma. *J Clin Oncol* 1996;14(3):859–868.
36. Davis AM, O'Sullivan B, Bell RS, et al. Function and health status outcomes in a randomized trial comparing preoperative and postoperative radiotherapy in extremity soft tissue sarcoma. *J Clin Oncol* 2002;20(22):4472–4477.
37. Lin PP, Boland PJ, Healey JH. Treatment of femoral fractures after irradiation. *Clin Orthop Relat Res* 1998(352):168–178.
38. Lin PP, Schupak KD, Boland PJ, et al. Pathologic femoral fracture after periosteal excision and radiation for the treatment of soft tissue sarcoma. *Cancer* 1998;82(12):2356–2365.
39. DeLaney TF, Spiro IJ, Suit HD, et al. Neoadjuvant chemotherapy and radiotherapy for large extremity soft-tissue sarcomas. *Int J Radiat Oncol Biol Phys* 2003;56(4):1117–1127.

40. Peat BG, Bell RS, Davis A, et al. Wound-healing complications after soft-tissue sarcoma surgery. *Plast Reconstr Surg* 1994;93(5):980–987.
41. Rutkowski P, Ruka W. Emergency surgery in the era of molecular treatment of solid tumours. *Lancet Oncol* 2009;10(2):157–163.
42. Dematteo RP, Ballman KV, Antonescu CR, et al. Adjuvant imatinib mesylate after resection of localised, primary gastrointestinal stromal tumour: a randomised, double-blind, placebo-controlled trial. *Lancet* 2009;373(9669):1097–1104.
43. Gerrand CH, Wunder JS, Kandel RA, et al. The influence of anatomic location on functional outcome in lower-extremity soft-tissue sarcoma. *Ann Surg Oncol* 2004;11(5):476–482.
44. Chang AE, Steinberg SM, Culnane M, et al. Functional and psychosocial effects of multimodality limb-sparing therapy in patients with soft tissue sarcomas. *J Clin Oncol* 1989;7(9):1217–1228.
45. Ben Abraham R, Marouani N, Weinbroum AA. Dextromethorphan mitigates phantom pain in cancer amputees. *Ann Surg Oncol* 2003;10(3): 268–274.
46. Russo P, Kim Y, Ravindran S, et al. Nephrectomy during operative management of retroperitoneal sarcoma. *Ann Surg Oncol* 1997;4(5): 421–424.
47. Heslin MJ, Lewis JJ, Nadler E, et al. Prognostic factors associated with long-term survival for retroperitoneal sarcoma: implications for management. *J Clin Oncol* 1997;15(8):2832–2839.
48. Ballo MT, Zagars GK, Pollock RE, et al. Retroperitoneal soft tissue sarcoma: an analysis of radiation and surgical treatment. *Int J Radiat Oncol Biol Phys* 2007;67(1):158–163.
49. Feng M, Murphy J, Griffith KA, et al. Long-term outcomes after radiotherapy for retroperitoneal and deep truncal sarcoma. *Int J Radiat Oncol Biol Phys* 2007;69(1):103–110.

hematoma. The incidence of lymphedema after axillary dissection was 6% (13).

SLNB is widely accepted as an accurate, minimally invasive technique of assessing axillary lymph node status in patients with clinically negative axillary nodes and isolated or multifocal breast cancer tumors in the same quadrant. The premise for this technique is based on the theory that the sentinel lymph node, the first lymph node to receive the blue dye marker or technetium-99 sulfur colloid radioactive marker, is the first lymph node to be involved with axillary nodal metastatic disease. Multiple studies that validate SLNB as accurate with a low false-negative rate have been reported (1).

Patients with sentinel lymph nodes positive for cancer subsequently undergo a completion axillary dissection. The axillary dissection may be performed as a second surgery or during the same operation if the diagnosis is made on frozen section or touch prep analysis. An accuracy rate of 94% in diagnosing positive sentinel lymph nodes on frozen section was reported by Burak et al. (4). Diagnosis on intraoperative frozen section can prevent the patient's anxiety associated with a second surgery for axillary dissection. However, the immunohistochemical analysis performed in melanoma patients cannot be completed intraoperatively. Those who have sentinel nodes negative for metastatic disease do not require further surgery and can be spared of the risk of complications associated with axillary dissection.

SLNB injections for breast cancer patients may be performed in the retroareolar area or peritumoral. The retroareolar injection is based upon the premise that the retroareolar plexus of lymphatics consistently demonstrates the drainage of the breast to the sentinel node. Peritumoral injection is performed to demonstrate directly the lymphatic flow from the site of the tumor. There is no consensus regarding the optimal site of injection. Suami et al. (14) have demonstrated in a study of the lymphatic anatomy of the breast that while the majority of the breast does drain to a sentinel lymph node, as would be demonstrated by a subareolar injection, each area of the breast can be drained by more than one first-tier node, which does not involve the subareolar plexus. This may contribute to the incidence of false-negative sentinel lymph node biopsies, which may be 5% to 10% in breast cancer patients (14).

Multiple studies have demonstrated that SLNB significantly reduces the incidence of complications associated with lymphadenectomy. Burak et al. (4) reported a prospective, nonrandomized, controlled study of 96 patients in which they compared 48 patients who underwent SLNB and were found to have negative sentinel nodes to 48 patients who underwent SLNB, were found to have positive nodes, and subsequently underwent axillary dissection. Ninety-four percent of the patients undergoing axillary dissection had that procedure during the same surgery as the SLNB based upon positive frozen section diagnosis. Six percent had a separate procedure performed because the permanent SLNB specimen was read as positive. The axillary dissection group was found to have significantly more edema as determined by arm circumference at the mid-bicep and antecubital fossa when measured at a minimum of 6 months after surgery. Significantly more axillary dissection patients complained of arm numbness (81%); however, 17% of SLNB patients had complaints of arm numbness. The authors note that no attempts were made to spare the intercostobrachial nerve. Significantly fewer SLNB patients had axillary drains placed (16% vs. 100%). The length of drain duration was also highly significantly less among SLNB patients (0.5 vs. 13 days for axillary dissection). Eighty-seven percent of SLNB patients had outpatient procedures and 70% returned to normal activities <3 days after surgery versus 100% of axillary dissection patients staying overnight and 73% of patients returning to normal activities >7 days after surgery (4).

Schrenk et al. (7) reported a prospective, nonrandomized trial comparing 35 SLNB patients with 35 axillary dissection patients with negative nodes. No SLNB patients had drains placed and none required aspiration after surgery. All of the axillary dissection patients had drains placed, and 43% required aspiration after their drains were removed. SLNB patients had no lymphedema based upon arm circumference before and after surgery. Axillary dissection patients had a significantly increased arm circumference in the forearm and upper arm after surgery and a highly significant incidence of postoperative complaints of lymphedema. None of the SLNB patients had complaints of numbness, whereas 69% of axillary dissection patients had complaints of numbness after surgery. SLNB patients also had significantly fewer complaints of pain and restricted arm mobility (7).

The aforementioned Sunbelt Melanoma Trial compared complications of regional lymphadenectomy with those of SLNB in melanoma patients. A highly significant difference was found between total complications with axillary SLNB (4%) versus axillary dissection (20%). Lymphedema was less likely to occur after SLNB (<1%) compared to axillary dissection (5%). The overall complication incidence with SLNB was nearly 5% (vs. 23% with lymphadenectomy). Hematoma/seroma formation (2%) and wound infection (1%), however, were more common among SLNB patients (12).

Schijven et al. (5) reported a retrospective study of 213 axillary dissection patients and 180 SLNB patients who were evaluated by their answers on a quality-of-life questionnaire. Axillary dissection patients had significantly more complaints of postoperative pain, lymphedema, numbness or tingling in the arm and hand, impaired range of motion, and impaired use of the affected arm (5).

Though the incidence of complications is decreased with SLNB causes fewer complications than lymph node dissection, however, some complications still occur. One complication specific to SLNB is reaction to the dye-injected. Patent blue dye is the preferred dye in Europe for SLNB. It has been estimated that nearly 3% of the population may be allergic to patent blue dye. Patients have been reported to have reactions ranging from rashes and urticaria to anaphylaxis (15,16). In the United States, isosulfan blue is the preferred dye marker for SLNB. The incidence of allergic reactions is 1.5%, and as many as 1% may have anaphylaxis. In the Sunbelt Melanoma Trial of over 1,600 SLNB, there were no cases of reactions to isosulfan blue or technetium (12,15). Radiation safety precautions should be observed when using technetium as a radioactive marker for SLNB. Methylene blue dye has also been popularly received as a marker for SLNB. In a retrospective study reported by Stradling et al. (17), 5 of 24 consecutive patients had severe erythematous, ulcerated, or necrotic lesions where methylene blue dye was injected intradermally. No complications were associated with intraparenchymal injection of methylene blue.

One technique proposed to preserve the lymphatic drainage of the arm during axillary dissection and possibly reduce the incidence of lymphedema is axillary reverse mapping. This procedure, described by Klimberg's group involves identifying the lymphatics draining the arm by injecting blue dye subcutaneously in the upper arm. Subareolar injection of technetium is used to identify the sentinel lymph node. In this study including 220 patients, the axillary reverse mapping lymphatics draining the arm were within the area of dissection of the sentinel lymph node in 40.6% of cases. The axillary reverse mapping nodes were the same as the sentinel nodes in 2.8% of cases. All axillary reverse mapping nodes excised were negative for metastases. The incidence of lymphedema in this study was 5.4% overall; there were no cases of lymphedema in patients who had preservation of the axillary reverse mapping nodes (18).

INGUINAL

Inguinal lymphadenectomy (also called groin dissection) is performed for regional control of melanoma, vulvar carcinoma, and penile carcinoma. Anatomically, the superficial inguinal lymph node dissection specimen includes the soft tissue deep to the subcutaneous fascia extending several centimeters above the inguinal ligament superiorly, medially to the middle of the adductor longus muscle, inferiorly to the apex of the femoral triangle, and laterally to the middle of the sartorius muscle; the deep margin is the fascia overlying the quadriceps and sartorius muscles. A femoral dissection includes opening the deep fascia, identifying the femoral vein, and removing the deep nodes medial to it. A deep inguinal dissection is performed for extensive nodal involvement of a superficial dissection, palpable inguinal lymphadenopathy, radiologically positive pelvic nodes, or biopsy-proven deep inguinal nodal metastases. The boundaries of a deep dissection are from the inguinal ligament inferiorly to the common iliac vessels superiorly with the peritoneum reflected medially and superiorly. Dissection may be carried out up to the bifurcation of the aorta and vena cava.

Complications with inguinal lymphadenectomy are significantly more frequent than other regional lymphadenectomy procedures. Complications from inguinal lymphadenectomy tend to be the rule rather than the exception, and patients should be carefully informed of this preoperatively. The Sunbelt Melanoma Trial reported a 51% incidence of total complications with inguinal lymphadenectomy and an incidence of nearly 32% for lymphedema (12). Serpell et al. (13) reported an overall complication incidence of 71% associated with inguinal lymphadenectomy for melanoma with a 25% incidence of infection, 25% incidence of delayed wound healing, and 46% incidence of seroma. The incidence of lymphedema was 29% (13).

In a retrospective review from M.D. Anderson of 106 inguinal lymphadenectomy procedures in 53 patients with invasive penile cancer, Bevan-Thomas et al. (19) reported an overall complication rate of 57%. Prophylactic and therapeutic dissections had similar complication rates of approximately 35%. Palliative dissections had a significantly higher incidence of complications at 67% (19).

Gaarenstroom et al. (20) reported a retrospective study of 187 inguinal dissections in 101 patients for diagnosed vulvar carcinoma. The complication rate per inguinal dissection was 52%. Specific complication incidences noted were lymphedema (21%), lymphocyst (27%), wound breakdown (11%), wound infection (27%), hematoma (2%), deep venous thrombosis (2%), and pulmonary embolism (2%). A significant association was made between early postoperative complications and late lymphedema. No significant association was found between overall complication rate and postoperative radiation therapy (20).

In contrast, Gould et al. (21) reported a retrospective study of 112 inguinal lymphadenectomies in 67 patients with vulvar carcinoma in which they found that early complications (<30 days after surgery) did not predict late complications. Postoperative radiation therapy demonstrated a trend, though not statistically significant, toward late lymphedema. Early complications included cellulitis (35%), wound breakdown (19%), lymphedema (5%), and lymphocyst (13%). Late complications included cellulitis (22%), wound breakdown (3%), lymphedema (30%), and lymphocyst (5%) (21).

Rouzier et al. (22) reported a retrospective study of 194 patients who underwent inguinal lymphadenectomy for vulvar carcinoma. Logistic regression analysis found significant associations between lymphedema and radiation therapy, technique of lymphadenectomy, and sartorius muscle transposition; between cellulitis and obesity; and between wound breakdown and patient age 70 years and technique of lymphadenectomy (22).

The technique of saphenous vein preservation in modified inguinal lymphadenectomy has been associated with a lower incidence of lymphedema, the most debilitating complication of lymphadenectomy. Saphenous vein sparing is possible in patients with minimal nodal metastatic disease (e.g., microscopic sentinel lymph node metastasis in a grossly negative nodal basin). Saphenous vein sparing is not advised in patients with grossly positive nodes, which tend to cluster around the saphenous bulb.

PART VII

Complications of Transplantation

Laparoscopic donor nephrectomy, introduced in the mid-1990s (6–8), is now used for >90% of living donor renal procurement procedures. While a learning curve was initially described, as was a slight increase in delayed graft function (DGF), this has largely been overcome with experience. As with open nephrectomy, attention to renal perfusion through adequate intravenous fluid administration and avoidance of excessive manipulation, accompanied by the use of mannitol or a loop diuretic, is recommended to minimize this problem. Disadvantages with reduced renal vessel and ureter length have largely been eliminated with experience and advances in the laparoscopic stapler technology, but at any rate do not present an undue challenge for the recipient procedure.

Recipient-related complications

Arterial Thrombosis

Arterial thrombosis has a reported incidence of 0.5% to 2% (9,10). In rare instances, acute occlusion of the allograft renal artery may be noted at the time of transplantation, when potentially remediable lesions, such as intimal tears, native or donor renal artery dissection, improper construction of the arterial anastomosis, or acute angulation of the vessel, should be identified and corrected. Multiple renal arteries (particularly if they are not on a common aortic patch), severe atherosclerotic vascular disease in the recipient, and recipient thrombophilia may all contribute to an increased risk of arterial compromise. It should be noted that not all vascular thrombosis is technical. Arterial thrombosis may represent the endpoint of accelerated or hyperacute rejection, or severe ischemic reperfusion injury. An unusual cause of intraoperative problems is compression of the proximal iliac artery or vein by a retractor. Hypoperfusion or venous engorgement of the transplanted kidney may result, leading to an ill-advised exploration of the anastomotic sites until the offending device is discovered and removed.

Renal dysfunction in the immediate postoperative phase suggests the possibility of arterial thrombosis. Prompt diagnosis is imperative because the transplanted kidney has no collateral circulation to support the renal parenchyma. Although absence or abrupt cessation of urine output is perhaps the most suggestive sign of arterial thrombosis, the differential diagnosis includes other far more common causes.

The initial approach to the patient with anuria or oliguria following transplantation, once obstruction of the urinary catheter is ruled out by irrigation, is to perform ultrasonographic examination of the renal allograft to assess the adequacy of renal perfusion. While renal arteriography may be helpful in planning an operative intervention, under most circumstances, the delay in treatment is not justified if flow in the kidney cannot be identified by ultrasound.

Once the diagnosis of arterial thrombosis is suspected, immediate exploration offers the only hope for salvage. If identified early enough (within hours), salvage of the graft is possible, with thrombectomy and reconstruction of the arterial anastomosis or via interventional radiology techniques (11–13). The graft should be assessed for viability if a thrombectomy is to be considered. Unfortunately, removal of an infarcted graft is the outcome in most cases. If the problem is with the recipient iliac artery, significant iliac arterial reconstruction may be necessary.

Polar Artery Occlusion

Careful attention to the details of organ procurement should prevent missed or inadvertently ligated polar vessels. These circumstances are usually evident at the time of revascularization, with sharp demarcation of the involved segment. If the segment is sufficiently large, vascular reconstruction should be carried out if possible to maximize viable nephron mass and to prevent possible sequelae of segmental parenchymal infarction, which may include infection, urine leak, ureteral infarction, and post-transplant hypertension. If repair is not possible or the parenchyma involved comprises <10% of the renal volume, treatment may be expectant. In most of these cases, no problems develop.

Hemorrhage

Secondary hemorrhage from anastomotic leak or mycotic aneurysm is a relatively rare complication of renal transplantation, occurring with an incidence of 0.3% to 3.5% (14–16). Although arterial thrombosis and hemorrhage are equally uncommon, the latter is associated with an extremely high mortality. Hemorrhage that occurs within the first 12 to 24 hours of operation is most likely due to surgical error or incomplete hemostasis, and return to the operating room is indicated. Patients with thrombophilia are at risk for vascular thrombosis following kidney transplantation, and perioperative anticoagulation is required in these individuals. Depending on the severity of the prothrombotic state and the intensity of anticoagulation, significant postoperative hemorrhage may occur in as many as 65% of these patients (14,17). Under these circumstances, operative intervention is less likely to control the bleeding, and reduction or temporary cessation of anticoagulation may be necessary to stop the bleeding. Since postoperative hemorrhage is so common in these patients, careful attention must be paid to other comorbidities, particularly cardiovascular disease, when selecting patients with thrombophilia for transplantation.

Later hemorrhage is often related to an infectious complication. Leakage of infected urine, mycotic aneurysm, or necrosis of renal parenchyma secondary to a thrombosed polar artery may be responsible. Attempted repair of an infected, leaking anastomosis can only be described as foolhardy because bleeding invariably recurs. It is far safer to remove the allograft. Because the arterial anastomosis is usually performed end to side to the external iliac artery, ligation of the ipsilateral native vessel may be necessary. While acute limb-threatening lower extremity ischemia is fortunately rare in this situation (18), extraanatomic bypass to the affected extremity may be required if ischemia ensues. Because the donor may be the source of contamination that may later lead to life-threatening hemorrhage, administration of prophylactic antibiotics to all recipients of renal allografts is recommended (19).

Renal Vein Thrombosis

The overall incidence of venous thrombosis is about 0.5% to 4% (20–24). Allograft renal vein thrombosis can occur via a number of mechanisms. Improper placement of the graft in the iliac fossa may result in kinking or twisting of the venous anastomosis, especially if the renal vein is left too long. Attention to the orientation of the renal vein and the choice of anastomotic site on the iliac vein are important. Allograft renal vein thrombosis may also be encountered in association with severe rejection or concomitantly with arterial thrombosis. In these cases, the venous thrombosis is a secondary occurrence.

The usual presentation is heralded by sudden pain at the transplant site, accompanied by swelling and tenderness of the graft. Hematuria, markedly decreased urinary output, and proteinuria may be noted. Renal vein thrombosis may occur in the presence of extensive iliofemoral venous thrombosis, often months after transplantation. Paradoxically, the presentation may include hemorrhage from the transplant incision due to secondary venous rupture of the graft (20). There are very few successful outcomes when renal vein thrombosis occurs in the early post-transplant period (20,21,23). Therefore, prevention is of paramount importance. However, as in arterial thrombosis, prompt recognition and immediate operative intervention are essential for graft salvage.

Deep venous thrombosis

In general, thrombotic complications following renal transplantation are rare, especially considering the fact that systemic heparinization is usually not employed during vascular clamping, which is unusual for vascular surgical procedures. Uremic platelet dysfunction in transplant recipients typically prevents both arterial and venous complications from occurring. Nevertheless, the incidence of post-transplant Deep Vein Thrombosis (DVT) has ranged from <1% to 2%, and some form of DVT prophylaxis, either lower extremity compression devices or low-dose heparin, or both are recommended (24,25). Hypercoagulable states, DGF, and proteinuria all predispose to venous thrombosis, and, as mentioned earlier, extension of an iliofemoral DVT to the renal vein can threaten the function of the allograft.

Vascular Complications of Percutaneous Biopsy

Although percutaneous allograft biopsies are generally safe, hemorrhage is always a possible complication (26,27). The incidence of bleeding requiring transfusion has been reported as between 0.1% and 1% (28,29). Rarely, transplant nephrectomy may be required due to uncontrolled post-biopsy retroperitoneal hemorrhage. Postbiopsy hemorrhage may also occur in the setting of late chronic rejection, where fibrosis may prevent contraction around the needle tract. The use of antiplatelet agents such as clopidogrel or aspirin may increase this risk, although data on the incidence in patients taking these drugs are limited and the safety of biopsy without discontinuation is controversial. This is an increasingly important management consideration, as more and more recipients with coronary stets and cardiovascular disease are using these agents, and the implications of stopping these agents with respect to both stent reocclusion and delay in diagnosis of kidney rejection are significant.

Arteriovenous fistulae have also been reported following percutaneous biopsy. Most are peripheral arteriovenous fistulae, remain small and asymptomatic, and spontaneously regress (30). Thus, management is expectant for these arteriovenous fistulae. Central hilar fistulae are usually larger, present with a continuous high-pitched bruit, and are associated with evidence of renal dysfunction, hypertension, hemolytic anemia, and, occasionally, heart failure. Larger, symptomatic fistulae may be treated by ligation, embolization, or nephrectomy (30–32).

Transplant renal artery stenosis

Transplant renal artery stenosis is a well-characterized late complication of renal transplantation, usually presenting with hypertension and a variable degree of allograft dysfunction. Since the long-term effects of uncontrolled hypertension are significant for both allograft and patient, it is important to differentiate transplant renal artery stenosis from other causes of post-transplant hypertension.

Incidence and Etiology

The etiology of transplant renal artery stenosis is multifactorial. Injury to the intima of the renal artery during organ procurement, perfusion, or implantation may lead to anastomotic or postanastomotic stenosis. Kinking, angulation, and torsion of the artery may be contributing factors in some cases. Chronic rejection or progressive atherosclerotic vascular disease has also been noted. Because many renal transplant patients are hypertensive at baseline and are not studied completely, the true incidence of transplant renal artery stenosis is unknown. The reported incidence has ranged from 0.9% to as high as 23% in a series of 100 patients studied with routine post-transplant arteriography (33). Most surgical series report an incidence of 2% to 5% (21,33–38).

Diagnosis

Clinically important hypertension due to transplant renal artery stenosis may become manifest from several weeks to several years after transplant, but most present within 6 to 8 months with either new onset of hypertension or exacerbation of preexisting hypertension. Since most kidney transplant recipients experience some degree of hypertension, the pattern of blood pressure control must be assessed carefully. A bruit may often be heard over the graft. Renal

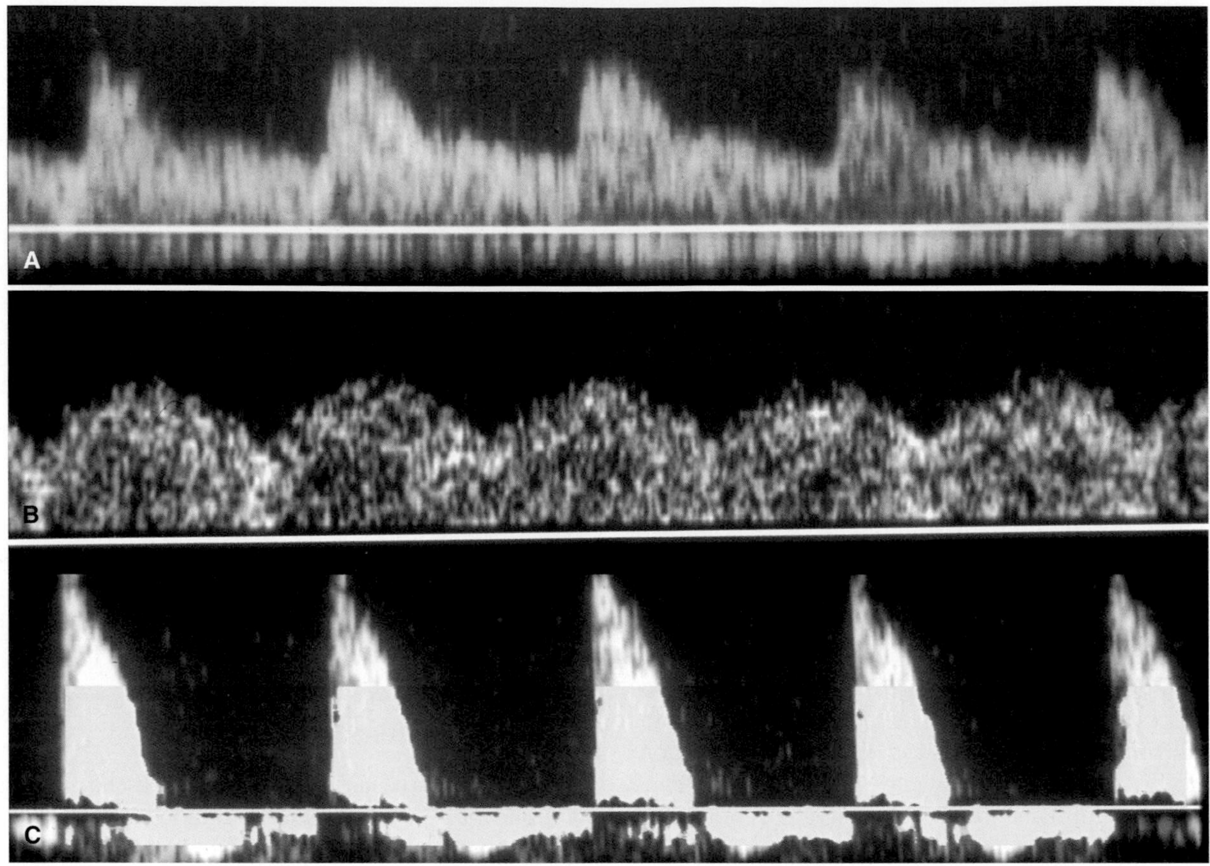

FIGURE 47.1. **A:** Normal Doppler ultrasound tracing from a transplanted kidney. **B:** Transplant renal artery stenosis showing a tardus waveform. **C:** Doppler ultrasound appearance of reversed diastolic flow associated with allograft rejection or venous obstruction.

dysfunction may be noted but is often a late sign. Angiotensin- converting enzyme inhibitors may cause severe, usually reversible renal dysfunction in the presence of transplant renal artery stenosis (39).

Screening is accomplished by Doppler ultrasonography, which in experienced hands is highly accurate in determining the presence or absence of transplant renal artery stenosis and can differentiate this entity from other causes of post-transplant allograft dysfunction (40) (Fig. 47.1). Some centers confirm the diagnosis by magnetic resonance angiography (MRA) (41). The MRA is noninvasive and uses a non-nephrotoxic dye load but is generally lower resolution than a conventional angiogram. The diagnosis of transplant renal artery stenosis should be confirmed by either selective biplane angiography or CT angiography to delineate the anatomy and the location, characteristics, and severity of the responsible lesion. Figure 47.2A is an MRA and Figure 47.2B is a conventional angiogram (digital subtraction technique) that shows a tight stenosis at the renal artery anastomosis. The patient had developed increasing hypertension and renal dysfunction 20 months after transplant from a living related donor. The lesion was successfully dilated with percutaneous transluminal angioplasty at the time of angiography (Fig. 47.2C).

There are two basic patterns of stenosis in transplant recipients, either an anastomotic lesion or postanastomotic narrowing. A short segment of stenosis suggests technical problems, such as injury from the tip of a perfusion cannula or extrinsic compression by fibrous bands, whereas a longer segment may be related to rejection, the so-called immunologic stenosis (37).

Treatment

Before the 1980s, the treatment of transplant renal artery stenosis consisted primarily of surgical intervention. The transabdominal approach was preferred because of the relative ease of dissection of the involved blood vessels compared with the extraperitoneal technique. Identification of the ureter is important during the dissection, as it may lie in close proximity to the renal vasculature. Surgical options include autogenous vein patch angioplasty or bypass, endarterectomy, and excision and reanastomosis. Transplant nephrectomy is only rarely indicated. Among several combined series, the overall success rate for operative treatment was 77% (21,33,34,38). The overall mortality was 3.6%, and up to 15% of grafts were lost as a result of surgical intervention.

Percutaneous transluminal angioplasty with or without stenting has now largely replaced operative intervention as

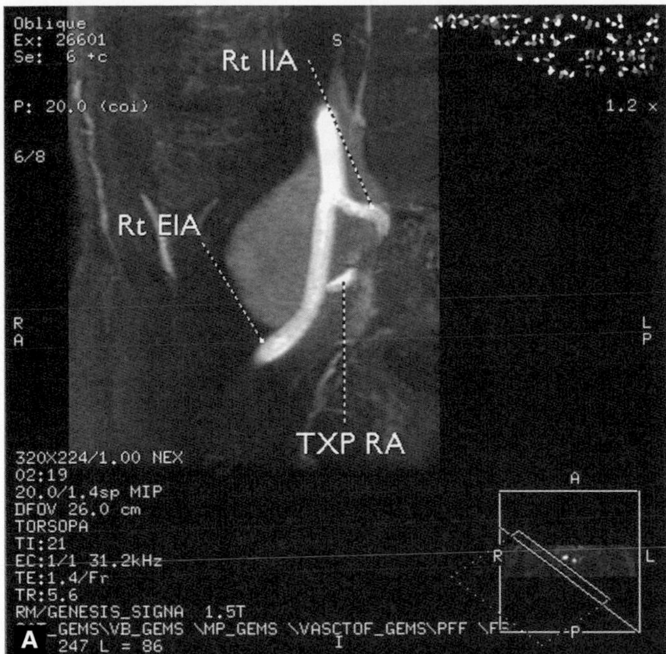

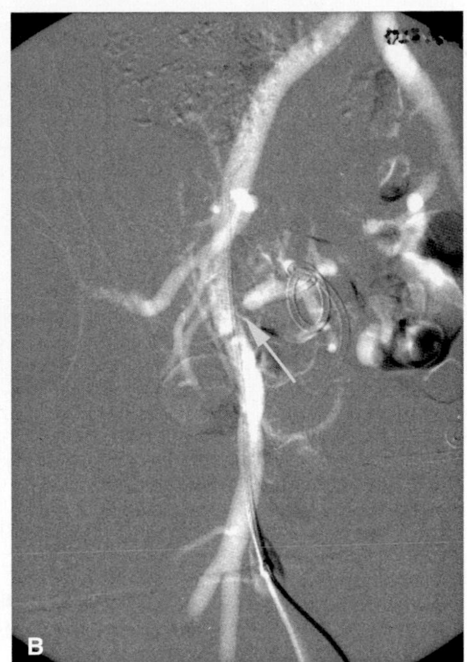

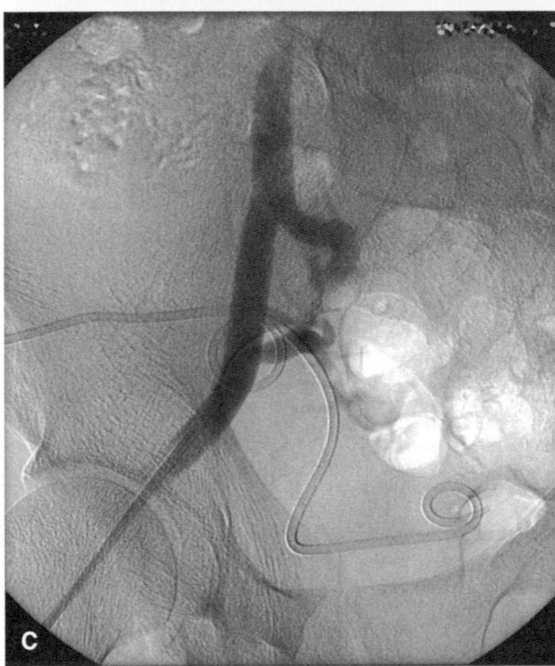

FIGURE 47.2. **A:** Magnetic resonance angiogram demonstrating a critical stenosis at the anastomosis between the transplant renal artery and the recipient external iliac artery. **B:** Conventional digital subtraction angiogram demonstrating the anastomotic stenosis (*arrow*). **C:** The lesion following transluminal balloon angioplasty with resolution of the pressure gradient across the anastomosis (22 mm Hg–8 mm Hg).

definitive therapy in most cases. Despite occasional complications, the majority of studies show a rate of success as high as 92%, as judged by angiographic and hemodynamic improvement, reduction in systemic blood pressure, improvement in renal function, and lower morbidity and mortality when compared with open surgical techniques (42–46). In the largest report so far, 88% of 55 patients had a successful angioplasty by both arteriographic and blood pressure criteria (43). No grafts were lost, and there was one death. Graft function was improved in half of the cases, and recurrences were rare.

EARLY POST-TRANSPLANT RENAL DYSFUNCTION

Oligoanuric renal failure following transplantation is a common occurrence; the incidence ranges from <10% up to 60% in reported series (47–51).

Delayed graft function

DGF secondary to acute tubular necrosis is by far the most common cause and is considered not a complication per se, but an only partially avoidable consequence of ischemic injury to the kidney. DGF is most commonly defined as the need for dialysis in the first week following transplant; however, it should be recognized that occasionally dialysis is required immediately following transplant for severe hyperkalemia despite acceptable urine output and subsequent graft function. DGF rates vary by type of deceased donor: they are typically 20% or less after standard deceased donor transplants. Expanded criteria donors (ECDs) are defined as kidneys from donors aged 60 years or older, or from donors aged 50 to 59 years with at least two of the following: cerebrovascular accident as cause of death, terminal serum creatinine >1.5 mg/dL, or a history of hypertension. DGF occurs in approximately 30% of ECD transplants (52). Approximately 9% of deceased donor kidneys come from donors after cardiac death (DCD, as opposed to donors that are brain dead, BDD); these kidneys have similar graft survival to those from BDD, but have a 40% rate of DGF. Living donor kidneys rarely experience DGF; this is attributable to the hemodynamic stability of the live donor and the extremely short cold ischemia times, which is a risk factor for DGF.

Etiology

Extrinsic Causes

Many factors may be responsible for post-transplant renal dysfunction. These include vascular thrombosis, lower urinary tract obstruction, and hyperacute or accelerated rejection. Meticulous attention to the surgical technique during organ procurement and transplantation prevents most cases of acute vascular compromise and urinary obstruction. Modern immunologic crossmatch testing has nearly eliminated hyperacute rejection. The diagnosis and management of these entities are discussed elsewhere.

Intrinsic Causes

Donor factors that may contribute to an increased incidence of post-transplant oligoanuria after deceased donor transplant include hypovolemia secondary to hemorrhage or diabetes insipidus, hypotension, hypoxemia, high-dose vasoconstrictor therapy, and prolonged warm ischemia time. These may lead to renal injury either prior to or during the renal recovery. Skilled donor maintenance is necessary until the time of nephrectomy to minimize the impact of these factors. As mentioned earlier, the use of in situ aortic perfusion results in virtually no warm ischemia time. In general, longer periods of cold preservation, whether by simple hypothermia or by pulsatile perfusion, result in higher rates of post-transplant DGF (53).

In the recipient, long anastomotic time may contribute to delayed function (54). Adequate hydration and the use of osmotic diuretics have been shown to reduce the incidence of DGF in recipients of kidneys from deceased donors. For most recipients without preexisting cardiomyopathies, this can be accomplished without the need for central venous pressure monitoring. Volume loading of 3 to 4 L prior to reperfusion in generally sufficient, although this can be modified as the patient's cardiac and volume/dialysis status may warrant. Mannitol is given at a dose of 0.5 to 0.75 g/kg just prior to release of the vascular clamps, and systolic blood pressure is kept at least 100 mm Hg. Additional intravenous fluid is given postoperatively, and urine output is replaced volume for volume for the first 12 to 24 hours. Because of the synergistic nephrotoxic effect of calcineurin inhibitors on ischemically damaged kidneys (55), these agents are frequently withheld until diuresis is established and the serum creatinine has fallen. Until then, patients receive immunosuppression with an antimetabolite, such as mycophenolate mofetil, corticosteroids, and, if DGF is prolonged, administration of an antilymphocyte antibody.

Diagnosis

The approach to the patient who exhibits intrinsic renal dysfunction immediately following transplantation should focus on the rapid identification of correctable underlying causes to reduce the chances of ultimate graft loss. The diagnosis of preservation-associated acute tubular necrosis or DGF is one of exclusions.

Urinary Drainage

The first priority should be the assurance of a freely draining urinary catheter. Blood clots in the bladder or in the catheter can frequently be removed by gentle irrigation with sterile saline solution. When doubt exists about the patency of the urinary catheter, it should be replaced.

Hydration

Inadequate hydration or failure to maintain normovolemia after an initial diuresis may contribute to renal dysfunction in the postoperative period. Immediate restoration of hydrational status may result in reinstitution of urine flow, and administration of crystalloid boluses is generally the first intervention in the treatment of post-transplant oligoanuria. In this situation, attention must be paid to the patient's cardiovascular risk profile. If no increase in urine output occurs, subsequent fluid management must be undertaken with the recognition that many ischemically injured kidneys are not responsive to volume resuscitation, and the potential for volume overload, congestive heart failure, and need for early dialysis exists if fluid is administered too aggressively.

Perfusion

Failure of the previously mentioned strategies to generate urinary output demands investigation of the adequacy of allograft perfusion. The diagnostic modality of choice is ultrasonography with Doppler interrogation of the renal vessels and determination of the resistive index (RI), which is a measure of allograft perfusion (56). Since normally renal blood flow continues during diastole, the ratio of systolic-to-diastolic flow can be assessed using the Doppler measurements of flow velocity in the transplant renal artery and its branches. Defined by the formula [1– (systolic flow – diastolic flow)/systolic flow], the RI is increased at low diastolic flow velocities; the normal values are approximately 0.6 to 0.8. Values approaching 1 (no diastolic flow) are suggestive of increased renal resistance, and can be seen in Acute Tubular Necrosis (ATN), rejection, or renal vein stenosis. Reversal of diastolic flow is an ominous sign and suggests renal vein thrombosis. Low RIs are suggestive of renal artery stenosis; however, this finding is not uncommon early after transplant, and may represent anastomotic edema.

Radionuclide scanning with examination of time–activity curves can demonstrate perfusion abnormalities and identify failure of excretory function compatible with acute tubular necrosis (57). In occasional cases, such studies may suggest urinary extravasation or obstruction.

Rejection

During the course of post-transplant DGF, it is challenging to identify concomitant allograft rejection, since urine output and creatinine are not reliable indicators in this setting. Therefore, percutaneous biopsy is indicated at 7- to 14-day intervals. In this way, histologic evidence of tubular regeneration can be seen and occult rejection can be diagnosed and appropriately treated.

Treatment

The management of post-transplant acute tubular necrosis is primarily supportive. Dialysis therapy is continued as necessary. If oliguria is established, which is not responsive to fluid challenge, fluid administration should be restricted to measured losses plus 500 mL/day. Protein and potassium restrictions may be necessary until allograft function improves.

The underlying factors leading to acute tubular necrosis may be more important prognostically than the renal dysfunction itself. Overall, the incidence of DGF appears to be lower among kidneys preserved by pulsatile perfusion than among those preserved with simple hypothermia (52,58). Among kidneys preserved by pulsatile perfusion, however, higher incidences of DGF have been noted with higher final pump systolic pressures or terminal resistance measurements (48). While graft survival rates are significantly lower if early dysfunction occurs (47,48,59), this is less true for kidneys from DCD donors.

UROLOGIC COMPLICATIONS

In comparison with immunologic barriers, the apparent simplicity of the renal transplant operation may at times lull the operating surgeon into a sense of complacency regarding this procedure. It is particularly frustrating, however, to lose a kidney for technical reasons in the absence of rejection. Fortunately, this is a relatively rare occurrence. Urologic problems account for a large percentage of the technical complications that are encountered in renal transplantation. The reported incidence ranges from 3% to 14% (60–65).

Ureteral obstruction

Incidence

Obstruction of the transplant ureter is a rare complication of renal transplantation, with reported incidence ranging from <1% to 7%. Although a rare complication, ureteral obstruction greatly complicates the management of the transplant patient, adds enormously to the expense of the procedure, and may ultimately result in allograft loss or patient death. Mundy et al. (62) reported a high operative mortality rate, as high as 19%, when operative intervention was more common, primarily due to sepsis. Urine in the obstructed system may become infected, or the obstructed ureter may become necrotic; if infected urine is spilled into the peritransplant space, the resultant local infection may be difficult to diagnose and treat. The use of ultrasonography to diagnose obstruction and localized fluid collections has markedly improved the diagnosis and management of the transplant patient with a urologic complication, and the use of percutaneous interventional techniques has reduced the associated morbidity and mortality (66–70).

Etiology

A wide variety of operative and postoperative conditions may result in obstruction of the renal transplant ureter. The most common problem encountered is stenosis of the distal ureter (Fig. 47.3A) (62). This problem may be due to surgical error in placement of ureteral sutures, ischemia of the distal ureter, improper closure of the submuscular tunnel, hematoma in the submuscular tunnel, or angulation of the ureterovesical anastomosis. Obstructive fibrosis of the distal ureter occurs as a late sequela of ischemia; which, in turn, results from damaged or atherosclerotic blood supply of the ureter or occasionally from rejection. Lymphocele is a frequent cause of renal transplant ureter obstruction (62). The mechanism of obstruction typically involves angulation of the ureterovesical junction or compression of the collecting system. Peritransplant hematoma may have the same effect, and ureteral blood clots secondary to trauma incurred at either kidney recovery harvesting or implantation have also been reported as a cause of early post-transplant obstruction (62). Rarely, the operating surgeon may inadvertently position the ureter anterior to the spermatic cord (71), round ligament (62), or inferior epigastric vessels, resulting in obstruction. Finally, stones in the transplanted ureter (62) and a fungus ball, usually secondary to candidal infection of the urine (72,73), have been reported as rare causes of obstruction.

Diagnosis

Ultrasonography is the mainstay of initial diagnosis of urologic complications following transplantation because it is accurate, noninvasive, and does not rely on function of the transplant. Routine screening of all transplant patients with ultrasonography has, however, highlighted some pitfalls in interpretation that should be emphasized. First, it is not at all

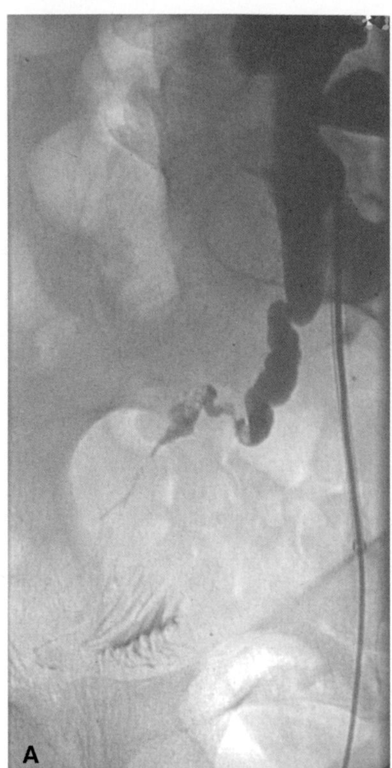

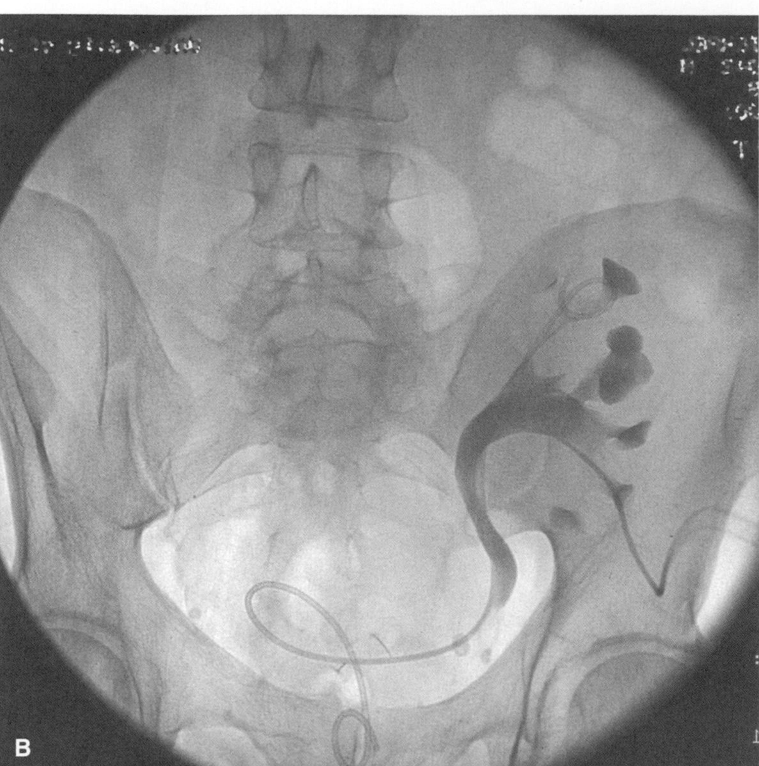

FIGURE 47.3. **A**: Percutaneous nephrostogram demonstrating a tight stenosis at the ureteral anastomosis to the bladder. **B**: Treatment of the stenosis with a percutaneously placed stent.

uncommon to diagnose mild hydronephrosis in the early post-transplant period in a normal kidney transplant; the ultrasonographic appearance of dilated calyces and renal pelvis probably results from the profound diuresis occurring after transplantation. Further evaluation is warranted only if this finding persists or worsens in a setting of unsatisfactory renal function. A second pitfall is that an obstructed ureter occasionally does not produce obvious hydronephrosis by ultrasonographic examination. In these cases, the obstruction is high, at the ureteropelvic junction, or prolonged obstruction has resulted in poor function with small volumes of urine. In this difficult situation, obstruction usually becomes a diagnosis by exclusion. In the absence of dilated calyces, antegrade pyelography is more difficult.

Treatment

Treatment of the obstructed renal transplant ureter may be simple or complex, depending on the cause and timing of the obstruction. However, improvements in interventional genitourinary radiology have made this complication less emergent. Patients most frequently have a percutaneous nephrostomy tube placed at the time of diagnosis and, therefore, are not likely to be septic or uremic if surgery is necessary (Fig. 47.3B). Under these conditions, the operating surgeon is more able to evaluate the problem carefully, map out a strategy, and proceed with all available resources.

Under the simplest of circumstances, the obstruction is at the level of the distal ureter. A nonoperative technique involves percutaneous antegrade dilatation of the ureteral stricture (74). Newer techniques include endoscopic ureterostomy, or cutting of the stricture, either through the percutaneous nephrostomy or through a cystoscopic approach. Standard operative repair, which is indicated for long segmental strictures or those refractory to nonoperative management, involves creation of a new ureterovesical anastomosis, usually with mobilization and resection of the involved ureter. If the operative findings are such that sufficient viable transplant ureter is not available to reach the bladder, the bladder can be extensively mobilized and fixed to the psoas muscle to provide additional length, or a Boari flap of bladder can be advanced to replace the resected ureteral segment. A difficult but common situation may arise when a patient's bladder is found to be contracted, nonpliable, and trabeculated. In this circumstance, it may be preferable to mobilize and remove the ipsilateral kidney and anastomose the remaining transplant ureter or renal pelvis to native ureter.

Extensive local drainage, nephrostomy, and urinary catheter drainage are usually indicated after reoperation. Stenting the anastomosis with a soft double-J internal stent is also helpful. Despite these measures, further morbidity following treatment of the obstruction is frequent. In one large series (62), 49% of patients developed a further urologic complication (usually urinary fistula) after operative repair of a primary urologic complication. This alarming statistic underscores the importance of preventing urinary complications through the use of proper technique during the organ procurement and the primary renal transplant operation.

Urinary leak

The first few postoperative weeks after renal transplantation are usually characterized by rapid reduction in the serum creatinine and rapid elevation of the patient's mood. Sometimes, however, the large urine volume of the first few postoperative days falls off dramatically. The patient may report clear drainage from the operative site and suprapubic pain or discomfort; fever and systemic sepsis may supervene. This clinical situation, which is suggestive of a urinary leak, requires rapid and accurate diagnosis and effective treatment.

Urinary extravasation may occur anywhere from the bladder to the renal transplant calyx. The incidence of extravasation following transplant has varied from 0.1% (64) to 8.5% (63). The most common site is the distal ureter at the ureteroneocystostomy. Predisposing factors relate primarily to the blood supply at this site and thus involve the degree of trauma at the time of procurement, operative handling of the ureter at the time of the transplant procedure, the presence of multiple renal arteries, and possibly the intensity of the rejection process (2).

The ureter usually leaks because it is ischemic. The relatively tenuous blood supply of the distal ureter is vulnerable to operative trauma at the time of procurement and at reimplantation. Also, the ureter may become ischemic if a lower polar artery has been inadvertently tied off or improperly anastomosed to the recipient blood vessels. Whether acute rejection commonly results in ureteral ischemia is not established, but it seems a possibility because reduction in blood flow to the transplant in general is well documented during acute rejection, and the delicate nature of the ureteral blood supply makes it particularly vulnerable.

Adequate bladder drainage with a urinary catheter is important in preventing postoperative leaks because the profound diuresis that often follows transplantation may put enormous pressure on the new suture line if the bladder cannot empty properly. To avoid this problem, most centers regularly irrigate the catheter with sterile saline solution in the immediate postoperative period. However, prolonged catheter drainage is not necessary and predisposes to bacterial colonization of the bladder and later urethral stricture (75,76). It is necessary in the preoperative evaluation of the transplant recipient to establish that prostatic hypertrophy or urethral stricture does not impair bladder emptying because these factors might also contribute to early postoperative suture line dehiscence.

Diagnosis

Accurate diagnosis is important because another renal transplant complication, lymphocele, also may be manifested by reduced urine output and a peritransplant fluid collection. A peritransplant fluid collection observed on ultrasonography should be aspirated if it is large (>5 cm in diameter) and accessible (Fig. 47.4). Patients should be placed on broad-spectrum antibiotics prior to this procedure. The fluid specimen is sent for a creatinine determination. If a sufficient concentration gradient exists between fluid and serum creatinine, the diagnosis of urinary leak is

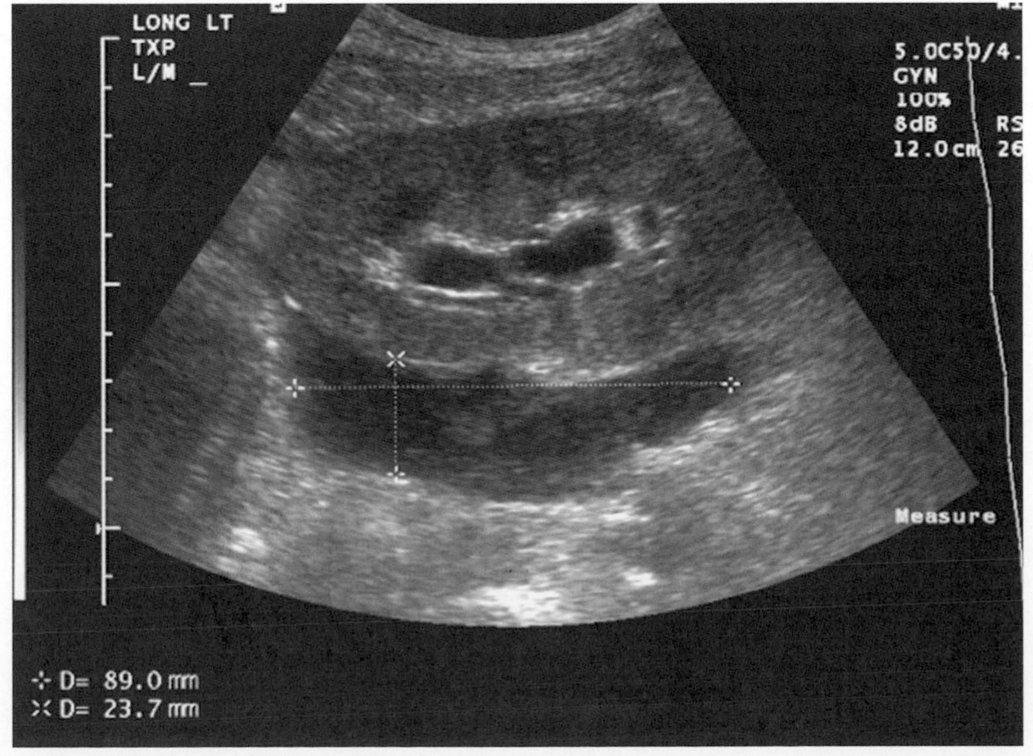

FIGURE 47.4. Ultrasound image of a urinoma inferior to the renal allograft.

established and further diagnostic steps are undertaken to define the extent of the problem. If the fluid creatinine is identical to that of serum, it can be assumed that the fluid is lymph rather than urine. Confirmatory cell counts and differential analysis may be done. An exception may occur if the degree of renal function is such that the kidney makes urine but does not clear creatinine, in which case this differentiation is more difficult.

If urinary extravasation is suspected, a cystogram or percutaneous nephrostomy is obtained. This may localize the leak to the bladder, the ureterovesical anastomosis, or a higher leak may be identified. Percutaneous nephrostograms are the procedure of choice at the author's institution, as the approach offers diagnostic and therapeutic value—if a leak is identified, a nephrostomy tube with nephroureteral stent can be placed at the same time. Flexible fiberoptic cystoscopy with retrograde cannulation of the ureter is usually not an attractive option because most cases of urinary leak occur in the early post-transplant period, when distension of the bladder with a new suture line would not be advisable. Also, when the ureteroneocystostomy is performed to the dome of the bladder, as in the popular Lich technique, it is technically difficult to cannulate the ureteral orifice even if it can be identified. For equivocal cases where the pretest likelihood of a leak is low, radionuclide scintigraphy (renal scan) is less invasive and can be used to rule out the possibility of a leak (77).

Nonoperative management of urinary leaks is successful in a majority of cases without further sequelae. Patients require temporary nephrostomy for 2 to 6 months, depending on the size of the leak and the pace of healing. However, stricture formation requiring further therapy or late operative intervention occurs in up to 30% of cases where the initial management is nonoperative (2). Any significant peritransplant urinoma should be separately drained. If ischemia of the ureter has resulted in distal tissue loss and a large leak, operative repair is necessary. Resection of the involved segment with reanastomosis or use of a Boari flap to reestablish urinary continuity is usually performed. Cutaneous ureterostomy might theoretically be used, but in the context of renal transplantation, this procedure is not usually a satisfactory long-term solution to the problem of ureteral necrosis.

Bladder leak

The incidence of leakage from the urinary bladder is 0% to 4% (2,63,64). The opportunity for leakage is higher when the Ledbetter–Politano ureterovesical anastomosis is employed because this procedure involves a large cystostomy not required for the external ureteroneocystostomy. Our group has reported a low rate of ureterovesical leak, approximately 3%, in (>1,600 of the latter procedures (2). Another factor of importance is the prior condition of the recipient bladder. If there have been multiple previous operative procedures, the risk of leakage is higher. Most bladder leaks can be repaired primarily or treated conservatively with local drains and prolonged urinary catheterization.

Pelvicalyceal leak

Urinary extravasation at the calyx is rare and usually the result of trauma to or occlusion of subsegmental arteries. Because there is no effective collateral arterial circulation in the kidney, the result may be either loss of renal parenchyma with subsequent fibrosis or necrosis and urinary extravasation. There is an association between this complication and the presence of multiple renal arteries in the donor kidney. Calyceal leaks tend to occur later than ureteral or bladder leaks and thus may be harder to diagnose and treat effectively. In one report, seven of eight patients with this complication ultimately lost the transplant and three died (78). Treatment is prolonged nephrostomy tube drainage through the infarct into the involved calyx if possible. Leakage from the renal pelvis is encountered very rarely, probably owing to its rich capillary blood supply. This complication may be associated with operative trauma or, rarely, as a spontaneous complication after transplantation (79). In one series, spontaneous rupture of the renal pelvis presented from 5 to 46 days after transplantation and was not associated with mechanical obstruction. The cause of this complication was not obvious in any case. One case was successfully treated with prolonged nephrostomy drainage, but transplant nephrectomy was required in three cases.

LYMPHOCELE

Incidence

A lymphocele is an extralymphatic collection of lymphatic fluid. Owing to the pelvic location of the renal transplant, an area rich in lymphatics, lymphocele is a common complication of renal transplantation. It is not clear what percentage of peritransplant fluid accumulations develop into clinically significant lymphoceles requiring intervention. Most transplant surgeons prefer to follow asymptomatic collections expectantly until symptoms or deterioration of renal function mandate operative intervention. Clinically oriented series (80–84) have reported this complication to occur in 0% to 22% of patients. A lymphocele typically presents later in the postoperative period than urinary extravasation. The most common clinical presentation is abdominal mass (72%), ipsilateral leg edema (58%), hypertension (26%), clear drainage from the wound (19%), fever (19%), and decreasing urine output (15%) (85). The patient occasionally presents with rapid progression to anuria (86). The origin of the lymphatic accumulation may be from recipient lymphatics severed at the time of surgery, a conclusion drawn by lymphoradiographic studies involving injection of radionuclide into the ipsilateral leg of patients with this condition (87). However, a universal clinical observation is that lymphoceles either present or greatly enlarge during a rejection episode, suggesting that renal hilar lymphatics of the allograft contribute lymph to the lymphocele as well (88).

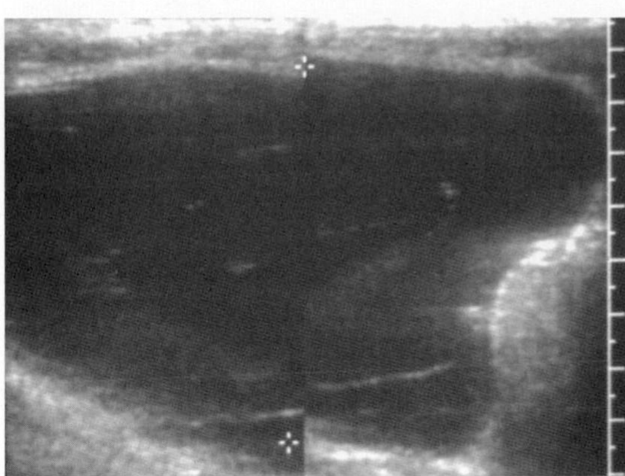

FIGURE 47.5. High-magnification ultrasound image of a lymphocele that demonstrates fine linear septations not typically seen in ultrasound imaging of urinoma or abscess.

Diagnosis

The diagnosis of lymphocele has been greatly facilitated by the widespread use of diagnostic ultrasonography. Lymphoceles typically demonstrate fine linear septations not seen with urinoma or abscess (Fig. 47.5). Careful aspiration under sterile conditions with antibiotic coverage is routinely performed to establish the diagnosis and rule out urinoma.

Treatment

The treatment of lymphocele may be conservative at first, consisting of complete aspiration under ultrasonographic guidance. Occasionally, this therapy is all that is required. Aspiration should not be repeated as infection may result. External drainage will usually require a prolonged course and carries the risk of infection. The use of sclerosing agents as an adjunct to external drainage, which dramatically shortens the period of drainage, has been reported (89,90). The mean duration from external drainage to complete cessation of drainage was 4.5 weeks. Internal drainage is the treatment of choice in most centers. A peritoneal window from the lymphocele cavity into the peritoneum is created either with open or laparoscopic technique so that peritransplant lymph has free egress into, and can be reabsorbed by, the peritoneal membrane. Care should be taken to make the window large enough so that bowel cannot become incarcerated in it, and to minimize the risk of reperitonealization of the defect and recurrence of the lymphocele. Also, the transplant ureter frequently is incorporated into the medial (operated) wall of the lymphocele, and ureteral injury during this procedure has been reported (84).

Certain technical maneuvers at the original transplant procedure may be helpful in preventing lymphoceles. First, most of the large lymphatics coursing from the leg follow the external iliac artery and vein. These can be easily moved out of harm's way. If division of large visible lymphatics is necessary, ligation may be preferable to electrocautery because lymphatics do not coagulate well as do blood vessels. While meticulous ligation of lymphatics near the transplant hilum was employed by some surgeons in the era of open nephrectomy to decrease lymph leakage from this source, this is impractical for laparoscopic nephrectomy.

SUPERFICIAL WOUND INFECTION

With the increasing success and availability of kidney transplantation, infection of the superficial transplant wound is increasing in incidence, as the spectrum of predisposing factors grouping kidney recipients has expanded over time. When the urine is sterile preoperatively, the transplant wound is considered a clean-contaminated wound. While Belzer et al. (91) in the 1970s reported an infection rate of (<1%, more recent reviews report higher infection rates, as high as 15% (92–94). The increase in wound infection rates, despite the existence of more specific immunosuppression, is likely a consequence of increased level of comorbidities present in current kidney transplant recipients, especially with respect to obesity and diabetes, although higher infection rates have been reported with the use of sirolimus (94). In a recent large single center study, obesity, recipient age, and DGF were associated with an infectious wound complication (92). When infection does occur, Gram-positive organisms are most commonly cultured.

Prevention of superficial wound infection relies on the meticulous operative technique and administration of prophylactic antibiotics. Tissue should be handled gently, and care should be taken to avoid hematoma in the subcutaneous tissue. Copious irrigation of the wound with warm saline before closure of the skin may be beneficial. Diagnosis of superficial wound infection obligates the surgeon to investigate the possibility that a perinephric infection exists as well.

PERINEPHRIC ABSCESS

Subfascial peritransplant infection is an unusual but potentially grave complication of renal transplantation. The clinical presentation with fever and oliguria mimics rejection, and catastrophic results are certain if an underlying abscess is treated with increased immunosuppression. Aggressive and thorough evaluations of patients with a suggestive history are important.

Peritransplant abscess has been reported to be associated with peritransplant hematoma (95–98), post-transplant urinary fistula (95), the presence of infected urine at the time of transplantation (99), and the use of an ileal conduit (100,101) for urinary diversion. Other factors predisposing to abscess formation are more general and include the use of immunosuppressive drugs, poor nutritional status of the transplant recipient, obesity, and the location of the transplant incision in the groin area. The diagnosis is made by ultrasonography-guided needle aspiration of fluid collections in the appropriate clinical context. The ultrasonographic appearance of the abscess itself is not particularly characteristic, but particulate debris is occasionally noted (68) and multiple linear septations such as those that would be seen in a lymphocele are not present.

Immediate transplant nephrectomy with wide wound drainage may be required if sepsis is extensive, but percutaneous or operative drainage alone is usually satisfactory if the infection is localized and not associated with systemic sepsis. Although the location may raise concern about the development of a pseudoaneurysm at the arterial anastomosis, this, in fact, rarely occurs. Immunosuppression can generally be drastically reduced in the setting of sepsis without immediate loss of the allograft. Long-term treatment with broad-spectrum antibiotics is indicated. The offending organisms are Gram positive in one-half of cases (99). Multiple organisms may be cultured from as many as 30%. The most common organisms encountered are coagulase-positive *Staphylococcus aureus* and *Escherichia coli.*

Measures to avoid this complication should be undertaken at several levels. Transplant donors with generalized sepsis and active urinary tract infections should be adequately treated with antibiotics prior to donation. Donors and recipients should receive preoperative antibiotics, and serious attempts at eradicating recipient urinary tract infection should be made preoperatively, either with long-term antibiotics or pretransplant native nephrectomy if the source of infection is within the kidney. The bladder should be irrigated with povidone–iodine or antibiotic solution just prior to opening the bladder intraoperatively, and the transplant wound should be thoroughly irrigated on completion of all anastomoses. In many cases, the organism isolated from the peritransplant infection is identical to the organism cultured preoperatively from the recipient urine (99).

A very unusual presentation of peritransplant abscess is rupture of the infected fluid into the peritoneal cavity with the development of peritonitis (99,102). This development has an associated mortality of 80% (102).

ALLOGRAFT FRACTURE

Fracture of the renal allograft is rare. Fracture historically has occurred late in the course of an episode of acute rejection when the patient has returned to dialysis (103–108). The patient presents with pain at the site of the transplant and with hypotension. Operative findings vary, but in most reported series, the fracture is linear, shallow, and located on the convex surface of the kidney.

The incidence of allograft fracture ranges from 0.14% to 8.5%, with the true figure likely very low, and the incidence has decreased as rates of severe rejection have dropped over the decades. This complication is related to severe swelling of the kidney during acute rejection, but it has been suggested that anticoagulation during hemodialysis may contribute to the bleeding as well. It is interesting that fracture of the native kidney has been reported in conditions such as hydronephrosis and pregnancy, in patients receiving anticoagulant therapy, and in association with renal vein thrombosis, indicating that the mechanisms involved are not solely related to immunologic aspects of the rejection process.

Whether the transplant can be saved following fracture depends on the clinical circumstances and operative findings. If the fractured area is shallow, there may be some merit in repairing the kidney with pledgeted sutures or mesh, as has been reported (108,109). However, in most circumstances, rejection is advanced at the time of rupture and transplant nephrectomy is the wisest alternative, in conjunction with careful and thorough evacuation of the resultant peritransplant hematoma.

HYPERCALCEMIA

Virtually all patients with chronic renal failure have secondary hyperparathyroidism as the result of inability to produce 1,25-di-hydroxyvitamin D, renal phosphate retention, and extracellular complexing of circulating calcium. After successful renal transplantation, postoperative hypercalcemia is not uncommon. When the hypercalcemia is resistant to phosphate repletion, this condition has been referred to as tertiary post-transplant hyperparathyroidism, suggesting that the hypertrophic parathyroid glands have become autonomous. True adenomatous degeneration is rare (110) but parathyroid hyperplasia may persist for prolonged periods of time even with a well-functioning transplant.

Early post-transplant hypercalcemia occurs in up to 28.6% of renal transplant recipients (111). The most important etiologic factor appears to be slow resolution of hyperactive parathyroid function in combination with increased absorption of calcium as the result of restored 1,25-dihydroxyvitamin D activity (112). In addition, renal transplant recipients are commonly phosphate depleted in the postoperative period, a factor that contributes to hypercalcemia. Current practice is to treat conservatively with aggressive diuresis and elimination of phosphate-binding antacids.

In most cases, excess parathyroid function subsides enough in the post-transplant period to avoid long-term hypercalcemia. Some patients do develop long-term hypercalcemia if the hypertrophic glands fail to involute (111). This condition may persist and, depending on the severity of the hypercalcemia, may adversely influence transplant function (112). Subtotal parathyroidectomy should be reserved for those hyperparathyroid patients who have serum calcium in excess of 12.5 mg per dL or who experience persistent symptoms (113).

REFERENCES

1. Garcia-Rinaldi R, Lefrak EA, Defore WW, et al. In situ preservation of cadaver kidneys for transplantation. *Ann Surg* 1975;182:576.
2. Englesbe MJ, Dubay DA, Gillespie BW, et al. Risk factors for urinary complications after renal transplantation. *Am J Transplant* 2007;7:1536–1541.
3. Rosenthal JT, Shaw BW Jr, Hardesty RL, et al. Principles of multiple organ procurement from cadaver donors. *Ann Surg* 1983;198:617.
4. Sahani DV, Rastogi N, Greenfield AC, et al. Multi-detector row CT in evaluation of 94 living renal donors by readers with varied experience. *Radiology* 2005;235(3):905–910.
5. Kawamoto S, Montgomery RA, Lawler LP, et al. Multidetector CT angiography for preoperative evaluation of living laparoscopic kidney donors. *Am J Roentgenol* 2003;180:1633–1638.

6. Ratner LE, Kavoussi LR, Schulam PG, et al. Comparison of laparoscopic live donor nephrectomy versus the standard open approach. *Transplant Proc* 1997;29:138.
7. Flowers JL, Jacobs S, Cho E, et al. Comparison of open and live donor nephrectomy. *Ann Surg* 1997;226:483.
8. Wolf JS Jr, Marcovich R, Merion RM, et al. Prospective, case-matched comparison of hand-assisted laparoscopic and open surgical live donor nephrectomy. *J Urol* 2000;163:1650–1653.
9. Smith JM, Stablein D, Singh A, et al. Decreased risk of renal allograft thrombosis associated with interleukin-2 receptor antagonists: a report of the NAPRTCS. *Am J Transplant* 2006;6(3):585–588.
10. Englesbe MJ, Punch JD, Armstrong DR, et al. Single-center study of technical graft loss in 714 consecutive renal transplants. *Transplantation* 2004;78(4):623–626.
11. Iwami D, Harada H, Miura M, et al. Successfully rescued renal graft artery thrombosis by ex vivo thrombectomy: a case report. *Transplant Proc* 2009;41(5):1951–1953.
12. Libicher M, Radeleff B, Grenacher L, et al. Interventional therapy of vascular complications following renal transplantation. *Clin Transplant* 2006;20(Suppl 17):55–59.
13. Rouviere O, Berger P, Beziat C, et al. Acute thrombosis of renal transplant artery: graft salvage by means of intra-arterial fibrinolysis. *Transplantation* 2002;73(3):403–409.
14. Kusyk T, Verran D, Stewart G, et al. Increased risk of hemorrhagic complications in renal allograft recipients receiving systemic heparin early posttransplantation. *Transplant Proc* 2005;37(2):1026–1028.
15. Osman Y, Shokeir A, Ali-el-Dein B. Vascular complications after live donor renal transplantation: study of risk factors and effects on graft and patient survival. *J Urol* 2003;169(3):859–862.
16. Potti A, Danielson B, Sen K. True mycotic aneurysm of a renal artery allograft. *Am J Kidney Dis* 1998;31(1):E3.
17. Mathis AS, Dave N, Shah NK, et al. Bleeding and thrombosis in high-risk renal transplantation candidates using heparin. *Ann Pharmacother* 2004;38(4):537–543.
18. Sienko J, Tejchman K, Cnotliwy M, et al. Crossed bypass femorofemoralis in patient with external iliac artery occlusion in the course of septic hemorrhage after renal graft explantatation. *Ann Transplantation* 2006;11(3):12–14.
19. Pfundstein J, Roghmann MC, Schwalbe RS, et al. A randomized trial of surgical antimicrobial prophylaxis with and without vancomycin in organ transplant patients. *Clin Transplant* 1999;13:245–252.
20. Merion RM, Calne RY. Allograft renal vein thrombosis. *Transplant Proc* 1985;17:1746.
21. Salehipour M, Salahi H, Jalaeian H, et al. Vascular complications following 1500 consecutive living and cadaveric donor renal transplantations: a single center study. *Saudi J Kid Dis Transplant* 2009;20(4): 570–572.
22. Melamed ML, Kim HS, Jaar BG, et al. Combined percutaneous mechanical and chemical thrombectomy for renal vein thrombosis in kidney transplant recipients. *Am J Transplant* 2005;5(3):621–626.
23. Sterrett SP, Mercer D, Johanning J, et al. Salvage of renal allograft using venous thrombectomy in the setting of iliofemoral venous thrombosis. *Nephrol Dial Transplant* 2004;19(6):1637–1639.
24. Alkhunaizi AM, Olyaei AJ, Barry JM. Efficacy and safety of low molecular weight heparin in renal transplantation. *Transplantation* 1998;66(4):533–534.
25. Allen RD, Michie CA, Murie JA, et al. Deep venous thrombosis after renal transplantation. *Surg Gynecol Obstet* 1987;164(2):137–142.
26. Matas AJ, Sibley R, Mauer M, et al. The value of needle renal allograft biopsy. I. A retrospective study of biopsies performed during putative rejection episodes. *Ann Surg* 1983;197:226.
27. Rohr MS. Renal allograft acute tubular necrosis. II. A light and electron microscopic study of biopsies taken at procurement and after revascularization. *Ann Surg* 1983;197:663.
28. Manno C, Strippoli GFM, Arnesano L, et al. Predictors of bleeding complications in percutaneous ultrasound-guided renal biopsy. *Kidney Int* 2004;66:1570–1577.
29. Hergesell O, Felten H, Andrassy K, et al. Safety of ultrasound-guided percutaneous renal biopsy—retrospective analysis of 1090 consecutive cases. *Nephrol Dial Transplant* 1998;13:975–977.
30. Debruyne FMJ, Koene RAP, Moonen WA, et al. Intrarenal arteriovenous fistula following renal allograft biopsy. *Eur Urol* 1978;4: 435.
31. Baquero A, Morris MC, Cope C, et al. Selective embolization of vascular complications following renal biopsy of the transplant kidney. *Transplant Proc* 1985;17:1751.
32. Guz G, Yuksel A, Onal B, et al. Selective embolization in the management of arteriovenous fistula after renal allograft biopsy preserves renal allograft function. *Int Urol Nephrol* 2005;37(1):207–208.
33. Lacombe M. Arterial stenosis complicating renal allotransplantation in man: a study of 38 cases. *Ann Surg* 1975;181:283.
34. Dimitroulis D, Bokos J, Zavos G, et al. Vascular complications in renal transplantation: a single-center experience in 1367 renal transplantations and review of the literature. *Transplant Proc* 2009;41(5):1609–1614.
35. Polak WG, Jezior D, Garcarek J, et al. Incidence and outcome of transplant renal artery stenosis: single center experience. *Transplant Proc* 2006;38(1):131–132.
36. Fernandez-Najera JE, Beltran S, Aparicio M, et al. Transplant renal artery stenosis: association with acute vascular rejection. *Transplant Proc* 2006;38(8):2404–2405.
37. Dickerman RM, Peters PC, Hull AR, et al. Surgical correction of post-transplant renovascular hypertension. *Ann Surg* 1980;192:639.
38. Ridgway D, White SA, Nixon M, et al. Primary endoluminal stenting of transplant renal artery stenosis from cadaver and non-heart-beating donor kidneys. *Clin Transplant* 2006;20(3):394–400.
39. VanSon WJ, VanderSlikke LB, Hoorntje SJ. Captopril-induced deterioration of graft function in patients with a transplant renal artery stenosis. *Proc Eur Dial Transplant Assoc* 1983;20:325.
40. Gao J, Ng A, Shih G, et al. Intrarenal color duplex ultrasonography: a window to vascular complications of renal transplants. *J Ultrasound Med* 2007;26(10):1403–1418.
41. Lanzman RS, Voiculescu A, Walther C, et al. ECG-gated nonenhanced 3D steady-state free precession MR angiography in assessment of transplant renal arteries: comparison with DSA. *Radiology* 2009;252(3): 914–921.
42. Pappas P, Zavos G, Kaza S, et al. Angioplasty and stenting of arterial stenosis affecting renal transplant function. *Transplant Proc* 2008;40(5): 1391–1396.
43. Peregrin JH, Stribrna J, Lacha J, et al. Long-term follow-up of renal transplant patients with renal artery stenosis treated by percutaneous angioplasty. *Eur J Radiol* 2008; 66(3):512–518.
44. Peregrin JH, Burgelova M. Restoration of failed renal graft function after successful angioplasty of pressure-resistant renal artery stenosis using a cutting balloon: a case report. *Cardiovasc Intervent Radiol* 2009;32(3):548–553.
45. Henning BF, Kuchlbauer S, Boger CA. Percutaneous transluminal angioplasty as first-line treatment of transplant renal artery stenosis. *Clin Nephrol* 2009;71(5):543–549.
46. Hagen G, Wadstrom J, Magnusson M, et al. Outcome after percutaneous transluminal angioplasty of arterial stenosis in renal transplant patients. *Acta Radiologica* 2009;50(3):270–275.
47. Moers C, Kornmann NS, Leuvenink HG, et al. The influence of deceased donor age and old-for-old allocation on kidney transplant outcome. *Transplantation* 2009;88(4):542–552.
48. Cecka JM. Kidney Transplantation in the United States. In: Clinical Transplants 2008, Cecka JM, Terasaki PI, Eds. *UCLA Tissue Typing Laboratory*, pp 1–18.
49. Barlow AD, Metcalfe MS, Johari Y, et al. Case-matched comparison of long-term results of non-heart beating and heart-beating donor renal transplants. *Br J Surg* 2009;96(6):685–691.
50. Yarlagadda SG, Coca SG, Formica RN Jr, et al. Association between delayed graft function and allograft and patient survival: a systematic review and meta-analysis. *Nephrol Dial Transplantat* 2009;24(3):1039–1047.
51. Nogueira JM, Haririan A, Jacobs SC, et al. The detrimental effect of poor early graft function after laparoscopic live donor nephrectomy on graft outcomes. *Am J Transplant* 2009;9(2):337–347.
52. Sung RS, Christensen LL, Leichtman AB, et al. Determinants of discard of expanded criteria donor kidneys: Impact of biopsy and machine perfusion. *Am J Transplant* 2008;8:783–792.
53. Hetzel GR, Klein B, Brause M, et al. Risk factors for delayed graft function after renal transplantation and their significance for long-term clinical outcome. *Transpl Int* 2002;15:10–16.
54. Shimshak RR, Hattner RS, Tucker C, et al. Segmental acute tubular necrosis in kidneys with multiple renal arteries transplanted from living-related donors. *J Nucl Med* 1977;18:1074.
55. Provoost AP, Kaptein L, VanAken M. Nephrotoxicity of cyclosporine A in rats with a diminished renal function. *Clin Nephrol* 1986;25:S162.
56. Baxter GM. Ultrasound of renal transplantation. *Clin Radiol* 2001;56: 802–818.
57. Diethelm AG, Dubovsky EV, Whelchel JD. Diagnosis of impaired renal function after kidney transplantation using renal scintigraphy, renal plasma flow and urinary excretion of hippurate. *Ann Surg* 1980;191:604.

58. Wight J, Chilcott J, Holmes M, et al. The clinical and cost-effectiveness of pulsatile machine perfusion versus cold storage of kidneys for transplantation retrieved from heart-beating and non-heart-beating donors. *Health Technol Assess* 2003;7:1–94.
59. Geddes CC, Woo YM, Jardine AG. The impact of delayed graft function on the long-term outcome of renal transplantation. *J Nephrol* 2002; 15:17–21.
60. Li Marzi V, Filocamo MT, Dattolo E, et al. The treatment of fistulae and ureteral stenosis after kidney transplantation. *Transplant Proc* 2005;37(6): 2516–2517.
61. Karam G, Maillet F, Parant S, et al. Ureteral necrosis after kidney transplantation: risk factors and impact on graft and patient survival. *Transplantation* 2004;78(5):725–729.
62. Mundy MR, Podesta ML, Bewick M, et al. The urological complications of 1000 renal transplants. *Br J Urol* 1981;53:397.
63. Laughlin KR, Tilney NL, Richie JP. Urologic complications in 718 renal transplant patients. *Surgery* 1984;95:297.
64. Santiago-Delpin EA, Baquero A, Gonzalez Z. Low incidence of urologic complications after renal transplantation. *Am J Surg* 1986;151:374.
65. Ohl DA, Konnak JW, Campbell DA Jr, et al. Extravesical ureteroneocystostomy in renal transplantation. *J Urol* 1988;139:499.
66. Koehler PR, Kanenafo HH, Maxwell JC. Ultrasonic "B" scanning in the diagnosis of complications in renal transplant patients. *Radiology* 1976;119:661.
67. Morley P, Barnett E, Bell PRF, et al. Ultrasound in the diagnosis of fluid collections following renal transplantation. *Clin Radiol* 1975;26:199.
68. Silver TM, Campbell DA Jr, Wicks JD, et al. Peritransplant fluid collections: ultrasonic evaluation and clinical significance. *Radiology* 1981; 138:145.
69. Bhagat VJ, Gordon RL, Osorio RW. Ureteral obstructions and leaks after renal transplantation: outcome of percutaneous antegrade ureteral stent placement in 44 patients. *Radiology* 1998;209(1):159–167.
70. Alcaraz A, Bujons A, Pascual X. Percutaneous management of transplant ureteral fistulae is feasible in selected cases. *Transplant Proc* 2005; 37(5):2111–2114.
71. Karmi SA, Dagher FJ, Ramos E, et al. Spermatic cord: cause of ureteral obstruction in renal allograft recipients. *Urology* 1978;11:380.
72. Ireton RC, Krieger JN, Rudd TG, et al. Percutaneous endoscopic treatment of fungus ball obstruction in a renal allograft. *Transplantation* 1985;39:453.
73. Walzer Y, Bear RA. Ureteral obstruction of renal transplant due to ureteral candidiasis. *Urology* 1983;21:295.
74. Lieberman RP, Glass NR, Crummy AB, et al. Non-operative percutaneous management of urinary fistulas and strictures in renal transplantation. *Surg Gynecol Obstet* 1982;155:667.
75. Loening SA, Banowsky LH, Braun WE, et al. Bladder neck contracture and ureteral stricture as complications of renal transplantation. *J Urol* 1975;114:688.
76. Nerstrom B, Brix E, Clausen E, et al. Late urological complications following human kidney transplantation. *Acta Clin Scand Suppl* 1973; 433:113.
77. Rosenberg RJ, Schweizer RT, Spencer RP. Ureteral leak after renal transplantation. *Clin Nucl Med* 1999;24(6):440–442.
78. Goldman MN, Burleson RL, Tilney NL. Calyceal–cutaneous fistulae in renal transplant patients. *Ann Surg* 1976;184:679.
79. Kogan BA, Konnak JW, MacGregor RJ, et al. Spontaneous rupture of renal pelvis after renal transplantation. *Urology* 1981;18:456.
80. Saidi RF, Wertheim JA, Ko DS, et al. Impact of donor kidney recovery method on lymphatic complications in kidney transplantation. *Transplant Proc* 2008;40(4):1054–1055.
81. Derweesh IH, Ismail HR, Goldfarb DA, et al. Intraoperative placing of drains decreases the incidence of lymphocele and deep vein thrombosis after renal transplantation. *BJU Int* 2008;101(11):1415–1419.
82. Zietek Z, Sulikowski T, Tejchman K. Lymphocele after kidney transplantation. *Transplant Proc* 2007;39(9):2744–2747.
83. Smyth GP, Beitz G, Eng MP, et al. Long-term outcome of cadaveric renal transplant after treatment of symptomatic lymphocele. *J Urol* 2006;176(3):1069–1072.
84. Hamza A, Fischer K, Koch E, et al. Diagnostics and therapy of lymphoceles after kidney transplantation. *Transplant Proc* 2006;38(3):701–706.
85. Brooks JG, Hulbert JC, Patel AS, et al. The diagnosis and treatment of lymphoceles associated with renal transplantation. A report of six cases and a review of the literature. *Br J Urol* 1978;50:307.
86. Diethelm AG. Anuria secondary to perirenal lymphocele: a complication of renal transplantation. *South Med J* 1972;65:350.
87. Ward K. The origin of lymphoceles following renal transplantation. *Transplantation* 1978;25:346.
88. Cockett ATK, Netto KV. Increased lymphatic drainage from renal transplant. *Urology* 1973;2:571.
89. Tasar M, Gulec B, Saglam M. Posttransplant symptomatic lymphocele treatment with percutaneous drainage and ethanol sclerosis: long-term follow-up. *Clin Imaging* 2005;29(2):109–116.
90. Silas AM, Forauer AR, Perrich KD, et al. Sclerosis of postoperative lymphoceles: avoidance of prolonged catheter drainage with use of a fibrin sealant. *J Vasc Interv Radiol* 2006;17(11 Pt 1):1791–1795.
91. Belzer FO, Salvatierra O, Schwerzer RT, et al. Prevention of wound infection by topical antibiotics in high risk patients. *Am J Surg* 1973; 126:180.
92. Lynch RJ, Ranney DN, Shijie C, et al. Obesity, surgical site infection, and outcome following renal transplantation. *Ann Surg* 2009;250(6): 1014–1020.
93. Menezes FG, Wey SB, Peres CA, et al. Risk factors for surgical site infection in kidney transplant recipients. *Infect Control Hosp Epidemiol* 2008;29(8):771–773.
94. Troppmann C, Pierce JL, Gandhi MM, et al. Higher surgical wound complication rates with sirolimus immunosuppression after kidney transplantation: a matched-pair pilot study. *Transplantation* 2003;76(2): 426–429.
95. Kyriakides GK, Simmons RL, Najarian JS. Wound infections in renal transplant wounds: pathogenetic and prognostic factors. *Ann Surg* 1975;182:770.
96. Lee HM, Madge GE, Mendez-Picon G, et al. Surgical complications in renal transplant recipients. *Surg Clin North Am* 1978;58:285.
97. Schwerzer RT, Kountz SL, Belzer FO. Wound complications in recipients of renal transplants. *Ann Surg* 1973;177:58.
98. Starzl TE, Groth CG, Putnam CW, et al. Urologic complications in 216 human recipients of renal transplants. *Ann Surg* 1970;172:1.
99. Lorber MI, Campbell DA Jr, Konnak JW, et al. Etiology and management of early and late peritransplant infections. *J Urol* 1982;127: 870.
100. Lartro JE, Mustapha N, Mee AD, et al. Ileal urinary diversion in patients with renal transplants. *Br J Urol* 1975;47:603.
101. Markland C, Kelly WD, Buselmeier T, et al. Renal transplantation into iliac urinary conduits. *Transplant Proc* 1972;4:629.
102. Han T, VanHook EJ, Simmons RL, et al. Prognostic factors of peritoneal infections in transplant patients. *Surgery* 1978;84:403.
103. Martinez Mansur R, Piana M, Codone J, et al. The rupture of the renal graft. *Archivos Espanoles de Urologia* 2006;59(5):489–492.
104. Shahrokh H, Rasouli H, Zargar MA, et al. Spontaneous kidney allograft rupture. *Transplant Proc* 2005;37(7):3079–3080.
105. Lee HM. Surgical techniques of renal transplantation. In: Morris PJ, ed. *Kidney transplantation, principles and practice.* New York: Grune & Stratton; 1979.
106. Sanchez de la Nieta MD, Sanchez-Fructuoso AI, Alcazar R, et al. Higher graft salvage rate in renal allograft rupture associated with acute tubular necrosis. *Transplant Proc* 2004;36(10):3016–3018.
107. Richardson AJ, Higgins RM, Jaskowski AJ. Spontaneous rupture of renal allografts: the importance of renal vein thrombosis in the cyclosporin era. *Br J Surg* 1990;77(5):558–560.
108. Gandy R, Asthana S, Menon KV, et al. The use of polyglactin 910 mesh to obtain haemostasis and prevent further splitting in a fractured transplant kidney. *Ann R Coll Surg Engl* 2006;88(6):590–591.
109. Dryburgh P, Porter KA, Krom RAF, et al. Should the ruptured renal allograft be removed? *Arch Surg* 1979;114:850.
110. Diethelm AG, Edwards RP, Whelchel JD. The natural history and surgical treatment of hypercalcemia before and after renal transplantation. *Surg Gynecol Obstet* 1982;154:481.
111. Parfitt AM. Hypercalcemic hyperparathyroidism following renal transplantation and complications for population control in the parathyroid gland. *Miner Electrolyte Metab* 1982;8:92.
112. McCarron DA, Bennett WM, Muther RS, et al. Post-transplant hyperparathyroidism demonstration of retained control of parathyroid function by ionized calcium. *Am J Clin Nutr* 1980;33: 1536.
113. David DS, Sakai S, Brennan L. Hypercalcemia after renal transplantation. Long-term follow-up data. *N Engl J Med* 1973;289:398.

Complications of Liver Transplantation

Shawn J. Pelletier

INTRODUCTION

Liver transplantation is the treatment of choice for patients with end-stage liver disease due to a variety of disorders as well as for patients with severe acute liver failure. This life-saving procedure is primarily limited by the number of available organs. Graft and patient survival rates have increased gradually since the 1980s (1). At present, the average 1-year patient survival rate in the United States is approaching 90% (2). Patients who survive the first year typically have relatively low mortality rates thereafter (3,4) and current 10-year patient survival is >60% (2). Early death and graft loss can largely be traced to complications that occur at the time of transplantation or in the perioperative period, whereas late death is usually due to the cardiovascular disease or the development of immunosuppression-related infection or malignancy (3,4). Much of the improvement in early mortality can be attributed to improved immunosuppression and advances in the diagnosis and management of complications.

COMPLICATIONS DURING DECEASED DONOR ORGAN PROCUREMENT

The liver transplant procedure truly begins with the donor organ. Despite the recent development of living donor liver transplantation, the vast majority of liver grafts in the United States continue to derive from deceased donors. Complications that occur during procurement of the liver graft from deceased donors include intraoperative cardiac arrest and injury to the portal vascular structures. Donors who suffer intraoperative cardiac arrest can be considered to be similar to controlled donation following cardiac death (DCD) donors. As such, cardiac arrest of the donor should not be considered a contraindication to donation (5). Nijkamp et al. (6) reported that almost one in three donor livers had some injury related to procurement. While most were minor, 7% were clinically relevant and 17% were vascular in nature (6). Injury to the portal vascular structures should not generally preclude use of a donor graft for transplantation given the multiple options that are available for vascular reconstruction. Laceration of the portal vein can be repaired using a segment of donor iliac vein or inferior vena cava (IVC), while injuries to the arterial supply may be salvaged using donor iliac arterial grafts (7). Injury to the suprahepatic IVC cuff may occur and can be reconstructed with an end-to-end extension graft using the infrahepatic IVC from the same donor (8). Although embarrassing, the need to reconstruct the hepatic arterial circulation of a donor liver should not cause undue concern, given that reconstruction of a replaced right hepatic artery or other aberrant vessel is frequently necessary despite the finest surgical technique and a satisfactory outcome can be expected (7).

Shawn J. Pelletier: University of Michigan Health System, 1500 East Medical Center, Ann Arbor, MI 48109-5300

PRIMARY NONFUNCTION

Primary nonfunction of the allograft is the single most disastrous complication following orthotopic liver transplantation (OLT). Primary nonfunction is diagnosed by the presence of profound coagulopathy, metabolic acidosis, and hepatic transaminase values that are >3,000 U/mL. The etiology of primary nonfunction is thought to be primarily preservation injury, although recipient factors are important as well (9–11). Patients rapidly become exceedingly ill with progressive renal, pulmonary, neurologic, and cardiac failure. Survival beyond the fifth postoperative day is uncommon, and the only available therapy is retransplantation. An effective method of temporary hepatic support continues to be elusive despite decades of research (12). Initial reports suggested that prostaglandin E1 may improve immediate liver function (13). Later studies of prostaglandin E1 therapy failed to demonstrate a clinically significant decrease in the rate of primary nonfunction (14). To date, no pharmacologic therapy aimed at preventing primary nonfunction has been shown to be effective in controlled studies.

The best means of dealing with primary nonfunction in liver transplantation is avoiding its occurrence. Numerous factors have been associated with primary nonfunction including steatosis of the liver graft, older donor age, prolonged cold ischemia, DCD donors, split livers, need for portal vein reconstruction, donor hypernatremia, and transplantation of high-risk recipients (9,15–22). Despite intensive scrutiny, objective variables fail to provide strong predictive value about whether a donor liver will function in the recipient. In fact, the factor with the highest predictive value has been the subjective impression of the surgeon who removed the graft from the donor (23).

At present, patients in the United States with primary nonfunction are eligible to be re-listed as United Network for Organ Sharing (UNOS) Status 1A. This emergency transplant status is reserved for patients who received a transplanted liver within 7 days with an aspartate transaminase (AST) ≥3,000 along with either coagulopathy (INR ≥2.5) or an acidosis (defined as having an arterial pH ≤7.30, venous pH <7.25, or lactate ≥4 mmol/L) or if the recipient is anhepatic (24). One-year patient survival following retransplant for primary nonfunction has been reported at 66% and is not unlike survival rates for retransplantation for other indications (25).

Status 1A patients receive regional priority over less ill patients. Despite this advantage, some patients deteriorate during the waiting process. Total hepatectomy with temporary portacaval shunt has been advocated as a possible means of avoiding the adverse effects associated with the effluent from the nonviable liver graft (26). There is insufficient experience with this technique to evaluate whether it offers a survival benefit.

GRAFT REJECTION

Liver transplantation was revolutionized in the early 1980s by the introduction of cyclosporine and refined in the 1990s by the availability of tacrolimus (27). Triple immunosuppression therapy, including a calcineurin inhibitor, mycophenolate, and prednisone, has been demonstrated to have lower rejection rates when compared with dual therapy (28). Despite this success, acute rejection remains relatively common following liver transplantation, with an incidence between 7% and 60% (29–31). The majority of acute cellular rejection episodes occur early, usually within 6 weeks post-transplantation. Early episodes usually resolve with antirejection treatment (29). Acute rejection following liver transplantation may be difficult to diagnose definitively because recurrent disease such as hepatitis C virus infection (HCV) may have similar clinical signs and ambiguous histopathology (32). Assays to evaluate immune function (33) to aid in the diagnosis of acute rejection are available but their utility has yet to be validated in randomized clinical trials.

Unlike kidney transplantation, the sharing of human leukocyte antigens (HLAs) does not appear to decrease rejection rates (34). Also, unlike kidney transplantation, the occurrence of an episode of acute rejection in the first year is not associated with worsened long-term outcome (35). Even late rejection does not carry an adverse prognosis as long as rejection is detected and treated (36). Chronic hepatic graft rejection, a rare phenomenon, manifests as ductopenia, or the "vanishing bile duct syndrome" (37). Once ductopenic rejection manifests, the only effective treatment to date has been retransplantation.

INCISIONAL COMPLICATIONS

Compared with other solid organ transplant procedures, liver transplantation has one of the highest rates of surgical site infection, developing in 10% to 38% of patients (38–42). Liver recipients that develop surgical site infections have been found to have almost a three-fold increased risk for graft loss or death (40). Predisposing factors include poor wound healing due to corticosteroid therapy, malnutrition, a high incidence of wound hematomas secondary to thrombocytopenia and coagulopathy, attenuated musculature due to ascites and cachexia, use of Roux-en-Y biliary reconstruction, small graft to recipient mass ratio, obesity, and prolonged operative times (40,43). Although corticosteroids are currently being greatly reduced, rapidly weaned, or eliminated from immunosuppressive regimens altogether, it is likely that incisional hernias will remain a significant problem following this procedure. Newer immunosuppressive agents, such as everolimus and sirolimus, that profoundly inhibit smooth muscle cellular proliferation have been reported to increase the incidence of incisional complications if used perioperatively in liver transplant recipients (44–46) but remains controversial (47).

Incisional hernia repair should be deferred until the patient has stable graft function and has been withdrawn from corticosteroids or is taking a stable, low dose. Repair of large hernias of the bilateral subcostal incision often entails the use of a large piece of mesh. Investigators report success using laparoscopic techniques to repair incisional hernias following liver transplantation (48,49).

Abdominal wall closure following liver transplantation may not always be possible due to a large liver allograft or bowel edema from prolonged clamping of the portal vein or massive resuscitation if excess bleeding was encountered. In this setting, abdominal closure may lead to unacceptable intrathoracic or abdominal pressure. Acute renal failure is associated with excessive increases in intraabdominal pressure postoperatively (50). This observation suggests that some instances of acute renal failure may be avoided by recognition of intraabdominal hypertension, defined as >25 mm Hg (51), and treatment by reexploration and closure of the incision with prosthetic or biological material if necessary (52). This approach has been successful with trauma patients, where the abdominal compartment syndrome has become a widely recognized phenomenon (53).

Fasciitis may lead to dehiscence and an open abdomen. Numerous techniques have been described for temporary wound closure in liver transplant recipients (54–56). Recently, the use of biological mesh has been described and can allow early closure with avoidance of abdominal compartment syndrome (57). Figure 48.1 depicts a liver recipient who developed fasciitis and was closed with human acellular dermal matrix after extensive fascial debridement. Use of the nonvascularized fascia from deceased donor rectus muscle has also been described with a low incidence of postoperative hernia (58).

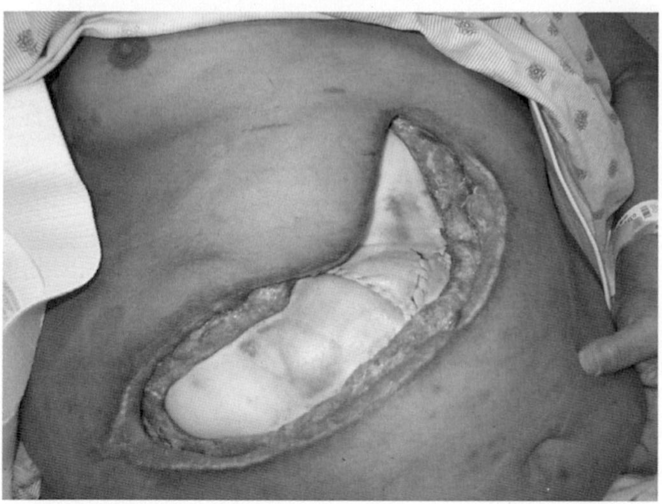

FIGURE 48.1. Closure of an abdominal liver transplant incision with human acellular dermal matrix (AlloDerm®) after extensive fascial debridement for fasciitis complicating a wound infection.

RENAL FAILURE

Renal failure may occur either acutely or chronically following the procedure. Acute renal failure is usually due to acute tubular necrosis. This complication is most often the result of poor renal perfusion during the operation due to intraoperative blood loss, clamping of the suprarenal vena cava, or insufficient replacement of fluid losses during the procedure. Liver transplant patients are predisposed to the development of acute tubular necrosis because of the physiologic derangements associated with cirrhotic liver disease. These include decreased blood pressure, increased cardiac output, and decreased peripheral vascular resistance. These hemodynamic disturbances are believed to be caused by peripheral shunting of blood due to vasoactive substances that are improperly metabolized in the liver. Together, these factors mean that patients with advanced chronic liver disease are universally prerenal before the operation begins. In addition, many liver transplant patients have preexisting renal insufficiency due to hepatorenal syndrome at the time of transplantation.

Current liver allocation is based on the Model for End-stage Liver Disease (MELD) score in which an elevated serum creatinine or a requirement for dialysis leads to a higher MELD score, increasing the likelihood for receiving a liver offer. Liver candidates requiring renal replacement therapy for acute renal failure have been identified to have a waiting list mortality of up to 65% and have posttransplant 1-year mortality almost three times higher (30% vs. 9.7%) when compared with recipients not requiring renal replacement therapy (59). Consideration should be given to combined liver kidney transplantation for appropriate candidates.

The influence of surgical technique on postoperative renal failure remains controversial. Cabezuelo et al. reported a decreased incidence of postoperative renal failure with use of the piggyback technique (18%) for caval reconstruction when compared with a bicaval technique with (50%) or without (39%) venovenous bypass (60). The side-to-side caval anastomosis (61) has also been suggested to result in improved inferior vena caval flow with partial clamping (62) and to potentially further decrease the risk for postoperative renal insufficiency. For 500 patients undergoing liver transplant utilizing a cavocavostomy, the incidence of renal failure was reported at 6.2% (63).

Postoperative immunosuppression may also have an effect on early renal function. Cyclosporine has been demonstrated to decrease renal blood flow and lower glomerular filtration rates acutely by up to 43% (64). Interleukin (IL)-2 receptor inhibitor (65–68) or antithymocyte globulin (69–71) induction may improve postoperative renal function by safely allowing a delay in starting a calcineurin inhibitor as well as a decreased dosage post-transplantation.

Chronic renal failure is also a significant problem long term, affecting 18% and 27% of liver recipients at 5 and 10 years post-transplantation, respectively (72–74). Chronic renal failure has been associated with a 4.6-fold increased risk of mortality for nonrenal solid organ transplant recipients (74). The use of nephrotoxic immunosuppressive agents, such as tacrolimus and cyclosporine, that induce progressive loss of renal function is assumed to be the primary cause of most renal insufficiency in this setting. Nephrotoxicity associated with chronic calcineurin inhibitor therapy may be partially abrogated by institution of mycophenolate, sirolimus, or everolimus therapy and withdrawing or lowering the dosage of the calcineurin inhibitor without increasing the risk of either acute or chronic graft rejection (75–78). Improvement in renal function appears to be related to the duration of dysfunction. Withdrawal of calcineurin inhibitors after renal insufficiency has reached an advanced stage is not associated with the same degree of improvement in renal function (79–81). However, attempts at avoiding calcineurin inhibitors altogether have been disappointing due to an increase in early acute rejection (82).

Interestingly, patients who are treated with combined liver/kidney transplantation for chronic liver disease associated with renal failure have fewer episodes of graft rejection compared with recipients of the contralateral grafts from the same donor who received only the kidney grafts or combined kidney/pancreas graft (83). This phenomenon is believed to be due to the immunological advantage conferred by the liver graft on the kidney grafts. The basis for this apparent immunological phenomenon is not understood.

RECURRENT DISEASE

Recurrence of the primary etiology for liver failure has become an increasingly recognized long-term complication of liver transplantation. Hepatitis C virus infection, now the leading cause of cirrhosis in the United States, recurs in the vast majority of cases and leads to cirrhosis within

5 years in 25% of liver recipients (84). The incidence of severe, early recurrence of hepatitis C following liver transplantation appears to be increasing, perhaps due to the increased use of older liver donors (85). While retransplantation for graft loss related to hepatitis C recurrence remains an option, retransplantation of liver recipients with HCV has been demonstrated to have a significantly decreased 1-year survival when compared with those retransplanted for other indications (2,86).

The possibility of recurrent alcoholism has been a concern for liver transplant surgeons since the inception of the procedure. Fortunately, the incidence of recurrent alcohol use in patients receiving liver transplant for alcohol-induced cirrhosis is low, at approximately 15% (87). The incidence of serious liver damage due to recurrent alcohol use is even lower. Given that recidivism rates following conventional alcohol rehabilitation are generally >50%, it appears that liver transplantation is truly the "ultimate eye-opening experience."

For many years, it was believed that autoimmune diseases did not recur because of the immunosuppression used to suppress graft rejection. However, careful follow-up of large cohorts of liver recipients has demonstrated that autoimmune diseases do recur in some patients. Primary biliary cirrhosis, primary sclerosing cholangitis, and autoimmune hepatitis each recur in 15% to 20% of patients within 5 years of the transplant (88–90). It is unclear whether maintenance immunosuppression can be manipulated in such a way as to minimize recurrent autoimmune disease. This possibility seems unlikely given that immunosuppression does not play a role in forestalling the development of cirrhosis in these conditions—with the possible exception of autoimmune hepatitis.

It is currently unclear whether cryptogenic cirrhosis, an indication for transplantation in approximately one-sixth of liver transplant candidates, recurs. Although chronic inflammation is commonly seen on post-transplant biopsies, the incidence of graft failure is low (91).

Hepatocellular carcinoma is the fifth most common cancer worldwide (92) with the number of HCC candidates on the liver transplant waiting list increased by 108% from 2002 to 2008 (2). Transplant of appropriate candidates with stage II or earlier HCC simultaneously treats the malignancy and underlying liver disease and can result in a 4-year patient survival rate of 75% and a recurrence-free survival of 83% (93). If recurrent HCC is identified on post-transplant surveillance, standard treatment includes minimization of immunosuppression. Because of their antineoplastic effects, the use of sirolimus (94) or everolimus (95) has been reported with variable success. Surgical resection may be possible for isolated areas of recurrence and has been associated with reasonable long-term survival (96). Recent reports have suggested a possible benefit of sorafenib (97). Overall, mean survival rates vary between 5 months for recipients with unresectable recurrent disease and 65 months for those undergoing resection (96).

GRAFT VERSUS HOST DISEASE

Graft versus host disease (GVHD) occurs when passenger lymphocytes from the donor that are within the graft are transferred to an immunosuppressed host. The transferred cells colonize the recipient and recognize recipient antigens as foreign. Typically, the skin, intestines, and bone marrow are involved. Since the liver itself is not foreign relative to the lymphocytes, it is not involved. Despite the large number of donor lymphocytes that are present in a liver graft, GVHD is a very uncommon problem following liver transplantation, with an incidence of <1% (98). This low incidence is probably because donor lymphocytes are usually very immunogenic and are promptly destroyed by the recipient immune system. The incidence of GVHD is higher when the donor is both haploidentical to the recipient and also homozygous at several HLA alleles. In this situation, the recipient's immune system does not recognize the donor lymphocytes as foreign. Diagnosis is usually made by tissue biopsy of the affected organ and confirmed by the finding of circulating donor lymphocytes using flow cytometry. Treatment of GVHD consists of intensified immunosuppression. Antitumor necrosis factor alpha therapy has been widely used for the treatment of steroid-resistant acute GVHD in the hematopoietic stem cell transplant setting and etanercept was recently reported to be successful in a liver transplant recipient with GVHD (99). Despite therapy, mortality is high (80%), with most patients dying of infection (100).

INFECTION

Since liver transplantation requires suppression of normal immunological responses, infection is an unavoidable complication, affecting as many as 83% of liver transplant recipients with the majority of severe infections occurring within the first 2 months post-transplantation (101–103). Because of immunosuppression, the signs and symptoms of severe, post-transplant infection may or may not be subtle or abated (104) and a high level of suspicion must be maintained for early diagnosis and improved outcomes. Infections that occur during the initial transplant admission are associated with a mortality rate of 30% compared with 8% for those occurring in subsequent admissions (102).

In addition to the usual bacterial infections that are associated with postoperative patients, liver transplant recipients are also prone to viral and fungal infections. Acute rejection, obesity, and prolonged hospitalization are clear risk factors for clinically important infections (105,106). Biliary complications also dramatically increase the risk of infection. Approximately 20% of late graft loss (after 1 year) in pediatric liver recipients is attributable to infection (107). Cytomegalovirus (CMV) infection, once a common problem, has become much less common due to the routine use of prophylactic oral ganciclovir and valganciclovir.

Fungal infections may be minimized by prophylaxis with topical mycostatin or oral fluconazole or itraconazole (108). Newer agents may offer improved efficacy against aspergillosis and other fungi, rare but deadly opportunistic post-transplant infections (109).

VASCULAR COMPLICATIONS

Vascular complications in general occur at a rate of approximately 10% of all liver transplant recipients and are a frequent cause of early graft loss. Diagnosis is usually suggested by graft dysfunction and confirmed by Doppler examination of the hepatic vasculature. Extensive ascites, hematoma, body habitus, and bowel gas can make the interpretation of Doppler studies difficult in some patients (110). Many centers advocate contrast computed tomography (CT), and it can be an alternative noninvasive technique. Magnetic resonance evaluation is the choice if patients have allergic reactions to contrast or impaired renal function due to the use of iodinated contrast material (111). Magnetic resonance scanning may also be useful for confirmation of ultrasound studies and for the evaluation of hepatic outflow problems. Selective angiography remains the gold standard for diagnosing vascular complications.

HEPATIC ARTERY THROMBOSIS

Hepatic artery thrombosis (HAT), the most common vascular complication of OLT, has an incidence of 4% to 12% in adult patients and up to 40% in children, with a mortality rate of as high as 50% to 60% (112). The clinical presentation of HAT varies from mild transaminase elevation due to ischemic changes in the liver parenchyma to delayed bile leak, bile duct strictures, and relapsing bacteremia and sepsis. Acute thrombosis in the first week following a liver transplant is associated with biliary necrosis and graft failure and invariably requires retransplantation if thrombectomy cannot be performed (113). In contrast, late HAT has a variable clinical course with one-third of patients not requiring intervention (114).

Multiple risk factors for HAT have been identified. Technical factors include a difference in the caliber of donor and recipient arteries, preexisting lesions such as hepatic artery dissection in the donor or recipient and celiac stenosis. A recipient to donor weight ratio of >1.25 is a clear risk factor. The need for reconstructive arterioplasty in the presence of nonstandard donor anatomy, present in as many as 50% of donor livers, is known to predispose to HAT. Nontechnical factors also predispose to hepatic artery problems, most likely because they are associated with graft edema and poor flow. Nontechnical factors include prolonged cold ischemia time, ABO-type incompatibility, biopsy-proven rejection within the first week post-transplant, donor positive/recipient negative CMV status, and the G20210 A prothrombin polymorphism (112,115). Recently, a strong association between cigarette smoking and increased incidence of arterial thrombosis has been found in OLT recipients. Smoking cessation at least 2 years before OLT decreased the risk (116).

While successful thrombectomy and thrombolysis has been reported using an endovascular approach (117–119), there is limited experience and few prospective studies reported in the literature with this approach. Urgent intraoperative thrombectomy with intraoperative thrombolysis and arterial reconstruction can restore arterial flow in up to 88% of recipients with early HAT with a 17-month graft survival of 65% (120). In the pediatric population, immediate surgical thrombectomy for HAT may lead to long-term graft salvage in approximately one of three recipients while others may lose their graft to biliary complications related to ischemia. In contrast, immediate retransplantation may have an improved 5-year patient survival (approximately 70%) but requires the utilization of a second donor organ. Because of the donor organ shortage, attempts at thrombectomy should be made when possible.

HEPATIC ARTERY STENOSIS

In some instances, hepatic artery stenosis is diagnosed because of an elevation of hepatic enzymes, because of new onset biliary complications, or on the basis of a Doppler study obtained for some other, unrelated reason. Although Doppler ultrasonography may suggest this problem, confirmation with angiography is usually required (Fig. 48.2A). Most stenoses occur at either the anastomotic site or because of clamp injury on the native vessel. When detected early in the postoperative period, abdominal exploration with takedown and thrombectomy may be an effective therapeutic option (121). In some instances when recipient inflow is the problem, the use of additional donor arterial graft is necessary to reestablish arterial flow. In cases of late arterial stenosis, selective angiography and balloon angioplasty may be successful (Fig. 48.2B) (122). When the donor arterial system is damaged and after a revision there is absence of flow, retransplantation is necessary.

HEPATIC ARTERY PSEUDOANEURYSM

Hepatic artery pseudoaneurysm is an uncommon but life-threatening complication after OLT. It occurs more commonly in the presence of infected biloma or after using arterial graft reconstruction. Hepatic artery pseudoaneurysms can rupture intraperitoneally and lead to massive hemorrhage. The possibility of a mycotic pseudoaneurysm should be considered (123). Treatment options include surgical resection and reconstruction using homograft, embolization, or exclusion with stent placement (124).

PORTAL VEIN THROMBOSIS OR STENOSIS

Portal vein complications following OLT are relatively uncommon, occurring at a rate of only 1% to 3% (125). Portal venous complications are usually the result of a technical surgical problem, such as size discrepancy, misalignment,

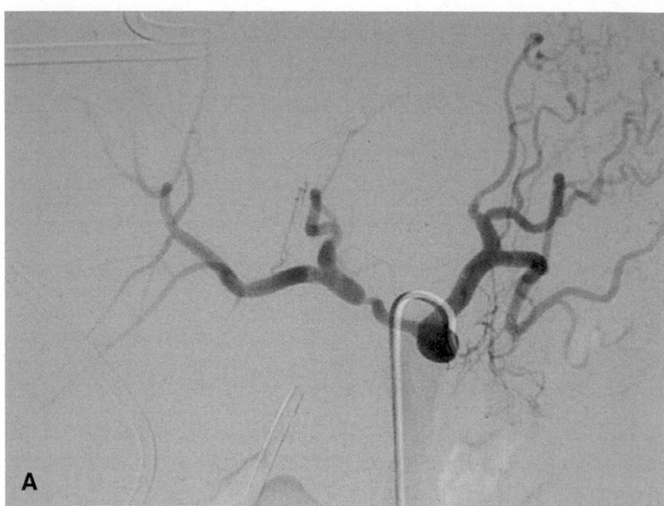

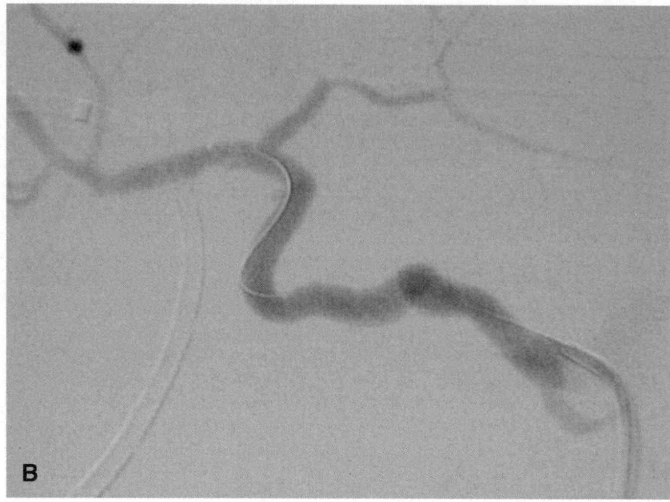

FIGURE 48.2. **A:** Selective hepatic arteriogram demonstrating anastomotic narrowing of the hepatic artery. **B:** Arteriogram following balloon angioplasty showing resolution of the narrowing.

or purse-stringing causing turbulent flow. A higher incidence of portal vein problems is seen in patients who have had previous portal vein operations or prior thrombosis of the portal system and are at an increased risk for post-transplant mortality (126). Patients with portal vein thrombosis or stenosis typically present with complications of portal hypertension, including variceal bleeding and ascites.

Doppler ultrasound examination is usually the first diagnostic tool, but it is inadequate to assess portal pressure gradients across a stricture or focal narrowing. Percutaneous transhepatic direct portography allows the measurement of pressures across a stenotic area, with values of >5 mm Hg being considered significant. Percutaneous transluminal angioplasty with or without stent placement may also be a good choice for this particular problem (Fig. 48.3) (127–129). In cases where there is a recalcitrant stricture, surgical intervention, including thrombectomy, placement of a venous jump graft, use of the left renal vein (130), or creation of a porto-systemic shunt, may be necessary. In very severe cases in which frank hepatic decompensation occurs, retransplantation may be the only option.

COMPLICATIONS OF THE IVC ANASTOMOSIS

Complications arising from the vena cava anastomosis, either stenosis or occlusion, account for a small percentage of all complications. Vena cava problems that take place intraoperatively relate to venous tears in the recipient's cava, which may lead to catastrophic hemorrhage or air embolism. Rapid sternotomy and control of the intrapericardial portion of the IVC may be life-saving in this situation. Post-transplant complications can relate to size discrepancy between the donor and recipient, allowing for rotation of the graft and kinking at the level of the suprahepatic vena cava anastomosis (Fig. 48.4). This circumstance is particularly problematic when the donor is small relative to the recipient. IVC thrombosis can be caused by a hypercoagulable state or by technical errors, such as including the back wall of the anastomosis when suturing the front wall. Hepatic outflow problems usually present with lower extremity edema or severe ascites, or both.

The incidence of outflow problems appears to be related to surgical technique. The traditional bicaval anastomotic technique involves resection of the intrahepatic portion of the recipient vena cava and separate suprahepatic and infrahepatic anastomosis of the donor vena cava to the recipient (Fig. 48.5A). The incidence of caval obstruction using this technique is 1% to 2% (131). The "piggyback technique," involving preservation of the recipient cava, oversewing of the donor infrahepatic cava, and end-to-side anastomosis between the donor and recipient suprahepatic cava, has been advocated as a means of obviating venovenous bypass (Fig. 48.5B) (132,133). The incidence of caval complications using the piggyback technique appears to be higher, at approximately 4% (134). Outflow stenosis appears to be more common if the combined orifice of two, rather than three, hepatic veins is used for the anastomotic site on the recipient (134). More recently, a side-to-side cavocavostomy, where the recipient vena cava is partially clamped in a longitudinal fashion, the supra- and infrahepatic donor IVC is stapled or oversewn, and a venotomy on the posterior aspect of the donor vena cava is sutured to a longitudinal venotomy on the anterior aspect of the recipient IVC, has been described (Fig. 48.6) (61–63). The side-to-side cavocavostomy appears to have a lower rate of IVC complications similar to the bicaval technique without the requirement of complete caval occlusion during anastomosis.

In many cases, hepatic vein or suprahepatic caval stenosis can be successfully treated noninvasively with the use of balloon angioplasty, or stenting, or both (135,136).

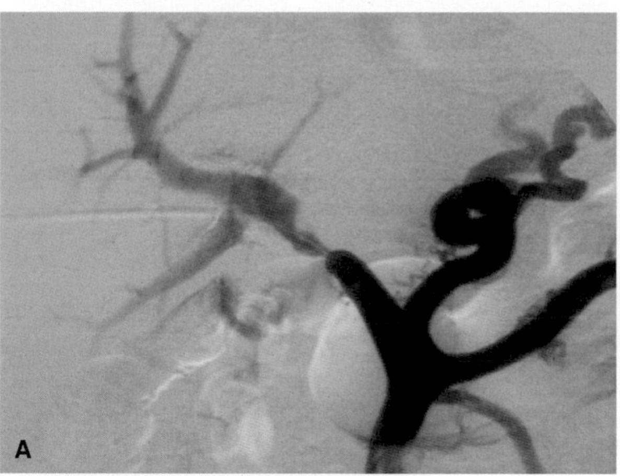

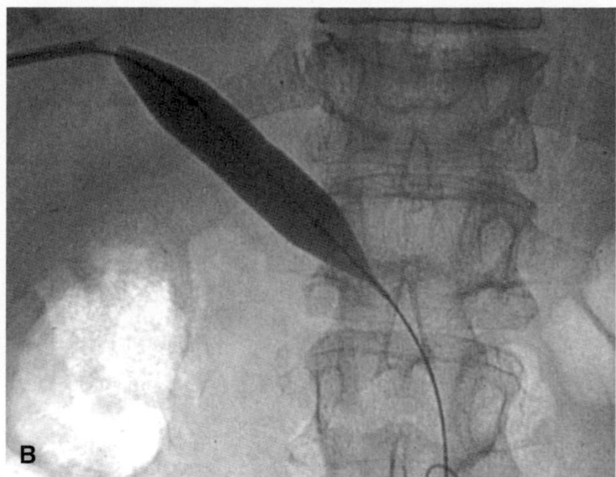

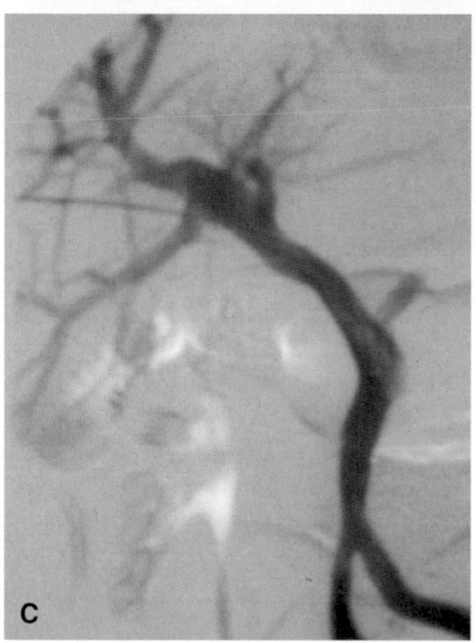

FIGURE 48.3. **A:** Transhepatic portal venogram showing narrowing of the portal vein anastomosis. **B:** Balloon angioplasty of the portal vein at the area of narrowing. **C:** Portal venogram following angioplasty showing resolution of the anastomotic narrowing.

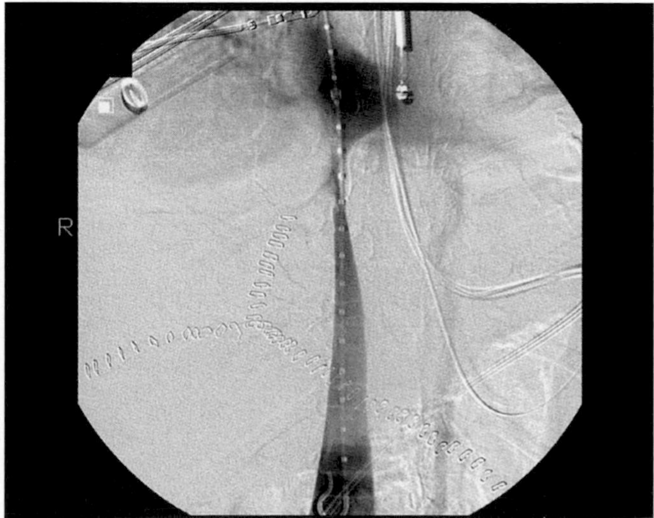

FIGURE 48.4. Venogram of the IVC performed 2 weeks after liver transplantation of a relatively small allograft into a larger recipient using a piggyback technique. The suprahepatic vena cava is stenotic at the junction of the right atrium, likely as a result of rotation of the graft and kinking of the vena cava. This stenosis was successfully treated with venoplasty and stenting of the IVC and right hepatic vein.

BILIARY COMPLICATIONS

Biliary complications following liver transplantation continue to cause substantial morbidity in both the early and late perioperative periods (137). In general, biliary complications can be divided into (a) anastomotic leaks, (b) anastomotic strictures, and (c) intrahepatic biliary strictures. Both anastomotic leaks and strictures are often amenable to endobiliary, percutaneous, or surgical therapy while intrahepatic biliary strictures tend to be more diffuse and progressive, possibly leading to graft loss. In spite of better understanding of the biliary blood supply, improved surgical technique, and the use of absorbable suture material, the reported biliary complication rate varies from 10% to 41% (137,138). The pathogenesis of biliary complications is multifactorial. The single most important factor appears to be poor or absent arterial flow. The transected donor bile duct is totally dependent on arterial flow from the liver graft. Factors that have been associated with biliary problems include prolonged cold and warm ischemia time, sphincter of Oddi dysfunction, CMV infection, vascular rejection, and ABO incompatibility. Recipients with a

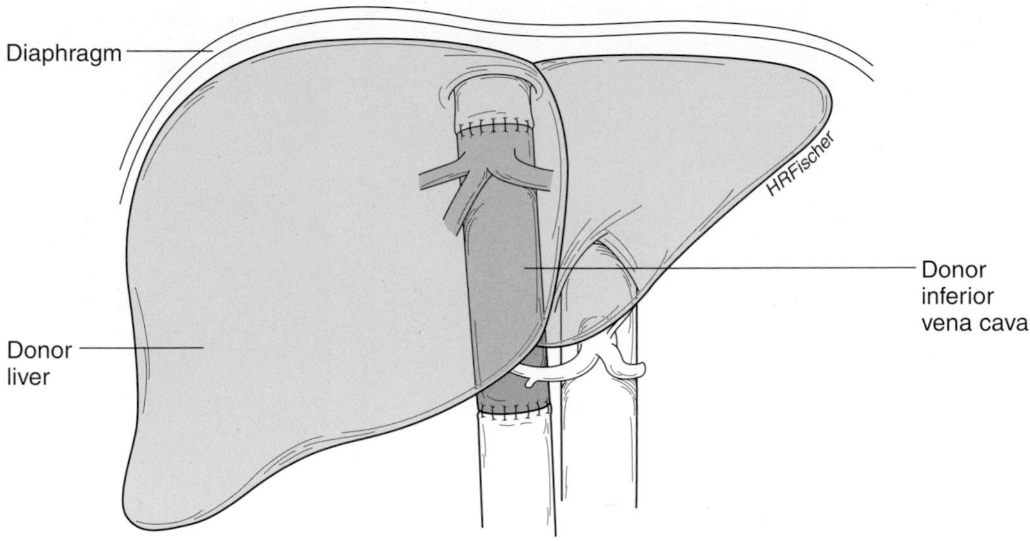

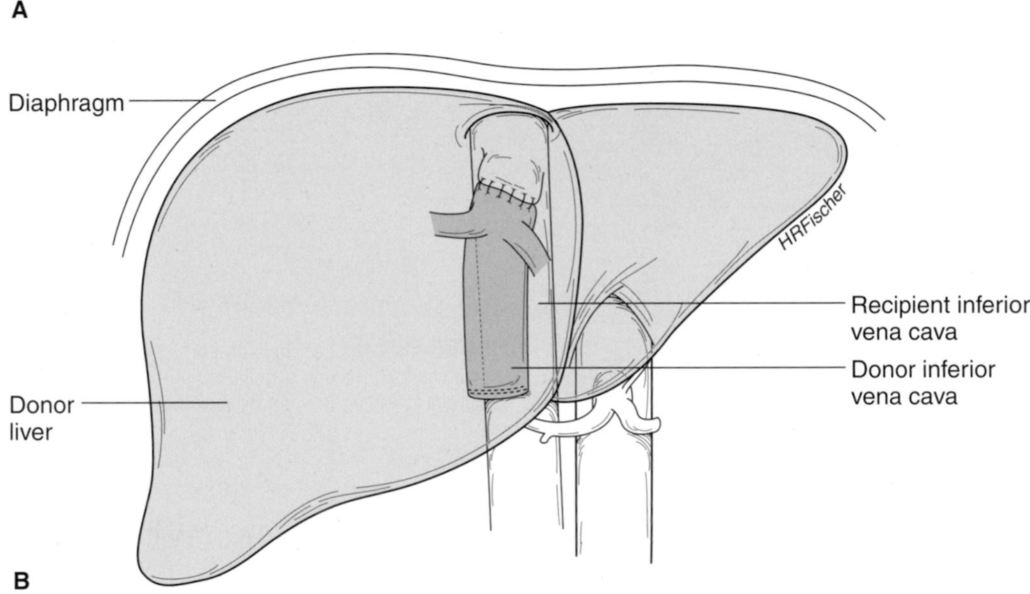

FIGURE 48.5. **A:** Liver transplant using bicaval technique showing the relationship between the donor liver, the donor cava, and the recipient cava. **B:** Liver transplant using the piggyback technique, showing the relationship between the donor liver, the donor cava, and the recipient cava.

diagnosis of primary sclerosing cholangitis have a higher rate of biliary complications.

Early diagnosis and treatment of biliary complications is paramount. Diagnostic procedures should take place urgently when bilirubin or alkaline phosphatase levels remain abnormally elevated in the perioperative period or when these values rise after a period of decline. Biliary leak or stricture is suggested by the development of abdominal pain, nausea, or persistent fever and by the development of ascites with a bilirubin level greater than serum or the presence of frank bile in a surgically placed drain. Whenever a biliary complication is identified, it is important to rule out hepatic arterial thrombosis with a Doppler ultrasound examination.

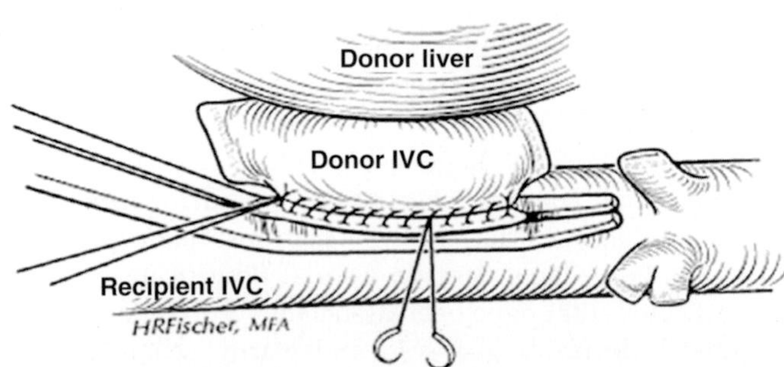

FIGURE 48.6. Liver transplant using a side-to-side cavocavostomy technique. The relationship between the donor liver, inferior vena cava (IVC), and recipient IVC is shown.

Two general techniques, namely, duct to duct and Roux-en-Y hepatico-jejunostomy, are used for biliary anastomosis in liver transplantation. In addition, a T-tube or other external biliary stent (139) may be placed, allowing for monitoring of bile production and for contrast injection for diagnostic purposes. When a T-tube or external biliary stent is in place and a biliary complication is suspected, a cholangiogram through the stent is the first diagnostic test that should be performed. Use of an internal biliary stent has been demonstrated to decrease the risk of biliary complications (137).

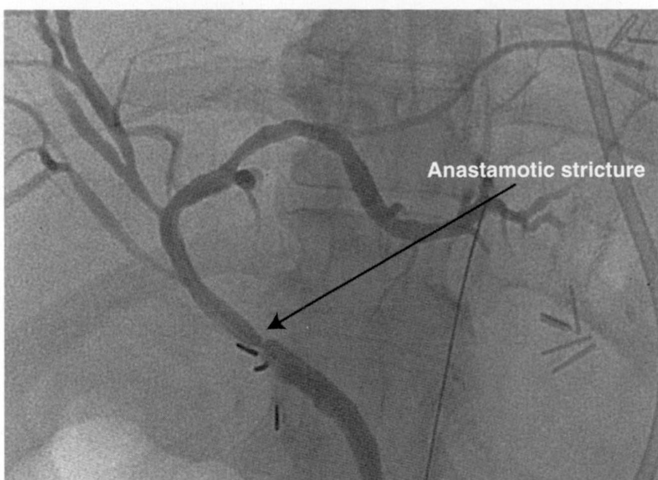

FIGURE 48.7. Transhepatic cholangiogram showing severe stenosis of the bile duct at the duct to duct anastomosis that responded to balloon dilatation.

In the absence of an external stent, an ultrasound examination followed by endoscopic retrograde cholangiopancreatography (ERCP) is appropriate. ERCP has the advantage of being potentially both diagnostic and therapeutic when combined with sphincterotomy and the insertion of an internal stent. Percutaneous transhepatic cholangiography is a more invasive alternative, which is usually reserved for cases where ERCP is not possible, such as patients with Roux-en-Y bile duct reconstruction.

The initial management of biliary complications can generally be nonoperative. Management should include intraluminal and external drainage, antibiotic administration as indicated, and reevaluation at 4 to 6 weeks. In cases where initial studies show a large defect and in cases where the leak is not controlled through percutaneous measures, operative repair using a Roux-en-Y hepatico-jejunostomy is indicated. Similarly, anastomotic strictures can generally be managed nonoperatively using ERCP or percutaneous cholangioplasty (Fig. 48.7). When anastomotic strictures persist beyond two attempts at balloon dilatation and stent replacement, operative repair should be performed (140,141).

Late leaks, following 1-month post-transplant, are associated with T-tube removal. The incidence of this problem is ~35%, but episodes are usually short-lived and resolve after a period of observation with antibiotic therapy. In some instances, it may be advisable to insert a small feeding tube or other drain through the previously formed tract to serve as a drain until symptoms resolve. ERCP or percutaneous transhepatic cholangiogram injection and ultrasound or CT-guided placement of drains is necessary in cases where abdominal pain and/or fluid collections persist. Surgical intervention is only rarely necessary when a large defect is identified, which cannot be controlled noninvasively (142). Because of the increased rate of complications directly related to the tube itself, T-tube placement is rarely utilized.

Diffuse intrahepatic strictures or intrahepatic cholangiopathy is often related to donor ischemia, poor organ preservation, HAT, immunologic injury, or recurrent disease (primary sclerosing cholangitis) and can be refractory to treatment, progressive, and lead to graft loss (143). The highest incidence of intrahepatic cholangiopathy, ranging from <10% (144) up to 50% (145), occurs following the transplantation of DCD livers (Fig. 48.8). Attempts at percutaneous drainage can occasionally be successful, but retransplantation is often required.

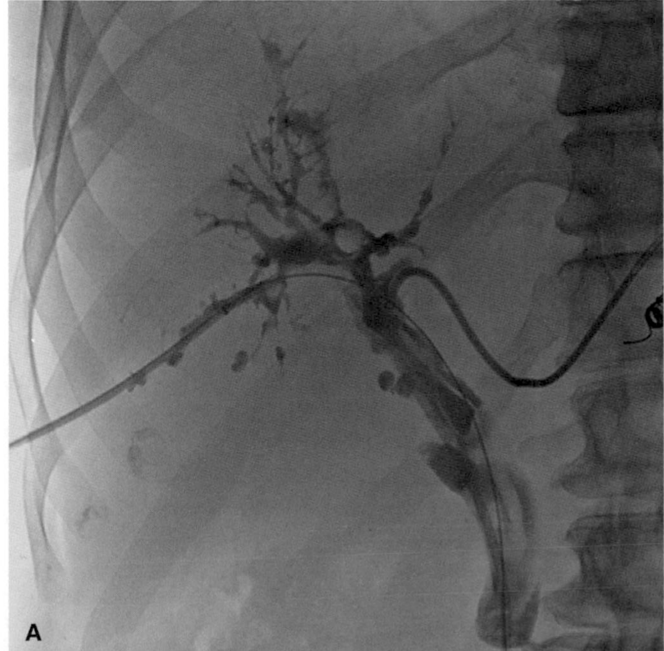

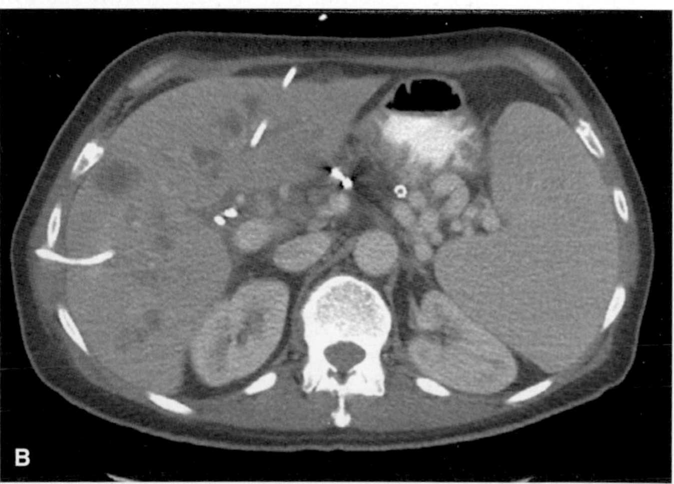

FIGURE 48.8. A: Bilateral percutaneous cholangiogram 6 weeks after transplantation of a liver from a donation following cardiac death (DCD) donor. Diffuse intrahepatic strictures and pruning of the intrahepatic biliary tree are noted. **B:** Abdominal CT scan of the same DCD liver recipient demonstrating bilateral, diffuse bile lakes.

COMPLICATIONS OF LIVING DONOR LIVER TRANSPLANTATION

Since its inception in 1989, living donor liver transplantation has gradually become a standard treatment for patients with liver failure. Originally developed to overcome the inadequate number of organ donors for children, the technique has more recently been applied to adult liver transplantation for the same reason (142). Several complications are relatively unique to living donor transplantation. It has been said that living donor transplantation is the only surgical procedure that has a potential mortality of 200%, causing the death of both the donor and the recipient. It is interesting to compare living donor liver transplantation, which has only recently been developed, to living donor kidney transplantation. In the 1950s, the first successful kidney transplants used living donors (identical twins) (146). Since that time, living donor kidney transplantation has become increasingly accepted to the point that living kidney donors now outnumber deceased kidney donors. The mortality of donating a kidney is approximately 0.03% (147). The long-term consequences of donating a kidney appear to be minimal (148). In contrast, the risk of donating the right hepatic lobe is estimated at 0.2% to 0.8% (149,150), leading some experts to question the development of the practice of adult-to-adult donation (151).

In addition to ethical issues related to donor mortality, the morbidity of the procedure is significant, with >12% to 67% of donors experiencing major complication (152–156). The risk of donor morbidity appears to be higher for right lobe donors than for left lateral segment donors. In right lobe donors, biliary complications occur in approximately 15% of cases (157). Although most biliary problems can be treated nonoperatively with ERCP or percutaneous drainage, some require operative repair. Although the donor liver regenerates, the long-term consequences of the donor operation are unknown (158).

Biliary complications are particularly common following living donor liver transplantation, with an incidence of between 16% and 38% (159). Biliary reconstruction is usually performed in living donor liver transplantation using either Roux-en-Y hepatico-jejunostomy or duct-to-duct anastomosis. Depending on the plane of transection, a single or double anastomosis may be necessary. The use of intrabiliary stenting is common practice. Most programs evaluate the duct anatomy at the time of abdominal exploration with either intraoperative cholangiography or probe exploration through the cystic duct after cholecystectomy. When the two ducts are in close proximity, a ductoplasty can be performed, allowing the creation of a single orifice and a larger anastomotic opening (160).

One of the major difficulties during the development of the living donor technique has been the choice of graft. For pediatric recipients the left lateral segment comprising segments 2 and 3 has usually been selected. However, when the recipient is large (<30 kg), it may be necessary to use an extended left graft that includes segment 1 (the caudate lobe), or segment 4, or both. Adult recipients generally require a right lobe graft to supply sufficient hepatic mass for the recipient. The mass of the donor graft should be at least 0.8% of the recipient's body mass to support the recipient until a normal hepatic mass can regenerate, a process that takes several weeks. Grafts that are <1% of recipient body weight exhibit risk of post-transplant graft dysfunction (161). Graft dysfunction is manifested by prolongation of prothrombin time, necessitating continued infusions of fresh frozen plasma and persistent elevation of total bilirubin that may require retransplantation in some cases. Morbidity and mortality due to septic complications are also more common. Recipient factors are also known to play a role, as the small-for-size syndrome is observed more commonly when the recipient is extremely ill (162). One theory regarding the etiology of the graft dysfunction in small-for-size syndrome is that the hepatic dysfunction relates to "hyperperfusion" of the graft with portal blood, which causes a compensatory decrease in hepatic arterial flow. Methods to attenuate graft dysfunction with small-for-size grafts by temporarily shunting portal blood away from the graft have been suggested and are currently being evaluated (163).

Because of the complexity of the procedure and the severity of illness of those with acute or chronic liver failure, complications following liver transplantation are anticipated in nearly all recipients. Signs and symptoms of complications may be abated or delayed and a high index of suspicion must be maintained to aid in the early diagnosis to limit morbidity and mortality. Continued advancements in perioperative patient management, immunosuppression, and surgical techniques have improved outcomes so that 90% 1-year patient survival has become the norm.

REFERENCES

1. Roberts JP, Brown RS Jr, Edwards EB, et al. Liver and intestine transplantation. *Am J Transplant* 2003;3(Suppl 4):78–90.
2. Thuluvath PJ, Guidinger MK, Fung JJ, et al. Liver transplantation in the United States, 1999–2008. *Am J Transplant* 2010;10:1003–1019.
3. Pruthi J, Medkiff KA, Esrason KT, et al. Analysis of causes of death in liver transplant recipients who survived more than 3 years. *Liver Transpl* 2001;7:811–815.
4. Rabkin JM, de La Melena V, Orloff SL, et al. Late mortality after orthotopic liver transplantation. *Am J Surg* 2001;181:475–479.
5. Moon JI, Nishida S, Butt F, et al. Multi-organ procurement and successful multi-center allocation using rapid en bloc technique from a controlled non-heart-beating donor. *Transplantation* 2004;77:1476–1477.
6. Nijkamp DM, Slooff MJ, van der Hilst CS, et al. Surgical injuries of postmortem donor livers: incidence and impact on outcome after adult liver transplantation. *Liver Transpl* 2006;12:1365–1370.
7. Goldstein RM, Secrest CL, Klintmalm GB, et al. Problematic vascular reconstruction in liver transplantation. Part I. Arterial. *Surgery* 1990;107:540–543.
8. Nicolini D, di Francesco F, Cautero N, et al. Technical solutions for venous outflow reconstruction in damaged liver grafts during procurement: case reports. *Transplant Proc* 2008;40:1941–1943.
9. Strasberg SM, Howard TK, Molmenti EP, et al. Selecting the donor liver: risk factors for poor function after orthotopic liver transplantation. *Hepatology* 1994;20:829–838.
10. Abt PL, Desai NM, Crawford MD, et al. Survival following liver transplantation from non-heart-beating donors. *Ann Surg* 2004;239:87–92.
11. Oh CK, Sawyer RG, Pelletier SJ, et al. Independent predictors for primary non-function after liver transplantation. *Yonsei Med J* 2004;45:1155–1161.
12. Adham M. Extracorporeal liver support: waiting for the deciding vote. *ASAIO J* 2003;49:621–632.

13. Takaya S, Doyle H, Todo S, et al. Reduction of primary nonfunction with prostaglandin E1 after clinical liver transplantation. *Transplant Proc* 1995;27:1862–1867.
14. Henley KS, Lucey MR, Normolle DP, et al. A double-blind, randomized, placebo-controlled trial of prostaglandin E1 in liver transplantation. *Hepatology* 1995;21:366–372.
15. Johnson SR, Alexopoulos S, Curry M, et al. Primary nonfunction (PNF) in the MELD Era: an SRTR database analysis. *Am J Transplant* 2007;7:1003–1009.
16. Marsman WA, Wiesner RH, Rodriguez L, et al. Use of fatty donor liver is associated with diminished early patient and graft survival. *Transplantation* 1996;62:1246–1251.
17. Kim DY, Cauduro SP, Bohorquez HE, et al. Routine use of livers from deceased donors older than 70: is it justified? *Transpl Int* 2005;18: 73–77.
18. Busquets J, Xiol X, Figueras J, et al. The impact of donor age on liver transplantation: influence of donor age on early liver function and on subsequent patient and graft survival. *Transplantation* 2001;71: 1765–1771.
19. Totsuka E, Dodson F, Urakami A, et al. Influence of high donor serum sodium levels on early postoperative graft function in human liver transplantation: effect of correction of donor hypernatremia. *Liver Transpl Surg* 1999;5:421–428.
20. Abt P, Crawford M, Desai N, et al. Liver transplantation from controlled non-heart-beating donors: an increased incidence of biliary complications. *Transplantation* 2003;75:1659–1663.
21. Foley DP, Fernandez LA, Leverson G, et al. Donation after cardiac death: the University of Wisconsin experience with liver transplantation. *Ann Surg* 2005;242:724–731.
22. Sharma R, Kashyap R, Jain A, et al. Surgical complications following liver transplantation in patients with portal vein thrombosis—a single-center perspective. *J Gastrointest Surg* 2010;14:520–527.
23. Zamir GA, Markmann JF, Abrams J, et al. The fate of liver grafts declined for subjective reasons and transplanted out of a local organ procurement organization. *Transplantation* 2000;70:1149–1154.
24. Health Resources and Services Administration and Organ Procurement and Transplantation Network. Policy 3.6 Organ Distribution: Allocation of Livers. Vol. 2010. UNOS Liver Allocation Policy; 2010. http://optn.transplant.hrsa.gov/PoliciesandBylaws2/policies/pdfs/policy_8.pdf. Accessed January 18, 2011.
25. Uemura T, Randall HB, Sanchez EQ, et al. Liver retransplantation for primary nonfunction: analysis of a 20-year single-center experience. *Liver Transpl* 2007;13:227–233.
26. Oldhafer KJ, Bornscheuer A, Fruhauf NR, et al. Rescue hepatectomy for initial graft non-function after liver transplantation. *Transplantation* 1999;67:1024–1028.
27. Calne RY. Immunosuppression in liver transplantation. *N Engl J Med* 1994;331:1154–1155.
28. Wiesner RH, Steffen BJ, David KM, et al. Mycophenolate mofetil use is associated with decreased risk of late acute rejection in adult liver transplant recipients. *Am J Transplant* 2006;6:1609–1616.
29. Demetris AJ, Ruppert K, Dvorchik I, et al. Real-time monitoring of acute liver-allograft rejection using the Banff schema. *Transplantation* 2002;74:1290–1296.
30. Jain A, Kashyap R, Dodson F, et al. A prospective randomized trial of tacrolimus and prednisone versus tacrolimus, prednisone and mycophenolate mofetil in primary adult liver transplantation: a single center report. *Transplantation* 2001;72:1091–1097.
31. Ramirez CB, Doria C, di Francesco F, et al. Basiliximab induction in adult liver transplant recipients with 93% rejection-free patient and graft survival at 24 months. *Transplant Proc* 2006;38:3633–3635.
32. Burton JR Jr, Rosen HR. Acute rejection in HCV-infected liver transplant recipients: the great conundrum. *Liver Transpl* 2006;12:S38–S47.
33. Cabrera R, Ararat M, Soldevila-Pico C, et al. Using an immune functional assay to differentiate acute cellular rejection from recurrent hepatitis C in liver transplant patients. *Liver Transpl* 2009;15:216–222.
34. Toyoki Y, Renz JF, Mudge C, et al. Allograft rejection in pediatric liver transplantation: comparison between cadaveric and living related donors. *Pediatr Transplant* 2002;6:301–307.
35. Wiesner RH, Rakela J, Ishitani MB, et al. Recent advances in liver transplantation. *Mayo Clin Proc* 2003;78:197–210.
36. Ramji A, Yoshida EM, Bain VG, et al. Late acute rejection after liver transplantation: the Western Canada experience. *Liver Transpl* 2002;8:945–951.
37. Ludwig J, Wiesner RH, Batts KP, et al. The acute vanishing bile duct syndrome (acute irreversible rejection) after orthotopic liver transplantation. *Hepatology* 1987;7:476–483.
38. Gomez R, Hidalgo M, Marques E, et al. Incidence and predisposing factors for incisional hernia in patients with liver transplantation. *Hernia* 2001;5:172–176.
39. Janssen H, Lange R, Erhard J, et al. Causative factors, surgical treatment and outcome of incisional hernia after liver transplantation. *Br J Surg* 2002;89:1049–1054.
40. Hellinger WC, Crook JE, Heckman MG, et al. Surgical site infection after liver transplantation: risk factors and association with graft loss or death. *Transplantation* 2009;87:1387–1393.
41. Hollenbeak CS, Alfrey EJ, Souba WW. The effect of surgical site infections on outcomes and resource utilization after liver transplantation. *Surgery* 2001;130:388–395.
42. Iinuma Y, Senda K, Fujihara N, et al. Surgical site infection in living-donor liver transplant recipients: a prospective study. *Transplantation* 2004;78:704–709.
43. Sawyer RG, Pelletier SJ, Pruett TL. Increased early morbidity and mortality with acceptable long-term function in severely obese patients undergoing liver transplantation. *Clin Transplant* 1999;13: 126–130.
44. Guilbeau JM. Delayed wound healing with sirolimus after liver transplant. *Ann Pharmacother* 2002;36:1391–1395.
45. Toso C, Meeberg GA, Bigam DL, et al. De novo sirolimus-based immunosuppression after liver transplantation for hepatocellular carcinoma: long-term outcomes and side effects. *Transplantation* 2007;83: 1162–1168.
46. Mehrabi A, Fonouni H, Wente M, et al. Wound complications following kidney and liver transplantation. *Clin Transplant* 2006;20(Suppl 17):97–110.
47. Molinari M, Berman K, Meeberg G, et al. Multicentric outcome analysis of sirolimus-based immunosuppression in 252 liver transplant recipients. *Transpl Int* 2010;23:155–168.
48. Andreoni KA, Lightfoot H Jr, Gerber DA, et al. Laparoscopic incisional hernia repair in liver transplant and other immunosuppressed patients. *Am J Transplant* 2002;2:349–354.
49. Mekeel K, Mulligan D, Reddy KS, et al. Laparoscopic incisional hernia repair after liver transplantation. *Liver Transpl* 2007;13:1576–1581.
50. Biancofiore G, Bindi ML, Romanelli AM, et al. Postoperative intra-abdominal pressure and renal function after liver transplantation. *Arch Surg* 2003;138:703–706.
51. Kron IL, Harman PK, Nolan SP. The measurement of intra-abdominal pressure as a criterion for abdominal re-exploration. *Ann Surg* 1984;199: 28–30.
52. Biancofiore G, Bindi L, Romanelli AM, et al. Renal failure and abdominal hypertension after liver transplantation: determination of critical intra-abdominal pressure. *Liver Transpl* 2002;8:1175–1181.
53. Ivatury RR, Sugerman HJ, Peitzman AB. Abdominal compartment syndrome: recognition and management. *Adv Surg* 2001;35:251–269.
54. Jones WT, Ratner I, Abrahamian G, et al. Use of a silastic silo for closure of the abdominal wall in a pediatric patient receiving a cadaveric split liver. *J Pediatr Surg* 2003;38:E20–E22.
55. Seaman DS, Newell KA, Piper JB, et al. Use of polytetrafluoroethylene patch for temporary wound closure after pediatric liver transplantation. *Transplantation* 1996;62:1034–1036.
56. Jafri MA, Tevar AD, Lucia M, et al. Temporary silastic mesh closure for adult liver transplantation: a safe alternative for the difficult abdomen. *Liver Transpl* 2007;13:258–265.
57. Singh MK, Rocca JP, Rochon C, et al. Open abdomen management with human acellular dermal matrix in liver transplant recipients. *Transplant Proc* 2008;40:3541–3544.
58. Gondolesi G, Selvaggi G, Tzakis A, et al. Use of the abdominal rectus fascia as a nonvascularized allograft for abdominal wall closure after liver, intestinal, and multivisceral transplantation. *Transplantation* 2009;87:1884–1888.
59. Wong LP, Blackley MP, Andreoni KA, et al. Survival of liver transplant candidates with acute renal failure receiving renal replacement therapy. *Kidney Int* 2005;68:362–370.
60. Cabezuelo JB, Ramirez P, Acosta F, et al. Does the standard vs piggyback surgical technique affect the development of early acute renal failure after orthotopic liver transplantation? *Transplant Proc.* 2003;35: 1913–1914.
61. Belghiti J, Panis Y, Sauvanet A, et al. A new technique of side to side caval anastomosis during orthotopic hepatic transplantation without inferior vena caval occlusion. *Surg Gynecol Obstet* 1992;175:270–272.
62. Sonnenday CJ, Mathur AK, Lee DS, et al. The side-to-side cavocavostomy technique eliminates hepatic venous outflow stenosis in orthotopic liver transplantation. *Liver Transpl* 2009;15:S168.
63. Mehrabi A, Mood ZA, Fonouni H, et al. A single-center experience of 500 liver transplants using the modified piggyback technique by Belghiti. *Liver Transpl* 2009;15:466–474.

64. Murray BM, Paller MS. Beneficial effects of renal denervation and prazosin on GFR and renal blood flow after cyclosporine in rats. *Clin Nephrol* 1986;25(Suppl 1):S37–S39.
65. Lin CC, Chuang FR, Lee CH, et al. The renal-sparing efficacy of basiliximab in adult living donor liver transplantation. *Liver Transpl* 2005; 11:1258–1264.
66. Emre S, Gondolesi G, Polat K, et al. Use of daclizumab as initial immunosuppression in liver transplant recipients with impaired renal function. *Liver Transpl* 2001;7:220–225.
67. Eckhoff DE, McGuire B, Sellers M, et al. The safety and efficacy of a two-dose daclizumab (zenapax) induction therapy in liver transplant recipients. *Transplantation* 2000;69:1867–1872.
68. Calmus Y, Kamar N, Gugenheim J, et al. Assessing renal function with daclizumab induction and delayed tacrolimus introduction in liver transplant recipients. *Transplantation* 2010;89:1504–1510.
69. Soliman T, Hetz H, Burghuber C, et al. Short-term induction therapy with anti-thymocyte globulin and delayed use of calcineurin inhibitors in orthotopic liver transplantation. *Liver Transpl* 2007;13: 1039–1044.
70. Tchervenkov JI, Tzimas GN, Cantarovich M, et al. The impact of thymoglobulin on renal function and calcineurin inhibitor initiation in recipients of orthotopic liver transplant: a retrospective analysis of 298 consecutive patients. *Transplant Proc* 2004;36:1747–1752.
71. Bajjoka I, Hsaiky L, Brown K, et al. Preserving renal function in liver transplant recipients with rabbit anti-thymocyte globulin and delayed initiation of calcineurin inhibitors. *Liver Transpl* 2008;14:66–72.
72. Cohen AJ, Stegall MD, Rosen CB, et al. Chronic renal dysfunction late after liver transplantation. *Liver Transpl* 2002;8:916–921.
73. Gonwa TA, Mai ML, Melton LB, et al. End-stage renal disease (ESRD) after orthotopic liver transplantation (OLTX) using calcineurin-based immunotherapy: risk of development and treatment. *Transplantation* 2001;72:1934–1939.
74. Ojo AO, Held PJ, Port FK, et al. Chronic renal failure after transplantation of a nonrenal organ. *N Engl J Med* 2003;349:931–940.
75. Nair S, Eason J, Loss G. Sirolimus monotherapy in nephrotoxicity due to calcineurin inhibitors in liver transplant recipients. *Liver Transpl* 2003;9:126–129.
76. Raimondo ML, Dagher L, Papatheodoridis GV, et al. Long-term mycophenolate mofetil monotherapy in combination with calcineurin inhibitors for chronic renal dysfunction after liver transplantation. *Transplantation* 2003;75:186–190.
77. Masetti M, Montalti R, Rompianesi G, et al. Early withdrawal of calcineurin inhibitors and everolimus monotherapy in de novo liver transplant recipients preserves renal function. *Am J Transplant* 2010;10:2252–2262.
78. Karie-Guigues S, Janus N, Saliba F, et al. Long-term renal function in liver transplant recipients and impact of immunosuppressive regimens (calcineurin inhibitors alone or in combination with mycophenolate mofetil): the TRY study. *Liver Transpl* 2009;15:1083–1091.
79. Neau-Cransac M, Morel D, Bernard PH, et al. Renal failure after liver transplantation: outcome after calcineurin inhibitor withdrawal. *Clin Transplant* 2002;16:368–373.
80. Rogers CC, Johnson SR, Mandelbrot DA, et al. Timing of sirolimus conversion influences recovery of renal function in liver transplant recipients. *Clin Transplant* 2009;23:887–896.
81. Watson CJ, Gimson AE, Alexander GJ, et al. A randomized controlled trial of late conversion from calcineurin inhibitor (CNI)-based to sirolimus-based immunosuppression in liver transplant recipients with impaired renal function. *Liver Transpl* 2007;13:1694–1702.
82. Hirose R, Roberts JP, Quan D, et al. Experience with daclizumab in liver transplantation: renal transplant dosing without calcineurin inhibitors is insufficient to prevent acute rejection in liver transplantation. *Transplantation* 2000;69:307–311.
83. Fong TL, Bunnapradist S, Jordan SC, et al. Analysis of the United Network for Organ Sharing database comparing renal allografts and patient survival in combined liver-kidney transplantation with the contralateral allografts in kidney alone or kidney-pancreas transplantation. *Transplantation* 2003;76:348–353.
84. Ghobrial RM. Retransplantation for recurrent hepatitis C. *Liver Transpl* 2002;8:S38–S43.
85. Charlton M. The impact of advancing donor age on histologic recurrence of hepatitis C infection: the perils of ignored maternal advice. *Liver Transpl* 2003;9:535–537.
86. Pelletier SJ, Schaubel DE, Punch JD, et al. Hepatitis C is a risk factor for death after liver retransplantation. *Liver Transpl* 2005;11:434–440.
87. Jauhar S, Talwalkar JA, Schneekloth T, et al. Analysis of factors that predict alcohol relapse following liver transplantation. *Liver Transpl* 2004;10:408–411.
88. Kugelmas M, Spiegelman P, Osgood MJ, et al. Different immunosuppressive regimens and recurrence of primary sclerosing cholangitis after liver transplantation. *Liver Transpl* 2003;9:727–732.
89. Molmenti EP, Netto GJ, Murray NG, et al. Incidence and recurrence of autoimmune/alloimmune hepatitis in liver transplant recipients. *Liver Transpl* 2002;8:519–526.
90. Sylvestre PB, Batts KP, Burgart LJ, et al. Recurrence of primary biliary cirrhosis after liver transplantation: histologic estimate of incidence and natural history. *Liver Transpl* 2003;9:1086–1093.
91. Heneghan MA, Zolfino T, Muiesan P, et al. An evaluation of long-term outcomes after liver transplantation for cryptogenic cirrhosis. *Liver Transpl* 2003;9:921–928.
92. Parkin DM, Bray F, Ferlay J, et al. Estimating the world cancer burden: Globocan 2000. *Int J Cancer* 2001;94:153–156.
93. Mazzaferro V, Regalia E, Doci R, et al. Liver transplantation for the treatment of small hepatocellular carcinomas in patients with cirrhosis. *N Engl J Med* 1996;334:693–699.
94. Kornberg A, Kupper B, Tannapfel A, et al. Adjuvant conversion to sirolimus in liver transplant patients with recurrent hepatocellular carcinoma—preliminary results. *Transpl Int* 2008;21:96–99.
95. Gomez-Camarero J, Salcedo M, Rincon D, et al. Use of everolimus as a rescue immunosuppressive therapy in liver transplant patients with neoplasms. *Transplantation* 2007;84:786–791.
96. Kornberg A, Kupper B, Tannapfel A, et al. Long-term survival after recurrent hepatocellular carcinoma in liver transplant patients: clinical patterns and outcome variables. *Eur J Surg Oncol* 2010;36:275–280.
97. Yeganeh M, Finn RS, Saab S. Apparent remission of a solitary metastatic pulmonary lesion in a liver transplant recipient treated with sorafenib. *Am J Transplant* 2009;9:2851–2854.
98. Burdick JF, Vogelsang GB, Smith WJ, et al. Severe graft-versus-host disease in a liver-transplant recipient. *N Engl J Med* 1988;318:689–691.
99. Thin L, Macquillan G, Adams L, et al. Acute graft-versus-host disease after liver transplant: novel use of etanercept and the role of tumor necrosis factor alpha inhibitors. *Liver Transpl* 2009;15:421–426.
100. Sanchez-Izquierdo JA, Lumbreras C, Colina F, et al. Severe graft versus host disease following liver transplantation confirmed by PCR-HLA-B sequencing: report of a case and literature review. *Hepatogastroenterology* 1996;43:1057–1061.
101. Kusne S, Dummer JS, Singh N, et al. Infections after liver transplantation. An analysis of 101 consecutive cases. *Medicine (Baltimore)* 1988;67: 132–143.
102. Pelletier SJ, Crabtree TD, Gleason TG, et al. Characteristics of infectious complications associated with mortality after solid organ transplantation. *Clin Transplant* 2000;14:401–408.
103. Kibbler CC. Infections in liver transplantation: risk factors and strategies for prevention. *J Hosp Infect* 1995;30(Suppl):209–217.
104. Sawyer RG, Crabtree TD, Gleason TG, et al. Impact of solid organ transplantation and immunosuppression on fever, leukocytosis, and physiologic response during bacterial and fungal infections. *Clin Transplant* 1999;13:260–265.
105. Nair S, Cohen DB, Cohen MP, et al. Postoperative morbidity, mortality, costs, and long-term survival in severely obese patients undergoing orthotopic liver transplantation. *Am J Gastroenterol* 2001;96: 842–845.
106. Wade JJ, Rolando N, Hayllar K, et al. Bacterial and fungal infections after liver transplantation: an analysis of 284 patients. *Hepatology* 1995;21:1328–1336.
107. Wallot MA, Mathot M, Janssen M, et al. Long-term survival and late graft loss in pediatric liver transplant recipients—a 15-year single-center experience. *Liver Transpl* 2002;8:615–622.
108. Sharpe MD, Ghent C, Grant D, et al. Efficacy and safety of itraconazole prophylaxis for fungal infections after orthotopic liver transplantation: a prospective, randomized, double-blind study. *Transplantation* 2003;76:977–983.
109. Linden PK, Coley K, Fontes P, et al. Invasive aspergillosis in liver transplant recipients: outcome comparison of therapy with amphotericin B lipid complex and a historical cohort treated with conventional amphotericin B. *Clin Infect Dis* 2003;37:17–25.
110. Huang DZ, Le GR, Zhang QP, et al. The value of color Doppler ultrasonography in monitoring normal orthotopic liver transplantation and postoperative complications. *Hepatobiliary Pancreat Dis Int* 2003;2: 54–58.

111. Glockner JF, Forauer AR, Solomon H, et al. Three-dimensional gadolinium-enhanced MR angiography of vascular complications after liver transplantation. *AJR Am J Roentgenol* 2000;174:1447–1453.
112. Oh CK, Pelletier SJ, Sawyer RG, et al. Uni- and multi-variate analysis of risk factors for early and late hepatic artery thrombosis after liver transplantation. *Transplantation* 2001;71:767–772.
113. Sheiner PA, Varma CV, Guarrera JV, et al. Selective revascularization of hepatic artery thromboses after liver transplantation improves patient and graft survival. *Transplantation* 1997;64:1295–1299.
114. Bhattacharjya S, Gunson BK, Mirza DF, et al. Delayed hepatic artery thrombosis in adult orthotopic liver transplantation—a 12-year experience. *Transplantation* 2001;71:1592–1596.
115. Mas VR, Fisher RA, Maluf DG, et al. Hepatic artery thrombosis after liver transplantation and genetic factors: prothrombin G20210 A polymorphism. *Transplantation* 2003;76:247–249.
116. Pungpapong S, Manzarbeitia C, Ortiz J, et al. Cigarette smoking is associated with an increased incidence of vascular complications after liver transplantation. *Liver Transpl* 2002;8:582–587.
117. Singhal A, Stokes K, Sebastian A, et al. Endovascular treatment of hepatic artery thrombosis following liver transplantation. *Transpl Int* 2010;23:245–256.
118. Singhal A, Mukherjee I, Stokes K, et al. Continuous intraarterial thrombolysis for early hepatic artery thrombosis following liver transplantation: case report. *Vasc Endovasc Surg* 2010;44:134–138.
119. Kim BW, Won JH, Lee BM, et al. Intraarterial thrombolytic treatment for hepatic artery thrombosis immediately after living donor liver transplantation. *Transplant Proc* 2006;38:3128–3131.
120. Pinna AD, Smith CV, Furukawa H, et al. Urgent revascularization of liver allografts after early hepatic artery thrombosis. *Transplantation* 1996;62:1584–1587.
121. Abbasoglu O, Levy MF, Vodapally MS, et al. Hepatic artery stenosis after liver transplantation—incidence, presentation, treatment, and long term outcome. *Transplantation* 1997;63:250–255.
122. Maruzzelli L, Miraglia R, Caruso S, et al. Percutaneous endovascular treatment of hepatic artery stenosis in adult and pediatric patients after liver transplantation. *Cardiovasc Intervent Radiol* 2010;33:1111–1119.
123. Johnston T, Jeon H, Gedaly R, et al. Importance of local infection in hepatic artery pseudoaneurysms. *Liver Transpl* 2008;14:388.
124. Bonham CA, Kapur S, Geller D, et al. Excision and immediate revascularization for hepatic artery pseudoaneurysm following liver transplantation. *Transplant Proc* 1999;31:443.
125. Sieders E, Peeters PM, TenVergert EM, et al. Early vascular complications after pediatric liver transplantation. *Liver Transpl* 2000;6:326–332.
126. Englesbe MJ, Kubus J, Muhammad W, et al. Portal vein thrombosis and survival in patients with cirrhosis. *Liver Transpl* 2010;16:83–90.
127. Bhattacharjya T, Olliff SP, Bhattacharjya S, et al. Percutaneous portal vein thrombolysis and endovascular stent for management of post-transplant portal venous conduit thrombosis. *Transplantation* 2000;69:2195–2198.
128. Cherukuri R, Haskal ZJ, Naji A, et al. Percutaneous thrombolysis and stent placement for the treatment of portal vein thrombosis after liver transplantation: long-term follow-up. *Transplantation* 1998;65:1124–1126.
129. Gonzalez-Tutor A, Abascal F, Cerezai L, et al. Transjugular approach to treat portal vein stenosis after liver transplantation—a case report. *Angiology* 2000;51:511–514.
130. Perumalla R, Jamieson NV, Praseedom RK. Left renal vein as an option for portal inflow in liver transplant recipients with portal vein thrombosis. *Transpl Int* 2008;21:701–703.
131. Glanemann M, Settmacher U, Langrehr JM, et al. Results of end-to-end cavocavostomy during adult liver transplantation. *World J Surg* 2002;26:342–347.
132. Navarro F, Le Moine MC, Fabre JM, et al. Specific vascular complications of orthotopic liver transplantation with preservation of the retrohepatic vena cava: review of 1361 cases. *Transplantation* 1999;68:646–650.
133. Nemec P, Cerny J, Hokl J, et al. Hemodynamic measurement in liver transplantation. Piggyback versus conventional techniques. *Ann Transplant* 2000;5:35–37.
134. Parrilla P, Sanchez-Bueno F, Figueras J, et al. Analysis of the complications of the piggy-back technique in 1,112 liver transplants. *Transplantation* 1999;67:1214–1217.
135. Borsa JJ, Daly CP, Fontaine AB, et al. Treatment of inferior vena cava anastomotic stenoses with the Wallstent endoprosthesis after orthotopic liver transplantation. *J Vasc Interv Radiol* 1999;10:17–22.
136. Frazer CK, Gupta A. Stenosis of the hepatic vein anastomosis after liver transplantation: treatment with a heparin-coated metal stent. *Australas Radiol* 2002;46:422–425.
137. Welling TH, Heidt DG, Englesbe MJ, et al. Biliary complications following liver transplantation in the model for end-stage liver disease era: effect of donor, recipient, and technical factors. *Liver Transpl* 2008;14:73–80.
138. Feller RB, Waugh RC, Selby WS, et al. Biliary strictures after liver transplantation: clinical picture, correlates and outcomes. *J Gastroenterol Hepatol* 1996;11:21–25.
139. Sawyer RG, Punch JD. Incidence and management of biliary complications after 291 liver transplants following the introduction of transcystic stenting. *Transplantation* 1998;66:1201–1207.
140. Roumilhac D, Poyet G, Sergent G, et al. Long-term results of percutaneous management for anastomotic biliary stricture after orthotopic liver transplantation. *Liver Transpl* 2003;9:394–400.
141. Sung RS, Campbell DA Jr, Rudich SM, et al. Long-term follow-up of percutaneous transhepatic balloon cholangioplasty in the management of biliary strictures after liver transplantation. *Transplantation* 2004;77:110–115.
142. Marcos A, Fisher RA, Ham JM, et al. Right lobe living donor liver transplantation. *Transplantation* 1999;68:798–803.
143. Nishida S, Nakamura N, Kadono J, et al. Intrahepatic biliary strictures after liver transplantation. *J Hepatobiliary Pancreat Surg* 2006;13:511–516.
144. Grewal HP, Willingham DL, Nguyen J, et al. Liver transplantation using controlled donation after cardiac death donors: an analysis of a large single-center experience. *Liver Transpl* 2009;15:1028–1035.
145. Maheshwari A, Maley W, Li Z, et al. Biliary complications and outcomes of liver transplantation from donors after cardiac death. *Liver Transpl* 2007;13:1645–1653.
146. Murray JE, Merrill JP, Harrison JH. Kidney transplantation between seven pairs of identical twins. *Ann Surg* 1958;148:343–359.
147. Starzl TE. Living donors: con. *Transplant Proc* 1987;19:174–175.
148. Johnson EM, Anderson JK, Jacobs C, et al. Long-term follow-up of living kidney donors: quality of life after donation. *Transplantation* 1999;67:717–721.
149. Miller C, Florman S, Kim-Schluger L, et al. Fulminant and fatal gas gangrene of the stomach in a healthy live liver donor. *Liver Transpl* 2004;10:1315–1319.
150. Trotter JF, Adam R, Lo CM, et al. Documented deaths of hepatic lobe donors for living donor liver transplantation. *Liver Transpl* 2006;12:1485–1488.
151. Cronin DC II, Millis JM, Siegler M. Transplantation of liver grafts from living donors into adults–too much, too soon. *N Engl J Med* 2001;344:1633–1637.
152. Brown RS Jr, Russo MW, Lai M, et al. A survey of liver transplantation from living adult donors in the United States. *N Engl J Med* 2003;348:818–825.
153. Umeshita K, Fujiwara K, Kiyosawa K, et al. Operative morbidity of living liver donors in Japan. *Lancet* 2003;362:687–690.
154. Broering DC, Wilms C, Bok P, et al. Evolution of donor morbidity in living related liver transplantation: a single-center analysis of 165 cases. *Ann Surg* 2004;240:1013–1024; discussions 1024–1026.
155. Ghobrial RM, Freise CE, Trotter JF, et al. Donor morbidity after living donation for liver transplantation. *Gastroenterology* 2008;135:468–476.
156. Yi NJ, Suh KS, Cho JY, et al. Three-quarters of right liver donors experienced postoperative complications. *Liver Transpl* 2007;13:797–806.
157. Ito T, Kiuchi T, Egawa H, et al. Surgery-related morbidity in living donors of right-lobe liver graft: lessons from the first 200 cases. *Transplantation* 2003;76:158–163.
158. Shiffman ML, Brown RS Jr, Olthoff KM, et al. Living donor liver transplantation: summary of a conference at The National Institutes of Health. *Liver Transpl* 2002;8:174–188.
159. Lo CM. Complications and long-term outcome of living liver donors: a survey of 1,508 cases in five Asian centers. *Transplantation* 2003;75:S12–S15.
160. Egawa H, Inomata Y, Uemoto S, et al. Biliary anastomotic complications in 400 living related liver transplantations. *World J Surg* 2001;25:1300–1307.
161. Inomata Y, Uemoto S, Asonuma K, et al. Right lobe graft in living donor liver transplantation. *Transplantation* 2000;69:258–264.
162. Kiuchi T, Tanaka K, Ito T, et al. Small-for-size graft in living donor liver transplantation: how far should we go? *Liver Transpl* 2003;9:S29–S35.
163. Boillot O, Mechet I, Le Derf Y, et al. Portomesenteric disconnection for small-for-size grafts in liver transplantation: preclinical studies in pigs. *Liver Transpl* 2003;9:S42–S46.

CHAPTER

49

Complications of Pancreatic Transplantation

Dixon B. Kaufman

RATIONALE OF PANCREATIC TRANSPLANTATION FOR PATIENTS WITH TYPE 1 DIABETES MELLITUS

The prevalence of type 1 diabetes in the United States is estimated to be 1,000,000 individuals, and 35,000 new cases are diagnosed each year. The discovery of insulin as a therapeutic agent in 1927 revolutionized the treatment of diabetes mellitus by changing it from a rapidly fatal disease into a chronic illness. Unfortunately, this increased longevity brought to the fore serious secondary complications, including nephropathy, neuropathy, retinopathy, and macrovascular and microvascular complications in survivors 10 to 20 years after disease onset. The metabolic, microvascular, and macrovascular complications of diabetes are responsible for increased mortality in patients with type 1 diabetes compared with the general US population (1). In 2002, the national direct and indirect costs of type 1 and type 2 diabetes, including hospital and physician care, laboratory tests, pharmaceutical products, and patient workdays lost because of disability and premature death, exceeded $130 billion (2).

Hyperglycemia is the most important factor in the development and progression of secondary complications of diabetes. The Diabetes Control and Complication Trial demonstrated that the microvascular and, possibly, macrovascular complications of diabetes may be prevented by maintaining euglycemia (3,4). This realization has led to a search for alternative methods of treatment designed to achieve better glycemic control so that the progression of long-term complications can be altered.

Currently, there is no practical artificial endocrine pancreas, a mechanical insulin-delivery device coupled with an automated glucose-sensory system that could administer insulin with the degree of control necessary to produce a near-constant euglycemic state without risk of hypoglycemia. Since severe hypoglycemia is life threatening, persons with type 1 diabetes are resigned to manually regulating blood glucose levels by various forms of insulin administration. As a consequence, patients with type 1 diabetes typically exhibit wide deviations of plasma glucose levels from hour to hour and from day to day. Because hypoglycemia is intolerable, glucose control must err on the high side. Therefore, patients must live with relative chronic hyperglycemia.

The only treatments that influence the progression of secondary complications include β-cell replacement therapy with pancreas or islet transplantation and intensive insulin therapy. Since diabetes is not a rapidly fatal disease, and because transplant procedures require the patient to receive life-long immunosuppression, the results of islet or pancreas transplantation must be sufficiently efficacious and safe to warrant application in place of standard medical management of the primary disease. Currently, islet transplantation is an experimental procedure for highly selective cases. Pancreas transplantation is a proven therapeutic treatment option for diabetes and is superior to manual intensive insulin therapy with regard to the efficacy of achieving glycemic control and beneficial effects on diabetic secondary complications.

A successful pancreas transplant produces an immediate normoglycemic and insulin-independent state that normalizes hemoglobin A1C levels for as long as the graft functions. Transplantation also has the added physiological properties of proinsulin and C-peptide release not possible with intensive insulin therapy (5). Through improved metabolic control, many secondary complications of diabetes, including diabetic neuropathy (6), autonomic neuropathy-associated sudden death (7), and diabetic nephropathy in both uremic and nonuremic patients (8,9) may be markedly improved. A successful pancreas transplant significantly improves quality of life (10) and life expectancy (11,12).

Approximately 1,300 pancreas transplants are performed annually in the United States. Of these, 65% to 70% involve a simultaneous pancreas and kidney (SPK) transplant for patients with type 1 diabetes and chronic renal failure. These individuals are excellent candidates for an SPK transplant from the same donor because the immunosuppressive medications that are needed are similar to those for a kidney transplant alone and the surgical risk of adding the pancreas is low. The benefits of adding a pancreas transplant to ameliorate diabetes are profound—transplantation saves lives (11,12). The second category for pancreas transplantation consists of patients with type 1 diabetes who

Dixon B. Kaufman: Department of Surgery. Division of Transplantation, University of Wisconsin (Madison).

have received a previous kidney transplant from either a living or deceased donor. This group accounts for approximately 20% of patients receiving pancreas transplants. The important consideration is that of surgical risk, since the risk of immunosuppression has already been assumed.

The third category for pancreas transplantation is composed of nonuremic patients with type 1 diabetes. In this situation, one assesses the risk of immunosuppression to be less than the risk of diabetes treated with conventional exogenous insulin. Some of these patients with diabetes have extremely labile disease, such that there is difficulty with day-to-day living associated with frequent emergency room visits and inpatient hospitalizations for hypoglycemia or diabetic ketoacidosis. Other patients have significant difficulty with hypoglycemic unawareness that results in unconsciousness without warning. For select patients, this state can be a devastating problem that affects their employment and their ability to keep a driver's license and creates concern about lethal hypoglycemia while asleep. Pretransplant evaluation often incorporates an assessment of the Clarke Score (13) to semiquantitatively determine the severity of hypoglycemic complications in an effort to more fully understand the risk–benefit relationship for undergoing a pancreas or islet transplant.

OUTCOME MEASURES OF PANCREATIC TRANSPLANTATION

The most important outcome measures of pancreas transplantation are defined in terms of patient and graft survival and rejection. The definition of patient survival is obvious. Pancreas graft losses are defined as (a) patient death with a functioning graft or (b) loss of insulin independence irrespective of whether the pancreas allograft is in place or removed. Rejection is an immunologic host response to the foreign graft that will destroy it unless antirejection medications are effectively administered. The definition of a rejection episode usually requires tissue biopsy confirmation. Patients are treated with a short course of anti-T-cell antibody, often in conjunction with corticosteroids.

The most valuable and complete information on the results of pancreas transplantation comes from two sources, namely, the International Pancreas Transplant Registry (IPTR) and the Scientific Registry of Transplant Recipients (SRTR) of the Organ Procurement and Transplant Network (OPTN). The SRTR is the scientific arm of the OPTN, where data on all transplants in the United States have been collected since 1987. The SRTR supports ongoing evaluation of the scientific and clinical status of solid-organ transplantation, including pancreas transplants. Funding comes from the Health Resources and Services Administration, a division of the U.S. Department of Health and Human Services. The SRTR is administered by Arbor Research, a nonprofit health research organization, based in Ann Arbor, MI.

In addition to the national databases, multicenter studies and single-center experiences with pancreas transplantation have also been valuable in reporting results of specific technical and immunosuppressive protocols.

Figure 49.1 shows patient, kidney, and pancreas graft survival rates in SPK transplant recipients in the most recent era analyzed (2000 to 2006) by the IPTR. These are the best outcomes reported to date, with 1-year patient, kidney, and pancreas graft survival rates of 95%, 92%, and 85%, respectively.

Figure 49.2 shows the comparative survival rates of the pancreas graft among the three transplant groups [SPK, pancreas after kidney (PAK), and pancreas transplant alone (PTA)] for the current era analyzed. These results demonstrate that pancreas allograft loss commonly occurs.

General causes and incidence of pancreas graft loss

The two most important general categories of graft loss are technical and immunological. The most common cause of

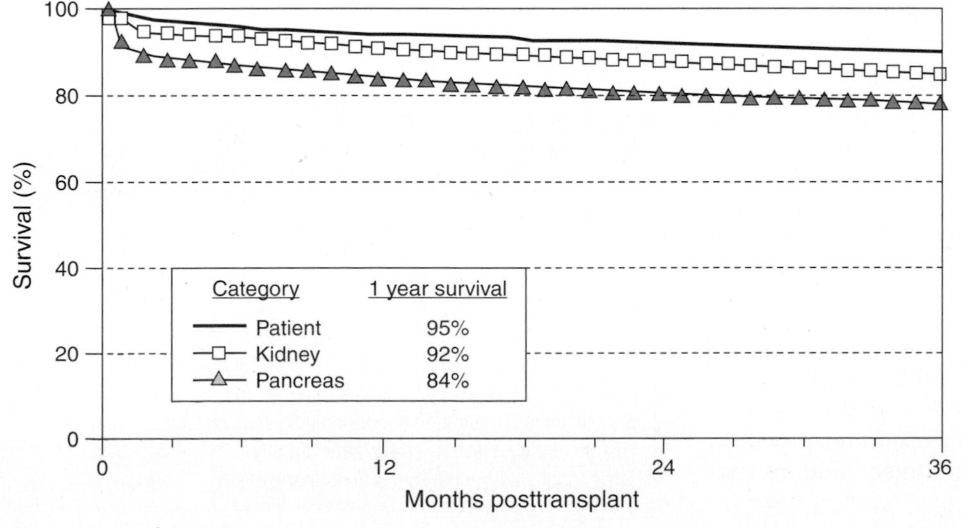

FIGURE 49.1. Patient, kidney, and pancreas survival rates of simultaneous pancreas–kidney transplant recipients (n = 6102, January 1, 2000, to December 31, 2006). (Adapted from International Pancreas Transplant Registry, 2007.)

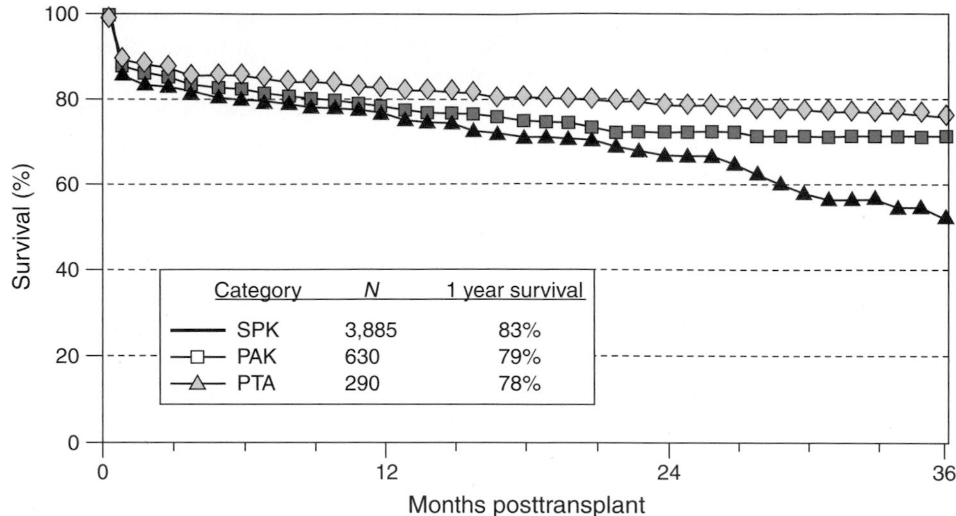

FIGURE 49.2. Pancreas transplant survival rates according to transplant category (2000 to 2006). SPK, simultaneous pancreas and kidney; PAK, pancreas after kidney; PTA, pancreas transplant alone. (Adapted from International Pancreas Transplant Registry, 2007.)

pancreas graft failure within the first 6 months post-transplant in all three recipient categories is technical. The absolute rate of pancreas graft loss within the first 6 months post-transplant is approximately 10% in SPK transplant recipients and 20% in PAK transplant and PTA recipients. Technical failures account for >60% of the cases of pancreas graft loss within this early time period. Knowledge of the technical aspects of the surgical procedures pertaining to pretransplant organ procurement and pancreas graft implantation shed light on the potential complications of pancreas transplantation. The most important cause of technical failure is pancreas graft thrombosis. It occurs in approximately 4% to 9% of cases. SPK transplant recipients are at the lowest risk, and PTA recipients are at the highest risk. Graft losses due to infection, pancreatitis, bleeding, or a duodenal leak are relatively rare.

Immunologic causes of graft loss, acute and chronic rejection, become more important after the 6-month period. The absolute rate of pancreas graft loss from rejection within the first year post-transplant is actually very low. The current rate of immunologic loss in SPK transplant recipients is only 2% at 1 year. The immunologic risk for graft loss for the technically successful cases of PAK transplant and PTA has been reduced to only 3% to 5% at 1 year. Patient death at a time when the transplanted organs are functional is another important cause of graft loss, especially in the SPK and PAK transplant category.

COMPLICATIONS OF PANCREATIC TRANSPLANTATION

Pancreas transplant recipients may experience several common and potentially life-threatening complications. Complications may be anticipated and averted in the settings of recipient selection, donor selection and procurement, and pancreas transplantation surgery and in the postoperative management setting.

Pancreas transplant recipient selection

In the evaluation phase of a pancreas transplant candidate, the history of disease, the review of systems, and the physical examination are conducted in a manner that focuses on specific comorbid conditions that may compromise transplant outcome. Contraindications to solitary pancreas transplantation include patients with type 1 diabetes who have normal renal function and do not exhibit a brittle course, hypoglycemic unawareness, or evidence of nephropathy. Often times the Clarke Score is utilized to determine the threshold of severity of hypoglycemic complications that might justify a solitary pancreas transplant. For patients who have an indication for pancreas transplantation, it is important to exclude significant medical contraindications, including recent malignancy, active or chronic untreated infection, advanced forms of major extrarenal disease (i.e., coronary artery disease), life expectancy of <1 year, sensitization to donor tissue, noncompliance, active substance abuse, and uncontrolled psychiatric disorder (Table 49.1).

Preexisting morbidities have direct implications for predicting and, therefore, avoiding postoperative complications. Premature cardiovascular disease and advanced coronary

Table 49.1 Contraindications to pancreas transplantation

1. Omission of consent for organ donation from family
2. Incompatible blood group
3. Donor HLA class I antigen generating a positive immunological crossmatch
4. History of type 1 or type 2 diabetes mellitus in donor
5. Donor viral infectious disease of HIV, hepatitis B and/or C
6. Significant bacterial and/or fungal infection of the donor
7. Significant and prolonged donor hemodynamic instability
8. History of previous donor pancreatic surgery
9. Intra-abdominal trauma to the donor pancreas

artery disease are the most important comorbidities in patients with type 1 diabetes, especially those with diabetic nephropathy (14–16). There is a fourfold elevation in cardiovascular mortality in type 1 diabetics without proteinuria compared with the general population. In type 1 diabetics with proteinuria, cardiovascular mortality is 37 times higher than it is in the general population (15). The diabetic, uremic patient has several risk factors in addition to diabetes for the development of coronary artery disease, including hypertension, hyperlipidemia, and smoking. Because of the neuropathy associated with diabetes, patients are often asymptomatic because ischemia-induced angina is not perceived. The prevalence of significant (>50% stenosis) coronary artery disease in patients with diabetes starting treatment for end-stage renal disease is estimated to be 45% to 55%.

The interventional screening studies to detect significant, treatable coronary artery disease require a uniform methodology. Noninvasive screening that has high sensitivity and specificity for significant coronary artery disease can be used in low-risk patients. Patients considered at moderate or high risk for significant coronary artery disease should undergo coronary arteriography to determine the severity and location of the lesions. A liberal policy of coronary angiography is reasonable because the current noninvasive tests are relatively insensitive. Also, the techniques of coronary angiography have changed in the past few years, allowing for selected arteriography with very low-dose, less toxic contrast agents using biplanar imaging techniques. The nephrotoxic risk of angiography has been reduced considerably, if a left ventriculogram is omitted, in a preuremic patient with creatinine clearance >20 mL/min.

Patients with coronary lesions amenable to angioplasty with stenting or bypass grafting should be treated, re-evaluated, and then reconsidered for transplantation. The goal of revascularization is to diminish the perioperative risk of the transplant procedure and to prolong the duration of life post-transplant. Patients who have experienced long waiting periods before pancreas transplantation should have their cardiac status assessed at regular intervals.

Autonomic neuropathy is prevalent and may manifest as neurogenic bladder dysfunction, gastropathy, and orthostatic hypotension. Neurogenic bladder dysfunction is an important consideration in patients receiving a bladder-drained, pancreas-alone transplant or an SPK transplant (17). Inability to sense bladder fullness and to empty the bladder predisposes to urine reflux and high postvoid residuals. These problems may adversely affect renal allograft function, increase the incidence of bladder infections and pyelonephritis, and predispose to graft pancreatitis.

Impaired gastric emptying, gastroparesis, is an important consideration with significant implications in the post-transplant period. Patients with severe gastroparesis may have difficulty tolerating the oral immunosuppressive medications that are essential to prevent rejection of the transplants.

The combination of orthostatic hypotension and recumbent hypertension results from dysregulation of vascular tone. This condition has implications for blood pressure control post-transplant, especially in patients with bladder-drained pancreas transplants that are predisposed to volume depletion. Careful reassessment of post-transplant antihypertensive medication requirement is important.

Diabetic retinopathy is a nearly ubiquitous finding in patients with diabetes and end-stage renal disease. Blindness is not an absolute contraindication to transplantation since many blind patients lead very independent life styles. Although rarely a problem, it should be confirmed that a patient with significant vision loss has an adequate support system to ensure help with travel and immunosuppressive medications.

Lower extremity peripheral vascular disease is significant in patients with diabetes. Uremic diabetic patients are at risk for amputation of a lower extremity. These problems typically begin with a foot ulcer associated with advanced somatosensory neuropathy. The risk is further complicated by sensory and motor neuropathies in patients with long-standing diabetes. Vascular disease may have implications for the rehabilitation post-transplant and is an indicator for potential risk for injury to the feet and subsequent diabetic foot ulcers.

Mental or emotional illnesses, including neuroses and depression, are common. Diagnosis and appropriate treatment of these illnesses is an important pretransplant consideration with important implications for ensuring a high degree of medical compliance.

Deceased donor pancreas selection and procurement

Identification of suitable deceased donor organs for pancreas transplantation is an important and often underappreciated determinant of outcome. Misjudgment regarding the quality of the transplantable organs may result in significant adverse consequences post-transplant. The transplant operation begins with organ procurement.

In general, the criteria that determine an appropriate donor for pancreas transplantation are more stringent than for kidney or liver donors. Development of a pancreas donor risk index (PDRI) has been published that identifies factors associated with an increased risk of allograft failure in the context of SPK transplant, PAK transplant, or PTA (18). Ten donor variables and one transplant factor (ischemia time) have been combined into the PDRI. These DRIs include factors that can be identified at the time of organ allocation that also predict the risk of early graft failure. Increased PDRI was associated with a significant, graded reduction in 1-year pancreas graft survival (Fig. 49.3). The cause of failure appeared similar across DRI categories for SPK transplant recipients. In the isolated pancreas transplant recipients (PAK and PTA), however, there was a trend toward higher rates of technical early loss among recipients of high DRI organs.

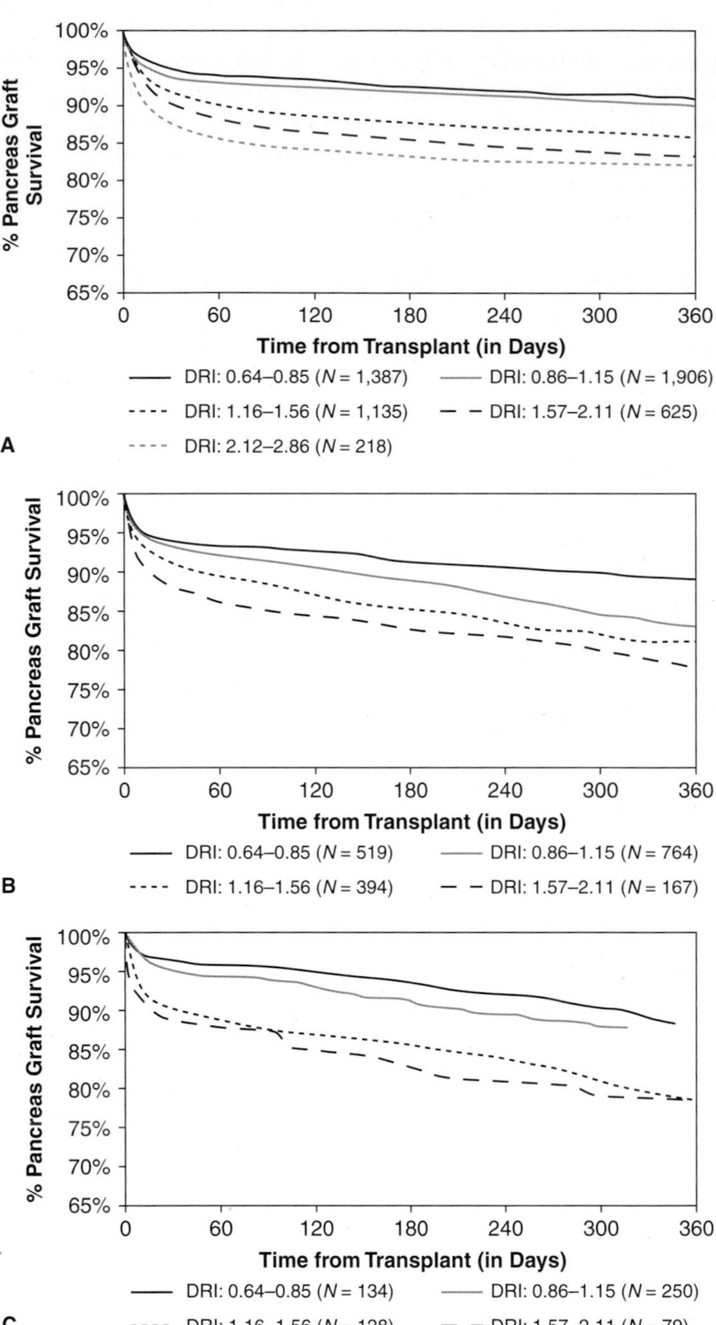

FIGURE 49.3. Adjusted 1-year graft survival following **(A)** simultaneous kidney-pancreas (SPK) transplant, **(B)** pancreas after kidney (PAK) transplant, and **(C)** pancreas transplant alone (PTA), as a function of the pancreas donor risk index (PDRI).

Deceased pancreas organ donors are typically between the ages of 10 and 55. The lower age limit does not relate to the metabolic efficiency of the pediatric endocrine pancreas to regulate blood sugar control in an adult. Rather, the lower age limit of a pediatric donor pancreas reflects the anticipated small size of the splenic artery, which may preclude successful construction of the arterial Y-graft needed for pancreas allograft revascularization. With respect to upper age limits, the use of pancreata from older donors has been associated with increased technical failure due to pancreas graft thrombosis, a higher incidence of post-transplant pancreatitis, and decreased pancreas graft survival rates.

The body weight of the deceased organ donor is an important consideration. Obese donors >100 kg are frequently found not to be suitable pancreas donors. Obese patients may have a history of type 2 diabetes, or the pancreas may be found to be unsuitable for transplantation because of a high degree of adipose infiltration of the pancreas.

Donor hemodynamic stability and need for inotropic support are important considerations. Hemodynamic stability has more influence on the anticipated function of the kidney allograft than it does on initial endocrine function of the pancreas allograft in the case of an SPK transplant. Deceased donors who have experienced a significant period of cardiac arrest or who require high doses of prolonged inotropic support frequently exhibit slow deterioration of renal function that may result in delayed renal allograft function in the SPK transplant recipient.

The most important determinant of suitability of the pancreas for transplantation is direct examination of the organ during surgical procurement. The experience of the procurement team is important. During procurement that judgment regarding the degree of fibrosis, adipose tissue infiltration into the parenchyma, trauma, and specific vascular anomalies can be made. Pancreata with heavy infiltration of adipose tissue are believed to be relatively intolerant of cold preservation and the potential of a high degree of saponification due to reperfusion pancreatitis following revascularization. These organs may be more suitable for islet isolation.

The important vascular anomaly that must be evaluated during procurement is the occurrence of a replaced or accessory right hepatic artery originating from the superior mesenteric artery (SMA). The presence of a replaced right hepatic artery is no longer an absolute contraindication for the use of the pancreas for transplantation. Experienced procurement teams will be able to successfully separate the liver and the pancreas either in situ or on the backbench, without sacrificing quality of either organ for transplantation.

A few important caveats determine whether this maneuver is possible. The replaced right hepatic artery must be dissected to the junction with the SMA. If the replaced right hepatic artery traverses deep into the parenchyma of the head of the pancreas, requiring extensive dissection, this circumstance may preclude the pancreas for transplantation. The SMA is divided distal to the origin of the replaced right hepatic artery, preserving intact a short length of SMA with a carrel patch for the liver graft. Occasionally, there is a large inferior pancreaticoduodenal arterial branch vascularizing the head of the pancreas that originates proximal to the origin of the replaced right hepatic artery. The inferior pancreaticoduodenal vessels are critical to vascularization of the head of the pancreas because the gastroduodenal artery is routinely ligated during the process of hepatic artery mobilization for the liver transplant. In the case of a very proximal origin of the inferior pancreaticoduodenal artery, dividing the SMA at the appropriate location for proper liver procurement would significantly impair vascularization of the head of the pancreas and preclude its use for transplantation. Evaluation of the arterial vascularity of the pancreaticoduodenal allograft can be tested on the backbench by several methods: (a) injection of Renografin into the SMA or Y-graft and obtaining an x-ray; (b) intra-arterial injection of fluorescein, with visualization using a Wood lamp; and (c) performing a methylene blue angiogram.

The use of marginal and nonheartbeating donors for pancreas transplantation has been reported. If the pancreas is deemed suitable, there is the added consideration of the effect of delayed kidney graft function in a uremic SPK transplant candidate. The use of marginal and nonheartbeating donors for pancreas-alone transplantation is a selective decision made on a case-by-case basis.

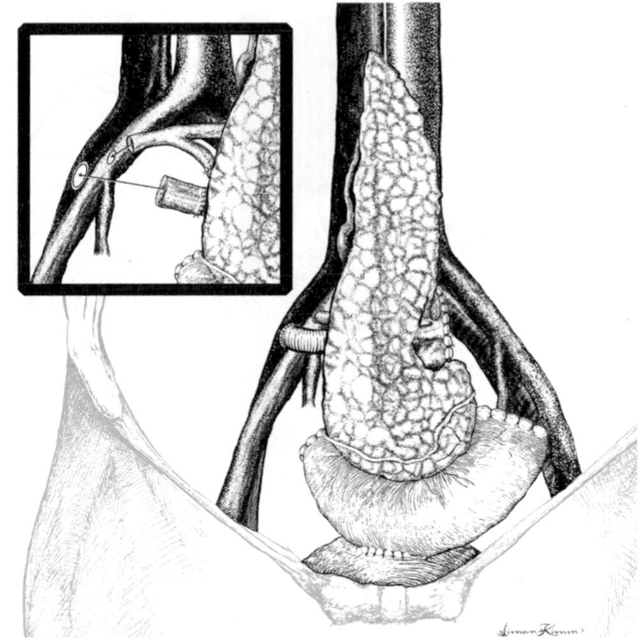

FIGURE 49.4. Pancreaticoduodenal allograft with exocrine bladder drainage and systemic venous drainage. (Adapted from Stuart FP, Abecassis MM, Kaufman DB. *Organ transplantation*, 2nd ed. Georgetown: Landes Bioscience; 2003:166.)

The use of living related and unrelated pancreas donors has also been described. A distal pancreatectomy is performed for a segmental pancreas transplant. Anecdotal cases of combined live donor partial pancreatectomy and nephrectomy have also been reported. These procedures are not widely performed and are confined to one or two pancreas transplant programs.

Pancreas transplantation surgery

The surgical techniques for pancreas transplantation are diverse (Figs. 49.4 to 49.6). The principles are consistent, however, and include providing adequate arterial blood flow to the pancreas and duodenal segment, adequate venous outflow from the pancreas, and management of the pancreatic exocrine secretions. The native pancreas is not removed.

Pancreas graft arterial revascularization is typically accomplished using the recipient right common or external iliac artery. The Y-graft of the pancreas is anastomosed end to side. Positioning of the head of the pancreas graft cephalad or caudad is not relevant with respect to successful arterial revascularization. There are two choices for venous revascularization—systemic and portal. Systemic venous revascularization commonly involves the right common iliac vein, or right external iliac vein. If portal venous drainage is used, it is necessary to dissect the superior mesenteric vein at the root of the mesentery. The pancreas portal vein is anastomosed end to side to a branch of the

Urine leak from breakdown of the duodenal segment can occur and is usually encountered within the first 2 to 3 months post-transplant, but it can occur years postoperatively. Leak is the most serious postoperative complication of the bladder-drained pancreas. The onset of abdominal pain with elevated serum amylase, which can mimic reflux pancreatitis or acute rejection, is a typical presentation. Supporting imaging studies utilizing a cystogram or CT scanning are necessary to confirm the diagnosis. Operative repair is usually required. The degree of leakage can be best determined intraoperatively and proper judgment made about whether direct repair is possible or more aggressive surgery involving enteric diversion (25) (Fig. 49.12) is indicated.

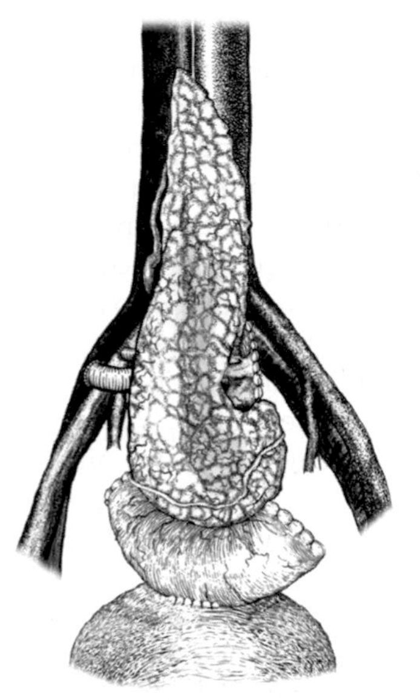

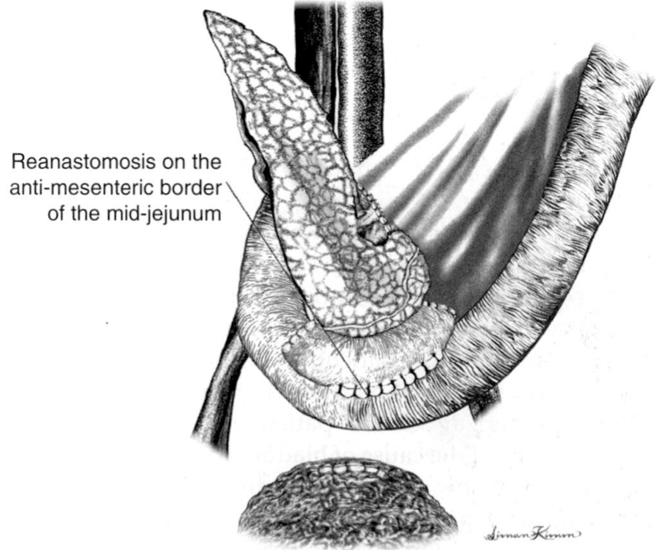

FIGURE 49.12. Surgical procedure of enteric conversion of the bladder-drained pancreaticoduodenal transplant.

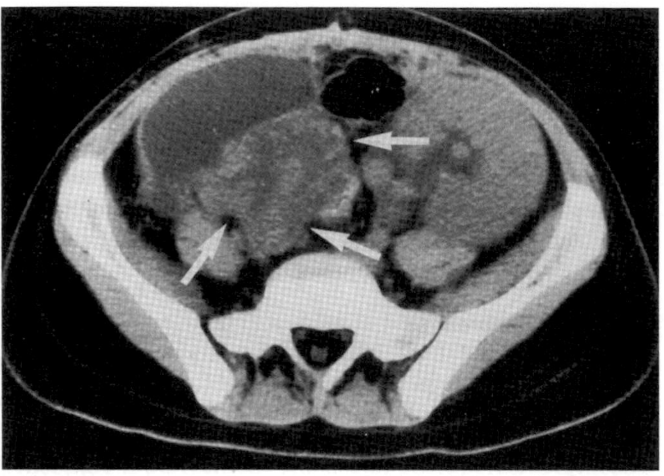

FIGURE 49.13. Computed tomographic study of a well-marginated, low-density fluid collection anterior to the pancreas transplant (*arrows*). (Reprinted from Letourneau JG, Day DL, Ascher NL. *Radiology of organ transplantation.* St Louis: Mosby, 1991:278, with permission.)

Infection

The most serious complication of pancreas transplantation is leak and intra-abdominal abscess. Patients present with fever, abdominal discomfort, and leukocytosis. Computed tomographic study of the abdomen is helpful to confirm clinical suspicion and to localize infected peripancreatic fluid collections (Fig. 49.13). Duodenoenteric anastomotic leak occurs as a result of an ischemic duodenal stump, technical error, or duodenal stump blowout. Percutaneous access of intra-abdominal fluid collections for Gram stain and culture is essential. The flora is typically mixed with bacteria and possibly fungus (26), particularly *Candida*. Broad-spectrum antibiosis is essential. Surgical exploration is required if conservative methods of percutaneous drainage do not adequately control established infection.

Intraoperative findings usually reveal fibrinous adhesive disease with interloop abscess. Exploration and repair of a duodenal graft leak is necessary. A decision must be made on whether the infection can be eradicated without removing the pancreas allograft. Incomplete eradication of the infection will result in progression to sepsis and multiple organ system failure. Peripancreatic infections can result in development of a mycotic aneurysm at the arterial anastomosis that could cause arterial rupture. Transplant pancreatectomy is indicated if mycotic aneurysm is diagnosed.

The occurrence of intra-abdominal abscess has been greatly reduced with greater recognition of the suitability of cadaveric pancreas grafts for transplantation. Improved perioperative antibiosis, including antifungal agents, has contributed to the decreased incidence of intra-abdominal infection as well. There is no convincing evidence that a Roux-en-Y intestinal reconstruction decreases incidence. Perhaps the most significant contribution to reducing intra-abdominal abscesses is the efficacy of the immunosuppressive agents in reducing acute rejection and thereby minimizing the need for intensive antirejection immunotherapy.

The most important threat to loss of a functioning pancreas allograft is acute rejection. The graft's fate is intimately linked to the efficacy and safety of immunosuppressive agents and the recipient's medical compliance. Through judicious application of immunosuppression, both rejection and infectious complications may be avoided. Pancreatic allograft monitoring to diagnose acute rejection in a timely manner is essential to achieve long-term survival. Overtreatment of a suspected rejection episode can be a serious cause of infectious morbidity and mortality in pancreas transplant recipients.

Pancreas allograft rejection can be characterized as hyperacute, acute, and chronic. Hyperacute rejection occurs minutes to hours following revascularization of the pancreas graft. Hyperacute rejection occurs when preformed anti-HLA (Histocompatibility Leukocyte Antigens) antibodies bind to graft endothelium, activate the compliment cascade, and produce capillary microthrombi. Hyperacute rejection is rare if the pretransplant screening crossmatch is nonreactive. This form of rejection can be a difficult diagnosis because of the relatively high incidence of early organ failure due to vascular thrombosis. The few cases published describe negative crossmatches in recipients with high panel-reactive antibody levels (27).

Acute pancreatic graft rejection typically occurs 3 to 12 months post-transplant but can happen later if medical noncompliance occurs. Acute rejection is primarily a function of cell-mediated cytotoxicity. The initial cellular targets of rejection are endothelial cells, acinar, and ductal epithelial cells. Islets and β cells are not primary targets of alloimmune rejection (27). Islets may be involved late in rejection and may also stop functioning before becoming involved with inflammatory cells (28,29).

Chronic rejection is a more indolent process that occurs relatively late in the course of transplantation. The most notable contributing factor includes multiple acute rejection episodes (30). Chronic rejection in the pancreas is characterized by arterial narrowing and interstitial fibrosis with variable loss of acinar and islet tissue (29,31). Arteriopathy causes progressive ischemic damage to the acinar and islet tissues, resulting in extensive pancreatic fibrosis.

Diagnosis

The clinical presentation of pancreas allograft rejection can be subtle. Only 5% to 20% of patients with pancreatic graft rejection present with obvious clinical symptoms. The pancreatic graft undergoing acute rejection becomes inflamed. Patients experience pain and discomfort due to surrounding peritoneal irritation, but rejection is difficult to distinguish clinically from benign graft pancreatitis. Fever as a clinical symptom of rejection is uncommon, partly due to maintenance immunosuppressive therapy with prednisone. If the workup for infection is negative, fever is highly suspicious for rejection. A paralytic ileus or acute abdomen rarely occurs but can be caused by rejection-induced pancreatitis. Inflammation of the surrounding organs, such as the small and large intestine, may result in a dynamic ileus or diarrhea, respectively.

Laboratory markers are commonly relied on to guide subsequent imaging studies or biopsy. Profound destruction of exocrine pancreatic tissue occurs before significant deterioration in endocrine pancreatic function (32). Hyperglycemia is a late parameter of rejection and is usually apparent only after extensive destruction of the islets has taken place. Hyperglycemia is not useful to diagnose acute rejection that is likely to be reversed. Hyperglycemia is also a sign of development of peripheral insulin resistance (type 2 diabetes). Differentiation of loss of β cell insulin production (rejection) is accomplished by measurement of C-peptide levels. Using pancreas-specific serum markers to detect rejection is problematic due to the pathophysiology of the exocrine pancreas. Rejection, as well as pancreatitis, infection, or preservation injury, leads to damage of acinar tissue, with subsequent enzyme and cytokine release. The causes of destruction of pancreas acinar tissue are multiple and, with pancreas-specific serum parameters only, difficult to differentiate.

An increase in serum amylase usually occurs with rejection and precedes a decline in urinary amylase (in recipients with bladder-drained pancreas) (33,34). Post-transplant hyperamylasemia can be caused by any process inducing pancreatic inflammation. In addition, serum amylase is also derived in large part from other tissues, including salivary glands and intestine. Several studies on SPK transplant recipients showed elevated human anodal trypsinogen (HAT) levels during clinically diagnosed rejection episodes (35). HAT levels are frequently elevated in the early post-transplant period, which may reflect preservation or procurement injury rather than rejection. Renal dysfunction, pancreatitis, trauma, and bladder outlet obstruction may also influence HAT levels. One study performed on SPK and PAK transplant recipients included both renal biopsies and HAT levels, finding HAT as a reliable marker of pancreas rejection in all cases (36).

In the context of SPK transplantation, the kidney allograft is the best indicator of a rejection episode. Rejection of the kidney allograft will manifest as a rise in serum creatinine. Increased serum creatinine will prompt ultrasound and biopsy of the kidney allograft, and if rejection is diagnosed, antirejection therapy is instituted. If there is a concurrent pancreas graft rejection process, the antirejection therapy will reverse the process in both organs.

Bladder drainage is a widely used technique for management of exocrine secretion in pancreatic transplantation because it also allows graft exocrine function to be monitored by measuring pancreatic enzymes secreted directly into the urine (37). Bladder drainage is mostly used in recipients of PAK transplant and PTA. The technique is becoming less frequently used in SPK transplant recipients because monitoring renal allograft function serves as a better indication of rejection (and a surrogate marker of pancreas graft rejection) and there is less morbidity with enteric drainage. Serial urine amylase measurement has emerged as a very common surveillance and diagnostic laboratory test. A reduction in urinary amylase activity, relative hypoamylasuria, is the most commonly used biochemical marker of acute rejection in the PAK transplant and PTA recipient categories. By monitoring urinary amylase levels, antirejection treatment can begin before hyperglycemia occurs. Urinary amylase measurements are simple, without morbidity, and relatively inexpensive, and most laboratories can perform them. One of the limitations of urinary amylase monitoring is that a decrease in activity does not necessarily mean rejection. Reduced urinary amylase levels may be caused by other factors, such as preservation injury in the early posttransplant period, pancreatitis, fibrosis, thrombosis, ductal obstruction, prolonged fasting, hydration status, and diuresis (38).

Core Needle biopsy is the standard for the diagnosis of pancreas allograft rejection in the context of PAK transplant and PTA. For most solid organ transplants, histologic evaluation of graft biopsies became the standard assessment for rejection early on. For pancreas transplantation, the development was different for two reasons. It is rare that isolated pancreatic rejection occurs in SPK transplant recipients without simultaneous renal allograft rejection. In these patients, most rejection episodes involve either the kidney alone or the kidney and the pancreas simultaneously (39). This observation has promoted the perception that pancreatic graft rejection can be monitored indirectly by relying on serum creatinine changes or kidney graft biopsies. For SPK transplants, the kidney serves as an excellent surrogate marker for rejection. In solitary pancreas transplant recipients (PAK and PTA), serum creatinine levels or kidney biopsies cannot be used as markers of rejection, and, given the inadequacies of laboratory parameters, biopsies are therefore essential for monitoring solitary pancreas transplants. In SPK transplant recipients, isolated pancreatic graft rejection can occur and pancreatic graft biopsies may become necessary if a change in exocrine or endocrine laboratory parameters occurs without an elevation in serum creatinine.

Currently, the vast majority of pancreatic graft biopsies are obtained either percutaneously or cystoscopically and only rarely by laparotomy or laparoscopy. Most centers prefer ultrasound-guided, percutaneous biopsy, performed under local anesthesia. If it is impossible to obtain tissue for histology or if overlying bowel prohibits sampling, the cystoscopic approach is employed for bladder-drained grafts. Laparotomy or laparoscopy and biopsy are reserved for grafts inaccessible by the aforementioned approaches when the risks of empiric antirejection therapy outweigh those of surgery.

Immunosuppression

Over the past decade, pancreas transplantation results have improved significantly due to advances in immunosuppression. The principles of immunosuppressive therapy for pancreas recipients are similar to those applied to recipients of other solid-organ allografts. The advent of more effective immunomodulating agents has reduced the frequency and severity of pancreatic allograft rejection episodes. However, acute rejection continues to be the most challenging event in the course of pancreatic graft recipients.

The use of induction therapy has been shown to significantly improve pancreas graft survival rates in several subgroups. According to data from the IPTR, the use of induction therapy in SPK transplant recipients with systemic venous–enteric exocrine drainage significantly improves pancreas graft survival rates (40,41). Interestingly, pancreas graft survival is not improved with induction therapy in the subgroups with portal venous-enteric or bladder drainage. Furthermore, SPK transplant recipients who receive induction therapy benefit from a reduced incidence and severity of biopsy-confirmed, treated, acute kidney rejection episodes. For solitary pancreas transplant recipients (PAK and PTA), the addition of induction therapy is associated with a clinically significant improvement in pancreas graft survival rates.

Maintenance immunosuppressive agents used for pancreas transplantation fall into the following categories: (a) corticosteroids, (b) calcineurin inhibitors (cyclosporine and tacrolimus), (c) antimetabolites (azathioprine and mycophenolate mofetil), and (d) cell cycle inhibitors (sirolimus). In 2002, solitary pancreas transplant recipients received corticosteroids in approximately 90% of cases, tacrolimus in 91% (cyclosporine 8%), mycophenolate mofetil in 70% (azathioprine 1%), and sirolimus in 18%. Therefore, in 2002, the most frequently used combination of maintenance therapy at discharge was tacrolimus, mycophenolate mofetil, and corticosteroids.

Trends in the uses of maintenance therapies over the past 10 years for solitary pancreas transplant recipients (PAK and PTA) are depicted in Figure 49.14. The dominant use of tacrolimus today represents a marked shift from earlier eras. The U.S. Food and Drug Administration (FDA) approved tacrolimus for marketing for kidney transplantation in 1994. In 1993, cyclosporine accounted for virtually 100% of the calcineurin inhibitor use in pancreas transplantation. Since that time, tacrolimus use has increased yearly and reached 91% in 2002. The FDA approved mycophenolate mofetil for marketing for kidney transplantation in 1995, and it was used in only 14% of solitary pancreas transplant cases that year (azathioprine was used in 72% of cases). However, within 1 year, nearly 80% of solitary pancreas transplant recipients received mycophenolate mofetil, with only 12% receiving azathioprine. The use of azathioprine has diminished yearly and dropped to 1% usage in 2002. In 1999, the FDA approved the use of sirolimus for marketing for kidney transplantation. For pancreas transplantation, this agent is usually used in combination with a calcineurin inhibitor and as a substitute for an antimetabolite. The use of sirolimus has been relatively slow to penetrate

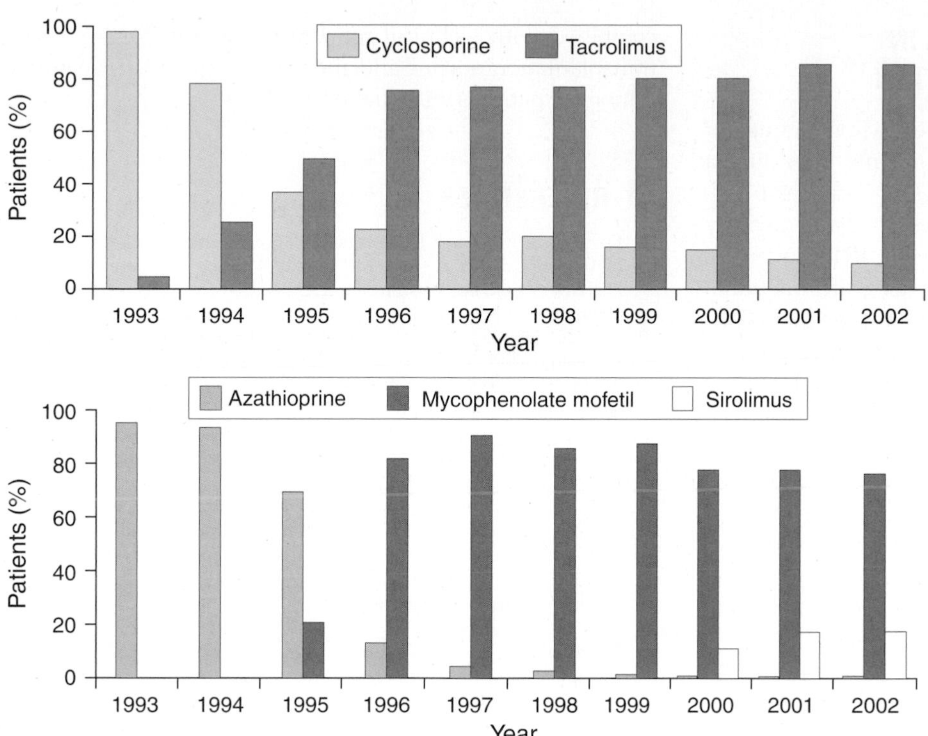

FIGURE 49.14. Trends in maintenance immunosuppression in recipients of solitary pancreas transplants. (Adapted from 2005 OPTN/SRTR Annual Report.)

the market, compared with the rapid spread of tacrolimus and mycophenolate mofetil. In 2002, sirolimus was used for 18% of solitary pancreas transplant cases.

Similar trends in maintenance immunosuppression were also observed for SPK transplant recipients. The changes in uses of specific maintenance immunotherapies over the past 10 years for SPK transplant recipients are depicted in Figure 49.15. The use of tacrolimus rose from 55% in 1995 to 85% in 2004. Cyclosporine usage has dropped from 35% of cases in 1994 to only 10% of cases in 2004. Similar trends in the use of antimetabolites are seen with respect to azathioprine and mycophenolate mofetil. In 1995, azathioprine was used in 60% of cases, dropping to 1% in 2004; mycophenolate mofetil usage grew from 25% in 1995 to 80% in 2004. From 2000 to 2004, sirolimus usage rose from 12% to 20% of cases.

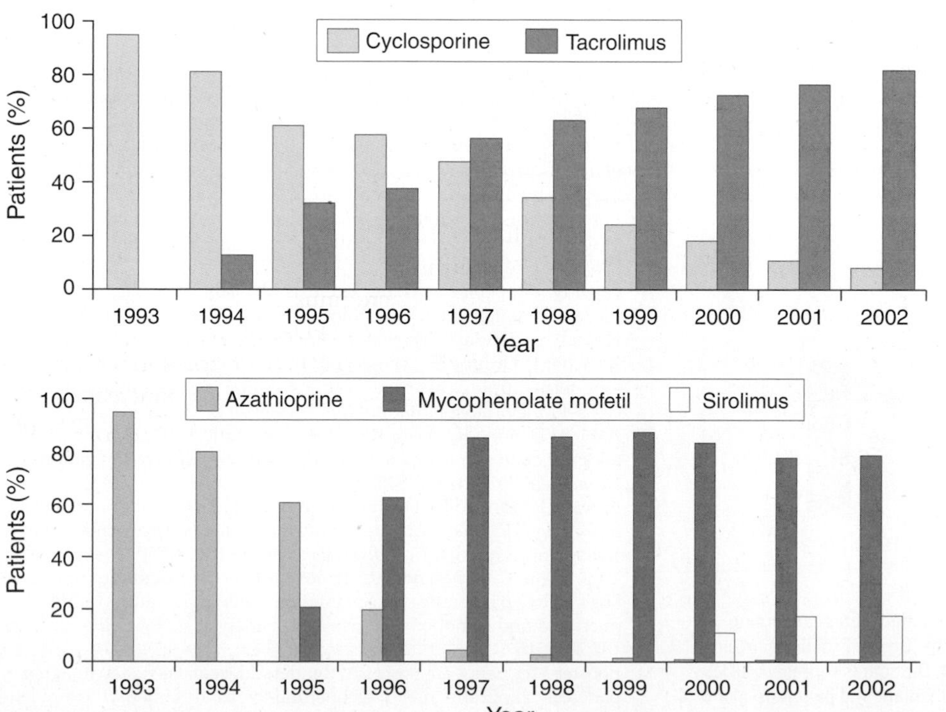

FIGURE 49.15. Trends in maintenance immunosuppression in recipients of simultaneous pancreas-kidney transplants. (Adapted from 2005 OPTN/SRTR Annual Report.)

IMMUNOLOGICAL PROGRESS IN PANCREATIC TRANSPLANTATION

Changes in clinical practice patterns regarding the use of the maintenance immunosuppressive agents have had a significant beneficial effect on outcomes of pancreas transplantation (40). Pancreas transplant results have steadily improved. According to the SRTR and the IPTR, over the 10-year period from 1995 to 2004, pancreas graft functional survival (enteric drainage) in SPK transplant recipients has increased from 76% to 86% (42). For PAK transplantation, pancreas graft functional survival (enteric drainage) has shown steady improvement over the 10-year interval from 1995 to 2004 from a 1-year patient survival rate of 67% to 77%. For patients receiving a PTA, the pancreas graft functional survival (enteric drainage) rates over the past 10 years has improved from 67% to 84%. The period 1995 reflects use of today's "second-line" immunosuppressants (cyclosporine and azathioprine), whereas 2004 reflects the period of mature integration of the new "first-line" immunosuppressive agents (tacrolimus, mycophenolate, and sirolimus) into mainstream use. In addition to graft survival improvements, there have been substantial improvements in controlling the risk of graft rejection. Figure 49.16 shows 1-year rejection rates according to transplant era. Rejection rates decreased from 59% to 20% in SPK transplant recipients and decreased from 56% to 23% in solitary pancreas transplant recipients.

Aggregate outcome information from national databases and single-center reports (43) also demonstrate that improvements in the technical and immunologic approaches to pancreatic transplantation have moved the field forward. However, further refinements are needed to decrease complication rates. Continued advances in immunotherapy combined with technical refinements will make pancreatic transplantation a safer and more widely applied treatment option for patients with diabetes.

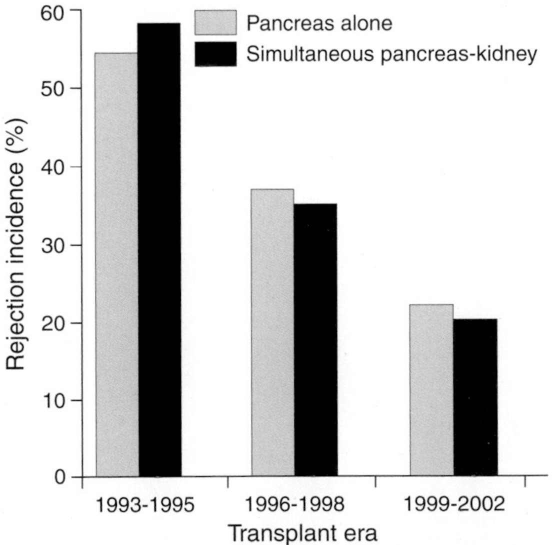

FIGURE 49.16. Pancreas allograft 1-year rejection rates according to transplant era. Outcomes based on data from the Organ Procurement and Transplant Network (OPTN) as of January 2, 2004. Outcomes represent all US cases of simultaneous pancreas-kidney (SKP) transplant and pancreas-alone transplants performed from January 1993 to December 2002.

REFERENCES

1. Portuese E, Orchard T. Mortality in insulin-dependent diabetes. In: Harris MI, Cowie CC, Stern MP, Boyko EJ, Reiber GE, Bennett PH, eds. *Diabetes in America*. Washington, DC: US Government Printing Office; 1995:221–232.
2. National Diabetes Data Group, National Institutes of Health. *Diabetes in America*, 2nd ed. Bethesda, MD: National Institutes of Health; 1995. NIH Publication No. 95-1468.
3. Epidemiology of Diabetes Interventions and Complications (EDIC) Research Group. Effect of intensive diabetes treatment on carotid artery wall thickness in the epidemiology of diabetes interventions and complications. *Diabetes* 1999;48:383–390.
4. DCCT/EDIC Research Group. Effect of intensive therapy on the microvascular complications of type 1 diabetes mellitus. *JAMA* 2002;287: 2563–2569.
5. Morel P, Goetz F, Moudry-Munns KC, et al. Long term metabolic control in patients with pancreatic transplants. *Ann Intern Med* 1991;115: 694–699.
6. Navarro X, Kennedy WR, Loewenson RB, et al. Influence of pancreas transplantation on cardiorespiratory reflexes, nerve conduction, and mortality in diabetes mellitus. *Diabetes* 1990;39:802–806.
7. Kennedy WR, Navarro X, Goetz FC, et al. Effects of pancreatic transplantation on diabetic neuropathy. *N Engl J Med* 1990;322:1031–1037.
8. Fioretto P, Mauer SM, Bilous RW, et al. Effects of pancreas transplantation on glomerular structure in insulin-dependent diabetic patients with their own kidneys. *Lancet* 1993;342:1193–1196.
9. Bilous RW, Mauer SM, Sutherland DE, et al. The effects of pancreas transplantation on the glomerular structure of renal allografts in patients with insulin-dependent diabetes. *N Engl J Med* 1989;321:80–85.
10. Zehr PS, Milde FK, Hart LK, et al. Pancreas transplantation: assessing secondary complications and life quality. *Diabetologia* 1991;34(Suppl 1): S138–S140.
11. Ojo AO, Meier-Kriesche HU, Hanson JA, et al. Impact of simultaneous pancreas–kidney transplantation on long-term patient survival. *Transplantation* 2001;71:82–90.
12. Mohan P, Safi K, Little DM, et al. Improved patient survival in recipients of simultaneous pancreas–kidney transplant compared with kidney transplant alone in patients with type 1 diabetes mellitus and end-stage renal disease. *Br J Surg* 2003;90:1137–1141.
13. Clarke WL, Cox DJ, Gonder-Frederick LA, et al. Reduced awareness of hypoglycemia in adults with IDDM. A prospective study of hypoglycemic frequency and associated symptoms. *Diabetes Care* 1995;18: 517–522.
14. Kroslewski AS, Kosinski EJ, Warram JH, et al. Magnitude and determinants of coronary artery disease in juvenile-onset, insulin-dependent diabetes mellitus. *Am J Cardiol* 1987;59:750–755.
15. Borch-Johnsen K, Kreiner S. Proteinuria: value as predictor of cardiovascular mortality in insulin dependent diabetes mellitus. *Br Med J* 1987;294:1651–1654.
16. Grundy SM, Benjamin IJ, Burke GL, et al. Diabetes and cardiovascular disease: a statement for healthcare professionals from the American Heart Association. *Circulation* 1999;100:1134–1146.
17. Blanchet P, Droupy S, Eschwege P, et al. Urodynamic testing predicts long-term urological complications following simultaneous pancreas–kidney transplantation. *Clin Transplant* 2003;17:26–31.
18. Axelrod D, Sung R, Meyer KH, et al. Systematic evaluation of pancreas allograft quality, outcomes, and geographic variation in utilization. *Am J Transplant* 2010;10:837–845.
19. Pirsch JD, Odorico JS, D'Alessandro AM, et al. Intra-abdominal infection in enteric versus bladder-drained simultaneous pancreas–kidney transplant recipients. *Transplantation* 1998;66:1746–1750.
20. Troppmann C, Gruessner AC, Benedetti E, et al. Vascular graft thrombosis after pancreatic transplantation: univariate and multivariate operative and nonoperative risk factor analysis. *J Am Coll Surg* 1996; 182:285–316.
21. Booster MH, Schoenmakers EA, Rijnders AJ, et al. Perfusion imaging of pancreas allografts using technetium-99 m hexamethyl propylene amine oxime. *Transplant Int* 1992;5(Suppl. 1):S265–S267.

22. Gilabert R, Fernandez-Cruz L, Real MI, et al. Treatment and outcome of pancreatic venous graft thrombosis after kidney—pancreas transplantation. *Br J Surg* 2002;89:355–360.
23. Barone GW, Webb JW, Hudec WA. The enteric drained pancreas transplant: another potential source of gastrointestinal bleeding. *Am J Gastroenterol* 1998;93:1369–1371.
24. Sollinger HW, Messing EM, Eckhoff DE, et al. Urologic complications in 210 consecutive simultaneous pancreas–kidney transplants with bladder drainage. *Ann Surg* 1993;218:561–568.
25. West M, Gruessner AC, Metrakos P, et al. Conversion from bladder to enteric drainage after pancreaticoduodenal transplantations. *Surgery* 1998;124:883–893.
26. Benedetti E, Gruessner AC, Troppmann C, et al. Intra-abdominal fungal infections after pancreatic transplantation: incidence, treatment, and outcome. *J Am Coll Surg* 1996;183:307–316.
27. Sibley RK. Pancreas transplantation. In: Sale GE, ed. *The Pathology of organ transplantation.* Boston, MA: Butterworth–Heineman; 1990:179–215.
28. Nakhleh RE, Gruessner RWG, Swanson PE, et al. Pancreas transplant pathology: a morphologic immunohistochemical, and electron microscopic comparison of allogeneic grafts with rejection, syngeneic grafts, and chronic pancreatitis. *Am J Surg Pathol* 1991;15:246–256.
29. Nakhleh RE, Sutherland DER. Pancreas rejection: significance of histopathologic findings with implication of classification for rejection. *Am J Surg Pathol* 1992;16:1098–1107.
30. Humar A, Khwaja K, Ramcharan T, et al. Chronic rejection: the next major challenge for pancreas transplant recipients. *Transplantation* 2003; 76:918–923.
31. Papadimitriou JC, Drachenberg CB, Klassen DK, et al. Histological grading of chronic pancreas allograft rejection/graft sclerosis. *Am J Transplant* 2003;3:599–605.
32. Dragstedt LR. Some physiologic problems in surgery of the pancreas. *Ann Surg* 1943;118:576–593.
33. Tyden G, Gunnarsson R, Ostman J, et al. Laboratory findings during rejection of segmental pancreatic allografts. *Transplant Proc* 1984;16:715–717.
34. Cheng SS, Munn SR. Posttransplant hyperamylasemia is associated with decreased patient and graft survival in pancreas allograft recipients. *Transplant Proc* 1994;26:428–429.
35. Marks WH, Borgstrom A, Sollinger H, et al. Serum immunoreactive anodal trypsinogen and urinary amylase as biochemical markers for rejection of clinical whole-organ pancreas allografts having exocrine drainage into the urinary bladder. *Transplantation* 1990;49:112–115.
36. Perkal M, Marks C, Lorber MI, et al. A three-year experience with serum anodal trypsinogen as a biochemical marker for rejection in pancreatic allografts. False positives, tissue biopsy, comparison with other markers, and diagnostic strategies. *Transplantation* 1992;53:415–419.
37. Prieto M, Sutherland DE, Fernandez-Cruz L, et al. Experimental and clinical experience with urine amylase monitoring for early diagnosis of rejection in pancreas transplantation. *Transplantation* 1987;43: 73–79.
38. Munn SR, Engen DE, Barr D, et al. Differential diagnosis of hypoamylasuria in pancreas allograft recipients with urinary exocrine drainage. *Transplantation* 1990;49:359–362.
39. Gruessner RWG, Dunn DL, Tzardis PJ, et al. Simultaneous pancreas and kidney transplants versus single kidney transplants and previous kidney transplants in uremic patients and single pancreas transplants in nonuremic diabetic patients: comparison of rejection, morbidity and long-term outcome. *Transplant Proc* 1990;22:622–623.
40. Gruessner AC, Sutherland DE. Pancreas transplant outcomes for United States (US) and Non-US cases as reported to the United Network for Organ Sharing (UNOS) and the International Pancreas Transplant Registry (IPTR) as of October, 2002. In: Cecka JM, Terasaki PI, eds. *Clinical Transplants 2002.* Los Angeles, CA: UCLA Tissue Typing Laboratory, 2002:41–77.
41. Kaufman DB. Induction therapy. In: Gruessner RWG, Sutherland DE, eds. *Transplantation of the pancreas.* New York: Springer; 2004:267–300.
42. Gruessner AC, Sutherland DE. Analysis of United States (US) and Non-US pancreas transplants reported to the United Network for Organ Sharing (UNOS) and the International Pancreas Transplant Registry (IPTR) as of October, 2001. In: Cecka JM, Terasaki PI, eds. *Clinical transplants 2001.* Los Angeles, CA: UCLA Tissue Typing Laboratory, 2001: 41–72.
43. Kaufman DB, Leventhal JR, Gallon LG, et al. Technical and immunological progress in simultaneous pancreas–kidney transplantation. *Surgery* 2002;132:545–555.

reduced level of flow through the anastomosis. Open exploration is occasionally necessary to confirm the diagnosis and conduct appropriate repair.

Sternal Complications

Historically, bilateral lung transplantation has been done through a median sternotomy and more recently through the so-called "clam-shell" incision or bilateral transsternal thoracotomy (transverse thoracosternotomy) (9,10). This technique provides extensive exposure to the hila and bilateral pleural spaces and access to the great vessels (11–14). However, this technique has some drawbacks and is associated with a series of complications.

The incidence of sternal complications after lung transplantation can range from 32% to 46% and in some lung transplant recipients leads to significant morbidity and even mortality. Sternal complications after lung transplantation can include sternal override, dehiscence or disruption, infection, and pseudoartrosis. Lung transplant recipients may be particularly prone to poor sternal healing because of their debilitated state (osteoporosis, poor nutritional status, diabetes mellitus, obesity, and heavy smoking) and the routine use of perioperative corticosteroids and postoperative immunosuppression (12,13).

Sternal disruption, commonly called "sternal overriding," is a common complication in sternal healing. Brown et al. (15) report a prevalence of 36% for sternal disruption in transverse bilateral thoracosternotomy for lung transplantation at their institution, and they cite disruption rates of 20% to 60% at institutions worldwide. Sternal overriding occurs because of the tendency toward angulation and anterior displacement of the distal sternum, and it appears to be unique to the bilateral transsternal thoracotomy (16). There is a translational movement that is not prevented by sternal wires. The solution to sternal override has been the addition of coaxial stabilization: either by long, thin Kirschner wires or short, stout Steinmann pins, placed within the cancellous bone of the sternum to help prevent sternal override and translational movement at the bony closures. However, these wires have a tendency to migrate and have been removed in patients after migration from the sternum to various locations in the body. Such retrievals have required interventions ranging from local anesthetic to liberate a wire eroding through the anterior chest wall to general anesthesia with laparoscopy to remove a Kirschner wire from the pouch of Douglas. Sternal dehiscence is defined as "the total disruption of surgical sutures with or without infection" (11), and it is associated with significant morbidity (34%) and mortality (26%) (12,17). Sternal (deformed or angled healing), nonunion (persistent sternal fracture at least 3 months after surgery or 6 months after trauma without evidence of infection or healing), wound infection and/or broken fixation wires can precede sternal dehiscence (11).

Sternal disruption or overriding and sternal dehiscence can lead to both restrictions in chest wall movement and compliance (16), resulting in lower forced vital capacity and forced expiratory volume in 1 second after lung transplantation (12). These complications can be associated with prolonged need for ventilatory support, mediastinitis, osteomyelitis, and even death (18). Many groups have developed methods to improve fixation in the transsternal bilateral thoracotomy incision from single (11) and double plating (15) to different wiring techniques (12,13); however, complications continue to pose a challenge. Meyers et al. and other groups advocate avoiding sternal division altogether with bilateral anteriolateral thoracotomies, which have been demonstrated to provide adequate exposure in most circumstances (2,12,14,19). Additionally, in rare selected cases, the use of modified approaches, such as a combined left posterolateral and right anterior thoracotomy, is advocated to optimize the left hilar exposure without the need for either sternal division or for a separate positioning, preparing, and draping.

A deep sternal wound infection is a notorious complication after open-heart surgery, and patients undergoing lung transplantation are not an exemption. Bacterial infections account for the majority of sternal wound infections, *Staphylococcus* being the most common pathogen (20); however, fungal infections have been reported (21). The incidence of sternal wound infections can vary, but typically range from 0.4% to 8.8% (22–24). They classically occur within the first 30 days after transplantation. The presentation of sternal wound infections can occur along a spectrum from sterile wound dehiscence to mediastinitis and sternal osteomyelitis. Patients usually present with fever, elevated white blood cell counts, tachycardia, and an erythematous, edematous, tender wound site with or without drainage. The diagnosis is further confirmed with chest radiographs, cultures, and computed tomographic scans. Treatment requires operative and bedside wound debridement with antibiotics and possible reconstruction procedures in the future. Sternal wound infections are associated with prolonged hospital course, increased hospital costs, and significant morbidity and mortality for the patient. Long-term effects include chronic pain, sternal instability, and cosmetic defects (20).

POSTOPERATIVE COMPLICATIONS

The numerous complications that can occur after transplantation often occur along a predictable time course. Detailed discussion of the most important complications follows.

Ischemia–reperfusion injury

Ischemia–reperfusion injury is one of the most important complications of lung transplantation, affecting 10% to 25% of all lung transplant recipients (25–28). It represents the most frequent cause of early mortality and prolonged ICU stay. Ischemia–reperfusion injury encompasses an array of definitions, including primary graft dysfunction, implantation response, acute lung injury, and hyperacute rejection

(29). Mortality rates are significantly higher in recipients with ischemia–reperfusion injury, and those who do survive have significantly impaired physical function (26) and an increased risk of chronic rejection or bronchiolitis obliterans syndrome (BOS) (30).

A variety of donor, recipient, and operative factors play a role in the development of ischemia–reperfusion injury. Some inherent donor risk factors include older age, female sex, African-American race, and history of smoking. Acquired donor risk factors include prolonged mechanical ventilation, aspiration, trauma, and hemodynamic stability (31). Whitson et al. (32) found that increasing donor age, donor smoking history, increasing preoperative pulmonary arterial pressure, and recipient diagnosis were significant risk factors for primary graft dysfunction. Operative variables associated with primary graft dysfunction include use of cardiopulmonary bypass and blood production transfusion (31). Hyperacute rejection is exceedingly rare, but it must be a consideration in cases of early severe lung dysfunction.

Ischemia–reperfusion injury is characterized by noncardiogenic pulmonary edema and progressive lung injury over the first few hours following implantation. In its most severe form, ischemia–reperfusion injury is described as primary graft failure that pathologically appears as diffuse alveolar damage (Fig. 50.1). Irrespective of the cause, it is important to establish a diagnosis of early graft dysfunction and rule out other treatable conditions. One may perform open lung biopsy at the time of implantation if graft dysfunction is immediately apparent in the operating room. Additionally, serological evaluation for anti-HLA antibodies may reveal evidence for hyperacute rejection in some of these patients.

Fortunately, severe reperfusion injury has not commonly been encountered in recent years. Superior strategies of lung preservation have evolved (33). It is clear from experimental (34) and clinical work (35–38) that low potassium dextran solution provides superior preservation relative to the high potassium preservation solutions previously in use. In addition, experimental work suggests

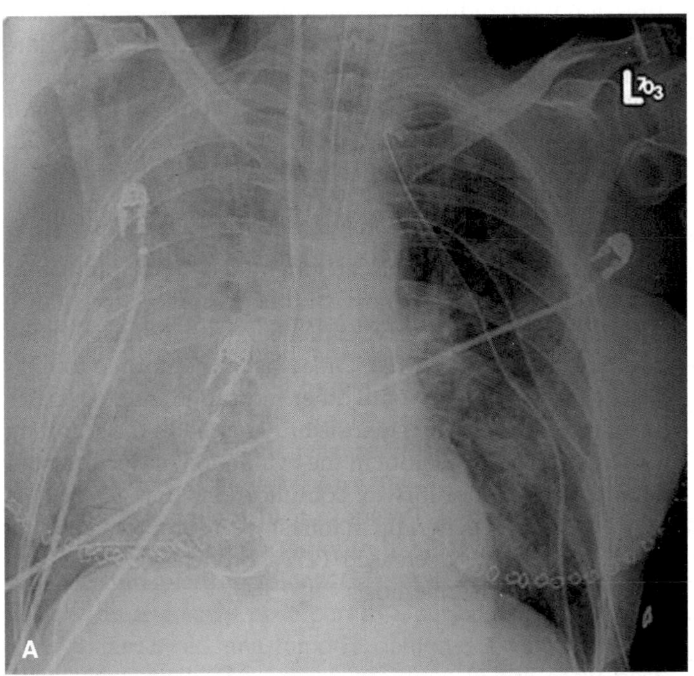

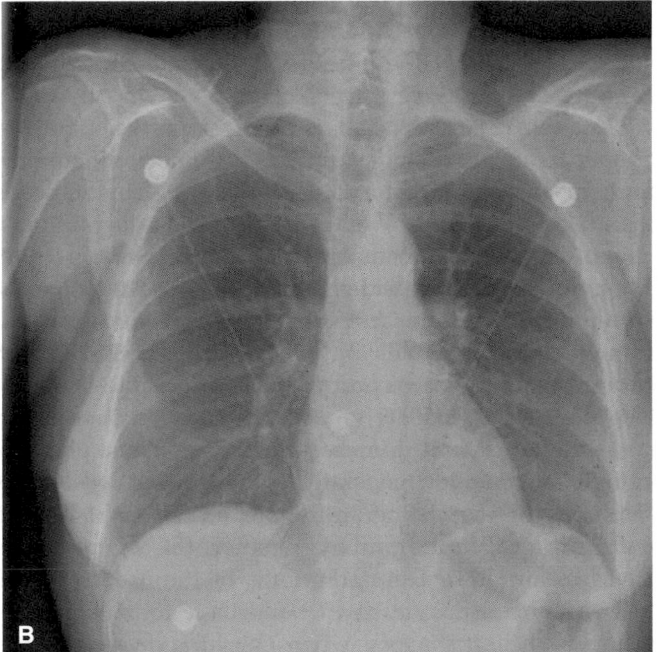

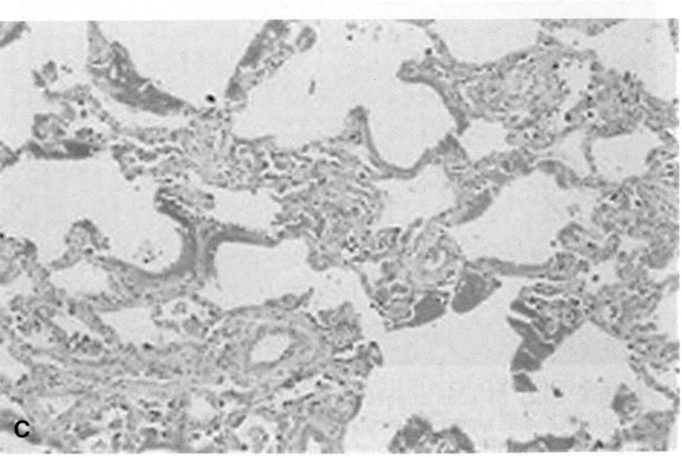

FIGURE 50.1. A: Chest radiograph showing severe right-sided ischemia–reperfusion injury following bilateral lung transplantation. Right lung was implanted first. **B:** Chest radiograph of the same patient after resolution of ischemia–reperfusion injury. **C:** Transbronchial biopsy showing diffuse alveolar damage characteristic of ischemia–reperfusion injury.

in lung transplant recipients with viral respiratory infections indicate severe infection and are a marker for poor prognosis (77). Symptomatic adenoviral infection, in particular, is typically associated with new radiologic abnormalities and is frequently fatal (77).

Treatment options for respiratory viral infections are limited. Aerosolized ribavirin has shown benefit in the treatment of RSV and parainfluenza infection in children (81). Intravenous immunoglobulin to RSV has been used in prevention and treatment of RSV infections in infants (80). Although the efficacy of these agents in lung transplant recipients remains unclear, it has been recommended that all patients with severe symptomatic RSV or parainfluenza infection receive aerosolized ribavirin. Ribavirin is also recommended in patients with radiographic abnormalities in the setting of RSV or parainfluenza infection given the increased potential to progress to respiratory failure. Care for adenovirus is currently supportive as no definitive therapies are currently available. A trial of reduced immunosuppression appears worthwhile, although the risk for rejection must be considered. Reports of the use of intravenous ribavirin or immunoglobulin have suggested potential value in adenoviral infections in pediatric, bone marrow recipient, and AIDS patients (38,82–84). Intravenous ribavirin has also been used with some success in a pediatric patient with adenoviral infection after liver transplantation (85). Treatment for influenza in nonimmunocompromised patients includes several potential drugs, including amantadine, rimantadine, and the newer neuraminidase inhibitors such as zanamivir and oseltamivir (86,87). The use of these agents in lung transplant recipients requires further study.

Because treatment options for community-acquired viral infections in lung transplant recipients are limited, the main goal in this population is prevention. It is routine for all lung transplant recipients to receive yearly influenza vaccines. Unfortunately, the response to influenza vaccine in solid-organ transplant recipients is impaired and revaccination does not seem to improve the vaccine response (81). In a series of heart transplant patients, the efficacy of the influenza vaccine was significantly impaired. Although vaccination was less effective compared to nonimmunosuppressed individuals, 50% of patients still reached protective serum antibody titers against two of three virus strains (88). Therefore, routine influenza immunization is still recommended, but serologic testing may be indicated (75). Importantly, all close contacts should receive influenza vaccination with the intended goal of decreasing the risk of infection to the transplant patient. Lung transplant recipients should avoid contact with family and friends with respiratory symptoms, especially children, to minimize risks of acquiring community viral infection. Frequent hand washing should be encouraged after contact with infected patients.

Fungal Infections

Fungal infections are a major problem after lung transplantation and occur early and late after transplant. *Aspergillus* and *Candida* account for >80% of these infections (89,90) (Fig. 50.5). Risk factors for fungal infections include complicated postoperative course, early fungal colonization, frequent bacterial infections, CMV infection, chronic rejection, renal failure, and age of recipient (91).

Candida accounts for the majority of fungal infections during the first month after transplantation. *Candida albicans* is commonly isolated from bronchial washings after transplant and its presence usually represents colonization (66), but it may also be invasive (92). Although *C. albicans* is the most common, there has been a recent shift toward non-*albicans* species.

Aspergillus infections are categorized into infections of the bronchial anastomosis, tracheobronchial tree, pneumonia, or disseminated disease (90,91). *Aspergillus* can also represent colonization, but because of the potential for invasive life-threatening infections, strong consideration needs to be given for treatment. More than 50% of cases of *Aspergillus* colonization and infection occur within 6 months after transplantation. Mortality rates associated with invasive *Aspergillus* pneumonia approach 40% to 80% and 90% to

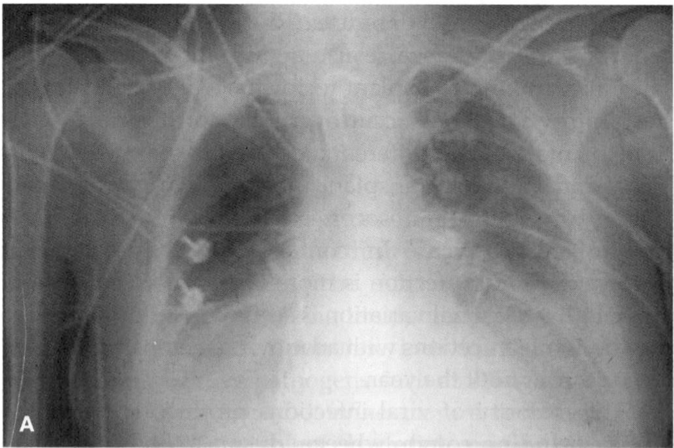

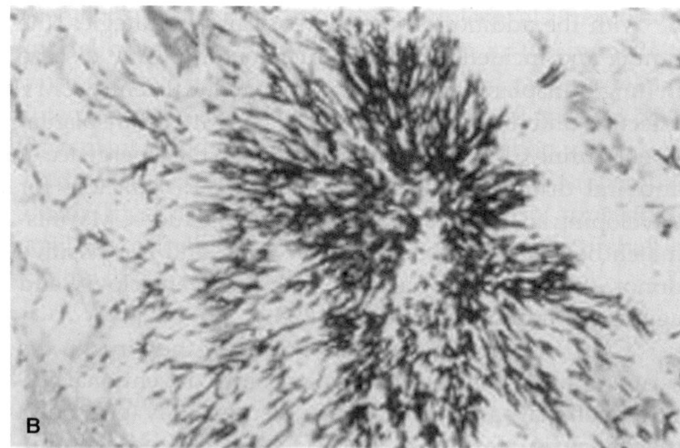

FIGURE 50.5. **A:** Transbronchial lung biopsy showing Cytomegalovirus (CMV) pneumonitis with demonstration of CMV inclusion bodies (hematoxylin and eosin). **B:** Demonstration of CMV inclusion bodies by immunoperoxidase staining.

100% with disseminated infection in one series of lung transplant recipients (90,93). Risk factors for post-transplant fungal infection are well defined; single-lung transplant, CMV infection, renal failure, chronic rejection, and pre-transplant colonization or prior treated infection may identify patients at higher risk for post-transplant infection (90). In patients with a single-lung transplant, one obvious potential reservoir of persistent *Aspergillus* is the native lung (66,94). Aspergilloma lesions found in the recipient-explanted lungs have been associated with reduced post-transplant survival (95). Patients with cystic fibrosis and positive preoperative sputum cultures for *Aspergillus* are at higher risk for postoperative infections (96).

Nocardia infections are increasingly recognized as complications of lung transplantation (97). Although *Nocardia asteroides* accounts for the most transplant-related nocardiosis, a case of disseminated infection with *N. brasiliensis* (98) in a single-lung transplant recipient has been reported. Although the mortality is high for immunocompromised patients with *N. brasiliensis*, prompt diagnosis and early initiation of appropriate therapy may improve outcome.

Reports of other fungal infections such as Histoplasma, Coccidiomycosis, Mucormycosis, Zygomycetes, and Cryptococcus are also documented (66). *Scedosporium apiospermum* is an uncommon cause of disseminated infection, and importantly, it is resistant to amphotericin B (99). *Pneumocystis carinii*, now classified as a fungus, remains a rare cause of infection because of the routine use of effective prophylaxis in all lung transplant recipients. Dematiaceous fungi, such as Mucormycosis, are also infrequent causes of postoperative infection.

Treatment for fungal infection is based on the specific organism causing the infection; amphotericin B has been the drug of choice for *Aspergillus* and *Fusarium*. Newer options that may be as effective with less toxicity include liposomal formulations of amphotericin, voriconazole, and caspofungin. Voriconazole must be used with caution in lung transplant recipients because of its extensive list of known drug interactions. High-dose azole therapy (itraconazole and voriconazole) may be used for Scedosporium. *Nocardia* infections are treated with trimethoprim–sulfamethoxazole. Most candidal infections can be treated with fluconazole. Non-*albicans Candida* species, however, are increasingly resistant to Diflucan but can be effectively treated by new drugs such as voriconazole. Single-lung transplant should probably not be performed in patients with mycetomas as adequate removal of fungal organisms cannot be achieved and the newly transplanted lung will be at increased risk of colonization and infection (95). Prolonged therapy is required for all fungal infections.

Because of the potential morbidity and mortality associated with fungal infections, several antifungal prophylactic strategies have been used in lung transplant recipients, often employing either systemic or inhaled antifungal agents, or both (100). However, enthusiasm for the use of systemic antifungal therapies is limited by the lack of in vitro activity against some infections, drug interactions, and significant treatment-limiting toxicities. Furthermore, the use of inhaled amphotericin B has been associated with significant subjective intolerance leading to treatment discontinuation in up to 50% of patients (101).

One lung transplant group has recently demonstrated the safety and tolerability of inhaled amphotericin B lipid complex (ABLC) in >50 lung transplant recipients. Because of the lipid properties, it was hypothesized that ABLC would be more effectively nebulized with greater pulmonary deposition than conventional amphotericin B. Consistent with this hypothesis, very low rates of intolerance and very low rates of fungal infection were seen in patients who received nebulized ABLC (102). Although further study is needed, nebulized ABLC seems a promising approach to prevent fungal infections without systemic toxicities after lung transplantation.

PLEURAL SPACE COMPLICATIONS

Hyperinflation

Acute Native Lung Hyperinflation

Acute native lung hyperinflation is defined as mediastinal shift toward the transplanted lung with flattening of the ipsilateral diaphragm causing graft compression. This is associated with respiratory dysfunction, possible weaning difficulties, or hemodynamic instability (103). Acute native lung hyperinflation can occur after single-lung transplantation, especially in patients with chronic obstructive pulmonary disease. The incidence of acute native lung hyperinflation ranges from 26% to 64% (103–105), with an associated mortality rate of 42% (103). Patients with an obstructive component, high mean pulmonary artery pressures, FEV1 <15%, residual volume >200%, and a left lung transplant may have a greater tendency toward acute native lung hyperinflation (103,104).

Conservative treatment consists of supportive therapy with vasopressors, ventilatory strategies aimed at prolonging expiration, and early extubation. Patients can be placed in a lateral decubitus position, with the graft in a nondependent position, to reduce hyperinflation in the native lung. However, this is not effective as a long-term strategy or in the weaning process. Differential ventilation allows for a decrease in ventilation of the hyperinflated lung; however, the use of a double-lumen tube and the need for deep sedation also hinders the weaning process. Surgical treatment could include lung volume reduction surgery of the native lung or retransplantation. Prevention strategies in patients with emphysematous lungs can include double-lung transplant, single-lung transplant with contralateral lung volume reduction surgery, or exclusive right-sided single-lung transplants (104,105).

Lung Hyperinflation in Undersized Grafts

Routinely after lung transplantation, patients are temporarily maintained on positive pressure ventilation with thoracostomy tubes in place. In lung transplant recipients with undersized grafts, the negative pleural pressure that occurs from thoracostomy tubes on suction can lead to altered respiratory mechanics. Presumably, in the enlarged pleural space, the negative pleural pressure inhibits the lung's elastic recoil and leads to detrimental hyperinflation. With the hyperinflation, alveoli do not completely decompress during exhalation, resulting in an increase in functional residual capacity. As more mechanical breaths are delivered, a stacking of the breaths occurs and the lungs function on a flatter portion of the volume–pressure curve. This can manifest as increased airway pressures with a higher potential for barotrauma. In extreme cases, this can lead to detrimental alveolar hyperexpansion and hemodynamic instability. Awareness of the potential for acute hyperinflation can lead to preventive measures such as avoidance of thoracostomy tube suction or by placing thoracostomy tubes on water seal while the patient is on positive pressure ventilation (106).

Pneumothorax

The most frequent pleural complication after lung transplantation is pneumothorax (107,108). Any new, persistent, or enlarging pneumothoraces should be promptly evaluated to identify the cause of the air leak. Any significant pneumothoraces should be initially treated with the insertion of a thoracostomy tube until further evaluation. In a retrospective review of their lung transplant recipients, Herridge et al. (108) found that the majority of pneumothoraces resolved spontaneously or with chest tube thoracostomy and there was no associated increase in mortality.

A pneumothorax is encountered primarily in two circumstances. The most common circumstance is the development of insignificant pneumothoraces in patients with obstructive lung disease, either emphysema or cystic fibrosis, who have undergone bilateral replacement and have received lungs smaller than the pleural space into which they were implanted. Often a minimal degree of bilateral pneumothorax occurs subsequent to chest tube removal. In general, these pneumothoraces can be ignored and the pleural air will eventually reabsorb and any remaining space will fill with fluid. Pneumothorax can occur infrequently as a result of airway dehiscence with communication into the pleural space. This is a rare occurrence and is usually readily managed by intercostal tube drainage with appropriate re-expansion of the underlying lung.

Pleural Effusion

Pleural effusions are common, with a reported incidence of 25%, after lung transplantation (108,109). Effusions occur because of increased capillary permeability due to ischemia–reperfusion injury of the allograft, disruption of lymphatic flow, hemorrhage, and acute lung rejection or infection. Early in the postoperative period, these effusions are usually exudative and bloody and commonly small to moderate in size. Most effusions resolve within 9 days in single-lung transplant recipients (110) and 14 days in bilateral lung transplant recipients (111). Most groups have reported that early postoperative pleural effusions are not concerning if the fluid output is steadily decreasing, and the remainder of the clinical course is appropriate.

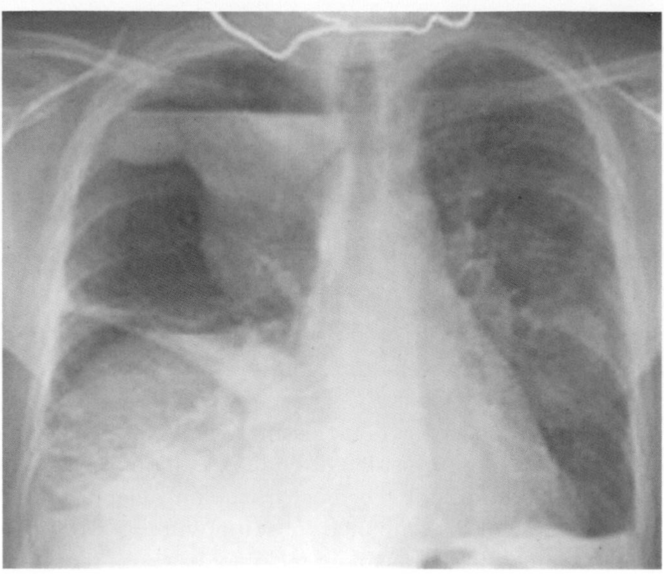

FIGURE 50.6. Chest radiograph showing empyema of the native lung following single-lung transplantation.

Empyema

Pleural empyema is an uncommon complication following lung transplantation, but its occurrence is associated with a significant mortality (Fig. 50.6). Spontaneous development of an empyema is rare. More commonly, an empyema develops after a prolonged air leak or as a result of open lung biopsy performed on a patient receiving high-dose corticosteroids. Persistent air leak and failure to achieve reexpansion of the lung and subsequent pleurodesis result in a chronic pleural space that eventually will become infected. Nunley et al. (112) performed a retrospective review of 392 transplant recipients and found empyema documented in 14 patients (3.6%). In this series, empyemas tended to occur early in the post-transplant period and 28.6% (4 patients) with empyemas died secondary to related infectious complications. No predominant organism was isolated in empyemic fluid with Gram-positive, Gram-negative, and saprophytic organisms seen. There was no relationship between the development of an empyema and the type of transplant performed or whether the transplant was done for a septic or nonseptic lung diagnosis. Surgeons have treated a number of patients who developed empyemas by open drainage by rib resection or by creation of a Clagett window or Eloesser flap. Interestingly, an empyema rarely occurs as a result of bronchial dehiscence in communication with the pleural space.

REJECTION

Both acute lung allograft rejection and chronic lung allograft rejection contribute substantially to morbidity in lung transplant recipients. Chronic lung rejection remains the major limitation to long-term success in lung transplantation today. Hyperacute rejection has only anecdotally been reported in the literature (113–115). Saint Martin et al. (116) performed immunofluorescence with C3, immunoglobin M, and immunoglobin G and found no evidence of humoral rejection in 106 biopsies. In this report, only one patient had a high reactivity pretransplant panel of reactive antibodies (PRA), suggesting a low risk for hyperacute rejection. Conversely, others have reported immunohistochemical findings of humoral injury in some recipients with high PRA (117). Interestingly, investigators have recently reported evidence suggesting that a frequently occurring septal capillary injury syndrome may represent humoral injury in lung allografts (118).

Acute rejection

Acute allograft rejection is one of the most common complications following lung transplantation. Most recipients experience at least one episode of acute rejection within the first year following transplant (119,120). In 1990, the Lung Rejection Study Group developed a system to characterize lung allograft rejection based on histologic criteria detected in lung biopsy specimens, with emphasis on perivascular and interstitial infiltration of mononuclear cells. Note is also made of the coexistence of airway inflammation (121). Modest revisions in this system were described in 1995 (122). In recent years, airway-centered inflammation (lymphocytic bronchitis/bronchiolitis) has been associated with subsequent development of chronic lung allograft dysfunction characterized by the pathologic lesion of bronchiolitis obliterans (123). In addition, it is clear that there is an association between frequency and severity of acute rejection episodes and the subsequent development of bronchiolitis obliterans (123). Thus, early detection of acute rejection and alteration of immunosuppression to deal with this problem may have a significant impact in the subsequent reduction of chronic lung allograft dysfunction.

In the early years of lung transplant experience, clinical parameters were often used to establish a clinical diagnosis of acute rejection. Unfortunately, dyspnea, low-grade fever, perihilar infiltrates, leukocytosis, hypoxia, and the clinical response to intravenous bolus doses of corticosteroid are nonspecific findings. Pathologic assessment of multiple transbronchial biopsy specimens has proven to be the "gold" standard for the diagnosis of acute lung allograft rejection (121,124,125). Indeed, many programs have adopted a program of prophylactic surveillance transbronchial biopsy (119,125–129). However, this strategy is controversial and a number of active lung transplant programs have abandoned it (130,131).

Since acute rejection is a predictor of BOS, induction and maintenance immunosuppression regimens, as well as treatment strategies for documented acute rejection, are subjects of intense interest. Induction therapy with either a cytolytic agent or an interleukin-2 receptor (IL-2R) blocker has been shown to reduce early rejection rates (132). Because of ease of administration, a low rate of side effects, similar efficacy, and fewer secondary infections, the IL-2R blockers are becoming the induction agents of choice for centers adhering to such a protocol.

Treatment of acute rejection has two goals: to treat the acute problem and to reduce the likelihood of further acute rejection episodes. Conventional therapy has been intravenous methylprednisolone in a dose of 10 to 15 mg/kg for 3 to 5 days (133). Although this strategy often accomplishes resolution of perivascular infiltrates, airway-centered inflammation has been more refractory to therapy. Depending on the maintenance steroid dose, 2 to 3 weeks of an oral steroid taper is usually prescribed. As acute therapy is initiated, the maintenance immunosuppression regimen should be scrutinized. A frequent first adjustment is a switch from maintenance cyclosporine to tacrolimus in the event of cyclosporine toxicity or acute rejection episodes despite adequate cyclosporine dosage (134,135). The roles of newer agents such as sirolimus or leflunomide, a pyrimidine synthesis inhibitor, are evolving in lung transplantation based on success in other solid-organ transplants (136–139). Low calcineurin inhibitor drug levels warrant investigation, especially for new medications activating the cytochrome P450 enzyme pathway and enhancing calcineurin inhibitor metabolism (e.g., dilantin, rifampin, and nafcillin) (140).

Chronic Allograft Rejection/BOS

The descriptive term "bronchiolitis obliterans syndrome" has been used to describe a late decline from a postoperative baseline forced expiratory volume in 1 second (FEV_1) that is not attributable to acute rejection, infection, or mechanical obstruction due to a bronchial anastomotic complication. The pathologic lesion associated with this decline is bronchiolitis obliterans (Fig. 50.7). A working formulation was created to characterize and grade BOS (141) and has been recently revised (142). BOS is a very common condition following lung transplantation (143).

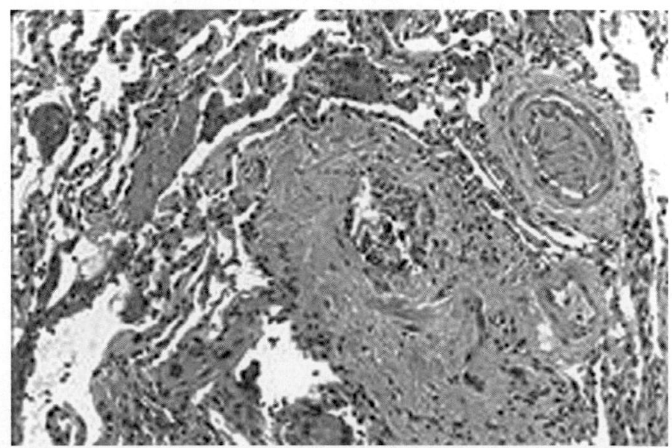

FIGURE 50.7. Transbronchial lung biopsy showing bronchiolitis obliterans with scarring and fibrosis of the small airways (hematoxylin and eosin).

Most observers believe that every recipient will develop some degree of BOS with long-term follow-up. Actuarial freedom from BOS at 1, 3, and 5 years post-transplant is 82%, 42%, and 25%, respectively (144).

The specific causes of BOS are not clear. Evidence suggests that both alloimmune and nonalloimmune mechanisms are important (145). Recipients who have more frequent and severe episodes of acute allograft rejection are more likely to develop subsequent BOS (123). Nonimmune mechanisms are also important. These include airway injury from primary graft dysfunction, allograft infections (CMV), airway ischemia, single-lung transplantation, noncompliance with immunosuppression, and gastroesophageal reflux disease (GERD). Lung transplant recipients appear to have a high incidence of GERD. Patients without GERD have a much lower incidence of BOS than those with uncorrected GERD. Improvement of BOS has been noted in recipients with GERD who underwent corrective fundoplication (146). In one series, the United Network for Organ Sharing database was reviewed for donor factors associated with the development of BOS in lung transplant recipients. Female donors, donors who were not current smokers, donors without a history of myocardial infarction, and donors with immunologic similarity to their recipients had longer BOS-free survival. Recipients who received lungs with higher partial pressures of oxygen in arterial blood developed more BOS (147).

Currently, the link between acute cellular rejection and BOS has made augmentation or changing immunosuppressive medication the mainstay of therapy (148). Until we have a better understanding of the molecular and cellular mechanisms of BOS, we are not likely to make much progress in its treatment. This goal is hampered by the lack of a suitable experimental model of the bronchiolitis obliterans lesion. A definitive solution for chronic allograft rejection may come through the development of strategies to promote immune tolerance or permanent acceptance of the graft by the recipient without the need for immunosuppression.

NONPULMONARY COMPLICATIONS

GI complications

GI complications are frequent in lung transplant recipients, occurring in as many as 50% of patients in some series (149). Frequently reported nonsurgical GI complications include esophagitis, pancreatitis, gastric atony, adynamic colonic ileus, gastroesophageal reflux, peptic ulcer disease, gastritis, GI bleeding, CMV hepatitis, CMV colitis, diverticulitis, cholecystitis, and Clostridium difficile colitis/diarrhea. Nausea is the most common GI compliant, which is likely secondary to medication side effects (150). The majority of these nonsurgical GI complications occur in the first month postoperatively and most respond to conservative therapy (149). Acute abdominal processes requiring surgical intervention have a reported incidence of 4% to 17% in lung transplant recipients and include, in decreasing occurrence, bowel perforation, appendicitis, cholecystitis, colitis, and pneumatosis intestinalis (151). Post-transplant lymphoproliferative disease (PTLD) may present as an acute abdominal process, secondary to intussusception or bowel perforation. Recipients with cystic fibrosis are at increased risk for additional abdominal complications such as gastric bezoars and distal intestinal obstruction syndrome (152). Surgical GI complications can occur at any time after transplantation, and immunosuppression may initially mask their severity. When emergent operative exploration is required, such an intervention has significant associated [u5]morbidity and mortality. Elective abdominal surgical procedures can be performed safely in this population with acceptable morbidity (153).

More recently, GERD has received significant attention because of its association with chronic lung rejection or bronchiolitis obliterans. Although prevalent in end-stage lung patients, its occurrence is very common after lung transplantation. Up to 75% of recipients have some degree of reflux based on pH studies (154). Factors causing post-transplant GERD include vagal damage, impaired cough and airway mucociliary clearance, an immunosuppression drug effect or the preexisting presence of GERD (146). Treatment with proton pump inhibitors has not shown to be promising in the prevention of BOS when associated with GERD (154). Nissen fundoplication has successfully been used to treat lung transplant patients with documented GERD. Antireflux surgery in lung transplant recipients has shown a survival benefit and a delay in onset of BOS, particularly if performed before the late stages of the BOS (146,155).

Post-transplant lymphoproliferative disease

PTLD is a well-recognized complication after solid-organ and bone marrow transplantation with an incidence between 4% and 10% after lung transplantation (156–159). Investigators have reported a 6.1% incidence of PTLD after lung transplantation in the adult population (159). The incidence of PTLD is reported to be two to six times higher in lung transplant recipients than other solid organ transplants (160,161). PTLD includes a spectrum of disease entities ranging from atypical lymphoid proliferation to malignant non-Hodgkin lymphoma (162,163). Most commonly, the neoplastic cells are of B-cell origin and there are often associations between PTLD and the presence of Epstein–Barr virus (EBV) (164). Cytotoxic T cells are involved in destroying cells presenting EBV in the context of MHC I. It has been proposed that an immunocompromised recipient experiencing a primary EBV infection may not be capable of destroying the virus-infected B cells, resulting in EBV-driven B-cell proliferation. In lung transplant recipients, a strong correlation has been reported between negative EBV serology prior to transplantation and the subsequent development of PTLD. Studies have reported a 6.8- to 20-fold increased risk of development of PTLD in recipients who had EBV-negative pretransplantation (156,165). Some have proposed that EBV carried in the donor lung lymphocytes results in a primary infection in the recipient. However, some reports have shown the recipient to be the origin of the lymphocytes in PTLD (112,166). The use of induction therapy (167) and the presence of CMV infection (168) have both been suggested as contributing factors to the development of PTLD.

PTLD often occurs in the first year after transplantation and shows a predilection for the thorax, most commonly the lung allograft (156–159). Cases of PTLD that present after the first year, in contrast, are usually extrathoracic, commonly arising in the abdomen and pelvis (159). In one series, of the 16 reported cases of PTLD that occurred after the first year, 14 of 16 (88%) were extrathoracic. Late cases of PTLD in the abdomen and pelvis occur at a median time of 5.8 years after transplantation (169). Interestingly, in all late cases occurring in the abdomen and pelvis, the recipients were EBV positive prior to transplant. Late-occurring abdominal and pelvic PTLD cases were most commonly malignant non-Hodgkin lymphomas, and despite aggressive therapy the prognosis was poor. In contrast, the patients who presented with early PTLD, unless disseminated at diagnosis, had a favorable prognosis and often responded to simply decreasing the level of immunosuppression (169).

Treatment of PTLD is based on the stage and progression of disease. Initially, a trial of reduction of immunosuppression is attempted, particularly with disease limited to the allograft. Many investigators have recommended the simultaneous use of antiviral therapy (165). Although chemotherapy has been used in patients with widespread disease or who have progression of disease, treatment-related mortality is considerable. In one reported study, 75% of PTLD patients treated with chemotherapy died as a result of sepsis (165). Recently, rituximab, a humanized anti-CD20 monoclonal antibody, has shown promise as a treatment option (170). Verschuuren et al. (170) reported complete remission in three lung transplant patients treated with rituximab. Complications occurred in two, one relapsed with a partial CD20-negative PTLD and the other developed hypogammaglobulinemia with subsequent sepsis and death. Another series used rituximab as first-line treatment in six lung transplant recipients with PTLD and demonstrated complete remission in four patients (171).

Preventative strategies have been contemplated. In adult lung transplantation, it does not appear prudent to match recipient and donor EBV status because >90% of the population is EBV positive by the time they are 35 years old. This strategy may have more value in children who have a higher percentage of EBV-negative recipients. Malouf et al. (172) reported that prophylactic use of antiviral therapy might reduce the incidence of PTLD.

Atrial dysrhythmias

Atrial dysrhythmias occur frequently after lung transplantation and have been shown to increase hospital stay and perioperative mortality (173). Prevalence ranges from 20% to 40% in multiple series (173–175) with a peak of onset at day 2 to 3 postoperatively with 70% occurring by postoperative day 4 (176,177). Dysrhythmias likely occur secondary to operative trauma and surgical dissection of the atrium, local inflammation, and catecholamine production (175).

Mason et al. (175) reported that 68 of their 333 lung transplant recipients developed postoperative atrial fibrillation. Risk factors for atrial fibrillation were older age, primary pulmonary hypertension, and extremes of weight. Rate-controlling drug agents were successfully used in 27% of recipients, while 7.5% required antiarrhythmics and 66% required both agents. Cardioversion was required in 36% of lung transplant recipients (175). Another series reported that patients with atrial dysrhythmias had higher rates of reintubation, additional operative intervention, and longer ICU and hospital stays. Use of cardiopulmonary bypass, age of recipient, and time on the waiting list were identified as significant risk factors for atrial dysrhythmias (178).

Renal Failure

Renal failure is a common complication following lung transplantation that carries a significant morbidity and mortality. In our recent review of our 346 lung transplant recipients, 9.5% developed acute postoperative renal failure with 4.6% of those requiring dialysis. None of the patients who required dialysis had recovery of their renal function, and of those requiring dialysis, 75% died during initial hospitalization versus only 5.8% of patients who did not progress to dialysis. Ishani et al. (179) reviewed the course of 219 lung and heart–lung transplant recipients surviving at least 6 months post-transplant and found that by 6 months 200 patients (91.3%) had a decrease in renal function. Doubling of creatinine from pretransplant baseline occurred in 34%, 43%, and 53% at 1, 2, and 5 years, respectively. End-stage renal disease occurred in 16 lung transplant recipients (7.3%) at a median duration of 28 months. The majority of recipients who developed ESRD had received cyclosporine (13 of 16), compared to only three who had received tacrolimus. Of the patients who developed ESRD, 44% (33) received hemodialysis alone and 56% (35) received kidney transplants. Risk factors associated with time to doubling of creatinine by multivariate analysis were serum creatinine at 1-month post-transplant and the number of cumulative follow-up periods with the diastolic blood pressure 90 mm Hg. Compared with cyclosporine, the use of tacrolimus in the first 6 months following transplantation was associated with a decreased risk for doubling of serum creatinine.

Risk factors include perioperative hemodynamic instability, infections, use of calcineurin inhibitors, and use of nephrotoxic antibiotics (180). It is apparent that prevention of subsequent renal failure in lung transplant recipients requires preserving renal function early in the course of transplantation. Early identification of high-risk recipients for renal dysfunction should prompt aggressive blood pressure control in these recipients and

80. Wandstrat TL. Respiratory syncytial virus immune globulin intravenous. *Ann Pharmacother* 1997;31(1):83–88.
81. Blumberg EA, Albano C, Pruett T, et al. The immunogenicity of influenza virus vaccine in solid organ transplant recipients. *Clin Infect Dis* 1996;22(2):295–302.
82. Jurado M, Navarro JM, Hernández J, et al. Adenovirus-associated haemorrhagic cystitis after bone marrow transplantation successfully treated with intravenous ribavirin. *Bone Marrow Transplant* 1995;15(4): 651–652.
83. Maslo C, Girard PM, Urban T, et al. Ribavirin therapy for adenovirus pneumonia in an AIDS patient. *Am J Respir Crit Care Med* 1997;156(4 Pt 1): 1263–1264.
84. McCarthy AJ, Bergin M, De Silva LM, et al. Intravenous ribavirin therapy for disseminated adenovirus infection. *Pediatr Infect Dis J* 1995; 14(11):1003–1004.
85. Shetty AK, Gans HA, So S, et al. Intravenous ribavirin therapy for adenovirus pneumonia. *Pediatr Pulmonol* 2000;29(1):69–73.
86. The MIST (Management of Influenza in the Southern Hemisphere Trialists) Study Group. Randomised trial of efficacy and safety of inhaled zanamivir in treatment of influenza A and B virus infections. *Lancet* 1998;352(9144):1877–1881.
87. Cox NJ, Subbarao K. Influenza. *Lancet* 1999;354(9186):1277–1282.
88. Dengler TJ, Strnad N, Bühring I, et al. Differential immune response to influenza and pneumococcal vaccination in immunosuppressed patients after heart transplantation. *Transplantation* 1998;66(10):1340–1347.
89. Grossi P, Farina C, Fiocchi R, et al. Prevalence and outcome of invasive fungal infections in 1,963 thoracic organ transplant recipients: a multicenter retrospective study. Italian Study Group of Fungal Infections in Thoracic Organ Transplant Recipients. *Transplantation* 2000;70(1):112–116.
90. Sole A, Salavert M. Fungal infections after lung transplantation. *Curr Opin Pulm Med* 2009;15(3):243–253.
91. Remund KF, Best M, Egan JJ. Infections relevant to lung transplantation. *Proc Am Thorac Soc* 2009;6(1):94–100.
92. Kanj SS, Welty-Wolf K, Madden J, et al. Fungal infections in lung and heart–lung transplant recipients. Report of 9 cases and review of the literature. *Medicine (Baltimore)* 1996;75(3):142–156.
93. Mehrad B, Paciocco G, Martinez FJ, et al. Spectrum of *Aspergillus* infection in lung transplant recipients: case series and review of the literature. *Chest* 2001;119(1):169–175.
94. Westney GE, Kesten S, De Hoyos A, et al. *Aspergillus* infection in single and double lung transplant recipients. *Transplantation* 1996;61(6): 915–919.
95. Hadjiliadis D, Sporn TA, Perfect JR, et al. Outcome of lung transplantation in patients with mycetomas. *Chest* 2002;121(1):128–134.
96. Nunley DR, Ohori P, Grgurich WF, et al. Pulmonary aspergillosis in cystic fibrosis lung transplant recipients. *Chest* 1998;114(5):1321–1329.
97. Husain S, McCurry K, Dauber J, et al. *Nocardia* infection in lung transplant recipients. *J Heart Lung Transplant* 2002;21(3):354–359.
98. Palmer SM Jr, Kanj SS, Davis RD, et al. A case of disseminated infection with *Nocardia brasiliensis* in a lung transplant recipient. *Transplantation* 1997;63(8):1189–1190.
99. Raj R, Frost AE. *Scedosporium apiospermum* fungemia in a lung transplant recipient. *Chest* 2002;121(5):1714–1716.
100. Calvo V, Borro JM, Morales P, et al. Antifungal prophylaxis during the early postoperative period of lung transplantation. Valencia Lung Transplant Group. *Chest* 1999;115(5):1301–1304.
101. Erjavec Z, et al. Tolerance and efficacy of Amphotericin B inhalations for prevention of invasive pulmonary aspergillosis in haematological patients. *Eur J Clin Microbiol Infect Dis* 1997;16(5):364–368.
102. Palmer SM, et al. Safety of aerosolized amphotericin B lipid complex in lung transplant recipients. *Transplantation* 2001;72(3):545–548.
103. Yonan NA, et al. Single lung transplantation for emphysema: predictors for native lung hyperinflation. *J Heart Lung Transplant* 1998;17(2): 192–201.
104. Angles R, et al. Lung transplantation for emphysema. Lung hyperinflation: incidence and outcome. *Transpl Int* 2005;17(12):810–814.
105. Weill D, et al. Acute native lung hyperinflation is not associated with poor outcomes after single lung transplant for emphysema. *J Heart Lung Transplant* 1999;18(11):1080–1087.
106. Kozower BD, et al. Potential for detrimental hyperinflation after lung transplantation with application of negative pleural pressure to undersized lung grafts. *J Thorac Cardiovasc Surg* 2003;125(2):430–432.
107. Ferrer J, et al. Acute and chronic pleural complications in lung transplantation. *J Heart Lung Transplant* 2003;22(11):1217–1225.
108. Herridge MS, et al. Pleural complications in lung transplant recipients. *J Thorac Cardiovasc Surg* 1995;110(1):22–26.
109. Wahidi MM, et al. Diagnosis and outcome of early pleural space infection following lung transplantation. *Chest* 2009;135(2):484–491.
110. Judson MA, Handy JR, Sahn SA. Pleural effusions following lung transplantation. Time course, characteristics, and clinical implications. *Chest* 1996;109(5):1190–1194.
111. Chiles C, et al. Heart–lung transplantation: the postoperative chest radiograph. *Radiology* 1985;154(2):299–304.
112. Nunley DR, et al. Empyema complicating successful lung transplantation. *Chest* 1999;115(5):1312–1315.
113. Bittner HB, et al. Hyperacute rejection in single lung transplantation–case report of successful management by means of plasmapheresis and antithymocyte globulin treatment. *Transplantation* 2001;71(5):649–651.
114. Choi JK, et al. Hyperacute rejection of a pulmonary allograft. Immediate clinical and pathologic findings. *Am J Respir Crit Care Med* 1999; 160(3):1015–1018.
115. Frost AE, Jammal CT, Cagle PT. Hyperacute rejection following lung transplantation. *Chest* 1996;110(2):559–562.
116. Saint Martin GA, et al. Humoral (antibody-mediated) rejection in lung transplantation. *J Heart Lung Transplant* 1996;15(12):1217–1222.
117. Lau CL, et al. Influence of panel-reactive antibodies on posttransplant outcomes in lung transplant recipients. *Ann Thorac Surg* 2000;69(5): 1520–1524.
118. Magro CM, et al. Humorally mediated posttransplantation septal capillary injury syndrome as a common form of pulmonary allograft rejection: a hypothesis. *Transplantation* 2002;74(9):1273–1280.
119. Hopkins PM, et al. Prospective analysis of 1,235 transbronchial lung biopsies in lung transplant recipients. *J Heart Lung Transplant* 2002; 21(10):1062–1067.
120. Husain AN, et al. Analysis of risk factors for the development of bronchiolitis obliterans syndrome. *Am J Respir Crit Care Med* 1999;159(3): 829–833.
121. Berry GJ, et al. A working formulation for the standardization of nomenclature in the diagnosis of heart and lung rejection: Lung Rejection Study Group. The International Society for Heart Transplantation. *J Heart Transplant* 1990;9(6):593–601.
122. Yousem SA, et al. Revision of the 1990 working formulation for the classification of pulmonary allograft rejection: Lung Rejection Study Group. *J Heart Lung Transplant* 1996;15(1 Pt 1):1–15.
123. Sharples LD, et al. Risk factors for bronchiolitis obliterans: a systematic review of recent publications. *J Heart Lung Transplant* 2002;21(2): 271–281.
124. Higenbottam T, et al. Transbronchial lung biopsy for the diagnosis of rejection in heart–lung transplant patients. *Transplantation* 1988;46(4): 532–539.
125. Trulock EP, et al. The role of transbronchial lung biopsy in the treatment of lung transplant recipients. An analysis of 200 consecutive procedures. *Chest* 1992;102(4):1049–1054.
126. Baz MA, et al. Diagnostic yield of bronchoscopies after isolated lung transplantation. *Chest* 1996;110(1):84–88.
127. Boehler A, et al. Prospective study of the value of transbronchial lung biopsy after lung transplantation. *Eur Respir J* 1996;9(4):658–662.
128. Guilinger RA, et al. The importance of bronchoscopy with transbronchial biopsy and bronchoalveolar lavage in the management of lung transplant recipients. *Am J Respir Crit Care Med* 1995;152(6 Pt 1): 2037–2043.
129. Sibley RK, et al. The role of transbronchial biopsies in the management of lung transplant recipients. *J Heart Lung Transplant* 1993;12(2): 308–324.
130. Tamm M, et al. Bronchiolitis obliterans syndrome in heart–lung transplantation: surveillance biopsies. *Am J Respir Crit Care Med* 1997;155(5): 1705–1710.
131. Valentine VG, et al. Success of lung transplantation without surveillance bronchoscopy. *J Heart Lung Transplant* 2002;21(3):319–326.
132. Brock MV, et al. Induction therapy in lung transplantation: a prospective, controlled clinical trial comparing OKT3, anti-thymocyte globulin, and daclizumab. *J Heart Lung Transplant* 2001;20(12):1282–1290.
133. Trulock EP. Lung transplantation. *Am J Respir Crit Care Med* 1997;155(3): 789–818.
134. Horning NR, et al. Tacrolimus therapy for persistent or recurrent acute rejection after lung transplantation. *J Heart Lung Transplant* 1998; 17(8):761–767.
135. Vitulo P, et al. Efficacy of tacrolimus rescue therapy in refractory acute rejection after lung transplantation. *J Heart Lung Transplant* 2002;21(4): 435–439.
136. Hong JC, Kahan BD. Sirolimus rescue therapy for refractory rejection in renal transplantation. *Transplantation* 2001;71(11):1579–1584.

137. Kahan BD. Efficacy of sirolimus compared with azathioprine for reduction of acute renal allograft rejection: a randomised multicentre study. The Rapamune US Study Group. *Lancet* 2000;356(9225): 194–202.
138. Snell GI, et al. Rescue therapy: a role for sirolimus in lung and heart transplant recipients. *Transplant Proc* 2001;33(1/2):1084–1085.
139. Williams JW, et al. Experiences with leflunomide in solid organ transplantation. *Transplantation* 2002;73(3):358–366.
140. Chakinala MM, Trulock EP. Acute allograft rejection after lung transplantation: diagnosis and therapy. *Chest Surg Clin N Am* 2003;13(3): 525–542.
141. Cooper JD, et al. A working formulation for the standardization of nomenclature and for clinical staging of chronic dysfunction in lung allografts. International Society for Heart and Lung Transplantation. *J Heart Lung Transplant* 1993;12(5):713–716.
142. Estenne M, Hertz MI. Bronchiolitis obliterans after human lung transplantation. *Am J Respir Crit Care Med* 2002;166(4):440–444.
143. Hertz MI, et al. The registry of the international society for heart and lung transplantation: nineteenth official report—2002. *J Heart Lung Transplant* 2002;21(9):950–970.
144. Meyers BF, et al. Lung transplantation: a decade of experience. *Ann Surg* 1999;230(3):362–370; discussion 370–371.
145. Estenne M, et al. Bronchiolitis obliterans syndrome 2001: an update of the diagnostic criteria. *J Heart Lung Transplant* 2002;21(3):297–310.
146. Davis RD Jr, et al. Improved lung allograft function after fundoplication in patients with gastroesophageal reflux disease undergoing lung transplantation. *J Thorac Cardiovasc Surg* 2003;125(3):533–542.
147. Hennessy SA, Swenson BR, Kozower BD, et al. Donor hyperoxia is associated with development of bronchiolitis obliterans following lung transplantation. Presented at the 56th Annual Meeting of Southern Thoracic Surgical Association, Marco Island, FL, November 4–7, 2009.
148. Belperio JA, et al. Chronic lung allograft rejection: mechanisms and therapy. *Proc Am Thorac Soc* 2009;6(1):108–121.
149. Lubetkin EI, et al. GI complications after orthotopic lung transplantation. *Am J Gastroenterol* 1996;91(11):2382–2390.
150. Bravo C, et al. Prevalence and management of gastrointestinal complications in lung transplant patients: MITOS study group. *Transplant Proc* 2007;39(7):2409–2412.
151. Hoekstra HJ, et al. Gastrointestinal complications in lung transplant survivors that require surgical intervention. *Br J Surg* 2001;88(3):433–438.
152. Gilljam M, et al. GI complications after lung transplantation in patients with cystic fibrosis. *Chest* 2003;123(1):37–41.
153. Pollard TR, et al. Abdominal operations after lung transplantation. Indications and outcome. *Arch Surg* 1997;132(7):714–717; discussion 717–718.
154. Robertson AG, et al. A call for standardization of antireflux surgery in the lung transplantation population. *Transplantation* 2009;87(8):1112–1114.
155. Cantu E III, et al. J. Maxwell Chamberlain Memorial Paper. Early fundoplication prevents chronic allograft dysfunction in patients with gastroesophageal reflux disease. *Ann Thorac Surg* 2004;78(4):1142–1151; discussion 1142–1151.
156. Aris RM, et al. Post-transplantation lymphoproliferative disorder in the Epstein–Barr virus-naive lung transplant recipient. *Am J Respir Crit Care Med* 1996;154(6 Pt 1):1712–1717.
157. Armitage JM, et al. Posttransplant lymphoproliferative disease in thoracic organ transplant patients: ten years of cyclosporine-based immunosuppression. *J Heart Lung Transplant* 1991;10(6):877–886; discussion 886–887.
158. Levine SM, et al. A low incidence of posttransplant lymphoproliferative disorder in 109 lung transplant recipients. *Chest* 1999;116(5):1273–1277.
159. Paranjothi S, et al. Lymphoproliferative disease after lung transplantation: comparison of presentation and outcome of early and late cases. *J Heart Lung Transplant* 2001;20(10):1054–1063.
160. Angel LF, et al. Posttransplant lymphoproliferative disorders in lung transplant recipients: clinical experience at a single center. *Ann Transplant* 2000;5(3):26–30.
161. Dharnidharka VR, et al. Post-transplant lymphoproliferative disorder in the United States: young Caucasian males are at highest risk. *Am J Transplant* 2002;2(10):993–998.
162. Schaar CG, et al. Successful outcome with a "quintuple approach" of posttransplant lymphoproliferative disorder. *Transplantation* 2001;71(1): 47–52.
163. Swerdlow SH. Classification of the posttransplant lymphoproliferative disorders: from the past to the present. *Semin Diagn Pathol* 1997; 14(1):2–7.
164. Montone KT, et al. Analysis of Epstein-Barr virus-associated posttransplantation lymphoproliferative disorder after lung transplantation. *Surgery* 1996;119(5):544–551.
165. Wigle DA, et al. Epstein–Barr virus serology and posttransplant lymphoproliferative disease in lung transplantation. *Transplantation* 2001;72(11):1783–1786.
166. Wood BL, et al. The recipient origin of posttransplant lymphoproliferative disorders in pulmonary transplant patients. A report of three cases. *Cancer* 1996;78(10):2223–2228.
167. Swinnen LJ, et al. Increased incidence of lymphoproliferative disorder after immunosuppression with the monoclonal antibody OKT3 in cardiac-transplant recipients. *N Engl J Med* 1990;323(25):1723–1728.
168. Walker RC, et al. Pretransplantation assessment of the risk of lymphoproliferative disorder. *Clin Infect Dis* 1995;20(5):1346–1353.
169. Hachem RR, et al. Abdominal-pelvic lymphoproliferative disease after lung transplantation: presentation and outcome. *Transplantation* 2004;77(3):431–437.
170. Verschuuren EA, et al. Treatment of posttransplant lymphoproliferative disease with rituximab: the remission, the relapse, and the complication. *Transplantation* 2002;73(1):100–104.
171. Knoop C, et al. Post-transplant lymphoproliferative disorders after lung transplantation: first-line treatment with rituximab may induce complete remission. *Clin Transplant* 2006;20(2):179–187.
172. Malouf MA, et al. Anti-viral prophylaxis reduces the incidence of lymphoproliferative disease in lung transplant recipients. *J Heart Lung Transplant* 2002;21(5):547–554.
173. Nielsen TD, et al. Atrial fibrillation after pulmonary transplant. *Chest* 2004;126(2):496–500.
174. Kogan A, et al. Atrial fibrillation after adult lung transplantation. *Transplant Proc* 2003;35(2):679.
175. Mason DP, et al. Atrial fibrillation after lung transplantation: timing, risk factors, and treatment. *Ann Thorac Surg* 2007;84(6):1878–1884.
176. Aranki SF, et al. Predictors of atrial fibrillation after coronary artery surgery. Current trends and impact on hospital resources. *Circulation* 1996;94(3):390–397.
177. Roselli EE, et al. Atrial fibrillation complicating lung cancer resection. *J Thorac Cardiovasc Surg* 2005;130(2):438–444.
178. Lau CL, Trulock E, Guthrie T. Post-operative atrial dysrhythmias after lung transplantation. *J Heart Lung Transplant* 2004;23:150A.
179. Ishani A, et al. Predictors of renal function following lung or heart–lung transplantation. *Kidney Int* 2002;61(6):2228–2234.
180. Mason DP, et al. Dialysis after lung transplantation: prevalence, risk factors and outcome. *J Heart Lung Transplant* 2007;26(11):1155–1162.
181. Soccal PM, et al. Improvement of drug-induced chronic renal failure in lung transplantation. *Transplantation* 1999;68(1):164–165.
182. Broekroelofs J, et al. Long-term renal outcome after lung transplantation is predicted by the 1-month postoperative renal function loss. *Transplantation* 2000;69(8):1624–1628.
183. Lichtenstein GR, et al. Fatal hyperammonemia following orthotopic lung transplantation. *Gastroenterology* 1997;112(1):236–240.
184. Lichtenstein GR, et al. Fatal hyperammonemia after orthotopic lung transplantation. *Ann Intern Med* 2000;132(4):283–287.
185. Tuchman M, et al. Hepatic glutamine synthetase deficiency in fatal hyperammonemia after lung transplantation. *Ann Intern Med* 1997; 127(6):446–449.
186. Berry GT, et al. Successful use of alternate waste nitrogen agents and hemodialysis in a patient with hyperammonemic coma after heart–lung transplantation. *Arch Neurol* 1999;56(4):481–484.
187. Singh N, Gayowski T, Marino IR. Hemolytic uremic syndrome in solid-organ transplant recipients. *Transpl Int* 1996;9(1):68–75.
188. Hachem RR, et al. Thrombotic microangiopathy after lung transplantation. *Transplantation* 2006;81(1):57–63.
189. George JN. How I treat patients with thrombotic thrombocytopenic purpura–hemolytic uremic syndrome. *Blood* 2000;96(4):1223–1229.

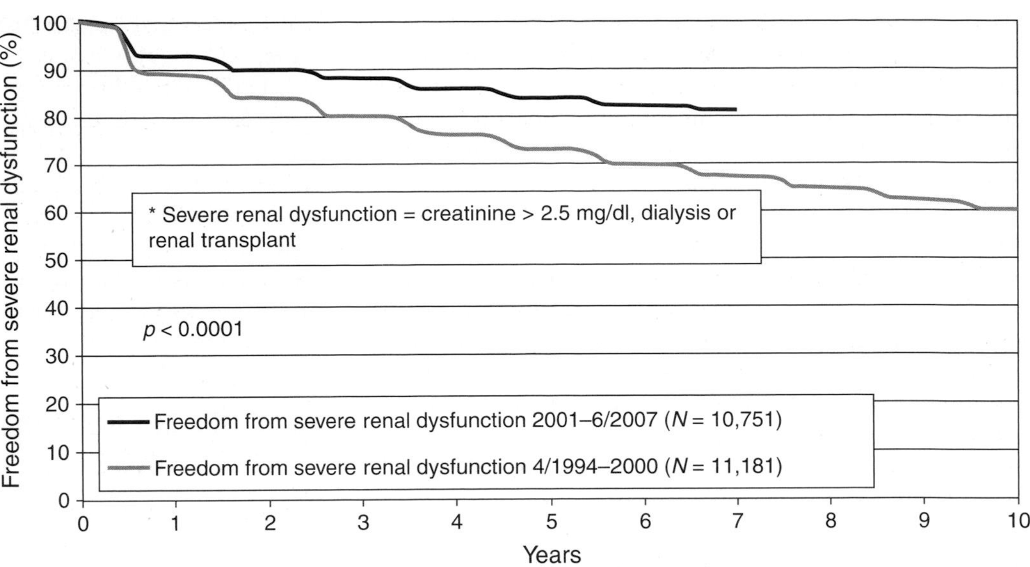

FIGURE 51.15. Kaplan–Meier freedom from severe renal dysfunction, stratified by era, for transplants performed from April 1994 to June 2007. (Reprinted from Taylor DO, Stehlik J, Edwards LB, et al. Registry of the International Society for Heart and Lung Transplantation: twenty-sixth official adult heart transplant report—2009. *J Heart Lung Transplant* 2009;28(10):1020 (Fig. 16).)

inhibitors are thought to be irreversible and dose independent (186,192). Risk factors for the development of renal insufficiency with calcineurin inhibitors use following heart transplantation have not been clearly defined but may include recipient age at the time of heart transplantation and glomerular-filtration rate at 1 year following heart transplantation. Vossler et al. (193) conducted a 5-year retrospective analysis of heart transplant recipients who survived for >1 year following operation. Patients were divided into three groups based on perioperative renal function: (1) preoperative creatinine concentration <1.5 mg/dL and a postoperative (first 4 days) creatinine <2.0 mg/dL; (2) preoperative creatinine of <1.5 mg/dL but a postoperative creatinine of >2.0 mg/dL; (3) preoperative creatinine of >1.5 mg/dL. Nearly 30% of patients experienced chronic renal insufficiency (serial serum creatinine >2.0 mg/dL) on two or more monthly examinations. The mean preoperative serum creatinine was 1.6 mg/dL in patients who experienced chronic renal insufficiency, whereas it was 1.3 mg/dL in patients who did not ($p = 0.01$). The fraction of patients in whom chronic renal insufficiency developed was highest in Group 3 (55.3%), lower in Group 2 (25.5%), and lowest in Group 1 (18.7%) ($p = 0.01$). After adjusting for multiple potential confounding variables, including cyclosporine dosage, the risk of chronic renal insufficiency linearly decreased in the three groups, stratified by perioperative renal function (relative risk, 1.82; 95% confidence interval, 1.23–2.7). Although pretransplant serum creatinine was the best predictor of the development of chronic renal insufficiency in the study by Vossler et al. (193), the pathophysiology of chronic renal insufficiency appears more complex and probably results from multiple interacting factors. These factors include the acute and chronic nephrotoxic effects of calcineurin inhibitors, the abnormal renal function in patients with advanced heart failure, transplant operation with associated cardiopulmonary bypass, recipient age, immunologic factors, and other risk factors for chronic renal insufficiency such as hypertension, diabetes mellitus, and hypercholesterolemia. This concept is supported by the finding that although there was a strong association between preoperative serum creatinine and development of chronic renal insufficiency in the study by Vossler et al. (193), 19% of patients with normal preoperative creatinine also experienced chronic renal insufficiency following heart transplantation. Renal functional reserve before transplantation is probably an important factor in determining whether a patient will tolerate long-term treatment with calcineurin inhibitors. Histologic evidence of progressive glomerulosclerosis and loss of functioning glomeruli is present in patients treated with calcineurin inhibitors despite maintaining a stable serum creatinine (194). Thus, all patients treated with calcineurin inhibitors are likely to have some renal damage, but that the degree of functional impairment is highly dependent on the degree of pretransplant renal disease.

There is no effective treatment to reverse progressive renal dysfunction following heart transplantation. Alterations in cyclosporine dosing regimens have been proposed but have not been consistently demonstrated to have a significant impact (195). There are no consistent data to suggest that treatment with calcium channel blockers, statins, or ACE inhibitors has a significant benefit on long-term renal function (180,196). Calcineurin-sparing immunosuppressive protocols have been proposed as one alternative to reduce the risk of chronic renal insufficiency secondary to calcineurin inhibitors. Alternative strategies involve reduction of doses of calcineurin inhibitors with introduction of non-nephrotoxic immunosuppressants such as mycophenolate mofetil and sirolimus. This strategy is currently being investigated extensively in renal transplantation, and it has been shown to improve renal function, at least in the short term (197,198). More recently, some benefit has been shown with calcineurin-free protocols utilizing sirolimus in combination with mycophenolate mofetil (199). The substitution of mycophenolate mofetil for azathioprine, with a concomitant reduction in the dose of calcineurin inhibitors, has been reported to improve renal function, without increasing the rate of allograft rejection (200,201). In addition to changes in immunosuppressive therapy, continued long-term management of nonimmunologic factors, (i.e., hypertension and diabetes mellitus) remain important.

Hypertension

The development of systemic hypertension is a significant complication following heart transplantation. The incidence of hypertension has been reported to range from 40% to 90% in the era of calcineurin inhibitors (202). The overwhelming factor responsible for the development of hypertension following heart transplantation is the use of calcineurin inhibitors. Additional risk factors thought to be important include male gender, a family history of hypertension, and recipient age >20 years (203). However, the additional influence of these factors in the setting of calcineurin use may be relatively minor (203,204). Calcineurin inhibitors are thought to contribute to the development of hypertension by a direct effect on sympathetic stimulation (205), neurohormonal activation (189), and peripheral vasoconstriction through release of endothelin-1 (206). Corticosteroids may also contribute to the development of hypertension secondary to their mineralocorticoid effect; however, heart transplant recipients on steroid-free immunosuppressive regimens have a similar degree of postoperative hypertension. Recently, several studies have demonstrated the development of less-severe hypertension with the use of tacrolimus when compared with cyclosporine in heart transplant recipients (207–209). Patients receiving tacrolimus-based immunosuppression have been shown to have a lower incidence of new onset hypertension and require fewer antihypertensive agents for management (207).

The treatment of post-transplant hypertension is similar to that of essential hypertension. Calcium channel–blocking agents are usually the first line of therapy for hypertension in patients treated with cyclosporine. Diltiazem has the advantage of decreasing the cyclosporine dose and therefore decreasing immunosuppression costs. Angiotensin-converting enzyme (ACE) inhibitors are also used for treatment of hypertension in transplant recipients. A randomized trial comparing diltiazem and lisinopril in the treatment of post-transplant hypertension demonstrated equal efficacy (210). Monotherapy is effective in <50% of patients. Therapy with both agents is generally required to obtain adequate blood pressure regulation, and peripheral alpha-adrenergic blocking agents such as doxazosin, peripheral arterial dilators such as hydralazine and minoxidil, and centrally acting sympathetic inhibitors such as clonidine may be useful adjuvants to therapy with calcium channel blockers and ACE inhibitors if first-line therapy is not sufficient in controlling blood pressure.

METABOLIC AND ENDOCRINE DISORDERS

Hyperlipidemia

The incidence of hyperlipidemia following heart transplantation has been reported to be as high as 60% to 80% of heart transplant recipients and is manifest by elevated serum levels of total cholesterol, low-density lipoprotein (LDL) cholesterol, apolipoprotein B, and triglyceride (211). The etiology of hyperlipidemia following heart transplantation is attributable to several factors that include diets high in fat, familial predisposition, and immunosuppressive therapy with corticosteroids and calcineurin inhibitors (212,213). Cyclosporine blood levels have been shown to correlate directly with total plasma cholesterol, LDL cholesterol, and apoB and inversely with high-density lipoprotein (HDL) cholesterol and apoA-I (the antiatherogenic protein component of HDL). In addition, significant correlation with the total cholesterol/HDL ratio and cyclosporine levels have been reported (213). Tacrolimus appears to have less adverse effects on lipid metabolism when compared with cyclosporine (207).

The benefits of cholesterol reduction in patients with coronary artery disease and in high-risk patients without established coronary artery disease are well established. All-cause mortality is significantly reduced due to a dramatic reduction in coronary end points. The benefit of treatment of hyperlipidemia in heart transplant recipients has been demonstrated by Kobashigawa et al. (156) in a study of 97 heart transplant recipients randomized to therapy with or without pravastatin. Pravastatin at doses of 20 to 40 mg daily produced a 22% lowering of total plasma cholesterol. There was no change in the number of episodes of rejection, but there was a dramatic reduction in episodes of rejection associated with hemodynamic compromise, as well as a marked improvement in survival. There was also a lower incidence of coronary vasculopathy, as determined by angiography or IVUS. The mechanism of this effect was most likely related to cholesterol reduction. However, a significant decrease was noted in the cytotoxicity of natural killer cells, suggesting that an immunologic mechanism may contribute to the effectiveness of this intervention. Despite the potential for rhabdomyolysis in patients receiving pravastatin together with cyclosporine, no elevation in creatine kinase, transaminases, myositis, or rhabdomyolysis were documented over the 12 months of study.

Hyperglycemia

The reported incidence of diabetes mellitus following transplantation has varied widely (from 2% to 46%), largely due variations in the criteria used to define diabetes mellitus after transplantation. The onset of diabetes mellitus after organ transplantation is related to exogenous glucocorticoid administration. Glucocorticoids impair hepatic and extrahepatic actions of insulin, probably at the postreceptor level as neither binding of insulin to its receptor nor the number of insulin receptors is affected by glucocorticoid

103. Kobashigawa JA, et al. Benefit of immune monitoring in heart transplant patients using ATP production in activated lymphocytes. *J Heart Lung Transplant* 29(5):504–508.
104. Mancini D, et al. Use of rapamycin slows progression of cardiac transplantation vasculopathy. *Circulation* 2003;108(1):48–53.
105. Eisen HJ, et al. Everolimus for the prevention of allograft rejection and vasculopathy in cardiac-transplant recipients. *N Engl J Med* 2003;349(9):847–858.
106. De Marco T, et al. Successful immunomodulation with intravenous gamma globulin and cyclophosphamide in an alloimmunized heart transplant recipient. *J Heart Lung Transplant* 1997;16(3):360–365.
107. Miller LW, et al. Infection after heart transplantation: a multiinstitutional study. Cardiac Transplant Research Database Group. *J Heart Lung Transplant* 1994;13(3):381–392; discussion 393.
108. Hunt SA, Current status of cardiac transplantation. *JAMA* 1998;280(19):1692–1698.
109. Hunt SA, Haddad F. The changing face of heart transplantation. *J Am Coll Cardiol* 2008;52(8):587–598.
110. Robbins RC, et al. Thirty years of cardiac transplantation at Stanford university. *J Thorac Cardiovasc Surg* 1999;117(5):939–951.
111. Fishman JA, Rubin RH. Infection in organ-transplant recipients. *N Engl J Med* 1998;338(24):1741–1751.
112. Fishman JA. Infection in solid-organ transplant recipients. *N Engl J Med* 2007;357(25):2601–2614.
113. Haddad F, et al. Changing trends in infectious disease in heart transplantation. *J Heart Lung Transplant* 29(3):306–315.
114. Smart FW, et al. Risk factors for early, cumulative, and fatal infections after heart transplantation: a multiinstitutional study. *J Heart Lung Transplant* 1996;15(4):329–341.
115. Macdonald PS, et al. A double-blind placebo-controlled trial of low-dose ganciclovir to prevent cytomegalovirus disease after heart transplantation. *J Heart Lung Transplant* 1995;14(1 Pt 1):32–38.
116. Potena L, Valantine HA. Cytomegalovirus-associated allograft rejection in heart transplant patients. *Curr Opin Infect Dis* 2007;20(4):425–431.
117. Potena L, et al. Prophylaxis versus preemptive anti-cytomegalovirus approach for prevention of allograft vasculopathy in heart transplant recipients. *J Heart Lung Transplant* 2009;28(5):461–467.
118. Montoya JG, et al. Infectious complications among 620 consecutive heart transplant patients at Stanford University Medical Center. *Clin Infect Dis* 2001;33(5):629–640.
119. Rubin RH. Prevention and treatment of cytomegalovirus disease in heart transplant patients. *J Heart Lung Transplant* 2000;19(8):731–735.
120. Potena L, et al. Acute rejection and cardiac allograft vascular disease is reduced by suppression of subclinical cytomegalovirus infection. *Transplantation* 2006;82(3):398–405.
121. Kalil AC, et al. Meta-analysis: the efficacy of strategies to prevent organ disease by cytomegalovirus in solid organ transplant recipients. *Ann Intern Med* 2005;143(12):870–880.
122. Hodson EM, et al. Antiviral medications to prevent cytomegalovirus disease and early death in recipients of solid-organ transplants: a systematic review of randomised controlled trials. *Lancet* 2005;365(9477):2105–2115.
123. Merigan TC, et al. A controlled trial of ganciclovir to prevent cytomegalovirus disease after heart transplantation. *N Engl J Med* 1992;326(18):1182–1186.
124. Wedemeyer H, et al. Long-term outcome of chronic hepatitis B in heart transplant recipients. *Transplantation* 1998;66(10):1347–1353.
125. Wachs ME, et al. The risk of transmission of hepatitis B from HBsAg(−), HBcAb(+), HBIgM(−) organ donors. *Transplantation* 1995;59(2):230–234.
126. Lake KD, et al. Outcomes of hepatitis C positive (HCV+) heart transplant recipients. *Transplant Proc* 1997;29(1/2):581–582.
127. Ong JP, et al. Outcome of de novo hepatitis C virus infection in heart transplant recipients. *Hepatology* 1999;30(5):1293–1298.
128. Israelski DM, Remington JS. Toxoplasmosis in the non-AIDS immunocompromised host. *Curr Clin Top Infect Dis* 1993;13:322–356.
129. Luft BJ, Billingham M, Remington JS. Endomyocardial biopsy in the diagnosis of toxoplasmic myocarditis. *Transplant Proc* 1986;18(6):1871–1873.
130. Wreghitt TG, et al. Efficacy of pyrimethamine for the prevention of donor-acquired *Toxoplasma gondii* infection in heart and heart-lung transplant patients. *Transpl Int* 1992;5(4):197–200.
131. Schmauss D, Weis M. Cardiac allograft vasculopathy: recent developments. *Circulation* 2008;117(16):2131–2141.
132. Kapadia SR, et al. Development of transplantation vasculopathy and progression of donor-transmitted atherosclerosis: comparison by serial intravascular ultrasound imaging. *Circulation* 1998;98(24):2672–2678.
133. Gould DS, Auchincloss H Jr. Direct and indirect recognition: the role of MHC antigens in graft rejection. *Immunol Today* 1999;20(2):77–82.
134. Avery RK. Viral triggers of cardiac-allograft dysfunction. *N Engl J Med* 2001;344(20):1545–1547.
135. Young JB. Allograft vasculopathy: diagnosing the nemesis of heart transplantation. *Circulation* 1999;100(5):458–460.
136. Mehra MR, et al. The prognostic impact of immunosuppression and cellular rejection on cardiac allograft vasculopathy: time for a reappraisal. *J Heart Lung Transplant* 1997;16(7):743–751.
137. Kobashigawa JA, et al. Does acute rejection correlate with the development of transplant coronary artery disease? A multicenter study using intravascular ultrasound. Sandoz/CVIS Investigators. *J Heart Lung Transplant* 1995;14(6 Pt 2):S221–S226.
138. Stovin PG, et al. Lack of association between endomyocardial evidence of rejection in the first six months and the later development of transplant-related coronary artery disease. *J Heart Lung Transplant* 1993;12(1 Pt 1):110–116.
139. Liu Z, et al. Contribution of direct and indirect recognition pathways to T cell alloreactivity. *J Exp Med* 1993;177(6):1643–1650.
140. Liu Z, et al. Indirect recognition of donor HLA–DR peptides in organ allograft rejection. *J Clin Invest* 1996;98(5):1150–1157.
141. Tugulea S, et al. New strategies for early diagnosis of heart allograft rejection. *Transplantation* 1997;64(6):842–847.
142. Vanderlugt CJ, Miller SD. Epitope spreading. *Curr Opin Immunol* 1996;8(6):831–836.
143. Rose EA, et al. Relation of HLA antibodies and graft atherosclerosis in human cardiac allograft recipients. *J Heart Lung Transplant* 1992;11(3 Pt 2):S120–S123.
144. Reed EF, et al. Monitoring of soluble HLA alloantigens and anti-HLA antibodies identifies heart allograft recipients at risk of transplant-associated coronary artery disease. *Transplantation* 1996;61(4):566–572.
145. Dunn MJ, et al. Anti-endothelial antibodies and coronary artery disease after cardiac transplantation. *Lancet* 1992;339(8809):1566–1570.
146. Rickenbacher PR, et al. Coronary artery intimal thickening in the transplanted heart. An in vivo intracoronary ultrasound study of immunologic and metabolic risk factors. *Transplantation* 1996;61(1):46–53.
147. Lowry RW, et al. What are the implications of cardiac infection with cytomegalovirus before heart transplantation? *J Heart Lung Transplant* 1994;13(1 Pt 1):122–128.
148. Mehra MR, et al. International Society for Heart and Lung Transplantation working formulation of a standardized nomenclature for cardiac allograft vasculopathy—2010. *J Heart Lung Transplant* 29(7):717–727.
149. Mehra MR, et al. The prognostic significance of intimal proliferation in cardiac allograft vasculopathy: a paradigm shift. *J Heart Lung Transplant* 1995;14(6 Pt 2):S207–S211.
150. Tuzcu EM, et al. Intravascular ultrasound evidence of angiographically silent progression in coronary atherosclerosis predicts long-term morbidity and mortality after cardiac transplantation. *J Am Coll Cardiol* 2005;45(9):1538–1542.
151. Kobashigawa JA, et al. Multicenter intravascular ultrasound validation study among heart transplant recipients: outcomes after five years. *J Am Coll Cardiol* 2005;45(9):1532–1537.
152. Kao J, et al. Elevated serum levels of the CXCR3 chemokine ITAC are associated with the development of transplant coronary artery disease. *Circulation* 2003;107(15):1958–1961.
153. Mehra MR, et al. An intravascular ultrasound study of the influence of angiotensin-converting enzyme inhibitors and calcium entry blockers on the development of cardiac allograft vasculopathy. *Am J Cardiol* 1995;75(12):853–854.
154. Lamich R, et al. Efficacy of augmented immunosuppressive therapy for early vasculopathy in heart transplantation. *J Am Coll Cardiol* 1998;32(2):413–419.
155. Schroeder JS, et al. A preliminary study of diltiazem in the prevention of coronary artery disease in heart-transplant recipients. *N Engl J Med* 1993;328(3):164–170.
156. Kobashigawa JA, et al. Effect of pravastatin on outcomes after cardiac transplantation. *N Engl J Med* 1995;333(10):621–627.
157. Wenke K, et al. Simvastatin reduces graft vessel disease and mortality after heart transplantation: a four-year randomized trial. *Circulation* 1997;96(5):1398–1402.

158. Marx SO, et al. Rapamycin-FKBP inhibits cell cycle regulators of proliferation in vascular smooth muscle cells. *Circ Res* 1995;76(3):412–417.
159. Poon M, et al. Rapamycin inhibits vascular smooth muscle cell migration. *J Clin Invest* 1996;98(10):2277–2283.
160. Sehgal SN. Rapamune (RAPA, rapamycin, sirolimus): mechanism of action immunosuppressive effect results from blockade of signal transduction and inhibition of cell cycle progression. *Clin Biochem* 1998;31(5):335–340.
161. Poston RS, et al. Rapamycin reverses chronic graft vascular disease in a novel cardiac allograft model. *Circulation* 1999;100(1):67–74.
162. Gallo R, et al. Inhibition of intimal thickening after balloon angioplasty in porcine coronary arteries by targeting regulators of the cell cycle. *Circulation* 1999;99(16):2164–2170.
163. Sousa JE, et al. Lack of neointimal proliferation after implantation of sirolimus-coated stents in human coronary arteries: a quantitative coronary angiography and three-dimensional intravascular ultrasound study. *Circulation* 2001;103(2):192–195.
164. Luo Y, et al. Rapamycin resistance tied to defective regulation of p27Kip1. *Mol Cell Biol* 1996;16(12):6744–6751.
165. Marx SO, Marks AR. Bench to bedside: the development of rapamycin and its application to stent restenosis. *Circulation* 2001;104(8):852–855.
166. Kahan BD, et al. Immunosuppressive effects and safety of a sirolimus/cyclosporine combination regimen for renal transplantation. *Transplantation* 1998;66(8):1040–1046.
167. Groth CG, et al. Sirolimus (rapamycin)-based therapy in human renal transplantation: similar efficacy and different toxicity compared with cyclosporine. Sirolimus European Renal Transplant Study Group. *Transplantation* 1999;67(7):1036–1042.
168. Raichlin E, et al. Conversion to sirolimus as primary immunosuppression attenuates the progression of allograft vasculopathy after cardiac transplantation. *Circulation* 2007;116(23):2726–2733.
169. Hunt SA. Malignancy in organ transplantation: heart. *Transplant Proc* 2002;34(5):1874–1876.
170. Penn I. Incidence and treatment of neoplasia after transplantation. *J Heart Lung Transplant* 1993;12(6 Pt 2):S328–S336.
171. Haldas J, Wang W, Lazarchick J. Post-transplant lymphoproliferative disorders: T-cell lymphoma following cardiac transplant. *Leuk Lymphoma* 2002;43(2):447–450.
172. Johnson WM, Baldursson O, Gross TJ. Double jeopardy: lung cancer after cardiac transplantation. *Chest* 1998;113(6):1720–1723.
173. Couetil JP, et al. Malignant tumors after heart transplantation. *J Heart Transplant* 1990;9(6):622–626.
174. Penn I, Porat G. Central nervous system lymphomas in organ allograft recipients. *Transplantation* 1995;59(2):240–244.
175. Everly MJ, et al. Posttransplant lymphoproliferative disorder. *Ann Pharmacother* 2007;41(11):1850–1858.
176. Swinnen LJ, et al. Increased incidence of lymphoproliferative disorder after immunosuppression with the monoclonal antibody OKT3 in cardiac-transplant recipients. *N Engl J Med* 1990;323(25):1723–1728.
177. Armitage JM, et al. Posttransplant lymphoproliferative disease in thoracic organ transplant patients: ten years of cyclosporine-based immunosuppression. *J Heart Lung Transplant* 1991;10(6):877–886; discussion 886–887.
178. Ippoliti G, et al. Incidence of cancer after immunosuppressive treatment for heart transplantation. *Crit Rev Oncol Hematol* 2005;56(1):101–113.
179. van Gelder T, et al. Renal insufficiency after heart transplantation: a case-control study. *Nephrol Dial Transplant* 1998;13(9):2322–2326.
180. Lindelow B, et al. Predictors and evolution of renal function during 9 years following heart transplantation. *J Am Soc Nephrol* 2000;11(5):951–957.
181. Goldstein DJ, et al. Cyclosporine-associated end-stage nephropathy after cardiac transplantation: incidence and progression. *Transplantation* 1997;63(5):664–668.
182. Ojo AO, et al. Chronic renal failure after transplantation of a nonrenal organ. *N Engl J Med* 2003;349(10):931–940.
183. Boyle JM, et al. Risks and outcomes of acute kidney injury requiring dialysis after cardiac transplantation. *Am J Kidney Dis* 2006;48(5):787–796.
184. Granerus G, Aurell M. Reference values for 51Cr-EDTA clearance as a measure of glomerular filtration rate. *Scand J Clin Lab Invest* 1981;41(6):611–616.
185. Myers BD, et al. Cyclosporine-associated chronic nephropathy. *N Engl J Med* 1984;311(11):699–705.
186. Bennett WM. Insights into chronic cyclosporine nephrotoxicity. *Int J Clin Pharmacol Ther* 1996;34(11):515–519.
187. Andoh TF, Burdmann EA, Bennett WM. Nephrotoxicity of immunosuppressive drugs: experimental and clinical observations. *Semin Nephrol* 1997;17(1):34–45.
188. Grieff M, et al. Cyclosporine-induced elevation in circulating endothelin-1 in patients with solid-organ transplants. *Transplantation* 1993;56(4):880–884.
189. Julien J, et al. Cyclosporine-induced stimulation of the renin–angiotensin system after liver and heart transplantation. *Transplantation* 1993;56(4):885–891.
190. Feutren G, Mihatsch MJ. Risk factors for cyclosporine-induced nephropathy in patients with autoimmune diseases. International Kidney Biopsy Registry of Cyclosporine in Autoimmune Diseases. *N Engl J Med* 1992;326(25):1654–1660.
191. Young EW, et al. A prospective study of renal structure and function in psoriasis patients treated with cyclosporin. *Kidney Int* 1994;46(4):1216–1222.
192. Waser M, et al. Irreversibility of cyclosporine-induced renal function impairment in heart transplant recipients. *J Heart Lung Transplant* 1993;12(5):846–850.
193. Vossler MR, et al. Pre-operative renal function predicts development of chronic renal insufficiency after orthotopic heart transplantation. *J Heart Lung Transplant* 2002;21(8):874–881.
194. Falkenhain ME, Cosio FG, Sedmak DD. Progressive histologic injury in kidneys from heart and liver transplant recipients receiving cyclosporine. *Transplantation* 1996;62(3):364–370.
195. Furlanut M, et al. Effect of fluctuations of blood cyclosporine concentrations on renal function. *Transplant Proc* 1994;26(5):2574–2575.
196. Chan C, et al. A randomized controlled trial of verapamil on cyclosporine nephrotoxicity in heart and lung transplant recipients. *Transplantation* 1997;63(10):1435–1440.
197. Pascual M, et al. Strategies to improve long-term outcomes after renal transplantation. *N Engl J Med* 2002;346(8):580–590.
198. Pascual M, et al. A prospective, randomized clinical trial of cyclosporine reduction in stable patients greater than 12 months after renal transplantation. *Transplantation* 2003;75(9):1501–1505.
199. Bestetti R, et al. Switch from calcineurin inhibitors to sirolimus-induced renal recovery in heart transplant recipients in the midterm follow-up. *Transplantation* 2006;81(5):692–696.
200. Tedoriya T, et al. Reversal of chronic cyclosporine nephrotoxicity after heart transplantation-potential role of mycophenolate mofetil. *J Heart Lung Transplant* 2002;21(9):976–982.
201. Soccal PM, et al. Improvement of drug-induced chronic renal failure in lung transplantation. *Transplantation* 1999;68(1):164–165.
202. Starling RC, Cody RJ. Cardiac transplant hypertension. *Am J Cardiol* 1990;65(1):106–111.
203. Ozdogan E, et al. Factors influencing the development of hypertension after heart transplantation. *J Heart Transplant* 1990;9(5):548–553.
204. Thompson ME, et al. The contrasting effects of cyclosporin-A and azathioprine on arterial blood pressure and renal function following cardiac transplantation. *Int J Cardiol* 1986;11(2):219–229.
205. Scherrer U, et al. Cyclosporine-induced sympathetic activation and hypertension after heart transplantation. *N Engl J Med* 1990;323(11):693–699.
206. Ong AC, et al. Effect of cyclosporin A on endothelin synthesis by cultured human renal cortical epithelial cells. *Nephrol Dial Transplant* 1993;8(8):748–753.
207. Reichenspurner H. Overview of tacrolimus-based immunosuppression after heart or lung transplantation. *J Heart Lung Transplant* 2005;24(2):119–130.
208. Taylor DO, et al. A randomized, multicenter comparison of tacrolimus and cyclosporine immunosuppressive regimens in cardiac transplantation: decreased hyperlipidemia and hypertension with tacrolimus. *J Heart Lung Transplant* 1999;18(4):336–345.
209. Pham SM, et al. A prospective trial of tacrolimus (FK 506) in clinical heart transplantation: intermediate-term results. *J Thorac Cardiovasc Surg* 1996;111(4):764–772.
210. Brozena SC, et al. Effectiveness and safety of diltiazem or lisinopril in treatment of hypertension after heart transplantation. Results of a prospective, randomized multicenter trail. *J Am Coll Cardiol* 1996;27(7):1707–1712.
211. Ballantyne CM, et al. Hyperlipidemia after heart transplantation: report of a 6-year experience, with treatment recommendations. *J Am Coll Cardiol* 1992;19(6):1315–1321.

CHAPTER

52

Surgical Complications in Newborns

Samir Gadepalli and Ronald B. Hirschl

OVERVIEW

Disease processes manifested by newborns are almost always related to an underlying birth anomaly. The complications associated with such anomalies are related to the effects that the birth defect has upon cardiopulmonary physiology or organ system function. For example, depending on the associated cardiopulmonary compromise, a congenital pulmonary airway malformation (CPAM) or congenital diaphragmatic hernia (CDH) may prove to be lethal at birth or manifest only in the ensuing months or years.

In most cases, the outcome of newborns and infants following operative intervention is determined by the associated direct cardiopulmonary effects, such as with CDH, or related to the presence of other anomalies, especially neurologic or cardiac defects. Although there are a few exceptions, correction of a gastrointestinal (GI), pulmonary, abdominal wall, or diaphragmatic anomaly is straightforward, with little morbidity and mortality associated with the procedure itself; rather, it is other associated anomalies and the effect of the birth defect upon the heart, lungs, or nervous system that adversely affect outcome.

INTESTINAL OBSTRUCTION IN THE NEWBORN

Bilious vomiting is the hallmark of bowel obstruction that requires operative intervention in the newborn. Newborns with bowel obstruction should have an orogastric or nasogastric tube placed to continuous suction to prevent vomiting and pulmonary aspiration and to decompress the GI tract. Fluid resuscitation should be performed until appropriate urine output is noted (1 to 2 mL/kg/h). The electrolyte status should be evaluated and any aberrancies corrected prior to administration of anesthetics. The newborn should be placed in a warm environment since the surface-to-mass ratio of the newborn is high and the ability to maintain normothermia is limited. Radiographic evaluation typically begins with an abdominal flat plate and either a cross-table lateral or left lateral decubitus assessment. Further radiographic evaluation varies depending on the specific clinical picture and abnormalities observed.

Samir Gadepalli, Ronald B. Hirschl: University of Michigan, Ann Arbor, MI 48109.

Typically, an upper GI contrast series allows assessment of the presence, etiology, and location of a proximal obstruction, whereas a contrast enema is frequently performed to rule out obstruction in the colon or terminal ileum. A contrast enema may also be performed to rule out a second colonic obstruction downstream from the primary anomaly that the surgeon otherwise might miss. In order to minimize the risk of ischemia and bowel necrosis, the workup of bowel obstruction in the newborn should be performed emergently until the diagnosis of malrotation with volvulus has been excluded.

Congenital duodenal obstruction

Congenital duodenal obstruction with duodenal dilation is due to atresia in 76% of cases and stenosis in 23% of cases. Causes include the presence of a duodenal web (18%), annular pancreas (36%), absence of a portion of the duodenum (10%), or a malrotation with either volvulus or the presence of Ladd bands (36%) (1). Annular pancreas coexists with duodenal atresia due to a common embryologic origin and is always treated in the same manner (2). The presence of a duodenal obstruction may be appreciated on prenatal ultrasound usually due to identification of polyhydramnios (41%) or a dilated stomach and duodenum (double bubble, 87%) (3). Finally, about half the patients with duodenal atresia are premature (<37 weeks gestation) (4); therefore, issues related to prematurity such as retinopathy, intracranial bleeding, and pulmonary difficulties must also be addressed when present (5).

Typical presenting symptoms in the first 1 to 2 days of life include feeding intolerance and emesis, which is usually bilious unless the obstruction is proximal to the ampulla of Vater, which is in 5% to 10% of cases. Plain abdominal radiographs demonstrate the classic "double bubble" of an air-filled, dilated stomach and proximal duodenum in 77% of patients (Fig. 52.1) (4). Air can be used as a contrast agent by injecting 20 mL through the nasogastric tube during performance of the radiograph. The distal small intestine and colon remain gasless with a duodenal atresia. In contrast, in the setting of a duodenal web with an opening or a malrotation with Ladd bands or volvulus, gas is often present in the downstream GI tract. The importance of the distinction is that the urgency with

Laparoscopy in neonates can be difficult due to the limited operating space; however, the decompressed distal bowel in duodenal atresia may allow for an easier visualization than most other laparoscopic procedures. In addition, the dissection required to mobilize the duodenum up into the field is limited with the laparoscopic approach, thus simplifying the operation.

Malrotation

At approximately 8 to 10 weeks of development, the midgut, which consists of the intestines oriented on the blood supply of the superior mesenteric artery, rotates 270 degrees counterclockwise (from the perspective of the surgeon looking toward the base of the mesentery), which leads to fixation of the proximal small bowel at the ligament of Treitz, attachment of the cecum and right colon in the right lower quadrant, and broad fixation of the base of the small-bowel mesentery to the retroperitoneum. If this rotation fails to occur, the small intestine remains on the right side of the abdomen, the cecum is typically at a location other than the right lower quadrant, and the bowel overall remains unfixed. The entire midgut is thus mobile and prone to a twist, or volvulus, which is the form of presentation in 31% of patients but 85% of newborns (16,17). Volvulus may compromise superior mesenteric artery inflow and venous blood outflow, leading to ischemia or necrosis of the entire small intestine and transverse colon (Fig. 52.3). In addition, peritoneal bands, known as Ladd bands, that cross over the distal portions of the duodenum and the proximal jejunum are residue of the failed rotation and may partially obstruct the duodenum and small bowel.

Eighty-nine percent of patients with symptomatic malrotation present in the first year of life, with 50% in the first week and 65% in the first month, leaving only 11% to present after the first year (18). An occasional older patient presents with intermittent midgut volvulus and recurrent abdominal pain.

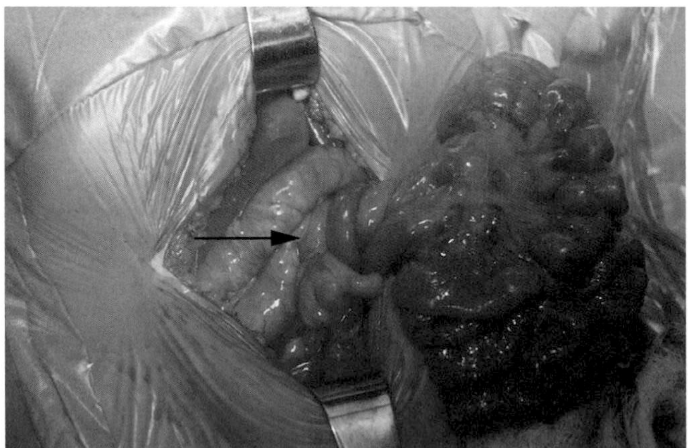

FIGURE 52.3. Malrotation with volvulus. The arrow demonstrates the site of the volvulus. Note that the volvulus is in a clockwise direction and that the small bowel is ischemic.

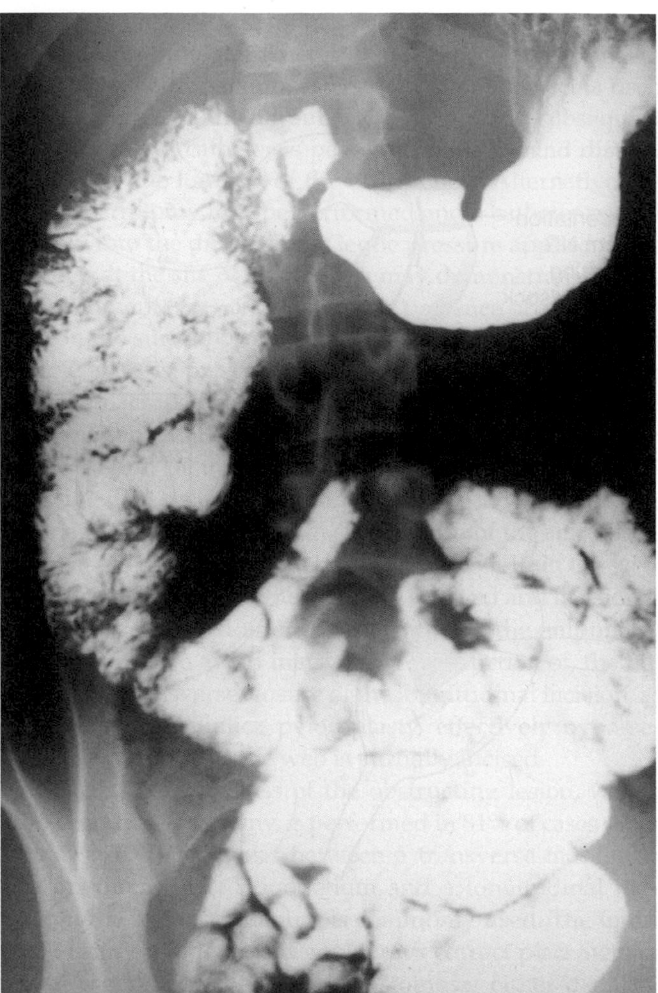

FIGURE 52.4. Classic upper GI with small-bowel follow-through in a patient with malrotation. Note that the duodenojejunal junction never passes to the left of the midline (spine) and the jejunum is on the right side of the abdomen.

One of the most common complications of treatment for malrotation and acute midgut volvulus is the failure to recognize this entity promptly, with ensuing loss of the entire midgut. The primary symptom of acute midgut volvulus is sudden onset of bilious vomiting (19). It is incumbent upon clinicians to pursue the diagnosis of malrotation in infants with bilious vomiting. With midgut volvulus, as the distal bowel empties, the abdomen is often scaphoid rather than distended. Physical examination is surprisingly unremarkable until later in the process when intestinal ischemia and necrosis develop. At that point, abdominal distension, tenderness, and hematochezia are often present. As the course progresses, hypovolemia, shock, and acidosis ensue. Contrast radiography evaluation of the course of the duodenum demonstrates that the duodenojejunal junction remains to the right of the midline and the normal posterior and cephalad fixation of the duodenum at the ligament of Treitz is absent (Fig. 52.4) (20). If volvulus is present, a corkscrew appearance of the duodenojejunal junction is noted. Ultrasound is proving to be of value in the diagnosis of this anomaly (21).

Midgut volvulus is one of the most serious emergencies in the neonate. Once the diagnosis of malrotation is made in the symptomatic patient, immediate laparotomy is indicated even if radiologic and clinical signs of volvulus are absent. The child should be rapidly resuscitated either in the operating room or while the operating room is being readied. Ladd procedure consists of the following: (a) exploration of the midgut; (b) counterclockwise derotation of a midgut volvulus (if present); (c) performance of a Kocher maneuver with division of Ladd bands (which may be causing the obstruction); (d) broadening of the mesentery of the proximal jejunum and the transverse colon, which, along with subsequent adhesion formation, will prevent recurrent volvulus; (e) return of the intestine to the abdomen without any twists in the mesentery and placement of the cecum in the left lower quadrant to further broaden the mesentery; and (f) appendectomy because of the potential of a difficult diagnosis of appendicitis in the future with the inappropriate location of the appendix (22). Failure to detorse the bowel completely or to lyse all Ladd bands may result in persistent obstruction or recurrence of volvulus. Since the volvulus is almost always clockwise from the surgeon's perspective, two or more counterclockwise rotations of the bowel may be required, and the process of derotation can be very confusing. One must continue to derotate until the entire mesentery can be broadly followed to the base.

There is no value in fixing—or need to fix—the intestines to the retroperitoneum. If compromised bowel is noted, a second look at 24 hours is an option. Another approach may entail resection of clearly necrotic bowel with either reanastomosis if the status of the remaining bowel is certain or staple closure of the ends in areas of compromise with re-exploration at 24 hours. If possible, sufficient length of intestine is maintained to avoid the short gut syndrome. Performance of an ileostomy is usually necessary only if there is continued question of intestinal viability at re-exploration. Necrosis of the entire midgut makes survival unlikely and excessive morbidity a likely outcome with requirement for life-long parenteral nutrition or small-bowel transplantation (23).

Postoperative complications are relatively few. Recurrence of midgut volvulus occurs in <2% of patients and is thought to be related to a failure to lyse all the Ladd bands. Adhesive bowel obstruction occurs in 1% to 10% of patients and can be treated with nasogastric decompression, although lysis of adhesions, sometimes via a laparoscopic approach, may be required. Malrotation is associated with a duodenal atresia or a partially obstructing web in 11% of patients (18). To exclude this, one option is to pass a Foley catheter through the duodenum via a small gastrotomy and withdraw it with the balloon gently inflated in order to ensure that a duodenal web or other obstruction does not exist.

In those with short bowel syndrome (SBS), complications are associated with long-term parenteral nutrition, fluid and electrolyte abnormalities, and liver failure. The length of bowel sufficient for enteral nutrition traditionally has been considered to be 15 cm with an intact ileocecal valve and 40 cm without, although recent data suggest that it is not just the length, but also the character of the bowel that determines successful provision of enteral feeding (24).

Perioperative mortality is 4% and is primarily associated with sepsis from massive intestinal necrosis (17). Mortality is at least 50% in those with extensive (>75%) small-bowel infarction (20). Mortality may also be increased in those with congenital heart disease (25). A recent review of patients with malrotation and heterotaxy identified nearly 10% in-hospital mortality, due to cardiac causes, in those who underwent a Ladd procedure, although the authors note that the deaths were not due to the Ladd procedure (26). Of interest, 27% of the patients with heterotaxy and symptomatic malrotation had midgut volvulus. In another study, 18% of patients with heterotaxy died after a Ladd procedure and 14% developed postoperative small-bowel obstruction requiring an operation (27). However, all deaths occurred more than 1 month after the operation and were due to the underlying cardiac disease. Therefore, the surgeon must partner with the cardiologist in considering the risk benefit of a Ladd procedure in patients with congenital heart disease and asymptomatic malrotation.

Laparoscopic approaches to the Ladd procedure, even in the neonate, have been described for malrotation with and without midgut volvulus (28–31). Case series with historical controls have suggested that laparoscopic approaches are equally safe and effective as open techniques, with improved cosmesis, quicker return to bowel function, and decreased pain (32,33).

Jejunoileal obstruction

Among cases of jejunoileal obstruction, atresia occurs in 95% while stenosis occurs in 5% (8). The diagnosis of bowel obstruction is made on the basis of fetal ultrasound in 29% of cases via identification of enlarged loops of bowel in conjunction with maternal polyhydramnios, although about 50% of positive scans are false-positive studies (4,34). Associated *in utero* causes of jejunoileal atresia include volvulus in 27%, malrotation in 19%, gastroschisis in 17%, and intussusception in 2%. Other anomalies are unusual with jejunoileal atresia (7%) (4). Familial causes of intestinal atresias have also been postulated (35).

The diagnosis can be made by plain radiography when a large loop of dilated, air-filled bowel is noted. The enlarged loops are usually thumb-sized or greater on the newborn radiograph (rule of thumb). If such large, dilated loops are noted, further preoperative diagnostic studies are not required except for a contrast enema, which often demonstrates a diminutive and unused colon and rules out colonic pathology, which can be missed during exploration. Peritoneal calcification is noted in 12% of patients, indicating prior *in utero* perforation and saponification of fat from pancreatic enzymes in the extruded meconium.

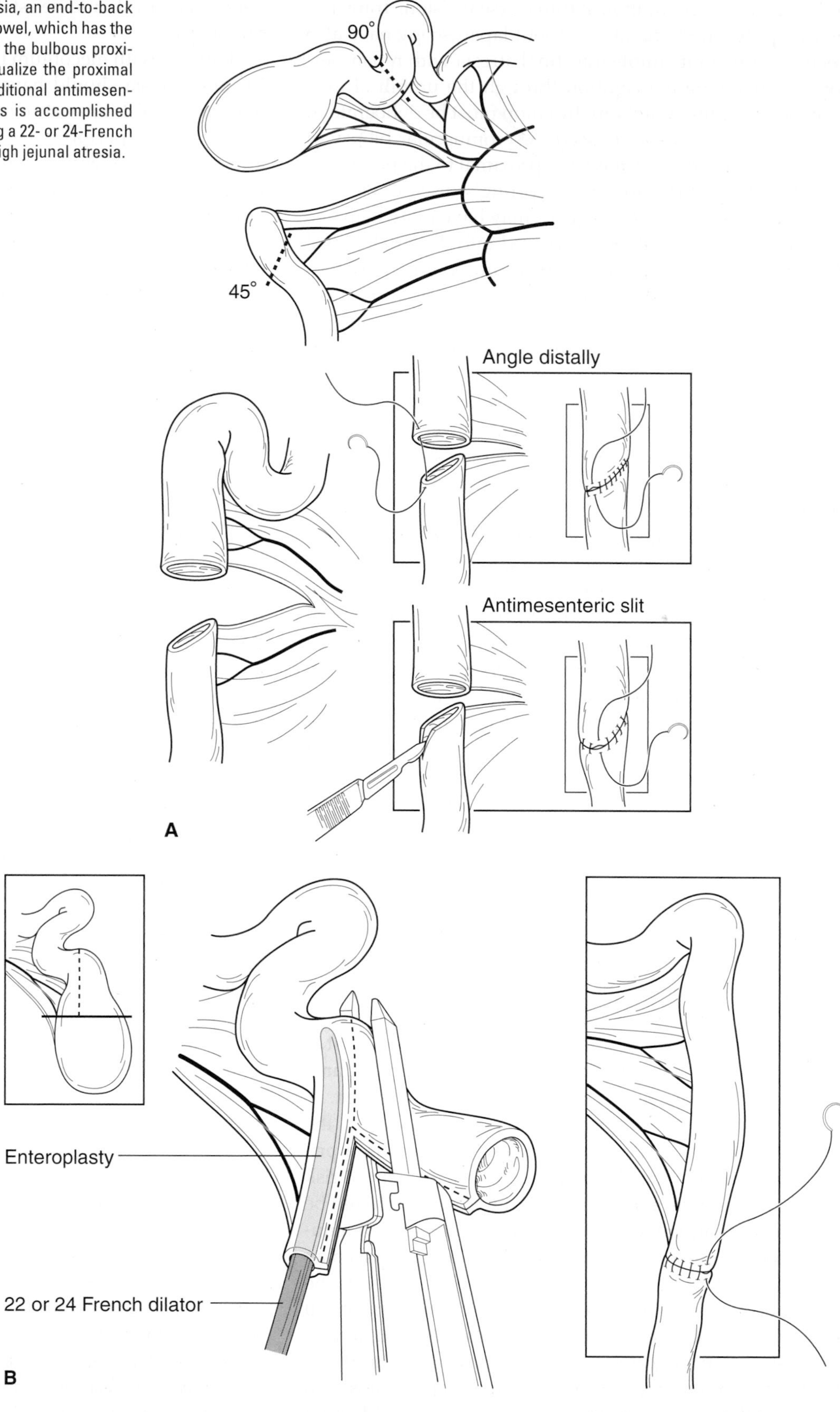

FIGURE 52.6. **A:** For jejunoileal atresia, an end-to-back anastomosis is performed. The distal bowel, which has the smaller caliber even after resection of the bulbous proximal end, is divided on an angle to equalize the proximal and distal bowel caliber. Often, an additional antimesenteric slit is required. The anastomosis is accomplished with 5–0 Vicryl. **B:** An enteroplasty using a 22- or 24-French catheter stent and staples is used for high jejunal atresia.

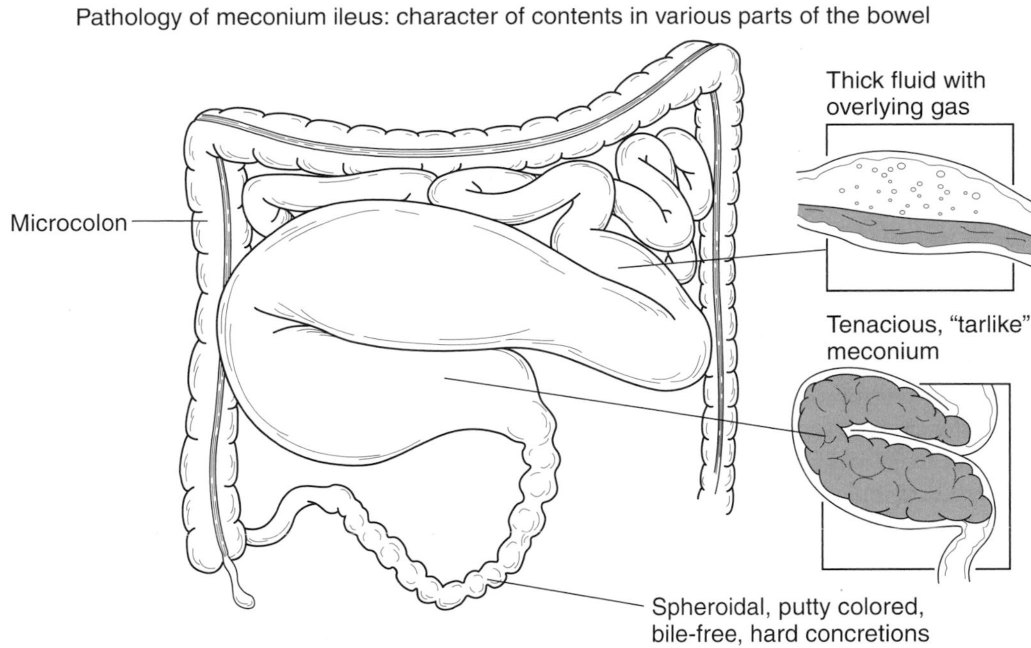

FIGURE 52.7. Typical intestinal findings in the setting of meconium ileus.

with associated liver failure is a potentially lethal complication in infants that is not as prevalent in adults. Liver and small bowel transplantation have not yet had a consistent impact upon outcome in those with this complication. Vitamin deficiencies can also occur and levels should be evaluated regularly.

Meconium ileus

Meconium ileus is present in approximately 20% of newborns with cystic fibrosis (43). With meconium ileus, secretion of viscous intestinal mucus, an abnormal concentrating process in the proximal bowel, and impaired pancreatic enzyme secretion together result in bowel obstruction because of the presence of thick, tenacious meconium in the mid-ileum and pellets of gray, inspissated meconium in the distal ileum (Fig. 52.7). The hallmark of the newborn with meconium ileus is abdominal distention at birth, with multiple doughy loops of dilated bowel noted on palpation. Bilious emesis occurs and the newborn fails to pass meconium in the first 24 to 48 hours of life. Meconium ileus is divided into uncomplicated and complicated. The uncomplicated meconium ileus is simple obstruction of the terminal ileum and occurs in 55% of cases (44,45). In contrast, meconium-filled bowel may twist and produce a volvulus, resulting in ischemic necrosis with associated perforation (19%) and/or atresia (48%) (46). Perforation, with intraperitoneal dissemination of sterile meconium, may lead to isolated regions of calcification (meconium peritonitis) or even the development of a large meconium-containing pseudocyst (19%). Extra intestinal anomalies are uncommon with meconium ileus, other than its association with cystic fibrosis and related sequelae.

For uncomplicated meconium ileus, a contrast enema can be both diagnostic and therapeutic (Fig. 52.8). Gastrografin, Hypaque, or Conray may be used to perform the study; the osmolarity of the contrast agent does not appear to be of significance. A small, unused microcolon is noted with thick, inspissated meconium in the terminal ileum. The distal small bowel must be filled or the therapeutic aspect of the study

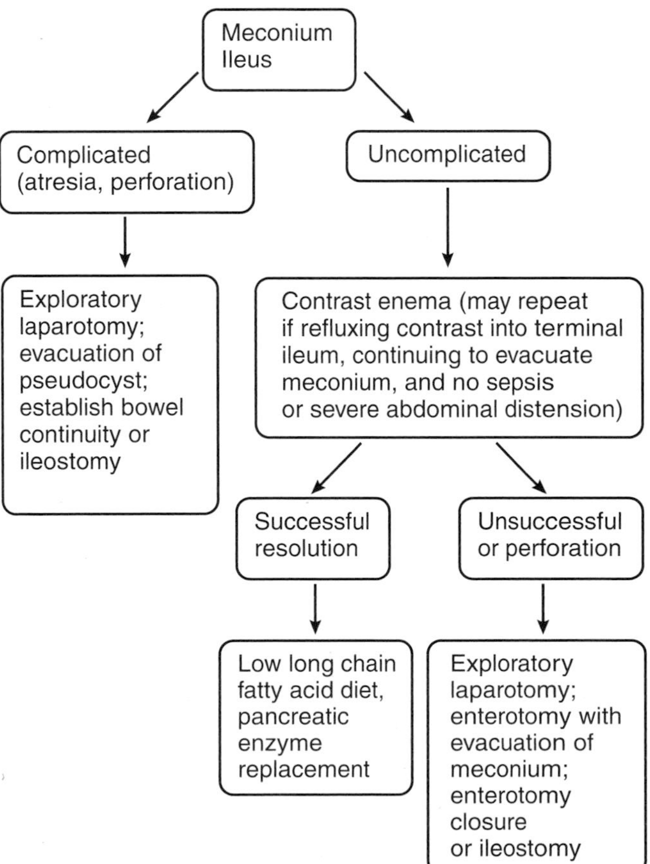

FIGURE 52.8. Management approach to the newborn with meconium ileus.

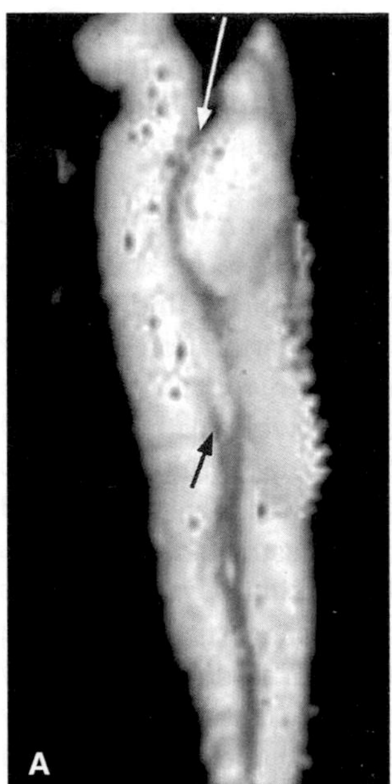

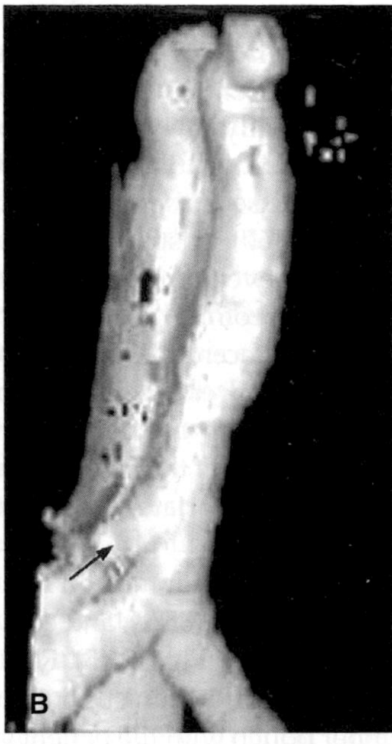

FIGURE 52.16. **A:** Three-dimensional CT reconstruction of the trachea and esophagus. White arrow on proximal tracheoesophageal fistula, which was missed at the initial operation; black arrow on remnant pouch. **B:** Similar reconstruction from different rotational angle depicts accessory bronchus (*arrow*). (From Islam S, Cavanaugh E, Honeke R, et al. Diagnosis of a proximal tracheoesophageal fistula using three-dimensional CT scan: a case report. *J Pediatr Surg* 2004;39(1):100–102, with permission.)

operating room prior to repair of the EA/TEF (168). However, bronchoscopy may miss small proximal fistulas, and contrast study of the proximal pouch appears to be an equally useful adjunctive test, when appropriately performed, though the risks of aspiration must be weighed.

Since 64% of patients have associated anomalies, a search for congenital defects should be undertaken (169). Approximately 15% of patients with EA and TEF have a constellation of findings compatible with the VATER or VACTERL association (vertebral defects, anal atresia, cardiac anomalies, TEF and EA, renal defects, and limb abnormalities). The most common anomalies are cardiac (38%) and are responsible for many of the deaths associated with EA and TEF. Renal anomalies (17%) should also be identified so that further damage is not incurred (170).

In general, patients with EA and a distal TEF have adequate esophageal length to allow primary reconstruction. Thus, a repair is undertaken within the first 24 to 48 hours unless contraindicated by prematurity, the presence of congenital heart disease, or another physiologically compromising situation. In that case, temporizing with proximal pouch Replogle suction and a gastrostomy tube with plans for delayed repair may be the best strategy. Otherwise, an approach through the right chest using a muscle-sparing incision is performed with access via the fourth intercostal space. The presence of a right aortic arch, found in 2% of patients with the EA/TEF anomaly, should be identified on echocardiography so that a left thoracic approach can be used (171). Anastomosis via a right thoracotomy in the presence of a right aortic arch is associated with a high anastomotic leak rate (42%) and often requires a left thoracotomy for completion of the operation (172). A double aortic arch makes division of the TEF and esophagoesophagostomy difficult via either approach. The distal TEF is identified in the region of the carina and is divided (Fig. 52.17). Prior to division of the fistula, maintenance of oxygenation may be tenuous and requires that the

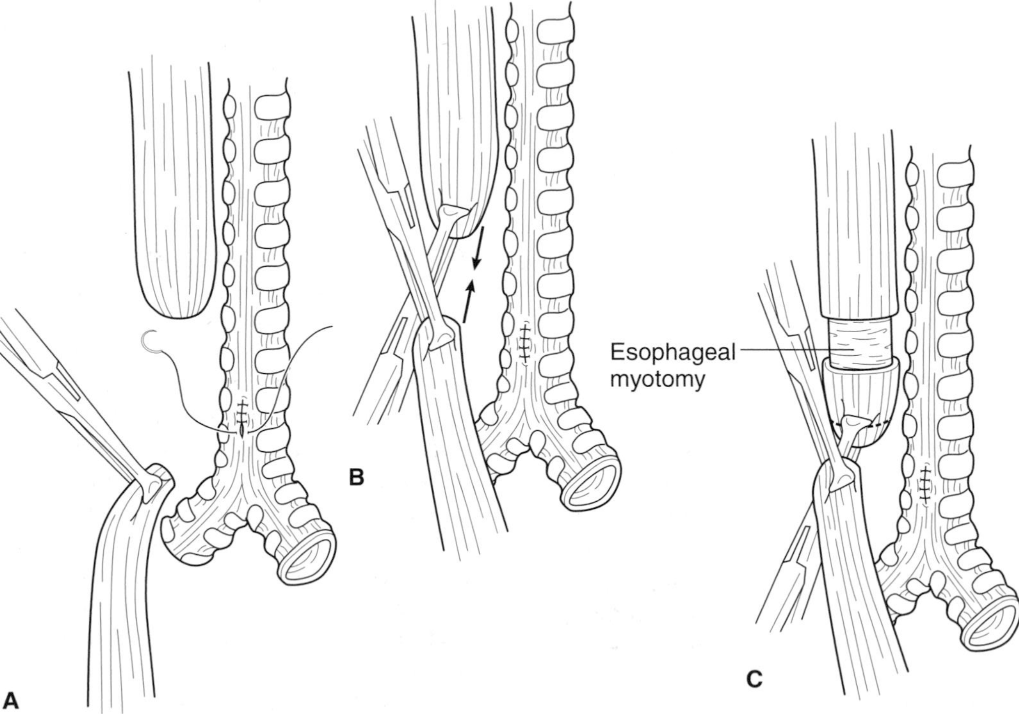

FIGURE 52.17. Repair of esophageal atresia (EA) and tracheoesophageal fistula (TEF) **A:** The TEF has been divided and the tracheal opening closed with 5–0 or 6–0 PDS suture. **B:** The feasibility of primary anastomosis between the two esophageal segments is being assessed. **C:** A circumferential proximal esophagomyotomy is being used to gain additional length.

surgeon intermittently allow expansion of the right lung; this problem usually resolves once the fistula is ligated. A few millimeters of esophageal tissue are left on the trachea during division of the TEF in order to avoid compromise of the tracheal lumen. In contrast, leaving too much esophagus on the trachea can compromise the length of the distal esophageal segment and result in an airway diverticulum, which can serve as a source of ongoing airway contamination. The tracheal closure is checked for an air leak while under saline with application of sustained airway pressure. The distal esophagus can be mobilized with little fear of it being devascularized. The proximal esophageal pouch is best identified by having the anesthesiologist advance a catheter placed through the mouth into the pouch. A suture is placed in the apex of the proximal pouch for manipulation in order to avoid trauma due to repeated grasping of the tissue. The pouch is mobilized in the upper mediastinum; care is taken while mobilizing the anterior esophagus because of the risk of entry into the membranous trachea. Use of cautery should be limited, especially in the apex of the thorax, because of the risk of thermal injury to the recurrent laryngeal nerve. An esophagoesophagostomy is performed in most cases under mild to moderate levels of tension. Care must be taken to ensure that sutures include the full thickness of the esophagus since the mucosa can easily retract. A nasogastric tube is passed through the anastomosis into the stomach to ensure patency of the distal esophagus. Gastrostomy tubes are done only if the presence of other anomalies suggests that tube feeding will be required. Most surgeons use a retropleural approach and place a drainage tube near, but not on, the anastomosis at the end of the operation to contain a postoperative anastomotic leak, which occurs in 16% of cases (169). Small openings in the pleura are unimportant and should not be closed when a retropleural approach is used. Silk sutures are associated with a two- to three-fold increase in the incidence of anastomotic leak (173). A leak, along with tension and GER, can result in postoperative strictures, found in up to 40% of cases (174). Oropharyngeal suctioning is limited to <6 cm from the lips in order to avoid trauma to the anastomosis. An esophageal contrast study is performed approximately 1 week after operation. If the anastomosis appears intact, feedings are initiated, antibiotics are discontinued, and the retropleural chest tube is removed.

In patients with isolated EA without a TEF (pure EA), the distal esophagus is typically short (approximately two vertebral bodies), which precludes immediate repair. Some patients with EA and a distal TEF will have a longer gap between the proximal and distal esophagus (more than two vertebral bodies). Some of the latter situations can still be repaired via a primary approach. Patients with pure EA or those with long-gap atresias that are not amenable to a primary approach can still be repaired at 8 to 12 weeks with a delayed primary anastomosis (175). The management involves placement of a gastrostomy tube and allowing for growth of the proximal and distal pouch over the ensuing 3 months prior to an attempt at a primary repair (176). At times, the fistula may need to be ligated if respiratory effects of pulmonary soilage are observed. Daily dilation of the proximal pouch may enhance lengthening. Another option is to mobilize the entire distal and proximal esophagus, to perform the anastomosis under considerable tension, and to maintain the patient sedated with the head in the flexed position to decrease postoperative anastomotic tension (177). Alternatively, a proximal or distal pouch circular myotomy of Livaditis may be performed, which increases the length by 1 to 2 cm (Fig. 52.16) (178,179). With this technique, the muscularis is divided circumferentially while the mucosa is carefully maintained intact. Two or three proximal myotomies may be used to enhance length. Unfortunately, complications such as leaks, stricture, outpouching of the esophagus at the site of the myotomy, and esophageal dysfunction are associated with this technique (180). A spiral myotomy may be used to decrease the outpouching associated with myotomy. All these situations present a challenge to the surgeon where a decision must be made on whether to attempt to salvage the native esophagus. In patients with very long gaps (greater than six vertebral bodies), replacement of the esophagus with a natural conduit might be the best option (175).

Other innovative techniques for lengthening the esophagus when the proximal and distal segments cannot be brought together include a multistaged approach in which an esophagostomy is formed on the chest and sequentially lengthened every 2 to 3 weeks by advancing the esophagostomy inferiorly along the chest wall (181). This technique allows sham feedings, which are important for normal feeding development, to take place. Another approach promoted by Scharli involves transverse division of the lesser curvature of the stomach along with ligation of the left gastric artery (182). Similar to a Collis procedure, except performed along the lesser curvature, the technique is effective at lengthening the distal esophagus (183).

Foker et al. have suggested placing externalized sutures on the ends of the esophagus to apply tension with eventual approximation of the ends (184). With this approach, continuous traction is used to slowly approximate the ends of the esophagus followed by performance of an anastomosis. Postoperative strictures and reflux may occur with this approach and can be managed with dilations and Thal fundoplication, respectively (185). At times, the sutures may pull through the ends of the esophagus with potential leak from the ends of the esophagus. Options when this complication occurs are to replace the sutures with repair of the leak (if present) or to convert to a cervical esophagostomy with plans for esophageal reconstruction at a later date.

Finally, an intriguing approach developed by Gough (186) suggests formation of a flap from the dilated proximal fistula, which is then tubularized in order to enhance proximal esophageal length. Whatever approach is used, a long gap adversely affects the outcome with regard to death (18%), anastomotic leak (31%), stricture (44%), and GER (56%) (187).

In general, all attempts are made at salvaging the native esophagus (188). However, when the esophagus cannot be approximated or if complications of stricture, recurrent GER, or esophageal dysfunction persist, esophageal replacement is an alternative. Right or left colon, jejunum, or the stomach, either as a reversed gastric tube or as a gastric transposition, can be used (189–193). Although an effective solution to establishing esophageal continuity, the complication rate with esophageal replacement is substantial and includes an anastomotic leak rate of approximately 30%, stricture formation in 20% to 60%, and a mortality of 5% (189–191,194,195). Anastomotic leaks almost always resolve spontaneously. When a colon conduit is used, it can be placed behind the hilum of the lung on either side or in a substernal position, although the latter is associated with a higher stenosis rate (189). A vagotomy is effective in preventing the development of ulcers when a colon conduit is used. The colon may become redundant in the chest, leading to dysfunction and stasis (16%). Reoperation is necessary in approximately 50% of patients and is most often performed to redo the esophagocolic or cologastric anastomoses due to strictures (194,196). Gastrocolic reflux may also occur, and approximately 20% will ultimately require replacement of the colon graft, which is best managed by performance of a gastric transposition or a free jejunal graft (194,196).

Another option for esophageal replacement is the reverse gastric tube, which is formed by creating a tube from the greater curvature of the stomach. This is most often brought up to the neck through what would have been the esophageal bed. Complications are similar to those of the colonic substitutes with the addition of leak from the long suture line. In addition, compromise of the stomach size in newborns may be a problem. Finally, gastric transposition is a successful option since the blood supply to the stomach is excellent and the operation is technically easier than other alternatives. This option can be used even when previous operations have been performed on the stomach (193). The right and left gastroepiploic arteries are maintained intact while the stomach is otherwise mobilized. The distal esophageal segment is excised and the fundus preferably brought through the posterior mediastinum, which limits the potential complication of gastric distension. The posterior aspect of the stomach must be anchored to the sternocleidomastoid muscles in the infant and to the prevertebral fascia in the older patient to prevent retraction of the stomach into the thorax. A pyloromyotomy should be performed to enhance gastric emptying. The dumping syndrome occurs in a minority of patients in the postoperative period but typically resolves over the first year. Care must be taken to avoid a twist in any of the conduits performed, which may result in ischemia or obstruction (197). Dissection must be maintained on the proximal esophagus to avoid injury to the recurrent laryngeal nerves.

The simultaneous presentation of EA/TEF and duodenal atresia is a difficult clinical situation. Duodenal atresia occurs in 10% of patients with isolated EA, and the lack of air in the GI tract can delay diagnosis of the duodenal atresia until a gastrostomy tube is placed. An intraoperative contrast study at the time of gastrostomy tube placement helps to identify this combined anomaly (176). Imperforate anus should be addressed by performing a colostomy unless a primary, laparoscopic repair of the imperforate anus is to be performed.

Patients with a TEF but no EA (4%) often have episodes of gastric distention during crying and choking, recurrent pneumonia, and cyanotic spells during feeding. The diagnosis is best made by a contrast swallow, bronchoscopy, or esophagoscopy, which may demonstrate the H-type fistula between the trachea and esophagus. A Fogarty catheter may be placed through the fistula at the time of bronchoscopy to help with identification of the fistula at operation. Ligation of the fistula is usually performed via a right cervical approach. The recurrent laryngeal nerve must be identified to prevent injury, the most common complication of this procedure. Recurrence of the fistula is rare.

Overall survival rate is 95% (169). Mortality is usually secondary to associated anomalies and is associated with the presence of major cardiac disease and birth weight <1,500 g (Table 52.1) (198). One of the most difficult decision-making situations involves the premature newborn with respiratory distress syndrome and EA/TEF since the associated ventilator leak through the fistula increases with airway pressure escalation; therefore, ligation of the fistula is ideally performed before compromised respiratory status precludes a safe operation, requiring close monitoring. Early thoracotomy and ligation of the fistula provides an ability to ventilate and prevents gastric distension though this decision must weighed against the overall clinical status of the neonate (199).

Immediate postoperative complications include small anastomotic leaks on postoperative contrast study in 15% of EA/TEF patients with primary repair. Almost all small leaks will resolve spontaneously with continuation of IV antibiotics and chest tube drainage. A repeat study is performed 1 week later, and oral feedings are held until the leak resolves. Disruption of the anastomosis occurs in approximately 5% due to excess tension, ischemia, or poor surgical technique and presents with persistent pneumothorax, respiratory distress, pleural fluid, and/or sepsis. The

Table **52.1** **Predictors of survival from an esophageal atresia anomaly**

Group	Total (*n*)	Dead (*n*)	Survival Rate (%)
I. Birth weight >1,500 g without major congenital heart disease	293	10	97
II. Birth weight <1,500 g or major congenital heart disease	70	29	59
III. Birth weight <1,500 g and major congenital heart disease	9	7	22

disruption should be managed with either direct repair of the anastomosis, preferably with reinforcement with an intercostal muscle flap or a pleural or pericardial patch, or with formation of a cervical esophagostomy and placement of a gastrostomy tube with subsequent esophageal replacement (200). Stricture formation occurs in approximately 15% of cases and is often associated with a prior anastomotic leak. Most strictures are responsive to repeated antegrade dilatation initially at a frequency of approximately every 2 to 3 weeks. Esophagoscopy should be performed before dilatation to assess the anastomotic caliber and after dilatation to ensure that full-thickness perforation has not occurred. In narrow strictures, a wire passed under endoscopic and/or fluoroscopic guidance will allow safe passage of sequentially larger Savory dilators under fluoroscopic guidance to safely enlarge the anastomosis. Contrast injection at the end of the dilatation can be performed to identify a leak at the site of the stricture. Rarely, strictures that are refractory to routine dilatation require placement of a gastrostomy tube with maintenance of a silicone "string" from the nares internally to the gastrostomy tube. The ends of the string can be tied externally and taped on the infant's back, leaving adequate laxity to prevent ulceration at the nose or gastrostomy sites while maintaining enough tension to keep from pulling out the string. Vigorous dilations with Tucker dilators can then be performed on a recurring basis. Occasionally, refractory strictures may require resection or even esophageal replacement; although refractory strictures are most often due to the presence of reflux and usually respond to dilatation once a fundoplication has been performed. Thus, the presence of GER should be investigated if a stricture does not respond after two or three dilatations.

Leak from the trachea or compromise of the tracheal lumen is unusual but requires operation in the former and bronchoscopic evaluation in the latter. Recurrent TEF occurs in 3% of cases, is usually associated with a postoperative leak, and requires reoperation, with division and ligation of the fistula (169). Recurrent pneumonia, coughing, and choking are frequently noted. Esophagoscopy with the patient prone or balloon catheter obstruction of the distal esophagus during esophageal contrast administration can enhance identification of the fistula. High-resolution CT may help to identify a recurrent fistula or a missed proximal fistula (201). Thoracotomy with fistula ligation is required. A 2-French balloon catheter should first be passed through the fistula under bronchoscopic guidance to allow intraoperative identification of the fistula. Once the fistula is ligated, a pleural or pericardial flap should be interposed between the trachea and esophagus to help prevent recurrence. Injection of fibrin glue into the fistula may result in closure of the communication without thoracotomy (202).

The most common long-term problems associated with EA include GER (40% to 60%), tracheomalacia (16%), and esophageal dysfunction (169,203). GER is likely due to the tension placed on the distal esophagus with compromise of the native antireflux mechanisms and shortening of the intra-abdominal esophagus. Recurrent pneumonia, reactive airway disease, cyanotic spells, and persistent anastomotic stricture can be symptoms/signs of GER in the EA/TEF patient. GER symptoms are present in at least 20% to 40% of adult patients with previous EA/TEF (204,205). Evaluation with upper GI contrast study and/or 24-hour pH probe may document the diagnosis (206). GER is typically first managed with prokinetic agents and proton pump inhibitors, although approximately 30% to 40% of patients require a fundoplication (169,203). A 360-degree Nissen fundoplication is most frequently performed, although a Nissen fundoplication may exacerbate the esophageal dysfunction associated with EA/TEF (207). Under those circumstances, recurrent reflux, esophageal dilation and dysfunction, and dysphagia may result in an adverse outcome (208). A Thal fundoplication is a reasonable alternative because of the partial nature of the wrap, but the failure rate has been too high. As a result, the optimal approach is to perform a "floppy" Nissen fundoplication. Since studies have demonstrated a relatively high incidence of Barrett's esophagitis among patients with repaired EA/TEF (5% to 7%), long-term endoscopic surveillance of these patients is important (205,209).

Tracheomalacia results in stridor and a barking cough in newborns, although some patients may present with apnea, as the result of a weakness in the tracheal wall such that the anterior and posterior tracheal walls coapt during expiration. Bronchoscopy during spontaneous breathing demonstrates the collapse in the distal third of the trachea. Mild symptoms in most patients can be followed with expected resolution as the patient grows. Life-threatening symptoms require operation in 6% (169). An aortopexy, in which the anterior aspect of the aortic arch is approximated to the posterior sternum, is effective in almost all patients at resolving the symptoms of tracheomalacia (210). A Palmaz airway stent or tracheostomy may be of benefit should the aortopexy fail (211). Frequently, it is difficult to determine whether the symptoms observed are due to tracheomalacia, stricture, or GER (212).

Esophageal dysmotility is present in the majority of EA/TEF children, and 40% to 75% of adult EA/TEF patients have mild-to-severe dysphagia and esophageal dysmotility (204,205,213,214). In most cases, the dysphagia is tolerable and in infants can be managed by feeding while the patient is sitting up. An occasional patient develops a diverticulum proximal to the anastomosis that requires resection. Scoliosis develops in 8% of patients, probably due to fusion of the ribs at the site of the thoracotomy, which prevents ipsilateral spine growth and results in anterior chest wall deformities in 20%, though a muscle-sparing or thoracoscopic (see below) approach may decrease the incidence of this complication. Foreign body impaction occurs in 13% of patients with corrected EA/TEF usually during the child's first 5 years of life (215).

A thoracoscopic approach has been advocated by some centers to avoid the complications associated with the thoracotomy (216). In a multi-institutional retrospective review

(217) of 104 patients who underwent thoracoscopic EA/TEF repair, 11.5% developed an early leak or stricture and a third needed esophageal dilation at least once. Two infants developed a recurrent fistula and 24% required a subsequent laparoscopic fundoplication. In another retrospective comparison of the thoracoscopic and open techniques (218), a minimally invasive approach allowed decreased postoperative narcotic use, shorter time to extubation, earlier feeding by mouth, and decreased length of stay, without an increase in operative time, anastomotic leaks, strictures, or mortality. Anesthetic considerations and potential complications during thoracoscopic EA/TEF repair are significant (219).

Congenital diaphragmatic hernia

CDH occurs due to failure of the pleuroperitoneal canal to close at 6 to 8 weeks of development. The diaphragmatic defect is in the posterolateral aspect and is referred to as Bochdalek hernia. The CDH is left sided in 78% and typically contains the small and large intestine and the spleen and may contain the stomach and the left lobe of the liver (220). With a right CDH, the liver and the abdominal viscera are typically in the hemithorax. CDH remains one of the most challenging for pediatric surgeons, though the relatively high inpatient mortality rate of approximately 50% has improved over the years to a survival of 69% even though the survival of those that require ECLS has decreased to 51% (221,222). The high mortality rate is related to the effect of the herniated abdominal viscera on the developing heart and lungs, although developmental studies in animals suggest that the lung hypoplasia may precede the diaphragmatic defect and serve as the primary insult (223,224).

By whatever mechanism, both the ipsilateral and contralateral lungs are hypoplastic, with the alveolar number on the ipsilateral side decreased by at least 90% and the contralateral lung decreased by 60% (Fig. 52.18) (225). There is a marked reduction in the number of alveoli and pulmonary arterial branches. In addition, pulmonary arteries in newborns with CDH demonstrate a thickened media with the presence of abnormal smooth muscle in small arterioles (226). As a result of a decrease in the total cross-sectional area of the pulmonary arterial vessels, along with increased muscularization of small arteries, which promotes vasospasm, pulmonary hypertension persists in the perinatal period when it is necessary for pulmonary pressures to drop in order to transition from fetal to newborn circulation. Thus, pulmonary hypoplasia is represented by abnormal development of the airways (decreased number of alveoli and airways), vasculature (decreased number of vessels and thickened media), and interstitium (increased tissue density), affecting pulmonary compliance, gas exchange, and pulmonary arterial pressures (227).

Furthermore, postnatal fetal circulation persists with right-to-left shunting of blood across the foramen ovale and patent ductus arteriosus. This shunting, in conjunction with the presence of pulmonary hypoplasia, which inhibits gas exchange, results in further increases in $Paco_2$ and reductions in Pao_2 and pH. All these variables augment pulmonary arterial vasospasm, further increasing the right-to-left shunt and reducing pulmonary blood flow. A vicious cycle as described above persists, which, if not interrupted, can result in severe respiratory failure and death. Outcome in CDH appears to depend on the degree of pulmonary hypoplasia and reactive pulmonary hypertension (228,229).

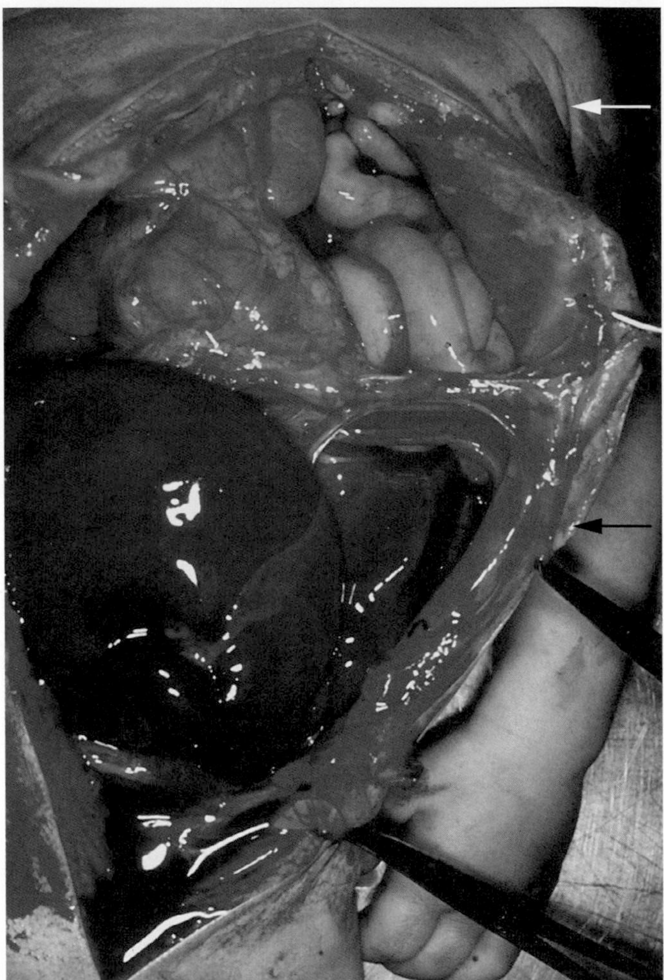

FIGURE 52.18. Congenital diaphragmatic hernia (CDH). Note the lip of the diaphragmatic defect (*black arrow*) and the left lobe of the liver that is at the opening of the defect. In some cases, the left lobe of the liver may actually reside in the left chest. The small bowel is seen in the left hemithorax. The heart is shifted to the right. The major complications in patients with CDH are pulmonary hypertension and lung hypoplasia. The latter is demonstrated in this image by the small lung to the right of the heart and a diminutive lung on the left (*white arrow*).

Most patients with CDH present in the first 24 hours, although approximately 10% to 20% present later (230). The diagnosis of CDH is typically made on chest radiograph where bowel in the chest, along with mediastinal shift to the side opposite the hernia, is noted. An upper GI contrast study can be confirmatory if there is question of a hiatal hernia, a congenital cystic lesion of the lung, or an eventration. Survival is related to the size of the diaphragmatic defect, and the stomach's location may act as a surrogate for defect size. Thus, the presence of the stomach in the chest is associated with 30% survival, but survival is nearly 100% if it is in the abdomen (231,232). The ability to reduce $PaCO_2$ <40 mm Hg with reasonable levels of ventilation also predicts survival (233).

In ~60% of fetuses with CDH, the defect is identified prenatally during initial ultrasound screening, though right-sided CDH is diagnosed far less frequently (234). Those infants who are identified *in utero* should be delivered at a center that has capabilities of performing state-of-the art care for the newborn with CDH, including ECLS. Amniocentesis should be performed to establish the karyotype since trisomy 13, 18, and 21 may be associated with CDH. The fetuses are screened for associated anomalies using ultrasound, and an assessment of the liver position is made. Lack of liver herniation is associated with excellent survival (93%) without the need for ECLS in most instances (235). At an increasing rate, fetal MRI is used to assess lung volumes, as these measurements have been shown to correlate with prognosis postnatally (236,237). The lung-to-head ratio (LHR = multiplication of the length and width of the right lung divided by the value of the head perimeter) can be calculated using prenatal ultrasound, but is of higher predictive value when assessed with MRI (238). An LHR of <1 portends a poor prognosis with values <0.97 representing the severest form of CDH and an LHR >1.4 indicating an excellent prognosis (239–241). Unfortunately, these calculations have dramatically decreased predictive value for patients with a right-sided CDH.

A strategy employed for prenatally diagnosed severe CDH involves ex-utero intrapartum treatment (EXIT) with initiation of ECMO (ECMO/ECLS, EXIT-to-ECMO). With this approach, patients are delivered by Cesarean section, but maintained on placental support while cannulae are placed and ECMO initiated. Survival has been demonstrated to be an impressive 64% using an EXIT-to-ECMO strategy in patients with prenatal LHR <1.4 (242). Proponents of this approach favor the associated gentle ventilation, stability of the fetus during delivery and cannulation, and controlled, planned approach to delivery. However, opponents of the strategy question whether survival is indeed enhanced by this approach, which requires high resource use and cost. Furthermore, current prenatal outcome predictions are sufficiently inaccurate such that the mother and fetus might be placed at increased risk and complications of Cesarean section, ECMO, and the EXIT-to-ECMO approach when such invasive strategies might not otherwise have been required.

Another approach to the prenatal treatment of CDH involves *in utero* fetal endoscopic tracheal occlusion (FETO). With this technique, an occlusive balloon is inserted via transuterine bronchoscopy into the fetal trachea at 26 to 28 weeks with planned removal at 34 weeks. In patients with left-sided CDH and low LHR, the associated tracheal occlusion has demonstrated an improvement in LHR from 0.7 to 1.8 over a 2-week period and an increase in survival from <15% to approximately 50% (234,243). One of the major complications of *in utero* CDH repair or open tracheal ligation is early onset of labor, which may be reduced by the less-invasive FETO endoscopic approach (244,245).

At the time of birth, a nasogastric tube should be inserted to avoid GI distension. An endotracheal tube should be placed for ventilation. Bag mask ventilation should be avoided because of the risk of gaseous distension of the viscera both in the abdomen and the chest. An umbilical arterial line is placed and intravenous access established. An umbilical venous catheter may result in vessel disruption due to the angulation of the vessels in the rotated liver if the left lobe is in the chest (246). After stabilization, a right radial artery blood gas should be evaluated. Conventional mechanical ventilation techniques should be applied while avoiding ventilator-induced lung injury, which can result in acute lung deterioration and chronic lung disease. An arterial oxygen saturation >85% and a $PaCO_2$ <60 mm Hg are acceptable. High-frequency oscillatory ventilation can be applied, although it is questionable whether this enhances survival (247,248). Application of inhaled nitric oxide in newborns with CDH may actually increase the need for ECLS (249). Echocardiography should be performed to evaluate for congenital heart disease.

If gas exchange cannot be enhanced, ECLS is instituted, preferably prior to marked cardiopulmonary deterioration (250). An oxygenation index [(mean airway pressure × FIO_2/PaO_2) × 100] of >25 is an indication for ECLS. ECLS allows for lung rest, resolution of pulmonary hypertension, and avoidance of ventilator-induced lung injury while providing adequate gas exchange. Venoarterial access via the right carotid artery and the right internal jugular vein is often used because this configuration provides cardiac support. Patients with CDH who require ECLS have lower left ventricular mass and associated hemodynamic compromise and, therefore, may require cardiac support (251). However, a double-lumen venovenous configuration provides adequate support in most CDH patients and has the advantages of avoiding carotid artery ligation, providing well-oxygenated blood to the lungs and the heart, and minimizing the risk for arterial embolization (252).

Hemorrhagic complications are the most common clinical complications, due to anticoagulation, occurring in 43% of patients overall. The most common locations for bleeding are a surgical repair site (24%), head (11.5%), cannulation site (7.5%), and GI site (5%) (253). Bleeding complications are most common in those undergoing diaphragmatic hernia repair while on ECLS (58%). When controlling for factors associated with severity of CDH, delayed repair after ECMO therapy has been associated with increased survival (254). As a result, it is generally preferred that diaphragmatic hernia repair be delayed until the patient has weaned from ECLS or is just about to be removed from extracorporeal support, although some surgeons are recommending early repair on ECMO. When operation on ECLS is required, administration of aminocaproic acid may reduce bleeding complications (255). Factors influencing survival of patients with CDH on ECMO include initial blood gases, cardiac defects, and renal failure, but not the timing of surgery (256).

The operation for CDH is no longer an emergency. In fact, survival may be increased and the need for ECLS decreased if a delayed approach to the repair of the diaphragmatic defect is taken, although some studies dispute this approach (257–259). Either way, a delay in repair does not appear to be detrimental, and thus, in most centers, the diaphragm is repaired once the physiologic issues have resolved. Typically, the defect is approached via a subcostal incision, although a thoracic approach can be used. In approximately 20% of patients, a sac consisting of peritoneum and pleura that contains the herniated viscera is present and must be excised to allow full lung expansion. The viscera are carefully reduced. If the patient has been on ECLS, the spleen and liver are enlarged and prone to injury. Extralobar sequestration is observed in some patients with CDH and should be resected with care to control the systemic arteries extending through the inferior pulmonary ligament from the aorta to the sequestered lobe. The posterior leaf of the diaphragm typically has to be freed from the peritoneum, after which an assessment is made of whether sufficient diaphragm is present for primary repair. If so, 3–0 Prolene mattress sutures are used for the repair. In approximately 50% of patients, a patch is required to complete the diaphragmatic closure (220). Typically, inadequate muscle is present posterolaterally. Use of prosthetics such as Goretex (W.L. Gore and Assoc., Inc., Newark, DE) or small intestinal submucosa mesh (Surgisis ES; Cook Tissue Engineering Products, Bloomington, IN) allows a loose repair but may be associated with high rates (40% to 80%) of diaphragmatic hernia recurrence, especially when little or no diaphragmatic muscle is present (260–262). In addition, with use of a prosthetic, the risk of infection is low but present. Posterior sutures of 3–0 Prolene are all placed and then tied to approximate the prosthesis to the muscle. The patch is approximated to the ribs where the native diaphragm is absent. The needle is passed around individual ribs to provide a strong closure. One must be careful to ensure that bowel does not get entrapped between the sutures or the patch and the rib.

An alternative is to use an internal oblique and transversalis muscle flap to close the diaphragmatic defect, which may reduce the risk of recurrence (263). To do this, the muscle is separated from the external oblique at the upper aspect of the subcostal incision and folded downward. Division of the posterior lower ribs aids in creating the flap; however, extensive dissection should only be undertaken if the risk for imminent initiation of ECLS and associated anticoagulation is low. Likewise, correction of the typical malrotation with a Ladd procedure is performed only if it appears unlikely that ECLS will be required. An appendectomy is specifically not performed if a prosthesis has been placed because of the risk of infection. A chest tube may be placed, although one must be careful to avoid application of excess negative pressure, which can induce a shift in the mediastinum with associated hemodynamic compromise (151).

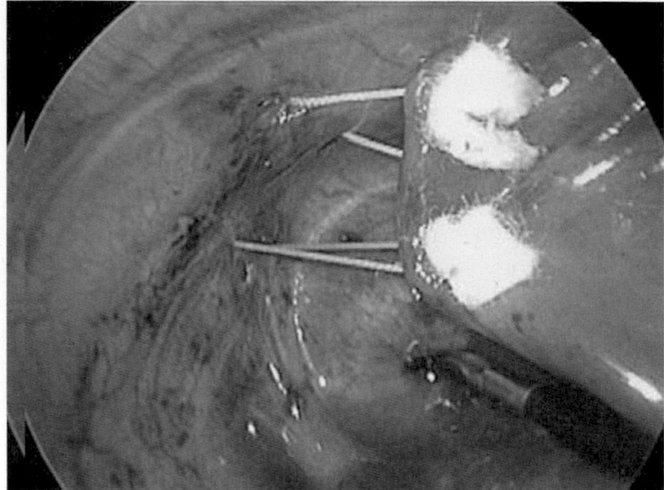

FIGURE 52.19. A thoracoscopic congenital diaphragmatic hernia repair begins by using pledgets sutured to anchor the lateral border to the ribs. Medial sutures were placed later to complete the repair.

In general, the abdomen is closed primarily. Alternatively, abdominal wall closure may not be possible because the peritoneal cavity is poorly developed. Mesh closure of the abdominal wall or even placement of a silo may be necessary to avoid the complications associated with increased intra-abdominal pressure (see section on abdominal wall defects) and compromise of diaphragmatic excursion in a patient with concomitant CDH and respiratory insufficiency (264).

Thoracoscopic approach to CDH repair is an effective strategy in patients after stabilization, though 20% were converted to open repair (265). Most conversions to open repair are due to hypercarbia, cardiopulmonary instability of the CDH patient with already compromised heart and lung function, or need for patch closure, which may be performed via the thoracoscope, but may be technically challenging (266). Ideal candidates for the thoracoscopic repair include preoperative factors such as minimal ventilatory support, presence of the stomach in the abdomen, and the lack of pulmonary hypertension (Fig. 52.19) (267). Laparoscopy is ideal for repair of patients with Morgagni-type diaphragmatic hernias with a high success rate (268,269).

Postoperative complications are predominantly associated with the cardiorespiratory sequelae associated with CDH. Chylothorax occurs in 10% of patients after repair and is increased among those patients requiring ECLS (270). In one series (271), those patients who developed chylothorax were left sided and associated with patch repair. Nearly half the patients were refractory to octreotide and required pleurectomy for management, with one death occurring from septic complications. Recurrent hernias are managed with transabdominal reoperation and generous use of a patch to decrease tension on the repair. The survival rate for patients with CDH is 63% (220). Associated anomalies are present in 40% of newborns with CDH and most commonly involve heart defects (63%) (271). The combination of CDH and congenital heart disease confers a worse prognosis (41%), especially in those with univentricular disease (5%) (272).

The long-term morbidity in patients with CDH is substantial. Chronic lung disease is present in 50% of survivors at 1 year of age (273). In most patients, pulmonary function normalizes over time, although pulmonary blood flow to the ipsilateral side remains reduced, especially in those patients who required ECLS (274,275). GER is evident in up to 81% of patients at the time of discharge and in 50% at 1 year (276). The esophagus is ectatic in 70% of patients with CDH, likely related to kinking of the gastroesophageal junction when the stomach is in the hemithorax (277). Tube feedings are required in over half of the patients at the time of discharge, but most are tolerating oral feeds within the first few years. Malrotation is present in most patients with CDH. The incidence of subsequent volvulus is 3% to 9% (278,279). Bowel obstruction occurs in approximately 10%.

Spinal and chest wall abnormalities are potential long-term problems in children with CDH and include pectus deformities in 33% and thoracic spine scoliosis in 12% (279). A thoracoscopic approach to the repair may ameliorate problems with scoliosis, which appears to be related to the thoracotomy incision (268).

Developmental delay classified as mild or moderate is evident in 45% of patients, but these findings tend to improve over time. Those managed with ECLS demonstrate severe neurologic abnormalities in 20% to 40% of patients. Hearing deficits are observed in 21%.

ABDOMINAL WALL DEFECTS

Gastroschisis

The newborn with gastroschisis has a smooth 2- to 5-cm opening almost always to the right of an intact umbilical cord through which the stomach, small intestine, and colon are typically herniated. The liver is almost never eviscerated, and associated anomalies are mostly limited to those of the GI tract where the bowel is often short and intestinal atresia occurs in 10% to 15% (280).

Prenatal diagnosis via ultrasound occurs in most infants (281). Controversy exists as to whether newborns diagnosed *in utero* should be delivered early by Cesarean section to prevent injury to and swelling of the exposed bowel (282,283). However, there is evidence to suggest that there is minimal, if any, advantage to preterm or Cesarean section delivery (284–289). At this point, the optimal timing of delivery is uncertain, although most clinicians are convinced that Cesarean section is not required for gastroschisis.

At the time of delivery, a nasogastric tube should be placed to prevent vomiting and aspiration. The bowel should be examined and any twists in the mesentery or constriction of the viscera from a small opening relieved immediately to avoid vascular compromise. Dehydration and hypothermia from insensible fluid and heat losses are prevented by administration of intravenous fluids, wrapping of the viscera with a gauze dressing, and placement of the lower portion of the newborn's body in a bowel bag. The viscera should be supported by the gauze so that they remain on top of the abdomen, rather than falling over to the side, to avoid vascular obstruction, especially venous outflow obstruction, which can lead to increased bowel edema. Broad-spectrum antibiotics should be administered to prevent infection.

After resuscitation, the newborn is taken to the operating room. The size of the peritoneal cavity is often limited and can make safe reduction of the viscera challenging. Rectal irrigation is performed, along with manual massage of the intestines, to evacuate as much meconium as possible, thus reducing the volume of the intra-abdominal contents. Likewise, a Foley catheter is inserted to decompress the bladder. After establishing a sterile field, the fingers are used to stretch the anterior abdominal fascia in an attempt to enlarge the peritoneal cavity if needed. The small and large bowels are typically matted together with a peel on the surface; they can be edematous, thickened, foreshortened, and, at times, ischemic-appearing. The bowel should be handled gently and operations on the bowel generally avoided. Any attempt to remove peel risks bowel injury, including perforation, and development of an enterocutaneous fistula. When jejunoileal atresia is identified, a primary anastomosis should be performed only if the edema and peel are minimal. Otherwise, there is a reasonable risk of anastomotic leak and stricture. In most cases (80%), the atresia should be left intact at the initial operation (280). The bowel should be re-explored at 3 to 4 weeks with repair of the atresia. If a silo was placed initially, the bowel should be evaluated at the time of fascial closure and a primary resection of the atresia with anastomosis performed if the thickening has resolved. In some circumstances, an enterostomy is required, especially in the setting of colonic atresia.

Primary closure of the abdominal wall is successful in approximately 80% of newborns (281,290). The viscera are gently reduced while avoiding twists in the mesentery. The edge of the opening is incised and the fascia identified circumferentially. Vicryl sutures are then placed to close the fascia; this is often done in a horizontal fashion because the tension is less than with a vertical fascial closure. Communication between the surgeon and the anesthesiologist allows recognition of adverse effects of the closure: significant increase in airway pressures, compromise of hemodynamics, or development of acidosis due to excess intra-abdominal pressure. Examination of the newborn's thighs may demonstrate cyanosis due to venous congestion. Intra-abdominal pressure may be measured via the nasogastric or bladder catheter. If signs of increased abdominal pressure are observed, the bowel should be removed to decompress the abdomen and a silo placed (see below). At times, the viscera may be successfully reduced, but fascial closure leads to physiologic compromise. In that case, a Vicryl or small intestinal submucosa mesh (Surgisis ES; Cook Tissue Engineering Products, Bloomington, IN) may

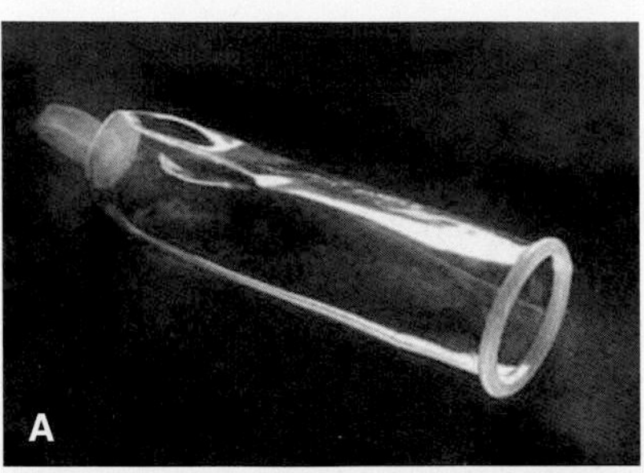

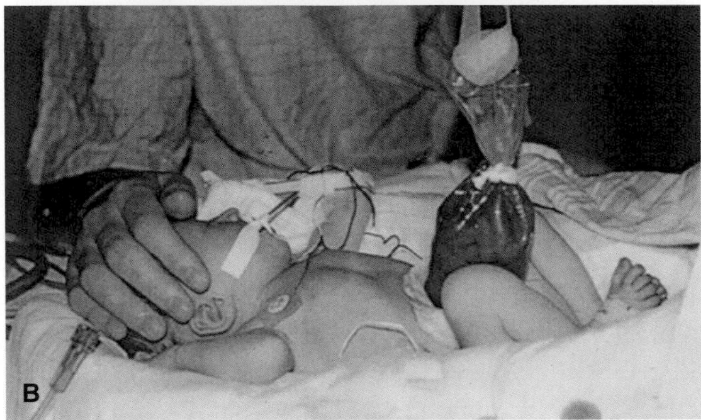

FIGURE 52.20. **A:** A preformed, spring-loaded silo (Specialty Surgical Products, Victor, MT) used to contain the bowel in patients with gastroschisis. **B:** The silo is in place with the round, spring-loaded base inside the peritoneal cavity. The umbilical tapes are tied sequentially lower to reduce the bowel into the abdomen over a period of days.

be used to augment the fascia, although a ventral hernia may result. Failure to recognize the signs of increased intra-abdominal pressure may lead to reduced visceral and renal blood flow and associated bowel necrosis and renal failure.

If the bowel cannot be safely reduced, a staged closure using a prosthesis is useful. Spring-loaded preformed silos are now available in different sizes and are easy to place, which precludes the need to manually construct the silo and to sew the silo to the relatively tenuous fascia (Fig. 52.20) (291). In some cases, the abdominal wall defect is enlarged to avoid a funnel-type configuration of the silo, which could lead to compression of the bowel at the base of the silo with ischemia and necrosis. The silo is wrapped in Betadine-moistened gauze to prevent infection and suspended from the overbed warmer to encourage gravity-assisted reduction of the remaining viscera. Over the ensuing days, the viscera are gradually reduced by compressing or twisting the silo and tying an umbilical tape sequentially lower on the silo every 12 to 24 hours. One must be careful to avoid injury to the bowel during these maneuvers; the silo is constructed of a transparent material specifically to allow monitoring of the bowel's status. The viscera are usually reduced within a week such that the base of the silo is flat. The patient is then taken back to the operating room and the fascia closed as described earlier.

Postoperative mechanical ventilation is required in most newborns, and care should be taken to avoid ventilator-induced lung injury as a result of high intra-abdominal pressure. Oliguria unresponsive to fluid administration, cyanosis and edema of the legs and lower abdomen, and compromised ventilation are all indications for silo placement or release of the umbilical tape on the silo. Patients with gastroschisis have an approximately 50% increase in fluid requirements when compared with other newborns (292).

There is a growing trend toward placement of a silo rather than attempting to close the abdomen primarily (293). It has been suggested that primary closure may be traumatic to the bowel and place the newborn at risk for physiologic compromise and pulmonary barotrauma (294). Spring-loaded silo placement can be performed at the bedside in the newborn intensive care unit (ICU). Closure of the gastroschisis defect can then occur once the viscera are reduced. This approach may be associated with a decrease in time on the mechanical ventilator, time to initial and full feedings, and complication rate (293). However, one must monitor the bowel in the silo for venous congestion with removal and readjustment of the silo to prevent bowel infarction when such is observed (295). In addition, it is important to avoid a funnel shape into a small abdominal wall opening during reduction of the intestinal contents of the silo as this can lead to bowel ischemia. Rather, a cylindrical shape, with expansion of the gastroschisis opening when necessary, can allow for gradual reduction without compression the of bowel contents at the base and resultant bowel ischemia.

Postoperative complications, in addition to those mentioned earlier, include delay in return of GI function (median time to initiation of feedings is 15 days with full enteral intake achieved by 22 days) (296). Support with parenteral nutrition is required in most patients. As such, central access should be achieved early in the course, although catheter-related sepsis is a potential complication. Postoperative bowel obstruction is relatively uncommon and an upper GI contrast study is performed only after approximately 3 weeks without return of GI function. Patients with gastroschisis are also at risk for infection as long as the silo is in place; as a result, broad-spectrum antibiotics are administered while the silo is in place. The complication of silo separation from the fascia, which often occurred after 7 to 10 days, has diminished with application of the spring-loaded silo. If this complication occurs, a pseudomembrane has usually formed beneath the silo, which can be allowed to granulate. Skin graft closure of the abdominal wall is possible once infection has been resolved using topical silver sulfadiazine.

Necrotizing enterocolitis (NEC, see below) is a complication that may be observed during advancement of enteral feeds after gastroschisis closure (297). The risk for NEC in the setting of gastroschisis may be increased due to enhanced mucosal permeability of the bowel, which is thickened and inflamed as a result of exposure to the amniotic fluid *in utero* or due to intestinal dysmotility or intestinal atresia. Those with gastroschisis who develop NEC have a lower birth weight and are more likely to be formula-fed (298). An enterocutaneous fistula may develop from an anastomotic leak or a suture-induced intestinal injury. Malrotation, if not corrected at the time of the initial operation, may result in jejunal obstruction due to Ladd bands or volvulus. SBS may occur as a result of bowel dysfunction or loss of bowel due to atresia or associated with many of the complications outlined previously. By 6 months of age, intestinal function, in general, has returned to normal. GER is observed in 16% of patients with gastroschisis, likely related to the presence of increased intra-abdominal pressure (299). Survival is >90% (281,300).

Omphalocele

In contrast to gastroschisis, an omphalocele consists of an abdominal wall defect at the umbilicus, a peritoneal and amnion covering or sac, a normal umbilical cord that attaches to the sac, and umbilical vessels that radiate over the defect. These characteristics of an omphalocele allow differentiation from a gastroschisis, even when the sac ruptures in approximately 10% of cases (301). The liver is present in approximately half of the defects.

Associated anomalies are present in approximately 30% to 60% of newborns with omphalocele and are a source of major morbidity and mortality for such patients (302). Congenital heart disease occurs in 20% and may increase operative risk (303). Abnormal karyotypes are observed in 29% and the Beckwith–Wiedemann syndrome in 10% (304). The latter patients have macroglossia, which can obstruct the airway, and may have hypoglycemia, which requires preoperative recognition and treatment.

The initial management of omphalocele is similar to that previously described for gastroschisis. Prevention of hypothermia and dehydration is paramount. Treatment with broad-spectrum antibiotics is initiated. Endotracheal intubation and mechanical ventilation are frequently required. The sac is left intact and is covered with moist nonadherent gauze to prevent desiccation and to decrease heat and fluid losses. Multiple layers of wrapping may be necessary to prevent heat loss; however, it is important to keep the underlying sac intact and prevent its rupture. Evaluation for other chromosomal and developmental anomalies, especially those that are cardiac, is undertaken.

If the defect is <4 cm in size, it is considered a hernia of the umbilical cord. Closure of a defect of this size is fairly straightforward and primary closure should be performed. The management of omphaloceles >4 cm is more challenging and complicated and is associated with a poorly developed peritoneal cavity. Coverage of the omphalocele defect is the primary goal. The skin–amnion junction is incised circumferentially and the fascia mobilized; caution should be exercised when dissecting over the superior aspect of the liver since the hepatic veins are often superficial in this location because of the downward position of the liver in the omphalocele. Injury to and bleeding from the hepatic veins can result. Examination of the diaphragm should be performed in case an associated defect is present.

With a large omphalocele, primary closure is rarely possible. Thus, staged reductions are typically employed. Traditionally, the omphalocele sac is excised during staged reduction except for where it is adherent to the liver. To excise the sac in that location could result in liver injury and bleeding. Should bleeding occur, pressure- and clot-enhancing agents should be applied. Unfortunately, once the sac is excised, reduction must be achieved within a reasonable period of time to avoid septic complications. Some surgeons have recommended leaving the sac intact and sequentially gathering the sac to achieve reduction (305). Alternatively, mesh can be sutured to the skin–amnion junction and progressively tightened to reduce the bowel and liver within the abdomen (306). Once reduction is accomplished, the linea alba is approximated, leaving the amnion intact, allowing staged reduction without a commitment to rapid closure. If the mesh separates, the sac is still in place.

Most recently, surgeons have approached giant omphaloceles by compressing the omphalocele via wrapping with ace bandages and simply allowing the sac to epithelialize over a number of months (307–309) (Fig. 52.21). Application of Silvadene, rather than mercurochrome, which can cause mercury poisoning, results in eschar formation of the sac. To

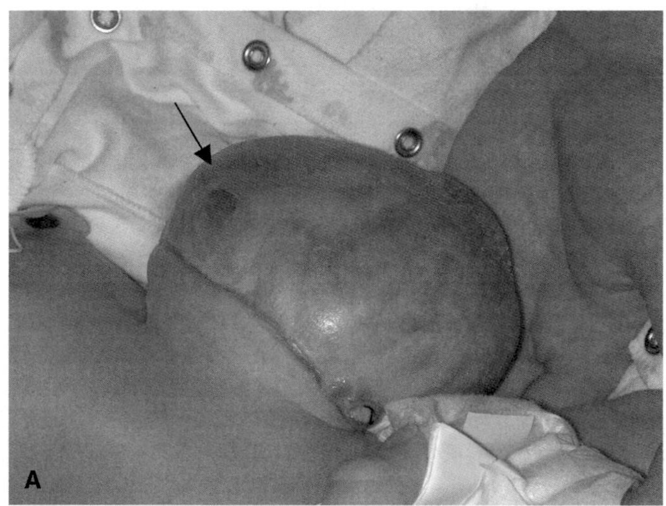

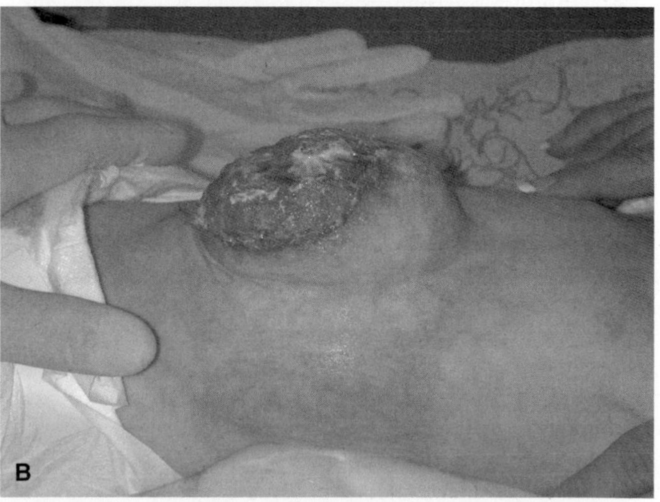

FIGURE 52.21. **A:** An omphalocele at birth. Note the dark area on the superior aspect (*arrow*), which denotes the liver in the omphalocele. The omphalocele was treated expectantly with compression wrapping and Silvadene. **B:** Note the reduction in the size of the omphalocele over the ensuing months.

decrease the incidence of neutropenia with chronic Silvadene use, bacitracin can be used on alternating days. It is imperative that the omphalocele wrapping should "not distort the sac, be too tight at the base, or restrict ventilation" (310). Contraction and flattening of the omphalocele are often the result, although a massive ventral hernia usually remains. One may be trading complications associated with immediate attempts at fascial closure with other challenges in the future.

Another approach is the creation of a silo from Dacron-reinforced silastic or Goretex (W. L. Gore and Assoc., Newark, DE) and suturing it to the fascial edges. The mesh is sequentially gathered in the midline every 12 to 24 hours until the fascial edges are nearly approximated. During this process, one must balance aggressively tightening the mesh with avoiding undue tension on the mesh; excess tension could lead to premature separation of the mesh from the fascia. The patient should also be monitored for evidence of high intra-abdominal pressure resulting in hypercarbia, oliguria, hemodynamic compromise, and acidosis. Such high pressures could compromise ventilation, renal blood flow, cardiac output, intestinal perfusion, and venous drainage from the lower extremities. The intra-abdominal pressure can be assessed using a nasogastric tube or a bladder catheter and should be maintained <20 cm H_2O. Once it is nearly approximated, the fascia can then be closed with removal of the mesh, although a reasonable option is to close the skin while leaving part of the mesh in place. If the mesh remnant is substantial, subsequent staged operations may be performed to remove the mesh and to approximate the fascia in the midline. If fascia or skin closure is not achieved within 7 to 10 days, the mesh is at risk for becoming infected and may separate, leaving granulation tissue underneath and presenting a challenging wound care problem that may be complicated by the development of enterocutaneous fistulae and sepsis. Application of homograft and other artificial wound coverings should be considered. One option is to allow the wound to epithelialize (311). An alternative is split-thickness skin graft placement, which is often effective once wound infection is controlled.

Return of GI function is often delayed in patients with a large omphalocele. Parenteral nutrition support will uniformly be required. Mechanical obstruction can occur, but is unusual. Lung and chest wall hypoplasia and chronic respiratory insufficiency are reasonably common among patients with giant omphaloceles, and tracheostomy tube placement may be required. Staged reduction, with its associated effect upon the diaphragm, is frequently complicated by the lung dysfunction. A few patients, at the point of delayed ventral hernia closure, developed severe pulmonary hypertension requiring ECLS postoperatively even though no evidence for pulmonary hypertension was found on preoperative echocardiograms.

Survival is 80% to 90% and is mostly related to the impact of associated anomalies (302,312). Most patients do well in the long term and have a good quality of life (304,313). In children with an omphalocele, the incidence of GER is high (43%), likely due to the effects of elevated intra-abdominal pressure (300). Ventral hernias frequently need to be addressed, especially in those in whom a nonoperative approach was undertaken. A staged approach to closure of the ventral hernia is required in those with massive ventral hernias. The incidence of cryptorchidism is increased in patients with omphalocele (16%), presumably because of the decreased intra-abdominal pressure present during the usual *in utero* testicular descent (314).

ACQUIRED NEWBORN SURGICAL PROBLEMS

Pyloric stenosis

Hypertrophic pyloric stenosis typically presents with projectile nonbilious vomiting in the newborn at 2 to 8 weeks of age. Palpation of the upper abdomen reveals the classic "olive" rolling under the examining hand in 72% of patients and in and of itself is an indication for operation (315). The olive can be easily missed unless a nasogastric tube is placed to decompress the stomach and the infant is quieted with feeding of 5% dextrose water. An ultrasound demonstrating a pylorus longer than 15 to 19 mm or with a wall thickness >3 mm is considered diagnostic, although the patient's age and prematurity should be taken into account to avoid misdiagnosis (316,317). The ultrasound is operator dependent and may not be accurate if the radiologist is inexperienced (318). An upper GI contrast study should demonstrate an elongated, narrowed pyloric channel and "shouldering" of the pyloric mass upon the antrum. The barium should be evacuated from the stomach after the study via a nasogastric tube to prevent aspiration.

Patients with pyloric stenosis have been vomiting and must be sufficiently resuscitated before operation. Many patients will have a degree of hypochloremic, hypokalemic, metabolic alkalosis (319). Bicarbonate levels >30 mEq/L are of concern and >35 mEq/L are even more so. Preoperative resuscitation is advised in most patients unless the bicarbonate is <30 mEq/L, the chloride normal, and urine output excellent by history.

The stomach should be aspirated before induction of anesthesia to prevent aspiration even if a nasogastric tube was in place prior to operation (320). The pyloric musculature is divided via a Ramstedt pyloromyotomy while the mucosa is maintained intact. The operation was typically performed using a right upper quadrant transverse incision, though the supraumbilical and laparoscopic approaches are now increasingly more popular (321,322). The laparoscopic approach uses a 5-mm umbilical port for the scope and both a right and left upper quadrant stab wound for placement of 3-mm instruments. With the open technique, the antrum is first delivered, followed by "rocking" the pylorus out through the incision. Failure to make an incision of adequate size will make delivery of the pylorus difficult and potentially result in trauma to the serosa of the antrum or even perforation. From this point, the open and laparoscopic techniques are similar. Vessels on the surface of the pylorus are scored with the electrocautery since deeper use of cautery may lead to potential injury to the mucosa. An incision with a knife is then performed from a point just proximal to the duodenum up onto the antrum. With the laparoscopic technique, it is important to make the incision long enough and deep enough to facilitate subsequent spreading of the pyloric muscle. The back of a knife blade (open) or the sheathed arthrotomy knife (laparoscopic) is then insinuated into the incision and twisted to further spread the edges of the pyloric muscle. The pyloromyotomy spreader is then used to engage the edges and complete the pyloromyotomy. The first spread should be generous to crack the pylorus and expose the underlying mucosa. It is important to engage the spreader equally between the edges of the pylorus so that the edges are perpendicular rather than oblique, which makes completion of the pyloromyotomy difficult. In order to avoid perforation, the pyloromyotomy should not extend onto the duodenum. There is a color change at the pyloroduodenal junction, which, along with palpation with a finger or instrument, allows identification of the distal end of the pylorus. The pyloromyotomy should extend proximally onto the antrum for approximately 1 cm until the circular muscles of the antrum are identified. Failure to extend the pyloromyotomy proximally to this point risks an incomplete pyloromyotomy and postoperative feeding intolerance. The mucosa should be visible for the entire length of the pyloromyotomy, and the two halves of the pylorus should be tested to see that they easily move longitudinally separately from each other. A volume of 30 to 60 mL of air is injected through a nasogastric (NG) tube, the duodenum occluded just distal to the pylorus, and the stomach compressed while observing for leak of air or bile from the pyloromyotomy site. Perforation of the mucosa occurs in 2% to 4% of patients and is usually at the duodenal end of the pyloromyotomy. The mucosa can be closed directly with a 5–0 Vicryl suture. A better alternative is to approximate the gastric side of the opening to the pyloric muscle at the duodenal end with interrupted 5–0 Vicryl sutures (Fig. 52.22). Consideration should be given to suturing the omentum to the pyloromyotomy site to reinforce the closure. Alternatively, the serosa of the pyloromyotomy site can be closed with 4–0 Vicryl sutures and the pylorus turned 90 or 180 degrees, where another pyloromyotomy is performed. The results of either approach appear to be equivalent (323). NG suction should be maintained for 48 hours after such a repair. Small amounts of bleeding from the surface or edges of the pyloromyotomy may be seen and will uniformly stop without cautery. Cauterizing the mucosa should never be attempted because of the risk of perforation.

The laparoscopic approach has decreased complication rates, especially wound infections, shorter time to full feeds, reduced postoperative emesis, and reduced lengths of stay compared with the open pyloromyotomy (324,325). However, the laparoscopic approach is also associated with an increased incidence of incomplete myotomy and mucosal perforation (325–327). A learning curve exists with laparoscopy and may contribute to the increased complication rates, as the majority of perforations and incomplete myotomies occurred in the first 2 to 3 years at high-volume hospitals (328,329).

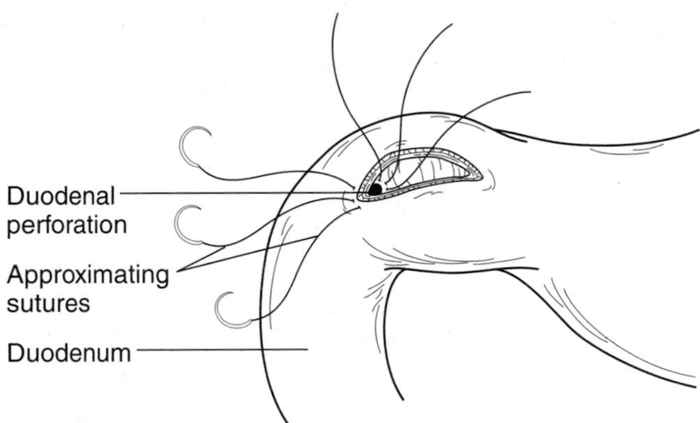

FIGURE 52.22. Repair of a duodenal perforation following pyloromyotomy. The opening in the mucosa is almost always adjacent to the duodenum. Three or four sutures are placed approximating the mucosa to the seromuscular layer of the duodenum. Note that the pyloromyotomy is carried proximally onto the antrum until the gastric circular fibers are encountered in order to ensure that the pyloromyotomy is adequate.

Feedings are often initiated 4 to 6 hours after the procedure and can be given ad libitum (330). Emesis in the first day or two after the operation occurs in 44% of patients and is thought to be secondary to gastritis (331). Persistent vomiting occurs in approximately 5% and usually resolves, although vomiting that persists beyond 3 to 5 days should raise concern for an incomplete pyloromyotomy (332). An upper GI study will not be helpful in distinguishing an incomplete pyloromyotomy because changes in the pylorus are not observed for many weeks after adequate pyloromyotomy. In the case of prolonged feeding intolerance, parenteral nutrition should be initiated. If gastric outlet obstruction persists over the next 1 to 2 weeks, reoperation should be considered. Administration of intravenous or oral atropine may treat the symptoms of pyloric stenosis and serve as an alternative to reoperation in this setting (333). Unrecognized perforation can be devastating; the incidence should be <1%. Any infant manifesting fever, lethargy, and/or physiologic instability should undergo upper GI contrast study to evaluate for a leak. The incidence of wound infections may be higher than expected for a clean case (4%), and for that reason, it is recommended that antibiotics such as Cephazolin be administered in the perioperative period (334). Postoperative wound fascial dehiscence, which used to be a concern when operations were performed in malnourished infants, is now an unusual complication.

Necrotizing enterocolitis

The etiology of NEC is unclear, but the result is hypoperfusion of the mesenteric blood supply with intestinal ischemia leading to bacterial invasion and necrosis. Although it can occur in full-term newborns, the risk of NEC increases with gestational age <35 to 36 weeks (335). Administering enteral feeds, especially with hyperosmolar solutions, appears to augment the risk of NEC; however, neonates who have never been fed are also susceptible. NEC may be associated with either a single site of perforation in 50% of cases or multiple, discontinuous segments with bowel thinning, pneumatosis, and even frank necrosis, in contrast to idiopathic spontaneous intestinal perforation (SIP), in which a perforation without associated necrosis is noted on the antimesenteric border of the terminal ileum (336).

The most difficult aspect of the surgical treatment of NEC is the decision on when to intervene operatively. In the absence of pneumoperitoneum or evidence for bowel necrosis, the patient is managed with nasogastric suction, broad-spectrum antibiotics, fluid resuscitation, and frequent monitoring of hemodynamics, urine output, platelet count, white blood cell count, blood gas values, electrolytes, and abdominal radiographs. Clinical signs and symptoms consistent with ongoing sepsis (lethargy, temperature instability, apnea, bradycardia, and shock) despite antibiotic therapy, an erythematous or discolored abdomen, palpable loops of bowel, a falling platelet count or one that remains <150,000 cells/mm^3, oliguria, neutropenia, and metabolic acidosis are all relative indications for operation (337). Portal vein gas, which occurs in 9% to 20% of patients with NEC, and a gasless, distended abdomen are harbingers of advanced disease likely to require operative intervention. Pneumoperitoneum is a firm indication for operative intervention in the setting of NEC. Up to 56% of patients will require operation at some point during their course (338).

Operation is undertaken following resuscitation, usually in the newborn ICU to avoid the hypothermia and deterioration in hemodynamics, oxygenation, and ventilation parameters observed during transport of the critically ill premature newborn (339). It is critical to keep the newborn warm. A tense abdomen may require drainage prior to laparotomy if it is physiologically embarrassing. Venous access for parenteral nutrition is required postoperatively; as such, central access is obtained at the time of the exploratory laparotomy. A supraumbilical, transverse incision is created and a finger used to eviscerate the bowel, which may be matted with adhesions. The entire GI tract is examined and areas of necrosis identified and resected. Cases in which an isolated area of perforation is identified in the terminal ileum may be treated with a primary anastomosis. Otherwise, an ileostomy is created during operation in almost all cases of NEC (89%), although some studies have demonstrated the safety of immediate anastomosis even in those selected newborns with NEC <1000 g in weight (340,341). When performed, an ileostomy is created by bringing the bowel out through either the supraumbilical incision or a separate 1-cm incision in the right lower quadrant while carefully maintaining the mesenteric blood supply. The former facilitates subsequent ostomy closure, while the latter is advantageous should a dehiscence of the supraumbilical incision occur. The bowel is sutured to the external oblique fascia at four points around the circumference of the enterostomy in order to prevent the frequent complication of peristomal hernia. Typically, a mucous fistula is created along with the enterostomy, which allows a local operation at the time of takedown of the enterostomy. Stoma and wound complications occur in 39% of patients operated upon for NEC and include wound infection, dehiscence, and stomal prolapse, retraction, necrosis, or stricture (342).

In cases in which the extent of disease is patchy but involves a minority of the small bowel, all ischemic and necrotic regions are excised. In contrast, if the majority of the bowel is compromised, then only frankly necrotic, but not ischemic, areas should be resected because of the risk of SBS. The ends of the bowel may be ligated with re-exploration in 24 to 48 hours. Alternatively, if an enterostomy is created that is proximal to all ischemic regions such that all distal areas are defunctionalized, then re-exploration may be required only if refractory sepsis develops. Multiple enterostomies or anastomoses distal to the most proximal enterostomy may be required. Alternatively, multiple segments distal to the enterostomy may be placed over a feeding tube "stent" in hopes of preserving bowel length and preventing the SBS (343). These segments may even autoanastomose. A proximal jejunostomy may be associated with fluid management challenges and electrolyte imbalance.

Pan-involvement with necrosis of the majority of the small bowel occurs in 12% of patients and occurs equally in both premature and full-term newborns (344). Resection would be uniformly associated with the development of SBS. Mortality in patients with pan-involvement is nearly 100%, especially in premature newborns. As such, most surgeons do not perform resection but instead choose to withdraw support.

An alternative strategy to operation in the newborn with NEC is peritoneal drainage (345). This involves placement of a Penrose drain under local anesthesia via a 1-cm incision placed in the right lower quadrant, which is the most likely site of perforated NEC. During drain placement, the bowel is examined locally for viability and a catheter is passed to the left upper and lower quadrants in order to irrigate the abdomen. A drain is then placed through the right lower quadrant incision toward the left side of the abdomen.

Interestingly, studies suggest that using this approach, 32% of patients with perforated NEC survive and require no further operations while 24% succumb soon after drainage. Laparotomy is required within 24 hours in 24%, and operation for delayed strictures becomes necessary in an additional 19%. The survival among those with perforated NEC appears to be equivalent among those undergoing laparotomy when compared with those managed with peritoneal drainage and may depend more on the underlying comorbidities than on the operative approach (346,347). Others have suggested that peritoneal drainage is most effective in patients with isolated SIP, while most patients with NEC require subsequent laparotomy (348). Assignment of patients to SIP versus NEC preoperatively by the attending pediatric surgeon was confirmed to be accurate intraoperatively approximately 95% of the time (349). Randomized controlled trials among premature infants of low birth weight with perforated NEC demonstrated no difference in survival, bowel length, hospital stay, or mortality following abdominal drain placement or laparotomy (350,351). NEC, overall, is associated with compromised neurodevelopmental outcomes (352). However, neurodevelopmental morbidity may be increased in those patients managed with peritoneal drainage when compared with initial exploratory laparotomy (353). Currently, most practitioners apply peritoneal drainage to the premature newborn with perforated NEC and perform laparotomy if physiologic parameters do not improve in the ensuing 24 hours, although the salvage rate for laparotomy following peritoneal drainage is low (346).

An extraordinary and potentially devastating complication of operation for NEC is spontaneous liver hemorrhage (354). The liver in premature newborns has less stromal components and is prone to laceration and bleeding. As such, extreme care should be taken to avoid liver injury to patients with NEC. If bleeding does occur, packing with application of hemostatic agents and correction of coagulopathy should be undertaken rather than attempts at suture ligation (355).

It is rare for newborns with enterostomies to tolerate full feedings unless the stoma is in the terminal ileum and the amount of bowel resected was minimal. Administration of Imodium may decrease gut motility, enhance the success of feeding, and limit fluid and electrolyte losses. The urine sodium and serum bicarbonate should be followed and repleted when deficient. In general, the enterostomy is closed at 4 to 6 weeks after the operation but preferably not until the premature newborn reaches approximately 2 kg in weight. Closure of an enterostomy may be challenging for the surgeon because of the presence of dense adhesions and physiologically disruptive for the premature newborn. Early closure of the ostomy (<10 weeks following the operation for NEC) is associated with increased ventilator days, days of total parenteral nutrition, days required to reach full oral intake, and length of stay (356). However, delayed closure of the ostomy requires refeeding into the distal bowel via the mucus fistula and may present challenges such as dislodgement or erosion of the refeeding catheter, potential injury to the liver from total parental nutrition if oral intake is not fully tolerated, and failure to thrive due to electrolyte losses and dehydration.

Anastomotic leaks are rare but do occur, although they often close spontaneously given conservative management for a number of weeks. If the newborn is thriving with enteral feedings despite the presence of an ostomy, closure can be postponed. Factors such as the onset of cholestatic jaundice, the presence of excessive stoma output, failure to thrive, and development of a stricture at the site of the stoma may indicate early stoma closure. Stoma strictures may be prevented by intermittent dilation of the stoma opening with a small blunt-tipped catheter.

Recurrent NEC occurs in approximately 5% of patients and can frequently be treated nonoperatively (357). Abscess development is rare in newborns, although it can occur and may be diagnosed and drained readily by abdominal ultrasound. Multiple operations are required in 55% of patients with NEC (342). Strictures occur in 29% of patients with NEC, most commonly in those treated without laparotomy, and are most often seen in the large intestine (70%) and the terminal ileum, with the splenic flexure being most common (Fig. 52.23). Most patients with strictures demonstrate feeding intolerance, bowel obstruction, or Hemoccult positive stools. A contrast enema is usually diagnostic for the most common large intestinal strictures, though routine diagnostic contrast enemas are not recommended over clinical follow-up (358). Strictures may resolve and repeat contrast studies to confirm persistence of the stricture

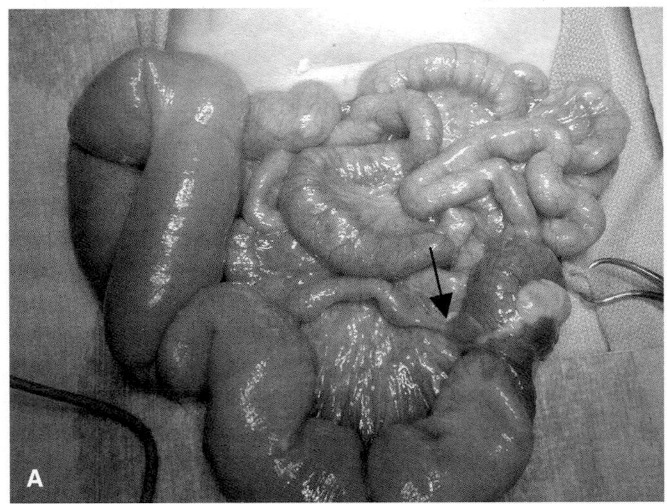

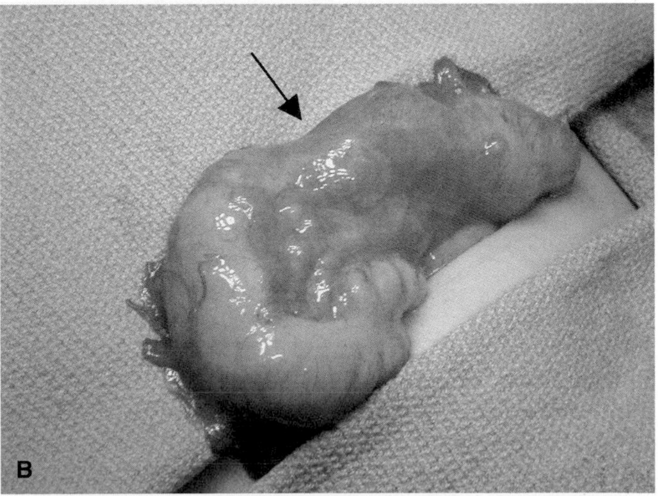

FIGURE 52.23. Strictures following necrotizing enterocolitis in the newborn in the **(A)** terminal ileum (*arrow*) and the **(B)** distal transverse colon (*arrow*).

should be considered (359). Because of the risk of distal stricture, a contrast enema is performed before enterostomy closure in all patients.

The mortality associated with NEC is related to the prematurity and associated comorbidities as well as complications of the SBS (360). Overall survival among patients with NEC is 87% and is decreased (68%) among those patients whose weight is <1,000 g, in those who have diffuse intestinal involvement, and in premature newborns with four or more comorbidities (30%) (340,344,347). Those patients with SIP have a higher survival rate (88%) even though they have lower gestational age and increased incidence of respiratory distress syndrome (361). Limited ileal resection for NEC is associated with a subsequent increased prevalence of cholelithiasis and a risk of vitamin B_{12} deficiency (362). Otherwise, limited ileocecal resection is not associated with increased morbidity or mortality (363). Intestinal problems occur in 25% of patients over the long term and are mostly associated with development of the SBS (344).

Neurodevelopment is significantly delayed in infants with NEC such that 55% have severe neurologic deficit when compared with 23% of non-NEC controls (364). Specifically, extremely low birth weight (<1000 g) infants with NEC that required surgery, drainage or laparotomy, had low mental development index and psychomotor development index scores, high rates of cerebral palsy, and high rates of vision impairment and deafness (353). Long-term growth, though, does not differ between infants with and without NEC when matched for their initial gestational age.

The best approach to NEC is prevention. NEC occurs more frequently in formula-fed babies (365) and in those with prolonged periods without feeding when feeding is ultimately initiated. In contrast, trophic feeds, feeding with human milk, the addition of arginine to the diet, and oral antibiotics have been shown to reduce the incidence of NEC (366–370). Prophylaxis for NEC with antibiotics has not become commonplace because of concerns for increasing antibiotic resistance. Probiotics are a promising concept (371,372), although using *Lactobacillus* has been shown to have an increased incidence of sepsis (373).

Short bowel syndrome

SBS occurs in approximately 1% of live births with development of liver disease in 40% to 60% of patients and a mortality rate of almost 30% (374,375). SBS occurs due to motility disorders (e.g., Hirschsprung disease and pseudo-obstruction), congenital diseases of absorption (e.g., microvillous atrophy), and loss of bowel (e.g., NEC, malrotation and midgut volvulus, intestinal atresia, and gastroschisis) (376,377).

When assessing the potential severity of SBS, the length of remnant small bowel must be considered in conjunction with the presence of the ileocecal valve and length of functioning colon (378). Measurement of the small intestine should proceed from the ligament of Treitz to the ileocecal junction along the antimesenteric border (379). At birth, the expected small bowel length for a term infant is approximately 240 cm with an additional 40 cm associated with the colon. By 1 year of age, the small bowel has grown to an estimated 380 cm. For preterm infants, nomograms for normal ball length are available; total length (small and large bowel) increases from about 140 cm at 19 to 27 weeks to almost 300 cm by 35 weeks (380). A small bowel length ≥10% of predicted and the presence of the ileocecal valve are associated with weaning from parenteral nutrition (PN) (381). Patients who wean off PN have a 95% survival at 5 years with or without transplantation when compared with a 52% survival for those who remained on PN (375).

Fluid and electrolyte problems along with micronutrient abnormalities are usually present and treated with meticulous monitoring of stool and urine output along with supplementation of electrolyte and nutrient deficiencies when present. Prevention of dehydration is crucial to the growth of SBS patients. Liberal utilization of agents to decrease gastric and intestinal secretion and transit time is helpful to control ostomy or stool output. Use of antimicrobials, as prevention for bacterial overgrowth, and weekly cycling to prevent resistance, has also been advocated (377).

The major complications of SBS are related to the need for PN and potential for bacterial overgrowth. Associated complications include recurrent infections (catheter related and otherwise), venous thrombosis and lack of vascular access, malnutrition, metabolic bone disease, and liver failure (379). About 40% to 60% of patients on long-term IV nutrition develop PN-associated liver disease (PNALD), presenting initially with cholestasis in childhood or steatosis as an adolescent (377). Prematurity, duration of PN, and sepsis have all been correlated with faster development of cholestasis (382). Measures to prevent PN-associated cholestasis in infancy include avoiding overfeeding by limiting total calories to <100 kcal/kg/d, discontinuing PN 2 to 6 hours each day and thus allowing cyclical GI hormone release, aggressively treating bacterial infections or overgrowth, and optimizing enteral nutrition. Intravenous fish oil supplementation may also decrease progression of PNALD (377). Omegaven (Fresenius Kabi, Bad Homburg, Germany), an artificial omega-3 fatty acid supplement, may decrease progression of PNALD. The potential fatty acid deficiency associated with Omegaven may be avoided by also administering Intralipid (Fresenius Kabi), which is an omega-6 fatty acid fish-oil derivative (383).

Although the approach to SBS commonly involves primary medical strategies to improving nutrition and preventing the complications outlined earlier, surgical efforts to increase bowel length and function are part of the management armamentarium available. Most bowel-lengthening procedures take advantage of the fact that the small bowel in the patient with SBS is typically dilated. In the occasional cases where the bowel caliber is normal, controlled intussusception of the terminal ileum into the colon may produce the required small-bowel dilatation (384).

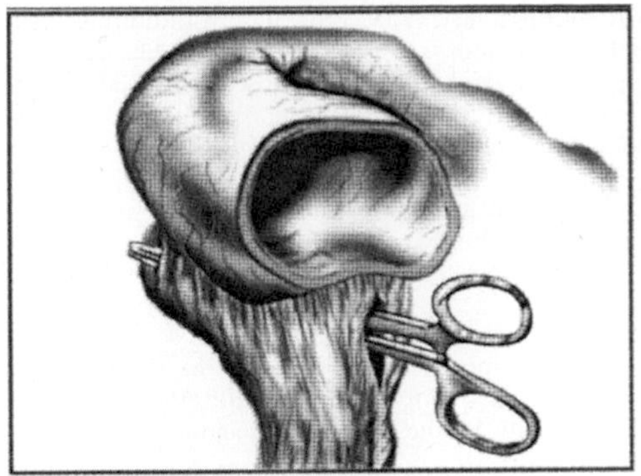
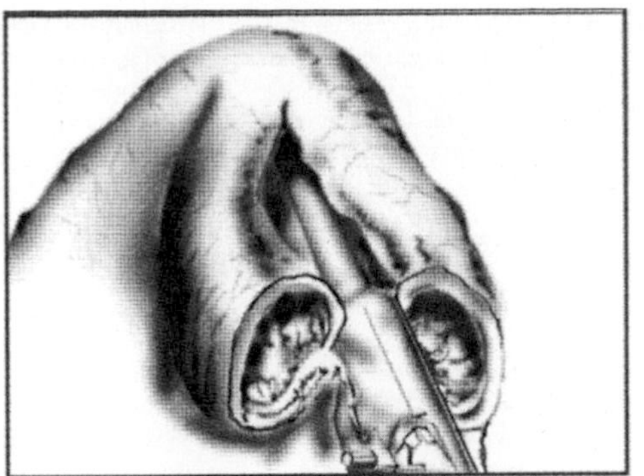
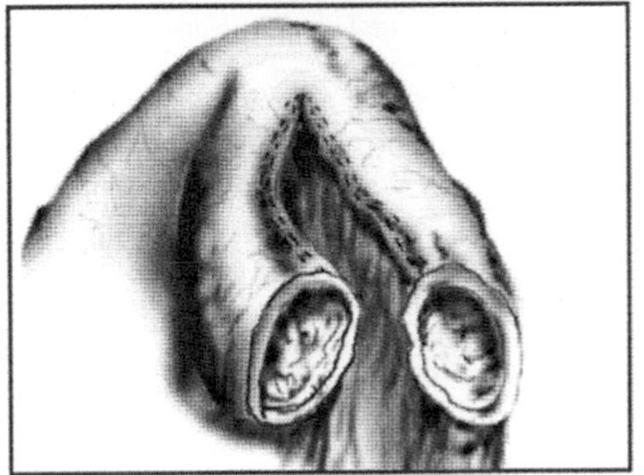
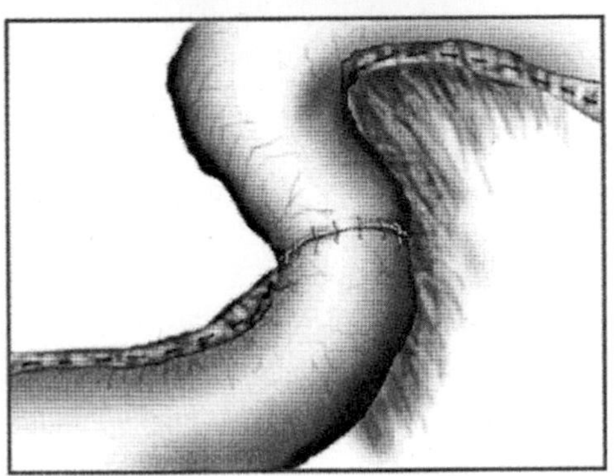

FIGURE 52.24. A Bianchi procedure separates the intestine longitudinally along with its individual leaf of mesentery and then reconnects them sequentially doubling the initial intestinal length.

The Bianchi procedure is an intestinal lengthening procedure in which the dilated bowel is stapled longitudinally within the leaves of the mesentery thereby creating two separate segments of bowel (Fig. 52.24). An isoperistaltic anastomosis is then performed between the two newly created loops of small bowel, thus, effectively, doubling the length. Serial transverse enteroplasty (STEP) is another bowel-lengthening procedure in which alternating mesenteric and antimesenteric dividing staple lines are placed perpendicular to and partially across the width of the bowel resulting in enhancement in bowel length and reduction in bowel caliber (Fig. 52.25) (379).

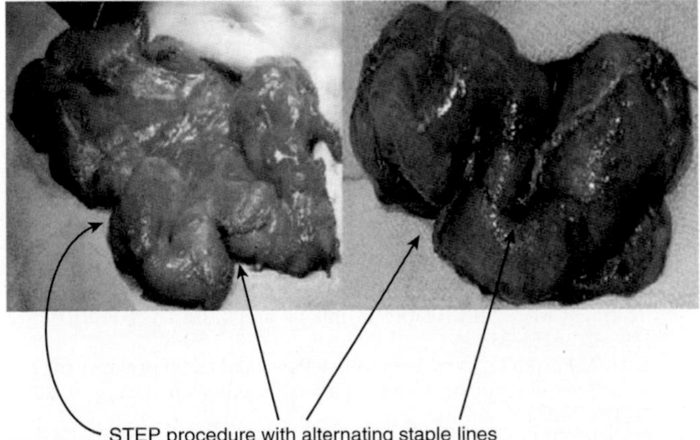

FIGURE 52.25. A Step procedure uses alternating partial staple lines to increase the overall surface area of the bowel and functional intestinal length for absorption of nutrients.

Enteropexy of the small intestine to the exposed abdominal wall, specifically the rectus abdominus muscle, is another approach used to lengthen the small bowel. The enteropexy allows development of a parasitic blood supply to the loop of small bowel that can be used in subsequent intestinal lengthening procedures (385). Studies evaluating bowel-lengthening procedures have shown that these procedures slow transit time and increase fat and carbohydrate absorption: enteral feeds are better tolerated and catheter infections are decreased (386). Complications following bowel-lengthening procedures are significant and include postoperative bowel obstruction and staple line leaks, which often require reoperation.

Medical and surgical options should be maximized before considering bowel and/or liver transplantation. Intestinal lengthening procedures, such as the Bianchi and STEP, can be used as a bridge to transplantation (379). Although the 1-year survival after intestinal transplantation is 80% to 90% and PN is costly and burdensome, the morbidity of life-long immunosuppression and the 5-year survival of approximately 50% must be taken into account before committing a patient to bowel and/or liver transplantation (374).

REFERENCES

1. Grosfeld JL, Rescorla FJ. Duodenal atresia and stenosis: reassessment of treatment and outcome based on antenatal diagnosis, pathologic variance, and long-term follow-up. *World J Surg* 1993;17:301–309.
2. Hajivassiliou CA. Intestinal obstruction in neonatal/pediatric surgery. *Semin Pediatr Surg* 2003;12(4):241–253.
3. Lawrence MJ, Ford WD, Furness ME, et al. Congenital duodenal obstruction: early antenatal ultrasound diagnosis. *Pediatr Surg Int* 2000;16:342–345.

4. Dalla Vecchia LK, Grosfeld JL, West KW, et al. Intestinal atresia and stenosis: a 25-year experience with 277 cases. *Arch Surg* 1998;133: 490–496; discussion 496–497.
5. Escobar MA, Ladd AP, Grosfeld JL, et al. Duodenal atresia and stenosis: long-term follow-up over 30 years. *J Pediatr Surg* 2004;39(6): 867–871.
6. Rothenberg SS. Laparoscopic duodenoduodenostomy for duodenal obstruction in infants and children. *J Pediatr Surg* 2002;37:1088–1089.
7. Soutter AD, Askew AA. Transumbilical laparotomy in infants: a novel approach for a wide variety of surgical disease. *J Pediatr Surg* 2003;38: 950–952.
8. Rescorla FJ, Grosfeld JL. Intestinal atresia and stenosis: analysis of survival in 120 cases. *Surgery* 1985;98:668–676.
9. Spigland N, Yazbeck S. Complications associated with surgical treatment of congenital intrinsic duodenal obstruction. *J Pediatr Surg* 1990;25:1127–1130.
10. Arnbjornsson E, Larsson M, Finkel Y, et al. Transanastomotic feeding tube after an operation for duodenal atresia. *Eur J Pediatr Surg* 2002;12:159–162.
11. Upadhyay V, Sakalkale R, Parashar K, et al. Duodenal atresia: a comparison of three modes of treatment. [see comment]. *Eur J Pediatr Surg* 1996;6:75–77.
12. Adzick NS, Harrison MR, deLorimier AA, et al. Tapering duodenoplasty for megaduodenum associated with duodenal atresia. *J Pediatr Surg* 1986;21:311–312.
13. Kokkonen ML, Kalima T, Jaaskelainen J, et al. Duodenal atresia: late follow-up. *J Pediatr Surg* 1988;23:216–220.
14. Bax NM, Ure BM, van der Zee DC. Laparoscopic duodenoduodenostomy for duodenal atresia. *Surg Endosc* 2001;15(2):217.
15. Georgeson KE, Robertson DJ. Minimally invasive surgery in the neonate: review of current evidence. *Semin Perinatol* 2004;28(3):212–220.
16. Seashore JH, Touloukian RJ. Midgut volvulus. An ever-present threat. *Arch Pediatr Adolesc Med* 1994;148:43–46.
17. Prasil P, Flageole H, Shaw KS, et al. Should malrotation in children be treated differently according to age? *J Pediatr Surg* 2000;35:756–758.
18. Ford EG, Senac MO, Srikanth MS Jr, et al. Malrotation of the intestine in children. *Ann Surg* 1992;215:172–178.
19. Millar AJ, Rode H, Cywes S, et al. Malrotation and volvulus in infancy and childhood. *Semin Pediatr Surg* 2003;12:229–236.
20. Long FR, Kramer SS, Markowitz RI, et al. Radiographic patterns of intestinal malrotation in children. *Radiographics* 1996;16:547–556; discussion 556–560.
21. Orzech N, Navarro OM, Langer JC. Is ultrasonography a good screening test for intestinal malrotation? *J Pediatr Surg* 2006;41(5):1005–1009.
22. Torres AM, Ziegler MM. Malrotation of the intestine. *World J Surg* 1993;17:326–331.
23. Severijnen R, Hulstijn-Dirkmaat I, Gordijn B, et al. Acute loss of the small bowel in a school-age boy. Difficult choices: to sustain life or to stop treatment? *Eur J Pediatr* 2003;162:794–798.
24. Wilmore DW. Factors correlating with a successful outcome following extensive intestinal resection in newborn infants. *J Pediatr* 1972;80: 88–95.
25. Messineo A, MacMillan JH, Palder SB, et al. Clinical factors affecting mortality in children with malrotation of the intestine. *J Pediatr Surg* 1992;27:1343–1345.
26. Yu DC, Thiagarajan RR, Laussen PC. Outcomes after the Ladd procedure in patients with heterotaxy syndrome, congenital heart disease, and intestinal malrotation. *J Pediatr Surg* 2009;44(6):1089–1095.
27. Tashjian JB, Weeks B, Brueckner M. Outcomes after a Ladd procedure for intestinal malrotation with heterotaxia. *J Pediatr Surg* 2007;42(3): 528–531.
28. van der Zee DC, Bax NM. Laparoscopic repair of acute volvulus in a neonate with malrotation. *Surg Endosc* 1995;9(10):1123–1124.
29. Gross E, Chen MK, Lobe TE. Laparoscopic evaluation and treatment of intestinal malrotation in infants. *Surg Endosc* 1996;10(9):936–937.
30. Waldhausen JH, Sawin RS. Laparoscopic Ladd's procedure and assessment of malrotation. *J Laparoendosc Surg* 1996;6(Suppl 1):S103–S105.
31. Bass KD, Rothenberg SS, Chang JH. Laparoscopic Ladd's procedure in infants with malrotation. *J Pediatr Surg* 1998; 33(2):279–281.
32. Matzke GM, Dozois EJ, Larson DW. Surgical management of intestinal malrotation in adults: comparative results for open and laparoscopic Ladd procedures. *J Pediatr Surg* 2005;19(10):1416–1419.
33. Palanivelu C, Rangarajan M, Shetty AR. Intestinal malrotation with midgut volvulus presenting as acute abdomen in children: value of diagnostic and therapeutic laparoscopy. *J Laparoendosc Adv Surg Tech A* 2007;17(4):490–492.
34. Phelps S, Fisher R, Partington A, et al. Prenatal ultrasound diagnosis of gastrointestinal malformations. *J Pediatr Surg* 1997;32:438–440.
35. Shorter NA, Georges A, Perenyi A, et al. A proposed classification system for familial intestinal atresia and its relevance to the understanding of the etiology of jejunoileal atresia. *J Pediatr Surg* 2006;41(11): 1822–1825.
36. Zerella JT, Martin LW. Jejunal atresia with absent mesentery and a helical ileum. *Surgery* 1976;80:550–553.
37. Miller RC. Complicated intestinal atresias. *Ann Surg* 1979;189(5): 607–611.
38. Yamataka A, Koga H, Shimotakahara A, et al. Laparoscopy-assisted surgery for prenatally diagnosed small bowel atresia: simple, safe, and virtually scar free. *J Pediatr Surg* 2004;39(12):1815–1818.
39. Thomas CG Jr. Jejunoplasty for the correction of jejunal atresia. *Surg Gynecol Obstet* 1969;129:545–546.
40. Lally KP, Chwals WJ, Weitzman JJ, et al. Hirschsprung's disease: a possible cause of anastomotic failure following repair of intestinal atresia. *J Pediatr Surg* 1992;27:469–470.
41. Touloukian RJ. Diagnosis and treatment of jejunoileal atresia. *World J Surg* 1993;17:310–317.
42. Waldhausen JH, Sawin RS. Improved long-term outcome for patients with jejunoileal apple peel atresia. *J Pediatr Surg* 1997;32:1307–1309.
43. Lai HJ, Cheng Y, Cho H, et al. Association between initial disease presentation, lung disease outcomes, and survival in patients with cystic fibrosis. *Am J Epidemiol* 2004;159:537–546.
44. Murshed R, Spitz L, Kiely E, et al. Meconium ileus: a ten-year review of thirty-six patients. *Eur J Pediatr Surg* 1997;7:275–277.
45. Mushtaq I, Wright VM, Drake DP, et al. Meconium ileus secondary to cystic fibrosis. The East London experience. *Pediatr Surg Int* 1998;13:365–369.
46. Rescorla FJ, Grosfeld JL, West KJ, et al. Changing patterns of treatment and survival in neonates with meconium ileus. *Arch Surg* 1989;124:837–840.
47. Kao SC, Franken EA Jr. Nonoperative treatment of simple meconium ileus: a survey of the society for pediatric radiology. *Pediatr Radiol* 1995;25:97–100.
48. Fuchs JR, Langer JC. Long-term outcome after neonatal meconium obstruction. *Pediatrics* 1998;101:E7.
49. Del Pin CA, Czyrko C, Ziegler MM, et al. Management and survival of meconium ileus. A 30-year review. *Ann Surg* 1992;215:179–185.
50. Jawaheer J, Khalil B, Plummer T, et al. Primary resection and anastomosis for complicated meconium ileus: a safe procedure? *Pediatr Surg Int* 2007;23(11):1091–1093.
51. Wong KK, Lan LC, Lin SC, et al. Mucous fistula refeeding in premature neonates with enterostomies. *J Pediatr Gastroenterol Nutr* 2004;39(1): 43–45.
52. Fakhoury K, Durie PR, Levison H, et al. Meconium ileus in the absence of cystic fibrosis. *Arch Dis Child* 1992;67:1204–1206.
53. Mishra A, Greaves R, Massie J. The relevance of sweat testing for the diagnosis of cystic fibrosis in the genomic era. *Clin Biochem Rev* 2005;26(4):135–153.
54. Casaccia G, Trucchi A, Nahom A, et al. The impact of cystic fibrosis on neonatal intestinal obstruction: the need for prenatal/neonatal screening. *Pediatr Surg Int* 2003;19(1/2):75–78.
55. Farrell PM, Kosorok MR, Rock MJ, et al. Early diagnosis of cystic fibrosis through neonatal screening prevents severe malnutrition and improves long-term growth. Wisconsin Cystic Fibrosis Neonatal Screening Study Group. *Pediatrics* 2001;107(1):1–13.
56. Munck A, Gérardin M, Alberti C, et al. Clinical outcome of cystic fibrosis presenting with or without meconium ileus: a matched cohort study. *J Pediatr Surg* 2006;41(9):1556–1560.
57. Lloyd-Still JD, Beno DW, Kimura RM, et al. Cystic fibrosis colonopathy. *Curr Gastroenterol Rep* 1999;1:231–237.
58. Eggermont E. Gastrointestinal manifestations in cystic fibrosis. *Eur J Gastroenterol Hepatol* 1996;8(8):731–738.
59. Chan WK, Kay SM, Laberge JM, et al. Injection sclerotherapy in the treatment of rectal prolapse in infants and children. *J Pediatr Surg* 1998;33(2):255–258.
60. Shah A, Parikh D, Jawaheer G, et al. Persistent rectal prolapse in children: sclerotherapy and surgical management. *Pediatr Surg Int* 2005; 21(4):270–273.
61. O'Kelly TJ, Davies JR, Tam PK, et al. Abnormalities of nitric-oxide-producing neurons in Hirschsprung's disease: morphology and implications. *J Pediatr Surg* 1994;29:294–299; discussion 299–300.
62. Reding R, de Ville de Goyet J, Gosseye S, et al. Hirschsprung's disease: a 20-year experience. *J Pediatr Surg* 1997;32:1221–1225.

63. Polley TZ, Coran AG, Wesley JR Jr, et al. A ten-year experience with ninety-two cases of Hirschsprung's disease. Including sixty-seven consecutive endorectal pull-through procedures. *Ann Surg* 1985;202: 349–355.
64. Lewis NA, Levitt MA, Zallen GS, et al. Diagnosing Hirschsprung's disease: increasing the odds of a positive rectal biopsy result. *J Pediatr Surg* 2003;38:412–416; discussion 412–416.
65. Maia DM. The reliability of frozen-section diagnosis in the pathologic evaluation of Hirschsprung's disease. *Am J Surg Pathol* 2000;24: 1675–1677.
66. Pierro A, Fasoli L, Kiely EM, et al. Staged pull-through for rectosigmoid Hirschsprung's disease is not safer than primary pull-through. *J Pediatr Surg* 1997;32:505–509.
67. Wilcox DT, Bruce J, Bowen J, et al. One-stage neonatal pull-through to treat Hirschsprung's disease. *J Pediatr Surg* 1997;32:243–245; discussion 245–247.
68. Minford JL, Ram A, Turnock RR, et al. Comparison of functional outcomes of Duhamel and transanal endorectal coloanal anastomosis for Hirschsprung's disease. *J Pediatr Surg* 2004;39:161–165; discussion 161–165.
69. Sherman JO, Snyder ME, Weitzman JJ, et al. A 40-year multinational retrospective study of 880 Swenson procedures. *J Pediatr Surg* 1989;24: 833–838.
70. Moore SW, Albertyn R, Cywes S, et al. Clinical outcome and long-term quality of life after surgical correction of Hirschsprung's disease. *J Pediatr Surg* 1996;31:1496–1502.
71. Soper RT, Miller FE. Modification of Duhamel procedure: elimination of rectal pouch and colorectal septum. *J Pediatr Surg* 1968;3:376.
72. Teitelbaum DH, Cilley RE, Sherman NJ, et al. A decade of experience with the primary pull-through for Hirschsprung disease in the newborn period: a multicenter analysis of outcomes. *Ann Surg* 2000;232: 372–380.
73. Langer JC, Fitzgerald PG, Winthrop AL, et al. One-stage versus two-stage Soave pull-through for Hirschsprung's disease in the first year of life. *J Pediatr Surg* 1996;31:33–36; discussion 36–37.
74. Georgeson KE, Cohen RD, Hebra A, et al. Primary laparoscopic-assisted endorectal colon pull-through for Hirschsprung's disease: a new gold standard. *Ann Surg* 1999;229:678–682; discussion 682–683.
75. Langer JC, Durrant AC, de la Torre L, et al. One-stage transanal Soave pullthrough for Hirschsprung disease: a multicenter experience with 141 children. *Ann Surg* 2003;238:569–583; discussion 583–585.
76. Nasr A, Langer JC. Evolution of the technique in the transanal pull-through for Hirschsprung's disease: effect on outcome. *J Pediatr Surg* 2007;42(1):36–40.
77. Davies MR, Cywes S. Inadequate pouch emptying following Martin's pull-through procedure for intestinal aganglionosis. *J Pediatr Surg* 1983;18:14–20.
78. Ziegler MM, Royal RE, Brandt J, et al. Extended myectomy–myotomy. A therapeutic alternative for total intestinal aganglionosis. *Ann Surg* 1993;218:504–509; discussion 509–511.
79. Ruttenstock E, Puri P. A meta-analysis of clinical outcome in patients with total intestinal aganglionosis. *Pediatr Surg Int* 2009;25(10): 833–839.
80. Sauvat F, Grimaldi C, Lacaille F, et al. Intestinal transplantation for total intestinal aganglionosis: a series of 12 consecutive children. *J Pediatr Surg* 2008;43(10):1833–1838.
81. Becker L, Mashimo H. Further promise of stem cells therapies in the enteric nervous system. *Gastroenterology* 2009;136(7):2055–2058.
82. Metzger M, Caldwell C, Barlow AJ, et al. Enteric nervous system stem cells derived from human gut mucosa for the treatment of aganglionic gut disorders. *Gastroenterology* 2009;136(7):2214–2225.
83. Thapar N. New frontiers in the treatment of Hirschsprung disease. *J Pediatr Gastroenterol Nutr* 2009;48(Suppl 2):S92–S94.
84. Elhalaby EA, Hashish A, Elbarbary MM, et al. Transanal one-stage endorectal pull-through for Hirschsprung's disease: a multicenter study. *J Pediatr Surg* 2004;39:345–351; discussion 345–351.
85. Weber TR, Fortuna RS, Silen ML, et al. Reoperation for Hirschsprung's disease. *J Pediatr Surg* 1999;34:153–156; discussion 156–157.
86. Van Leeuwen K, Geiger JD, Barnett JL, et al. Stooling and manometric findings after primary pull-throughs in Hirschsprung's disease: perineal versus abdominal approaches. *J Pediatr Surg* 2002;37:1321–1325.
87. Elhalaby EA, Coran AG, Blane CE, et al. Enterocolitis associated with Hirschsprung's disease: a clinical–radiological characterization based on 168 patients. *J Pediatr Surg* 1995;30:76–83.
88. Marty TL, Seo T, Sullivan JJ, et al. Rectal irrigations for the prevention of postoperative enterocolitis in Hirschsprung's disease. *J Pediatr Surg* 1995;30(5):652–654.
89. Murphy F, Puri P. New insights into the pathogenesis of Hirschsprung's associated enterocolitis. *Pediatr Surg Int* 2005;21(10): 773–779.
90. Hackam DJ, Filler RM, Pearl RH, et al. Enterocolitis after the surgical treatment of Hirschsprung's disease: risk factors and financial impact. [see comment]. *J Pediatr Surg* 1998;33:830–833.
91. Wildhaber BE, Pakarinen M, Rintala RJ, et al. Posterior myotomy/myectomy for persistent stooling problems in Hirschsprung's disease. *J Pediatr Surg* 2004;39:920–926; discussion 920–926.
92. Langer JC, Birnbaum E. Preliminary experience with intrasphincteric botulinum toxin for persistent constipation after pull-through for Hirschsprung's disease. *J Pediatr Surg* 1997;32:1059–1061; discussion 1061–1062.
93. Wester T, Rintala RJ. Early outcome of transanal endorectal pull-through with a short muscle cuff during the neonatal period. *J Pediatr Surg* 2004;39:157–160; discussion 157–160.
94. Dasgupta R, Langer JC. Evaluation and management of persistent problems after surgery for Hirschsprung disease in a child. *J Pediatr Gastroenterol Nutr* 2008;46(1):13–19.
95. Hadidi A. Transanal endorectal pull-through for Hirschsprung's disease: experience with 68 patients. *J Pediatr Surg* 2003;38:1337–1340.
96. Blair GK, Murphy JJ, Fraser GC, et al. Internal sphincterotomy in post-pull-through Hirschsprung's disease. *J Pediatr Surg* 1996;31: 843–845.
97. Farrugia MK, Alexander N, Clarke S, et al. Does transitional zone pull-through in Hirschsprung's disease imply a poor prognosis? *J Pediatr Surg* 2003;38:1766–1769.
98. White FV, Langer JC. Circumferential distribution of ganglion cells in the transition zone of children with Hirschsprung disease. *Pediatr Dev Pathol* 2000;3:216–222.
99. Schmittenbecher PP, Sacher P, Cholewa D, et al. Hirschsprung's disease and intestinal neuronal dysplasia—a frequent association with implications for the postoperative course. *Pediatr Surg Int* 1999;15: 553–558.
100. Langer JC. Repeat pull-through surgery for complicated Hirschsprung's disease: indications, techniques, and results. *J Pediatr Surg* 1999;34:1136–1141.
101. van Leeuwen K, Teitelbaum DH, Elhalaby EA, et al. Long-term follow-up of redo pull-through procedures for Hirschsprung's disease: efficacy of the endorectal pull-through. *J Pediatr Surg* 2000;35:829–833; discussion 833–834.
102. Wilcox DT, Kiely EM. Repeat pull-through for Hirschsprung's disease. *J Pediatr Surg* 1998;33:1507–1509.
103. Ludman L, Spitz L, Tsuji H, et al. Hirschsprung's disease: functional and psychological follow up comparing total colonic and rectosigmoid aganglionosis. *Arch Dis Child* 2002;86:348–351.
104. Teitelbaum DH, Drongowski RA, Chamberlain JN, et al. Long-term stooling patterns in infants undergoing primary endorectal pull-through for Hirschsprung's disease. *J Pediatr Surg* 1997;32:1049–1052; discussion 1052–1053.
105. Bai Y, Chen H, Hao J, et al. Long-term outcome and quality of life after the Swenson procedure for Hirschsprung's disease. *J Pediatr Surg* 2002;37:639–642.
106. Martucciello G. Hirschsprung's disease, one of the most difficult diagnoses in pediatric surgery: a review of the problems from clinical practice to the bench. *Eur J Pediatr Surg* 2008;18(3):140–149.
107. Ghirardo V, Betalli P, Mognato G, et al. Laparotomic versus laparoscopic Duhamel pull-through for Hirschsprung disease in infants and children. *J Laparoendosc Adv Surg Tech A* 2007;17(1):119–123.
108. Rückauer KD, von Dobschuetz E. Laparoscopically assisted colorectal resection in Hirschsprung's disease. *Eur J Med Res* 2005;10(8):361–365.
109. Craigie RJ, Conway SJ, Cooper L, et al. Primary pull-through for Hirschsprung's disease: comparison of open and laparoscopic-assisted procedures. *J Laparoendosc Adv Surg Tech A* 2007;17(6): 809–812.
110. Sauer CJ, Langer JC, Wales PW. The versatility of the umbilical incision in the management of Hirschsprung's disease. *J Pediatr Surg* 2005;40(2):385–389.
111. Singh R, Cameron BH, Walton JM, et al. Postoperative Hirschsprung's enterocolitis after minimally invasive Swenson's procedure. *J Pediatr Surg* 2007;42(5):885–889.
112. Liu DC, Rodriguez J, Hill CB, et al. Transanal mucosectomy in the treatment of Hirschsprung's disease. *J Pediatr Surg* 2000;35(2):235–238.

113. El-Sawaf MI, Drongowski RA, Chamberlain JN, et al. Are the long-term results of the transanal pull-through equal to those of the trans-abdominal pull-through? A comparison of the 2 approaches for Hirschsprung disease. *J Pediatr Surg* 2007;42(1):41–47.
114. McHugh K, Dudley NE, Tam P, et al. Pre-operative MRI of anorectal anomalies in the newborn period. *Pediatr Radiol* 1995;25(Suppl 1): S33–S36.
115. Boocock GR, Donnai D. Anorectal malformation: familial aspects and associated anomalies. *Arch Dis Child* 1987;62:576–579.
116. Hassink EA, Rieu PN, Hamel BC, et al. Additional congenital defects in anorectal malformations. *Eur J Pediatr* 1996;155:477–482.
117. Rittler M, Paz JE, Castilla EE, et al. VACTERL association, epidemiologic definition and delineation. *Am J Med Genet* 1996;63:529–536.
118. Tsakayannis DE, Shamberger RC. Association of imperforate anus with occult spinal dysraphism. *J Pediatr Surg* 1995;30:1010–1012.
119. Cortes D, Thorup JM, Nielsen OH, et al. Cryptorchidism in boys with imperforate anus. *J Pediatr Surg* 1995;30:631–635.
120. Adeniran JO. One-stage correction of imperforate anus and rectovestibular fistula in girls: preliminary results. *J Pediatr Surg* 2002;37:E16.
121. Georgeson KE, Inge TH, Albanese CT. Laparoscopically assisted anorectal pull-through for high imperforate anus—a new technique. *J Pediatr Surg* 2000;35:927–930; discussion 930–931.
122. Rintala RJ, Pakarinen MP. Imperforate anus: long- and short-term outcome. *Semin Pediatr Surg* 2008;17(2):79–89.
123. De Filippo RE, Shaul DB, Harrison EA, et al. Neurogenic bladder in infants born with anorectal malformations: comparison with spinal and urologic status. [see comment]. *J Pediatr Surg* 1999;34:825–827; discussion 828.
124. Anderson KD, Newman KD, Bond SJ, et al. Diamond flap anoplasty in infants and children with an intractable anal stricture. *J Pediatr Surg* 1994;29:1253–1257.
125. Powell RW, Sherman JO, Raffensperger JG, et al. Megarectum: a rare complication of imperforate anus repair and its surgical correction by endorectal pullthrough. *J Pediatr Surg* 1982;17:786–795.
126. Nixon HH, Puri P. The results of treatment of anorectal anomalies: a thirteen to twenty year follow up. *J Pediatr Surg* 1977;12:27–37.
127. Nakayama DK, Templeton JM, Ziegler MM Jr, et al. Complications of posterior sagittal anorectoplasty. *J Pediatr Surg* 1986;21:488–492.
128. Kulshrestha S, Kulshrestha M, Yadav A, et al. Posterior sagittal approach for repair of rectourethral fistula occurring after perineal surgery for imperforated anus at birth. *J Pediatr Surg* 2000;35: 1155–1160.
129. Tsugawa C, Hisano K, Nishijima E, et al. Posterior sagittal anorectoplasty for failed imperforate anus surgery: lessons learned from secondary repairs. *J Pediatr Surg* 2000;35:1626–1629.
130. Chowdhary SK, Chalapathi G, Narasimhan KL, et al. An audit of neonatal colostomy for high anorectal malformation: the developing world perspective. *Pediatr Surg Int* 2004;20:111–113.
131. Heikkinen M, Rintala R, Luukkonen P, et al. Long-term anal sphincter performance after surgery for Hirschsprung's disease. *J Pediatr Surg* 1997;32:1443–1446.
132. Javid PJ, Barnhart DC, Hirschl RB, et al. Immediate and long-term results of surgical management of low imperforate anus in girls. *J Pediatr Surg* 1998;33:198–203.
133. Fleming SE, Hall R, Gysler M, et al. Imperforate anus in females: frequency of genital tract involvement, incidence of associated anomalies, and functional outcome. *J Pediatr Surg* 1986;21:146–150.
134. Bliss DP Jr, Tapper D, Anderson JM, et al. Does posterior sagittal anorectoplasty in patients with high imperforate anus provide superior fecal continence? *J Pediatr Surg* 1996;31:26–30; discussion 30–32.
135. Ellsworth PI, Webb HW, Crump JM, et al. The Malone antegrade colonic enema enhances the quality of life in children undergoing urological incontinence procedures. *J Urol* 1996;155:1416–1418.
136. da Silva GM, Jorge JM, Belin B, et al. New surgical options for fecal incontinence in patients with imperforate anus. *Dis Colon Rectum* 2004;47:204–209.
137. Morotti RA, Cangiarella J, Gutierrez MC, et al. Congenital cystic adenomatoid malformation of the lung (CCAM): evaluation of the cellular components. *Hum Pathol* 1999;30:618–625.
138. Kim WS, Lee KS, Kim IO, et al. Congenital cystic adenomatoid malformation of the lung: CT-pathologic correlation. *AJR Am J Roentgenol* 1997;168:47–53.
139. Sauvat F, Michel JL, Benachi A, et al. Management of asymptomatic neonatal cystic adenomatoid malformations. *J Pediatr Surg* 2003;38: 548–552.
140. Roggin KK, Breuer CK, Carr SR, et al. The unpredictable character of congenital cystic lung lesions. *J Pediatr Surg* 2000;35:801–805.
141. Taguchi T, Suita S, Yamanouchi T, et al. Antenatal diagnosis and surgical management of congenital cystic adenomatoid malformation of the lung. *Fetal Diagn Ther* 1995;10:400–407.
142. Morin L, Crombleholme TM, D'Alton ME, et al. Prenatal diagnosis and management of fetal thoracic lesions. *Semin Perinatol* 1994;18: 228–253.
143. Miller JA, Corteville JE, Langer JC, et al. Congenital cystic adenomatoid malformation in the fetus: natural history and predictors of outcome. *J Pediatr Surg* 1996;31:805–808.
144. Adzick NS, Harrison MR, Flake AW, et al. Fetal surgery for cystic adenomatoid malformation of the lung. *J Pediatr Surg* 1993;28:806–812.
145. Atkinson JB, Ford EG, Kitagawa H, et al. Persistent pulmonary hypertension complicating cystic adenomatoid malformation in neonates. *J Pediatr Surg* 1992;27:54–56.
146. van Leeuwen K, Teitelbaum DH, Hirschl RB, et al. Prenatal diagnosis of congenital cystic adenomatoid malformation and its postnatal presentation, surgical indications, and natural history. *J Pediatr Surg* 1999;34:794–798; discussion 798–799.
147. Murphy JJ, Blair GK, Fraser GC, et al. Rhabdomyosarcoma arising within congenital pulmonary cysts: report of three cases. *J Pediatr Surg* 1992;27:1364–1367.
148. Hasiotou M, Polyviou P, Strantzia CM, et al. Pleuropulmonary blastoma in the area of a previously diagnosed congenital lung cyst: report of two cases. *Acta Radiol* 2004;45:289–292.
149. Coran AG, Drongowski R. Congenital cystic disease of the tracheobronchial tree in infants and children. Experience with 44 consecutive cases. *Arch Surg* 1994;129:521–527.
150. Gluer S, Scharf A, Ure BM, et al. Thoracoscopic resection of extralobar sequestration in a neonate. *J Pediatr Surg* 2002;37:1629–1631.
151. Becmeur F, Horta P, Christmann D, et al. Mediastinal stabilization by an expansion prosthesis in postoperative congenital diaphragmatic hernia with severe pulmonary hypoplasia. *Eur J Pediatr Surg* 1995;5: 295–298.
152. Audry G, Balquet P, Vazquez MP, et al. Expandable prosthesis in right postpneumonectomy syndrome in childhood and adolescence. *Ann Thorac Surg* 1993;56(2):323–327.
153. Podevin G, Larroquet M, Camby C, et al. Postpneumonectomy syndrome in children: advantages and long-term follow-up of expandable prosthesis. *J Pediatr Surg* 2001;36(9):1425–1427.
154. Halkic N, Cuenoud PF, Corthesy ME, et al. Pulmonary sequestration: a review of 26 cases. *Eur J Cardiothorac Surg* 1998;14:127–133.
155. Tsolakis CC, Kollias VD, Panayotopoulos PP, et al. Pulmonary sequestration. Experience with eight consecutive cases. *Scand Cardiovasc J* 1997;31:229–232.
156. Conran RM, Stocker JT. Extralobar sequestration with frequently associated congenital cystic adenomatoid malformation, type 2: report of 50 cases. *Pediatr Dev Pathol* 1999;2:454–463.
157. Bratu I, Flageole H, Chen MF, et al. The multiple facets of pulmonary sequestration. *J Pediatr Surg* 2001;36:784–790.
158. Nobuhara KK, Gorski YC, La Quaglia MP, et al. Bronchogenic cysts and esophageal duplications: common origins and treatment. *J Pediatr Surg* 1997;32:1408–1413.
159. Kim KW, Kim WS, Cheon JE, et al. Complex bronchopulmonary foregut malformation: extralobar pulmonary sequestration associated with a duplication cyst of mixed bronchogenic and oesophageal type. *Pediatr Radiol* 2001;31:265–268.
160. Di Lorenzo M, Collin PP, Vaillancourt R, et al. Bronchogenic cysts. *J Pediatr Surg* 1989;24:988–991.
161. Ribet ME, Copin MC, Gosselin BH, et al. Bronchogenic cysts of the lung. *Ann Thorac Surg* 1996;61:1636–1640.
162. Cohen SR, Geller KA, Birns JW, et al. Foregut cysts in infants and children. Diagnosis and management. *Ann Otol Rhinol Laryngol* 1982;91: 622–627.
163. Yerman HM, Holinger LD. Bronchogenic cyst with tracheal involvement. *Ann Otol Rhinol Laryngol* 1990;99:89–93.
164. Harle CC, Dearlove O, Walker RW, et al. A bronchogenic cyst in an infant causing tracheal occlusion and cardiac arrest. *Anaesthesia* 1999; 54:262–265.
165. Merry C, Spurbeck W, Lobe TE, et al. Resection of foregut-derived duplications by minimal-access surgery. *Pediatr Surg Int* 1999;15:224–226.
166. Langer JC, Hussain H, Khan A, et al. Prenatal diagnosis of esophageal atresia using sonography and magnetic resonance imaging. *J Pediatr Surg* 2001;36:804–807.

167. Maoate K, Myers NA, Beasley SW, et al. Gastric perforation in infants with oesophageal atresia and distal tracheo-oesophageal fistula. *Pediatr Surg Int* 1999;15:24–27.
168. Atzori P, Iacobelli BD, Bottero S, et al. Preoperative tracheobronchoscopy in newborns with esophageal atresia: does it matter? *J Pediatr Surg* 2006;41(6):1054–1057.
169. Engum SA, Grosfeld JL, West KW, et al. Analysis of morbidity and mortality in 227 cases of esophageal atresia and/or tracheoesophageal fistula over two decades. *Arch Surg* 1995;130:502–508; discussion 508–509.
170. Keckler SJ, St Peter SD, Valusek PA, et al. VACTERL anomalies in patients with esophageal atresia: an updated delineation of the spectrum and review of the literature. *Pediatr Surg Int* 2007;23(4): 309–313.
171. Bowkett B, Beasley SW, Myers NA, et al. The frequency, significance, and management of a right aortic arch in association with esophageal atresia. *Pediatr Surg Int* 1999;15:28–31.
172. Babu R, Pierro A, Spitz L, et al. The management of oesophageal atresia in neonates with right-sided aortic arch. [see comment]. *J Pediatr Surg* 2000;35:56–58.
173. Chittmittrapap S, Spitz L, Kiely EM, et al. Anastomotic leakage following surgery for esophageal atresia. *J Pediatr Surg* 1992; 27:29–32.
174. Chittmittrapap S, Spitz L, Kiely EM, et al. Anastomotic stricture following repair of esophageal atresia. *J Pediatr Surg* 1990;25(5):508–511.
175. Spitz L. Esophageal atresia: past, present, and future. *J Pediatr Surg* 1996;31(1):19–25.
176. Ein SH, Shandling B. Pure esophageal atresia: a 50-year review. *J Pediatr Surg* 1994;29:1208–1211.
177. Boyle EM, Irwin ED, Foker JE Jr, et al. Primary repair of ultra-long-gap esophageal atresia: results without a lengthening procedure. *Ann Thorac Surg* 1994;57:576–579.
178. Giacomoni MA, Tresoldi M, Zamana C, et al. Circular myotomy of the distal esophageal stump for long gap esophageal atresia. *J Pediatr Surg* 2001;36:855–857.
179. Sharma AK, Wakhlu A. Simple technique for proximal pouch mobilization and circular myotomy in cases of esophageal atresia with tracheoesophageal fistula. *J Pediatr Surg* 1994;29:1402–1403.
180. Lai JY, Sheu JC, Chang PY, et al. Experience with distal circular myotomy for long-gap esophageal atresia. *J Pediatr Surg* 1996;31:1503–1508.
181. Kimura K, Nishijima E, Tsugawa C, et al. Multistaged extrathoracic esophageal elongation procedure for long gap esophageal atresia: experience with 12 patients. *J Pediatr Surg* 2001;36:1725–1727.
182. Fernandez MS, Gutierrez C, Ibanez V, et al. Long-gap esophageal atresia: reconstruction preserving all portions of the esophagus by Scharli's technique. *Pediatr Surg Int* 1998;14:17–20.
183. Evans M. Application of Collis gastroplasty to the management of esophageal atresia. *J Pediatr Surg* 1995;30:1232–1235.
184. Foker JE, Linden BC, Boyle EM Jr, et al. Development of a true primary repair for the full spectrum of esophageal atresia. *Ann Surg* 1997;226:533–541; discussion 541–543.
185. Till H, Muensterer OJ, Rolle U, et al. Staged esophageal lengthening with internal and subsequent external traction sutures leads to primary repair of an ultralong gap esophageal atresia with upper pouch tracheoesophageal fistula. *J Pediatr Surg* 2008;43(6):E33–E35.
186. Gough MH. Esophageal atresia—use of an anterior flap in the difficult anastomosis. *J Pediatr Surg* 1980;15:310–311.
187. Brown AK, Tam PK. Measurement of gap length in esophageal atresia: a simple predictor of outcome. *J Am Coll Surg* 1996;182:41–45.
188. Rescorla FJ, West KW, Scherer LR III, et al. The complex nature of type A (long-gap) esophageal atresia. *Surgery* 1994;116:658–664.
189. Pompeo E, Coosemans W, De Leyn P, et al. Esophageal replacement with colon in children using either the intrathoracic or retrosternal route: an analysis of both surgical and long-term results. *Surg Today* 1997;27:729–734.
190. McCollum MO, Rangel SJ, Blair GK, et al. Primary reversed gastric tube reconstruction in long gap esophageal atresia. *J Pediatr Surg* 2003; 38:957–962.
191. Spitz L, Kiely E, Pierro A. Gastric transposition in children—a 21-year experience. *J Pediatr Surg* 2004;39:276–281; discussion 276–281.
192. Khan AR, Stiff G, Mohammed AR, et al. Esophageal replacement with colon in children. *Pediatr Surg Int* 1998;13:79–83.
193. Hirschl RB, Yardeni D, Oldham K, et al. Gastric transposition for esophageal replacement in children: experience with 41 consecutive cases with special emphasis on esophageal atresia. *Ann Surg* 2002;236: 531–539; discussion 539–541.
194. Ahmad SA, Sylvester KG, Hebra A, et al. Esophageal replacement using the colon: is it a good choice? *J Pediatr Surg* 1996;31:1026–1030; discussion 1030–1031.
195. Ruangtrakool R, Spitz L. Early complications of gastric transposition operation. *J Med Assoc Thai* 2000;83:352–357.
196. Dunn JC, Fonkalsrud EW, Applebaum H, et al. Reoperation after esophageal replacement in childhood. *J Pediatr Surg* 1999;34:1630–1632.
197. Chan KL, Saing H. Iatrogenic gastric volvulus during transposition for esophageal atresia: diagnosis and treatment. *J Pediatr Surg* 1996;31: 229–232.
198. Spitz L, Kiely EM, Morecroft JA, et al. Oesophageal atresia: at-risk groups for the 1990s. *J Pediatr Surg* 1994;29:723–725.
199. Templeton JM Jr, Templeton JJ, Schnaufer L, et al. Management of esophageal atresia and tracheoesophageal fistula in the neonate with severe respiratory distress syndrome. *J Pediatr Surg* 1985;20(4): 394–397.
200. Chavin K, Field G, Chandler J, et al. Save the child's esophagus: management of major disruption after repair of esophageal atresia. *J Pediatr Surg* 1996;31:48–51; discussion 52.
201. Islam S, Cavanaugh E, Honeke R, et al. Diagnosis of a proximal tracheoesophageal fistula using three-dimensional CT scan: a case report. *J Pediatr Surg* 2004;39:100–102.
202. Gutierrez C, Barrios JE, Lluna J, et al. Recurrent tracheoesophageal fistula treated with fibrin glue. *J Pediatr Surg* 1994;29:1567–1569.
203. Wheatley MJ, Coran AG, Wesley JR, et al. Efficacy of the Nissen fundoplication in the management of gastroesophageal reflux following esophageal atresia repair. *J Pediatr Surg* 1993;28:53–55.
204. Deurloo JA, Ekkelkamp S, Bartelsman JF, et al. Gastroesophageal reflux: prevalence in adults older than 28 years after correction of esophageal atresia. *Ann Surg* 2003;238:686–689.
205. Krug E, Bergmeijer JH, Dees J, et al. Gastroesophageal reflux and Barrett's esophagus in adults born with esophageal atresia. *Am J Gastroenterol* 1999;94:2825–2828.
206. Bergmeijer JH, Bouquet J, Hazebroek FW, et al. Normal ranges of 24-hour pH-metry established in corrected esophageal atresia. *J Pediatr Gastroenterol Nutr* 1999;28:162–163.
207. Bergmeijer JH, Tibboel D, Hazebroek FW, et al. Nissen fundoplication in the management of gastroesophageal reflux occurring after repair of esophageal atresia. *J Pediatr Surg* 2000;35:573–576.
208. Lindahl H, Rintala R. Long-term complications in cases of isolated esophageal atresia treated with esophageal anastomosis. *J Pediatr Surg* 1995;30:1222–1223.
209. Schier F, Korn S, Michel E, et al. Experiences of a parent support group with the long-term consequences of esophageal atresia. *J Pediatr Surg* 2001;36:605–610.
210. Vazquez-Jimenez JF, Sachweh JS, Liakopoulos OJ, et al. Aortopexy in severe tracheal instability: short-term and long-term outcome in 29 infants and children. *Ann Thorac Surg* 2001;72:1898–1901.
211. Tazuke Y, Kawahara H, Yagi M, et al. Use of a Palmaz stent for tracheomalacia: case report of an infant with esophageal atresia. *J Pediatr Surg* 1999;34:1291–1293.
212. Delius RE, Wheatley MJ, Coran AG, et al. Etiology and management of respiratory complications after repair of esophageal atresia with tracheoesophageal fistula. *Surgery* 1992;112:527–532.
213. Tomaselli V, Volpi ML, Dell'Agnola CA, et al. Long-term evaluation of esophageal function in patients treated at birth for esophageal atresia. *Pediatr Surg Int* 2003;19:40–43.
214. Dutta HK, Grover VP, Dwivedi SN, et al. Manometric evaluation of postoperative patients of esophageal atresia and tracheo-esophageal fistula. *Eur J Pediatr Surg* 2001;11:371–376.
215. Zigman A, Yazbeck S. Esophageal foreign body obstruction after esophageal atresia repair. *J Pediatr Surg* 2002;37:776–778.
216. Bax KM, van der Zee DC. Feasibility of thoracoscopic repair of esophageal atresia with distal fistula. *J Pediatr Surg* 2002;37: 192–196.
217. Holcomb GW III, Rothenberg SS, Bax KM, et al. Thoracoscopic repair of esophageal atresia and tracheoesophageal fistula: a multi-institutional analysis. *Ann Surg* 2005;242(3):422–430.
218. Lugo B, Malhotra A, Guner Y, et al. Thoracoscopic versus open repair of tracheoesophageal fistula and esophageal atresia. *J Laparoendosc Adv Surg Tech A* 2008;18(5):753–756.
219. Krosnar S, Baxter A. Thoracoscopic repair of esophageal atresia with tracheoesophageal fistula: anesthetic and intensive care management of a series of eight neonates. *Paediatr Anaesth* 2005;15(7): 541–546.

220. Clark RH, Hardin WD, Hirschl RB Jr, et al. Current surgical management of congenital diaphragmatic hernia: a report from the Congenital Diaphragmatic Hernia Study Group. *J Pediatr Surg* 1998;33:1004–1009.
221. Congenital Diaphragmatic Hernia Study Group. Defect size determines survival in infants with congenital diaphragmatic hernia. *Pediatrics* 2007;120(3):e651–e657.
222. Extracorporeal Life Support Organization (ELSO) Registry. The ELSO Registry Report. Ann Arbor, MI: Extracorporeal Life Support Organization; June 30, 2009.
223. Iritani I. Experimental study on embryogenesis of congenital diaphragmatic hernia. *Anat Embryol (Berl)* 1984;169:133–139.
224. Harrison MR, Jester JA, Ross NA, et al. Correction of congenital diaphragmatic hernia in utero. I. The model: intrathoracic balloon produces fatal pulmonary hypoplasia. *Surgery* 1980;88:174–182.
225. Bohn D, Tamura M, Perrin D, et al. Ventilatory predictors of pulmonary hypoplasia in congenital diaphragmatic hernia, confirmed by morphologic assessment. *J Pediatr* 1987;111:423–431.
226. Yamataka T, Puri P. Pulmonary artery structural changes in pulmonary hypertension complicating congenital diaphragmatic hernia. *J Pediatr Surg* 1997;32:387–390.
227. Laberge JM, Flageole H. Fetal tracheal occlusion for the treatment of congenital diaphragmatic hernia. *World J Surg* 2007;31(8):1577–1586.
228. Price MR, Galantowicz ME, Stolar CJ, et al. Congenital diaphragmatic hernia, extracorporeal membrane oxygenation, and death: a spectrum of etiologies. *J Pediatr Surg* 1991;26:1023–1026; discussion 1026–1027.
229. Dillon PW, Cilley RE, Mauger D, et al. The relationship of pulmonary artery pressure and survival in congenital diaphragmatic hernia. *J Pediatr Surg* 2004;39:307–312; discussion 307–312.
230. Manning PB, Murphy JP, Raynor SC, et al. Congenital diaphragmatic hernia presenting due to gastrointestinal complications. *J Pediatr Surg* 1992;27:1225–1228.
231. Burge DM, Atwell JD, Freeman NV, et al. Could the stomach site help predict outcome in babies with left sided congenital diaphragmatic hernia diagnosed antenatally? *J Pediatr Surg* 1989;24:567–569.
232. Hatch EI, Kendall J, Blumhagen J Jr, et al. Stomach position as an in utero predictor of neonatal outcome in left-sided diaphragmatic hernia. *J Pediatr Surg* 1992;27:778–779.
233. Bohn DJ, James I, Filler RM, et al. The relationship between $PaCO_2$ and ventilation parameters in predicting survival in congenital diaphragmatic hernia. *J Pediatr Surg* 1984;19:666–671.
234. Doné E, Gucciardo L, Van Mieghem T, et al. Prenatal diagnosis, prediction of outcome and in utero therapy of isolated congenital diaphragmatic hernia. *Prenat Diagn* 2008;28(7):581–591.
235. Kitano Y, Nakagawa S, Kuroda T, et al. Liver position in fetal congenital diaphragmatic hernia retains a prognostic value in the era of lung-protective strategy. *J Pediatr Surg* 2005;40(12):1827–1832.
236. Rypens F, Metens T, Rocourt N, et al. Fetal lung volume: estimation at MR imaging-initial results. *Radiology* 2001;219(1):236–241.
237. Cannie MM, Jani JC, Van Kerkhove F, et al. Fetal body volume at MR imaging to quantify total fetal lung volume: normal ranges. *Radiology* 2008;247(1):197–203.
238. Kilian AK, Schaible T, Hofmann V, et al. Congenital diaphragmatic hernia: predictive value of MRI relative lung-to-head ratio compared with MRI fetal lung volume and sonographic lung-to-head ratio. *AJR Am J Roentgenol* 2009;192(1):153–158.
239. Waag KL, Loff S, Zahn K, et al. Congenital diaphragmatic hernia: a modern day approach. *Semin Pediatr Surg* 2008;17(4):244–254.
240. Yang SH, Nobuhara KK, Keller RL, et al. Reliability of the lung-to-head ratio as a predictor of outcome in fetuses with isolated left congenital diaphragmatic hernia at gestation outside 24–26 weeks. *Am J Obstet Gynecol* 2007;197(1):110–111; discussion e1–e5.
241. Lipshutz GS, Albanese CT, Feldstein VA, et al. Prospective analysis of lung-to-head ratio predicts survival for patients with prenatally diagnosed congenital diaphragmatic hernia. *J Pediatr Surg* 1997;32(11):1634–1636.
242. Kunisaki SM, Barnewolt CE, Estroff JA, et al. Ex utero intrapartum treatment with extracorporeal membrane oxygenation for severe congenital diaphragmatic hernia. *J Pediatr Surg* 2007;42(1):98–106.
243. Jani JC, Nicolaides KH, Gratacós E, et al. Severe diaphragmatic hernia treated by fetal endoscopic tracheal occlusion. *Ultrasound Obstet Gynecol* 2009;34(3):304–310.
244. Harrison MR, Keller RL, Hawgood SB, et al. A randomized trial of fetal endoscopic tracheal occlusion for severe fetal congenital diaphragmatic hernia. *N Engl J Med* 2003;349(20):1916–1924.
245. Harrison MR, Adzick NS, Bullard KM, et al. Correction of congenital diaphragmatic hernia in utero VII: a prospective trial. *J Pediatr Surg* 1997;32(11):1637–1642.
246. Nakstad B, Naess PA, de Lange C, et al. Complications of umbilical vein catheterization: neonatal total parenteral nutrition ascites after surgical repair of congenital diaphragmatic hernia. *J Pediatr Surg* 2002;37:E21.
247. Cacciari A, Ruggeri G, Mordenti M, et al. High-frequency oscillatory ventilation versus conventional mechanical ventilation in congenital diaphragmatic hernia. *Eur J Pediatr Surg* 2001;11:3–7.
248. Azarow K, Messineo A, Pearl R, et al. Congenital diaphragmatic hernia—a tale of two cities: the Toronto experience. *J Pediatr Surg* 1997;32:395–400.
249. The Neonatal Inhaled Nitric Oxide Study Group (NINOS). Anonymous inhaled nitric oxide and hypoxic respiratory failure in infants with congenital diaphragmatic hernia. *Pediatrics* 1997;99:838–845.
250. Shanley CJ, Hirschl RB, Schumacher RE, et al. Extracorporeal life support for neonatal respiratory failure. A 20-year experience. *Ann Surg* 1994;220:269–280; discussion 281–282.
251. Schwartz SM, Vermilion RP, Hirschl RB, et al. Evaluation of left ventricular mass in children with left-sided congenital diaphragmatic hernia. *J Pediatr* 1994;125:447–451.
252. Heiss KF, Clark RH, Cornish JD, et al. Preferential use of venovenous extracorporeal membrane oxygenation for congenital diaphragmatic hernia. *Pediatr Surg* 1995;30:416–419.
253. Vazquez WD, Cheu HW. Hemorrhagic complications and repair of congenital diaphragmatic hernias: does timing of the repair make a difference? Data from the Extracorporeal Life Support Organization. *J Pediatr Surg* 1994;29:1002–1005; discussion 1005–1006.
254. Congenital Diaphragmatic Hernia Study Group. Congenital diaphragmatic hernia requiring extracorporeal membrane oxygenation: does timing of repair matter? *J Pediatr Surg* 2009;44(6):1165–1171; discussion 1171–1172.
255. Wilson JM, Bower LK, Lund DP, et al. Evolution of the technique of congenital diaphragmatic hernia repair on ECMO. *J Pediatr Surg* 1994;29:1109–1112.
256. Rozmiarek AJ, Qureshi FG, Cassidy L, et al. Factors influencing survival in newborns with congenital diaphragmatic hernia: the relative role of timing of surgery. *J Pediatr Surg* 2004;39(6):821–824.
257. Reickert CA, Hirschl RB, Schumacher R, et al. Effect of very delayed repair of congenital diaphragmatic hernia on survival and extracorporeal life support use. *Surgery* 1996;120:766–772; discussion 772–773.
258. Nio M, Haase G, Kennaugh J, et al. A prospective randomized trial of delayed versus immediate repair of congenital diaphragmatic hernia. *J Pediatr Surg* 1994;29:618–621.
259. de la Hunt MN, Madden N, Scott JE, et al. Is delayed surgery really better for congenital diaphragmatic hernia?: a prospective randomized clinical trial. [see comment]. *J Pediatr Surg* 1996;31:1554–1556.
260. Atkinson JB, Poon MW. ECMO and the management of congenital diaphragmatic hernia with large diaphragmatic defects requiring a prosthetic patch. *J Pediatr Surg* 1992;27:754–756.
261. Hajer GF, vd Staak FH, de Haan AF, et al. Recurrent congenital diaphragmatic hernia; which factors are involved? *Eur J Pediatr Surg* 1998;8:329–333.
262. Tsang TM, Tam PK, Dudley NE, et al. Diaphragmatic agenesis as a distinct clinical entity. *J Pediatr Surg* 1995;30:16–18.
263. Scaife ER, Johnson DG, Meyers RL, et al. The split abdominal wall muscle flap—a simple, mesh-free approach to repair large diaphragmatic hernia. *J Pediatr Surg* 2003;38:1748–1751.
264. Rana AR, Khouri JS, Teitelbaum DH, et al. Salvaging the severe congenital diaphragmatic hernia patient: is a silo the solution? *J Pediatr Surg* 2008;43(5):788–791.
265. Kim AC, Bryner BS, Akay B, et al. Thoracoscopic repair of congenital diaphragmatic hernia in neonates: lessons learned. *J Laparoendosc Adv Surg Tech A* 2009;19(4):575–580.
266. Guner YS, Chokshi N, Aranda A, et al. Thoracoscopic repair of neonatal diaphragmatic hernia. *J Laparoendosc Adv Surg Tech A* 2008;18(6):875–880.
267. Yang EY, Allmendinger N, Johnson SM, et al. Neonatal thoracoscopic repair of congenital diaphragmatic hernia: selection criteria for successful outcome. *J Pediatr Surg* 2005;40(9):1369–1375.
268. Arca MJ, Barnhart DC, Lelli JL Jr, et al. Early experience with minimally invasive repair of congenital diaphragmatic hernias: results and lessons learned. *J Pediatr Surg* 2003;38:1563–1568.
269. Shah SR, Wishnew J, Barsness K, et al. Minimally invasive congenital diaphragmatic hernia repair: a 7-year review of one institution's experience. *Surg Endosc* 2009;23(6):1265–1271.

270. Hanekamp MN, Tjin ADGC, van Hoek-Ottenkamp WG, et al. Does V-A ECMO increase the likelihood of chylothorax after congenital diaphragmatic hernia repair? *J Pediatr Surg* 2003;38:971–974.
271. Gonzalez R, Bryner BS, Teitelbaum DH, et al. Chylothorax after congenital diaphragmatic hernia repair. *J Pediatr Surg* 2009;44(6): 1181–1185.
272. Graziano JN. Cardiac anomalies in patients with congenital diaphragmatic hernia and their prognosis: a report from the Congenital Diaphragmatic Hernia Study Group. *J Pediatr Surg* 2005;40(6): 1045–1050.
273. Fauza DO, Wilson JM. Congenital diaphragmatic hernia and associated anomalies: their incidence, identification, and impact on prognosis. *J Pediatr Surg* 1994;29:1113–1117.
274. Bernbaum J, Schwartz IP, Gerdes M, et al. Survivors of extracorporeal membrane oxygenation at 1 year of age: the relationship of primary diagnosis with health and neurodevelopmental sequelae. *Pediatrics* 1995;96:907–913.
275. Nagaya M, Akatsuka H, Kato J, et al. Development in lung function of the affected side after repair of congenital diaphragmatic hernia. *J Pediatr Surg* 1996;31:349–356.
276. D'Agostino JA, Bernbaum JC, Gerdes M, et al. Outcome for infants with congenital diaphragmatic hernia requiring extracorporeal membrane oxygenation: the first year. *J Pediatr Surg* 1995;30:10–15.
277. Stolar CJ, Levy JP, Dillon PW, et al. Anatomic and functional abnormalities of the esophagus in infants surviving congenital diaphragmatic hernia. *Am J Surg* 1990;159:204–207.
278. Rescorla FJ, Shedd FJ, Grosfeld JL, et al. Anomalies of intestinal rotation in childhood: analysis of 447 cases. *Surgery* 1990;108:710–715; discussion 715–716.
279. Lund DP, Mitchell J, Kharasch V, et al. Congenital diaphragmatic hernia: the hidden morbidity. *J Pediatr Surg* 1994;29:258–262; discussion 262–264.
280. Snyder CL, Miller KA, Sharp RJ, et al. Management of intestinal atresia in patients with gastroschisis. *J Pediatr Surg* 2001;36:1542–1545.
281. Driver CP, Bruce J, Bianchi A, et al. The contemporary outcome of gastroschisis. *J Pediatr Surg* 2000;35:1719–1723.
282. Lenke RR, Hatch EI Jr. Fetal gastroschisis: a preliminary report advocating the use of cesarean section. *Obstet Gynecol* 1986;67:395–398.
283. Sakala EP, Erhard LN, White JJ. Elective cesarean section improves outcomes of neonates with gastroschisis. *Am J Obstet Gynecol* 1993; 169(4):1050–1053.
284. Dunn JC, Fonkalsrud EW, Atkinson JB, et al. The influence of gestational age and mode of delivery on infants with gastroschisis. *J Pediatr Surg* 1999;34:1393–1395.
285. Bethel CA, Seashore JH, Touloukian RJ, et al. Cesarean section does not improve outcome in gastroschisis. *J Pediatr Surg* 1989;24:1–3; discussion 3–4.
286. Huang J, Kurkchubasche AG, Carr SR, et al. Benefits of term delivery in infants with antenatally diagnosed gastroschisis. [see comment]. *Obstet Gynecol* 2002;100:695–699.
287. Adra AM, Landy HJ, Nahmias J, et al. The fetus with gastroschisis: impact of route of delivery and prenatal ultrasonography. *Am J Obstet Gynecol* 1996;174(2):540–546.
288. Strauss RA, Balu R, Kuller JA, et al. Gastroschisis: the effect of labor and ruptured membranes on neonatal outcome. *Am J Obstet Gynecol* 2003;189(6):1672–1678.
289. Abdel-Latif ME, Bolisetty S, Abeywardana S, et al. Mode of delivery and neonatal survival of infants with gastroschisis in Australia and New Zealand. *J Pediatr Surg* 2008;43(9):1685–1690.
290. Singh SJ, Fraser A, Leditschke JF, et al. Gastroschisis: determinants of neonatal outcome. *Pediatr Surg Int* 2003;19:260–265.
291. Minkes RK, Langer JC, Mazziotti MV, et al. Routine insertion of a silastic spring-loaded silo for infants with gastroschisis. [see comment]. *J Pediatr Surg* 2000;35:843–846.
292. Mollitt DL, Ballantine TV, Grosfeld JL, et al. A critical assessment of fluid requirements in gastroschisis. *J Pediatr Surg* 1978;13:217–219.
293. Schlatter M, Norris K, Uitvlugt N, et al. Improved outcomes in the treatment of gastroschisis using a preformed silo and delayed repair approach. *J Pediatr Surg* 2003;38:459–464; discussion 459–464.
294. Schwartz MZ, Tyson KR, Milliorn K, et al. Staged reduction using a Silastic sac is the treatment of choice for large congenital abdominal wall defects. *J Pediatr Surg* 1983;18:713–719.
295. Ryckman J, Aspirot A, Laberge JM, et al. Intestinal venous congestion as a complication of elective silo placement for gastroschisis. *Semin Pediatr Surg* 2009;18(2):109–112.
296. Molik KA, Gingalewski CA, West KW, et al. Gastroschisis: a plea for risk categorization. *J Pediatr Surg* 2001;36:51–55.
297. Oldham KT, Coran AG, Drongowski RA, et al. The development of necrotizing enterocolitis following repair of gastroschisis: a surprisingly high incidence. *J Pediatr Surg* 1988;23(10):945–949.
298. Jayanthi S, Seymour P, Puntis JW, et al. Necrotizing enterocolitis after gastroschisis repair: a preventable complication? *J Pediatr Surg* 1998; 33(5):705–707.
299. Koivusalo A, Rintala R, Lindahl H, et al. Gastroesophageal reflux in children with a congenital abdominal wall defect. *J Pediatr Surg* 1999;34:1127–1129.
300. Saxena AK, Hulskamp G, Schleef J, et al. Gastroschisis: a 15-year, single-center experience. *Pediatr Surg Int* 2002;18:420–424.
301. Mahour GH, Weitzman JJ, Rosenkrantz JG, et al. Omphalocele and gastroschisis. *Ann Surg* 1973;177:478–482.
302. Heider AL, Strauss RA, Kuller JA, et al. Omphalocele: clinical outcomes in cases with normal karyotypes. *Am J Obstet Gynecol* 2004; 190:135–141.
303. Greenwood RD, Rosenthal A, Nadas AS, et al. Cardiovascular malformations associated with omphalocele. *J Pediatr* 1974;85:818–821.
304. Boyd PA, Bhattacharjee A, Gould S, et al. Outcome of prenatally diagnosed anterior abdominal wall defects. *Arch Dis Child Fetal Neonatal Ed* 1998;78:F209–F213.
305. Hong AR, Sigalet DL, Guttman FM, et al. Sequential sac ligation for giant omphalocele. *J Pediatr Surg* 1994;29:413–415.
306. de Lorimier AA, Adzick NS, Harrison MR, et al. Amnion inversion in the treatment of giant omphalocele. *J Pediatr Surg* 1991;26: 804–807.
307. Brown MF, Wright L. Delayed external compression reduction of an omphalocele (DECRO): an alternative method of treatment for moderate and large omphaloceles. *J Pediatr Surg* 1998;33:1113–1115; discussion 1115–1116.
308. Barlow B, Cooper A, Gandhi R, et al. External silo reduction of the unruptured giant omphalocele. *J Pediatr Surg* 1987;22:75.
309. Hatch EI, Baxter R. Surgical options in the management of large omphaloceles. *Am J Surg* 1987;153:449–452.
310. Mann S, Blinman TA, Douglas Wilson R. Prenatal and postnatal management of omphalocele. *Prenat Diagn* 2008;28(7):626–632.
311. Krasna IH. Is early fascial closure necessary for omphalocele and gastroschisis? *J Pediatr Surg* 1995;30:23–28.
312. Dunn JC, Fonkalsrud EW. Improved survival of infants with omphalocele. *Am J Surg* 1997;173:284–287.
313. Koivusalo A, Lindahl H, Rintala RJ, et al. Morbidity and quality of life in adult patients with a congenital abdominal wall defect: a questionnaire survey. *J Pediatr Surg* 2002;37:1594–1601.
314. Koivusalo A, Taskinen S, Rintala RJ, et al. Cryptorchidism in boys with congenital abdominal wall defects. *Pediatr Surg Int* 1998;13: 143–145.
315. Godbole P, Sprigg A, Dickson JA, et al. Ultrasound compared with clinical examination in infantile hypertrophic pyloric stenosis. [see comment]. *Arch Dis Child* 1996;75:335–337.
316. Kovalivker M, Erez I, Shneider N, et al. The value of ultrasound in the diagnosis of congenital hypertrophic pyloric stenosis. *Clin Pediatr* 1993;32:281–283.
317. Haider N, Spicer R, Grier D, et al. Ultrasound diagnosis of infantile hypertrophic pyloric stenosis: determinants of pyloric length and the effect of prematurity. *Clin Radiol* 2002;57:136–139.
318. Neilson D, Hollman AS. The ultrasonic diagnosis of infantile hypertrophic pyloric stenosis: technique and accuracy. *Clin Radiol* 1994;49: 246–247.
319. Miozzari HH, Tonz M, von Vigier RO, et al. Fluid resuscitation in infantile hypertrophic pyloric stenosis. *Acta Paediatr* 2001;90: 511–514.
320. Cook-Sather SD, Tulloch HV, Liacouras CA, et al. Gastric fluid volume in infants for pyloromyotomy. *Can J Anaesth* 1997;44:278–283.
321. Karri V, Bouhadiba N, Mathur AB, et al. Pyloromyotomy through circumbilical incision with fascial extension. *Pediatr Surg Int* 2003;19: 695–696.
322. Campbell BT, McLean K, Barnhart DC, et al. A comparison of laparoscopic and open pyloromyotomy at a teaching hospital. *J Pediatr Surg* 37:1068–1071; discussion 1068–1071.
323. Royal RE, Linz DN, Gruppo DL, et al. Repair of mucosal perforation during pyloromyotomy: surgeon's choice. *J Pediatr Surg* 1995;30: 1430–1432.
324. Sola JE, Neville HL. Laparoscopic vs open pyloromyotomy: a systematic review and meta-analysis. *J Pediatr Surg* 2009;44(8):1631–1637.

325. Fujimoto T, Lane GJ, Segawa O, et al. Laparoscopic extramucosal pyloromyotomy versus open pyloromyotomy for infantile hypertrophic pyloric stenosis: which is better? *J Pediatr Surg* 1999;34(2):3 70–372.
326. Hall NJ, van der Zee J, Tan HL, et al. Meta-analysis of laparoscopic versus open pyloromyotomy. *Ann Surg* 2004;240(5):774–778.
327. Campbell BT, McLean K, Barnhart DC, et al. A comparison of laparoscopic and open pyloromyotomy at a teaching hospital. *J Pediatr Surg* 2002;37(7):1068–1071.
328. van der Bilt JD, Kramer WL, van der Zee DC, et al. Laparoscopic pyloromyotomy for hypertrophic pyloric stenosis: impact of experience on the results in 182 cases. *Surg Endosc* 2004;18(6):907–909.
329. Adibe OO, Nichol PF, Flake AW, et al. Comparison of outcomes after laparoscopic and open pyloromyotomy at a high-volume pediatric teaching hospital. *J Pediatr Surg* 2006;41(10):1676–1678.
330. Puapong D, Kahng D, Ko A, et al. Ad libitum feeding: safely improving the cost-effectiveness of pyloromyotomy. *J Pediatr Surg* 2002;37: 1667–1668.
331. Luciani JL, Allal H, Polliotto S, et al. Prognostic factors of the postoperative vomiting in case of hypertrophic pyloric stenosis. *Eur J Pediatr Surg* 1997;7:93–96.
332. Yagmurlu A, Barnhart DC, Vernon A, et al. Comparison of the incidence of complications in open and laparoscopic pyloromyotomy: a concurrent single institution series. *J Pediatr Surg* 2004;39:292–296; discussion 292–296.
333. Yamataka A, Tsukada K, Yokoyama-Laws Y, et al. Pyloromyotomy versus atropine sulfate for infantile hypertrophic pyloric stenosis. *J Pediatr Surg* 2000;35:338–341; discussion 342.
334. Poon TS, Zhang AL, Cartmill T, et al. Changing patterns of diagnosis and treatment of infantile hypertrophic pyloric stenosis: a clinical audit of 303 patients. *J Pediatr Surg* 1996;31:1611–1615.
335. Wilson R, Kanto WP, McCarthy BJ Jr, et al. Age at onset of necrotizing enterocolitis: an epidemiologic analysis. *Pediatr Res* 1982;16: 82–85.
336. Pumberger W, Mayr M, Kohlhauser C, et al. Spontaneous localized intestinal perforation in very-low-birth-weight infants: a distinct clinical entity different from necrotizing enterocolitis. *J Am Coll Surg* 2002;195:796–803.
337. Hutter JJ, Hathaway WE, Wayne ER Jr, et al. Hematologic abnormalities in severe neonatal necrotizing enterocolitis. *J Pediatr* 1976;88: 1026–1031.
338. Butter A, Flageole H, Laberge JM, et al. The changing face of surgical indications for necrotizing enterocolitis. *J Pediatr Surg* 2002;37: 496–499.
339. Frawley G, Bayley G, Chondros P, et al. Laparotomy for necrotizing enterocolitis: intensive care nursery compared with operating theatre. *J Paediatr Child Health* 1999;35:291–295.
340. de Souza JC, da Motta UI, Ketzer CR, et al. Prognostic factors of mortality in newborns with necrotizing enterocolitis submitted to exploratory laparotomy. *J Pediatr Surg* 2001;36:482–486.
341. Hall NJ, Curry J, Drake DP, et al. Resection and primary anastomosis is a valid surgical option for infants with necrotizing enterocolitis who weigh less than 1000 g. *Arch Surg* 2005;140(12):1149–1151.
342. Chwals WJ, Blakely ML, Cheng A, et al. Surgery-associated complications in necrotizing enterocolitis: a multiinstitutional study. *J Pediatr Surg* 2001;36:1722–1724.
343. Lessin MS, Schwartz DL, Wesselhoeft CW Jr, et al. Multiple spontaneous small bowel anastomosis in premature infants with multisegmental necrotizing enterocolitis. *J Pediatr Surg* 2000;35:170–172.
344. Chardot C, Rochet JS, Lezeau H, et al. Surgical necrotizing enterocolitis: are intestinal lesions more severe in infants with low birth weight? *J Pediatr Surg* 2003;38:167–172.
345. Ein SH, Shandling B, Wesson D, et al. A 13-year experience with peritoneal drainage under local anesthesia for necrotizing enterocolitis perforation. *J Pediatr Surg* 1990;25:1034–1036; discussion 1036–1037.
346. Dimmitt RA, Meier AH, Skarsgard ED, et al. Salvage laparotomy for failure of peritoneal drainage in necrotizing enterocolitis in infants with extremely low birth weight. *J Pediatr Surg* 2000;35: 856–859.
347. Ehrlich PF, Sato TT, Short BL, et al. Outcome of perforated necrotizing enterocolitis in the very low-birth weight neonate may be independent of the type of surgical treatment. *Am Surg* 2001;67:752–756.
348. Cass DL, Brandt ML, Patel DL, et al. Peritoneal drainage as definitive treatment for neonates with isolated intestinal perforation. *J Pediatr Surg* 2000;35:1531–1536.
349. Blakely ML, Lally KP, McDonald S, et al. Postoperative outcomes of extremely low birth-weight infants with necrotizing enterocolitis or isolated intestinal perforation: a prospective cohort study by the NICHD Neonatal Research Network. *Ann Surg* 2005;241(6): 984–994.
350. Moss RL, Dimmitt RA, Barnhart DC, et al. Laparotomy versus peritoneal drainage for necrotizing enterocolitis and perforation. *N Engl J Med* 2006;354(21):2225–2234.
351. Rees CM, Eaton S, Kiely EM, et al. Peritoneal drainage or laparotomy for neonatal bowel perforation? A randomized controlled trial. *Ann Surg* 2008;248(1):44–51.
352. Rees CM, Pierro A, Eaton S. Neurodevelopmental outcomes of neonates with medically and surgically treated necrotizing enterocolitis. *Arch Dis Child Fetal Neonatal Ed* 2007;92(3):F193–F198.
353. Blakely ML, Tyson JE, Lally KP, et al. Laparotomy versus peritoneal drainage for necrotizing enterocolitis or isolated intestinal perforation in extremely low birth weight infants: outcomes through 18 months adjusted age. *Pediatrics* 2006;117(4):e680–e687.
354. VanderKolk WE, Kurz P, Daniels J, et al. Liver hemorrhage during laparotomy in patients with necrotizing enterocolitis. *J Pediatr Surg* 1996;31:1063–1066; discussion 1066–1067.
355. Pumberger W, Kohlhauser C, Mayr M, et al. Severe liver haemorrhage during laparotomy in very low birthweight infants. [see comment]. *Acta Paediatr* 2002;91:1260–1262.
356. Al-Hudhaif J, Phillips S, Gholum S, et al. The timing of enterostomy reversal after necrotizing enterocolitis. *J Pediatr Surg* 2009;44(5): 924–927.
357. Stringer MD, Brereton RJ, Drake DP, et al. Recurrent necrotizing enterocolitis. *J Pediatr Surg* 1993;28:979.
358. Born M, Holgersen LO, Shahrivar F, et al. Routine contrast enemas for diagnosing and managing strictures following nonoperative treatment of necrotizing enterocolitis. *J Pediatr Surg* 1985;20(4): 461–463.
359. Tonkin IL, Bjelland JC, Hunter TB, et al. Spontaneous resolution of colonic strictures caused by necrotizing enterocolitis: therapeutic implications. *AJR Am J Roentgenol* 1978;130(6):1077–1081.
360. Stevenson DK, Kerner JA, Malachowski N, et al. Late morbidity among survivors of necrotizing enterocolitis. *Pediatrics* 1980;66:925–927.
361. Okuyama H, Kubota A, Oue T, et al. A comparison of the clinical presentation and outcome of focal intestinal perforation and necrotizing enterocolitis in very-low-birth-weight neonates. *Pediatr Surg Int* 2002;18:704–706.
362. Davies BW, Abel G, Puntis JW, et al. Limited ileal resection in infancy: the long-term consequences. *J Pediatr Surg* 1999;34:583–587.
363. Fasoli L, Turi RA, Spitz L, et al. Necrotizing enterocolitis: extent of disease and surgical treatment. *J Pediatr Surg* 1999;34:1096–1099.
364. Sonntag J, Grimmer I, Scholz T, et al. Growth and neurodevelopmental outcome of very low birthweight infants with necrotizing enterocolitis. *Acta Paediatr* 2000;89:528–532.
365. Lucas A, Cole TJ. Breast milk and neonatal necrotising enterocolitis. *Lancet* 1990;336(8730):1519–1523.
366. Schanler RJ, Lau C, Hurst NM, et al. Randomized trial of donor human milk versus preterm formula as substitutes for mothers' own milk in the feeding of extremely premature infants. *Pediatrics* 2005; 116(2):400–406.
367. McClure RJ. Trophic feeding of the preterm infant. *Acta Paediatr Suppl* 2001;90(436):19–21.
368. Amin HJ, Zamora SA, McMillan DD, et al. Arginine supplementation prevents necrotizing enterocolitis in the premature infant. *J Pediatr* 2002;140(4):425–431.
369. Egan EA, Nelson RM, Mantilla G, et al. Additional experience with routine use of oral kanamycin prophylaxis for necrotizing enterocolitis in infants under 1,500 grams. *J Pediatr* 1977;90(2):331–332.
370. Siu YK, Ng PC, Fung SC, et al. Double blind, randomised, placebo controlled study of oral vancomycin in prevention of necrotising enterocolitis in preterm, very low birthweight infants. *Arch Dis Child Fetal Neonatal Ed* 1998;79(2):F105–F109.
371. Bin-Nun A, Bromiker R, Wilschanski M, et al. Oral probiotics prevent necrotizing enterocolitis in very low birth weight neonates. *J Pediatr* 2005;147(2):192–196.
372. Lin HC, Su BH, Chen AC, et al. Oral probiotics reduce the incidence and severity of necrotizing enterocolitis in very low birth weight infants. *Pediatrics* 2005;115(1):1–4.
373. Kunz AN, Fairchok MP, Noel JM. Lactobacillus sepsis associated with probiotic therapy. *Pediatrics* 2005;116(2):517–518.

374. Duro D, Kamin D, Duggan C. Overview of pediatric short bowel syndrome. *J Pediatr Gastroenterol Nutr* 2008;47(Suppl 1):S33–S36.
375. Nucci A, Burns RC, Armah T, et al. Interdisciplinary management of pediatric intestinal failure: a 10-year review of rehabilitation and transplantation. *J Gastrointest Surg* 2008;12:429–436.
376. Goulet O, Ruemmele F. Causes and management of intestinal failure in children. *Gastroenterology* 2006;130(2, Suppl 1):S16–S28.
377. Ching YA, Gura K, Modi B, et al. Pediatric intestinal failure: nutrition, pharmacologic, and surgical approaches. *Nutr Clin Pract* 2007;22:653.
378. Koehler AN, Yaworski JA, Gardner M, et al. Coordinated interdisciplinary management of pediatric intestinal failure: a 2-year review. *J Pediatr Surg* 2000;35(2):380–385.
379. Sudan D, Thompson J, Botha J, et al. Comparison of intestinal lengthening procedures for patients with short bowel syndrome *Ann Surg* 2007;246(4):593–601; discussion 601–604.
380. Wessel JJ, Kocoshis SA. Nutritional management of infants with short bowel syndrome. *Semin Perinatol* 2007;31(2):104–111.
381. Spencer AU, Neaga A, West B, et al. Pediatric short bowel syndrome: redefining predictors of success. *Ann Surg* 2005;242(3):403–409; discussion 409–412.
382. Btaiche IF, Khalidi N. Parenteral nutrition-associated liver complications in children. *Pharmacotherapy* 2002;22(2):188–211.
383. Diamond IR, Sterescu A, Pencharz PB, et al. The rationale for the use of parenteral omega-3 lipids in children with short bowel syndrome and liver disease. *Pediatr Surg Int* 2008;24(7):773–778.
384. Georgeson K, Halpin D, Figueroa R, et al. Sequential intestinal lengthening procedures for refractory short bowel syndrome. *J Pediatr Surg* 1994;29(2):316–320; discussion 320–321.
385. Ienaga T, Kimura K, Hashimoto K, et al. Isolated bowel segment (Iowa Model 1): technique and histological studies. *J Pediatr Surg* 1990;25(8):902–904.
386. Figueroa-Colon R, Harris PR, Birdsong E, et al. Impact of intestinal lengthening on the nutritional outcome for children with short bowel syndrome. *J Pediatr Surg* 1996;31(7):912–916.

CHAPTER

53 Surgical Complications in Children

James D. Geiger

THORACIC SURGERY

Chest infections

The majority of serious pediatric chest infections are treated medically. However, several suppurative conditions can lead to surgical complications both in diagnosis and management.

Mediastinitis

Acute mediastinitis follows bacterial and chemical soiling of the mediastinum by perforation of the pharynx, trachea, or esophagus. Perforation usually results from external trauma, surgery, foreign bodies, or instrumentation (1–4). Because the mediastinum offers no anatomic barriers to the spread of infection within it, early diagnosis and treatment are critical to reducing morbidity and mortality.

Acute mediastinitis is usually heralded by a high fever, chest pain, dyspnea, cyanosis, and marked tachycardia and leukocytosis. In neonates, acute mediastinitis may present with more subtle signs of sepsis such as lethargy, temperature instability, and leukopenia. Radiographs show mediastinal emphysema, and crepitance is sometimes apparent on palpation of the neck or chest wall. If the diagnosis is delayed and sepsis develops, the mortality rate can be significant, though less frequent than in adults (5).

The management of mediastinitis depends on the etiology and whether there is ongoing contamination or leak into the mediastinum or pleural space. Drainage is essential for an abscess or continued contamination from an esophageal perforation. The mediastinum can be drained by a cervical, transthoracic, retropleural, or anterior route, depending on the site of ongoing contamination.

Cervical Esophageal Perforation

Perforations generally occur in low-birth-weight premature infants. Typically, a nasogastric tube perforates the hypopharynx and courses along the esophagus until it enters the medial parietal pleura into a pleural space (6). Tubes terminating in the pericardium and retroperitoneum have been reported. Less commonly, endotracheal tubes or suction catheters can lead to perforation of the pharynx or cervical esophagus.

The diagnosis of perforation is suspected if intubation is difficult or if excessive blood-tinged oropharyngeal secretions are noted. An abnormal course of the nasogastric tube on radiographic examination indicates the presence of the perforation. Pneumomediastinum occurs variably. The diagnosis is confirmed by esophagram and if delayed can lead to sepsis. Diagnostic errors can lead to unnecessary thoracic exploration. Esophageal perforation may be mistaken for esophageal atresia, or the injury may be misinterpreted to be intrathoracic when, in fact, a cervical injury is present (7). Perforation into the pleural space may produce a large-tension pneumothorax. When the diagnosis of pharyngoesophageal perforation is made quickly, evacuation of pneumothoraces, antibiotics, gastric decompression, and hyperalimentation are usually adequate therapy, leading to a high rate of survival (8,9). Surgical drainage is rare for these injuries and is usually reserved for extensive extravasation or an abscess.

Thoracic Esophageal Perforation

Perforation of the thoracic esophagus may follow trauma, endoscopic or dilation procedures, or disruption of an esophageal anastomosis. Most of these perforations are small contained leaks that commonly occur after dilation of an esophageal stricture and can be effectively treated nonoperatively. If a contrast esophagram demonstrates a contained perforation in the mediastinum with free drainage back into the esophagus, then intravenous antibiotics and hyperalimentation with close observation are often adequate therapy (1,5,10). Major perforation of the thoracic esophagus not contained within the mediastinum can sometimes be effectively treated by the placement of a coated esophageal stent (11), but may require thoracotomy, closure of the perforation site, pleural drainage, and intravenous antibiotics. In some cases, esophageal diversion is also required.

Lung Abscess

Lung abscess is primarily a medical disease with surgical implications. There are many causes of lung abscess in children, including bacterial and fungal pneumonias, cystic fibrosis (CF), foreign body aspiration, lung cysts,

James D. Geiger: University of Michigan, Ann Arbor, MI 48109.

bronchiectasis, immune deficiencies, sequestration, and chronic granulomatous disease. Aspiration of gastric contents occurs in children with neurologic deficits or in patients with abnormal esophageal motility such achalasia or esophageal atresia. This is a significant risk factor for the development of aspiration pneumonia and lung abscess.

The initial and often only treatment is specific antibiotics with postural drainage and chest physiotherapy (12,13). Whenever possible, a specific bacteriologic diagnosis should be made before treatment. In some cases, needle aspiration guided by computed tomography (CT), ultrasound, or bronchoscopy is helpful in the identification of the pathogen and can also provide drainage of the abscess (14,15). Bronchoscopy with removal of an obstructing foreign body can be curative for a distal abscess. The antibiotic therapy of choice depends on the results of Gram stain and culture findings. Empiric antimicrobial therapy should include a penicillinase-resistant agent active against *Staphylococcus aureus* and an agent active against anaerobic bacteria. A course of at least 3 weeks is usually required. Surgical intervention is reserved for the rare patient who does not respond to prolonged antibiotic therapy. This is more likely in a patient with centrally located, fungal or multiple abscesses, as well as those with an abscess within a congenital lung lesion. Thoracoscopy with drainage of the abscess has been successful in some patients (16), but in general lobectomy is the best approach with the lowest rate of complications (17). In some cases, a segmentectomy or wedge resection may be effective. Endobronchial spill with contralateral lung contamination is a possible and potentially significant complication of thoracotomy for lung abscess or severe pneumonia. Use of a selective bronchial blocker, minimal manipulation of the abscess, and needle aspiration of the abscess once the chest is opened may minimize the morbidity associated with thoracotomy in these circumstances.

Empyema

Pleural effusion and empyema can complicate up to 20% of bacterial pneumonias. Despite advances in antimicrobial therapy and the use of the pneumococcal conjugate vaccine, several studies have noted an increase in the incidence of empyema as well as an increase in resistant organisms (18,19). In some studies, methicillin-resistant staphylococcus is a frequent pathogen (20).

In addition to antibiotics, multiple treatment modalities exist for pleural effusion and empyema, including thoracentesis, chest tube drainage, instillation of fibrinolytic therapy into the pleural cavity, and decortication of solid material coating the lung (21,22). In the last 10 years, the use of video-assisted thoracic surgery (VATS) has dramatically changed the management of complicated pneumonia (23). The less invasive nature of VATS, as well as the excellent published results, has led to the recommendation of an early surgical approach to drain the pleural space effectively (Fig. 53.1) (24,25). Early intervention as opposed to a stepwise approach of thoracentesis followed by chest tube placement appears to lead to excellent outcomes with significantly shorter length of hospitalization (20,26,27). Chest CT is useful for identifying patients with loculated effusions who are more likely to fail a nonsurgical approach. Rarely is open thoracotomy with decortication required.

Bronchiectasis

Bronchiectasis is an abnormal dilation of the bronchi and bronchials that is associated with chronic suppurative disease of the airways (28). The disease usually develops as a result of bronchial obstruction or of an antecedent infection such as pneumonia. Bronchiectasis is more rare now than in the 1940s and 1950s when it ranked as one of the most frequent indications for pulmonary resection in children (29,30). Today, most children with bronchiectasis have an underlying congenital pulmonary anomaly, CF, or an immunologic deficiency.

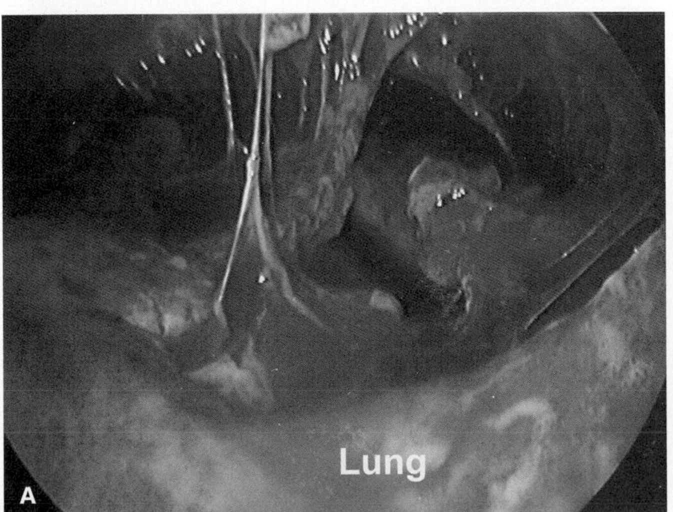

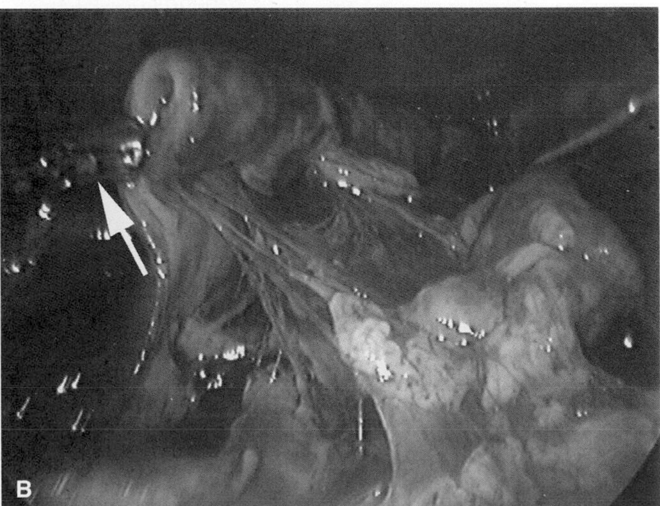

FIGURE 53.1. **A:** Thoracoscopic view of fibrinous empyema. **B:** Atraumatic grasper (*arrow*) removing the fibrinous peel and breaking down adhesions.

The preferred treatment for bronchiectasis is medical, consisting of antibiotics, postural drainage, and avoidance of inhaled toxins. Pulmonary resection is rarely required except when the disease is quite localized and contributes to chronic infection with contamination of the other lung fields (31,32). The decision to proceed with operation, especially in patients who have CF, must be made very carefully as it can be difficult to predict the benefit that lobectomy or segmental resection will provide (31,32).

Cystic Fibrosis

CF is hereditary and transmitted by a recessive gene, which was cloned and characterized in 1989 (33). There has been dramatic improvement in the medical management of the complications of CF. The median survival is now well over 30 years of age compared with less than a year when the disorder was first described in 1938 (34). Progressive infection and inflammation in the lower airways continues to limit the length and quality of life for most patients with CF and often leads to a number of pulmonary complications. Infection with an active host inflammatory response is present in CF airways from early in life. Infection is commonly caused *by S. aureus, Haemophilus influenzae, Pseudomonas aeruginosa,* and *Burkholderia cepacia.* Airway obstruction with viscous secretions is characteristic of CF and is the primary factor in perpetuating infection and inflammation. The course of the lung disease is inexorably progressive, although the rate of progression is variable depending on a number of factors, including genotype, nutritional status, exposure to environmental toxins, exposure to second-hand smoke, and aerobic activity (35,36). The earliest chest radiographic abnormality is hyperinflation, often with right upper lobe mucous retention (37). This progresses to widespread bronchial dilation, cyst, linear shadows, and infiltrates. The clinical course is marked by episodic exacerbations of the pulmonary infection and inflammation treated with antibiotic therapy, postural drainage, and physiotherapy. With intense oral and often intravenous antibiotic therapy as well as the intense airway clearance therapy, the length and frequency of these pulmonary exacerbations can be decreased. This in turn should delay scarring and loss of pulmonary function (38,39).

Pneumothorax occurs in 5% to 8% of patients with CF (40). It is one of the two acutely life-threatening complications of CF lung disease (hemoptysis is the other). Pneumothorax is more common in older patients with more severe lung disease. Patients present with sudden onset of chest pain and dyspnea; however, both the exam and initial x-ray may not be very impressive as the stiff CF lung may resist collapse. Simple tube thoracostomy is adequate treatment for most pneumothoraces, but there is a high rate of recurrence. The definitive treatment, both for prompt resolution and for prevention, involves ablating the pleural space with chemical pleurodesis or surgical pleurectomy and manual pleural abrasion (40). Ablative or surgical approaches should not be withheld because of the potential for future lung transplantation (41). Thoracoscopy is an effective approach for this group of patients. In some cases, oversewing or resection of surgical blebs is required to control a persistent air leak. Less commonly, a pulmonary resection may be needed.

Despite the advances in management, CF patients ultimately develop progressive respiratory failure. Lung transplantation is useful to correct irreversible respiratory failure, using either cadaveric or living lobar transplants. The outcome for lung transplantation has improved over time, with 5-year survival rates approaching 70% in a number of series (42–44).

Respiratory foreign bodies

Foreign body aspiration is a common and serious problem among children, accounting for 7% of lethal accidents in children aged 1 to 3 years (45). Foreign body aspiration may result in either airway compromise and death or serious sequelae such as recurrent pulmonary infection, atelectasis, and bronchiectasis (46). Early diagnosis and removal of the foreign body is critical to preventing complications (47). However, diagnosis can be delayed due to poor history and nonspecific findings on physical exam and chest x-ray. Lateral decubitus chest radiographs can at times be helpful in showing hyperinflation associated with a radiolucent foreign body. However, because of the risks of overlooked foreign body aspiration, there should be a low threshold to proceeding with bronchoscopy for both diagnosis and treatment (Fig. 53.2) (48).

Patients with chronic respiratory tract foreign body retention may present with a recent diagnosis of asthma, fever, hemoptysis, pneumonia, or pulmonary abscess. This group of patients should be considered for diagnostic bronchoscopy (49). When there is a relatively low suspicion for aspirated foreign body, then flexible bronchoscopy can be completed. When there is a high suspicion, rigid bronchoscopy is useful due to the broader array of instruments available for the removal of even difficult foreign bodies.

Complications of bronchoscopy are more common in patients with chronic foreign bodies due to the development of granulation tissue, stenosis, pneumonia, and bronchiectasis. Some patients who have bronchoscopy without identifying a foreign body may have a worsening of their symptoms following the procedure due to exacerbation of an underlying infectious process. It is important that these patients are monitored closely in the recovery room and admission considered if there are any persistent postprocedure respiratory symptoms. The rigid bronchoscope provides a protective sheath for the removal of many sharp foreign bodies. Pneumothorax and airway laceration are relatively uncommon complications (50).

When aspiration of peanuts is suspected, early bronchoscopy is critical for a good outcome. Peanuts that have been in the airway for some time become softer and an inflammatory reaction is initiated, making removal quite difficult (51). Fogarty catheters and ureteral stone baskets may facilitate removal of difficult foreign bodies.

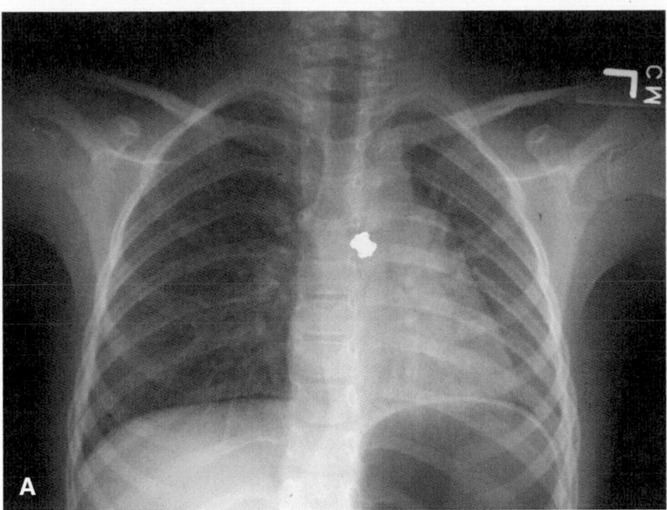

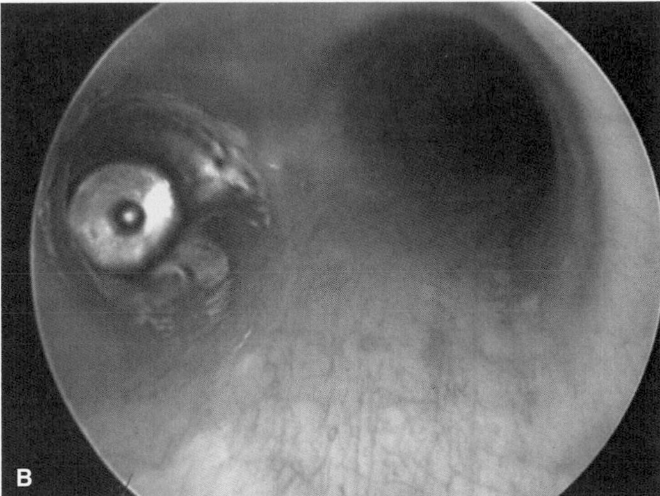

FIGURE 53.2. A: Chest x-ray showing aspirated metallic foreign body in left mainstem bronchus. **B:** Rigid bronchoscopic view of the foreign body obstructing the l mainstem bronchus.

Pectus excavatum

Pectus chest deformities are among the most common major congenital anomalies, occurring in approximately 1 in every 400 births (52). Pectus excavatum is commonly recognized during the first year of life. It is frequently asymptomatic until adolescent skeletal growth occurs, and the deformity becomes much more severe (53). There is evidence to indicate that pectus excavatum deformities cause physiologic impairment and limitations, and there is little controversy that the defects can lead to adverse cosmetic and psychologic effects (54–57).

Prior to 2000, most surgeons performed a small number of pectus operations for pectus excavatum each year primarily using modifications of the operation popularized by Ravitch (58), Welch (59), Haller et al. (60), and others. With the advent of the Nuss procedure first reported in 1998 (61), the number of pectus operations has significantly increased because of the reported lower morbidity, an easier to complete operation, and excellent outcomes. These two approaches accomplish the pectus excavatum repair in quite a different manner, and although studies suggest that the overall complication rate between the two procedures may not be significantly different (62), the pattern of complications is related to the procedure.

Complications of Ravitch Procedure

Although a number of variations of the operative technique have been reported, the major concepts of (a) resection of deformed costal cartilages with preservation of the perichondral sheaths, (b) wedge anterior sternal osteotomy with elevation of the lower sternum to the desired level, and (c) some type of internal or external fixation to support the sternum. Early complications following the Ravitch procedure are limited and generally include wound infection, pneumothorax, and pleural effusion (63,64). Most pneumothoraces can be observed unless there is associated pulmonary compromise. Recurrence of the pectus deformity has been reported in up to 5% of patients and appears to be more common in those who do not have at least temporary internal fixation of the sternum (65). Delaying repair until at least 10 years of age should minimize the extent of remodeling of the chest, which occurs with growth. Patients who have Marfan's syndrome have a higher risk of recurrence, and long-term internal fixation should be considered.

Jeune's disease (acquired thoracic chondrodystrophy syndrome) is a condition in which too extensive resection of the costal cartilages leads to failure of the subsequent chest wall growth (65). Although this can occur at any age, children who undergo pectus repair at younger ages seem to be at greater risk. Hypertrophic scar formation in the anterior chest incision can compromise an otherwise excellent cosmetic result. This complication can be prevented by minimizing trauma to the skin flaps and antiscar measures in the postoperative period. In some instances, excision of the hypertrophic scar is needed. Other complications, including a floating sternum and migration of the substernal fixation device, can occur (66,67).

Complications of the Nuss Procedure

Many pediatric surgeons now repair the majority of pectus excavatum defects with the Nuss procedure. This procedure, which is less invasive, avoids an anterior chest incision, cartilage resection, and sternal osteotomy by placing a carefully preformed, convex steel bar under the sternum through bilateral thoracic incisions (61). Early respiratory complications such as pneumothorax and pleural effusion appear to occur at a similar rate as the Ravitch procedure (68,69). Modification of the Nuss procedure with use of thoracoscopy to guide dissection of the anterior mediastinum and placement of the bar should significantly reduce the risk of cardiac perforation seen very early in the experience with this procedure when the dissection of the mediastinum was completed blindly (70). Pericarditis and

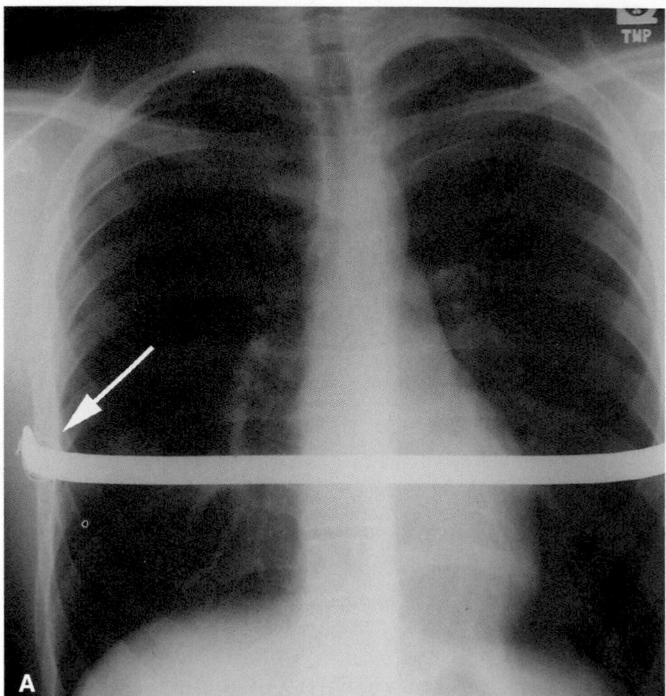

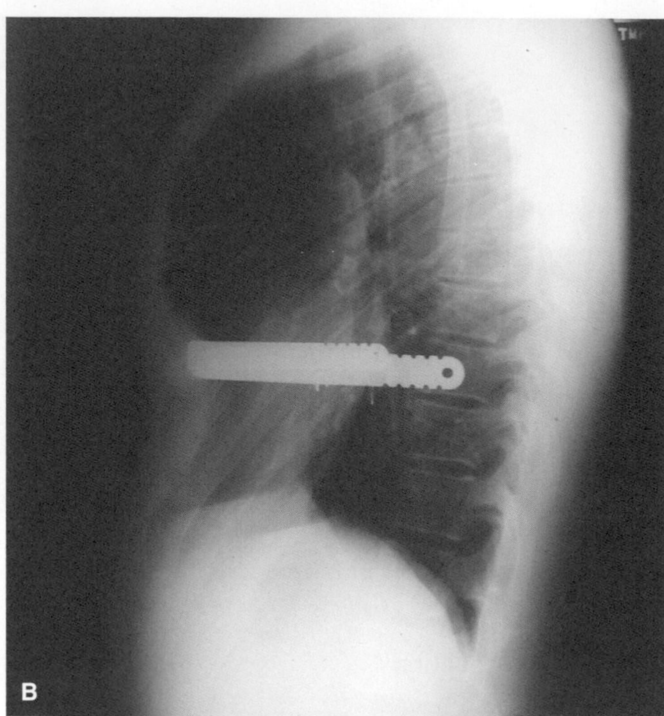

FIGURE 53.3. **A** and **B**: Anterior–posterior and lateral chest x-rays demonstrate Nuss bar position and use of heavy-gauge sternal wires around a rib for fixation.

pericardial effusion have been reported but in general do not require intervention. Wound infection occurs in roughly 2% to 3% of patients and may necessitate bar removal (71). Bar displacement occurs in 5% to 10% of patients, and a number of techniques to reduce this complication have now been described (72,73). Our preference is to use heavy gauge sternal wire placed around a rib to secure the bar (Fig. 53.3). Although postoperative pain is significant with both approaches necessitating epidural pain management, patients undergoing the Nuss procedure require longer courses of oral narcotics and in some cases the severe pain leads to early bar removal. The recurrence rate appears to be <10% and can be decreased by keeping the bar in place for a total of 3 years (70). The outcome of patients with severe asymmetric defects has been less satisfactory with the Nuss procedure, requiring either significant modifications or completion of a later Ravitch-type procedure. Other less common complications include allergic reactions to the bar (74), scoliosis, secondary rib deformities due to the bar (75), and extraosseous bone formation (76), which may make bar removal more difficult.

Gastric Surgery

Gastrostomy. Gastrostomy is a procedure used frequently in the care of pediatric surgical patients. Depending on the clinical variables, gastrostomy tube placement can be accomplished with an open laparotomy, percutaneous endoscopic approach, or a laparoscopic approach. As the indications for placement of gastrostomy tubes have broadened, the procedure is being completed on patients with significant comorbidities. Despite this, the complication rate overall is fairly low, but when complications do occur, they can lead to significant morbidity and even mortality (77). Minor complications such as gastrostomy site infections, granulation tissue, and leakage occur in a significant percentage of patients and postoperative care is important to preventing these problems (78).

Location of the gastrostomy tube on the abdominal wall is important and requires planning. During percutaneous endoscopic gastrostomy (PEG) or laparoscopic gastrostomy placement, it is important to mark the costal margin with a marking pen before insufflation of the stomach or abdomen is initiated. If this step is not completed, especially in small children, the gastrostomy tube may end up right on the costal margin, leading to significant gastrostomy site complications and the need to be repositioned.

Accurate placement of the gastrostomy tube into the stomach is not always straight forward even in open surgery, especially in neonates with pure esophageal atresia who have microgastria. In addition, PEG tube placement can lead to a development of gastroenteric, most commonly gastrocolic, fistulas in up to 3% of patients (79). Abnormal anatomy or previous surgery may contribute to this complication, and in this group of patients, a laparoscopic or laparoscopy-assisted approach is warranted. The diagnosis of a gastroenteric fistula following a PEG can be difficult and is often delayed (80). This problem often becomes apparent at the time of the first gastrostomy tube change.

A common complication of gastrostomy is inadvertent removal by either the patient or the treating medical personnel. If the tube was placed with an open or laparoscopic approach that included tacking sutures of the stomach to the posterior fascia, then replacement of the tube by an appropriately trained medical practitioner may be possible, but correct tube placement should be confirmed with a contrast study. In PEG placement, early dislodgement will require a redo PEG if recognized promptly or potentially a laparoscopic or open procedure if significant abdominal contamination has occurred. In chronically placed gastrostomy tubes, family members and caregivers can be trained in tube replacement. This should be done rapidly because the gastrostomy stoma can close quickly. At the very least, a smaller tube such as a Foley catheter can be placed until a new gastrostomy tube can be inserted.

In some patients, significant leakage from the gastrostomy site leading to enlargement of the gastrostomy wound and prolapse of gastric mucosa can occur. Delayed gastric emptying and increased intra-abdominal pressure, as can occur in patients with cerebral palsy with severe spasticity or patients with respiratory failure, increases the risk of this complication (78). In many patients, this can be managed by discontinuation of the gastrostomy tube for at least 24 hours to allow the stoma to close partially. A larger balloon catheter may also be of help in sealing the leak and allowing the site to heal. A number of topical agents may assist in protecting the skin and stimulating healing of the site. In difficult cases, the gastrostomy tube can be converted to a gastrojejunal feeding tube, and if this is unsuccessful, then this site can be surgically revised (81).

Gastrocutaneous fistula

When a patient no longer requires a gastrostomy, the tube is discontinued. Closure of the gastrostomy site occurs spontaneously in the majority of patients. In 20% to 40% of patients, a persistent gastrocutaneous fistula develops (82–84). The most important factor predisposing to the persistence of a gastrocutaneous fistula appears to be the length of time the tube was in place before removal (85). Local measures such as cautery of the epithelialized track, occlusive wound dressings, and installation of fibrin glue may facilitate closure of a gastrocutaneous fistula in some patients (86). A significant percentage of patients with a persistent gastrocutaneous fistula require surgical closure, which can be accomplished as an outpatient procedure. The gastrocutaneous fistula is mobilized, and the stomach is closed and physically separated from the facial closure.

Fundoplication

Gastroesophageal reflux disease (GERD) is a relatively benign condition in the younger infant. Most patients improve, at least symptomatically, during the first 18 months of life. In older children and adults, GERD is often a chronic disease, unlikely to resolve spontaneously. Some children, such as those with neurologic disorders or chronic pulmonary disease, are at particular risk for complications of poorly controlled GERD. In fact, in some patients, GERD may be the primary agent inducing respiratory disease such as asthma (87). In some infants, it may be a cause of sudden death (88). Medical treatment of GERD has traditionally involved administration of antisecretory and prokinetic agents (89). Proton pump inhibitors, widely used in children for the past few years, are effective in treating esophagitis. The loss of the use of cisapride has significantly depleted the armamentarium of prokinetic agents. Therefore, the management of other complications of reflux, including pulmonary aspiration of gastric contents (with subsequent pneumonia and reactive airway disease), apparent life-threatening events, and failure to thrive, may necessitate antireflux surgery.

The development of minimally invasive (laparoscopic) fundoplication increased the number of referrals for antireflux surgery, at least initially (90). Fundoplication remains one of the three most common major surgical procedures performed in infants and children by pediatric surgeons in the United States. In many studies, fundoplication has been shown to be highly effective in preventing reflux, emesis, and many of the complications associated with GERD. However, because of the alteration of the gastroesophageal anatomy and function, antireflux surgery may lead to a variety of side effects or complications. The Nissen fundoplication, either laparoscopic or open, is the most common procedure, but some surgeons prefer partial fundoplication such as the Thal fundoplication. In all procedures, fundoplication is designed to prevent GER by correcting hiatal herniation, lengthening the intra-abdominal portion of the esophagus, tightening the crura, and increasing the pressure at the level of the lower esophageal sphincter. Fundoplication is successful in abolishing GERD symptoms in 80% to 90% of patients in long-term follow-up studies (91). However, both short- and long-term complications occur and can at times be very difficult to manage.

Immediate complications of a primary laparoscopic fundoplication should be very rare events. In general, patients undergoing Nissen fundoplication have a short length of stay often <48 hours.

Failure of fundoplication to improve preoperative symptoms may be caused by erroneous diagnosis of GERD. Conditions commonly mimicking GERD and associated with a high incidence of problems after surgery include cyclic vomiting, rumination, gastroparesis, and eosinophilic esophagitis. It is critical that these conditions are considered before surgery (92).

Side effects directly related to antireflux surgery include dysphagia due to a tight fundoplication, herniation of the wrap through the hiatus, development of a periesophageal hernia, or a small-bowel obstruction from adhesions (93). There is an early experience with endoscopic, endoluminal fundoplication for GERD, but long-term data will be required to compare complications and outcomes (94).

Dysphagia

Dysphagia is a common problem especially in the early postoperative period (95). This is especially true in the toddler age group who often take longer to adjust to the fundoplication.

This early dysphagia, which is most likely made worse by the edema and inflammation associated with the normal healing process, resolves over the first few months in the vast majority of patients. In <15% of patients, dysphagia is persistent due to a tight fundoplication or overzealous closure of the hiatus. In this group, esophageal dilation may improve symptoms dramatically without compromising the fundoplication. The dilation should not be performed before 8 weeks postoperatively. In some patients, persistent dysphagia necessitates revision of the fundoplication.

Gas bloats

Dyspeptic symptoms such as fullness, early satiety, abdominal pain, and bloating occur in a significant number of patients after antireflux surgery. The "gas-bloat syndrome" may impair the symptomatic success of antireflux surgery. Patients with severe gas-bloat syndrome suffer episodes of retching and abdominal pain. The use of a venting gastrostomy is often helpful but may not relieve the symptoms completely. Patients with abnormal motility leading to delayed gastric emptying, impaired gastric accommodation, or gastric hypersensitivity are at increased risk for development of gas-bloat syndrome (96). Many pediatric surgeons use preoperative emptying studies to determine if a patient is at risk for gas-bloat syndrome, adding a pyloromyotomy or pyloroplasty to the antireflux procedure in children with delayed gastric emptying. Although some studies have demonstrated a benefit of this approach (97,98), other series failed to show benefit (99). It is well established that fundoplication improves the emptying of liquids. Gastric emptying scintiscans showing delay in emptying of a liquid meal is probably not the best indication for a drainage procedure, and use of solid phase emptying maybe more helpful. The treatment of gas-bloat symptoms is challenging, and there are no controlled studies evaluating the different pharmacological interventions available to treat these symptoms. Prokinetic agents such as metoclopramide, erythromycin, and octreotide have been used to treat gas-bloat symptoms. Metoclopramide is often the first prokinetic agent used, but the high prevalence of central nervous system side effects limits its use. New prokinetic agents are clearly needed. Anticholinergics, tricyclic antidepressants, and antagonist to $5HT_3$ receptors, such as ondansetron, may have some efficacy due to their effect on gastric hypersensitivity. Patients with severe gas-bloat syndrome and a gastrostomy tube in place may benefit from conversion of the gastrostomy to a gastro-jejunal feeding tube. In patients who have failed multiple fundoplications and still have chronic problems, esophagogastric dissociation with a Roux-en-Y esophagojejunostomy may be an option (100,101). Dumping syndrome, characterized by postprandial nausea, wretching, diaphoresis, diarrhea, and wide swings in serum glucose, have been reported to occur in up to 30% of children who undergo fundoplication (102). When suspected, dumping syndrome should be evaluated with a glucose tolerance test and treated with small feedings of complex carbohydrates.

Anatomic failure

Anatomic or physiologic failure of Nissen fundoplication occurs in 2% to 25% of patients and is more frequent in those with neurologic conditions. Herniation of the fundoplication into the hiatus is the most common cause of anatomic failure

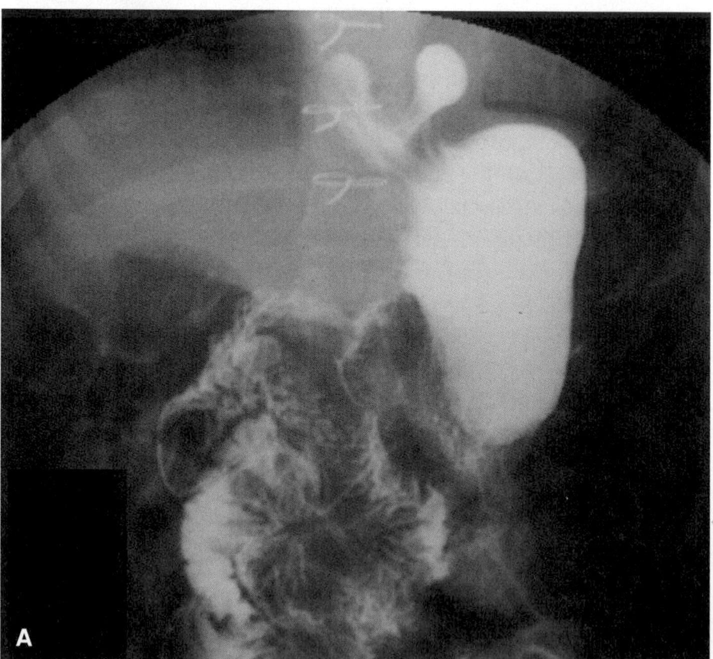

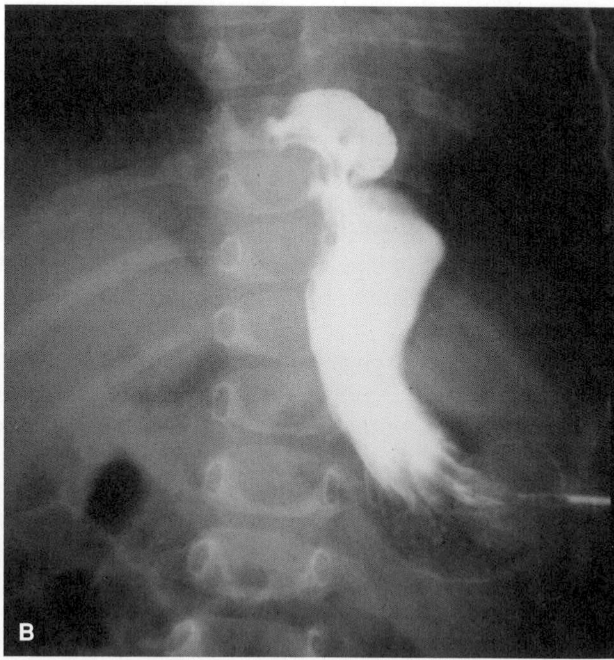

FIGURE 53.4. **A** and **B**: Upper gastrointestinal contrast studies showing transdiaphragmatic herniation after laparoscopic Nissen fundoplication.

and occurs at a higher frequency after laparoscopic approaches (103,104) (Fig. 53.4). Meticulous closure of the esophageal hiatus by crural approximation and securing the fundoplication by suturing the wrap to the crus or securing the intra-abdominal esophagus to the crura may help prevent a wrap migration. If only a small portion of the fundoplication is herniated, the wrap may still be functional and revision may not be needed. Loosening or complete breakdown of a fundoplication can occur and is more common in patients with repeated wretching and delayed gastric emptying. When a fundoplication still appears anatomically intact on upper GI study, the decision to complete a redo fundoplication is much more complex and definitive evidence of recurrent reflux by pH monitoring is required (93).

SMALL-BOWEL SURGERY

Meckel's diverticulum

Meckel's diverticulum is the most common congenital anomaly of the gastrointestinal tract with an incidence of approximately 2% (105). Although the incidence between men and women is nearly equal in asymptomatic patients, the symptomatic form occurs more frequently in men. Meckel's diverticulum is a remnant of the omphalomesenteric duct, which normally should regress between the fifth and seventh week of fetal life. Complications of a Meckel's diverticulum are obstruction, inflammation, perforation, or hemorrhage (106). The "rule of two" is often quoted in regards to Meckel's diverticulum: 2% incidence, two types of heterotopic mucosa (gastric and pancreatic) (Fig. 53.5), located within 2 ft of the ileocecal value, about 2 in. in length (and 2 cm in diameter), and usually symptomatic before 2 years of age. However, one detailed population study demonstrated a lifetime risk of developing complications from a Meckel's diverticulum at 6.4% and found that the risks were similar throughout all age groups (107).

The most common clinical presentations of Meckel's diverticulum are lower gastrointestinal bleeding, intestinal obstruction (usually due to intussusception or volvulus) (108), and inflammatory complications (106). In the case of lower

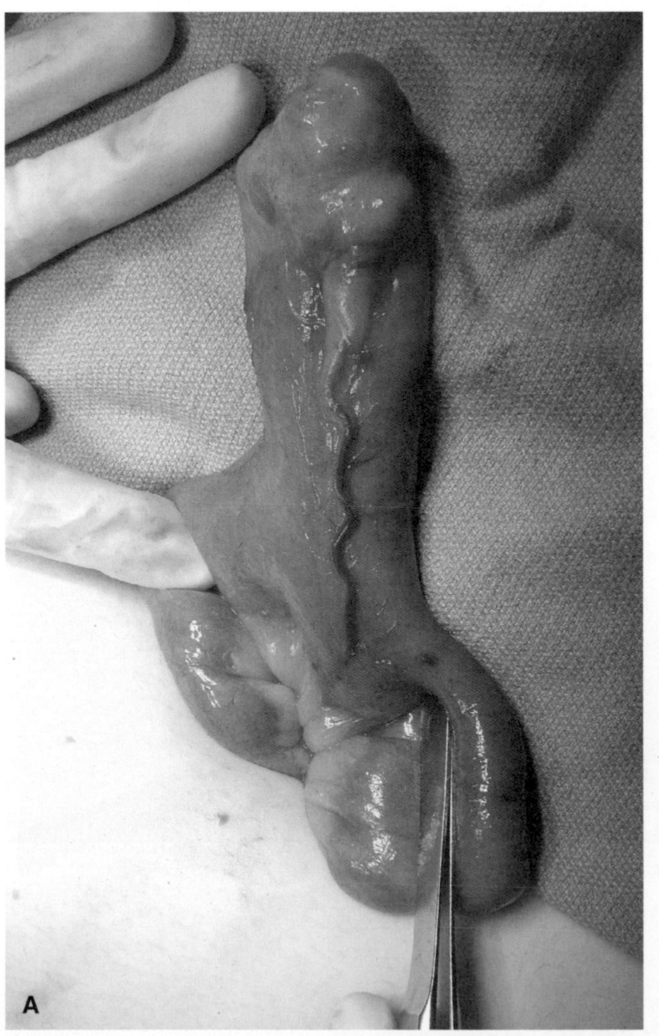

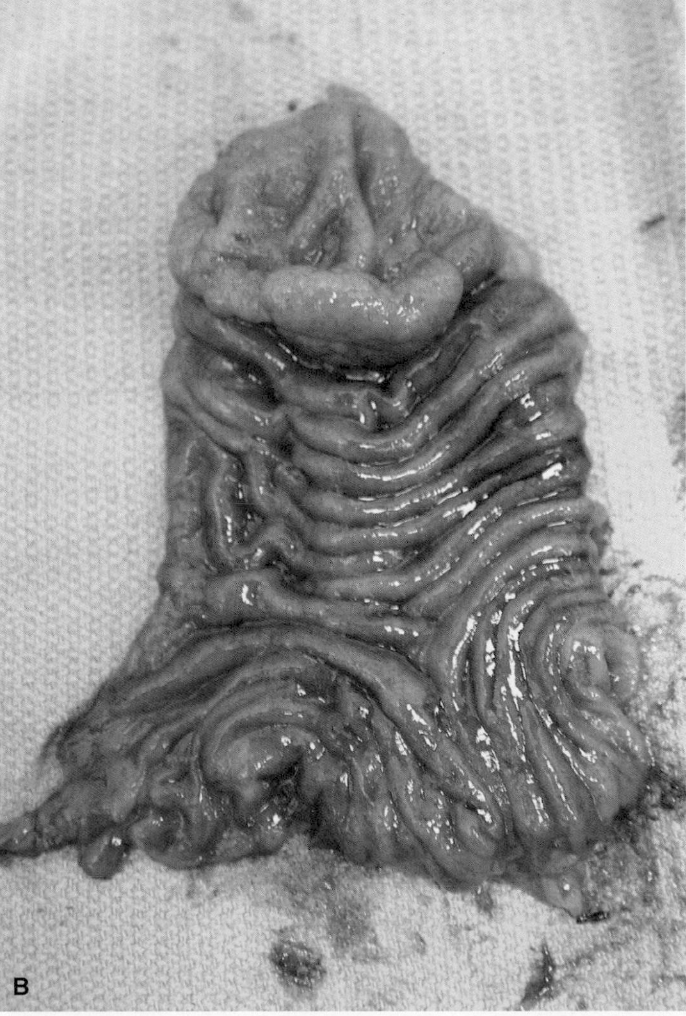

FIGURE 53.5. **A** and **B**: Operative photographs of bleeding Meckel's diverticulum. Opened Meckel's diverticulum demonstrates gastric mucosa in tip of diverticulum.

gastrointestinal hemorrhage, a technetium-pertechnetate or Meckel's scan is often used to demonstrate ectopic gastric mucosa in the Meckel's diverticulum. However, in a significant percentage of cases, diagnostic laparoscopy may ultimately be needed to evaluate for a bleeding Meckel's diverticulum (109,110).

Laparoscopy or a combination of laparoscopy and minilaparotomy can be used to manage most of the complications of Meckel's diverticulum (109,111). Whether an open resection with transverse suture closure or a mechanical stapling device is used, resection should be accomplished with a very low rate of complications. Anastomotic leak, partial obstruction due to narrowing of the ileum, bowel obstruction, and persistent GI bleeding are the major complications (112,113).

In general, when an asymptomatic Meckel's diverticulum is identified, resection should be performed, especially in younger patients who have a greater chance of developing complications (107,112,114). Resection in asymptomatic patients can be accomplished with very low morbidity; however, if the patient has abnormal bowel or distal obstruction, then resection may not be prudent.

Intussusception

Ileocolic intussusception is the most common form of intussusception of the intestine classically occurring at 4 to 12 months of age (115,116). An age-dependent risk of intussusception following rhesus-human reassortant rotavirus tetravalent vaccine has been reported (117). The diagnosis is often unsuspected and confused with other entities. Frequently, the infant may present with severe lethargy, obtundation, and nonspecific complaints and a workup for sepsis or meningitis is undertaken without considering the possibility of intussusceptions (118,119). The classic history includes awakening from sleep with severe spasms of pain during which the knees are drawn up onto the abdomen. The child recovers between spasm episodes but then the pain recurs eventually followed by vomiting and the passage of bloody mucous per rectum. Infants with unrecognized intussusception may go on to develop severe hypovolemic shock and intestinal ischemia. Before diagnostic evaluation begins, patients must be adequately rehydrated with intravenous fluids. Intravenous antibiotics are important prior to attempts at hydrostatic or air reduction of the intussusceptions (119).

Contrast enema or ultrasound is often used in the diagnosis of intussusceptions (120). Once intussusception is identified, nonoperative treatment using controlled hydrostatic reduction or air enema has a success rate of 85% to 90% (121) (Fig. 53.6). Contraindications to attempted enema reduction include clinical evidence of hypovolemia, shock, peritonitis, or radiographic evidence of perforation with free air. Patients with severe hypovolemia may be rehydrated and then undergo an attempt at reduction by enema. There are factors such as younger age, rectal bleeding, radiographic signs of intestinal obstruction, or longer duration of signs and symptoms that decrease the success rate of reduction. However, successful reduction can be achieved in the presence of any of these factors and none of them preclude an

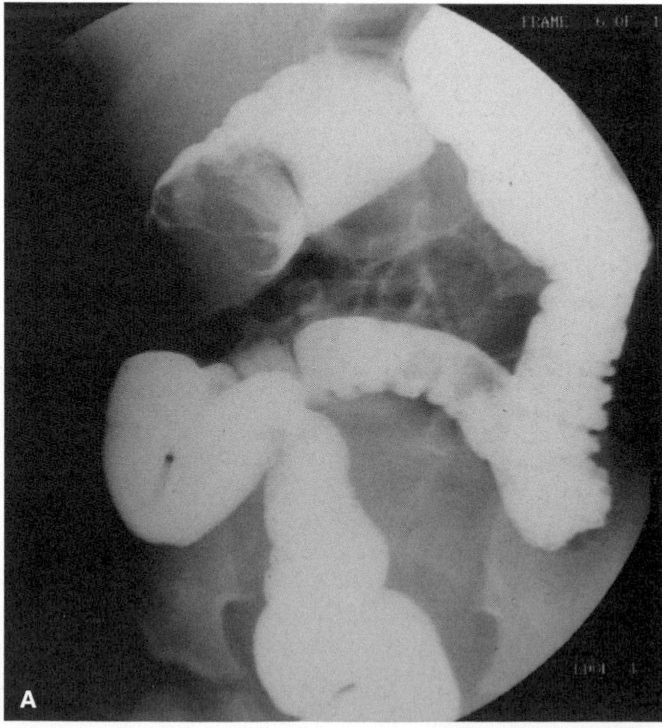

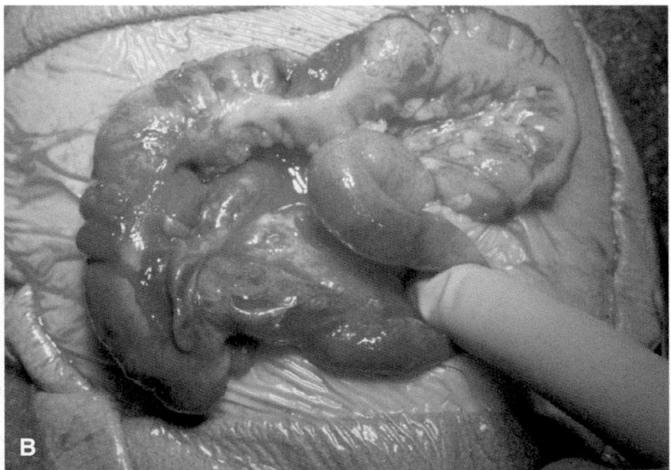

FIGURE 53.6. **A:** Barium enema demonstrates ileo-colic intussusception that would not reduce further. **B:** Intraoperative photograph shows the now-reduced ileo-colic segment, but section of bowel was necrotic, requiring resection.

attempted enema reduction if the patient is well hydrated and clinically stable (121).

The success rates of either hydrostatic reduction or pneumatic reduction using fluoroscopy are comparable. The perforation rate is <2% in nearly all of the series reported, and many large series have perforation rates <0.5% (121). Recurrence rates after radiologic reduction average approximately 10% (122,123). Patients who have a lead point such as a Meckel's diverticulum have a much lower rate of successful reduction.

Surgery for intussusception has improved due to advances in laparoscopic surgery. The conventional approach consists of a right transverse incision positioned just above the umbilicus. The intussusception is reduced by gentle finger pressure on the apex of the intussuscepted intestine in the descending or transverse colon. The intussusceptum should be gently pushed back from the distal end and usually not pulled. If a pathologic lead point is recognized, then resection is performed. A number of series indicate that laparoscopy may be the preferred approach for surgical reduction of classic ileocolic intussusception (124–126). In addition, some authors have reported a combined approach utilizing laparoscopy and pneumatic enema (127). If a pathologic lead point is recognized, then resection can be performed.

If the intussusception cannot be reduced, the involved segment is resected and a primary end-to-end anastomosis is completed. A decision regarding whether to remove the appendix at the time of laparotomy or laparoscopy is an arbitrary one, although many surgeons remove it. Feedings are usually started the day after surgery and patients are discharged from the hospital within 48 hours unless there is a persistent ileus. Immediate postoperative complications are rare, through long-term morbidity related to adhesions has been reported. The current mortality rate in children with intussusception in developed countries is <1% (119).

COLON SURGERY

Appendicitis

Appendectomy is one of the most common surgical procedures performed in children. Because of advances in the therapy of appendicitis including improved antibiotics, improved imaging both for diagnosis and treatment of complications, and improvement in the surgical techniques, the mortality of appendicitis in the United States is nearly zero. However, perforation rates over the last 70 years remain essentially unchanged (128) and appendicitis continues to lead to significant morbidity. A number of controversies regarding the management of acute appendicitis remain unresolved.

Since the introduction of laparoscopic appendectomy in 1983 by Semm (129), there have been numerous prospective randomized trials comparing laparoscopic and open appendectomies in adult patients (130–132). There have been no true randomized studies of laparoscopic versus open appendectomy in children. Clearly, laparoscopic appendectomy is technically feasible and safe and may offer some advantages related to a decreased rate of wound infection and shorter hospital stays. The complication rate between the two approaches seems to be similar in the retrospective series that have been reported (133–136). In cases where the diagnosis is uncertain, especially in teenage girls, laparoscopy offers the advantage of a complete view of the abdomen, especially the pelvic structures. One somewhat unique complication of the laparoscopic approach is the possibility of completing only a partial appendectomy and leaving an appendiceal stump (137). Care must be given to ensure that the base of the appendix at the cecum is clearly identified before removal of the appendix. The impact of new surgical approaches, including single-port surgery or natural orifice transluminal surgery, is still to be determined as experience with the procedures grows (138).

There is a wide range of clinical presentation in children with acute appendicitis, from mild inflammation of the appendix to ruptured appendicitis with diffuse peritonitis or localized abscess formation. The perforation rate varies significantly among different series but is often >50% for children <8 years of age (128). There is no consensus on the optimum timing of appendectomy in patients undergoing treatment for a perforated appendix. The complication rate of early appendectomy compared to delayed appendectomy does not appear to be dramatically different in the retrospective series that have been reported (128,139–141). The major complications, which are all higher in perforated appendicitis, include intra-abdominal abscess, prolonged ileus, small-bowel obstruction, wound infection, pneumonia, and urinary retention. Intra-abdominal abscess rates range from roughly 1.3% to 7% in pediatric series. Although some surgeons use closed suction drainage following appendectomy for perforated appendix, the utility remains unproven (142–145). Other variations in surgical technique, including the use of an endoscopic bag for removal of the appendix may help to decrease rates of intra-abdominal abscess and wound infections.

There has been concern that perforated appendix may lead to a higher rate of tubal infertility and ectopic pregnancy in women. This rate has been reported to range from 1.6% to 4.8% (146). However, because of confounding variables and other methodologic weaknesses of these studies, a causal relationship cannot definitively be supported (147). One potential advantage of interval laparoscopic appendectomy is the ability to assess the tubes and complete a tubal lysis if significant scaring is present.

Appendicitis continues to be a major challenge for surgeons in both diagnosis and treatment. Further studies will hopefully resolve some of the controversies and lead to even further lowering of the significant morbidity associated with appendicitis.

SURGERY FOR DEFECTS OF THE ABDOMINAL WALL

Umbilical hernia

Umbilical hernias are common in infants and young children. The natural history of umbilical hernia is spontaneous closure, usually in the first 3 years of life (148). African American infants have a high incidence of umbilical hernias and in particular large umbilical hernias (149,150). Expectant or nonoperative management is reasonable for the majority with umbilical hernias. Umbilical hernia defects with a small diameter (>1 cm) are more likely to close spontaneously than those with large diameters (<1.5 cm) (151). The incidence of umbilical hernia has been reported to be 18% to 20% in term babies weighing 2,500 g and as high as 84% in premature infants weighing 1,000 to 1,500 g (152). In general, it is common practice to wait until at least ~4 to 5 years of age before repairing umbilical hernia, and some defects may even close after 5 years of age (148). Defects >2 cm in diameter or those umbilical hernias that become symptomatic are indications for earlier operative intervention. It is important to distinguish an umbilical hernia from supraumbilical or epigastric hernias, which are caused by defects along the linea alba between the umbilicus and the xiphoid process.

Although the complications of umbilical hernia are believed to be rare (153), the frequency of incarceration and strangulation reported in the literature ranges from 6% to 37% (154–157). The frequency of incarceration appears to be increased for defects measuring 0.5 to 1.5 cm and does not appear to be dramatically different in infants >1 year of age compared with those <1 year of age.

Repair of an umbilical hernia is performed as an outpatient procedure with the patient under general anesthesia. Removal of the hernia sac down to a strong fascial edge and precise placement of interrupted sutures, usually in a transverse orientation, are important principals to reduce postoperative complications. The umbilical skin is tacked to the fascia to create a cosmetically acceptable umbilicus. In some instances, when there is significant redundant skin, this must be excised and a formal umbilicoplasty completed (158,159).

The most common postoperative complications include wound hematoma, which can be reduced with precise hemostasis and a pressure dressing (149). Wound infections are rare but should be treated with early wound drainage to avoid breakdown of the repair. Repair of very large umbilical defects or in patients <1 year of age increase the rate of recurrence. Visceral injuries are extremely rare, especially with an interrupted closure in which all of the sutures are tied after placement.

Inguinal hernia

Inguinal hernia repair is one of the most common general surgery operations performed by pediatric surgeons. The incidence of inguinal hernia in children ranges from 0.8% to 4.4% and is higher in infants, with approximately a third of hernias occurring in children >6 months of age (160). The incidence is highest in premature infants with reports ranging from 16% to 25% (161–163). An inguinal hernia does not resolve spontaneously and must be repaired due to the risk of incarceration particularly during the first few months of life (Fig. 53.7). Sixty-nine percent of incarcerated hernias occur before the age of 1 year and in these younger patients the hernia is often irreducible (164,165). In most patients, elective inguinal hernia repair is done as an outpatient with an extremely low risk of anesthetic complications. Premature infants and older children with cardiac, respiratory, or other disorders that increase the risk of anesthesia often require overnight hospitalization for monitoring (166).

Contralateral exploration

Among children undergoing hernia repair, there is up to a 30% chance that a hernia will develop on the contralateral side requiring subsequent repair (167). Routine contralateral exploration done frequently in the past is less common today, with surgeons either choosing observation alone or selective exploration based on the use of laparoscopy at the time of the repair of the symptomatic hernia. Those who advocate observation and repair of a metachronous hernia only if it becomes clinically apparent believe the approach leads to lower cost and complications (168,169). The alternative is to use laparoscopy through the symptomatic side hernia sac. The technique has been modified to allow an accurate determination of an open processus vaginalis, which is then repaired (170,171). This approach will identify a patent processus vaginalis in about 20% to 30% of children and can be accomplished rapidly and without complication (172).

Premature infants

There is strong evidence of an increased risk of postoperative life-threatening apnea in premature infants after repair of an inguinal hernia (173,174). Our current practice is to admit for overnight observation all premature infants who are <50 weeks postconceptional age. The timing of repair of inguinal hernia in premature infants when the hernia is recognized before discharge from the hospital is more controversial. Some advocate early repair when the baby is otherwise ready for discharge related to the issues surrounding the prematurity (175). These children are still at risk for significant respiratory complications and may require time on the ventilator postoperatively (176). Others advocate delayed herniorrhaphy when infants are older and have been out of the hospital for some time (177). Delayed surgery must be balanced against the risk of incarceration and development of testicular atrophy (178). Patients with Hunter syndrome, Hurler syndrome, Ehlers–Danlos syndrome, and Marfan syndrome frequently have

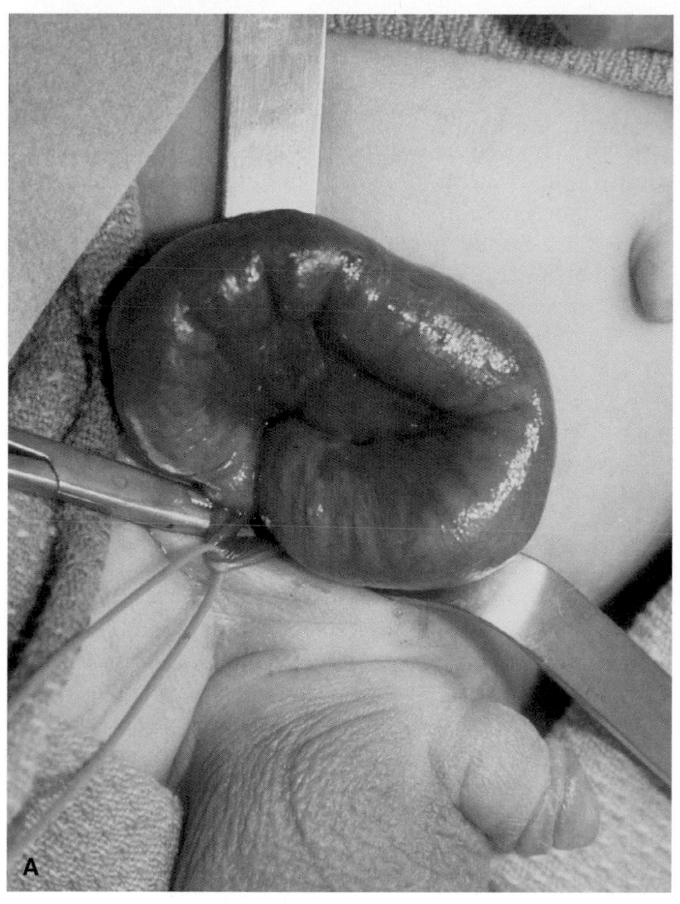

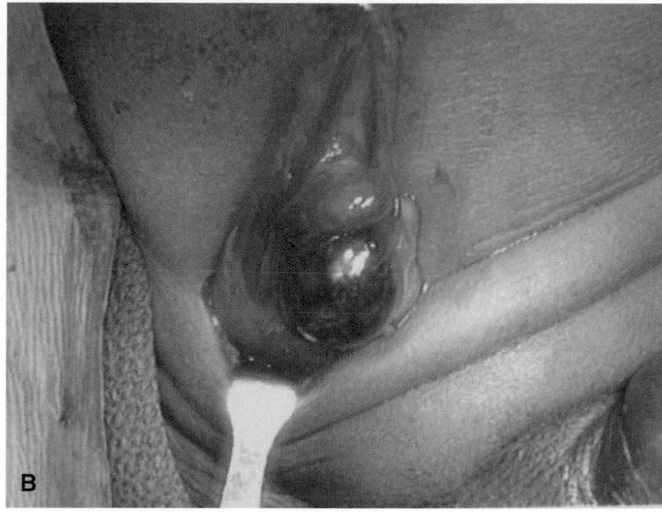

FIGURE 53.7. **A:** Strangulated bowel due to an incarcerated inguinal hernia in 4-week-old infant that necessitated resection. **B:** Ischemic testicle in same patient which at 3-month follow-up was no longer palpable due to atrophy.

inguinal hernias and are prone to recurrence unless the floor of the inguinal canal is repaired in addition to the usual high ligation of the sac. Use of prosthetic material at the initial repair may decrease the rate of recurrence in this high-risk population.

Cystic fibrosis

The incidence of inguinal hernia in children with CF is also increased to between 6% and 15% (179). The incidence of absent vas deferens in the general population is 5% to 1% based on vasectomy studies; however, in CF patients, abnormalities of the vas deferens are very common (180). These abnormalities range from obstruction to complete absence of the vas deferens and are usually symmetrical. Failure to identify the vas deferens at operation should, therefore, lead to investigation for CF.

Complications

A number of complications occur following inguinal herniorrhaphy and nearly all of these complications appear to occur at an increased rate in premature infants.

It is difficult to determine the precise incidence of recurrence after repair of an indirect inguinal hernia, but in general, the reported recurrence rate for uncomplicated hernias is 0% to 0.8% (181–183). The recurrence rate is increased in patients undergoing operations for incarcerated hernia and in premature infants. Most recurrent hernias are indirect and result from not identifying the process vaginalis during the initial operative procedure or due to improper ligation of the sac (183). Some patients recur with a direct hernia that results from failure to recognize a direct hernia at the initial operation, or due to new pathology as a result of damage to the posterior wall during the initial dissection. Injury to the vas deferens can occur by either transection (approximately 25% of vasal injuries) or compression (184). The exact incidence of vas deferens injury is difficult to quantify because this injury is unlikely to be recognized until adulthood and possibly only when the injury is bilateral. From a number of studies however, the incidence appears to be approximately 0.8% to 2% (184). Studies of male fertility and hernia sac pathology have helped to estimate the incidence of vas deferens injury (185,186). To reduce the incidence of injury to the vas deferens, it must be identified and protected throughout resection and division of the hernia sac. Crushing of the vas deferens with a clamp or forceps may also lead to permanent injury (187). Minimizing traction on the vas deferens during dissection of the processus vaginalis and careful ligation will also help to avoid injury. At the completion of inguinal herniorrhaphy, it is routine to palpate the testicles in the scrotum. Oversight of this maneuver can lead to an iatrogenic undescended testicle, which may ultimately require orchiopexy. Some premature infants have a very poorly developed gubernaculum, and if the testicle does not sit in the scrotum securely, then a simple orchiopexy should be considered.

Scrotal swelling is most commonly related to fluid accumulation or postoperative hydrocele and less commonly to hematoma. In general, postoperative hydrocele can be managed expectantly and resolves spontaneously (188). In some cases, aspiration or reoperation is needed.

Testicular atrophy can occur due to operative injury to the testicular vesicles or may occur preoperatively with incarcerated hernias in which the testicular blood supply is compromised by the incarcerated viscus (188–191).

Injury to the bladder can occur during mobilization of the cord structures when dissection is carried medially through the rectus muscle (181,192). The abdominal wall is extremely thin in infants, and the bladder, being mistaken for a hernia sac, can be mobilized in error. If the bladder is entered, the defect should be repaired in layers and decompression of the bladder considered.

Inadvertent trauma to bowel, ovary, or the fallopian tube can occur in the lumen of the hernia sac. This is avoided by opening the sac and inspecting the contents before transecting it if it is not absolutely clear that the hernia sac is empty. Wound infection after inguinal hernia repair is uncommon and may be minimized by the use of collodion or other tissue adhesive to seal the wound.

LIVER SURGERY

Biliary atresia

Biliary atresia is the most common neonatal cholestatic disorder, occurring in approximately 1 of 8,000 (Asian countries) to 1 of 15,000 (Western countries) live births, characterized by complete fibrotic obliteration of the lumen of all or part of the extrahepatic biliary tree within 3 months of life (193). The etiologic factors and pathogenesis of the obliteration of the biliary tree remain poorly understood (194). In approximately 20% of patients with biliary atresia, the presence of at least one other congenital anomalies suggest that defective development of the bile ducts plays a role in these cases (194,195). The more common form (found in 80% of patients) of biliary atresia is not associated with other congenital anomalies and has been termed the perinatal or acquired form. It is believed that various perinatal or postnatal events trigger progressive injury and fibrosis of a normally developed biliary tree (194,196). Despite these potential disparate etiologies, the clinical phenotype of these two forms of biliary atresia may be identical. The diagnosis of biliary atresia should be considered in any newborn whose jaundice persists after 14 days of age. Conjugated hyperbilirubinemia is present, and the majority of infants develop acholic stools and hepatomegaly. A number of diagnostic tests, including ultrasound, hepatic scintigraphy, and more recently magnetic resonance cholangiography, have been used to diagnosis biliary atresia. However, the diagnosis of biliary atresia is definitively established by intraoperative cholangiography and liver biopsy (197). This can often be accomplished with a laparoscopy-assisted or minilaparotomy approach. Intraoperative cholangiography that fails to demonstrate a lumen in some portion of the extrahepatic biliary tree, surgical findings of a fibrotic, non-patent bile duct, and characteristic findings on liver and bile duct histology confirm the diagnosis.

Kasai portoenterostomy

Optimal therapy for patients with biliary atresia is the Kasai procedure in which a Roux-en-Y loop of jejunum is connected to the portal plate identified during careful dissection of the fibrotic bile duct remnants (198). If performed by an experienced pediatric surgeon, the portoenterostomy yields bile drainage from the liver into the intestinal tract in approximately 70% to 80% of patients, resulting in resolution of the acholic stools and resolution of jaundice (199–201). Some studies report results comparable to a minimally invasive surgical Kasai procedure (202). Although some patients may have excellent bile drainage when undergoing the operation after 120 days of life (203), in general, the results in terms of both bile flow and longer term survival are improved if the operation is completed before 90 days of age (199).

Recently, there has been an interest in adjuvant medical therapy to enhance liver function and potentially decrease further fibrosis. Immunosuppression with corticosteroids or use of ursodeoxycholic acid to stimulate bile flow and as a cytoprotective agent has been utilized (204,205). Randomized studies will be needed to definitively prove the potential benefit of these agents. Antibiotic prophylaxis against cholangitis, as well as supplementation with fat-soluble vitamins, is indicated (206,207). The long-term outcome after the Kasai operation depends on several factors such as the time of the operation and the extent of liver fibrosis, as well as recurrent bouts of cholangitis (194, 199,200,208). If a portoenterostomy is not performed in patients with biliary atresia, 50% to 80% of children die (without liver transplantation) from biliary atresia by age 1 year and 90% to 100% die by age 3 years (209,210). Successful portoenterostomy, when performed at 60 to 90 days of age is associated with a 10-year survival rate ranging from 40% to 60% (199,210). If the portoenterostomy is not successful in establishing bile flow, survival without liver transplantation is similar to or worse than that of patients not undergoing surgery (211).

Liver transplantation has improved survival in patients with biliary atresia significantly and is indicated for patients with biliary atresia who do not undergo an attempt at portoenterostomy because of delayed diagnosis, those in whom portoenterostomy has failed to re-establish bile flow, and those with decompensated cirrhosis and endstage liver disease despite initial success of portoenterostomy. Long-term survival after liver transplantation for biliary atresia approaches 80% to 90% (212,213).

Complications

Failure to Achieve Bile Flow

If performed by an experienced pediatric surgeon, the portoenterostomy should yield bile drainage from the liver into the intestinal tract in approximately 70% to 80% of patients (199–201). It is always a concern of whether the operation was technically completed correctly in those patients who do not develop good bile flow. However, reoperation in this group of patients has not led to significantly improved outcome and further adhesions may complicate the later transplant procedure. In general, the only group of patients who may benefit from revision of a hepatic portoenterostomy are those who initially had good bile excretion but in whom the good bile flow suddenly ceases (195,214,215).

Cholangitis

In addition to the common postoperative complications associated with abdominal surgery in infancy, cholangitis is the most frequent and serious complication after portoenterostomy. The reported incidences range from 40% to 60% (206,214,216). The cause of postoperative cholangitis is not entirely clear but is thought to be due to reflux of intestinal contents toward the porta hepatis. Predisposing factors to infection are intrahepatic biliary stasis in patients with lower rates of bile flow. Attacks of cholangitis are manifested by fever, decreased quantity of bile, and a progressive increase in serum bilirubin levels. Early postoperative cholangitis may lead to a cessation of bile flow, and repeated attacks may cause a progressive deterioration of hepatic function. Prophylactic antibiotics are helpful in reducing the incidence of cholangitis. For recurrent cholangitis, Neomycin or Ciprofloxacin is beneficial (217,218). A number of modifications to the Roux-en-Y biliary construction have been reported to help prevent cholangitis. In a long-term study recently reported from the Japanese biliary atresia registry, complex modifications such as the Roux-en-Y with an intestinal valve and the Suruga-II in which a total biliary conduit is created and then later restored at a second operation did not lower the rate of cholangitis compared with the conventional Roux-en-Y procedure (199,219). Ascending cholangitis can develop during or after viral actions related to decreased bile flow and bile stasis. During the first 6 to 12 months after portoenterostomy, most fevers with any evidence of increased liver dysfunction or reduction in stool pigmentation should be treated as if cholangitis is present. In general, broad-spectrum IV antibiotics including anaerobic coverage is best. If there are no signs of sepsis, intravenous corticosteroid pulse therapy for 5 to 7 days utilizing intravenous methylprednisolone may increase drainage. Patients with persistent or recurring cholangitis can be evaluated with hepatic scintigraphy and ultrasonography to rule out a rare afferent limb obstruction.

Portal Hypertension

A variable degree of hepatic fibrosis is usually present in patients with biliary atresia at the time of initial surgery. In addition, many patients may continue to have some degree of bile stasis and progressive fibrosis, ultimately leading to the development of portal hypertension. Portal hypertension may become clinically manifest by the finding of progressive hepatosplenomegaly. Patients can also develop complications of portal hypertension, including gastrointestinal hemorrhage from esophageal or gastric varices, thrombocytopenia and/or pancytopenia related to hypersplenism, ascites, spontaneous bacterial peritonitis, portosystemic encephalopathy, or portopulmonary syndrome. Significant variceal hemorrhage has been reported in 20% to 60% of patients with biliary atresia (210,216). Patients with variceal hemorrhage are treated with both pharmacologic and endoscopic methods. In some patients, splenectomy and portosystemic shunts may be temporizing measures while the patient is being evaluated for liver transplantation (220).

Outcome

The Japanese Biliary Atresia Registry, a nationwide registry of children with biliary atresia in Japan, recently reported an overall 5- and 10-year survival rates of 75.3% (553 of 734) and 66.7% (72 of 108), respectively (199). A large multicenter review of the outcome of all children diagnosed with biliary atresia in France between 1986 and 1996 evaluated the combined results of portoenterostomy with liver transplantation and found that the 10-year survival for 472 patients with biliary atresia was 68%. The 10-year actuarial survival with the native liver after portoenterostomy was 29% and 5-year survival after liver transplantation was 71%. Prognostic factors predictive of overall 10-year survival were the performance of the portoenterostomy, age at portoenterostomy (survival of 80.4% with surgery at age >45 days vs. 68.5% at <45 days), anatomic pattern of atresia (100% for atresia of the common bile duct only vs. 65.4% for complete extrahepatic atresia), the presence of polysplenia syndrome (48.3% for yes vs. 69.9% for no), and the experience of the center performing the portoenterostomy (54% for (≤2 new patients per year, 59.8% for 3 to 5 per year, and 77.8% for >20 per year). The same factors predicted 5- and 10-year survival with the native liver after portoenterostomy. In the context of current therapeutic options, 70% to 80% of patients with biliary atresia in North America require liver transplantation during the first two decades of life, despite initial success with portoenterostomy. Consequently, biliary atresia accounts for 40% to 50% of all liver transplants performed in children. The Biliary Atresia Clinical Research Consortium has been funded by the National Institutes of Health (211). Through such multicenter collaborative approaches, major advances in our understanding of biliary atresia leading to improved outcomes may occur.

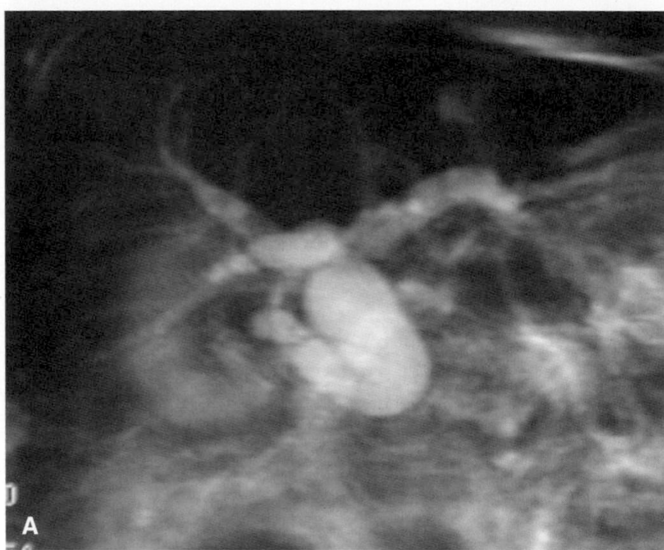

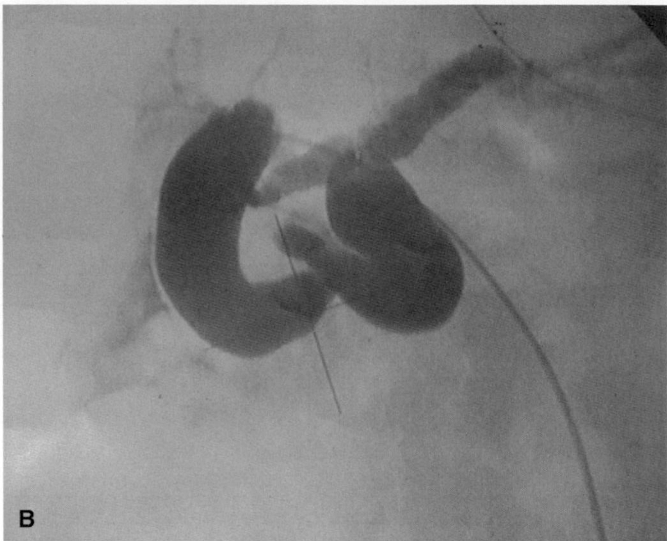

FIGURE 53.8. **A:** Magnetic resonance cholangiopancreatography demonstrates a type I choledochal cyst with excellent correlation with the intraoperative cholangiogram **(B)** in the same patient.

Choledochal cyst

Choledochal cyst is a rare congenital dilation of the bile ducts. The estimated incidence in western countries varies between 1 in 100,000 and 1 in 150,000. The incidence is significantly higher in Asia and occurs more commonly in girls (221). The most widely used subdivision of choledochal cyst is Todani's classification (222). Type 1 cysts are the most frequently encountered and may be caused by an abnormal arrangement of the pancreatic and biliary ducts, also known as "Common Channel," which occurs in up to 92% of patients with choledochal cyst (223–225) (Fig. 53.8).

If a choledochal cyst is not resected, a high incidence (20% to 30%) of cholangiocarcinoma has been reported, mainly after the second decade of life (226,227). The incidence of asymptomatic choledochal cyst identified both prenatally and in neonates has increased due to advances in diagnostic imaging (228,229). Choledochal cyst can present at any age; abdominal pain, jaundice, cholangitis, and pancreatitis are frequent presenting symptoms. Early diagnosis followed by cyst excision and Roux-en-Y reconstruction of the biliary tract is the treatment of choice, even in asymptomatic children. Early complications of complete cyst excision and Roux-en-Y hepatic reconstruction occur at a quite low rate. Biliary leak, Roux-en-Y anastomotic leak, afferent limb obstruction, pancreatitis and/or pancreatic duct injury, and early cholangitis have all been reported (222,230–232).

Long-term complications include cholangitis, and these patients should be evaluated for the possible development of intrahepatic bile duct stones or anastomotic stricture (231–233). Patients who have undergone complete cyst excision may still have an increased risk of development of cholangiocarcinoma at sites distant from the anastomosis, and long-term follow-up is necessary (234). Yamataka et al. have made recommendations for preventing complications related to Roux-en-Y hepatic-jejunostomy (235). These include completing an end-to-end anastomosis if possible, or if not minimizing the length of the end of the blind pouch in an end-to-side anastomosis. They recommend that the length of the Roux-en-Y limb be individualized based on the patient's size, as this may lengthen with age, and they recommend a long side-to-side jejunostomy.

Liver tumors

The most common indication for hepatic resection in children is hepatoblastoma (HB), followed by hepatocellular carcinoma (HCC) and then a number of other malignant and benign conditions as listed in Table 53.1 (236). There is general agreement that complete surgical resection is the cornerstone of treatment for patients with HB and HCC and the only opportunity for cure (237–239).

Table 53.1 Incidence of primary hepatic tumors in childhood

Tumor	Number of Patients	Percent
Hepatoblastoma	532	43
Hepatocellular carcinoma	284	23
Sarcoma	79	6
Benign vascular tumor	166	13
Mesenchymal hamartoma	75	6
Adenoma	22	2
Focal nodular hyperplasia	22	2
Miscellaneous	57	5

Adapted from Weinberg AG, Finegold MJ. Primary hepatic tumors of childhood. *Hum Pathol* 1983;14(6):512–537.

Hepatoblastoma

HB occurs most frequently in the first few years of life, whereas HCC usually occurs in older children and adolescents. Historically, only 30% of patients with HB were amenable to primary surgical resection. Currently, with the help of more sophisticated imaging and surgical techniques, the rate is probably closer to 50%. Approximately 50% of the tumors that are unresectable at the time of diagnosis can be made resectable with systemic chemotherapy (238). Cisplatin-based chemotherapy is capable of reducing tumor volume and treating pulmonary metastasis. Thus, roughly 75% of all tumors can be resected completely (240,241). Orthotopic liver transplantation can augment the percentage of patients who can undergo complete resection of their disease and should be considered early in patients with central tumors involving the portal structures, the hepatic veins or with multifocal disease in both lobes (242). Transplant for HB will be studied as part of the major cooperative group studies, but in pilot studies, it does appear to significantly improve survival in children with advanced HB (242,243).

Complications of hepatic resection

Most of the morbidity and mortality after hepatectomy is related to intraoperative blood loss and transfusion requirements (244). Therefore, control of intraoperative bleeding should be the cornerstone in any strategy for major liver resections and even in minor resections of centrally located tumors. Improved preoperative imaging with the use of CT 3D reconstructions of the tumor and vascular anatomy facilitates better preoperative planning (245,246). The use of intraoperative ultrasound is also beneficial for identification of the tumor and hepatic vasculature (247). A number of surgical techniques for vascular control during hepatectomy have been advocated and have led to reduced intraoperative blood loss. The Pringle maneuver, controlling only blood inflow, is effective and offers the advantage of simplicity, but patients are still exposed to the danger of retrograde bleeding from the hepatic veins and inferior vena cava (IVC), as well as air embolism. Total hepatic venous exclusion (THVE), consisting of both liver inflow and outflow occlusion provides a bloodless surgical field during hepatic transaction. However, because of the interruption of IVC blood flow, it is complicated by hemodynamic instability in 20% to 30% of patients (245,248). Selective hepatic venous exclusion appears to be as effective as THVE for controlling both inflow and outflow, with the advantage of not disturbing IVC patency. This technique involves disconnecting the liver from the retrohepatic IVC and meticulous dissection of the hepatic veins (249). This procedure is technically demanding and potentially hazardous, especially in children in whom the hepatic veins are short and intraparenchymal.

A number of other technical advances, including new devices for division of the liver parenchyma, local and systemic hemostatic agents, and understanding the effects of liver ischemia, should facilitate further reductions in liver resection morbidity and mortality (245,250). Normal liver parenchyma can safely tolerate continuous normothermic ischemia for as long as 90 minutes and intermittent ischemia for as long as 120 minutes (249). In addition to the major complications of hemorrhage and air embolism, a number of postoperative complications, including bile leak, abscess, pleural effusion, ascites, wound infection, and respiratory complications, have been reported (244). Most of these complications are directly related to the degree of intraoperative blood loss and the difficulty of the hepatic resection. Careful dissection of the bile ducts prior to parenchymal transection may reduce injury to the remaining hepatic duct.

PANCREAS SURGERY

Acute pancreatitis

Most cases of acute pancreatitis in children result from systemic infection, trauma, choledocholithiasis, anomalies of the pancreatobiliary duct system, and drugs (251). Other causes include idiopathic disease, metabolic disorders, familial pancreatitis, and Crohn's disease. Traumatic injury to the pancreas is often related to a direct impact to the epigastrium such as bicycle handle bar injuries (252). Diagnosis is confirmed by CT or ultrasound, but is sometimes delayed because of subtle clinical signs. More than 50% of patients develop pseudocysts; however, more than three-quarters resolve without surgery (251–253). Pancreatic transection can occur due to abdominal trauma. Although somewhat controversial, the majority of these patients can be managed without operation (254,255). In patients with pseudocysts that do not resolve with nonoperative management, cyst gastrostomy is the most common drainage option (256,257). In some patients, this can be accomplished endoscopically or even with a transgastric laparoscopic approach (258). Roux-en-Y cysto jejunostomy may be appropriate for a pancreatic pseudocyst that cannot be approached through the stomach.

The current medical management of pancreatitis is principally supportive, including aggressive hydration, management of metabolic complications and pain, and minimization of pancreatic stimulation by fasting, with nutritional support by parenteral or jejunoenteral feedings. The efficacy of pharmacologic interventions remains largely anecdotal and unproved (251).

Severe pancreatitis progressing to pancreatic necrosis is uncommon. When patients show signs of severe clinical pancreatitis, imaging studies should be obtained to evaluate for areas on pancreatic necrosis, which can lead to infection in 30% to 70% of patients. A fine needle aspiration can be used to diagnose infected necrotic pancreatic tissue. If this group of patients does not respond to supportive measures and broad-spectrum antibiotic coverage, then drainage of the infected material may be indicated (259). Surgery for chronic pancreatitis is indicated in small percentage of patients (260).

Hyperinsulinism

Congenital hyperinsulinism (CHI) is characterized by profound hyperglycemia related to inappropriate insulin secretion. The disease includes focal and diffuse forms, which share a similar presentation but appear to result from different molecular mechanisms (261,262).

The overall incidence of persistent hyperinsulinemia and hyperglycemia of infancy (PHHI) in 1 in 50,000 births and autosomal recessive inheritance with a risk of 1 in 2,500 has been recognized in Saudi Arabian and Ashkenazi Jewish people (with mutations in SUR gene) (261,263). Untreated or undertreated PHHI leads to almost certain neurologic impairment and often death. Historically, half of the infants surviving treatment for PHHI had neurologic impairment, with increased age at the time of surgery being associated with an increased incidence of neurologic damage. Even those who appear intact have been shown to have impaired head growth (261). It is now well recognized that neonates with CHI may have either diffuse involvement of the pancreatic B cells or focal adenomatous islet cell hyperplasia (264,265). Clinically, these two forms of CHI are indistinguishable, but imaging studies aid in identifying focal lesions (266). Patients with diffuse disease often required near-total pancreatectomy, which has the long-term risk of diabetes mellitus (267). Conversely, babies with focal disease potentially can be cured with a selective partial pancreatectomy with little risk of subsequent diabetes (264,262). A number of diagnostic tests have been evaluated for discriminating between these two forms of CHI, including transhepatic portal venous sampling, selection arterial stimulation with calcium with hepatic venous sampling, and 18-fluorodopa-PET scan (262). Patients who are identified to have focal lesions should undergo resection without significant delays. Diffuse disease is initially treated medically, but >50% of patients ultimately require surgical resection (262). The current recommendation for diffuse disease is a 95% resection, leaving only a rim of tissue on the duodenum and bile duct. Although a 95% pancreatectomy successfully controls hyperinsulinism in the majority of the infants, it can be associated with major intra- and postoperative morbidity (268). This can include hemorrhage, injury to the splenic vein and/or spleen, and bile duct injuries. Inadvertent splenic injuries should be treated by splenorrhaphy if technically feasible to avoid the risk of postsplenectomy sepsis in this young group of patients.

SPLEEN SURGERY

Splenectomy

Splenectomy is indicated for a variety of hematologic disorders, severe hypersplenism, occasionally trauma, and other causes as indicated in Table 53.2. The laparoscopic approach has been adopted for many of the hematologic indications for splenectomy. Overall, in the retrospective studies reported, the complications of the two approaches seem equivalent. Laparoscopic splenectomy offers improved cosmesis and possibly shorter hospital stay (269–271). Excellent results with a lateral open approach have also been reported, and it is unlikely that the two procedures will ever be compared directly (272). Careful dissection of the splenic hilum after complete mobilization of the spleen is required to avoid injury to the pancreas, leading to postoperative pancreatitis and pseudocyst formation. Injury to the greater curve of the stomach must be avoided during ligation or coagulation of the short gastric vessels. With preoperative antibiotics and careful attention to hemostasis, the risk of subphrenic abscess is low. When this does occur, it can usually be treated by percutaneous drainage. Accessory spleens are identified in 20% to 30% of patients and should be removed (273,274).

Table 53.2 Potential indications for splenectomy in children

Chronic Hemolytic Anemias
Hereditary spherocytosis
Autoimmune hemolytic anemia
Thalassemia intermedia
β-Thalassemia
Chronic Thrombocytopenias
Idiopathic thrombocytopenic purpura
Thrombotic thrombocytopenic purpura
Severe Hypersplenism
Severe cytopenia, pain, and splenic infarction
Myeloproliferative disorders
Myeloid metaplasia
Chronic myelogenous leukemia
Congestive splenomegaly (portal hypertension)
Storage diseases (Gaucher's disease)
Parasitic diseases
Primary Malignant Conditions
Splenic lymphoma
Angiosarcoma
Splenic Lesions
Cysts: Posttraumatic, congenital, and echinococcal
Hodgkin's disease (rarely for staging)
Trauma
Irreparable ruptured spleen
Ruptured spleen with other abdominal trauma requiring operation

Postsplenectomy sepsis

The most lethal complication of splenectomy is postsplenectomy sepsis caused by encapsulated organisms such as *Pneumococcus*, *Haemophilus influenza*, or *Meningococcus* (275). In elective hematologic cases, patients should be immunized with *Pneumococcus*, *Haemophilus type B*, and *Meningococcus* vaccines before splenectomy (276). The